D1461685

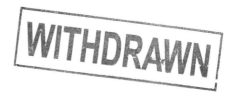

Patient Care in Neurology

Patient Care in Neurology

Edited by

Adrian C. Williams

Birmingham Neuroscience Centre,
Queen Elizabeth Hospital, Birmingham

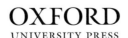

OXFORD
UNIVERSITY PRESS

OXFORD
UNIVERSITY PRESS

Great Clarendon Street, Oxford OX2 6DP

Oxford University Press is a department of the University of Oxford
and furthers the University's aim of excellence in research, scholarship,
and education by publishing worldwide in

Oxford New York

Athens Auckland Bangkok Bogotá Buenos Aires Calcutta
Cape Town Chennai Dar es Salaam Delhi Florence Hong Kong Istanbul
Karachi Kuala Lumpur Madrid Melbourne Mexico City Mumbai
Nairobi Paris São Paulo Singapore Taipei Tokyo Toronto Warsaw

and associated companies in Berlin Ibadan

Oxford is a registered trade mark of Oxford University Press
in the UK and in certain other countries

Published in the United States
by Oxford University Press Inc., New York

British Library Cataloguing Publication Data
Data available

Library of Congress Cataloging in Publication Data
Patient care in neurology / edited by Adrian C. Williams.
Includes bibliographical references and index.
1. Nervous system–Diseases–Patients–Care. 2. Neurology.
I. Williams, A. C. (Adrian C.)
[DNLM: 1. Nervous System Diseases–diagnosis. 2. Nervous System
Diseases–therapy. 3. Neurology. WL 140P298 1999]
RC346.P36   1999   616.8–dc21   98–39264

ISBN 0 19 262857 7

1 3 5 7 9 10 8 6 4 2

Typeset in Baskerville
by Alliance Phototypesetters, Pondicherry, India
Printed in Great Britain
on acid-free paper by
The Bath Press, Avon

Preface

We have taken a much wider view of care than is covered in other books on neurology to reflect the true aims of a service neurologist's job and its necessary concerns, over and above seeing patients, for teamwork, resources, the efficient delivery of neurological health care, contracting, and other aspects including teaching. Within the clinical chapters, we have attempted to emphasize a modern attitude to and management of the commoner situations rather than spend too much space on abstruse aspects of differential diagnosis. Neurology has, after all, shifted in the last decade or two from being a largely diagnostic service and has been extended into treatment and long-term support and education of our patients. At the end of a long day one is more likely to be proud of having managed well a potentially difficult situation with patients, staff, or institution, than having made some brilliant diagnosis.

Diagnosis of serious disease has, under most circumstances, become less difficult. However, clinical skills remain of great importance particularly given that the vast majority of our patients with more minor ailments are diagnosed on clinical grounds with either no assistance or attempted confusion from tests unwisely ordered. No one can deny that advances in imaging and other diagnostic tests have not made our life easier and with the slow but steady increase in number of consultants, more time is now available for following up patients and developing specialist clinics as the trend continues towards more management on an outpatient basis rather than during inpatient ward rounds.

A triage style for outpatients previously adopted by some of us, served to demonstrate the need for better staffing but is now a thing of the past and the entire structure of outpatients is rightly being questioned. Let us hope the diagnostic skills learnt during this earlier period can be retained and are not lost to wholesale investigation and an inability to see the wood for the trees.

Other themes that we have tried to incorporate into this book are the close working relationships we now have with other specialties including psychiatry, neurosurgery, and rehabilitation. Despite improvements in training, it remains a surprise that most neurologists do not spend more time studying psychiatry or a spell carrying out neurosurgery, although most practitioners nowadays will rotate through a certain amount of rehabilitation. Not only does a period spent in these specialties give one added insight into a somewhat different population but also into the different pressures these doctors experience, and may go some way towards understanding, for example, how the surgical or psychiatric mind 'thinks'. Hence, there are chapters on these topics as well as on more acute subjects, such as stroke, where our communal experience remains limited. We still have much to learn as we have in other emergency situations. Many of us have learnt the hard way the vagaries of diagnosis and management when not protected by long waiting lists.

Preventive neurology is fortunately upon us, so that genetics, always an intrinsically intriguing subject, is worthy of emphasis, in particular the way neurogenetic clinics function, remembering that some conditions, such as Huntington's chorea, will almost become things of the past in future generations. Prevention of some genetic disorders is only the beginning. This area will expand into trigger prevention and gene therapy in multifactorial disease and secondary prevention to reduce progression after early warnings of disease, will become an increasingly important aspect of management that we should not shirk.

Finally, and still on a preventive and treatment-orientated theme, the proper management and ideas about psychological aspects of the conditions we deal with are important. Most of us spend most of our time seeing patients with psychosomatic disease and many of these with proper handling and reassurance can be improved or cured, although given the frequency of such conditions, hard facts and active research into this area is woefully lacking. Also, the secondary psychological sequelae of organic neurological disease can be major and it is largely to minimize such reactions that good management including education of and feedback from patients should be encouraged and bad management, usually related to an unnecessarily drawn out investigative process side-tracked by 'red herrings', coupled with poor communication, will make matters worse. In today's evidence-based medicine, it may take years before such assertions are proved. However, we cannot afford to wait for trials to prove that the art and intuitive aspects of medicine are alive and necessary. The most important thing for most patients with a neurological problem is to see a smart up-to-date neurologist with a straightforward and empathetic demeanour accompanied by a friendly, efficient, and spirited team.

Birmingham
1999

Adrian Williams

Contents

List of contributors   xi

1 Loss of vision   1
Gordon T. Plant

2 Vestibular and auditory problems and falls   21
Linda M. Luxon

3 Chronic pain   43
Munseng S. Chong and Michael Tai

4 Epilepsy and blackouts   59
Nick Davies

5 Headache   93
Richard Peatfield

6 Neuromuscular disease   105
John Winer

7 Multiple sclerosis   111
David A. Francis

8 Involuntary movements   127
Hardev S. Pall

9 Parkinson's disease   145
Christopher Ward and Piers Newman

10 Dementia and delerium   161
Christopher McWilliam and Kenneth Barrett

11 Motor neurone disease   173
Adrian Williams

12 Stroke and subarachnoid haemorrhage   179
Peter Humphrey

13 Spinal cord diseases   197
Edmund M. R. Critchley

14 Controversies in the management of common tumours   213
Spiros Sgouros and A. Richard Walsh

15 Infectious diseases   233
Milne Anderson

16 The value of a clinical genetics unit   247
Sarah Bundey

17 Neurological problems in the elderly   259
Douglas G. MacMahon

18 Particular neurological problems of ethnic minority groups   281
Bashir Qureshi

19 The relationship between neurology and psychiatry   297
Tim Betts

20 Neuro-rehabilitation   311
Stephen Sturman and Jim Unsworth

21 Respiratory and swallowing disorders   325
C. M. Wiles

22 Muscle spasticity   345
Richard J. Hardie

23 Bladder, bowel, and sexual problems   355
Michael Swash

24 Neurological disease and driving   367
C. J. Earl

25 Dying from a neurological disease   373
David Oliver

26 Neurologists as useful providers of health care   383
Michael Donaghy

27 Coping with contracting in a changing National Health Service   391
Ian Williams

28 Commissioning   399
Jonathan R. Cook and Daphne I. Austin

29 Translating clinical research and technological developments into changes in practice   417
S. B. Blunt and C. Kennard

30 Medical education and the patient   425
I. M. S. Wilkinson

31 A team approach to neurological disease   433
Marie Oxtoby

x   *Contents*

32 Going behind the consultation   441
    Ruth Pinder

33 An outreach service for neurological
    disease   451
    Melesina Goodwin and Amanda Powell

34 Linking with lay societies   457
    Mary G. Baker and Bridget McCall

35 Organizing neurology outpatient services 463
    David L. Stevens

    Index   479

List of Contributors

Milne Anderson Consultant Neurologist, Birmingham Neuroscience Centre, Queen Elizabeth Hospital, Edgbaston, Birmingham, B15 2TH, UK

Daphne I. Austin Consultant in Public Health, Department of Public Health, Shrubhill Road, Worcester, WR4 3RW, UK

Mary G. Baker National and International Development Consultant, The Parkinson's Disease Society, 22 Upper Woburn Place, London, WC1H 0RA, UK

Kenneth Barrett Consultant Psychiatrist, The Wayward Hospital, High Lane, Burslem, Stoke-on-Trent, Staffordshire, ST6 7AG, UK

Tim Betts Consultant Neuropsychiatrist, Queen Elizabeth Hospital, Mindelson Way, Edgbaston, Birmingham, B15 2Q2 UK

S. Blunt Consultant Neurologist, Department of Neurology, Royal Postgraduate Medical School, Hammersmith Hospital, Du Cane Road, London, W12 0NN, UK

Sarah Bundey It is with regret that we record the death of Professor Sarah Bundey prior to publication of this book. Professor of Clinical Genetics, Department of Clinical Genetics, Birmingham Women's Hospital, Edgbaston, Birmingham, B15 2TH, UK

Munseng S. Chong Consultant Neurologist, Kings College Hospital, Denmark Hill, London SE5 9RS, UK

Jonathan R. Cook Christchurch House, Greyfriars Road, Coventry, CV1, UK

Edmund M. R. Critchley Emeritus Professor of Clinical Neurology, University of Central Lancashire, 18 Merlin Road, Blackburn, Lancashire, BB2 7BA, UK

Nick Davies Specialist Registrar, Birmingham Neuroscience Centre, Queen Elizabeth Hospital, Edgbaston, Birmingham, B15 2TH, UK

Michael Donaghy Reader in Clinical Neurology, University of Oxford and Consultant Neurologist, Radcliffe Infirmary, Oxford, OX2 6HE, UK

C. J. Earl Consultant Physician, National Hospital for Neurology and Neurosurgery, Queen Square, London WCIN 3BG, UK

David A. Francis Consultant Neurologist, Birmingham Neuroscience Centre, Queen Elizabeth Hospital, Edgbaston, Birmingham, B15 2TH, UK

Melesina Goodwin Epilepsy Specialist Nurse, Northampton District General Hospital, Northampton, UK

Richard J. Hardie Consultant Neurologist, St. George's and Atkinson Morley's Hospitals and Medical Director, Wolfson Rehabilitation Centre, Copse Hill, London, SW20 0NE, UK

Peter Humphrey Consultant Neurologist, The Walton Centre for Neurology and Neurosurgery, Lower Lane, Liverpool, L9 7LJ, UK

C. Kennard Professor, Department of Neuroscience, Charing cross and Westminster Medical School, Fulham Palace Road, London, W6 8RF, UK

Linda M. Luxon Professor of Audiological Medicine, University College London, 330/332 Gray's Inn Road, London, WC1X 8EE, UK, and Consultant Audiological Physician, National Hospital for Neurology and Neurosurgery, Queen Square, London WC1

Douglas G. MacMahon Consultant Physician, Cornwall Healthcare Trust, Camborne/Redruth Community Hospital, Barncoose Terrace, Redruth, Cornwall, TR15 3ER, UK

Bridget McCall Information Manager, National and International Development Consultant, The Parkinson's Disease Society, 22 Upper Woburn Place, London, WC1H 0RA, UK

Christopher McWilliam Consultant Psychiatrist to the Elderly, Ribbleton Hospital, Miller Road, Preston, Lancashire, PR2 6LS, UK

Piers Newman Specialist Registrar in Neurology, Birmingham Neuroscience Centre, Queen Elizabeth Hospital, Edgbaston, Birmingham, B15 2TH, UK

David Oliver Medical Director, The Wisdom Hospice, St. Williams Way, Rochester, Kent, ME1 2NU, UK

Mary Oxtoby Chairman, Bolton Branch of the Parkinson's Disease Society, Oaklands, Sweetloves Lane, Bolton, Lancashire, BL1 7ET, UK

Hardev S. Pall Consultant Neurologist, Birmingham Neuroscience Centre, Queen Elizabeth Hospital, Edgbaston, Birmingham, B15 2TH, UK

Richard Peatfield Consultant Neurologist, Regional Neuroscience Centre, Charing Cross Hospital, Fulham Palace Road, London, W6 8RF, UK

Ruth Pinder Associate Research Fellow and Education Consultant, Brunel—The University of West London, Uxbridge, Middlesex, UB8 3PH, UK

Gordon T. Plant Consultant Neuro-Ophthalmologist, St Thomas' Hospital, Lambeth Palace Road, London, SEI 7EH, UK

Amanda Powell   Neurology Liaison Sister, Birmingham Neuroscience Centre, Queen Elizabeth Hospital, Edgbaston, Birmingham, B15 2TH, UK

Bashir Qureshi   32 Legrace Avenue, Hounslow, Middlesex, TW4 7RS

Spiros Sgouros   Senior Lecturer in Neurosurgery, Birmingham Neuroscience Centre, Queen Elizabeth Hospital, Edgbaston, Birmingham, B15 2TH, UK

David L. Stevens   Consultant Neurologist, Department of Neurology, Gloucester Royal Hospital, Great Western Road, Gloucester, GL1 3NN, UK

Steven Sturman   Consultant in Neurology and Rehabilitation Medicine, Regional Rehabilitation Centre, Oak Tree Lane, Selly Oak, Birmingham, B29 6JA, UK

Michael Swash   Professor of Neurology, St. Bartholemew's and The Royal London College of Medicine and Dentistry, The Royal London Hospital, London, E1 1BB, UK

Ian Sutton   Research Registrar in Neurology, Department of Neurology, Queen Elizabeth Hospital, Birmingham B15 2TH, UK

Michael Tai   Consultant Anaesthetist in Pain Relief, Thanet General Hospital, St. Peters Road, Margate, Kent, CT9 4AN, UK

Jim Unsworth   Director, Regional Rehabilitation Centre, Oak Tree Lane, Selly Oak, Birmingham, B29 6JA, UK

Richard A. Walsh   Consultant Neurosurgeon, Birmingham Neuroscience Centre, Queen Elizabeth Hospital, Edgbaston, Birmingham, B15 2TH, UK

Christopher Ward   Professor of Rehabilitation Medicine, Derby City General Hospital, Uttoxeter Road, Derby, DE22 3NE, UK

C. M. Wiles   Professor of Neurology, University of Wales College of Medicine, Heath Park, Cardiff, CF4 4XN, UK

I. M. S. Wilkinson   Consultant Neurologist, Addenbrooke's Hospital, Hills Road, Cambridge, CB2 2QQ, UK

Adrian Williams   Professor of Clinical Neurology, Birmingham Neuroscience Centre, Queen Elizabeth Hospital, Edgbaston, Birmingham, B15 2TH, UK

Ian Williams   Medical Director, The Walton Centre for Neurology and Neurosurgery, Lower Lane, Liverpool, L9 7LJ, UK

John Winer   Consultant Neurologist, Birmingham Neuroscience Centre, Queen Elizabeth Hospital, Edgbaston, Birmingham, B15 2TH, UK

1 | *Loss of Vision*

Gordon T. Plant

The focus of this chapter is the management of patients who present with visual symptoms due to disorders of the nervous system. Neurological disorders frequently present with visual symptoms and in order to avoid a 'Cook's tour' through virtually the whole of neurology I will concentrate particularly on the early management and differential diagnosis of cases that would commonly present with loss of vision. Such cases often present first to an ophthalmologist rather than a neurologist.

The author sees many patients who present to an eye casualty/primary care clinic at Moorfields Eye Hospital. It is my belief that there is a marked divergence in the training of ophthalmologists and neurologists at an early stage which results in many of these patients falling between the two disciplines. Many of them require expert evaluation by clinicians who have some familiarity with clinical skills normally associated with one or the other speciality. *Medical ophthalmology* is now a recognized speciality in the United Kingdom and the need for physicians who can carry out a competent eye examination is well recognized for the management of, for example, inflammatory eye disease. However, in most UK hospitals neuro-ophthalmological problems are managed jointly or separately by ophthalmologists and neurologists who may not have a particular interest in the field. The British neurologists practising a century ago, in particular William Gowers, realized the importance of the ophthalmoscope and perimetry in neurological diagnosis and MacDonald Critchley in his article 'The training of a neurologist' (Critchley 1975) recommended that all neurologists should spend time working in an eye clinic. He did, however, also suggest that the attachment should be honorary—a suggestion that may be difficult to incorporate into a modern Calman training programme!

What follows is an account of problems in the management of patients with neurological problems affecting vision that have taxed and interested me in recent years, many of which have prompted me to publish articles. In this chapter I have included unpublished case reports to emphasize certain aspects of the difficulty in diagnosis and management.

HOW MANY PEOPLE ARE VISUALLY DISABLED AS A RESULT OF NEUROLOGICAL DISEASE?

It is difficult to obtain an accurate assessment of the numbers of patients with visual disability due to disorders of the brain and nervous system. A recent critique of the data available from blind and partial sight registration in the United Kingdom has been published (Evans 1995) which includes a breakdown of the data for 1990–1. It is likely that there is under-registration of patients with neurological disorders, particularly if they have other disabilities and are partially sighted rather than blind. In those aged 15 or under optic atrophy accounted for 15.5% of registered cases of blindness (defined as: 3/60 or worse in the better eye, or 6/60 or worse with markedly constricted fields) and 7.3% of cases of partial sight (3/60 to 6/36 in better eye or 6/18 if visual field loss is 'gross'). The number of certifications per head rises steeply over the age of 65 and the proportion falls to 3.4% and 2.3% if all ages are considered together, largely because of the rise in the incidence of degenerative conditions of the macula and posterior pole. As a cause of blindness optic atrophy is equal numerically to both (untreatable) cataract and diabetic retinopathy from these data.

Since the Second World War there has been a considerable decline in the incidence of all infective causes of blindness, including cerebral infections and meningitis, and out of the total of 13 950 reported cases of blindness there were only two from cerebral infections in 1990–1. Cerebrovascular disease accounted for 159 cases of blindness and there were 13 cases registered as being due to giant cell arteritis. Only about 40 cases were registered as being due to benign or malignant tumours of the nervous system. The figures for partial sight registration were very similar in all these groups.

Cases of homonymous hemianopia can be registered as partially sighted on the criterion of field loss but it is not possible to determine which these are from the data as ophthalmologists would code these patients as '6/18 or better with gross visual field defects', without necessarily stating what the field defect is. However, as most cases of hemianopia are due to cerebrovascular disease and this accounted for only 168 cases of partial sight I would estimate that there must be considerable under-registration of hemianopia. These figures would suggest that the incidence of blindness due to cerebrovascular disease is similar to the incidence of hemianopia or other field defects which cannot be corrected. In fact, the benefits of partial sight registration are not great and many ophthalmologists or neurologists may not consider there to be any need to arrange registration in cases of hemianopia.

A disability issue of great significance for many individuals with neurological disorders affecting vision is the question of the ability to drive. In the United Kingdom, no visual test is required to obtain a provisional driving licence. The only test of visual acuity recognized for the driving test is the ability to read a vehicle licence plate at 20.2 metres. This vision standard was introduced in 1934 and is equivalent to a Snellen acuity of around 6/12. Patients who as a result of neurological disease cannot fulfil the vision standard should be advised that they are not permitted to drive. The test is administered, often for the first time, at the commencement of the driving test and if the candidate fails he/she is not permitted to take the test. I have recently seen patients with neurological disorders who have adequate vision on Snellen testing but cannot pass the 'number plate test' (Plant and Tripathy 1997). This appears to be due to the excessively close spacing of the figures on contemporary number plates (7 letters and figures as opposed to 4 or 5 in 1934!). This has caused some distress because the patients had invested time and money in driving lessons having been assured that they had adequate vision, only to be turned away at the 'starting post' on the day of their driving test.

Patients with hemianopia are not permitted to drive in the United Kingdom. There is no statutory requirement for a visual field test to be carried out before a candidate takes the driving test, however. I have seen numerous examples of patients with congenital hemianopia who have passed the driving test and been driving safely for years until the hemianopia is discovered and they are thenceforth prohibited from driving. Needless to say this does not come as good news and can be difficult to justify logically. Difficult cases are those with quadrantanopia because the regulations (Munton 1995) state that in addition to having 120 degrees of field preserved along the horizontal meridian the field defect must not encroach within 20 degrees of fixation and many homonymous quadrantanopias are borderline on this criterion. Patients who have had surgery for temporal lobe epilepsy often have field defects of this type, which can cause difficulties particularly if a subsidiary aim of the surgery has to render the patient seizure free and able to hold a driving licence, (Manji and Plant 1999)!

Case report 1

A 50-year-old man developed mild diabetes and because of this was referred to an ophthalmologist to look for evidence of diabetic retinopathy. Perimetry was carried out which revealed a right partial superior homonymous quadrantanopia [Fig. 1.1a]. On further enquiry it transpired that 25 years previously he had experienced an episode of severe headache followed by a right hemiparesis and hemianopia. Angiography found no underlying cause and the hemiparesis and hemianopia appeared to recover fully and the attack was ascribed to migraine. He had passed his driving test after that event and this was the first occasion that his visual fields had been checked since then. He was informed that he had to give up driving. However the Esterman binocular field test (which is approved by the UK Driver and Vehicle Licensing Authority) showed the field defect to be borderline [Fig. 1.1b]. Following an appeal he regained his driving licence two years later.

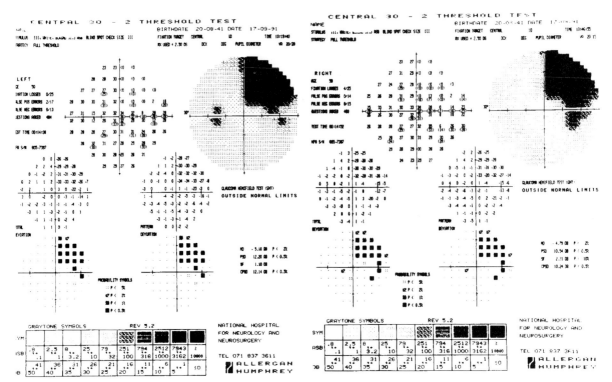

Fig. 1.1a Humphrey automated perimetric findings in a man who had been driving safely for 30 years with the homonymous superior quadrantanopia shown. When this was discovered he was told that he was no longer able to drive as according to the regulations a field defect must not encroach within 20 degrees of fixation.

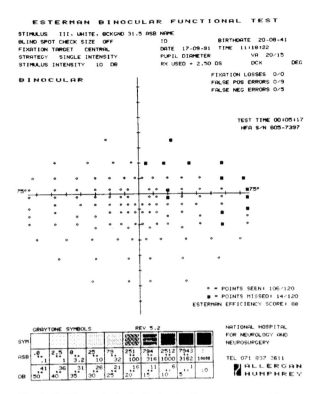

ESTERMAN BINOCULAR FUNCTIONAL TEST

```
STIMULUS   III, WHITE, BCKGND 31.5 ASB NAME
BLIND SPOT CHECK SIZE  OFF        ID              BIRTHDATE 20-08-41
FIXATION TARGET  CENTRAL          DATE 17-09-91  TIME 11:18:22
STRATEGY    SINGLE INTENSITY      PUPIL DIAMETER              VA 20/15
STIMULUS INTENSITY  10 DB         RX USED + 2.50 DS    DCX        DEG

BINOCULAR
                                        FIXATION LOSSES  0/0
                                        FALSE POS ERRORS 0/9
                                        FALSE NEG ERRORS 0/5

                                   TEST TIME 00:05:17
                                   HFA S/N 805-7397

75°                         875°

                           ° = POINTS SEEN: 106/120
                           ■ = POINTS MISSED: 14/120
                     ESTERMAN EFFICIENCY SCORE: 88
```

```
GRAYTONE SYMBOLS         REV 5.2          NATIONAL HOSPITAL
SYM                                       FOR NEUROLOGY AND
                                          NEUROSURGERY
ASB  .8  2.5  8   25  79  251  794  2512 7943
     .1    1  3.2  10  32 100  316 1000 3162 10000   TEL 071 837 3611
DB   .41  36  31  26  21  16  11   6    1
     50   40  35  30  25  20  15  10    5      :0    ALLERGAN
                                                     HUMPHREY
```

Fig. 1.1b The result obtained using the Esterman strategy (binocular viewing, high luminance target, and concentrating on the lower field). Using this strategy three points are missed which are on the 20 degree isopter. On appeal to the Driver and Vehicle Licensing Agency he was permitted to return to driving.

This case exemplifies both the difficulties that arise because there is no field test administered to prospective driving test candidates and the difficulties of dealing with homonymous field defects that are borderline.

Neurological disorders and cerebrovascular disease are a significant cause of visual disability at all ages. An understanding of how neurological disease can affect vision is essential for all neurologist and ophthalmologists. Clinical skills which the trainees might not acquire in their current training programs in either specialty are required to assess such patients with confidence.

OPTIC NERVE DISORDERS

OPTIC NEURITIS

Optic neuritis is familiar to neurologists as a manifestation of multiple sclerosis. Visual loss is subacute, progressing over a matter of days with recovery. Most of the recovery occurs within a few weeks although it may continue over many months. There is frequently orbital pain, exacerbated by eye movement or occurring only on eye movement, perhaps only on certain directions of eye movement, for a few days before

the onset of visual loss. The pain abates as the visual loss begins. Visual field defects at presentation are quite variable although central scotomata predominate and abnormal colour vision is universal. An interesting description of the subjective alterations in colour vision was published some years ago by an artist who had had the disorder (Mackarell 1986). Fundus examination may be entirely normal (retrobulbar neuritis), the optic disc may show mild swelling and haemorrhages may be seen on the disc occasionally. Abnormal colour vision will always be found using the Ishihara plates and there will always be a relative afferent pupillary defect if the disorder is unilateral or sufficiently asymmetric. There may be evidence of retinal venous sheathing or vitritis but these findings are not specific to optic neuritis and can be seen in multiple sclerosis with no evidence of current optic nerve involvement. In some patients, particularly in children, a macular star occurs and these cases are referred to as 'neuroretinitis' rather than pure optic neuritis, what exactly gives rise to this difference in the pathological process is unknown. Bilateral simultaneous optic neuritis is also more common in children. Childhood optic neuritis in general, and bilateral simultaneous optic neuritis and neuroretinitis at all ages are less commonly associated with multiple sclerosis.

When this typical story is heard the diagnosis is usually not in doubt. A careful history must be taken seeking evidence of previous neurological episodes and a careful clinical examination to look for evidence of lesions elsewhere in the nervous system which might point immediately towards a diagnosis of multiple sclerosis. If the optic neuritis is isolated then magnetic resonance imaging may demonstrate subclinical lesions and the number of lesions shows a clear positive correlation with the the likelihood of progression to *multiple sclerosis* (MS) (Morrisey *et al.* 1993).

My own management policy when confronted with a typical story and no clinical confirmation of multiple sclerosis on history or examination is to take blood for sedimentation rate, autoantibody screen and treponemal serology, and carry out a chest radiograph. Clinically indistinguishable stories can be heard from patients who prove to have other inflammatory conditions such as post-infectious disorders, sarcoidosis, systemic lupus erythematosis, or syphilis. If these investigations are normal I consider that it is reasonable to allow the passage of time to confirm the diagnosis. I ask the patient to return six weeks from the date of onset of visual symptoms and check that visual recovery has occurred. If so, then no further action is needed except that some discussion must take place warning the patient of the risk of further neurological episodes, usually mentioning multiple sclerosis specifically as a possibility. I warn patients to return if their vision continues to deteriorate and if visual loss reaches no perception of light or fails to show any indication of recovery 14 days following the onset of symptoms then I investigate further immediately because in such cases an alternative diagnosis is more likely and I will often treat with a three-day course of intravenous methylprednisolone if an inflammatory aetiology is confirmed which may be followed by high dose oral steroids if I suspect that I am dealing with a 'steroid-responsive' inflammatory cause (not demyelinating; *see below*).

Apart from steroid reponsive optic neuropathies the major treatable differential diagnosis which must not be missed is subacute optic nerve compression relating to sinus disease such as aspergillosis (Brown *et al.* 1994), other infections, or a mucocoel. The medial aspect of the optic canal is the lateral aspect of the posterior ethmoidal and sphenoid sinuses and the bone separating the nerve from the contents of the sinuses may be excessively thin or even deficient.

Treatment of demyelinating optic neuritis

The treatment of optic neuritis has continued to be a subject for debate. Until recently few clinicians have used steroid therapy routinely. Those patients with very severe visual loss, particularly if it is bilateral, may be selected for steroid therapy because of a poorer prognosis for visual outcome but the fact is that all studies of the use of steroids in the acute management of demyelinating optic neuritis have shown no evidence of any effect on the final visual outcome, including a recent double-blind study of the effect of intravenous methyl prednisolone on the visual outcome at six months (Kapoor *et al.* 1998). In a recent study (Beck *et al.* 1992) over 400 patients with isolated acute optic neuritis were randomly assigned to one of three treatment groups. One group received a 3-day course of high dose intravenous methylprednisolone followed by oral prednisolone reducing to zero over 15 days; a second group received the oral treatment alone and a third group oral placebo. Intravenous methylprednisolone accelerated visual recovery but did not affect visual outcome at one year. Oral prednisolone alone was associated with an increased risk of recurrent attacks of optic neuritis (double the risk in the fellow eye compared with the placebo treated group). Furthermore the intravenous methylprednisolone group had a lower incidence of subsequent attacks of demyelination by two years, this effect was particularly found in those patients with more abnormalities on magnetic resonance imaging (MRI) at presentation (the incidence of progression to multiple sclerosis was extremely low in the patients with normal imaging of the brain, Beck *et al.* 1993). After two years this beneficial effect decreased.

As a result of this study a management regimen has been advocated to the effect that all patients with acute optic neuritis should have MRI (e.g. see Wray 1995). If this shows evidence of disseminated lesions then a course of intravenous methylprednisolone followed by oral prednisolone therapy should be given. The reason for this treatment is to reduce the incidence of further episodes within two years.

There are some problems with the design of the study (Beck *et al.* 1992) in that it was designed principally to study the visual outcome. The progression to multiple sclerosis took into account subjective reports of symptoms and neither the investigators nor the subjects were blinded as to whether or not intravenous methylprednisolone had been given because there was no intravenous placebo. If the results are accepted, however, I still do not consider the proposed management regimen to be logical. Why should acute optic neuritis differ from any other isolated presentation—or indeed any symptomatic relapse—in the proposed protective effect of methylprednisolone? Optic neuritis, because of the location of the lesion, is the symptomatic 'iceberg tip' in patients with multiple lesions at presentation. If methylprednisolone does have a protective effect surely it is as likely to have the effect on patients with multiple sclerosis presenting in any manner—and perhaps if given at any time, not only during an acute symptomatic relapse. Before making a drastic change in the management of what is merely one manifestation of the disease I would prefer to see a trial of the effect of intravenous methylprednisolone on the progression of MS in general. The recent studies which have shown that beta-interferon is effective in reducing the number of relapses in MS have generated more studies of that and related treatments and I think it is unlikely that a study of the effect of methyl prednisolone treatment, such as I am suggesting, will ever be carried out.

OTHER CAUSES OF OPTIC NEUROPATHY OF SUBACUTE ONSET

If visual recovery does not occur then a diagnosis of Leber's hereditary optic neuropathy must be considered. The typical story is bilateral sequential visual loss in a young man. In most cases severe visual loss results (6/60 or worse). Typical fundus findings of dilated capillaries in the peripapillary region may be seen, the optic disc may be minimally swollen as may the nerve fibre layer, the disc does not leak on fluorescein angiography. It is now possible to confirm the diagnosis by analysis of mitochondrial DNA where four mutations have been described at positions 11778 (the most common), 3460, 15257, and 14484. No effective treatment is available and the major implications of making the diagnosis are genetic in that although the disease is not transmitted by affected males, male children of females in the family who have the mutation are at risk of developing the disease. The 11778 mutation carries the worst visual prognosis, the 14484 the best and very late recovery of vision has been reported in some cases. Since genetic tests have become available atypical manifestations of the disease—without typical fundus findings, in women, in older males, in cases thought to be examples of nutritional or toxic amblyopia—have been described.

Case report 2

A 23-year-old man presented with a history that for several weeks his vision had gradually deteriorated in both eyes. Central vision was predominantly affected and he had experienced no pain. Initially, he gave a history that an uncle on his mother's side had had poor vision since the age of 10 and had been seen then at Moorfields Eye Hospital. He was a non-smoker who drank about 40 units of alcohol per week. On examination he was found to have visual acuity of counting fingers on

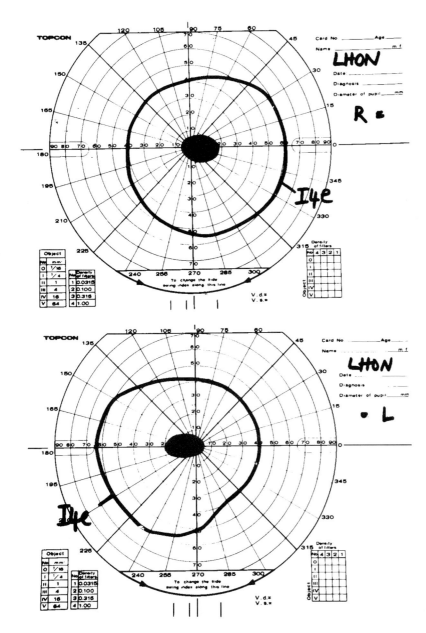

Fig. 1.2(a) The Goldman fields show the dense central scotomas and relatively preserved peripheral vision that are typical of Leber's hereditary optic neuropathy. Patients with field defects like this will never be functionally blind as they will be able to navigate unaided in most environments. Disability arises from the need for special aids to permit reading or any work requiring even moderate acuity levels. Once established, these field defects remain stable throughout the patient's life.

the right and 6/60 on the left. He was able to read N48 and no Ishihara plates on the right and N24 and only the control Ishihara plate with his left eye. He had bilateral dense central scotomas on perimetry [Fig. 1.2(a)]. The optic discs were hyperaemic with prominence of the nerve fibre layer except temporally where some nerve fibre loss was apparent [Fig. 1.2(b)]. Mitochondrial DNA analysis was positive for the 11778 mitochondrial DNA mutation. His uncle was examined and there was indeed a history of a diagnosis of optic atrophy being made at the age of 10. His vision had been at the 6/60 level since then. On examination, optic atrophy and bilateral central scotomas were found. It then emerged that his brother had had some problem with his vision in childhood and had multiple squint operations but that his vision was adequate for driving. He was also examined and found to have vision of 6/60 right and 6/6 left. With the right eye he could only read the control Ishihara plate and with the left 3 out of 17 plates. He had bilateral optic atrophy. The 11778 mutation was found in both uncles.

This case study illustrates the importance of taking a careful family history in young males with bilateral optic neuropathy. Particular importance lies in the identification of maternal uncles.

STEROID-DEPENDENT OPTIC NEUROPATHY

An important clinical problem concerns those patients who prove to have a steroid-dependent optic neuropathy. The

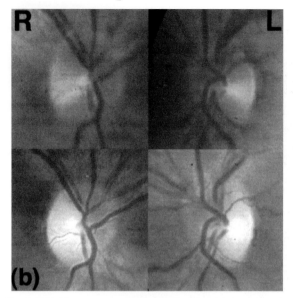

Fig. 1.2(b) The upper two panels show the left and right eye 6 weeks following the onset of symptoms. The optic discs are slightly hyperaemic, there was no leakage at the disc on fluorescein angiography. The lower panels show pictures taken 2 months later showing the loss of the nerve fibre layer corresponding to the caeco-central projection which subserves the scotoma shown in (a).

typical story is a patient with unilateral or bilateral visual loss whose vision continues to deteriorate for longer than expected in demyelinating optic neuritis, and a course of steroids is given with a favourable response. When the steroids are discontinued the patient may or may not relapse and if so, long-term immunosuppression is advisable. Some of these patients can be shown to have sarcoidosis, in many others there is no obvious underlying disease but a granulomatous optic neuropathy is presumed. I investigate them as thoroughly as possible but usually they are taking high doses of steroids when a diagnosis is being sought which can make a diagnosis of sarcoidosis difficult to confirm. Magnetic resonance imaging of the brain and optic nerves is important but there are no features that are characteristic of granulomatous optic neuropathy. The optic nerve may or may not be enlarged, it may or may not show gadolinium enhancement. I find spinal fluid examination to be useful because often in steroid responsive optic neuropathies there are oligoclonal bands in both cerebrospinal fluid and serum (which may not be identical). Steroid-responsive optic neuropathy may be a feature of HIV infection (Burton *et al.*, 1998).

The question of what alternative immunosuppression to use in patients who require high doses of steroids long term is unresolved. My personal preference is azathioprine but cylcophosphamide or cyclosporine may be useful in some cases and an important principle is that any vision is worth fighting for. This is a blinding disease and there is a considerable difference for the patient if he or she has any residual vision short of total blindness.

Case report 3

A 50-year-old woman presented with 6-week history of subacute visual loss in the right eye. Sixteen years previously she developed pain on moving the left eye, 20 days later she became aware that the vision was deteriorating and it progressively worsened over 3 weeks. She recalled being treated with oral steroids and that immediately the pain stopped and the vision returned to normal over 2 weeks. Steroids were discontinued and there was a rapid relapse and vision deteriorated again to 6/60. She was not given a second trial of steroids.

The first symptom of the new problem was pain on moving the right eye, vision deteriorated slightly to 6/9, and she took oral steroids at a moderately high dose for 5 days then gradually coming off them. Pain on eye movement returned and vision deteriorated to 6/24. She was recommenced on a low dose of steroids (prednisolone 20 mg daily) but her vision continued to deteriorate. On examination, she had left optic atrophy (vision was counting fingers in that eye) but the right fundus appeared normal.

MRI scan of brain and optic nerves showed no abnormality. Investigations revealed no evidence of a systemic inflammatory disorder such as sarcoidosis but CSF examination showed a moderate CSF lymphocytosis (8/mm³) and oligoclonal bands were present which were identical in CSF and serum. Although she was taking a small dose of steroids her vision was still getting worse and she was commenced on 80 mg prednisolone orally daily. Within a week her vision had begun to improve and within 3 weeks to near-normal (6/5, 50% of Ishihara plates read) [see Fig. 1.3 for perimetric findings]. Reduction in steroid dosage was carried out with great care and azathioprine added. One year later she is being treated with azathioprine alone and her vision is stable.

This story illustrates some characteristic features of the steroid responsive optic neuropathies. We presume these are 'granulomatous' because identical syndromes are seen in sarcoidosis although often there is no evidence of a systemic inflammatory disorder. The cardinal features are response to steroids and relapse when they are withdrawn. This subsequent relapse is often catastrophic. My policy is to treat with steroids until vision seems to be as good as it is going to get— oral prednisolone at 80 mg/day may need to be continued for 3–4 weeks—and then tail off very slowly warning the patient to report immediately if vision deteriorates in which case a high dose is recommended. I am thereafter in no hurry to stop them as I have seen a number of patients in whom this has resulted in severe and irrecoverable visual loss. There are no guidelines as to what alternative immunosuppression is most appropriate (as is the case with the treatment of neurosarcoidosis).

TOXIC AND NUTRITIONAL OPTIC NEUROPATHY

The hallmark of toxic and nutritional optic neuropathy is that both eyes are affected equally. It was recognized in the 19th century that smoking and alcoholism in developed countries and nutritional deficiencies in developing countries were associated with bilateral visual failure. The relative contributions of tobacco smoking, alcoholism, and nutritional deficiencies have been discussed throughout the 20th century but there is no established conclusion. The clinical presentation in all instances is rather similar in that there is the development of gradual visual loss (worsening over a matter of weeks) which affects particularly colour vision and later central acuity. There are bilateral central scotomata or, characteristically,

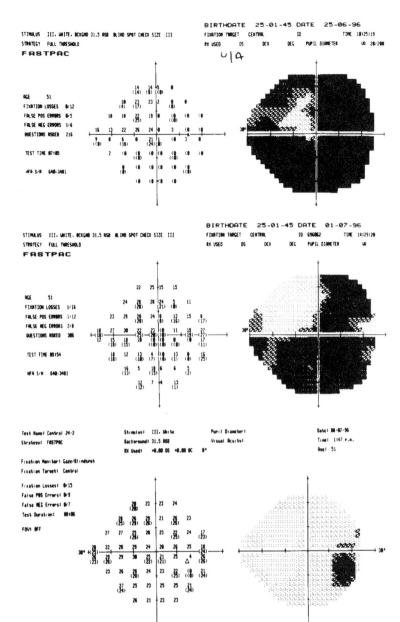

Fig. 1.3 This patient had perception of light vision in the left eye and presented with subacute loss of vision in the right eye. The upper panel shows her visual field following some months of inadequate treatment with 20 mg prednisolone daily, the lower panels show the improvement over three weeks treatment with 80 mg prednisolone daily.

caeco-central scotomata—that is, a scotoma that is not pericentric but encircles the fovea and the blind spot. In established cases it may be possible to identify nerve fibre loss in the caeco-central projection in the retinal nerve fibre layer. In the United Kingdom the typical patient has a high tobacco and alcohol consumption and a poor diet. Blood tests may reveal changes related to alcohol abuse such as a macrocytosis and abnormal liver function tests but it is, in fact, relatively unusual to demonstrate evidence of any specific nutritional deficiency. It is well known that a similar optic neuropathy can occur as a result of vitamin B_{12} deficiency, and cases of optic neuropathy have been attributed to deficiencies of B_1, B_2, B_6,

and folic acid but most of the patients we are discussing have marginal or no evidence of any specific micronutrient deficiency. This raises the question of whether tobacco smoking itself may contribute in some direct way to the pathogenesis.

This question, in relation to possible cyanide toxicity was investigated some years ago by Professor Foulds' group in Glasgow (at the time this was a fairly common diagnosis in the Glasgow Infirmary—although not as common as it had been in the 1920s when Traquair, the doyen of perimetry, stated that 1% of patients with visual failure attending the Glasgow Royal Infirmary had tobacco–alcohol amblyopia). Cyanide in tobacco smoke is detoxified by the enzyme rhodanese to thiocyanate which is excreted in the urine. The fascinating observation was made that although heavy smokers without visual symptoms have elevated thiocyanate levels in blood and urine they did not if they were also suffering from tobacco–alcohol amblyopia. This observation suggested that such cases are impaired in their ability to detoxify cyanide and very high blood cyanide levels indeed have been measured in some cases of tobacco–alcohol amblyopia (Jestico *et al.* 1984) this observation has never been repeated—similar high blood levels of cyanide have only been recorded in cases of smoke inhalation, acute Konzo (a spastic paraparesis occurring in Africa and thought to be caused by cyanide intoxication from the consumption of inadequately processed cassava), and in patients who were given cyanide as a treatment for cancer (the drug, laetrile).

Cases of nutritional optic neuropathy were described in prisoners of war largely in the tropics (e.g. Spillane 1947) and there were subsequently autopsy reports confirming the characteristic degeneration of the projection of the central retina in the optic nerve (Fisher 1955). In recent years there have been two important outbreaks of nutritional optic neuropathy in Cuba (Thomas *et al.* 1995) and Tanzania (Plant *et al.* 1997*a*). In the former there was a clear relationship with nutritional deficiency but smoking was a risk factor for the development of the optic neuropathy. Many cases also had a painful sensory peripheral neuropathy which was unrelated to smoking habits and which was seen independently. The combination of a painful sensory neuropathy associated with optic neuropathy and often sensorineural deafness is frequently referred to as Strachan's syndrome after the medical officer in Jamaica who described such cases over 100 years ago—although he attributed the polyneuropathy to malaria (Strachan 1888). In Cuba as many as 50 000 cases may have been affected although the precise numbers are difficult to establish. We have recently estimated that in 1997 there may be as many as 80 000 young Tanzanians affected in Dar es Salaam alone (Dolin *et al.*, 1998). Visual recovery has been documented in Tanzania and Cuba following treatment with vitamin supplements but a large number of cases are left with significant visual disability.

Do these disorders of distant lands have any relevance to cases in the United Kingdom? The author has seen in London cases of nutritional optic neuropathy associated with a painful peripheral neuropathy recently. These cases are clinically identical to those occurring in the tropics and occurred in non-smokers who were eating a largely vegetarian diet with a high carbohydrate intake but no meat: neither patient appeared malnourished. It seems likely that the major precipitating factor in all cases is a micronutrient deficiency but this has never been established, and certainly no specific micronutrient has ever been implicated—smoking plays a part as a risk factor and any contribution from alcohol abuse is very difficult to disentangle from a poor diet as the two are closely associated. A few cases may have mutations associated with Leber's hereditary optic neuropathy and there has been some

discussion as to whether these mutations may predispose to the development of optic neuropathy in heavy smokers or in nutritional deficiency, the evidence from Cuba and Tanzania is that they do not play a part (Newman *et al.* 1994; Plant *et al.* 1997*b*).

Case report 4

A 23-year-old man presented with a 2-month history of progressive bilateral loss of central vision and a 4-week history of painful feet, their 'burning' at night was keeping him awake. His parents were Cuban and he was born in Miami where he had lived until December 1994. He was a vegetarian and did not smoke tobacco (but occasionally cannabis). He told me that since moving to London he had experienced difficulty obtaining the variety of vegetables that his mother was accustomed to prepare for him in Florida and he was tending to subsist on rice. On examination, he had angular stomatits and his vision was reduced to 6/36 on the right and 6/60 on the left. Optic discs were initially hyperaemic and mildly swollen (later progressing to atrophy). There was sensory impairment to temperature and pin-prick distally in the lower limbs but tendon reflexes were preserved.

There was no evidence of a micronutrient deficiency on blood analysis. Nerve conduction studies were normal (compatible with a small fibre neuropathy) and screening for mutations associated with Leber's hereditary optic neuropathy were negative. [Fundus photographs and perimetric findings are shown in Fig. 1.4.] He was treated with vitamin supplements and his diet improved but unfortunately there was very little improvement in either his vision or neuropathic symptoms.

The immediate treatment of cases of tobacco–alcohol and nutritional amblyopia is to give B group vitamins, to encourage abstinence from tobacco and alcohol, and to take a varied diet. These instructions can prove difficult to enforce in many alcoholics or those with strict vegetarian ethics.

Other optic neuropathies caused by toxins are distinctly unusual. Only two cases were registered as blind and none partially sighted as a result of poisoning in 1990–1. Ethambutol treatment resulted in cases of visual failure when it was first introduced but when the importance of assessing vision during treatment was recognized this complication has fortunately become very rare. Cases do still occur and the usual problem is that patients have not been warned to report any visual symptoms immediately or, if they have, appropriate action (immediate cessation of the drug) has not been taken. Halogenated hydroxyquinolines have been identified as being responsible for the epidemic (10 000 cases) of subacute myelo-optic neuropathy (SMON) that occurred in Japan between 1956 and 1970. Most other examples of toxic optic neuropathies in the literature are limited to small numbers of case reports with the possible exception of quinine which has been a reasonably common cause of visual loss over the years—there is evidence of retinal toxicity rather than optic neuropathy from quinine.

Case report 5

A 38-year-old man inadvertently drank 150 mls of pure methyl alcohol mixed with orange juice (he was under the impression that he was drinking ethyl alcohol). Twenty-four hours later he complained of blurred vision, everything appeared tinged with yellow. He began vomiting and was taken to his local hospital's Accident and Emergency department. At first nothing was thought to be seriously wrong with him until he mentioned that he may have drunk some methyl alcohol.

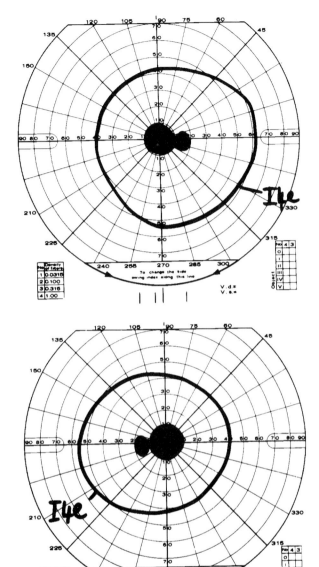

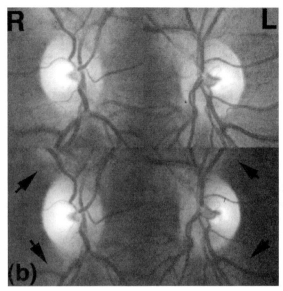

Fig. 1.4(b) The upper panels show the fundus appearances in a case of presumed nutritional optic neuropathy within a month of onset of symptoms. There is mild swelling of the optic nerve fibre layer. Four weeks later (lower panels) there is loss of the nerve fibres corresponding to the caeco-central projection. Note the similarity to Leber's hereditary optic neuropathy (Fig. 1.2), which this patient did not have.

TRAUMATIC OPTIC NEUROPATHY

Visual loss may be a sequel of injury. There are, of course, many ways that trauma can cause a visual disability but damage to the anterior visual pathways, in particular, optic neuropathy is not uncommon. Following a head injury or direct trauma to the orbit optic nerve avulsion may occur, there may be haemorrhage into the orbit or the optic nerve sheath itself. A skull fracture which passes through the optic canal may injure the nerve. In addition to this 'indirect' injury to the nerve may occur, that is, with no sign of haemorrhage or fracture, a head injury may cause a complete or partial optic neuropathy. The aetiology of such indirect injury is not known but it occurs particularly following a blow to the brow or a fall on to the brow (usually a fall from a bicycle or motor cycle). The optic nerve is mobile both in the orbit and intracranially but fixed in the optic canal and it may be that this particular type of injury gives rise to shearing forces which damage the optic nerve at that fixed point, perhaps shearing forces disrupt the vascular supply in the canal. The visual loss in these cases is immediate whereas following haemorrhage it may be delayed, and the prognosis for visual recovery is better in patients with such a 'lucid interval'. Examination of the fundus may reveal evidence of avulsion of the optic nerve, neuroimaging may show haemorrhage in the orbit or optic nerve sheath.

The management of optic nerve injury following trauma is controversial. Some groups advocate surgical decompression

Fig. 1.4(a) Central scotomas seen in a case of nutritional optic neuropathy.

Discussion with a local poisons unit reinforced the potential seriousness of the situation and an ethanol infusion was commenced. Not a moment to soon— within 12 hours he was unconscious requiring ventilatory support and heamodialysis.

Five days later he recovered consiousness and realized that his vision was impaired. When I saw him his vision was down to 6/36 bilaterally and has not recovered. [Visual fields are shown in Fig. 1.5(a)]. He also had a parkinsonian syndrome and the explanation for this is also shown in the Fig. 1.5(b).

This report points out the importance of thinking of an unusual toxic cause of acute bilateral visual failure and the extraordinarily selective neurological deficits found in those surviving methyl alcohol intoxication.

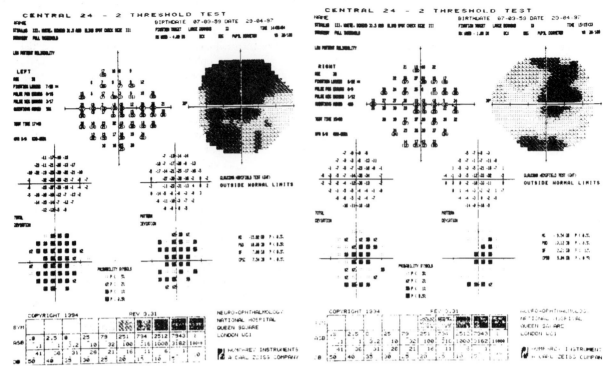

Fig. 1.5(a) Humphrey visual fields show caeco-central and, especially in the left eye, more generalized loss of vision, in a patient who survived methanol intoxication.

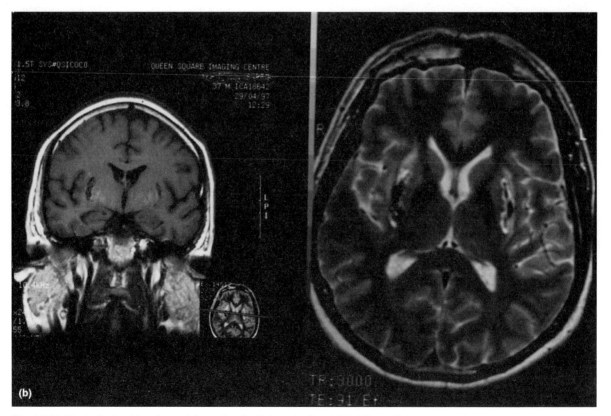

Fig. 1.5(b) He also had parkinsonism and the explanation is shown in these MRIs: bilateral haemorrhagic necrosis of the putamen.

of the optic canal in all cases, some only in those where there is evidence of haematoma or haemorrhage into the sheath. Others have suggested very high dose steroid therapy and a multi-centre trial of high dose steroids vs placebo has been initiated in the United States. Until the results of such trials are available it is impossible to give clear recommendations. Most centres give high dose steroids as soon as possible after the injury and some centres will proceed to optic nerve decompression if there is no return of vision within 48 hours. Fig. 1.6 shows examples of the frequently trivial permanent external signs of the injury.

OPTIC NERVE COMPRESSION

Tumours

Where visual failure is due to compression of the optic nerve or chiasm by tumour then the hallmark is gradually progressive visual loss. Monocular visual loss may go unnoticed by the patient until quite severe and peripheral visual loss, or bitemporal hemianopia, may not be noticed by the patient until central vision is involved.

In patients with progressive visual failure the visual field examination is of paramount importance. It is common experi-

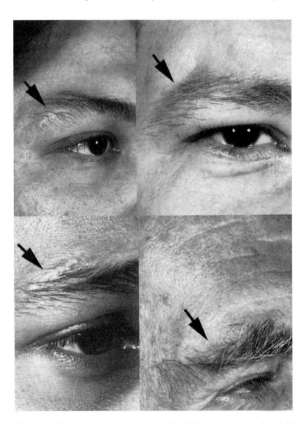

Fig. 1.6 These four right eyes are blind following relatively trivial trauma, falling from motor cycles and pedal cycles with the right brow receiving the focus of the impact. Note the similar tell-tale scars.

ence, for example, that patients with bitemporal hemianopia due to chiasmal compression may seek advice many times from physicians, ophthalmologists, and optometrists and be reassured because normal visual acuity is found. It is not until visual field examination is carried out that the diagnosis is suspected. I am sure that this seems too obvious to require stating here—but it is not. Patients in whom the diagnosis has been delayed for years simply for want of perimetry continue to present to me. Patients with bitemporal hemianopia may have some unusual symptoms such as diplopia when reading—which do not immediately suggest anterior visual pathway disease.

Apart from the neccessity of a careful clinical examination in patients complaining of progressive visual failure neuroimaging is clearly the mainstay of diagnosis and the author has seen many examples where the diagnosis has been missed because the neuroimaging carried out has been inadequate. There is now virtually no place for plain skull radiology in cases of visual failure. If nothing else is available then a normal sized pituitary fossa can almost totally exclude a pituitary macroadenoma and intracranial calcification may give other clues but many lesions will only be revealed by enhanced computerized tomographic (CT) scanning with high definition orbital cuts. Very few compressive lesions will be missed by a good quality enhanced CT scan. However I never accept the statement that a CT scan is normal without reviewing the images and assessing their quality—see Fig. 1.7 for an informative example.

In the author's view, the major advantage of MRI is that more information can be obtained about many lesions. In particular the relationship of the chiasm and optic nerves to a mass lesion is much better identified. For example, an important clue as to the underlying pathology can be obtained by observing whether a normal pituitary gland can be distinguished separately from a suprasellar tumour, if so then the tumour cannot have arisen from the pituitary.

The management of many of the common tumours which affect the optic nerve is controversial. In children, gliomas are the most common tumour affecting the anterior visual pathways and there is still no clear agreement as to whether they represent true neoplasms or hamartomas although recent histopathological evidence is in favour of a true neoplastic nature (Burnstine *et al.* 1993). In a meta-analysis of published cases (Dutton 1994) 70% were diagnosed in the first decade of life whether limited to the optic nerve, the chiasm, or both. Chiasmal gliomas often involve the hypothalamus and it is involvement of the brain that represents the life-threatening manifestation of these tumours. Unfortunately, there is no clear evidence that surgery, radiotherapy, or chemotherapy can influence the risk to life or vision. Fortunately, in the majority of patients visual function remains stable for many years. Around half of these tumours occur in patients with evidence of neurofibromatosis type I. Malignant glioma of the optic nerve and chiasm is a much rarer tumour of adult life which has a very poor prognosis—death in around 12

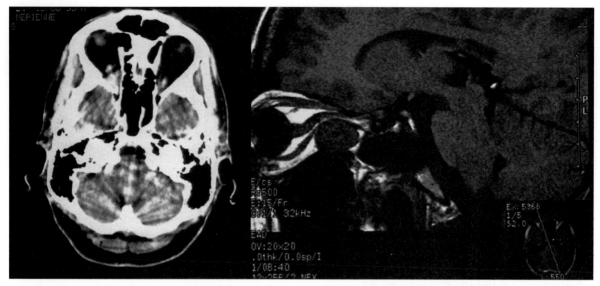

Fig. 1.7 This patient was referred as a case of optic neuritis, subacute visual loss without recovery and a normal CT scan. Review of the scan revealed an inadequate study for a case of visual failure and the pathology—a cavernoma—was revealed in keen detail on appropriate MR imaging (right panel).

months in the majority of cases—and for which no effective treatment is available.

About a third of all tumours found in the orbit are meningiomas and about half of these will have originated intracranially. Meningiomas can arise from meningoendothelial cells of the optic nerve sheath and these optic nerve sheath meningiomas are particularly common in older females. Visual loss is insidious and helpful clinical signs are swelling of the disc and retino-choroidal collateral vessels. Excision cannot be achieved without a deterioration in vision and in most patients they are best left alone. There is a suggestion that they may be more aggressive when they occur in younger patients (some of whom may have neurofibromatosis type II) and that excision should be considered in such cases as local morbidity from the orbital mass and intracranial extension may be prevented.

Case report 6

A 35-year-old woman presented with a history that 2 years previously she had noticed when closing her right eye vision was misty with the left. Her vision was 6/18 and she was referred to an ophthalmologist and then to a neurologist. Neuroimaging was carried out with both CT and MR scanning of the brain and anterior visual pathways showing no abnormality. A diagnosis of optic neuritis was made.

I first saw her 2 years later when I found that her vision had deteriorated to counting fingers in the periphery, there was a large central scotoma in which she was unable to see a moving finger, she had optic atrophy in that eye. The diagnosis of optic neuritis is excluded in a progressive optic neuropathy without spontaneous remission and I reinvestigated with MR imaging and CSF examination [Fig. 1.8]. These were both normal. A course of high dose steroids did not bring about any improvement in her vision. A year later I saw her again and found that her vision was down to no perception of light. I repeated the neuroimaging [Fig. 1.8] and on this occasion a small intercanalicular meningioma was found, just beginning to extend intracranially. She was referred for radiotherapy but declined because she was pregnant.

Cases like this, in the pre-CT era, were often followed up as 'tumour suspects'. Modern neuroimaging has almost rendered this clinical category obsolete, but not quite. Cases with progressive visual failure must be considered as 'tumour suspects' indefinitely unless some other cause is definitively demonstrated. Here, a small meningioma in the optic canal was missed despite state-of-the-art imaging.

Optic nerve compression: other pathology

Tumours are not the only cause of visual failure due to optic nerve compression. Disease of the closely associated sinuses, in particular, the ethmoid sinus may cause optic nerve compression—particularly if a mucocoel has formed.

Metastic disease can cause visual loss either by compression from a tumour mass or invasion of the optic nerve sheath as part of a neoplastic meningitis, in the latter case the optic disc is often swollen and the diagnosis can be difficult to establish because the imaging studies are relatively normal and a biopsy is difficult to achieve (although the diagnosis can sometimes be made by biopsy of the optic nerve sheath). Repeated lumbar punctures with careful cytological examination is usually the most effective means of confirming the diagnosis.

The optic nerves are in close proximity to the internal carotid arteries and compression can occur either by ectatic, tortuous vessels, or a supraclinoid aneurysm of the internal carotid artery or aneurysms of the ophthalmic and anterior communicating arteries. Giant aneurysms of the internal carotid occur usually in older females and are not life-threatening in the sense that rupture is extremely rare and if it does occur may not be fatal. Giant aneurysms more commonly affect the intracavernous portion of the internal carotid artery and in this situation cause ocular motor palsies without optic

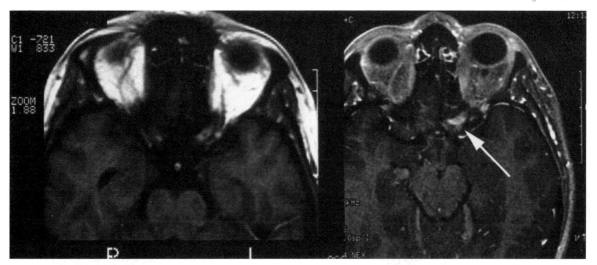

Fig. 1.8 This patient was also referred as a case of left optic neuritis, this time both CT-and MR-negative. My first scan (left) still did not reveal any pathology even with Gadolinium enhancement. A year later, however, a small meningioma arising from the optic canal and now extending intracranially was observed (right panel, arrow).

neuropathy but even these may enlarge to such an extent that they extend into the suprasellar cistern and cause chiasmal syndromes. The aneurysms are usually extradural and if they rupture, subarachnoid haemorrhage does not result but a carotid-cavernous fistula may form. Unless there is intractable pain the management is conservative but balloon embolization is more often contemplated where the aneurysm is causing visual failure.

VASCULAR DISORDERS

VASCULAR DISORDERS OF THE OPTIC NERVE

The most common vascular occlusive disorder of the optic nerve is non-arteritic anterior ischaemic optic neuropathy (NAION). The most common presentation is a lower altitudinal field defect and the patients will frequently relate that they suddenly were able to see only the top half of objects with the affected eye. There is no pain and usually no change in the symptom from the moment that the patient first notices it. Upper altitudinal defects, central and caeco-central defects, arcuate defects, and occasionally generalized loss of vision also occur. The important clinical finding is that the optic disc is swollen when the patient is seen acutely. Haemorrhages on the disc may be observed. These findings relate to the pathogenesis of NAION which is occlusion of one of the posterior ciliary arteries which supply the retrolaminar and laminar portions of the optic disc. The prelaminar portion of the disc is supplied by branches of the central retinal artery and is not ischaemic but swells because of delay of axonal transport. Later, the swelling is replaced by atrophy, often sectoral reflecting the portion of the disc affected by the occlusion of that particular posterior ciliary artery and corresponding to the visual field defect. There may or may not be evidence of

a systemic condition which may explain the event such as hypertension or diabetes but the pathogenesis is not clearly related to the presence of arteriosclerosis and it may be that anatomical variation in the vascular supply of the optic nerve head may predispose to the development of the condition. The disorder is also more common in patients with hypermetropia (small crowded discs). These two factors may explain the frequent subsequent involvement of the second eye—up to 50% of cases in some series—within a matter of months to many years later.

The most important task when confronted with a patient with anterior ischaemic optic neuropathy is to make sure that it is non-arteritic and not due to giant cell or cranial arteritis. The most important immediate clue is the age of the patient. Giant cell arteritis is unusual below the age of 70 while most patients with NAION are aged 50–70. The second feature is the severity of the visual loss which tends to be more profound in giant cell arteritis. General medical history taking and examination is of great importance because in giant cell arteritis there are almost invariably systemic symptoms of malaise, anorexia, and weight loss. In accord with its other name 'temporal arteritis' there may local pain and tenderness related to involvement of the temporal arteries which may be non-pulsatile and thickened, and in accordance with the name 'cranial arteritis' we find evidence of involvement of other arteries—pain on chewing (so-called jaw claudication) from ischaemia of the muscles of mastication—rarely ischaemia of the tongue which may lead to necrosis. The posterior cerebral circulation may be involved giving rise to brainstem symptoms and signs and non-cranial arteries giving rise to cervical radiculopathy or even coronary artery disease. The other ophthalmic manifestation which may be helpful are the fact that giant cell arteritis may affect the ophthalmic artery and thus give rise to retinal or prelaminar optic disc ischaemia—

these features are not seen in NAION and recently it has been pointed out that delay in the choroidal circulation in giant cell arteritis may also distinguish it from NAION.

However, the essential practical point is that although there is no effective treatment for NAION the treatment of giant cell arteritis with steroids is a medical emergency and if in doubt—treat with steroids. Rapid involvement of the fellow eye can occur and there is no reason for any delay in therapy if the diagnosis is suspected. High dose oral steroids must be given (80 mg daily). Intravenous hydrocortisone or methyl predisolone are used by some for the first dose but it is not known whether this confers any advantage. Some patients continue to lose vision in the first affected or the fellow eye after treatment with steroids has been initiated. I have treated some of these patients with low dose heparin anticoagulation but I do not know if this has any effect, particularly as the pathology of giant cell arteritis indicates that the vessel occlusion occurs without thrombosis.

As far as other aetiological factors are concerned patients will certainly be seen who have other forms of vasculitis, such as polyarteritis nodosum and systemic lupus erythematosis, but these are a very much smaller proportion than those found to have giant cell arteritis. Unlike central retinal artery occlusion there is virtually no point in looking for a source of emboli in cases of NAION although I have seen it occurring in the context of atrial myxoma. Episodes of severe hypotension and chronic anaemia may predispose to the development of NAION.

There may be some difficulty in confirming the diagnosis of NAION if the patient has not been examined acutely. An arcuate or altitudinal field defect found incidentally may represent a previous asymptomatic episode of NAION—the optic disc will show sectoral pallor corresponding to the field loss but no other specific features. Rarely, compressive disorders of the optic nerve may give rise to altitudinal or arcuate field defects and in this situation it is advisable to perform neuroimaging. Retrobulbar ischaemic optic neuropathies do occur but are decidedly rare, and in a patient who is seen acutely I have a general rule that I will never diagnose any form of visual loss as having a vascular cause unless there has been fundoscopic confirmation of AION (disc swelling) or central retinal artery occlusion (see below)—whatever the history. Confusion arises when a patient complains of abrupt loss of vision at some time in the past when, in fact, he/she is merely relating the moment at which the visual loss was first noticed (e.g. when the other eye was covered). In this situation the distinction between a previous NAION and normal tension glaucoma can be difficult unless there is obvious cupping of the disc. Where there is doubt, such patients should be followed up in a glaucoma clinic with serial perimetry and whether or not there is progressive loss of vision will give the pragmatic answer. Another reason for careful inspection of the optic disc in such patients is that occasionally the visual field defect is congenital and increasingly such defects are being detected incidentally by optometrists carrying out

perimetry on patients attending for refraction. The disc may show an anatomical change that could only occur if the defect were acquired very early in life—probably intrauterine in most cases—the disc itself may be unusually small (optic disc hypoplasia) or, if the field defect is altitudinal or arcuate there may be focal hypoplasia such that the main trunk of the central retinal artery is displaced.

In the case of NAION, typically the outcome with regard to visual acuity is favourable—about half will be left with 6/12 or better. It has been suggested that aspirin therapy may reduce the likelihood of involvement of the second eye. Unlike inflammatory optic neuritis the degree of impairment of colour vision is related to the acuity loss whereas in the case of optic neuritis the loss of colour vision tends to be out of proportion to acuity loss. The natural history of the disorder in terms of visual recovery has not been well defined until recently. Further work in this area has been prompted by the suggestion that optic nerve sheath fenestration was an effective therapy for a progressive form of NAION. This has led to some careful case reports showing that spontaneous recovery can occur and the US National Institutes of Health initiated a controlled trial of optic nerve sheath fenestration in anterior ischaemic optic neuropathy which was shown to be ineffective and possibly harmful.

VASCULAR DISORDERS OF THE RETINA

Occlusive disorders of the central retinal artery and its branches are important to neurologists because they may be a presenting feature of cerebrovascular disease for which other treatment is required. In a patient who has had a central retinal artery occlusion the retina appears cloudy and swollen and there is usually no perception of light. This applies to the appropriate sector of the retina in a branch artery occlusion. An embolus may be visible and if so can be very informative. Solitary emboli may be to cholesterol, platelet, or calcific. Multiple emboli are more likely to be cholesterol than the other two. As a broad generalization calcific emboli usually have a cardiac origin from calcified heart valves. Aspirin is the only treatment given to such patients unless the valvular heart disease has some haemodynamic problem. Where cholesterol or platelet emboli are found it is worthwhile investigating for a significant stenosis of the internal carotid artery but this is not commonly found. It has recently been shown that there is no need to investigate patients with no visual symptoms who are found to have cholesterol emboli in the retinal circulation as there is very little chance of finding any treatable abnormality of the carotid artery in these patients.

Transient visual loss can occur as a result of emboli passing through the retinal circulation. The most common complaint is of complete loss of vision the onset of which is over a second or so and is likened to a curtain or blind descending across the vision of one eye which recovers after several minutes. Similar arguments apply as in the management of arteriolar occlusions. It has been shown that the prognosis for the subsequent development of a completed stroke is much lower in the case of amaurosis fugax than in the case of transient ischaemic attacks affecting the cerebral hemispheres. A possible explanation for this is that small emboli, which would be unnoticed elsewhere in the cerebral circulation, cause symptoms when they pass through the retina. Nonetheless, patients with amaurosis fugax, if they are from other points of view suitable candidates for surgical treatment if a significant stenosis is, found should be investigated for the possibility of a significant stenosis in the light of the results of the trials of carotid endarterectomy which have shown a benefit of surgical treatment of stenoses of 70% or greater. In the prospective studies of carotid stenosis it has been shown that patients with ocular transient ischaemic attacks (TIAs) alone have a risk of stroke which is intermediate between cases of hemisphere TIAs and asymptomatic stenosis.

It is of great importance that a careful history is taken in cases of amaurosis fugax because patients are seen with transient visual symptoms which are not due to emboli. One clear example is visual loss related to posture (e.g. patients who lose vision in one eye when they get out of bed at night), such patients may have carotid stenosis but often nothing is found and quite young patients can experience postural visual loss of this type. It is always much briefer than true amaurosis fugax due to emboli and lasts perhaps 30 seconds or so. Secondly some young patients have attacks which are similar in duration to embolic disease which are ascribed to retinal migraine and there may be more positive symptoms. Spasm of the central retinal artery has been observed during attacks in some patients and calcium channel blockers have been effective in cases having very frequent attacks. In a young patient, say under 40, with no evidence of vascular disease and an otherwise typical story I do not carry out any investigations as they are invariably unrewarding. There is usually no history of any other type of migraine or of headache. This syndrome is not entirely benign and some cases have developed central or branch retinal artery occlusions, cilio-retinal artery occlusions or even NAION.

PAPILLOEDEMA AND OTHER CAUSES OF OPTIC DISC SWELLING

Optic disc swelling may be noticed incidentally in a patient who has no visual symptoms. In this situation the first problem is to decide whether the swelling is due to a congenital anomaly of the disc or a normal variant in the disc appearance, or whether it is due to a cause which requires further investigation—such as papilloedema. Hypermetropia is associated with a relatively small globe and a correspondingly small scleral canal through which the optic nerve must pass. Because of this the disc can appear swollen because of crowding of the optic nerve fibres at the optic nerve head. This should, of course, be immediately suspected if the patient has hypermetropia. The optic disc can also appear swollen if

there are buried drusen within the disc—these are hyaline bodies which may be visible on the surface of the disc or buried within it, in the latter situation the diagnosis is more difficult but can usually be confirmed by ultrasound or CT scanning. Drusen of the disc may present with visual loss—usually minor field defects, such as arcuate scotomas, but rarely the visual loss can be quite profound. Most patients with drusen present with unrelated symptoms and the disc appearance has alarmed someone who then initiates a specialist referral. Papilloedema due to raised intracranial pressure shows dilated capillaries on the surface of the disc and the nerve fibre layer around the disc is more opaque than usual because of axonal swelling. Haemorrhages and/or 'cotton wool' spots may also be seen on the disc if the papilloedema is decompensated and, if the papilloedema is longstanding, small hyaline bodies known as corpora amylacea. Radial folds may be visible in the retina (Paton's lines) or horizontal folds in the choroid. The former are directly related to the disc swelling the latter result from indentation of the globe posteriorly by the dilated optic nerve sheath—any orbital mass can produce this sign.

Papilloedema may cause no symptoms at all. The most typical symptom is transient visual obscuration. The patients notice very brief total or near total monocular visual loss when they stand suddenly or stoop or strain. This symptom, which may also be seen in patients with chronically low ophthalmic artery perfusion pressure, results from transiently increased compromise of the circulation at the disc due to a fall in arterial or rise in venous pressure in the circulation at the optic disc.

It is thought that papilloedema results from an increase in the pressure in the ophthalmic vein secondary to the raised cerebrospinal fluid pressure. After it exits the optic nerve the ophthalmic vein travels a short distance within the optic nerve sheath which is in direct communication with the cranial subarachnoid space and hence the pressure here reflects the intracranial cerebrospinal fluid pressure. Any process which increases the pressure in the venous drainage of the optic disc may cause swelling of the optic disc. A retinal vein occlusion, for example, is by far the most common but tumours of the optic nerve or arteriovenous fistulas in the orbit or cavernous sinus may give rise to optic disc swelling. Patients with optic neuritis, posterior uveitis, retinal vasculitis, or posterior scleritis can show swelling of the optic disc, in this case the venous pressure is probably normal and the swelling results from breakdown in the blood retinal barrier in the vessels at the optic nerve head secondary to the underlying inflammatory process.

In most cases, papilloedema results from an identifiable cause of raised intracranial pressure which may or may not be amenable to treatment. In a number of patients, however, the cause of the raised intracranial pressure is not revealed by imaging studies and the ventricles are normal in size. These patients have a 'pseudotumour' syndrome which may result from raised intracranial pressure secondary to certain drugs (e.g. tetracyclines) or due to thrombosis or obstruction of one of the intracranial venous sinuses. Some of these patients fall into the category of what has been called 'benign intracranial hypertension', however, 'idiopathic intracranial hypertension' is probably a better term because the visual outcome is not necessarily benign. Typically, such patients are young women who have recently put on weight (6–12 kg in 12–18 months is typical) and are overweight at the time that they are seen.

Patients with idiopathic intracranial hypertension may have persistent papilloedema for many years. There may be no decline in visual function or there may be an insidious loss of the peripheral visual field. It is of great importance that such patients are followed up regularly for as long as they continue to have papilloedema and that the visual fields are plotted. Visual acuity and colour vision may remain normal until vision is severely compromised and these tests cannot be regarded as a reliable means of checking whether or not the patient is losing vision. Neither is the appearance of the optic disc without its difficulties. The problem is that the optic disc swelling results from swelling of the optic nerve axons. As these axons are lost with insidious progression of papilloedema the swelling becomes less prominent. Patients occasionally presents with very advanced papilloedema and tiny fields with reasonably preserved acuity, the optic discs at this stage are pale and not dramatically swollen. Serial perimetry is therefore of great importance.

In cases of papilloedema due to idiopathic intracranial hypertension a number of treatments have been employed. As a general rule in medicine the more treatments there are available for any particular condition the less likely it is that any of them are effective. This is certainly true of idiopathic intracranial hypertension. Serial lumbar punctures are probably not of any great value because it is likely that the pressure returns to previous values very soon—possibly within hours—unless a long-term leak of cerebrospinal (CSF) has been induced by making a sufficiently large hole in the dura. Nonetheless, an initial measurement of the pressure is essential to document the fact that it is elevated and also to check that the CSF constituents are normal (a raised protein or cell count may indicate some other cause such as a chronic meningitis). If the diagnosis is idiopathic intracranial hypertension and visual function is good I advise weight loss but no other treatment unless the papilloedema is persistent, as in many of these patients the papilloedema resolves over 2–3 months. If the papilloedema persists diamox may be used in an attempt to lower the CSF pressure but some patients cannot tolerate diamox. If the papilloedema is severe and visual loss already advanced I readmit the patient after 2 weeks to see if the pressure has remained low or if it is high again, as such patients may require more aggressive management.

I have not found other medical treatment regimes (such as steroids or other diuretics) to be very useful. If such acute cases have persistent raised pressure or in chronic cases who are beginning to lose vision the choice is between CSF diversion by means of a lumbo-peritoneal shunt or fenestration

of the optic nerve sheath. The latter operation was shown in the last century to be effective in relieving papilloedema but has not been widely practised until the last 10 years or so. There is a very good chance that the papilloedema of the operated eye is relieved, with less certainty the swelling of the contralateral disc and symptoms of raised intracranial pressure may be relieved suggesting some long-term effect on intracranial pressure but there is no known mechanism for this. Early suggestions that the operation might produce a chronic fistula have not been substantiated in my experience. How this operation achieves what it does achieve is not understood and it may not always act in the same way. In some cases, chronic scarring and adhesions may occur in the optic nerve sheath thus protecting the disc from the effects of the raised CSF pressure which is not itself influenced by the procedure.

There is a small risk of damage to the optic nerve as a result of optic nerve sheath fenestration. But in the next few years we will obtain a clearer picture of the failure and recurrence rate associated with the operation. The alternative, lumbo-peritoneal CSF diversion is problematic because of the high incidence of complications. It has the advantage that it is virtually certain that the CSF pressure will be reduced immediately by the procedure but the shunts may give rise to *low pressure* headaches, they invariably block after an interval, they may fall out of position, or they may become infected. All else being equal I recommend optic nerve sheath fenestration as the initial treatment unless I consider the situation to be urgent, in which case CSF diversion is a more reliable technique in the short term if vision is deteriorating rapidly. I also continue to favour CSF diversion if the patient has disabling headache which I am convinced is due to the raised intracranial pressure. This usually applies to patients with very high CSF pressures (35–40 or higher). I prefer it to be confirmed that the headache is relieved by a lumbar puncture also. Very recently we have found ventriculo-peritoneal shunting may be preferable.

DISORDERS OF THE OPTIC CHIASM

Pituitary adenoma presents with visual failure less commonly than in the past—presumably because the endocrine manifestations are now detected earlier. Pituitary adenoma does, however, remain a significant cause of visual morbidity which is almost entirely preventible. The major reason for the continued existence of patients with significant visual loss is delay in diagnosis, as mentioned above. Many patients that I have seen with chiasmal compression due to pituitary adenoma without endocrine manifestations have very large tumours before they become aware of visual loss and there is sometimes a considerable delay before the diagnosis is made, even after the patient has noticed that there is a problem. Acuity may be normal and if visual fields are not checked carefully the diagnosis will be missed. Increasingly, 'high street' optometrists do have facilities for carrying out perimetry—particularly automated perimetric techniques—and it may well be that fewer cases will be missed.

Additional problems arise if patients are found to have some other common condition which may affect vision, such as glaucoma. Many ophthalmologists have expressed considerable concern that all patients with 'normal pressure' glaucoma should be investigated to exclude an underlying optic nerve or chiasmal compression. However, in the author's experience such errors are equally likely in patients with high tension glaucoma which is a common disorder and will by chance coexist with other causes of visual failure. When high tension glaucoma is diagnosed there may be less vigilance and a careful consideration of the visual field defects to exclude other conditions may not be undertaken.

TREATMENT OF SUPRASELLAR TUMOURS

Most prolactinomas can be treated successfuly with bromocriptine and this is now the treatment of choice even for quite large tumours associated with visual failure. Adenomas can reach a very large size and if they have extended laterally into the cavernous sinuses can be untreatable. Most operable tumours can be tackled surgically by the trans-sphenoidal route, some very large tumours may require a second procedure via a frontal craniotomy. Radiotherapy has an important part to play in the treatment of tumours which cannot be completed eradicated surgically or following bromocriptine therapy.

In marked contrast to orbital meningioma or those arising in the sphenoid wing and causing visual loss from optic nerve compression, suprasellar menigiomas are gratifyingly amenable to surgical treatment in many cases. Meningiomas causing chiasmal compression may arise from the clivus or the diaphragma sellae and frequently are capable of complete and curative excision.

The treatment of the third common suprasellar tumour, craniopharyngioma, is more controversial. These tumours are not as commonly cured by surgical treatment and the place of radiotherapy is uncertain. Many of these tumours are extremely slow growing and the author has followed up some patients conservatively for some years without deterioration in visual function or change in the appearance of the tumour on imaging. Particularly in older patients there may be occasion when it is better to do nothing and see if the visual loss is progressive before deciding on surgical treatment as these patients may remain stable for many years. This management strategy should never be adopted in cases of suprasellar meningioma or pituitary adenoma.

The aetiology and management of chiasmal gliomas follows similar considerations to those mentioned above in connection with optic nerve glioma with the exception that with involvement of the chiasm the risk of visual disability is, of course, greater than in the case of a unilateral optic nerve glioma. For this reason radiotherapy would be contemplated more readily in cases of chiasmal glioma than in optic nerve glioma. Patients should be followed up carefully with serial perimetry in order to determine the pace of visual deterioration, if any, before treatment is contemplated.

HIGHER VISUAL DISORDERS

The study of visual deficits resulting from damage to extrastriate visual areas of the brain is still in its infancy. It has been recognized for 100 years that bilateral deficits affecting occipitoparietal cortex (and hence usually associated with bilateral lower homonymous field defects) cause Bálint's syndrome (Bálint 1909) also known as the syndrome of visual disorientation (Holmes 1918). The projections to the parietal lobes from primary visual cortex are concerned with spatial localization and the control of eye movements and hence such patients have difficulty locating objects in space using vision alone—the so-called 'optic ataxia' of Bálint. Unilateral lesions cause defective localization in the contralateral visual hemifield and I have never known a patient to be aware of this, however, the bilateral syndrome is very disabling.

The major problem with such patients is that they may have normal visual acuity and apart from the field defects there is nothing to find on examination unless visual localization is tested specifically. I do this by asking the patients to reach into each hemifield to touch my moving finger within the preserved regions of the visual field. Optokinetic nystagmus is also useful as this will usually be abnormal with the stripes moving towards the side of the affected parietal lobe. This syndrome should be suspected if unexplained visual symptoms are reported following cardiac arrest or hypotension, as the occipitoparietal cortex concerned is in the watershed between the posterior and middle cerebral artery territories. It also occurs following sagittal sinus thrombosis. Patients may find it very difficult to find anyone who can explain their visual problems to them. Despite preserved acuity, reading can be problematic because of difficulty keeping track of the lines of text. Visual rehabilitation of such patients is arduous and it would be difficult to control for the effect of spontaneous recovery.

Some patients with Alzheimer's disease present with visual symptoms before they develop other features of dementia. Mean age of onset is 59 (45–70) in the 38 patients described since 1985. Typical history is slowly progressive difficulty with reading and repeated unhelpful visits to ophthalmologists and optometrists. There is no language disorder and the reading difficulty is related to visuospatial impairment. Features of Balint's syndrome eventually emerge. Simultanagnosia is particularly common. Imaging shows parieto-occipital atrophy out of proportion to other areas and as with this case usually by the time the diagnosis is made there is clear evidence of deteriorating memory and other cognitive functions. (Victoroff *et al.* 1994)

Case report 7

A 60-year-old woman complained of vague visual blurring for 5 years. She found it difficult to put letters in the correct spaces when doing crossword puzzles. For one year she had noticed difficulty identifying faces including her own husband and sister-in-law. When watching television she would see only one character when there should have been two. For 2 years she had also noticed deterioration in her memory and was losing her way when out shopping in familiar locations. In the past she had had a hysterectomy but had otherwise always been fit. Her father had had to retire at 55, he became gradually more immobile and uncommunicative but lived until age 72, his diagnosis was not known.

On examination, her best vision was 6/18 bilaterally and she was able to pick some letters at N5 but she was unable to read any Ishihara plates including the control. A neuropsychological assessment revealed a verbal IQ of 92 and a performance IQ of 76. There was evidence of dyslexia, dysgraphia, and acalculia but only mild impairment on the Farnsworth Munsell 100 hue test of colour discrimination. She had severe problems with visual localization of objects (visual disorientation, more marked in the right than the left hemifield). She was able to identify 3 of 12 famous faces. Neurological examination was otherwise normal. MRI showed cortical atrophy which was more marked posteriorly [Fig. 1.9].

This case illustrates the very long time that patients with the syndrome of visual disorientation may have to wait before a diagnosis is made.

Prosopagnosia, alexia, topographical disorientation, and impaired colour vision are often seen together in patients with damage to occipito-temporal cortex, usually bilaterally. The following patient was told that he probably had multiple sclerosis because of his impaired colour vision.

Case report 8

At the age of 44 the patient, a paediatrician, suddenly developed a right homonymous hemianopia. A CT scan suggested a left occipital lesion, presumed to be vascular but no predisposing cause was found. Four years later he suddenly became confused and his vision deteriorated further, he felt as though he was looking through frosted glass and since then was unable to perceive colour or to recognize faces. In addition to the right homonymous hemianopia he had now lost the superior quadrant of the left visual hemifield. Visual acuity was preserved. Because of the marked loss of colour vision he was thought to have bilateral optic nerve disease, *despite the homonymous nature of the field defects and the preserved acuity. He was told that in all probability he had MS. He was seen for a second opinion and the story was recognized to be typical of cerebral achromatopsia with prosopagnosia and topographical disorientation. The ventral location of the second infarction in the right hemisphere is suggested by the superior field defect and was confirmed on MRI [Fig. 1.10]. Recovery of his colour vision occurred over several years but his prosopagnosia remains profound.*

The message from both these case reports is to listen carefully to what the patients are telling you and test logically for the various submodalities of visual function.

Finally, cortical blindness usually occurs as a result of bilateral occipital infarction due to a basilar artery thrombosis or embolus. If the cortical blindness is isolated (with no attendant brainstem signs) then an embolus is the more likely of the two. These patients really do sometimes demonstrate no awareness of blindness (Anton's syndrome, a form of anosognosia) and may appear in casualty complaining that there is something wrong with their vision but at the same time confabulating as if experiencing an internally generated visual world. In view of the results of an eye examination (normal pupil light reflex, etc.) these patients may be thought to be in need of psychiatric attention.

In my experience, these patients usually do recover some useful vision and once they have done so it is worthwhile spending some time finding out what residual vision they have by carefully investigating each visual modality. On a number of occasions I have been sent patients because they are thought to have central impairment of colour vision because they cannot read the Ishihara plates. In fact they cannot read even the control plate and the essential problem is one of figure–ground discrimination. As it happens the Ishihara plates (including the control plates) can be used as a substitute for the fragmented letters test that is used to investigate the ability to identify what makes up a single object. Object identification is impossible if this early hurdle in visual

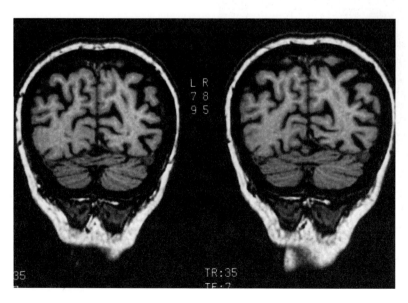

Fig. 1.9 MR scan showing posterior cortical atrophy in a patient who presented with progressive visual disorientation.

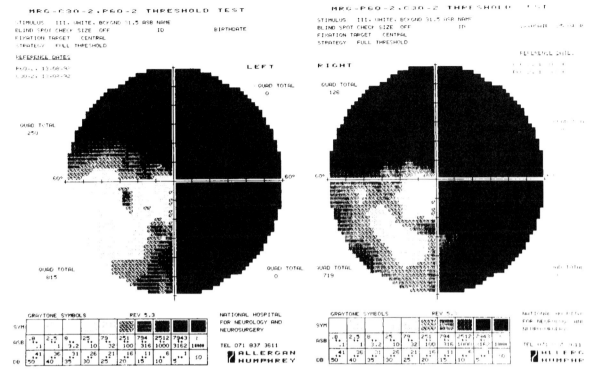

Fig. 1.10(a) This patient suffered a left occipital cerebral infarction giving a right homonymous hemianopia. Later he had a right occipital infarct giving him a left superior homonymous quadrantanopia.

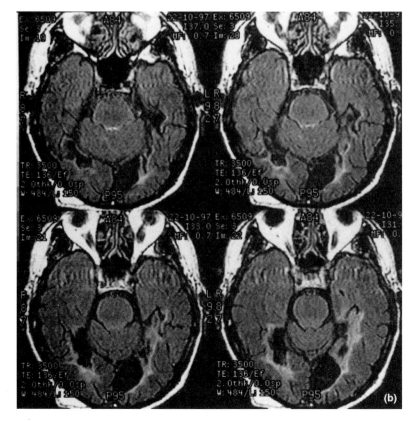

Fig. 1.10(b) Colour vision was absent in the surviving visual field and he also had prosopagnosia and topographical amnesia. The story is typical of bilateral ventral occipitotemporal lesions as shown in the MR scan.

processing cannot be crossed and it is essential to check that this and other early processes are intact before suggesting that there is a primary object recognition disorder (object agnosia).

CONCLUSION

I am fascinated by visual symptoms in neurological disorders and by the way such patients take me on a guided tour of the nervous system—but this fascination is not an end in itself. My intention in this chapter has been to demonstrate that the accurate diagnosis of such patients has a significant impact on issues of treatment and management.

REFERENCES

Bálint, R. (1909). Seelenlahmung des 'Schauens', optishce Ataxie, Räumliche storung der Aufmarksamkeit. *Monatschrift für Psychiatrie und Neurologie*, **25**, 51–181.

Beck, R. W., Cleary, P. A., Anderson, M. M., Jr, Keltner, J. L., Shults, W. T., Kaufman, D. I., *et al.* (1992). A randomised, controlled trial of corticosteroids in the treatment of acute optic neuritis. *New England Journal of Medicine*, **326**, 581–8.

Beck, R. W., Clear, P. A., Trobe, J. D., Kaufman, D. I., Kupersmith, M. J., Paty, D. W. *et al.* (1993). The effect of corticosteroids for acute optic neuritis on the subsequent development of multiple sclerosis. *New England Journal of Medicine*, **329**, 1764–9.

Brown, P., Demaerel, P. M., Revesz, T., Graham, E., Kendall, B. E., and Plant, G. T. (1994). The neuro-ophthalmological presentation of non-invasive aspergillus sinus disease in the non-immunocompromised host. *Journal of Neurology Neurosurgery and Psychiatry*, **57**, 234–7.

Burnstine, M. A., Levin, L. A., Louis, D. N., Hedley-Whyte, E. T., Kupsky, W. J., Doepner, D. *et al.* (1993). Nucleolar organiser regions in optic gliomas. *Brain*, **116**, 1564–76.

Burton, B. J. L., Leff, A. P., and Plant, G. T. (1998). Steroid-Responsive HIV optic neuropathy. *Journal of Neuro-ophthalmology*, **18**, 25–9.

Critchley, M. (1975). The training of a neurologist. *International Journal of Neurology*, **9**, 308–10.

Dolin, P. J., Mohamed, A. A., and Plant, G. T. (1998). Epidemic of optic neuropathy in Dar es Salaam, Tanzania. *New England Journal of Medicine*, **338**, 1547–8.

Dutton, J. J. (1994). Gliomas of the anterior visual pathway. *Survey of Ophthalmology*, **38**, 427–52.

Evans, J. (1995). *Causes of blindness and partial sight in England and Wales 1990–1991*, Studies on Medical and Population Subjects, No. 57. HMSO, London.

Fisher, C. M. (1955). Residual neuropathological changes in Canadians held prisoners of war by the Japanese. *Canadian Services Medical Journal*, **11**, 157–64.

Holmes, G. (1918). Disturbances of visual orientation. *British Journal of Ophthalmology*, **2**, 449–68; 506–16.

Jestico, J. V., O'Brien, M. D., Teoh, R., Toseland, P. A., and Wong, H. C. (1984). Whole blood cyanide levels in patients with tobacco amblyopia. *Journal of Neurology Neurosurgery and Psychaitry*, **47**, 573–578.

Kapoor, R., Miller, D. H., Jones, S. J., Plant, G. T., Brusa, A., Gass, A. *et al.* (1998). Effects of intravenous methylprednisolone on outcome in MRI-based prognostic subgroups in acute optic neuritis. *Neurology*, **50**, 230–7.

MacKarell, P. (1986). Interior journey and beyond: an artist's view of optic neuritis. In *Optic neuritis*, (ed. R. F. Hess and G. T. Plant), pp. 283–93. Cambridge University Press.

Manji, H. and Plant, G. T. (1999). Epilepsy surgery, visual fields and driving. *Journal of Neurology, Neurosurgery and Psychiatry*, **66** (in press).

Morrisey, S. P., Miller, D. H., Kendall, B. E., Kingsley, D. P. E., Kelly, M. A., Francis, D. A. *et al.* (1993). *Brain*, **116**, 135–46.

Munton, G. (1995). Vision. In *Medical aspects of fitness to drive*, (ed. J. F. Taylor), pp. 118–32. Medical Commission on Accident Prevention, London.

Newman, N. J., Torroni, M. D., Brown, M. T., Lott, M. T., Fernandez, M. M., and Wallace, D. C. (1994). Epidemic neuropathy in Cuba not associated with mitochondrial DNA mutations found in hereditary optic neuropathy patients. *American Journal of Ophthalmology*, **118**, 158–68.

Plant, G. T., Mtanda, A. T., Arden, G. B., and Johnson, G. J. (1997*a*). An epidemic of optic neuropathy in Tanzania: characterisation of the visual disorder and associated peripheral neuropathy. *Journal of the Neurological Sciences*, **145**, 127–40.

Plant, G. T., Dolin, P., Mohamed, A. A., and Mlingi, N. (1997*b*). Confirmation that neither cyanide intoxication nor mutations commonly associated with Leber's Hereditary Optic Neuropathy are implicated in Tanzanian Epidemic Optic Neuropathy. *Journal of the Neurological Sciences*, **145**, 107–8.

Plant, G. T., and Tripathy, S. P. (1997). Effect on vision of binocular foveal contour interactions. *Lancet*, **349**, 1296–7.

Spillane, J. D. (1947). *Nutritional disorders of the nervous system*. Livingstone, Edinburgh.

Strachan, H. (1888), Malarial multiple peripheral neuritis. *Sajou's Annual*, **1**, 139–47.

Thomas, P. K., Plant, G. T., Baxter, P., Bates, C., and Santiago-Luis, R. (1995). An epidemic of optic neuropathy and painful sensory neuroapathy in Cuba: clinical aspects. *Journal of Neurology*, **242**, 629–38.

Victoroff, J., Ross, G. W., Benson, F., Verity, F., and Vinters, H. V. (1994). Posterior cortical atrophy: neuropathological correlations. *Archives of Neurology*, **51**, 269–74.

Wray, S. H. (1995). Optic neuritis: guidelines. *Current Opinion in Neurology*, **8**, 72–6.

2 | *Vestibular and auditory problems and falls*

Linda M. Luxon

The symptoms of dizziness, tinnitus, and falls cause despair and disinterest for many doctors. The complaints are vague, a diagnosis is frequently elusive, and there is a preconception that there are no effective treatments. The aim of this chapter is to demonstrate that armed with some basic knowledge, a diagnostic strategy and some simple principles of management, much can be accomplished for patients with these symptoms, which not infrequently generate social and occupational dysfunction, quite out of proportion to the severity of the underlying problem.

The peripheral labyrinth is unique in that it subserves two systems: hearing and balance, while the auditory and vestibular pathways diverge within the central nervous system and interact with a multiplicity of information from other sensory inputs. The National Survey of Hearing (Davies 1989) has revealed that 17% of the population have a significant *hearing impairment*, but, by the seventh decade of life, this figure rises to 40%. The disability and handicap associated with hearing loss are well recognized, but a formal model of audiological rehabilitation is well established (Goldstein and Stephens 1981). *Tinnitus* is a universal perception, like headache, but in 10% of the population it becomes intrusive and symptomatic. Although the cause(s) of tinnitus are poorly understood, management strategies are well established (Luxon 1993), but in the United Kingdom they are not widely available and, in general, poorly provided.

Twenty percent of the working population report 'dizziness' in the previous month (Yardley *et al.* 1997), while by the age of 65, 35% of people have experienced episodes of *dizziness*. And by the age of 80 years, two-thirds of women and one-third of men have suffered episodes of disequilibrium. The economic and psychological morbidity of balance disorders have recently become the focus of research activity (Eagger *et al.* 1992; Yardley *et al.* 1992, 1997). However, it is only in the last five years that there has been a shift of emphasis away from vestibular diagnosis to include vestibular rehabilitation. Nonetheless, such facilities, like those for tinnitus, are still rare and poorly provided in the United Kingdom (Yardley and Luxon 1994).

Falls present a common yet difficult problem to investigate, as there is a continuum from trips and stumbles, when balance is regained, through near falls to completed falls. The risk of falling increases with age and most studies show that women are more likely to fall than men. While a variety of conditions may result in falls, it is usually possible to determine at least some of the factors that have caused the fall. Management of falls require a clear understanding of the mechanisms by which people fall, treatment of any specific medical condition, and advice about strategies that the faller may employ and changes that may be required in the environment in which they live.

VESTIBULAR DISORDERS

PATHOPHYSIOLOGY

Man has developed a sophisticated mechanism for maintaining balance, which is dependent on visual, vestibular, and proprioceptive inputs. This sensory information passes into the central nervous system (CNS), where it is modulated and integrated with activity from other neurological centres (Fig. 2.1). Normally, with the head in the anatomical position, the vestibular receptors generate neural activity, which is transmitted via the brainstem to the cerebral cortex. Head movements produce linear and/or angular accelerations within each labyrinth, which modulate this activity in an equal but opposite manner (Fig. 2.2) in each ear. This asymmetry of information is 'interpreted' by the CNS and allows cortical awareness of head and body position in space and provides the stimulus for compensatory eye and body movements (Savundra and Luxon 1998). However, vestibular pathology will also produce asymmetry of vestibular information, such that the subject experiences vertigo, feels unstable, and develops pathological vestibular nystagmus (Fig. 2.3).

The conditions causing dizziness may be divided into three main groups: (1) general medical; (2) neurological disorders; and (3) otological disorders (Table 2.1). Good management relies on accurate diagnosis and a single disorder (e.g. viral labyrinthitis, Ménière's disease, cardiac dysrhythmia) can often be identified, but certain generalizations are worthy of note. First, some pathologies may affect more than one site, for example, cerebrovascular disease may give rise to an ischaemic labyrinthitis, and brainstem dysfunction. Second, patients with peripheral vestibular disease (e.g. viral labyrinthitis), may make an excellent, initial recovery, but in the face of

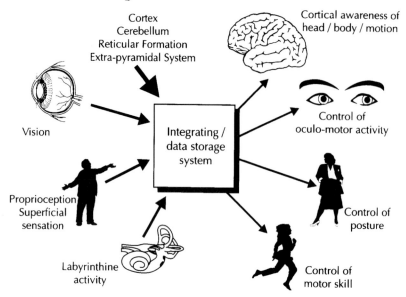

Fig. 2.1 Diagram of the mechanisms subserving balance. (Luxon, L.M.)

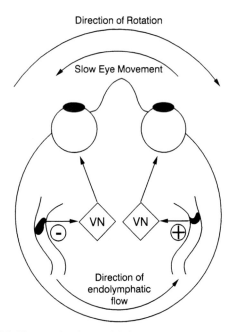

Fig. 2.2 Diagram showing modulation of vestibular activity in the horizontal semicircular canals in response to head movement (angular acceleration). (VN): vestibular nuclei; +: normal activity; –: reduced pathological input.

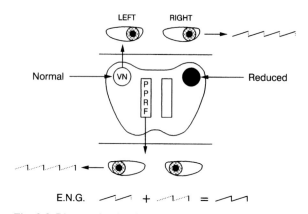

Fig. 2.3 Diagram showing the generation of pathological spontaneous vestibular nystagmus. (VN: vestibular nuclei, PPRF: Paropontine reticular formation, ENG: Electrony stagnography) [From Rudge, P. (1983). *Clinical Neuro-otology*. Churchill Livingstone, Edinburgh.]

physiological or psychological stress, decompensation may develop and their symptoms recur. In some patients, there may be a relapsing and remitting course of disequilibrium on this basis. Third, in the elderly patient, disequilibrium may result from different pathologies in a variety of sites, for example, visual impairment due to a cataract, altered proprioception, due to osteoarthritis, and decompensation from a pre-existing

peripheral vestibular disorder. Superimposed on these abnormalities, age-related degenerative or ischaemic changes, within the CNS, may impair the integration required for balance. Thus, a common presentation in the elderly is known as the *multisensory dizziness syndrome* (Drachman and Hart 1972) which is defined as disequilibrium resulting from sensory deficits on the basis of two or more of the following conditions: visual impairment (not correctable); neuropathy; vestibular deficit; cervical spondylosis; and orthopaedic disorders interfering with joint mechanoreceptors.

CLINICAL ASSESSMENT

Correct diagnosis of balance disorders relies heavily on a detailed and accurate clinical history and general medical

Table 2.1 Causes of dizziness

General medical	Otological
Haematological	Ménière's syndrome
Anaemia	Post-traumatic syndrome
Hyperviscosity	Positional nystagmus
Miscellaneous	Vestibular neuronitis
Cardiovascular	*a*infection
Postural hypotension	Otosclerosis and Paget's disease
Carotid sinus syndrome	Vascular accidents
Dysrhythmias, including:	Tumours
sick sinus syndrome	Autoimmune disorders
mitral leaflet prolapse	Drug intoxication
syndrome	
Mechanical dysfunction	
ventricular hypokinesis	
aortic stenosis	
Metabolic	
Hypoglycaemia	
Hyperventilation	
Neurological	**Mscellaneous**
Supratentorial	Ocular/visual
Epilepsy	Orthopaedic, including cervical
Syncope	Multisensory dizziness syn-
drome	
Infratentorial	
Multiple sclerosis	
Vertebrobasilar insufficiency	
subclavian steal syndrome	
Wallenberg's syndrome	
anterior inferior cerebellar	
artery syndrome	
Infective disorders	
Ramsay–Hunt	
neurosyphilis	
tuberculosis	
Degenerative disorders,	
including neuropathy	
Tumours, including acoustic	
neuroma	
Foramen magnum abnormalities	

examination, with special reference to the eyes, ears, and central nervous and cardiovascular systems. However, this account concentrates on the specific history and examination, relevant to neuro-otological disorders, which might otherwise be overlooked.

In the ***clinical history***, three aspects are of particular importance:

1. *Character of complaint*. Vertigo is defined as an hallucination of movement and is characteristic of vestibular dysfunction, while 'dizziness' is a lay term, defined by the Concise Oxford Dictionary as 'a feeling of being in a whirl, or in a daze, or as if about to fall'. Patients may volunteer readily understood symptoms such as 'dizziness', 'giddiness', 'swimmingess', or 'disorientation', to the more unusual complaints of 'I feel

my brain is sloshing around inside/lagging behind my head', 'I don't feel my head and eyes are synchronized', to the frankly bizarre, 'I feel spaced out', 'I feel as if I am standing outside myself and watching my life go by'. Such complaints, together with visually induced dysequilibrium produced by walking over highly patterned carpets, ironing striped material, walking down escalators, and scanning shelves in supermarkets, warrant specific vestibular investigation.

Classically, vertigo of peripheral labyrinthine origin is acute, unprecipitated, shortlived, and associated with nausea and vomiting; whereas vertigo of central vestibular origin is a more insidious and protracted sense of instability.

2. *Time course*. Acute rotational vertigo of less than one minute's duration is most commonly associated with a diagnosis of benign positional vertigo of paroxysmal type, associated with vascular disease, head trauma, and ageing. Acute rotational vertigo of more than one minute duration, but less than one hour duration, has been ascribed, particularly in the elderly, to vertebrobasilar insufficiency, but in the absence of other neurological symptoms and signs this is almost certainly incorrect (Luxon 1990).

Vertigo of several hours duration is commonly associated with Ménière's disease and migraine. In Ménière's disease, episodes of acute vertigo, with hearing loss (often fluctuating) and tinnitus are prerequisites (Pearson and Brackmann 1985), while in migraine, vertigo may occur with or without headache (Kayan and Hood 1984). It should be emphasized that in both conditions, the episodes tend to occur in clusters with intervals of months, or even years, of freedom.

A single, acute episode of vertigo with gradual resolution over days or weeks would suggest peripheral vestibular pathology, such as viral or ischaemic labyrinthitis. Cerebral plasticity brings about compensation over a period of a few days to many months, and although not fully understood, it is generally accepted that the cerebellum is of primary importance (1 to 1972), together with spontaneous regeneration of vestibular activity on the affected side (Yagi and Markham 1984). As noted above, compensation frequently brings about spontaneous resolution of vestibular symptoms, but subsequent physical or emotional stress can result in decompensation with a recurrence of symptoms which are usually milder, and of shorter duration, than the initial attack.

3. *Associated symptoms*. Within the labyrinth and VIIIth cranial nerve, the vestibular and cochlear elements are closely related anatomically and thus, hearing loss/tinnitus frequently occur with dysequilibrium arising in these sites. Neurological and general medical symptoms should be sought. In particular, vestibular dysfunction may contribute significantly to imbalance in cerebellar disease and peripheral neuropathies (Rinne *et al.* 1994).

A full ***general medical examination*** is essential, with particular assessment of the fundi, visual fields, visual acuity, general neurological, cardiovascular, and peripheral vascular systems. In all patients with vertigo, **otoscopy** to examine the tympanic membrane is essential to exclude active chronic middle ear disease, with labyrinthine erosion.

A detailed account of vestibular physiology and visuo-vestibular interaction is beyond the scope of this chapter, but a basic understanding of the principles involved is essential if an informed assessment of vestibular function and interpretation of vestibular investigations is to be made (Savundra and Luxon 1998). As outlined above, an asymmetry of vestibular activity brainstem is 'monitored' by the CNS. Via the pathways subserving the vestibulo-ocular reflex, there is a slow drift of the eyes in the same direction as a peripheral labyrinthine lesion. For reasons that are not fully understood, this slow drift is interrupted by a rapid saccadic eye movement, generated within the parapontine reticular formation, which tends to 're-centre' the eyes. This combination of slow and fast eye movements gives the characteristic sawtooth pattern of *spontaneous nystagmus* which is commonly observed in peripheral labyrinthine disease (see Fig. 2.3).

By definition, the direction of the nystagmus is defined by the fast phase and nystagmus should be sought in the primary position of gaze and with eyes deviated 30° to right, left, up and down. Eye deviation greater than 30° should be avoided as physiological end-point nystagmus may be confused with pathological spontaneous vestibular nystagmus. Peripheral vestibular lesions give rise to horizontal nystagmus beating in the contralateral direction, which obeys Alexander's law. This states that the intensity of the nystagmus is greatest when the eyes are deviated in the direction of the fast phase of the nystagmic response (Fig. 2.4).

Horizontal nystagmus which does not obey Alexander's law may be of central type, as is bidirectional nystagmus (e.g. right beating nystagmus on eye deviation to the right and left beating nystagmus on eye deviation to the left), vertical nystagmus, and dysconjugate nystagmus. Such findings require neurological investigation.

Spontaneous nystagmus is sought clinically in the presence of optic fixation (i.e in asking the patient to fixate on a target

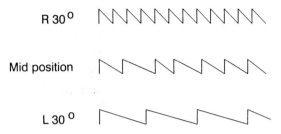

Fig. 2.4 Illustration of spontaneous vestibular nystagmus obeying Alexander's law, with eyes in three directions of gaze. (R, right; L, left.)

such as the point of a pen), but additional assessment in the absence of optic fixation (using either Frenzel's glasses or an infrared viewer in a darkened room; Fig. 2.5) provides valuable information. By observing the clinical characteristics of spontaneous nystagmus, it is usually possible to determine whether pathology is in the labyrinth and/or VIIIth nerve or in the CNS connections (Table 2.2).

Positional nystagmus is a valuable and frequently overlooked sign, which may be elicited by a briskly performed Hallpike manoeuvre (Fig. 2.6). The patient is sat on the edge of a flat examination couch, the head is turned 30–45° to the right or left and the patient is then rapidly taken backwards, so that the head is over the edge of the couch. The eyes are observed carefully to determine whether positional nystagmus develops. The characteristics of the nystagmus are observed to determine whether the nystagmus is of labyrinthine type (i.e.

Table 2.2 Characteristics of spontaneous vestibular nystagmus

	Peripheral type	Central type
Duration	Temporary	Permanent
Direction	Unilateral, horizontal	May be multidirectional
Character	Sawtooth	May be pendular
	Always conjugate	May be dysconjugate
Effect of removal of optic fixation	Enhances	Unchanged or inhibited

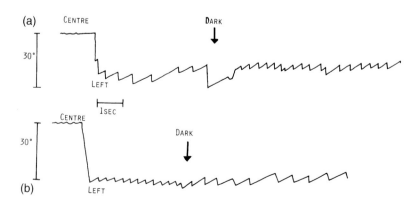

Fig. 2.5 Electronystagmographic recording of effect of optic fixation on: (a) peripheral spontaneous vestibular nystagmus; and (b) central spontaneous vestibular nystagmus. (arrow; point of introduction of optic fixation.)

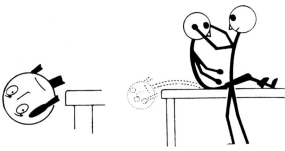

Fig. 2.6 Diagram showing the Hallpike manoeuvre for eliciting positional nystagmus.

Table 2.3 Characteristics of positional nystagmus

	Benign paroxysmal type	Central type
Latent period	2–20 s	None
Adaptation	Disappears in 50 s	Persists
Fatigue ability	Disappears on repetition	Persists
Vertigo	Always present	Typically absent
Direction of nystagmus	Rotational to undermost ear	Variable
Incidence	Relatively common	Relatively uncommon

benign paroxysmal) or CNS origin (Table 2.3). Harrison and Ozashinoglu (1975) found that 38% of patients with persistent positional nystagmus had CNS pathology, whereas only 4% of patients with benign paroxysmal positional nystagmus demonstrated such abnormalities.

Optokinetic nystagmus is a visually induced nystagmus of saw-tooth type, which can be elicited using a hand-held striped rotating drum or a small mechanically driven striped optokinetic drum. Optokinetic asymmetries and abnormalities are only observed in acute peripheral labyrinthine disorders, associated with florid spontaneous vestibular nystagmus, whereas in CNS disease persistent optokinetic asymmetries are common (Table 2.4).

An overall assessment of balance can be achieved using the *Romberg test* and an *assessment of gait*. In both tests, a tendency to sway or veer in one direction usually suggests ipsilateral peripheral vestibular pathology or, in the presence of neurological signs, ipsilateral cerebellar dysfunction. Anxious patients frequently tend to fall backwards like a wooden soldier

Table 2.4 The relationship between site of lesion and optokinetic abnormalities (*n* = 614)

Anatomical site	Normal (%)	Abnormal (%)
Brainstem	41	59
Cerebellum	28	72
Basal ganglia	43	57
Parietal lobe	26	74
Labyrinth	99	1

After Yee *et al.* (1982). Pathophysiology of optokinetic nystagmus. In *Nystagmus and vertigo: Clinical approaches to the patient with dizziness* (ed. Honrubia V. and Brazieu M.A.B). Academic Press, New York.

and this is indicative of a non-organic component to their symptoms, but it should be emphasized that such psychological overlay is almost always the result of underlying vestibular pathology. Gait testing, may provide additional information about neurological/orthopaedic disorders (e.g. foot drop, ataxia, parkinsonism), which are of significance in terms of the patient's overall balance disorder.

A variety of vestibular tests are available including caloric, rotation, and galvanic testing and posturography, but for practical purposes most centres rely on the *caloric* test. This test, introduced in 1942 by Fitzgerald and Hallpike, has become the cornerstone of vestibular diagnosis and has stood the test of time in terms of defining vestibular pathology and allowing identification of side and level of lesion. A thermal gradient across the two limbs of the horizontal semicircular canal is induced by means of irrigation of the external auditory canal with water 7° above and below body temperature. The thermal gradient generates a nystagmic response, which can be assessed in each ear independently of the other. The test is simple and cheap, although it does require a level of skill and understanding of vestibular physiology, if reproducible and reliable results are to be obtained. An asymmetry in the response generated from each ear (canal paresis) or an asymmetry of the nystagmic response (a directional preponderance) is assessed. In addition, the effect of optic fixation on the vestibular response is assessed to determine whether there is a peripheral labyrinthine or central neurological deficit.

Rotation testing with analysis of the resultant nystagmic response is invaluable for research purposes but is expensive, assesses both horizontal semicircular canals simultaneously, and is not widely available for clinical use. *Galvanic testing* allows differentiation of peripheral labyrinthine dysfunction from VIIIth nerve vestibular damage, but has not gained acceptance as a clinical tool. *Posturography* allows an overall assessment of balance, but it must be emphasized that the response is dependent on a multiplicity of sensory and motor activity and this technique cannot be considered a 'vestibular' test. Moreover, currently there is no evidence that it is a valuable diagnostic tool, although it is an excellent technique for assessing the efficacy of vestibular rehabilitation. A variety of *eye movement recording techniques* are available for documenting the vestibulo-ocular response and visually induced eye movement of relevance to vestibular function, including pursuit, saccades, and optokinetic nystagmus. The most widely available technique is electro-oculography, but it must be emphasized that this is not a vestibular test, merely a means of recording responses generated either by eye movements or vestibular stimuli, such as caloric and rotational testing.

MANAGEMENT

The clinical approach outlined frequently enables general medical, neurological, and otological balance disorders to be differentiated. Specific management of cardiovascular/ neurological disorders is undertaken as appropriate. This section is confined to the management of central and peripheral vestibular dysfunction, including specific disorders, such as Ménière's disease, and non-specific disorders, such as chronic peripheral vestibular dysfunction of undefined aetiology (Fig. 2.7).

The management of ***central vestibular dysfunction*** remains poorly understood and empirical in approach. Not infrequently, conditions giving rise to vertical nystagmus, such as the Arnold Chiari malformation and multiple sclerosis, give rise to persistent oscillopsia, with disequilibrium and nausea. The symptoms may be extremely distressing and, indeed, may appear out of proportion to the apparent clinical signs. In this situation, clonazepam, titrating the dose against sedative side-effects, may be of value, as may baclofen, again titrating the dose against the side-effect of muscular weakness. In patients with evidence of central vestibular dysfunction and 'dizziness', in the first instance a trial of cinnarizine is occasionally effective, but failing this carbamazepine or clonazepam may be of help. In patients with a sense of instability, associated with basal ganglion disorders and cerebellar disease, physiotherapy to teach alternative gait strategies may prove invaluable in improving the patient's sense of confidence and ability to cope.

Patients with ***peripheral vestibular disorders*** fall into two groups: (1) those with specific conditions for which there is a recognized treatment regime; and (2) those in whom there is evidence of a peripheral vestibular abnormality, but the precise aetiology remains unresolved.

Certain specific ***peripheral vestibular disorders*** deserve mention.

Ménière's disease is characterized by tinnitus, hearing loss, and episodic vertigo. The underlying pathological process is endolymphatic hydrops, although the mechanisms giving rise to this pathological entity are not clearly understood. Characteristically, Ménière's disease gives rise to recurrent attacks of symptoms during periods of relapse, but there may be periods of many months or even years of remission. Ultimately, the condition resolves spontaneously with residual subtotal or total auditory and/or vestibular failure. In up to 50% of cases, the disease may develop bilaterally.

The aim of treatment in Ménière's disease is to bring about remission and the therapeutic options in Ménière's disease are legion (Brookes 1996). However, a 60–80% success rate has been reported, regardless of treatment modality (Torak 1977). The fluctuant nature of the disease and the high rate of placebo effect makes the success of any treatment regime extremely difficult to evaluate. However, recent work has supported the value of salt restriction and diuretic therapy (Santos *et al.* 1993). Hydrochlorothiazide (Klockhoff and Lindblom 1967) and chlorthalidone (Klockhoff *et al.* 1974) have been convincingly demonstrated in double-blind crossover trials to improve hearing loss, vertigo, and general condition. However, no similarly convincing data for other treatments, such as prochlorperazine, betahistine, or cinnarizine, are available. Various surgical drainage procedures (e.g. endolymphatic sac decompression) have been advocated, and would appear to be helpful in individual cases, but lack definitive confirmation in well-controlled trials. In the face of disabling vertiginous attacks resistant to medical treatment, destructive surgical procedures may be considered. In the presence of useful auditory function, vestibular neurectomy is the treatment of choice while in a dead ear, labyrinthine ablation may be considered. It cannot be overemphasized that it is imperative that sophisticated vestibular investigations confirm the abnormal side and take into account the possibility of bilateral disease before any destructive procedure is undertaken.

Migraine

In 200 *migrainous* subjects, Kayan and Hood (1984) documented vestibular symptomatology in 39%, cochlear patho-

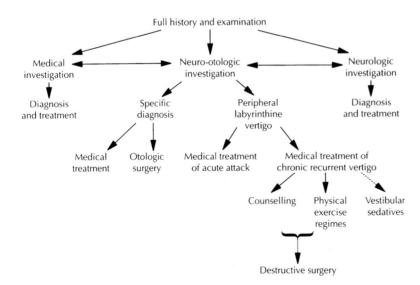

Fig. 2.7 Flow diagram showing the management of episodic vertigo.

logy in 4.5%, and combined auditory and vestibular dysfunction in 15.5%. Detailed neuro-otological investigation of 80 migrainous subjects, referred for assessment because of vestibulocochlear symptoms revealed that 77.5% had objective abnormalities and one-half of these suggested central vestibular pathology. Moreover, it is now clear that vestibular symptoms may occur as part of the aura, in the headache phase, or during the headache-free periods. Thus, in the presence of migrainous headaches, vestibular symptoms are common (Savundra *et al.* 1997) and appropriate management is comprised of standard antimigrainous treatment.

Syphilitic labyrinthitis

This may manifest as progressive hearing loss but vestibular symptoms are common. Vestibular manifestations include as episodes indistinguishable from Ménière's disease, or there may be progressive bilateral destruction of vestibular end organs resulting in imbalance and unsteadiness of gait, particularly in the dark. A high index of suspicion is required if this diagnosis is to be made and standard treatment with hospitalization to ensure adequate penicillin and steroid therapy are required, but despite adequate treatment progression of auditory and vestibular symptoms may continue.

Acoustic neurinoma

The majority of acoustic neurinoma arise on the superior division of the vestibular nerve, in the internal auditory meatus. The most common presentation is of an unilateral hearing loss with, or without, tinnitus and the frequency of isolated dizziness in this condition is low. Nonetheless, in a large series of acoustic neurinoma (Morrison 1975) reported that 10% of patients complained of vertigo and/or unsteadiness as the initial symptom.

Benign positional paroxysmal vertigo

This is a commonly misdiagnosed condition which is manifest as short-lived acute vertigo on assuming a critical head position. The diagnosis is made by observing nystagmus of characteristic type, as described above, on performing the Hallpike manoeuvre (Fig. 2.6). The underlying pathology has been attributed to cupulolithiasis (Schucknecht 1969) with degeneration of the otoconia of the utricular macula. Otoconia then fall on to the cupula of the posterior semicircular canal. However, this view has recently been challenged and the entity of canalithiasis is now considered to be the underlying pathophysiological mechanism (Parnes and McClure 1991).

Specific management of this condition is by means of particle repositioning procedures, the Semont manoeuvre (1988) and Epley manoeuvre (1992), which are highly effective with a reported 'cure' rate of 60–85% on the first attempt. Subsequent manoeuvres bring about resolution of symptoms in

an additional 10% of patients. Relapses may occur, but this management regime represents a significant improvement on the previous therapy of rehabilitative physical exercises regimes including the Brandt–Daroff exercises (1980). (For a detailed review see Luxon 1997*a*.)

The management of **peripheral vestibular disorders**, in which clear evidence of peripheral vestibular dysfunction has been detected on investigation, but no specific diagnosis amenable to treatment has been defined (e.g. viral labyrinthitis, ischaemic labyrinthitis, post-traumatic vestibular dysfunction), may be divided into treatment of the acute vertiginous attack and management of chronic vestibular symptoms.

Acute vertigo, associated with nausea and vomiting, requires immediate intervention and an antiemetic, such as prochlorperazine either intramuscularly or by suppository or metoclopramide intramuscularly, may alleviate nausea and vomiting, such that a vestibular sedative can be administered. Cinnarizine 15 mg 8-hourly by mouth is the preferred drug, although patients should be warned of the sedative side-effects. Cyclizine, dimenhydrinate, or promethazine may be given orally, intramuscularly, or by suppository. Such drugs are of value in acute vertigo, but should be avoided in the treatment of chronic peripheral labyrinthine disease as they may suppress vestibular activity which is crucial for compensation.

Chronic or recurrent vertigo due to poorly compensated vestibular dysfunction is a significant cause of morbidity, with restriction of both social and work activities. Frequently, the primary symptoms of dizziness and/or vertigo are associated with secondary symptoms of psychological origin (anxiety, depression, phobic symptoms), malaise, fatigue, and neck pain related to muscle tension as a result of conscious or subconscious limitation of head movements to reduce vertigo. Despite the prevalence of and morbidity associated with balance disorders, the value of vestibular rehabilitation is not widely recognized and the availability of trained personnel and appropriate facilities is very limited both within and outside the UK health service.

PHYSICAL EXERCISE REGIMES

In the mid 1940s, Cawthorne and Cooksey (1946) introduced physiotherapy for patients with vestibular injuries to counteract post-traumatic vestibular disorders leading to chronic invalidism. A graduated series of exercises aimed at encouraging head and eye movements was developed. This empirical approach to physical exercise regimes, was underpinned by more recent animal models. Courjon and co-workers (1977) identified the crucial role of vision in suppressing the vestibulo-ocular reflex in animals subjected to labyrinthectomy, while Lacour and co-workers (1976) demonstrated the value of active movements in the rehabilitation of baboons following unilateral vestibular nerve section.

Thus, a graded series of exercises has been refined to promote compensation within the CNS by a variety of mechanisms including central sensory substitution, rebalancing of chronic activity in central vestibular centres and physiological habituation. The work of Lacour and Xerri (1980) has suggested that following vestibular injury, there is a critical period of cerebral plasticity during which adaptive changes induced by multisensory inputs are required if full recovery is to be achieved.

An active rehabilitation programme, in which patients are encouraged to perform graded exercises to provoke dizziness in a controlled manner and safe environment is mandatory if effective rehabilitation is to occur. It is important to emphasize that the exercise regime is not an endurance test and that a gentle, systematic, consistent approach is more efficacious than infrequent bursts of aggressive exercises, which merely precipitate troublesome vertigo, associated with nausea and vomiting, and deter the patient from wishing to repeat the experience. Rarely, in patients who are extremely alarmed by their dizziness, it may be necessary to use a short course of an antivertiginous agent, such as cinnarizine, to enable the physical training regime to be started but such drugs should be discontinued as soon as possible.

The Cawthorne–Cooksey exercises have stood the test of time with respect to the management of peripheral vestibular lesions. However, recent workers have proposed that 'customized' as opposed to a standard exercise regime may be even more beneficial (Norre 1987; Shepard and Telian 1996). It is deemed that as balance is dependent on several sensory inputs, effective motor outputs, and general condition, the need for exercises specially aimed at improving one or more of these aspects may be more efficient in a given individual. To date, there is no definitive evidence that such an approach is superior, but further work is required in this area.

It is not completely understood why some patients with vestibular pathology seem to compensate more rapidly and effectively than others (Luxon 1997b). First, impaired compensation may result from the nature or severity of the disorder (e.g. recurrent impairment of the vestibular function) as seen in Ménière's disease may result in continually changing vestibular function for which the CNS cannot compensate. Second, disorders involving not only the peripheral vestibular labyrinth, but also the central vestibular connections, required for the process of compensation, result in damage to the very pathways required for recovery. Third, compensation requires multiple sensorimotor inputs and, thus, if senses other than the vestibular system are impaired, or the patient is immobilized, compensation is likely to be delayed or permanently impaired. A common problem is that patients with vestibular disorders tend to avoid moving their head to prevent dizziness. This imposes a strain on the neck muscles and neck pain develops, which may be mismanaged by the use of a cervical collar. This may inappropriately be assumed to support the neck, relieve pain, and reduce dizziness. However, the resultant immobilization fails to allow the provision of adequate information for vestibular compensation to take place. The rationale for abandoning the neck collar and undertaking a physical exercise regime must be emphasized in this group of patients.

PSYCHOLOGICAL SUPPORT

In addition to the improvement in disequilibrium achieved as a result of a vestibular exercise regime, significant psychological benefits accrue partly because an explanation of the regime is required in order for patients to understand their dizziness and secondly, the patients are encouraged to cope actively with their symptoms rather than avoid them (Yardley and Luxon 1994).

It is well recognized that patients with disequilibrium develop psychological symptoms, particularly panic attacks, anxiety disorders, and depression (Eagger et al. 1992). In a study of 54 patients with peripheral vestibular disorder, referred to a specialized neuro-otological centre, 35 developed a psychiatric illness based on DSMIIIR criteria. In nearly two-thirds, the psychiatric illness occurred during the first six months after the onset of neuro-otological problems. The commonest diagnoses were panic disorder, with or without agoraphobia, and phobic symptoms, including avoidance of crowds, enclosed spaces such as underground trains, buses and cars, together with the fear of going out alone, heights, and the dark. Patients feared being thought to be drunk and this lead to an avoidance of social situations. Recent work has suggested that active management of these psychological disturbances and, in particular, behavioural therapy is of considerable value in bringing about more rapid rehabilitation of these patients. Although there is no definitive study to assess the value of initial counselling in peripheral vestibular disorders it is the author's contention that appropriate explanation of the symptoms, early in the natural history of the disorder, would alleviate many of the long-term psychological sequelae. In particular, a patient with an inner ear disturbance, finds it hard to understand why he should feel 'spaced out', find shopping in a supermarket difficult, and feel his brain is 'disconnected' from his head. These types of symptoms frequently give rise to anxieties about sinister neurological diagnoses, such as brain tumours and, equally importantly, patients frequently report that they feel as though they 'are going mad'. These views are reinforced when they are seen by an inexperienced clinician, who dismisses their symptoms as psychological in origin. Such mismanagement must be avoided. Rehabilitation with psychological support and an active physical exercise regime with specific goals of returning to work and continuing to undertake social activities within realistic limits should be set.

DRUG THERAPY

As outlined above vestibular sedative drugs, such as cinnarizine, are invaluable in acute vertigo and have a limited role in certain patients in the early stages of vestibular rehabilitation for chronic disequilibrium. Antiemetics such as prochlorperazine, should not be prescribed long term, as there is no evidence that they are effective in the management of dysequilibrium and there is a danger of extrapyramidal side-effects. Psychotropic drugs should be avoided unless specifically required for psychiatric indications, as such drugs may interfere with vestibular compensation.

SURGICAL TREATMENT

Surgical intervention in the treatment of episodic vertigo is indicated in three main situations:

1. The treatment of complications of erosive middle ear disease.
2. To improve the quality of life in a patient suffering from severe recurrent vertigo in whom medical measures have failed.
3. To exclude the presence of a perilymph fistula.

It must be emphasized that before destructive surgery is undertaken detailed neuro-otological investigation to determine the exact site and severity of both auditory and vestibular dysfunction must be undertaken. Moreover, particularly in an elderly person, vestibular compensation may be prolonged or indeed incomplete as a consequent of age-related changes within the CNS. The concept that the subject will recover more effectively from labyrinthine destruction than a partial deficit is entirely misplaced. The risk of persisting imbalance must therefore be carefully weighed against any possible advantage.

AUDITORY DISORDERS

Hearing loss and tinnitus affect approximately one-fifth and one-tenth of the population, respectively. These symptoms may result from primary pathology of the outer, middle, or inner ear. Although tinnitus may result from central auditory dysfunction, significant hearing loss is rarely associated with brainstem or cortical disease, although loss of cochlear or VIIIth nerve origin is a common correlate of neurological conditions, and is seen in such conditions as inherited spinocerebellar degenerations, mitochondrial cytopathies, multiple sclerosis, vertebrobasilar ischaemia, and head injury.

HEARING IMPAIRMENT

PATHOPHYSIOLOGY

For clinical purposes the ear may be divided into three parts: the outer; middle; and internal ear (Fig. 2.8). Abnormalities in each of these sites may give rise to hearing impairment.

The outer ear is important in the localization of sound and funnels sound to the tympanic membrane. The middle ear

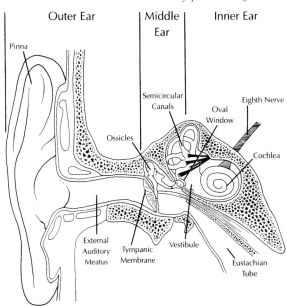

Fig. 2.8 Diagram of the anatomy of the ear.

ossicles connect the tympanic membrane to the oval window of the cochlea, such that airborne changes in sound pressure cause displacement within the fluid-filled compartment of the membranous labyrinth. Within the internal ear, the mechanical activity at the oval window is transduced into neural responses within the organ of Corti (Fig. 2.9).

Disorders of the outer ear and middle ear give rise to abnormalities of the mechanical transmission of sound from the environment to the inner ear, known as ***conductive hearing loss*** (i.e. bone-conducted sound applied to the mastoid bone is perceived normally by the cochlea), whereas air-conducted sounds, which are normally perceived more acutely by the cochlea as a result of the amplifying characteristics of the outer and middle ear are heard less well. Common examples include impacted wax, chronic middle ear disease, ossicular chain dysfunction (e.g. otosclerosis), and 'glue' ear in children.

Disorders of the inner ear and VIIIth cranial nerve characteristically give rise to a ***sensorineural hearing loss***, which is manifest as an inability to perceive either bone-conducted or air-conducted sounds in the normal way, and both the appreciation of the intensity of sound and the frequency resolution of complex sounds are impaired. A plethora of disorders may affect the cochlea ranging from inherited, congenital, or iatrogenic (e.g. thalidomide) malformations to ototoxic (e.g. aminoglycoside, antimalarial, loop diuretics) damage, ischaemia, infective agents (e.g. mumps, rubella, syphilis), autoimmune disorders, degenerative disorders, trauma, and idiopathic conditions such as Ménière's disease. Dysfunction of the VIIIth nerve has been documented in spinocerebellar degenerations, trauma, cerebellopontine angle tumours, bony disorders (e.g. Paget's disease) infective disorders (meningitis), and inflammatory conditions (sarcoidosis).

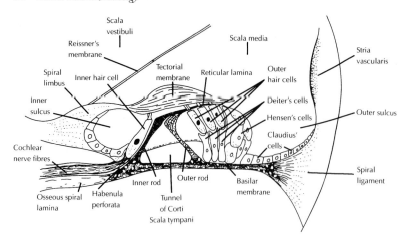

Fig. 2.9 Diagram to illustrate anatomical structure of one turn of the organ of Corti.

Lim and Stephens (1985) have shown that detailed investigation of elderly patients with so-called 'presbyacusis' reveal that 83% have evidence of conditions known to be associated with hearing loss and thus, auditory investigation of hearing loss in the elderly is appropriate.

INVESTIGATION

The investigation of hearing loss depends partly on a full audiological battery of tests to define the precise site of auditory dysfunction (Luxon 1988), but also on a broad knowledge of the plethora of general medical, neurological, and otological disorders associated with hearing loss (Yeoh 1997).

In order to differentiate a sensorineural hearing loss of cochlear origin from that of VIIIth nerve dysfunction or neurological origin, two pathophysiological phenomena are of important:

1. *Loudness recruitment* is defined as an abnormally rapid increase in loudness, with increase of intensity of stimulus, and is characteristic of disorders affecting the hair cells of the organ of Corti, but is absent in pathology of the VIIIth nerve.
2. *Abnormal auditory adaptation* is a decline in discharge frequency with time, observed following an initial burst of neural activity in response to an adequate continuing stimulus applied to the organ of Corti. This phenomenon is characteristic of VIIIth nerve and brainstem auditory dysfunction.

A battery of test procedures are required to facilitate accurate auditory diagnoses. **Pure tone audiometry** is the most widely available quantitative test of auditory thresholds. Electronically generated pure tones are delivered by an earphone and the subject is required to respond to the quietest tone, at a given frequency, either by air conduction (AC), or if the tones are delivered via a bone conductor on the mastoid process, by bone conduction (BC). As outlined above, bone-conduction thresholds significantly better than air-conduction

thresholds indicate a conductive hearing loss, whereas bone-conduction and air-conduction thresholds of approximately similar values are characteristic of sensorineural loss (Fig. 2.10).

The stapedius muscle in the middle ear, contracts bilaterally in response to loud sound directed into either ear (Fig. 2.11). Using an impedance bridge, the minimum intensity of sound at a given frequency, producing a contraction (known as the **acoustic reflex threshold**) can be measured. The acoustic reflex thresholds, enable recruitment and auditory adaptation to be measured and allow assessment of middle ear, cochlea, VIIIth nerve, and brainstem auditory function.

Speech audiometry requires a subject to repeat standard lists of words delivered at varying intensities through headphones. The responses are scored and provide an assessment of auditory discrimination, and are of particular value in assessing the efficacy of hearing aid provision.

Electrophysiological tests have provided a major means of assessing empirically auditory function and siting pathology in the auditory system. As a diagnostic tool, brainstem auditory-evoked responses are of particular value in discriminating between cochlear and VIIIth nerve dysfunction and are obtained by averaging a series of time-locked responses, which are generated by the major processing centres of the auditory system in response to a repetitive sound stimulus (Fig. 2.12). Analysis of the wave form should only be undertaken in conjunction with knowledge of pure tone thresholds, if appropriate and valid conclusions about auditory function are to be made. Cortical-evoked responses are the most effective method of defining auditory thresholds at each frequency in an uncooperative patient and are essential in legal cases, in which non-organic loss should be considered.

MANAGEMENT

Management of hearing loss requires a detailed history to define relevant factors, such as leisure (e.g. discos, shooting),

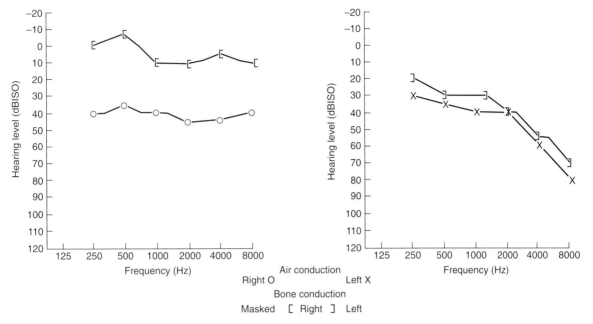

Air conduction

Right O   Left X

Bone conduction

Masked   [Right]   Left

Fig. 2.10 Diagram to illustrate pure tone audiometric thresholds. O, air conduction threshold *right* ear; X, air conduction threshold *left* ear; [, bone conduction threshold *right* ear;], bone conduction threshold *left* ear; A, bilateral sensorineural hearing loss; B, right conductive hearing loss.

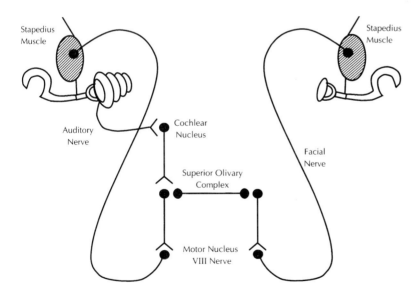

Fig. 2.11 Diagram showing the components of the ipsilateral and contralateral pathway of the stapedial reflex.

and occupational noise hazards; previous head injury; viral illnesses (e.g. mumps); a detailed family history and a general medical history to identify syndromes, in which hearing loss is a component feature (e.g. Alport's disorder, Pendred syndrome, Jervell–Lange–Neilsen syndrome); ototoxic damage (aspirin, quinine, aminoglyocide antibiotics); systemic disease, such as autoimmune disorders and vascular pathology. Of primary importance is the need to prevent deterioration of

hearing loss by such measures as ensuring adequate auditory protection in the workplace and early recognition of drug-induced ototoxicity. In the last decade, considerable advances have been made in the understanding of inherited hearing loss and genetic counselling may be required.

Auditory rehabilitation is well established in recognized centres throughout the United Kingdom and is directed at minimizing any disability experienced by an individual, as a

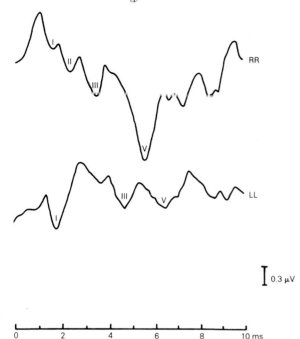

Fig. 2.12 Tracing of brainstem auditory-evoked potential illustrating a normal right ear response (RR) and an abnormal left ear response (LL) with a delayed wave V latency in a case of a left acoustic neurinoma. (With grateful thanks to Dr D. Prasher.)

result of their hearing loss, together with the prevention of any consequent handicap. Thus, it is a problem-solving exercise, which is centred around the particular needs of the individual concerned and must be approached within this framework (Fig. 2.13).

Despite the availability of health service provision in the United Kingdom, a number of studies have shown that only 20–25% of patients with significant auditory impairment obtain rehabilitative help. There are a number of reasons which explain this phenomenon. Hearing impairment is particularly common in the elderly, who may not be aware of any significant auditory disability, partly because of their lifestyle. Auditory impairment is often highlighted by social and/or occupational factors, which necessitate the patient seeking help. An elderly person living alone with little social contact, is therefore less likely to seek help, whereas a working man pres-

surized by family complaints and the necessity to function effectively at work, is more likely to seek help earlier. Clinicians' attitude is also important in a patient's decision to seek rehabilitative auditory help, for example, not infrequently patients are told 'you have nerve deafness and hearing aids will not help'. This negative advice deters patients from looking further for rehabilitation and reflects the clinician's lack of knowledge that auditory rehabilitation does not merely involve the provision of an hearing aid, but also relies heavily on the use of auditory tactics and the development of audiovisual communication skills. Financial factors are also important and, while not highly relevant in the United Kingdom, it has been shown that in countries where individuals are required to pay for the provision of an aid, the possession of a hearing aid is less common than in countries where they are provided free of charge.

A management model for the rehabilitation of the hearing impaired (Fig. 2.14) underlines the different components of the rehabilitative process which can be broadly divided into *evaluation* and *remediation* phases.

Evaluation depends on assessing the auditory disability of the individual and the implication of this for other important people in the patient's life. Thus, auditory impairment, communication skills (including lip-reading ability, visual cues, speech, and language), and psychological and sociological factors, including the patient's domestic circumstances, all require consideration. Moreover, assessment of the patient's response to his/her disability is essential, if appropriate rehabilitation is to be effective. The expectation from rehabilitation must be realistic, as either too low or too high an expectation may result in the patient failing to preserve and benefit from the measures introduced.

The *remediation* process is governed by the evaluations noted above. Patients are divided into 'straightforward' highly motivated cases in whom there is an uncomplicated hearing loss. In general, this group will be fitted with an appropriate hearing aid, given advice on relevant environmental aids and hearing tactics, with minimal need for ancillary help or communication training.

A second group of patients is comprised of similarly motivated people, but in whom complicating factors are present. Either the type of hearing loss from which they suffer is difficult to aid, or there are other complicating factors (e.g. arthritis), which makes hearing aid manipulation difficult, or

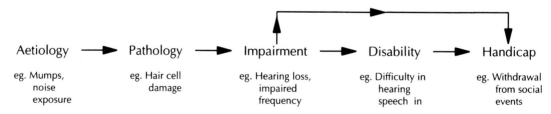

Fig. 2.13 World Health Organization schema for hearing loss disability. [From Stephens, S.D.G. (1987). Audiological rehabilitation. In *Scott-Brown's otolaryngology*, (5th edn), (ed. A. G. Kerr), Vol. 2. *Adult audiology*. Butterworth, London 1987.]

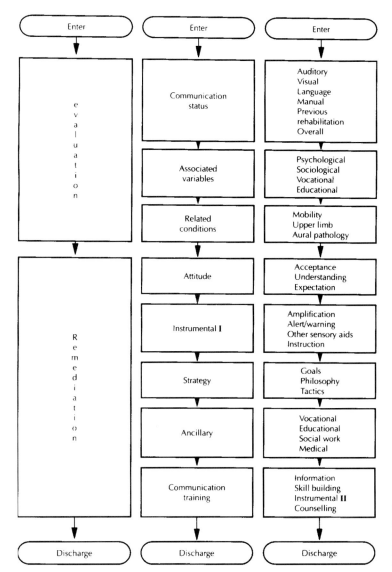

Fig. 2.14 Flowchart of a management model for auditory rehabilitation. [Reproduced with kind permission from Goldstein, D. and Stephens, S.D.G. (1981). Audiological rehabilitation: management model 1. *Audiology*, **20**, 432–52.]

inappropriate previous management has led to negative preconceptions, which must be overcome before success is likely to result from auditory rehabilitation. Considerably more care is required in the fitting of hearing aids for this group, with repeated reassessment in order to ensure the most appropriate instrumental fitting, together with integration of communication training, and optimal use of audiovisual training skills. Psychological problems may require specific psychological support.

A third group of patients are those who genuinely desire help, but are adamant that one or more major components of the rehabilitative process are not suitable for them. The most usual problem is a very negative view of hearing aids. In this

group, it may initially be helpful to gain the patient's confidence by providing environmental aids, teaching communication skills, and countering the patient's belief that 'nothing will help'. When such simple strategies are shown to be effective, the patient may then be introduced to the concept that an hearing aid could also be effective.

A final group of patients is those who do not desire help and have usually been brought along by well-meaning family members. In this situation, it is usually most profitable to discuss with the patient and his/her relatives the options available, explaining both the disadvantages and advantages, but emphasizing that no further follow-up will be made, unless the patient him/herself wishes to pursue matters further.

HEARING AIDS

These play a pivotal role in audiological rehabilitation. However, a detailed description of their function and selection are outside the scope of this chapter and consideration is restricted to the general principles involved.

The function of a hearing aid is to bring sound more effectively to the ear of an hearing-impaired person. The system, comprised of an hearing aid and the ear mould, should be cheap, either for the individual or the health service purchasing the equipment, as 'invisible' as possible, and with minimal requirements for repeated adjustments by the subject.

The ***ear mould*** must provide a comfortable, secure mounting for the aid and a good acoustic connection between the aid and the ear canal. The mould must fit perfectly to avoid the annoying whistle of acoustic feedback, but must not be too tight so as to be uncomfortable. To achieve this, an individual ear mould, made from an impression, is required. Ear mould modifications, partly for comfort, but more importantly to modify the sound path are important. A vent hole in the ear mould may be necessary, if the user complains of a blocked or sweaty sensation in the ear canal or complains of excessive background noise. Frequently, the vent acts as a low frequency cut, particularly if the diameter of the vent is greater than 1 mm. A variety of other modifications, such as 'dampers', to reduce the size of resonance peaks in the mid frequency region, the presence of a Libby horn to improve the transmission of high frequencies into the ear canal, and the siting of the ear mould's vent to alter the acoustic response of a hearing aid require consideration.

For most individuals, the most important need is to hear normal speech. ***Hearing aid selection*** involves matching the amplification required from the aid at specific frequencies with that required by the user. A particular disability experienced in most hearing-impaired subjects is that of hearing speech in a noisy environment and although programmable digital processing hearing aids are of some help in this situation, conventional aids provide selective amplification of the frequencies relevant to speech, with minimal amplification at the peak frequency of background noise.

Conventional hearing aids can be divided into *body-worn aids* and *head-worn aids*, which can be in spectacles, behind-the-ear, in-the-ear, or in-the-canal in design. The major advantage of body-worn aids is the very high gain and maximum output that can be achieved, whereas the disadvantage is the unsightly nature of the device and the poor microphone placement, with masking noise produced by rubbing of clothing on the microphone. Behind-the-ear aids are now the standard aid issued within the UK health service, whereas in-the-ear aids are the most commonly available commercial aid, although they are expensive and there is little scope for post-fitting modification.

Figure 2.15 shows the main components of a behind-the-ear aid. Immediately before the earphone, two features known as automatic gain control and peak clipping are noted.

Peak clipping prevents high amplitude peaks in the electric signal passing into the ear by reducing the current supply to the output stage. This prevents sudden loud noises distressing the user, but such 'clipping' produces distortion. Automatic gain control is a mechanism of limiting the output of the aid by compressing the gain of the response over a range of input sound levels, again to avoid excessively loud sounds being presented to the subject. The advantage of this technique also known as 'compression' is to avoid the distortion associated with peak clipping.

There is much evidence to show that binaural fitting of hearing aids has significant advantages, and as a general rule both ears should be fitted unless there is a valid reason for not fitting one ear, such as active discharge or total hearing loss. If a patient is resistant to the idea of aiding both ears, it may be worth asking him/her to try two aids in order to evaluate which ear to choose for the single hearing aid. This exposure to binaural fitting may convince the patient of the value of two aids.

In the fitting of hearing aids certain handling skills are required for the patient: ear mould insertion; volume control adjustment; and care of the aid. The patient must be competent in these skills before leaving the clinic. In elderly patients with poor manipulation skills, or an aversion to hearing aids, an ear trumpet may be of value, despite its 'low-tech' appearance.

In the past, instrumental help has largely focused on wearable hearing aids, but in recent years the value of ***environmental aids*** and ***sensory substitution systems*** has become more evident.

Environmental aids (assistive listening devices) may be subdivided into *amplification systems*, designed to help the individual hear speech or recorded speech more clearly and *alerting/warning devices* such as flashing lights connected to a door bell or an alarm clock (Table 2.5). Amplification systems can be used alone, or in association with a hearing aid system, and enable a person to listen to, for example, the television without turning it up so loudly as to disturb any other family members. An electromagnetic (loop) system containing the television sound system allows the hearing aid user to pick up the sound by setting the hearing aid on the 'T' or telecoil position. The major advantage of this facility is that the person can hear the television, uncontaminated by background noise, but the disadvantage is that he/she cannot take part in family conversation simultaneously. However, in certain hearing aids, it is now possible for the inputs from the telecoil and the microphone to be mixed within the aid and perceived simultaneously. Telephone aids provide the addition of an amplifier in the telephone handpiece, which generally gives an additional 15-decibel boost to the signal, or the use of an electromagnetic system which may be utilized by turning the hearing aid to the 'T' setting.

Sensory substitution systems include certain of the warning devices as noted above where visual signals are generated in response to auditory cues, such as the telephone

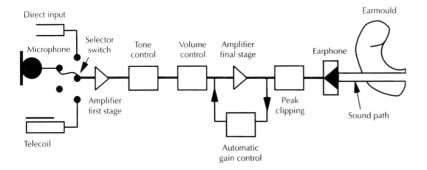

Fig. 2.15 Diagram showing the components of a behind-the-ear hearing aid. [Reproduced with kind permission from Corcoran, A. (1987). Hearing aids. In *Scott-Brown's otolaryngology*, (5th edn), (ed. A. G. Kerr), Vol. 2. *Adult audiology*. Butterworth, London.]

Table 2.5 Environmental aids and the approaches used

Approach	Additional amplification	Electro magnetic	FM radip	Infrared	Alternative acoustics	Visual	Vibrotactile
Amplification							
TV/radio/hi-fi	+	+	+	+	–	–	–
Telephone	+	+	–	–	–	–	–
Theatre/cinema	+	+	+	+	–	–	–
Station announcements	–	+	–	–	–	–	–
Banks/post offices	+	+	–	–	–	–	–
Alert/warning							
Telephone bell	+	+	–	–	+	+	+
Doorbell	+	+	–	–	+	+	+
Alarm clock	+	–	–	–	+	+	+
Baby alarm	+	–	–	–	+	+	+

Reproduced with kind permission from Stephens, S.D.G. (1987). Audiological rehabilitation. In *Scott-Brown's otolaryngology*, (5th edn), (ed. A. G. Kerr), Vol. 2. *Adult audiology*. Butterworths, London.

ringing, a door bell ringing, or a baby crying. In addition to providing such environmental information, sensory substitution systems provide additional information to supplement visual cues in the perception of speech and help patients monitor their own speech. Such systems have been available for many years and provide a vibrotactile signal to the mastoid or the wrist, with respect to sounds. Although having a role, particularly in blind–deaf individuals, vibrotactile stimulation is inferior in terms of transmitting meaningful speech information to the profoundly/totally deaf compared to modern cochlear implant technology.

COCHLEAR IMPLANTS

These are electronic devices that convert sound into electrical current for the purpose of directly stimulating residual auditory nerve fibres to produce hearing sensations (Rosen 1997). The devices are implanted in the cochlea, with either a single electrode or an electrode array with an externally worn microphone and processor. Acoustic signals detected by the microphone are electrically transduced and transmitting via cabling to the processor so they may be analysed and processed in a variety of ways. The application of an electrical signal to the electrode site(s) results in direct stimulation of neural fibres, such that auditory information proceeds up through the central auditory system and is interpreted as sound. Cochlear implants have been used in totally deaf adults and more recently in children, with good results. Within the last decade, a number of improvements in cochlear implant design have been introduced and the addition of more sophisticated speech-coding strategies has lead to improvement in the performance of many cochlear implant recipients. Following cochlear implantation, an individual programme of auditory training is initiated usually over a period of several months. A multisensory approach is adopted as individuals use cues available in everyday life. Thus, training often begins with speech stimuli presented in an auditory-visual context and after success at this level auditory only speech material may be introduced, initially in a closed set format progressing to an open set format.

Current research is aimed at determining whether patients' performance can be improved using an increased number of channels of electrical stimulation and higher stimulation rates to preserve the temporal structure of speech. Moreover, improvements in digital signalling processing may facilitate preservation of amplitude cues in speech and environmental sounds.

The value of ***counselling*** for the hearing-impaired by a skilled hearing therapist must be emphasized. Such simple hearing tactics as encouraging the individual to ensure that the light is always on the speaker's face, that he/she places him/herself so that the better ear is towards the speaker, that he/she sits close to the source of sound he/she wishes to hear and minimizes background noise, can greatly improve communication ability. For the profoundly hearing-impaired, psychological problems, associated with isolation, are significant and it is therefore essential that psychological, medical, and social support are readily available. Moreover, clinicians should be aware of other professionals with whom the hearing-impaired should be in contact: disablement resettlement officers/vocational guidance counsellors are of particular importance in helping disabled individuals to find and sustain suitable employment and specialist social workers for the deaf may help with specific housing/accommodation needs.

TINNITUS

PATHOPHYSIOLOGY

Tinnitus may be defined as the perception of sound, which originates from within the head rather than in the external world. Occasionally, the sound may have an externally detectable component, in which case it is termed 'objective tinnitus', as opposed to the more common 'subjective tinnitus'. It has been proposed that tinnitus needs no description, as it is a universal experience similar to headache and pain, but a distinction must be drawn between tinnitus experience and tinnitus complaint. It would appear that the prevalence of tinnitus complaint is increasing and in the United States, Vernon (1987) has estimated a population of 9 million cases of severe tinnitus, whereas in the United Kingdom, the British Tinnitus Association has estimated that 1 in 10 of the population suffer with this complaint, although the National Study of Hearing (Coles 1987) identified that only 8% of the population experience moderate to severe tinnitus. It is of note that tinnitus as a complaint is practically unknown in developing countries.

The conditions with which tinnitus is associated and the proposed mechanisms by which tinnitus originates are legion, but, nonetheless, in the majority of instances the pathophysiology of this symptom remains obscure. Tinnitus is frequently, but not always, associated with hearing impairment and the proposed pathophysiological mechanisms include the decoupling of the sterocilia of the hair cells, misinterpretation of auditory neural activity by higher auditory centres, and self-sustaining oscillation of the basilar membrane. Following Kemp's (1978) discovery of acoustic emissions from within the human auditory system, it was thought that spontaneous otoacoustic emissions might provide an explanation for many cases of tinnitus. Although such a link has been demonstrated (Penner 1989), this association has not proved to be common.

Various other theories of tinnitus generation depend on abnormalities of neural function. It has been proposed that an abnormality of the spontaneous resting activity of primary auditory nerve fibres, either secondary to hypo- or hyper-excitability of damaged hair cells, or as a direct consequence of derangement of the primary neurones themselves, may give rise to the symptom. Moller (1984) has proposed that damage to the myelin sheath between auditory nerve fibres, may allow ephaptic transmission ('cross-talk') between adjacent nerve fibres, while an alternative proposal is that derangement of efferent fibres of the vestibulocochlear nerve produce aberrant auditory behaviour. Nonetheless, it is necessary to address the fact that the majority of people who perceive tinnitus do not complain about it. A number of studies have demonstrated that tinnitus complaint does not correlate with psychoacoustical features of the tinnitus, while many studies have defined a significant correlation between tinnitus complaint and psychological symptoms (Hinchcliffe and King 1992). Moreover, the onset of tinnitus complaint may be associated with negative life events such as retirement, redundancy, bereavement, and divorce.

The diagnosis of tinnitus requires a detailed history and examination. The commonest causes of **objective tinnitus** include palatal myoclonus, temporomandibular joint abnormalities, whereas pulsatile tinnitus is associated with vascular abnormalities, such as arteriovenous fistula, and vascular bruit. Less commonly, a patulous auditory tube may give rise to a form of tinnitus, in which the patient complains of a sound of blowing, associated with respiration.

Subjective tinnitus requires a detailed assessment of hearing, but it must be emphasized that tinnitus may occur in the absence of any overt auditory deficit. Unilateral tinnitus, with or without an associated sensorineural hearing loss, must be fully investigated to exclude an underlying cerebellopontine angle lesion, in particular an acoustic neurinoma. Bilateral tinnitus, with evidence of a cochlear hearing loss, is associated most commonly with presbyacusis, endolymphatic hydrops, vascular labyrinthine lesions, and noise-induced hearing loss. In Barr's classic work characterizing occupational noise-induced hearing loss in 1886, he commented on the symptom of tinnitus: 'I have been surprised at its comparative infrequency in these men (boilermakers)'. This finding is in contrast to the current situation where many claimants of occupational noise-induced hearing loss complain frequently of tinnitus. Noise exposure due to gunfire, leisure activities, industrial exposure, and blast injuries may all give rise to noise-induced tinnitus. Tinnitus as a result of head injury is well recognized and may also result from direct mechanical or aural injury. Importantly, many patients complain of the onset of tinnitus after aural syringing, even in the absence of any obvious trauma. Tinnitus has also been reported after whiplash injury, electric shock, otic barotrauma, and surgical intervention, particularly stapedectomy.

Drug-induced tinnitus is an important entity and may result from an ototoxic effect (e.g. aminoglycoside antibiotics, salicylates, other non-steroidal anti-inflammatory drugs and loop diuretics), or as a result of side-effects of unknown pathophysiological mechanism (e.g. tricyclic antidepressants, certain tranquillizers, including the benzodiazepines, and cardiovascular agents).

Conductive hearing loss may rarely be associated with tinnitus directly, but more commonly will enhance an underlying tinnitus caused by sensorineural mechanisms.

INVESTIGATION

Empirically, there is no means of defining and thus diagnosing tinnitus. It is a subjective complaint for which there is no objective measure. Tinnitus may be matched and masked by standard audiometric techniques, but this in itself is subjective. A hearing loss may be defined, but the complaint of tinnitus is not directly correlated with the type or severity of any associated hearing impairment. Hoke and co-workers (1989) have reported that abnormalities of acoustically evoked magnetic fields of patients suffering from tinnitus are distinctly different from normally hearing individuals, but this is not a universal finding in tinnitus suffers and this work remains to be confirmed.

MANAGEMENT

The primary management of tinnitus is medical, with the rare exception of surgery for the correction of arterial stenosis giving rise to bruits, surgical intervention for glomus jugular tumours, and arteriovenous malformations. Destructive surgery (e.g. labyrinthectomy or nerve section) has no place in the management of tinnitus, as there is no evidence that destruction of the peripheral cochlear elements brings about an improvement in tinnitus complaint.

As clearly defined by Hinchcliffe and King (1992), the management of tinnitus can be considered under three headings: (1) psychological; (3) pharmacological; (2) and prosthetic.

The treatment of the *psychological* aspects of tinnitus is of paramount importance, as it has been shown that such an approach can reduce the stress caused by tinnitus, as distinct from the pitch of loudness (Hallam and Jakes 1985). Previous negative counselling, such as is commonly given by the non-specialist, for example, that there is no effective treatment and no known cause, must be countered by a clear and rational explanation of possible mechanisms of generation and modes of treatment for the management of tinnitus, together with the reassurance that the majority of cases improve and do not deteriorate with time (Rubinstein *et al.* 1992). Importantly, appropriate investigations must be conducted to exclude sinister cerebral pathology and to reassure the patient, as a commonly expressed fear is that of malignant brain tumours. Cognitive therapy aimed at helping the tinnitus sufferer by guidance of his/her thoughts, beliefs, attitudes, and images of the condition appears to offer the best psychological therapy (Jakes *et al.* 1986). Notwithstanding, a number of studies have documented the psychiatric morbidity in patients with tinnitus and the need for formal psychiatric referral must be considered (Erlandsson 1990). In addition, patients frequently find support from lay counselling and patients should be encouraged to join the British Tinnitus Association.

The *prosthetic* management of tinnitus include the provision of an hearing aid, which may improve the patient's hearing, lessen the attention given to hearing 'problems', and mask tinnitus by using amplification of desirable environmental sounds. However, recent work has suggested that hearing aids alone are not an effective device for managing tinnitus (Melin *et al.* 1987) and that the beneficial effects previously reported accrue from counselling and other non-specific rehabilitative measures, including an informed explanation of the symptom and management strategies as noted above (Coles *et al.* 1985). Furthermore, despite anecdotal evidence, controlled studies of tinnitus maskers have failed to demonstrate that they are unequivocally superior to a comparable placebo device (Erlandsson *et al.* 1987).

Pharmacologically, intravenous lignocaine has been shown to result in the disappearance or amelioration of tinnitus (Israel *et al.* 1982). However, various antidysrhythmic and anticonvulsant agents have been used, but double-blind placebo controlled studies have failed to define any drug of specific benefit (Hinchcliffe and King 1992). Formal psychiatric assessment with appropriate drug treatment is required in some patients, benzodiazepines have been the drug of choice in anxious patients, but they may make a depressed tinnitus sufferer more (Goodey 1987). In view of the association of tinnitus with depressive illness, treatment with tricyclic antidepressants has been proposed. Nonetheless, a double-blind control study of trimipramine in tinnitus complainers failed to reveal any advantage to a placebo (Mihail *et al.* 1988). However, there were flaws in the design of this study and a subsequent single-blind, non-randomized study using nortriptyline showed this particular drug to be effective (Sullivan *et al.* 1989).

In conclusion, for the patient with troublesome tinnitus the most important aspect of management is a positive medical approach, supported by an informed explanation based on appropriate tests and reassurance of the benign nature of the disorder. The patient should be reassured that this symptom will not deteriorate. Psychological support, together with informed counselling regarding coping strategies, form the basis of management.

FALLS

These present a difficult diagnostic dilemma. To elucidate the primary problem, it is necessary to consider normal mechanisms that maintain balance and age/disease related changes, which may predispose to falls. In addition, environmental factors are of particular importance, especially in the elderly.

The epidemiology of falls is difficult to evaluate partly because of the difficulty in defining a fall. The definition may relate to unprecipitated events, but may include slips, trips, and episodes of loss of consciousness. Data may be difficulty to collect as falls may be defined as events requiring medical intervention or help, but equally may relate to all events where the subject lands on the ground, whether or not medical help is sought. In this latter situation, subjects do not report the fall to anyone and thus accurate figures cannot be obtained, especially as it has been shown that accuracy of retrospective recall regarding falls, even within a period of 12 months, is unreliable. Environmental factors are highly relevant in the consideration of falls and would be quite different in, for example, an elderly population living at home, and a similar population who are institutionalized. Therefore, if comparisons between studies are to be made, it is necessary to consider similar groups of subjects or to ensure that the distribution of subjects within populations to be compared are similar.

Notwithstanding these difficulties, recent studies have shown that falls are a significant cause of injury in the young, with reduced incidence in the 15- to 25-year-old age range and then an increasing incidence above 55 years of age. In community-based studies, the frequency of falls has been shown to be approximately 28–35% for subjects aged 65 and over, rising to 32–42% for those 75 years of age and over (Downton 1992). It has been shown that of those who have fallen in the previous year, 60–70% are likely to fall again during the following 12 months.

RISK FACTORS

A number of factors have been identified as being associated with falls. As noted above, the elderly are more likely to fall and falls are more common in women.

Drug intake increases the risk of falling although it may be difficult to differentiate the effect of a drug from the effect of the disease for which the drug was prescribed. The changes in pharmacokinetics and pharmacodynamics render the elderly more liable to suffer side-effects from drug therapy and this may be of relevance with respect to falls, particularly with such drugs as psychotropic and cardiovascular agents, which may give rise to hypotension. Alcohol-related falls should be considered, particularly in the presence of associated head injury.

A number of neurological conditions are associated with falls including epilepsy, Parkinson's disease, cerebrovascular disease, peripheral neuropathies, cervical spondylosis, and dementia. An impairment of cognitive function is a significant factor in falls and subjects with dementia are three times more likely to fall than non-demented controls (Morris *et al.* 1987).

General medical conditions such as diabetes, cardiac dysrhythmia, carotid sinus syndrome, autonomic dysfunction, and postural hypotension are associated with falls. Musculoskeletal disease and disorders causing changes in posture and gait are also risk factors. Sensory impairment, particu-

larly of vision, and/or vestibular abnormalities, increase the risk of falling. In addition to medical factors, the environmental factors of particular note are uneven or slippery surfaces (e.g. paving stones or ice poor lighting, and unfamiliar environments).

The importance of falls lies in the morbidity and mortality of falling. Death following a fall may result directly from the injury sustained or indirectly from complications, such as pneumonia or hypothermia. In the elderly, there is an additional significant operative and post-operative mortality from surgical intervention for fractured neck of femur and other injuries, including wrist and vertebral crush fractures. The majority of deaths due to falls occur in the elderly (Fig. 2.16) and injury of some kind occurs in about one-half of those who fall.

INVESTIGATION

The management of falls includes a thorough general medical assessment with specific reference to vision, the cardiovascular, central nervous and musculoskeletal systems. In the elderly, a multidisciplinary assessment, including social and environmental factors is of benefit. The investigation of falls can be divided into two main areas: the assessment of the faller; and the evaluation of the interrelationship between the faller and his/her environment. This approach allows potentially treatable causes or predisposing factors for falls to be identified and corrected.

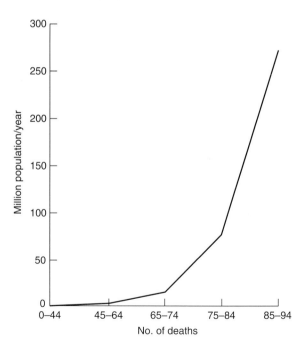

Fig. 2.16 Fatal accidental falls in the home: deaths per million per year. [Data reproduced with kind permission from Berfenstam *et al.* (1969). In *From falls in the elderly*, (ed. J. H. Downton). Edward Arnold, London.]

The uncomplicated fall with no sequelae should be identified such that the patient can be safely reassured and discharged. This group of subjects needs to be separated from those who require specific clinical intervention because of injuries, recurrent falls or because the fall is a marker of significant medical illness. Downton (1992) has emphasized that the essential question is: 'Why did this particular person fall at this particular time in this particular place?' Thus she defines internal, external (environmental) and situational factors which may be fixed but are more likely to be variable with time. Hence, for any particular fall, there is a *liability* to fall factor and an *opportunity* factor, and the relative importance of these two factors at different ages vary. However, a number of small studies have demonstrated that thorough assessment of elderly fallers and correction of alterable factors, predisposing to falls, can reduce the frequency of further falls (Morton 1989).

Initial assessment requires identification and appropriate management of any sustained injury. However, once the patient is comfortable, it is important to take a detailed history to determine the circumstances and nature of the fall or falls that have occurred (Fig. 2.17).

In the history several specific areas require clarification:

1. *Cause of fall.* An attempt should be made to define whether the patient tripped or fell, although very commonly people rationalize their falls and such remarks as 'I must have tripped', should be treated with caution, unless a clear description of uneven paving stones, a slippery patch on the pavement, or an uneven rug, is obtained. If several falls have occurred, details of the situation and circumstances may enable a single cause, or a number of mechanisms, underlying the falls to be defined.

2. *Description of the fall.* The patient should describe, in as much detail as possible, the exact set of circumstances that led to the fall (e.g. were they getting out of a chair/bed, walking, standing still, bending over, or turning their head?). Enquiries should be made as to how they felt immediately prior to and after the fall and whether they have clear recollection of the fall itself. If several falls have occurred, a typical fall and variable features should be described. The suggestion of any cognitive impairment or loss of consciousness, should prompt information from a witness, including the number of falls observed, similarities and differences of falls and circumstances, changes in colour of the faller, and complaints of associated symptoms. Information as to how the faller behaved before or after the event may also be of value.

3. *Contributory factors.* The patient should be specifically questioned about risk factors, including recent change of glasses (e.g. bifocals), balance disorders, medication, and changes in environment/activities.

4. *Associated illness.* Specific enquiry regarding cardiovascular, rheumatological/orthopaedic, vestibular/balance, and psychological illness must be made. In association with the

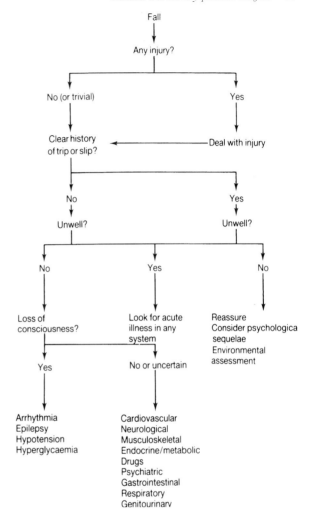

Fig. 2.17 Flowchart to aid the assessment and management of falls. [Reproduced with kind permission from Downton, J. H. (ed.) (1969). *Falls in the elderly*. Edward Arnold, London.

fall(s), dizziness, loss of awareness, loss of consciousness, epileptiform features, and/or disorientation should be identified.

5. *Drug treatment.* A detailed drug history must be obtained and in the elderly, the possibility of inadvertent overdose, in addition to side-effects and drug interactions, must be considered.

6. *Environmental factors.* A home visit to the faller's home or place of care may be invaluable to define environmental risk factors.

This specific information, together with a detailed general medical history, will usually identify a single factor or factors which are of importance in any one fall. If multiple falls are present, it is important to determine whether a pattern emerges, which may be explained on the basis of one or more factors, but if no pattern emerges it is likely that the falls are multifactorial in aetiology.

A general medical assessment is required to exclude the presence of any acute disorder (e.g. abnormalities of heart rate and rhythm, postural hypotension, and myocardial infarction). Cognitive function should be assessed, particularly to determine whether the history may be relied on. A neurological examination with particular reference to vestibular function, visual acuity and fields, and muscle power and symmetry is required. Orthopaedic/rheumatological abnormalities must be assessed and simple gait and mobility tests such as the 'get up and go' test in which the subject is asked to stand up from a chair, walk across the room, turn around and walk back to the chair and sit down again should be assessed (Mathias *et al.* 1986). Importantly, conditions which may be deemed to be trivial such as corns, ingrowing toenails, callosities, and hallux valgus may give rise to pain, which increases instability.

Detailed investigation varies depending upon the symptoms and signs elicited, but routine screening tests should include a full blood count, erythrocyle sedimentation rate (ESR), biochemical screen and thyroid function tests. An electrocardiogram (ECG) is mandatory and a chest X-ray should be performed if one is not available within the previous six months. Evidence of previous vascular disease, or dizziness, loss of consciousness and/or palpitations should prompt a 24-hour Holter monitor, although it may be necessary to repeat monitoring if symptoms do not occur during the 24-hour period. If necessary, cardiomemo equipment can be used.

MANAGEMENT

Thus, a general medical appraisal will dictate the need for *cardiological* investigation in the face of dizziness, palpitations, syncope, or chest pain, *neurological* investigation in the presence of dizziness, focal neurological signs, loss of consciousness, or gait disturbance, and orthopaedic/rheumatological assessment in the face of joint pain or deformity. Isolated falls in the absence of other symptoms with or without dizziness require *neuro-otological* investigation to exclude vestibular dysfunction, which is amenable to rehabilitation. 'Trivial' problems should be dealt with promptly (e.g. if the falls have occurred following the introduction of bifocal glasses, these should be abandoned to assess whether the falls improve), minor foot ailments should also be corrected. All drug regimes should be carefully reviewed and any new drug should be changed to determine whether improvement incurs.

The psychological impact of falling in the elderly is profound. There is a prolonged sense of vulnerability and many elderly people limit their activity for fear of falling. A 'postfall' syndrome has been described, including hesitancy of gait, irregularity of progress, a tendency to clutch and grab when walking, and symptoms of anxiety. The psychological aspects of falling are compounded by the fact that such symptoms may increase the rate of subsequent falls, and a vicious circle develops. The response of family and friends may compound the situation by demonstrating increased anxiety by the carer for the faller. The psychological impact of falls should not be underestimated and, if the fear of falling has become sufficiently incapacitating, intervention by a behavioural therapist and/or clinical psychologist should be encouraged.

Gait assessment and retraining by a physiotherapist may be helpful and measures aimed at improving general fitness and mobility are to be encouraged. Techniques for getting up following a fall are relatively simple and can be taught to elderly subjects at risk of falls. This serves to allay stress and promote confidence. The patient should be advised not to rush if he/she falls, but to relax and take his/her time. They should practise turning over from lying on their back and then getting on to their hands or knees. The patient can then crawl to a piece of furniture and used the raised surface to pull him/herself up gradually. Carers should also be taught how to assist in raising the faller. To date, physiotherapy advice is empirical rather than based on reliable experimental studies, but in the absence of such information it would appear sensible to adopt a pragmatic approach of support. As with balance disorders, a positive management approach with attention to perhaps minor problems aided by physiotherapy and psychological support can frequently make the difference between loss of confidence and gradual improvement, with gain in confidence.

Consideration of the patient's ***environment*** is important. Floor and floor coverings should have a non-slip surface with no irregularities, and carpets with underlay may reduce the risk of injury, if a fall occurs. Patterns and colours of floor coverings are also important and edges of stairs should be made as clearly visible as possible. Loose rugs and objects erratically scattered throughout a room should be removed. If bending or turning contribute to falls, devices to obviate these movements are of value, for example, raised electric points and a 'helping hand' device to pick things up from the floor without bending. Bright, glare-free lights are important to enhance vision, particularly in potentially dangerous areas such as corridors and staircases. Simple measures, such as a night light are effective for patients who need to regularly get up to go to the toilet at night. Bathrooms are particularly dangerous areas as the floors may be wet and slippery, loose bath mats may be on the floor and toilets may be too low for a patient with any muscular weakness. Similarly, kitchens should be designed to enable subjects to stand at the sink and reach utensils, washing-up liquid, dishcloths, etc., and a stool to prevent the need for constant standing while working in the kitchen may also help. A body-worn alarm if the faller lives alone may provide confidence and sensible consideration of footwear and clothing is necessary.

CONCLUSION

Vestibular and auditory problems, together with falls, are conditions which tend to engender despair in most clinicians.

They are often dismissed as 'trivial'; deemed extremely difficult to diagnose and there is a general misconception that there is little that can be done to ameliorate the symptoms, perhaps with the exception of providing an hearing aid to the hard of hearing. Such an approach is at best unhelpful and at worst ill-informed and dangerous. Active, constructive management of each of these symptoms can improve the quality of life for the patient and have significant economic and social benefits, both for the patient and society.

REFERENCES

Barr, T. (1886). Enquiry into the effects of loud sounds upon the hearing of boilermakers and others who work amid noisy surroundings. *Proceedings of the Glasgow Philosophical Society*, **17**, 223–39.

Brandt, T. and Daroff, R. B. (1980). Physical therapy for benign paroxysmal positional vertigo. *Archives of Otolaryngology*, **106**, 484–5.

Brookes, G. B. (1996). Pharmacological treatment of Meniere's disease. *Clinical Otolaryngology*, **21**, 3–11.

Coles, R. R. A. (1987). Tinnitus and its management. In *Scott-Brown's otolaryngology*, (5th edn), (ed. A. G. Kerr), Vol. 2. *Adult audiology*, (ed. S. D. G. Stephens), (pp. 368–414). Butterworth, London.

Coles, R. R. A., Davis, A., and Smith, P. (1985). Measurement and management of tinnitus. Part 2. *Journal of Laryngology and Otology*, **99**, 1010.

Cooksey, F. S. (1946). *Rehabilitation in vestibular injuries. Proceedings of the Royal Society*, **39**, 273–5.

Courjon, J. H., Jeannerod, M., Ossuzio, I., and Schmidt, R. (1977). The role of vision in compensation of vestibulo-ocular reflex after hemilabyrinthectomy in the cat. *Experimental Brain Research*, **28**, 235–48.

Davis, A. C. (1989). The prevalence of hearing impairment and reported hearing disability among adults in Great Britain. *International Journal of Epidemiology*, **18**, 901–7.

Downton, J. H. (1992). *Falls in the elderly*. Edward Arnold, London.

Drachman, D. A. and Hart, C. (1972). An approach to the dizzy patient. *Neurology*, **22**, 323–34.

Eagger, S., Luxon, L. M., Davies, R. A., Coehlo, A., and Ron, M. A. (1992). Psychiatric morbidity in patients with vestibular disorder: a clinical and neuro-otological study. *Journal of Neurology, Neurosurgery and Psychiatry*, **55**, 383–7.

Epley, J. M. (1992). The canalith repositioning procedure: For treatment of benign paroxysmal positional vertigo. *Otolaryngology Head and Neck Surgery*, **107**, 399–404.

Erlandsson, S. (1990). *Tinnitus: Tolerance or threat?* Göteborg: University of Göteborg.

Erlandsson, S., Ringdahl, A., Hutchins, T., and Carlsson, S. G. (1987). Treatment of tinnitus: a controlled comparison of masking and placebo. *British Journal of Audiology*, **21**, 37–44.

Fitzgerald, G. and Hallpike, C. S. (1942). Studies in human vestibular function: 1. Observations on the directional preponderance (*Nystagmusbereitschaft*) of caloric nystagmus resulting from cerebral lesions. *Brain*, **65**, 115–37.

Goldstein, D. P. and Stephens, S. D. G. (1981). Audiological rehabilitation: management model 1. *Audiology*, **20**, 432–52.

Goodey, R. J. (1987). Drug therapy in tinnitus. In *Tinnitus*, (ed. J. Hazell), Ch. 10. Churchill Livingstone, Edinburgh.

Hallam, R. S. and Jakes, S. C. (1985). Tinnitus: differential effects on a single case. *Behavioural Research and Therapy*, **23**, 691–4.

Harrison, M. S. and Ozsahinoglu, C. (1975). Positional vertigo. *Archives of Otolaryngology*, **101**, 675–8.

Hinchcliffe, R., and King, P. F. (1992). Medicolegal aspects of tinnitus: I. Medicolegal position and current stage of knowledge. *Journal of Audiological Medicine*, **1**, 38–58.

Hoke, M., Feldmann, H., Pantev, C., Lutkenhoner, B., and Lehnertz, K. (1989). Objective evidence of tinnitus in auditory evoked magnetic fields. *Hearing Research (Netherlands)*, **37**, 281–6.

Israel, J. M., Connelly, J. S., McTigue, S. T., Brummett, R. E., and Brown, J. (1982). Lidocaine in the treatment of tinnitus aurium: a double blind study. *Archives of Otolaryngology*, **108**, 471–3.

Ito, M. (1972). Neural design of the cerebellar motor control system. *Brain Research*, **40**, 81–4.

Jakes, S. C., Hallam, R. S., Rachman, S., and Hinchcliffe, R. (1986). The effects of reassurance, relaxation training and distracting on chronic tinnitus sufferers. *Behavioural Research and Therapy*, **24**, 497–506.

Kayan, A. and Hood, J. D. (1984). Neuro-otological manifestations of migraine. *Brain*, **107**, 1123–42.

Kemp, D. T. (1978). Stimulated acoustic emissions from within the human auditory system. *Journal of the Acoustical Society of America*, **64**, 1386–91.

Klockhoff, T. and Lindblom, U. (1967). Ménière's disease and hydrochlorthiazide: a critical analysis of symptoms and therapeutic effects. *Acta Oto-laryngologica*, **63**, 347–65.

Klockhoff, I., Lindblom, U., and Stahle, J. (1974). Diuretic treatment of Ménière's disease; longterm results with chlorthalidone. *Archives of Otolaryngology*, **100**, 262–5.

Lacour, M., Roll, J. P., and Appaiz, M. (1976). Modifications and development of spinal reflexes in the alert baboon (*Papio papio*) following a unilateral vestibular neurotomy. *Brain Research*, **113**, 255–69.

Lacour, M. and Xerri, C. (1980). Compensation of postural reactions to fall in the vestibular neuroectomized monkey. Role of the visual motion cues. *Experimental Brain Research*, **40**, 103–10.

Lim, D. and Stephens, S. D. G. (1985). *Clinical investigation of hearing loss in the elderly*. Paper presented to the British Society of Audiology, Hull, UK.

Luxon, L. M. (1988). Methods of examination: Audiological and vestibular. In *Edward Arnold's diseases of the ear*, (5th edn), (ed. H. Ludman and S. Mawson). Oxford University Press.

Luxon, L. M. (1990). Signs and symptoms of vertebrobasilar insufficiency. In *Vascular brain stem diseases*, (ed. B. Hofferberth). Karger, Basel.

Luxon, L. M. (1993). Tinnitus: its causes, diagnosis and treatment. *British Medical Journal*, **306**, 1490–1.

Luxon, L. M. (1997a). Theoretical basis of physical exercise regimes and manoeuvres. In *Handbook of vestibular rehabilitation*, (ed. L. M. Luxon and R. A. Davies). Whurr, London.

Luxon, L. M. (1997b). Vestibular compensation. In *Handbook of vestibular rehabilitation*, (ed. L. M. Luxon and R. A. Davies). Whurr, London.

Mathias, S., Nayak, U. S. L., and Isaacs, B. (1986). Balance in elderly patients: the 'get up and go' test. *Archives of Physical Medical Rehabilitation*, **67**, 387–9.

Melin, L., Scott, B., Lindberg, P., and Lyttkens, L. (1987). Hearing aids and tinnitus—an experimental study group. *British Journal of Audiology*, **21**, 91–7.

Mihail, R. C., Crowley, J. M., Walden, B. E., Fishburne, J., Reinwall, J. E., and Zajtchuk, J. T. (1988). The tricyclic trimipramine in the treatment of subjective tinnitus. *Annals of Otology, Rhinology and Laryngology*, **97**, 120–3.

Moller, A. R. (1984). Pathophysiology of tinnitus. *Annals of Otology, Rhinology and Laryngology*, **93**, 39–44.

Morris, J. C., Rubin, E. H., Morris, E. J., and Mandel, S. A. (1987). Senile dementia of the Alzheimer's type: an important risk factor for serious falls. *Journal of Gerontology*, **42**, 412–17.

Morrison, A. W. (1975) Endolymphatic hydrops. In *Management of sensorineural deafness*, (ed. A. W. Morrison). Butterworths, London. pp. 145–74.

Morton, D. (1989). Five years of fewer falls. *American Journal of Nursing*, **89**, 204–5.

Norré, M. E. (1987). Rationale of rehabilitation treatment for vertigo. *American Journal of Otolaryngology*, **8**, 31–5.

Parnes, L. S., and McClure, J. A. (1991). *Free floating endolymphatic particles. A new operative finding during posterior canal occlusion.* Presented at the Meeting of the Eastern Section of the American Laryngological, Rhinological and Otological Society, Philadelphia, PA.

Pearson, B. W. and Brackmann, D. E. (1985). Committee on hearing and equilibrium. Guidelines for reporting treatment results in Ménière's disease (editorial). *Otolaryngology, Head and Neck Surgery*, **93**, 579–81.

Penner, M. J. (1989). Empirical tests demonstrating two coexisting sources of tinnitus: a case study. *Journal of Speech and Hearing Research*, **32**, 458–62.

Rinne, R., Bronstein, A., Rudge, P., Gresty, M., and Luxon, L. M. (1994). Bilateral loss of vestibular function. *Proceedings of the Barany Society*, Uppsala, Sweden.

Rosen, S. (1997). Cochlear implants In *Scott-Brown's otolaryngology*, (6th edn), (ed. A. G. Kerr), Vol. 2. *Adult audiology*, (ed. S. D. G. Stephens). Butterworth–Heinemann, Oxford.

Rubinstein, B., Österberg, T., and Rosenhall, U. (1992). Longitudinal fluctuations in tinnitus as reported by an elderly population. *Journal of Audiological Medicine*, **1**, 149–55.

Santos, P. M., Hall, R. A., Snyder, J. M., Hughes, L. F., and Dobie, R. A. (1993). Diuretic and diet effect on Ménière's disease, evaluated by the 1985 Committee on Hearing and Equilibrium Guidelines. *Otolaryngology, Head and Neck Surgery*, **109**, 680–9.

Savundra, P. and Luxon, L. M. (1998). The physiology of equilibrium and its application in the dizzy patient. In *Scott-Brown's otolaryngology*, (6th edn) (ed. A. G. Kerr), Vol. 1. *Basic sciences*, (ed. M. Gleeson). Butterworth-Heinemann, Oxford.

Savundra, P., Carroll, J. D., Davies, R., and Luxon, L. M. (1997). Migraine associated with vertigo. *Cephalalgia*

Schuknecht, H. (1969) Cupulolithiasis. *Archives of Otolaryngology*, **90**, 765–78.

Semont, A., Freyss, G., and Vitte, E. (1988). Curing the BPPV with a Liberatory manoeuvre. *Advances in Otorhinolarngology*, **42**, 290–3.

Shepard, N. T., and Telian, S. A. (1996). *Practical management of the balance disorder patient*. Singular, San Diego & London.

Sullivan, M. D., Dobie, R. A., Sakai, C. S., and Katon, W. J. (1989). Treatment of depressed tinnitus patients with nortriptyline. *Annals of Otology, Rhinology and Laryngology*, **98**, 867–72.

Torak, N. (1977). Old and new in Ménière's disease. *The Laryngoscope*, **87**, 1870–7.

Vernon, J. (1987). Assessment of the tinnitus patient. In *Tinnitus*, (ed. J. W. P. Hazell), Ch. 4. Churchill Livingstone, Edinburgh.

Yagi, T. and Markhamm, C. H. (1984). Neural correlates of compensation after hemilabyrinthectomy. *Experimental Neurology*, **84**, 98–108.

Yardley, L. and Luxon, L. M. (1994). Treating dizziness with vestibular rehabilitation. *British Medical Journal*, **308**, 1252.

Yardley, L., Masson, E., Verschuur, C., Haacke, N., and Luxon, L. M. (1992). Symptoms, anxiety and handicap in dizzy patients: development of the Vertigo Symptom Scale. *Journal of Psychosomatic Research*, **36**, 731–41.

Yardley, L., Owen, N., Nazareth, I., and Luxon, L. (1998). Prevalence and presentation of dizziness in a general practice community sample of working age people. *British Journal of General Practice*, **48**, 1131–5.

Yeoh, L. H. (1997). Causes of hearing disorders. In *Scott-Brown's otolaryngology*, (6th ed.), (ed. A. G. Kerr), Vol. 2. *Adult audiology*, (ed. S. D. G. Stephens). Butterworth-Heinemann, Oxford.

3 | *Chronic pain*

Munseng S. Chong and Michael Tai

Chronic pain is variously defined as pain longer than three or six months in duration. Depending on the definition and the population studied, the exact prevalence of chronic pain is also variable and may be higher than is commonly recognized. In 1990, a survey carried out jointly by *Which* magazine and the College of Health in Britain reported that 11% of the population suffered chronic pain (Rigge 1990). In the United States approximately 1 in 5 individuals experience chronic pain and 3.3% of the population are permanently disabled by pain. At present, anaesthetists run most of the pain clinics in the United Kingdom. Yet some of the most complex chronic pain syndromes arise from dysfunction of neural processing—neuropathic pains. In the United Kingdom, about 1% of the population suffer from neuropathic pain (Bowsher 1991) and again, this may be underestimated. It is important that neurologists have an understanding of and develop an interest in treating and conducting research into pain. This chapter will begin with a description of pain physiology followed by an overview of treatment methods, then a discussion of some neurogenic pain syndromes commonly encountered by neurologists.

PHYSIOLOGY OF PAIN

Fundamental to any discussion about pain is the realization that pain after injury is different from physiological pain. Physiological pain arise from stimulation of Aδ and C fibre innervated nociceptors that have evolved as a protective reflex to prevent tissue damage. Once injury has occurred, changes to nociceptive sensory processing happen both at the periphery and in the spinal cord. Peripheral sensitization results from the release of substance P, neurokinins, CGRP (calcitonin gene related protein) from nociceptor nerve terminals as well as potassium, prostaglandins, hydrogen ions, reactive oxygen molecules, cytokines, and other peptides generated from inflammation at the wound site (Dray 1995). This increases signal transduction of stimuli by peripheral nociceptors. At the spinal cord and also more rostrally, there are changes in the pattern of activation of nociceptive transmission neurones. Signals from large myelinated fibres (e.g. afferent Aβ mechanoreceptors that normally signal touch and vibration) begin to evoke pain. This is central sensitization

and manifests as allodynia (i.e. touching, stroking, and other innocuous stimuli become painful). Both peripheral and central sensitization contribute to hyperalgesia (noxious stimulus becomes more painful) and hyperpathia (delayed and often prolonged pain). Central sensitization arises from afferent nociceptive stimuli reaching dorsal horn neurones. In experimental conditions, these afferent nociceptive stimuli cause 'wind-up' of dorsal horn neurones resulting in summation of signals and prolonged after-discharge (see Pockett 1995). Antagonists of the N-methyl-D-aspartate (NMDA) receptor blocks these changes (see Woolf 1995). Understanding these changes in nociceptive neurophysiology have already altered the management of post-operative acute pain. Pre-emptive analgesia using low dose analgesics and local anaesthetics given before surgical incision is commonly used. This prevents afferent nociceptive signals from causing wind-up of spinal dorsal horn neurones and significantly reduces post-operative pain (for a review see Woolf and Chong 1993).

Reduction of peripheral sensitization occurs with healing of the wound. The mechanism for termination of central sensitization is less clear. Rostral inhibitory control together with reduction of afferent nociceptive signals may cause a 'winding-down' of abnormal dorsal horn neurone activity. The inadequate suppression of central sensitization with healing may be one mechanism for the establishment of chronic pain.

The neurophysiology of nociceptive processing becomes more complicated when there is nerve injury. Abnormalities may arise from the periphery or the spinal cord. After peripheral nerve damage, spontaneous activity can originate from the regenerating nerve terminals, the dorsal root ganglion, and the nervi nervorum. Prolonged peripheral sensitization of nociceptors also occurs, with cycles of antidromic C fibre activation releasing nociceptive amines that further stimulate the terminals leading to more antidromic amine release (Ochoa 1994). Ephatic transmission between axons from demyelinated nerve segments contributes to spontaneous peripheral neural activation. In the spinal cord, nerve damage reduces central inhibition of nociceptive transmission. For example, the inhibitory neurotransmitter gamma-aminobutyric acid (GABA) is reported to be down-regulated in the spinal dorsal horn after peripheral nerve damage. Furthermore, nerve damage alters the whole cytoarchitecture of the spinal cord dorsal horn. Collateral sprouting from adjacent undamaged afferent neurones occupies empty synaptic sites left vacant by the degenerated central axons (Woolf *et al.* 1992). Similar structural changes after nerve injury that leads to chronic pain also occur more rostrally as the extent of central nervous system synaptic plasticity is increasingly recognized (Lee and van Donkelaar 1995). A more specific change occurs where there is damage to the spinothalamic tract causing central pain. This chronic pain syndrome may be explained by the disinhibition of non-nociceptive cold sensation over noxious input (see below). All these, in varying degrees, contribute to chronic pain after peripheral and central nerve damage. In addition, changes in the sympathetic nervous system after nerve damage should not be overlooked. For example, sympathetic nerves have been reported to sprout round large dorsal root ganglion cells after peripheral axotomy (McLachlan *et al.* 1993).

MANAGEMENT OF CHRONIC PAIN

The management of any medical condition begins with an attempt to make a diagnosis, formulating a treatment plan, followed by rehabilitation of any disabilities. In a broader perspective, prevention of the establishment of the condition would also be important. Chronic pain management is no different.

There is evidence from post-operative and phantom limb pain studies that inadequate pain control before surgery increases the incidence of chronic pain after the procedure (Bach *et al.* 1988; Jahangiri *et al.* 1994; Richardson *et al.* 1994). Clinically, there is anecdotal evidence to suggest greater efficacy of pain relief in central post-stroke pain and post-herpetic neuralgia when tricyclic antidepressants are initiated early. These effects of early treatment are predictable from greater understanding of pain neurophysiology. Therefore, one way of preventing chronic pain is to have adequate pain control in the early phase, preventing progression into a chronic problem.

Attempting to make a diagnosis is also important. There are many chronic pain syndromes that serve as useful labels but do not address the pathophysiology of the condition. Even when the aetiology is known, the pathogenesis of chronic pain may be quite different. In post-herpetic neuralgia for example, there may be varying degrees of damage to large myelinated or small myelinated and non-myelinated fibres. This may give rise to predominant mechanical, cold or very rarely, heat hyperalgesia with or without temporal summation to give varying degrees of continuous and evoked pain. A recent study, for example, has reported a correlation between the presence of severe allodynia and small diameter axonal damage (Morris *et al.* 1995). Yet, at present they are all grouped together as post-herpetic neuralgia. The response to treatment and meaningful results from future therapeutic trials will depend on the ability to reclassify neuropathic conditions according to their pathophysiology. More sophisticated assessments using dedicated sensory testing laboratories may be one way of bringing some scientific rationale to the treatment of neurogenic pain.

Continuously reviewing the diagnosis is also important. Any underlying treatable causes for the pain have to be excluded. Repeated guanethidine blocks, for example, will not permanently alleviate the pain from 'reflex sympathetic dystrophy' when there is non-union of a fracture. Patients seen in pain clinics may have already been seen and investigated by other medical specialities. This should not be a discouragement to repeat the whole clinical diagnostic process nor for a re-examination of the investigations already carried out.

For many chronic pain syndromes there is often no specific treatment. Symptomatic relief together with rehabilitation aiming to return back to normal function is all that can be offered. In selected patients, a multidisciplinary approach with the involvement of psychologists, physiotherapists, occupational therapists, and specialized nurse practitioners can produce good results. It is important that this team management strategy has defined and agreed goals. If properly implemented, the results can be suprisingly good. For example, the Centre for Pain Relief in Liverpool, UK, has been running four-week rehabilitation programmes since 1982. Half their patients managed to reduce drug intake and 29% were able to rejoin the job market (Wells and Miles 1991). Similar results have been reported from multidisciplinary pain management centres in the United States and, importantly, the functional improvement and reduction in analgesic intake in these patients were sustained (Deardoff *et al.* 1991; Maruta *et al.* 1990). In a meta-analysis of 65 studies with over 3000 patients, Flor *et al.* (1992) found that combination multidisciplinary pain rehabilitation programmes helped twice the number of chronic pain patients to get back to work compared to those which did not undergo any treatment, or had only unimodal therapy. Therefore, there is a strong argument for expanding multidisciplinary pain management services from an economical and humanitarian point of view.

MEDICAL TREATMENTS

Drug treatment of pain consists of the use of primary analgesics such as non-steroidal anti-inflammatory drugs (NSAIDs), opioids, and secondary analgesics like antidepressants, anticonvulsants, and membrane-stabilizing drugs. Primary analgesics are developed specifically for treating nociceptive pain and their efficacy has been carefully evaluated. Secondary analgesics, however, are used for treating neuropathic pain even though most of these drugs have not been rigorously tested. Their analgesic effects are often based on data collected from clinical series and case reports—unsatisfactory methods for evaluating any treatment. This adds to the difficulty of managing neuropathic pain clinically.

PRIMARY ANALGESICS

By the time patients are seen in the pain clinic, most would have tried NSAIDs, sold over-the-counter for pain relief.

Their response to treatment may be inconsistent. However, it may still be worthwhile prescribing NSAIDs when there is an inflammatory component to chronic pain. Slow release diclofenac, for example, is relatively potent, has a good side-effect profile, and has a long duration of action. NSAIDs may accelerate the underlying disease process in some conditions (e.g. degenerative arthritis). In these cases, the risk of earlier joint replacement is balanced against the need for pain relief. The mechanism of the analgesic effect of NSAIDs is unclear and does not correlate with potency of prostaglandin inhibition. Some non-steroidal drugs may act centrally and have been shown to affect nociceptive transmission in the spinal cord (Malmberg and Yaksh 1992).

Opioids are commonly prescribed for relieving acute pain and for terminal care. For chronic pain, especially neurogenic pain, this is more controversial (Fields 1988; Dubner 1991). It was claimed that opiates are inherently ineffective in treating neuropathic pain (Arner and Meyerson 1983). However, other physicians including Weir Mitchell have reported the beneficial effects of intravenous morphine in these patients. Pain arising from malignant and non-malignant peripheral nerve damage as well as central post-stroke pain syndromes may benefit from intravenous opioids (Portenoy *et al.* 1990; McQuay *et al.* 1992). Unfortunately, the side-effects, risk of addiction, and the legal system in some countries have restricted the use of opioids in chronic pain. This reduces our therapeutic options. At present, many pain physicians in the United Kingdom severely restrict the routine use of morphine and diamorphine for chronic non-malignant pain. Codeine or dihydrocodeine is used instead. The newly licensed drug, tramadol, may be an alternative. It is reported to be as potent as pethidine but has little tendency to cause respiratory depression, develop tolerance, or risk of abuse. Tramadol acts mainly on the μ-opiate receptor and have indirect α_2-adrenergic effect by reducing noradrenaline uptake (Eggers and Power 1995). Further experience and greater use will decide whether this drug is genuinely different. Pure peripherally acting opioids are also being developed. They have the potential of not causing any systemic side-effects or dependency.

NEUROLEPTICS

The effectiveness neuroleptics in treating chronic pain is not proven. Methotrimeprazine was reported to be as effective as morphine but only when administered parenterally (Lasagna *et al.* 1961). Chlorprothixene was reported to be effective for post-herpetic neuralgia pain (Nathan 1978*a*). It is not available on general prescription but is selectively used in some pain clinics. This probably increases its placebo effect. Haloperidol is sometimes prescribed for pain relief but was never adequately assessed (Portenoy 1990). On the whole, neuroleptic drugs possess little analgesic properties of their own. Their addition to analgesic regimes makes use of their antiemetic and antipsychotic effects

ANTIDEPRESSANTS

The main group of antidepressants used for treating chronic pain are the 'tricyclics'. Amitriptyline is the most commonly prescribed. It preferentially blocks the re-uptake of 5-hydroxytryptamine (5-HT) but also affects noradrenaline. Interestingly, the selective 5-HT re-uptake blocker fluoxetine possesses no secondary analgesic properties (Max *et al.* 1992). Paroxetine, however, has been reported to have superior analgesic properties to placebo for the treatment of painful diabetic neuropathy (Sindrup *et al.* 1992).

Amitriptyline is reported to be effective for treating painful diabetic neuropathy, post-herpetic neuralgia, myofascial pain, central post-stroke pain, psychogenic pain, and as a migraine prophylaxis. The analgesic effect is separate from any action as an antidepressant. The onset of pain relief is more rapid and the dose used is generally lower than when amitriptyline is prescribed as an antidepressant. Analgesic effect of amitriptyline has been reported in patients who are not depressed (Max *et al.* 1987), and useful pain relief may be obtained with no effect on depression. In a meta-analysis of 39 placebo controlled trials, Onghena and Van Houdenhove (1992) concluded that the average patient with chronic pain who receives a tricyclic antidepressant had less pain than 74% of those treated with placebo. Another more specific meta-analysis by McQuay *et al.* (1996) has reported antidepressant drugs, in general, and the tricyclics, in particular, to be more effective than placebo in treating neuropathic pain. The lowest possible dose (10 mg daily) of amitriptyline should be prescribed and the dose slowly increased over weeks to a maximum of 150 mg daily. This allows time for patients to adjust to its side-effects. There is also some evidence to suggest that amitriptyline has a therapeutic window (Watson *et al.* 1982) but others have reported a dose-dependent analgesic effect (McQuay *et al.* 1993). At doses in excess of 150 mg daily, drug level monitoring is necessary. The inability to tolerate side-effects rather than the lack of therapeutic response appears to be the commonest cause for discontinuing amitriptyline. If sedation is troublesome, imipramine is an alternative to amitriptyline. There is less published data on the use of imipramine in chronic pain. A few studies have reported good pain relief in diabetic neuropathy (Kvinsdahl *et al.* 1984) and arthritis (Gingras 1976). Other alternatives are nortriptyline, maprotiline, and dothiepin.

There are a few studies that have shown beneficial effects of monoamine oxidase inhibitors in psychogenic and atypical facial pain (Anthony and Lance 1969). However, their side-effects, especially reactions to certain foods, precludes their routine use.

ANTICONVULSANTS, ANTIARRYTHMICS, AND LOCAL ANAESTHETICS

Lancinating-evoked pains and dysaesthesiae are often treated with anticonvulsant drugs. However, there is a serious shortage of properly controlled trials to assess this (McQuay *et al.*

1995). Trigeminal neuralgia is the only painful condition in which anticonvulsants are effective, as judged by controlled trials (Rockliff and Davis 1968). Phenytoin was first used for this condition but is now the second line drug after carbamezepine. There are also small-scale studies and case reports of the efficacy of carbamezepine in treating post-herpetic neuralgia (Hatangdi *et al.* 1976), painful peripheral neuropathy including Fabry's disease (Filling-Katz *et al.* 1989), as well as multiple sclerosis (Espir and Millac 1970). It probably acts as a membrane stabilizer reducing neuronal excitability. Carbamezepine may cause a rash from drug reaction and its active metabolite oxcarbamezepine can be used instead. Sodium valproate is another useful alternative to carbamezepine. There are no full publications of placebo controlled trials of the newer anticonvulsants, such as gabapentin and lamotrigine, for treating pain but there are case reports of gabapentin use in treating reflex sympathetic dystrophy (Mellick and Mellick 1995; Rosner *et al.* 1996), post-herpetic neuralgia (Rosner *et al.* 1996; Segal and Rordorf 1996), and lamotrigine for trigeminal neuralgia (Canavero *et al.* 1995). In animal models, both these drugs possess intrinsic analgesic properties.

Antiarrhythmic drugs are prescribed for treating post-herpetic neuralgia and painful peripheral neuropathies. Tocainide, the orally active equivalent of lignocaine was useful for many painful peripheral neuropathies. Unfortunately, it has a tendency to cause bone marrow suppression and its use in treating chronic pain is severely restricted. Of the other drugs in this group, mexiletene has been reported to reduce pain, dysaesthesia, and paraesthesia of diabetic neuropathy (Dejgard *et al.* 1988; Stracke *et al.* 1992). Flecainide is another antiarrhythmic with secondary analgesic properties, mainly for treating pain from malignant nerve damage. The main difficulty with this group of drugs is their pro-arrhythmic tendency and hypotensive side-effect, making sudden cardiac death a rare but recognized complication (*ABPI datasheet compendium 1995–1996*). Consequently, flecainide is used for mainly for terminal care and treatment with high dose mexiletene may need to be initiated in hospital.

Topical anaesthetic creams such as EMLA (eutectic mixture of local anaesthetics) were used for treating post-herpetic neuralgia (Stow *et al.* 1989). The constituents of EMLA are usually 2.5% lignocaine and 2.5% prilocaine. Prilocaine, however, has a theoretical risk of inducing methaemoglobinaemia especially when absorption is increased when applied to large areas of damaged skin. The recently introduced 4% amethocaine gel is an alternative. A 5% lignocaine cream and gel patches were reported to cause prolonged alleviation of pain from post-herpetic neuralgia (Rowbotham *et al.* 1994). The effect of topical lignocaine may not be confined to the skin. When a 5% lignocaine cream is applied to skin, significant blood levels can be detected. In one experimental model of neuropathic pain, spontaneous discharges from dorsal root ganglion were reported to be silenced by similarly low levels of lignocaine (Devor *et al.* 1992). Intravenous low dose

lignocaine infusions to treat chronic pain is a logical translation of this into clinical practice. When this relieves pain, the patient is changed over to treatment with oral mexiletene. Unfortunately, the dose of lignocaine needed to the test for pain relief is uncertain: 100 mg of lignocaine infused intravenously over 1 hour is the usual method, but Boas *et al.* (1982) used 3 mg/kg bolus followed by a continuous 4 mg/min intravenous infusion. This high dose lignocaine test was also reported to be more effective in certain neuropathic pain conditions (Ferrante *et al.* 1996). Further studies in humans are necessary to determine not only the dose needed to do an adequate lignocaine challenge but also whether this is really predictive of whether mexiletene is likely to be effective in relieving pain.

MUSCLE RELAXANTS

Baclofen and dantrolene are routinely used by many neurologists to reduce muscle spasms. Where increased muscle tone is a cause of pain, they may relieve some of the discomfort. Baclofen is also effective for treating trigeminal neuralgia and post-herpetic neuralgia.

DRUGS ACTING ON THE NMDA RECEPTORS

NMDA (*N*-methyl-D-aspartate) receptor antagonists prevent increased excitability of dorsal horn neurones in experimental conditions. In human subjects, this group of drugs possesses secondary analgesic properties. They have the theoretical advantage of not affecting nociceptive pain but are able to suppress pathological pain. Ketamine binds to the phencyclidine site causing a non-competitive block of the NMDA receptor and was reported to be effective in treating post-herpetic neuralgia (Eide *et al.* 1994). Dextromethorphan is an antitussive but also an NMDA ionic channel blocker. In one study, it reduced intractable neurogenic cancer pain (Price *et al.* 1994). CPP [3-(2-carboxypiperazin-4-yl) propyl-1-phosphonic acid] another NMDA antagonist reduced mechanical hyperalgesia when administered intrathecally in a patient with neuropathic pain (Kristensen *et al.* 1992).

The NMDA receptor is important in the pathogenesis of chronic pain. Vast resources committed to finding therapeutically useful antagonists may not be successful because this receptor is widespread in the central nervous system, especially in the limbic system. Consequently, there are significant psychomimetic and motor side-effects of any drug which act on this site. In addition, unless there are irreversible antagonists acting on the NMDA receptor, continuous afferent nociceptive input will still cause wind-up of central neurones. The search for clinically useful NMDA antagonists should go on, but by itself is unlikely to fulfil the needs for treatment of all chronic pain syndromes.

OTHER DRUGS

A few studies have reported effective analgesia with intravenous naloxone infusions for central post-stroke pain. This was not replicated in a double-blind placebo controlled trial (Bainton *et al.* 1992). Post-stroke pain may resolve spontaneously anyway and this may explain the efficacy of naloxone in previous open trials. Propranolol was reported to reduce painful peripheral neuropathy and reflex sympathetic dystrophy but has not been found to be clinically effective.

Capsaicin is the active ingredient of hot chilli peppers. It depolarizes unmyelinated C fibres by opening a selective membrane ionic channel. This leads to the release of active amines at the periphery as well as central activation leading to burning pain. Prolonged application of capsaicin depletes these amines leading to functional desensitization of these nociceptors. Topical capsaicin cream was used in many conditions including post-mastectomy pain (Watson *et al.* 1989), post-herpetic neuralgia (Watson *et al.* 1988*a*), stump pain (Rayner *et al.* 1989), reflex sympathetic dystrophy (Sinoff and Hart 1993), and trigeminal neuralgia (Fusco *et al.* 1991). The beneficial effect was delayed for weeks after applying the cream. Most patients are unable to tolerate the initial burning from application of capsaicin and there is a high drop-out rate in trials. Where patients can overcome the initial irritation from capsaicin, the analgesic effect may last up to two years. Newer analogues of capsaicin that cause less initial irritation but still able to desensitize nociceptors are now being developed. The use of intranasal capsaicin in cluster headache (Sicuteri *et al.* 1989; Fusco *et al.* 1991) and topical application for itching from haemodialysis (Breneman *et al.* 1992), psoriasis (Kurkccugluo and Alaybeyi 1990), and even notalgia paraesthetica (Leibsohn 1992) is also reported.

REGIONAL DRUG INFILTRATIONS

The three drugs commonly infiltrated locally for treating pain are local anaesthetics, steroids, and sympathetic blocking agents. In rheumatology, a combination of local anaesthetics and steroids are commonly injected into joints, tendon sheaths, or bursae to treat musculoskeletal pains. For neuropathic pains, the injection of local anaesthetics is useful for short-term relief and sometimes to confirm the diagnosis. In many nerve entrapment syndromes (e.g. carpal tunnel syndromes, meralgia paraesthetica) the pain is from nervi nervorum and may be abolished by local blocks. The characteristic of pain often helps to point towards the diagnosis. The injection of steroids around nerves is more controversial. They may reduce soft tissue and peri-neural swelling. However, corticosteroids may retard nerve regeneration and the preservatives in some preparations (e.g. ethylene glycol in depomedrone) may theoretically cause damage. Other complications include both sterile and infective abscess formation and when injected near the spine, meningitis. It is also unclear what therapeutic function the steroids are expected to fulfil when injected near nerves. Epidural steroid injections, especially, are commonly performed for low back pain but as pointed out by Koes *et al.* (1995) in their meta-analysis of 12 randomized trials, there is

little evidence to support this practice. A recent Australian Government working party on this subject came to similar conclusions (Bogduk *et al.* 1993). Once again, further studies are suggested to test its efficacy but any properly designed trial to do so will need to delineate strictly where the pain is arising from. To administer epidural steroids for back pain without careful clinical evaluation to separate patients with predominant muscular, facet joint, radicular, or even psychogenic pain will not answer the question.

Sympathetic blocks either by injection into the sympathetic ganglia or regional guanethedine infusion are also extensively used for treating 'reflex sympathetic dystrophy' (RSD) and 'sympathetic maintained pain' (SMP). Whether these treatments work is unclear and controversial (see below). Where cold hyperalgesia predominates together with sympathetic over-reactivity (even from receptor hypersensitivity) it seems logical that warming the limb will reduce pain. Unfortunately, no such correlation has been found (see below) and sympathetic blocks have a theoretical risk of exacerbating the sympathetic receptor hypersensitivity. Therefore, when sympathetic blocks are performed, careful clinical evaluation after each procedure would seem sensible before embarking on further blocks indiscriminately.

STIMULATION ANALGESICS

TRANSCUTANEOUS ELECTRICAL NERVE STIMULATION (TENS)

The use of the electric torpedo fishes to treat headaches and arthritic pain was described in classical Greek literature. The present rationale for using electrical stimulation to treat pain originated from Melzack and Wall's gate theory of pain. Activation of large diameter nerve fibres by innocuous stimulation may inhibit the transmission of noxious signals. Although details of this theory were questioned (Nathan 1978*b*), the efficacy of low threshold nerve stimulation is reported in many studies of acute (Solomon *et al.* 1980; Nesheim 1981) and chronic pain (Wall and Sweet 1967; Bates and Nathan 1980). The mechanism of action of TENS is not clear. Pain relief using TENS cannot be reversed by naloxone. There is a suggestion that low threshold electrical nerve stimulation releases adenosine and this may be antagonized by methyxanthines. In a small study of experimental pain in normal volunteers, the analgesic effects of TENS were reduced after ingestion of a small amount of caffeine (Marchand *et al.* 1995).

TENS is effective for post-herpetic neuralgia (Nathan and Wall 1974), brachial plexus avulsion injuries (Wynn Parry 1980), as well as chronic back pain (Cauthen and Renner 1975) and arthritis (Taylor *et al.* 1981). It is less effective for central pain syndromes and is no better than placebo in 'psychogenic' pain. Low threshold TENS works on a segmental level, and for best effect the electrodes should be placed as close as possible to the site of pain. Consequently,

TENS is seldom effective for axial or diffuse pains and also where there is extensive loss of large myelinated fibres. Rarely, TENS may exacerbate existing pain and this may not be predictable from the amount of ongoing allodynia.

The low incidence of side-effects, ease of use, and the availability of so many small portable stimulators has resulted in TENS being tried for all forms of peripheral pain. What constitutes an adequate trial of TENS is, however, more difficult. Some pain physicians would recommend an inpatient trial for initiation of therapy. A long outpatient session with paramedical staff familiar with its use, for example, a clinical nurse specialist and a physiotherapist, together with a two- to four-week home trial and follow-up review may be enough. The main problem with use of TENS is the progressive decrement in effectiveness even when initial pain control is good. In the seven-year follow-up study reported by Bates and Nathan (1980), only 25% of patients who initially benefited from TENS continue to find it useful. In most studies, there is a rapid fall off in effectiveness followed by a slow gradual decline. Intermittent rather than continuous use may slow this decline in efficacy.

ACUPUNCTURE

This ancient treatment has been extensively studied but the scientific basis for analgesia is not clear. Even attempts to conduct trials are difficult as it is impossible to decide what constitutes 'sham' acupuncture. Very simplistically, the effect of acupuncture may be a form of tender point injection and also a counter-irritation analgesic. Melzack and co-workers in 1977 found a 70% correlation in points chosen by classical acupuncturists and that chosen by Travell, Simons, and Sola, practitioners of Western-style 'dry-needling'. Dry-needling originated from the practice of injecting local anaesthetics into tender trigger points for pain relief. Later, pain relief was seen whether saline, local anaesthetics, or indeed, when nothing was injected at all. Dry-needling was thought to work by destroying tender trigger areas and deliberately inducing fibrosis. Biopsies of these areas did not show any abnormal nerve collection to 'destroy' and it is still unclear how this works. A little more is known about the mechanism of action of counter-stimulation analgesia. In the same way, large fibre activation may modulate nociceptive transmission, simultaneous nociceptive signal at a different site is even more effective in reducing the first nociceptive input. Known as diffuse noxious inhibitory control (DNIC) this works at a suprasegmental level and depends on descending inhibitory control for modulating nociceptive transmission. Acupuncture has a low incidence of side-effects. Damage to viscera is rare and transmission of infection is reduced by using disposable needles. There are also many more medically qualified acupuncturists who, in theory, are less likely to cause tissue damage. The analgesic effects of acupuncture may be short-lived and repeated courses of weekly treatments lasting five to six weeks may be necessary.

NEUROSURGERY

DESTRUCTIVE NEUROSURGERY

The idea that destruction of nociceptive pathways will permanently alleviate chronic pain is outmoded and untrue. Nociceptive transmission is diffuse and the lateral spinothalamic tract is only one of many transmission pathways. Numerous techniques were developed in the 1960s for lateral spinothalamic tract destruction to treat chronic pain. Complications of such surgery include respiratory failure, limb paralysis, bladder and bowel dysfunction. More importantly, these procedures do not work and may induce anaesthesia dolorosa, which is often worse than the original pain. The lesions were often extensive, beyond the intended target. In one postmortem study, the corticospinal tract was clearly damaged in some patients (Nathan 1994). Cordotomies are now rarely used for non-malignant chronic pain. Even in cancer pain, whether such procedures should be carried out is controversial. Short-term pain relief from cordotomy in terminal care was preferable to using large doses of systemic opiates but indwelling intraspinal cathethers can now deliver smaller doses more effectively. More recently, dorsal root entry zone (DREZ) lesions were developed for pain relief. Thomas and Kitchen (1994), for example, reported good pain relief from DREZ lesions in 77% of their series of 44 patients with brachial plexus avulsion pain. However, nearly a quarter of their patients developed neurological deficit in the ipsilateral lower limb. For other painful conditions, the initial enthusiasm for this procedure has waned with time. For example, the initial reported efficacy of 75% pain relief for post-herpetic neuralgia is reduced to only 25% as more DREZ operations are performed (Friedman and Bullit 1988). The American Association of Neurological Surgeons has come to the conclusion that DREZ procedures have limited efficacy and high morbidity, making this unsuitable for treating post-herpetic neuralgia (quoted by Pappagallo and Campbell 1994).

Other destructive techniques tried for pain relief were lesions to spinal nerves, dorsal root, myelotomies, thalamotomies, destruction of many other subcortical structures including the pituitary gland, as well as lobotomies. None of these abolish chronic pain and all have serious side-effects. On the whole, destructive neurosurgery has a very limited role for the relieve of chronic pain.

SPINAL CORD STIMULATION (SCS)

SCS, like TENS was derived from the gate theory of pain. Dorsal column stimulation was first used but subsequent studies failed to show any difference when either the dorsal or ventral spinal cord was stimulated. The present use of extradural stimulation reduces the risk of infection and trauma of electrode placement. The three groups of patients that appear to gain most benefit from SCS are those with post-amputation pain (Neilson *et al.* 1975; Miles and Lipton 1987), ischaemic pain including angina (Tallis *et al.* 1983; Broseta *et al.* 1986; Mannheimer *et al.* 1993), and failed back surgery (Mittal *et al.* 1987; Kumar *et al.* 1991). Electrode placement is all important. To get the best result, the paraesthesia of stimulation should overlap with the site of pain. Trial placements using percutaneous electrodes under local anaesthetic increase the success rate but are not infallible. There are cases where initial trial stimulation has helped but subsequent permanent implantation failed to relief pain. Side-effects of this method are relatively few. In the series reported by Simpson *et al.* (1991), infection rate was 5% and the electrodes and stimulator had to be removed. Electrodes sometimes work loose and revisions are necessary to replace the power source. In the same series, 4 out of 60 patients reported exacerbation of pain from stimulation. The risk of this may possibly be reduced by initial careful assessment before implantation.

Approximately 40–60% of patients with implanted spinal cord stimulators obtain pain relieve (Neilson *et al.* 1975; Mittal *et al.* 1987; Kumar *et al.* 1991; Simpson 1991). This drops to as low as 8% after 3 years (Long *et al.* 1978). Persistence of benefit with over 30% deriving pain relief after 3 years was also reported when case selection was more rigorously applied (Long *et al.* 1981). Once again, intermittent rather than continuous use may also reduce the decline of pain relief with time (Simpson 1991). Improved electrode designs together with careful patient selection and work-up may increase the future long-term effectiveness of SCS.

PAINFUL CONDITIONS PRESENTING TO THE NEUROLOGIST

CENTRAL PAIN

In 1906, Dejerine and his students described patients with the 'thalamic syndrome'. All these patients suffer chronic pain after damage to their thalamus from either a stroke or haemorrhage. However, chronic pain from central nervous system damage may arise not only from thalamic damage but also anywhere along the neospinothalamic pathways and its projections up to the cerebral cortex (Andersen *et al.* 1995). Common sites of damage that give rise to chronic pain are the spinal cord, medulla, and thalamus. Referring to this group of patients as post-stroke pain is also strictly incorrect. Abscesses and tumours of the thalamus may also cause chronic pain similar to that in the thalamic syndrome. Moreover, the characteristics of post-stroke pain and pain from syringomyelia, syringobulbia, and even subarachnoid haemorrhage are remarkably similar (Boivie 1994). Central pain encompasses all these and is defined by the IASP as pain caused by a lesion or dysfunction anywhere in the central nervous system.

Neurophysiological recordings have reported burst activity in the thalamus of cats following transection of the spinothalamic tract. These have the characteristics of slow calcium channel activation probably linked to the NMDA receptor

(Koyama *et al.* 1993). There may also be a strong element of 'memory' in central pain syndromes. Thalamic stimulation can evoke pain from deafferented parts of the body as well as autonomic activation with palpitations, sweating, and feelings of panic (Lenz *et al.* 1995). Recently, the rediscovery of the Thunberg thermal grill has increased our understanding of the mechanism of central pain. In a series of experiments performed using this grill consisting of alternating hot and cold wires, the presence of non-nociceptive cold input carried by $A\delta$ fibres exerting an inhibitory effect on cold sensitive C nociceptors was demonstrated (Craig and Bushnell 1994). This explains the characteristics of central pain (see below) which is further supported by functional imaging (Craig *et al.* 1996). More importantly, this also suggests that the preservation of non-nociceptive cold sensation may be important for reducing other forms of cold burning pain, for example, complex regional pain syndromes (reflex sympathetic dystrophies).

Central pain is described as a superficial burning, lancinating pain and may arise months or even as long as two to three years after the initial injury (Boivie and Leijon 1991; see Bowsher 1996, for a more recent review). The pain is often associated with reduced sensation to temperature and pin-prick (Boivie *et al.* 1989) although, rarely, kinaesthetic sense and vibration are also affected. In about half, there is also allodynia and the cutaneous area involved may be more extensive than the area of chronic pain or motor deficit. Dystrophic changes may appear with time and sympathetic blocks are reported to be effective in relieving central pain (Loh *et al.* 1981). Unfortunately, this is not the general experience of other pain physicians (Boivie 1994; Bowsher 1995). Management once again relies on recognition of the problem followed by careful neurological examination to exclude any underlying painful conditions. Many stroke patients have communication difficulties and there is a tendency for all types of pain to be under-reported. A frozen shoulder, for example, is common after strokes and this may cause severe pain. There are few investigations to help with diagnosis. Patients with post-stroke pain are reported to have abnormal sensory evoked potentials using laser heat stimulators (Casey *et al.* 1990). This information can be obtained by questioning patients about temperature sensibility (e.g. the temperature of water while washing themselves) and the use of a cold tuning fork to check cutaneous cold sensation. Tricyclic antidepressants are the most effective drugs for central post-stroke pain (Leijon and Boivie 1989; Bowsher 1995). Early initiating treatment with amitriptyline is advisable as any delays may reduce the drug's efficacy. Anticonvulsants are disappointing and not been shown to be effective for continuous central pain (Leijon and Boivie 1989). The antiarrhythmic drug, mexiletene, is also reported to be effective (Awerbuch 1990), especially in conjunction with a tricyclic drug (Bowsher 1995). Intravenous opioids (Portenoy *et al.* 1990) or lignocaine may also alleviate post-stroke pain (Edwards *et al.* 1985). Spinal cord stimulation is only partially effective. In the series published by Simpson (1990), 3 each out of 10 patients with central pain gained significant or moderate benefit from spinal cord stimulation, whereas pain in the others was either unchanged or made worse. A less invasive method of stimulation is the use of TENS which is worth trying if there has not been extensive damage to the dorsal column/medial lemniscus pathways. Cortical stimulation was reported to be successful in some centres (Tsubokawa *et al.* 1993). At present, this remains an experimental form of treatment. Physiotherapy and occupational therapy are equally important in treating these patients. Disuse may set up a vicious cycle of pain leading to further disability and more pain. A careful rehabilitation programme with realistic goals is necessary for each patient.

POST-HERPETIC NEURALGIA (PHN)

The definition of post-herpetic neuralgia is persistence of pain one month after the onset of cutaneous eruption. This is not helpful for assessing different treatments as spontaneous resolution of pain after the first month is still quite common. Continuing pain three months after the appearance of the rash may be a more practical definition. In the study by Watson *et al.* (1988*b*), the incidence of PHN was 3% at 3 months and with a median follow-up of 3 years, over half had persistence of pain. The main risk factor for developing PHN is age. In a prospective study of patients over the age of 60, 13% had persistence of pain 6 months after herpes zoster (McKendrick *et al.* 1989).

The main pathological findings during acute infections are inflammatory infiltration with demyelination and secondary axonal loss. Fibrosis and cell loss in the dorsal root or Gasserian ganglion then appears (Watson *et al.* 1991). The damage is also seen in the ascending white matter tracts. There is no structural difference in the dorsal root ganglia, peripheral nerve, or dorsal root between those who develop PHN and those that do not. However, dorsal horn atrophy is only reported in those with pain (Watson *et al.* 1991). Chronic inflammation in the dorsal horn was found in one case of PHN and may be the underlying pathophysiology in a small number of patients where the pain actually gets worse with time after the initial eruption.

There are different types of pain in post-herpetic neuralgia. The area of persistent deep aching together with lancinating evoked pain over the site of the original rash is surrounded by an area of marked allodynia with coexisting cold and, very rarely, warm hyperalgesia (Watson *et al.* 1988*b*). Where PHN improves, there is usually initial shrinkage of the area of allodynia but the persistent pain may continue. The mechanism of pain is unknown. Inflammation and primary sensitization undoubtedly occur in the periphery during the initial acute phase reaction. This may be the cause of persistent vasodilatation that has been reported (Rowbotham and Fields, 1989). The peripheral release of vasoactive amines from C fibre terminals has been suggested as the cause for this (Bennet 1994). However, this cannot be the only explanation. The large area of surrounding allodynia extends beyond the normal cutaneous innervation of the affected nerve and implies central changes as well. The therapeutic implication of this is to encourage a dual central and peripheral approach for the treatment of PHN (Bennet 1994).

During acute attacks, a combination of non-steroidal analgesics and antiviricidal drugs are often used. Whether this reduces the incidence of post-herpetic neuralgia is unclear. Two studies have reported the effectiveness of topical aspirin in reducing pain from acute zoster and post-herpetic neuralgia (Debenedittis *et al.* 1992; King 1993). In some studies involving small number of patients, acyclovir reduces the incidence of PHN. In a large three-centre British study, no difference was initially found (McKendrick *et al.* 1989) but a later reanalysis from one centre reported a reduction in the incidence of post-herpetic neuralgia in patients with opthalmic zoster treated with acyclovir (McGill and White 1994). The results and conclusion from this study remain controversial (see the correspondence between these authors: *British Medical Journal* 1995, **310**, 1005). Combining the results of the smaller trials gives a statistical difference favouring acyclovir in the reduction of PHN risk (Crooks *et al.* 1991). The American famciclovir trial reported a more convincing result (Tyrings *et al.* 1995). This placebo controlled double-blind study recruited 400 patients who were treated within 72 hours of developing a herpes zoster rash. Famciclovir 500 mg or 750 mg 3 times a day for 1 week was compared to placebo. Pain one month after appearance of rash (one of the definitions for post-herpetic neuralgia) was the same in all three groups. The median time to disappearance of pain was 61 and 63 days for those treated with famciclovir but 119 days for those on placebo. Thus, famciclovir may not have reduced the incidence of PHN (if defined as persistent pain one month after appearance of the rash) but it significantly reduces the duration of pain.

Once post-herpetic neuralgia has developed, the most effective treatment is by using a 'tricyclic' antidepressant. Amitriptyline was superior to placebo in at least four trials (see Max 1994). It reduces the frequency of lancinating pain and lessens the allodynia. There is also an argument for the use of this group of medications prophylactically in PHN. Post-herpetic neuralgia is predictable, occurring after the cutaneous eruption and in the elderly who are most at risk, pre-emptive treatment may be justified. A large trial is needed to test the validity of this.

The peripheral component of the pain in post-herpetic neuralgia may respond to topical local anaesthetics or membrane stabilizing drugs. In one study, subcutaneous lignocaine injections halved the severity of pain in 75% of patients with PHN (Rowbotham *et al.* 1991). For oral treatment, mexiletene is an alternative and can be combined with amitriptyline.

Where amitriptyline (or one of its alternatives) in combination with mexiletene has not worked, a trial of opioids is worthwhile. In one study where lignocaine or morphine was infused sequentially, 11/19 favoured the opiate for pain relief as opposed to 4/19 for lignocaine (Rowbotham 1994). Obviously, this is a small uncontrolled study but demonstrates the effectiveness of opioids for treating PHN. Where a trial of short-acting opioids like fentanyl proves effective, conversion into sustained release fentanyl or morphine may provide longer pain relief.

Topical capsaicin is also effective for treating post-herpetic neuralgia (see above) but may need to be applied together with EMLA (eutectic mixture of local anaesthetics) cream. Inadvertent spread to mucosal surfaces (e.g. eyes) in opthalmic zoster is another drawback. The practical difficulties and the length of time needed before an effect is apparent rules out the use of capsaicin as a first line treatment for PHN. There are also studies reporting large-scale damage to C fibres in some patients with post-herpetic neuralgia (Morris *et al.* 1995). As capsaicin works exclusively on this group of neurones, it can be predicted to be ineffective in some patients.

TENS (transcutaneous nerve stimulation) is useful in some patients but may also exacerbate pain where there is severe allodynia. It does not work when there is extensive large fibre neuronal damage and insensibility to light touch is present. Destructive surgery has little to offer (see above). Spinal cord stimulation has not generally found to be effective. This may be due to damage to dorsal columns with herpes zoster. Therefore, there is a significant group of patients with severe pain from post-herpetic neuralgia who are not amenable to any treatment presently available. Psychological support together with practical help from paramedical services may be all that can be offered. This makes it more important to assess whether pre-emptive treatment with amitriptyline may work to prevent post-herpetic neuralgia.

TRIGEMINAL NEURALGIA

This is a condition commonly treated by neurologists. Typical attacks consist of repeated lancinating 'electric shock'-like pain lasting seconds with pain-free intervals in between confined to the cutaneous area of the trigeminal innervation. This is a condition of pure allodynia, the attacks often set off by innocuous mechanical stimuli, even in areas outside the trigeminal nerve innervation. Careful clinical assessment is important. There are no established criteria for diagnosis but the more typical the attacks, the more favourable the response to carbamezepine. Where there is residual pain between each lancinating attack or when there is permanent neurological deficit of trigeminal function, other underlying causes should be excluded. There have also been recent reports of a cluster–tic syndrome where there are coexisting features of trigeminal neuralgia and cluster headache. In these patients, carbamezepine alone is ineffective. The addition of amitriptyline sometimes helps to achieve pain relief. Most patients with 'idiopathic' trigeminal neuralgia present in their 5th to 7th decade. In younger patients, especially women, this may be the presenting feature of multiple sclerosis. Tumours, arteriovenous malformations, and many other structural lesions of the trigeminal nerve root and tract may cause symptoms similar to trigeminal neuralgia. The cause of 'idiopathic' trigem-

inal neuralgia is unknown. Aberrant loops of blood vessels—superior cerebellar artery impinging on the mandibular and maxillary divisions, and anterior inferior cerebellar artery on the opthalmic division of the trigeminal nerve has been implicated (Janetta 1980). Yet, at surgery, 10–15% of patients with trigeminal neuralgia have no visible vascular contact (Loeser 1994). More importantly, there are individuals with vascular contact who have never suffered from trigeminal neuralgia. In a post-mortem study of 50 cadavers not known to have trigeminal neuralgia, 60% had nerve–vascular contact. In 20%, this was bilateral (Hardy and Rhoton 1978). There have been endless arguments about the validity of this and other post-mortem studies, some carried in conjunction with neuroimaging (Hamlin and King 1992).

Allodynia in trigeminal neuralgia implies the establishment of central sensitization but where does the initial nociceptive signal originate from? There is no evidence of nociceptive input from the periphery via the trigeminal nerve itself. It is possible that nociceptive input comes from the nervi nervorum on the trigeminal nerve trunk activated by pulsating vascular loop(s). This convergence of nociceptive input into the spinal trigeminal nerve system may then cause 'wind-up' and allodynia. This may also explain why 'microvascular decompression' operations sometimes work even without partial rhizotomy when there is no vascular contact. Manipulation of the trigeminal nerve during operation may effectively 'denervate' it. Whatever the mechanism for the cause of trigeminal neuralgia, it needs urgent attention. The pain from attempting to eat and drink is often sufficiently severe to cause dehydration and malnourishment. The misery of trigeminal neuralgia is such that there is a definite risk of suicide among patients. The first line treatment is with carbamezepine. Approximately 70% will benefit from medical treatment. Around 10–15% are refractory to medications, and the same percentage will suffer intolerable side-effects (Tan *et al.* 1995). Therefore, approximately 20–30% are referred for surgical treatment.

The current investigation of choice before surgery is a 3-dimensional magnetic resonance tomography angiogram (MRTA). In the study using MRTA reported by Meaney *et al.* (1994), out of 40 patients with trigeminal neuralgia, 70% reported vascular contact on the appropriate side. Contrast enhancement in those who were initially negative identified a further 15%. In 114 controls, only 8% had asymptomatic nerve–vascular contact. In a similar study reported by Masur *et al.* (1995), 12/18 patients with trigeminal neuralgia had compression or dislocation of the nerve root by a vascular loop on the appropriate side. More interesting, 10/18 patients also had nerve–vascular contact on the asymptomatic side. Despite this, microvascular decompression can be very effective for trigeminal neuralgia. In his own series, Klun (1992) reported immediate relief in 171/178 patients he operated on. With a mean follow-up period of 5 years (range 6 months to 12 years) complete pain relief was permanent in 167/178 patients. Mendoza and Illingworth reported pain relief in 71%

of their series of 133 patients followed up for over 5 years. Similar results were reported by Barker *et al.* (1996) in their series of over 1000 microvascular decompression procedures for trigeminal neuralgia. Poor prognostic factors for pain relief were female gender, symptoms longer than 8 years pre-operatively, venous rather than arterial contact seen at operation, and the lack of immediate post-operative pain relief. Surgical mortality for this procedure is around 1% (range 0.2–2%) in most studies. Cranial nerve or cerebellar lesions occur in around 10% although the deficit is usually transient.

In patients without vascular contact or who are too infirm for microvascular decompression, trigeminal rhizotomy is an alternative surgical treatment. The relative merits of glycerol and radiofrequency rhizotomy were studied by Tan *et al.* (1995). Although strict comparison was not possible (because neither patients nor treatments were randomized between the two centres) some interesting results were reported. Immediate pain relief occurred in 80% of 50 patients who underwent glycerol rhizotomy compared to 88% of 80 patients who had radiofrequency rhizotomy. The procedure was repeated within one year in 42% of those who initially had glycerol as opposed to 25% that had radiofrequency rhizotomy. Sensory loss, however, was twice more likely in those who had radiofrequency rhizotomy. The overall result is that 24% of those treated with glycerol rhizotomy obtained pain relief at one year versus 12.5% of those treated with radiofrequency rhizotomy. Their conclusion was that glycerol rhizotomy was the treatment of choice because it can be easily repeated and has a lower morbidity.

The treatment for 'secondary' trigeminal neuralgia from multiple sclerosis can be more difficult. Drugs like carbamezepine, phenytoin, and baclofen are prescribed as for 'idiopathic' trigeminal neuralgia. Where they are ineffective or intolerable side-effects develop, misoprostol was found to be effective in one report (Reder and Arnasch 1995).

PAINFUL DIABETIC NEUROPATHY

Approximately 10–25% of all patients attending diabetic clinics suffer chronic pain. Diabetes may cause a painful radiculopathy, a painful plexopathy (diabetic amyotrophy), but most commonly, a painful symmetrical sensory and autonomic neuropathy. Spontaneous resolution of painful radiculopathy and plexopathy is often seen but the pain of symmetrical diabetic polyneuropathy usually persists. In the four year prospective study reported by Boulton *et al.* (1983), only one-third of diabetics with painful polyneuropathy noticed improvement. The remainder had pain that was either unchanged or worsened during the follow-up period.

The reasons why some diabetic neuropathies are painful whereas others are painless is unknown. Attempts to correlate different types of nerve fibre loss and propensities to pain have not proved to be useful. Morphologically, initial reports linking predominant unmyelinated and small myelinated axonal loss and pain failed to be repeated in later studies (Llewelyn *et al.* 1991). Physiologically, there is no definite correlation between painful neuropathy and defects in small sensory neuronal function (e.g. by testing thermal threshold) (Benbow *et al.* 1994).

The cause of pain is also unknown. In experimental studies, regenerating nerve sprouts may be a source of nociceptive signals but this cannot be confirmed in human studies (Britland *et al.* 1992). Thomas (1974) and subsequently Ashbury and Fields (1984) have suggested the nervi nervorum as another source for nociceptive signals in painful diabetic neuropathies. Once again, there is little evidence from human studies (Lincoln *et al.* 1993). More centrally, persistent high blood sugar may antagonize the analgesic effects of morphine. In rats, blood glucose interferes with physiological function of the opioid receptor (Simon and Dewey 1991). In humans, a defect in opioid signalling in patients with painful diabetic neuropathy was also reported (Tsigos *et al.* 1995). These theories are interesting but do not presently alter the treatment strategies for painful diabetic neuropathy.

The character of pain in peripheral diabetic neuropathy is described as shooting, sharp, nagging, or tingling (Masson *et al.* 1989). In numerous well-designed studies, 'tricyclic' antidepressants and amitriptyline, in particular, were the most effective treatments (Max *et al.* 1987, 1992). Desimipramine is an effective alternative for patients who are unable to tolerate the anticholinergic and sedating side-effects of amitriptyline (Max *et al.* 1991). Mexiletene also relieves painful diabetic neuropathy (Dejgard *et al.* 1988; Stracke *et al.* 1992). It may, however, exacerbate the orthostatic hypotension in patients with diabetic autonomic neuropathy and should be initiated with care. Intravenous lignocaine was also reported to work (Kastrup *et al.* 1986) but prolonged treatment would be difficult.

Carbamezepine is often used for treating painful diabetic neuropathy but the result is usually disappointing. The most commonly quoted placebo controlled study that assessed the effect of carbamezepine in diabetic neuropathy involved 30 patients and was reported in 1969 (Rull *et al.* 1969). Two further studies were also reported in the 1970s but the number of patients studied were similarly small (Wilton 1974; Chakrabaty and Samantary 1976). Overall, the evidence for the use of carbamezepine to treat painful diabetic neuropathy is at best tenuous and cannot be compared with the larger, more recent studies assessing amitriptyline.

A large multicentred placebo controlled trial involving 250 patients assessed the use of topical capsaicin to treat painful diabetic neuropathy (Capsaicin Study Group 1991). For those who were able to tolerate application of the cream, 20% obtained benefit after 8 weeks, compared to the placebo group. Patients on active treatment had to tolerate burning for at least 4 weeks before getting any relief. Even in untreated patients, the heat hyperalgesia is severe in painful diabetic neuropathy. Some patients attempt to alleviate this by immersing their painful limbs in cold water to the extent that their peripheral vascular disease becomes exacerbated (Harati 1992).

Therefore, those patients in this study that managed to finish the trial may be an atypical subgroup. In addition, it is questionable whether this was a truly double-blinded trial. A large number of patients on active treatment experienced coughing and sneezing from capsaicin cream. The role for capsaicin cream for routine use in patients with painful diabetic neuropathy remains controversial. Clonidine was also reported to be effective for painful diabetic neuropathy but only in a highly selected small subset of patients (Byas-Smith *et al.* 1995).

An important point in the management of pain in diabetic patients is to break down each component of pain, for example, muscle cramps, ischaemic pain from peripheral vascular insufficiency, painful neuropathy, etc. A modified shortened form of the McGill Pain Questionnaire is claimed to be able to reliably identify patients with painful diabetic neuropathy (Masson *et al.* 1989) but this cannot be a substitute for careful clinical evaluation. Once such an exercise has been carried out, it is theoretically easier to treat each component of the pain (i.e. amitriptyline or imipramine and mexiletene for deep pain, capsaicin for superficial pain) (Pfeifer *et al.* 1993), and sympathetic blocks, dorsal column stimulators for the ischaemic peripheral vascular pain.

Reflex sympathetic dystrophy (RSD)

RSD is defined by the IASP as 'a syndrome of continuous diffuse limb pain . . . consequent to injury or noxious stimulus with variable sensory, motor, autonomic and trophic changes'. Causalgia is a specific form of RSD associated with peripheral nerve damage. To diagnose RSD, the presence of pain or abnormal nociceptive perception would be a prerequisite. Yet there are authors who still include patients with sudomotor changes only and no pain (Christensen *et al.* 1982). Classical RSD is supposed to go through three stages with swelling and osteopaenia followed by dystrophy then atrophy of skin and integuments. However, in one of the largest reported study of 829 patients, 70% did not fulfil these criteria (Veldman *et al.* 1993). Even the term 'reflex sympathetic dystrophy' is controversial. Implicit with this is the assumption that reflex overactivation of the sympathetic system is present. This is now widely challenged. A recent suggestion to improve on this is to call RSD 'complex regional pain syndrome (CRPS) type 1' and causalgia, 'CRPS type 2' (Stanton-Hicks *et al.* 1995). Until these terms gain wider acceptance, most clinicians will continue to refer to 'RSD' and 'causalgia'.

The pathogenesis of RSD is unclear. A lot of research has concentrated on changes of the sympathetic system following nerve damage (e.g. the coupling of sympathetic nerves to damaged peripheral axons) (for a review see Janig and Koltenburg 1992), or the growth of sympathetic nerves around dorsal root ganglion cells after peripheral axotomy (McLachlan *et al.* 1993). Yet it is still unclear whether RSD, like causalgia, is a truly neuropathic pain condition. The character of pain and autonomic changes associated with both conditions may be very similar but even with careful testing, no somatic sensory loss can be found (Professor Per

Hansen Personal communication). However, to suggest that RSD is a purely psychogenic disorder is also too simplistic. First, the previous reports of rigidity and somatization traits in RSD patients were not supported by the thorough review by Lynch (1992) who concluded that there is not a predisposing 'RSD personality'. Second, the osteopaenia that is seen in many RSD patients is too rapid to be due to disuse alone. Third, the autonomic changes in the affected limb are similarly too rapid to be merely caused by sympathetic receptor hypersensitivity. Schott (1994, 1995) has argued for the concomitant block of visceral afferent fibres within the sympathetic nerve trunks to explain the effectiveness of sympathetic blocks for pain relief of both RSD and causalgia. Therefore, RSD may represent a form of neurogenic pain from damage to visceral afferent fibres which is not detectable by any test of somatic sensation. Further studies are needed to clarify this as well as the other numerous questions regarding the pathophysiology of RSD.

Recent research into the function of different primary afferent nerve fibres and their contribution to the development of RSD may help to delineate different subtypes of this condition. There may be predominant C fibre sensitization, causing antidromic activation and peripheral release of vasoactive peptides. This gives rise to erythralgia, described by Thomas Lewis, which is similar to Weir Mitchell's erythromelalgia and called the 'angry backfiring C fibres (ABC) syndrome' by Ochoa and colleagues (Cline *et al.* 1989). Clinically, this presents with heat hyperalgesia and hot skin. Alternatively, there may be small myelinated Aδ dysfunction giving rise to the CCC (cold hypoaesthesia, cold hyperalgesia, cold skin) syndrome (Ochoa and Yarnitsky 1994). Innocuous cold sensation is normally served by Aδ fibres. When there is a dysfunction of Aδ sensory processing normal cold sensation is lost. More importantly, this causes disinhibition of C cold nociceptors. Normal cold becomes painful and burning in character. This phenomenon has been reported in experimental Aδ fibre nerve blocks. In the CCC syndrome, the persistent cold limb arises from sympathetic overactivity causing vasoconstriction which presents a persistent stimulant to cause chronic pain. Abnormal signalling by Aβ afferent nerves causing pain has also been reported in patients whose pain were alleviated by sympathetic blocks (Price *et al.* 1989). This basic division of RSD into three types of altered afferent fibre sensory processing is obviously an oversimplification, as all three may coexist in varying and changeable degrees. There is also the further component of abnormal sympathetic hyperactivity and assays of noradrenaline breakdown products point to sympathetic receptor supersensitivity rather than increased neural activity to be responsible for this (Drummond *et al.* 1991; Harden *et al.* 1994).

With such a complicated proposed pathophysiology the approach to treatment is, not surprisingly, even more difficult and often needs to be individualized. Some general measures like physiotherapy and active mobilization should, however, be applied to all patients to prevent disuse and further atrophy of the affected limb. Exacerbation of symptoms is reported following physiotherapy but this is usually transient. Likewise, psychological assessment and supportive therapy, such as relaxation, biofeedback, and behavioural therapy, to deal with the chronic pain and disability is important. So is adequate pain control. TENS has a low side-effect profile and may be effective. Using a regime of TENS, physiotherapy, and psychological treatment, Wilder *et al.* (1992), reported encouraging results in their study of 70 children with RSD. In the same study, 56% of 41 patients who were prescribed amitriptyline, doxepin, or desimipramine reported an improvement of their pain. There have not been any placebo controlled trials of a tricyclic antidepressant for treating RSD or causalgia but its effectiveness in other neuropathic conditions merits a trial in most patients. Other drugs reported to alleviate pain from RSD include calcitonin (Salovarat and Kurev 1990) and steroids (Christensen *et al.* 1990). Their use is more controversial and until more extensive controlled studies are carried out, probably less justifiable.

Where cold hyperalgesia coexists with a cold limb, warming may alleviate pain. Local measures like providing a battery-powered warming glove sometimes work. More invasive methods to warm the affected limb, such as sympathetic blocks, are often carried out but are not always successful in alleviating the pain (Treede *et al.* 1992). Dellemijn *et al.* (1994) did not find any clinical parameters to be of predictive value for whether sympathetic blocks will relieve pain. Sometimes pain may actually be worse after sympathetic blocks. For example, it has been reported that ongoing pain when sympathetic blocks are performed is a risk factor for the development of post-sympathetic neuralgia or sympathalgia (Kramis *et al.* 1996). Also, there are two theoretical reasons why sympathetic blocks may be harmful. First, there is a risk of inducing further receptor hypersensitivity in patients with repeated sympathetic blocks so that the cold limb remains even colder. Second, the inhibitory effect of non-nociceptive cold may be unmasked (cf. CCC syndrome and burning cold pain of central origin). These potential complications should to be carefully considered and explained to patients before getting consent for sympathetic blocks. The 'reflex' action of the anaesthetist to perform a sympathetic block once 'reflex sympathetic dystrophy' is diagnosed must be curtailed. After every procedure, careful assessment is necessary before repeating sympathetic blocks.

There are few controlled studies testing the efficacy of sympathetic blocks. Jaddad *et al.* (1995) attempted to ameliorate this by performing an analysis of all the small controlled studies of regional sympathetic blocks in the treatment of RSD. They identified four reports where guanethedine intravenous sympathetic blocks were performed and found guanethedine to be no more effective than placebo for pain relief. One study each of bretylium and ketanserin were identified and both were better than placebo. None of these controlled studies involved sufficient numbers of patients to have any statistical power to determine whether any regional sympathetic blocks

were effective for treating RSD. There are uncontrolled series involving large numbers of patients where sympathetic blocks were successful in relieving pain in 62–80% of patients with RSD (Eulry *et al.* 1991). However, the methods used for patient selection is unclear and the clinical effect was not assessed in any systemic fashion. Verdugo and Ochoa (1994) have always argued that pain relief following sympathetic blocks is due to placebo alone (see also Price *et al.* 1996). However, some studies have reported recurrence of pain in RSD patients following iontophoretic application or cutaneous injection of noradrenaline, implicating the role of the sympathetic system in pathogenesis. Unfortunately, this is not dependent on whether previous sympathetic blocks alleviated pain and may be a dynamic phenomenon so that a rechallenge does not necessarily produce the same result (Torebjork *et al.* 1995).

Reflex sympathetic dystrophy is a difficult problem to treat. The management requires careful assessment and a multidisciplinary approach. Dramatic methods, such amputation of the affected limb, do not work (Dielissen *et al.* 1995). Physiotherapy and psychotherapy with adequate pain relief are the first line of treatment. Chemical sympathetic blocks may benefit a small number of patients when conservative measures fail. Permanent sympathetic blocks should be considered only in those who gain consistent relief from temporary blocks. At present, there is little scientific or clinical evidence on which to base any treatment regime and considerable work needs to be done. However, careful clinical assessment must form a mandatory part of these future studies. To ignore the diverse nature of this syndrome would handicap any attempts to investigate the methods of treatment.

CONCLUSION

Chronic pain is common and clinical management is difficult. This is especially true in neuropathic pain syndromes where careful assessment is important not only to exclude any underlying treatable causes but also to work out the diverse underlying pathophysiology. Any pain management strategy must be multidisciplinary in its approach. Pharmacotherapy is limited and most of the drugs have not undergone rigorous testing. Primary analgesics, such as NSAIDs and opioids, have a useful role and the dangers of using the latter are overemphasized. In addition, neuropathic pain may only be relatively rather than absolutely unresponsive to treatment with opioids. Adjunctive medications like tricyclic antidepressants and membrane stabilizing drugs are the mainstay of pharmacotherapy in neuropathic pain. Amitriptyline is the most widely tested and shown to be more effective than placebo for relieving the pain of diabetic neuropathy, central pain syndromes, and post-herpetic neuralgia. Mexiletene is also effective but less so as a monotherapy for treating these conditions. Anticonvulsants are of proven value only in trigeminal neuralgia. Transcutaneous nerve stimulation (TENS) may be tried in any form of localised pain. It has a low side-effect profile and is easy to use. Surgical pain management concentrates on implantation of dorsal column stimulators and microvascular decompression. The indications for destructive neurosurgery in treating pain are quite rightly diminishing. Surgical lesions along the nociceptive pathways have a high incidence of side-effects, and any benefit is often transient and may cause anaesthesia dolorosa. Of the neuropathic pain syndromes, reflex sympathetic dystrophy and causalgia are particularly difficult to treat. The pathophysiological mechanisms and management of these conditions are controversial. Conservative treatment is preferred. When this fails, sympathetic blocks may benefit selected patients. Chronic pain treatment as a whole need more rigorous methods of study, starting with more careful assessment of symptoms and better means of classification. The principles of pre-emptive analgesia should also be understood and translated into clinical practice by all health care workers dealing with patients.

ACKNOWLEDGEMENTS

We would like to thank Professor Clifford Woolf, Dr John Winer, and Dr Matthew Jackson for their helpful comments and our families for their patience and support in preparing this chapter.

REFERENCES

ABPI data sheet compendium 1995–1996. Datapharm, London

Andersen G, Vestergaard K, Ingeman-Nielsen M, Jensen TS. Incidence of central post-stroke pain. *Pain* 1995; **61**: 187–93.

Anthony M. Lance JW. MAO inhibition in the treatment of chronic pain. *Arch. Neurol.* 1969; **21**: 263–8.

Arner S, Meyerson BA. Lack of analgesic effects of opioids on neuropathic and idiopathic forms of pain. *Pain* 1983; **33**: 11–23.

Ashbury AK, Fields HL. Pain due to peripheral nerve damage: a hypothesis. *Neurology* 1984; **34**: 413–28.

Awerbuch G. Treatment of thalamic pain syndrome with mexiletene. *Ann. Neurol.* 1990; **28**: 233.

Bach S, Noreng MF, Tjellden NU. Phantom limb pain in amputees during the first 12 months following limb amputation after preoperative lumbar epidural block. *Pain* 1988; **33**: 297–307.

Bainton T, Fox M, Bowsher D, Wells C. A double-blind trial of naloxone in post-stroke pain. *Pain* 1992; **48**: 159–62.

Barker FG, Jannetta PJ, Bissonette DJ, Larkins MV, Jho HD. The long term outcome of microvascular decompression for trigeminal neuralgia. *N. Eng. J. Med.* 1996; **334**: 1077–83.

Bates JA, Nathan PW. Transcutaneous electrical nerve stimulation for chronic pain. *Anaesthesia* 1980; **35**: 817–22.

Benbow SJ, Chan AW, Bowsher D, MacFarlane IA, Williams G. A prospective study of painful symptoms, small-fibre function and peripheral vascular disease in chronic painful diabetic neuropathy. *Diabetic Medicine* 1994; **11**: 17–21.

Bennet GJ. Hypotheses on the pathogenesis of Herpes Zoster-associated pain. *Ann. Neurol.* 1994; **35**: S38–41.

Boas RA, Covino BG, Shahnarian A. Analgesic responses to i.v. lidocaine. *Brit. J. Anaesth.* 1982; **54**: 501–5.

Bogduk N, Christophidis N, Cherry D *et al. Epidural steroids in the management of back pain and sciatica of spinal origin: report of the working party on epidural use of steroids in the management of back pain.* Canberra, Australia: National Health and Medical Research Council. 1993.

Boivie J. Central pain. In Wall PD, Melzack R. ed. *Textbook of pain* (3rd edn). Churchill Livingstone, London. 1994. 871–901.

Boivie J, Leijon G. Clinical findings in patients with central post-stroke pain. In Casey KL ed. *Pain and central nervous system disease.* Raven, New York. 1991: 65–75.

Boivie J, Leijon G, Johansson I. Central post-stroke pain—a study of the mechanisms through analyses of sensory abnormalities. *Pain* 1989; **37**: 173–85.

Boulton AJM, Armstrong WD, Scarpello JHB, Ward JD. The natural history of painful diabetic neuropathy—a four year study. *Postgrad. Med. J.* 1983; **59**: 556–9.

Bowsher D. Neurogenic pain syndromes and their management. *Br. Med. Bull.* 1991; **47**: 644–6.

Bowsher D. The management of central post-stroke pain. *Postgrad Med J.* 1995; **71**: 598–604.

Bowsher D. Central pain: clinical and physiological characteristics. *J. Neurol. Neurosurg. Psychiatry.* 1996; **61**: 62–9.

Breneman DL, Cardone JS, Blumsack RF, Lather RM, Searle EA, Pollack VE. Topical capsaicin treatment for haemodialysis related pruritus. *Am. Acad. Dermatol.* 1992; **26**: 91–4.

Britland ST, Young RJ, Sharma AK, Clarke BF. Acute and remitting painful diabetic neuropathy: a comparison of peripheral nerve pathology. *Pain* 1992; **48**: 361–70.

Broseta J, Barbera J, de Vera JA *et al.* Spinal cord stimulation in peripheral arterial disease. A cooperative study. *J. Neurosurg.* 1986; **64**: 71–80.

Byas-Smith MG, Max MB, Muir J. Kingman A. Transdermal clonidine compared to placebo in painful diabetic neuropathy using a two stage 'enrichment enrollment' design. *Pain* 1995; **60**: 267–74.

Canavero S, Bonicalzi V, Ferroli P, Zeme S, Montalenti E, Benna P *et al.* control of idiopathic trigeminal neuralgia. *JNNP* 1995; **59**: 646.

Capsaicin Study Group. Treatment of painful diabetic neuropathy with topical capsaicin. *Arch. Neurol.* 1991; **151**: 2225–9

Casey KL, Boivie J, Holmgren H *et al.* Laser-evoked cerebral potentials and sensory function in patients with central pain. *Pain* 1990; **5**(suppl.): S204.

Cauthen JC, Renner EJ. Transcutaneius and peripheral nerve stimulation for chronic pain states. *Surgical Neurology* 1975; **4**: 102–4.

Chakrabaty AK, Samantary SK. Diabetic peripheral neuropathy: nerve conduction studies before, during and after carbamezepine therapy. *Australia NZ Med.* 1976; **6**: 565.

Christensen K, Jensen EM, Noer I. The reflex dystrophy syndrome: response to treatment with systemic corticosteroids. *Acta. Chir. Scand.* 1982; **148**: 653–5.

Cline MA, Ochoa JL, Torebjörk E. Chronic hyperalgesia and skin warming caused by sensitized C nociceptors. *Brain* 1989; **112**: 621–47.

Craig AD and Bushnell MC. The thermal grill illusion: unmasking the burn of cold pain. *Science* 1994; **265**: 252–5.

Craig AD, Reiman EM, Evans A, Bushnell MC. Functional imaging of an illusion of pain. *Nature* 1996; **384**: 258–60.

Crooks RJ, Jones DA, Fiddian AP. Zoster-associated chronic pain: an overview of clinical trials with acyclovir. *Scand. J. Inf. Dis.* 1991; **80**(suppl.): 62–8.

Deardorff WW, Rubin HS, Scott DW. Comprehensive multidisciplinary treatment of chronic pain: a follow-up study of treated and non-treated groups. *Pain* 1991; **45**: 35–43.

Debenedittis G, Besana F, Lorenzetti A. A new topical treatment for acute herpetic neuralgia and post-herpetic neuralgia-the aspirin diethyl-ether mixture—an open-label study plus a double-blind controlled clinical-trial. *Pain* 1992; **48**: 383–90.

Dellemijn PLI, Fields HL, Allen RR, McKay WR, Rowbotham MC. The interpretation of pain relief and sensory changes following sympathetic blockade. *Brain* 1994; **117**: 1475–87.

Dejgard A, Petersen P, Kastrup J. Mexiletene for treatment of chronic painful diabetic neuropathy. *Lancet* 1988; 9–11.

Devor M, Wall PD, Catalan N. Systemic lidocaine silences ectopic neuroma and DRG discharges without blocking nerve conduction. *Pain* 1992; **48**: 396–400.

Dielessen PW, Claasen ATPM, Veldman PHJM, Goris RJA. Amputation for reflex sympathetic dystrophy. *J. Bone and Joint Surg. (Brit).* 1995; **77B**: 270–3.

Dray A. Inflammatory mediators of pain. *Brit. J. Anaesth.* 1995; **75**: 125–31.

Drummond PD, Finch PM, Smythe GA. Reflex sympathetic dystrophy: the significance of differing cathecholamine concentrations in affected and unaffected limbs. *Brain* 1991; **114**: 2025–36.

Dubner R. A call for more science, not rhetoric, regarding opioids and neuropathic pain. *Pain* 1991; **47**: 1–2.

Edwards WT, Habib F, Burney RG, Begin G. Intravenous lidocaine in the management of various chronic pain states. *Regional. Anesth.* 1985; **10**: 1–6.

Eggers KA, Power I. Tramadol. *Brit. J. Anaesth.* 1995; **74**: 247–9.

Eide PK, Jorum E, Stubhung A, Brenner J, Breivik H. Reliefe of post-herpetic neuralgia with the N-methyl-D-aspartate receptor antagonist ketamine: a double blind, placebo controlled crossover comparison with morphine and placebo. *Pain* 1994; **58**: 347–54.

Espir MLE, Millac P. Treatment of paroxysmal disorders in multiple sclerosis with carbamezepine (Tegretol). *JNNP* 1970; **33**: 528–31.

Eulry F, Lechrvalier D, Pats B, Alliaume C, Crozes P, Vasseur P *et al.* Regional intravenous guanethedine blocks in algodystrophy. *Clinical Rheum.* 1991; **10**: 377–83.

Ferrante FM, Paggioli J, Cheruki S, Arthure GR. The analgesic response to intravenous lidocaine in the treatment of neuropathic pain. *Anesth. Analg.* 1996; **82**: 91–7.

Fields HL. Can opiates relieve neuropathic pain? *Pain* 1988; **35**: 365.

Filling-Katz MR, Merrick HF, Fink JK, Miles RB, Sokol J, Barton NW. Carbamezepine in Fabry's disease: effective analgesia with dose dependent exacerbation of autonomic dysfunction. *Neurology* 1989; **39**: 598–600.

Flor H, Fydrich T, Turk DC. Efficacy of multidisciplinary pain treatment centers: a meta-analytical review. *Pain* 1992; **49**: 221–30.

Friedman AH, Bullit E. Dorsal root entry zone lesions in the treatment of pain following brachial plexus avulsion, spinal cord injury and herpes zoster. *Appl. Neurophysiol.* 1988; **51**: 164–9.

Fusco BM, Geppetti P, Fanciullacci M, Sicuteri F. Local application of capsaicin for the treatment of cluster headache and trigeminal neuralgia. *Cephalalgia* 1991; **11**: 234–5.

Gingras MA. A clinical trial of tofranil in rheumatic pain in general practise. *J. Int. Med. Res.* 1976; **4**: 41–9.

Hamlin PJ, King TT. Neurovascular compression in trigeminal neuralgia: a clinical and anatomical study. *J. Neurosurg.* 1992; **76**: 948–54.

Harati Y. Frequently asked questions about diabetic peripheral neuropathies. *Neurologic Clinics* 1992; **10**: 783–807.

Harden RN, Duc TA, Williams TR, Coley D, Cate JC, Gracely RH. Norepinephrine and epinephrine levels in affected versus unaffected limbs in sympathetic maintained pain. *Clin. J. Pain* 1994; **10**: 324–30.

Hardy DG, Rhoton AL Jr. Microsurgical relationship of the superior cerebellar artery and the trigeminal nerve. *J. Neurosurg.* 1978; **49**: 669–78.

Hatangdi VS, Boas RA, Richards EG. Postherpetic-neuralgia: management with anti-epileptic and tricyclic drugs. In Bonica JJ ed.

Advances in pain research and therapy, Vol. 1 Raven, New York. 1976: 583–7.

Jaddad AR, Carroll D, Glynn CJ, McQuay HJ. Intravenous sympathetic blockade for pain relief in sympathetic dystrophy: a systemic review and a double-blind crossover study. *J. Pain Sympt. Man.* 1995; **10**: 13–20.

Jahangiri M, Bradley JWP, Jayatunga AP, Dark CH. Prevention of phantom limb pain after major lower limb amputation by epidural infusion of diamorphine, clonidine and bupivacaine. *Ann. Roy. Coll. Surg. England* 1994; **76**: 324–6.

Janig W, Koltenburg M. Possible ways of sympathetic afferent interactions. In Janig W and Schmidt RF ed. *Reflex sympathetic dystrophy. Pathophysiological mechanisms and clinical implications.* VCH Verlag, Weinheim. 1992: 213–45.

Jannetta PJ. Neurovascular compression in cranial nerve and systemic disease. *Ann. Surg.* 1980; **192**: 518–25.

Kastrup J, Angelo HR, Petersen P, Dejgard A, Hilsted J. Treatment of painful diabetic neuropathy with intravenous lidocaine infusion. *Lancet* 1986; **292**: 173.

King RB. Topical aspirin in chloroform and the relief of pain due to herpes zoster and post-herpetic neuralgia. *Arch. Neurol.* 1993; **50**: 1046–53.

Klun B. Microvascular decompression and partial sensory rhizotomy in the treatment of trigeminal neuralgia: a personal experience of 220 patients. *Neurosurg.* 1992; **30**: 49–52.

Koes BW, Scholten RJPM, Mens JMA, Bouter LM. Efficacy of epidural steroid injection for low-back pain and sciatica: a systematic review of randomised clinical studies. *Pain* 1995; **63**: 279–88.

Koyama S, Katayama Y, Maejima S, Hirayama T., Fujii M, and Tsubokawa T. Thalamic neuronal hyperactivity following transaction of the spinothalamic tract in the cat: involvement of N-methyl-D-aspartate receptor. *Brain Research* 1993; **612**: 345–50.

Kramis RC, Roberts WJ, Gillete RG. Post-sympathectomy neuralgia: hypotheses and central neuronal mechanisms. *Pain* 1996; **64**: 1–9.

Kristensen JD, Karlsen R, Gordh T, Berge OG. The NMDA receptor antagonist CPP abolishes neurogenic 'wind-up' pain after intrathecal administration in humans. *Pain* 1992; **51**: 249–53.

Kumar K, Nath R, Wyant GM. Treatment of chronic pain by epidural spinal cord stimulation: a 10 year experience. *J. Neurosurg.* 1991; **75**: 402–7.

Kurkccuoglu N, Alaybeyi F. Topical capsaicin for psoriasis. *Brit. J. Derm.* 1990; **123**: 1679–87.

Kvinsdahl B, Molin J, Froland A, Gram LF. Imipramine in the treatment of painful diabetic neuropathy. *JAMA* 1984; **251**: 1727–30.

Lasagna L, Dekornfeld TJ. Methotrimeprazine—a new phenothiazine derivative with analgesic properties. *JAMA* 1961; **178**: 119–22.

Lee RG and van Donkelaar P. Mechanisms underlying functional recovery following stroke. *Can. J. Neurosci.* 1995; **22**: 257–63.

Leibsohn E. Treatment of notalgia paraesthetica with capsaicin. *CUTIS* 1992; **49**: 335–6.

Leijon G, Boivie J. Central post-stroke pain—a controlled trial of amitriptyline and carbamezepine. *Pain* 1989; **36**: 27–36.

Lenz FA, Graceley RH, Romanoski AJ, Hope EJ, Rowland LH, Dougherty PM. Stimulation in the human somatosensory thalamus can reproduce both the affective and sensory dimensions of previously experienced pain. *Nature Medicine* 1995; **1**: 910–13.

Lincoln J, Milner P, Appenzeller G, Qualls C. Innervation of normal human sural and optic nerves by noradrenaline and peptide containing nervi nervorum: effect of diabetes and alcoholism. *Brain Res.* 1993; **632**: 48–56.

Llewelyn JG, Gilbey SG, Thomas PK, King RH, Muddle JR Watkins PJ. Sural nerve morphometry in diabetic autonomic and painful sensory neuropathy. A clinicopathological study. *Brain* 1991; **114**: 867–92.

Loeser JD. Tic douloureux and atypical facial pain. In Wall PD, Melzack R. ed. *Textbook of pain* (3rd edn). Churchill Livingstone London. 1994: 699–710.

Loh L, Nathan PW, Schott GD. Pain due to lesions of the central nervous system removed by sympathetic blocks. *BMJ* 1981; **282**: 1026–8.

Long DM, Erickson D, Campbell J, North R. Electrical stimulation of the spinal cord and peripheral nerves for pain control. A 10 year experience. *Appl. Neurophysiol.* 1981; **44**: 207–17.

Lynch ME. Psychological aspects of reflex sympathetic dystrophy: a review of the adult and paediatric literature. *Pain* 1992; **49**: 337–47.

Malmberg AB, Yaksh TL. Hyperalgesia mediated by spinal glutamate or substance P receptor blocked by spinal cycloxygenase inhibitor. *Science* 1992; **257**: 1276–9.

Mannheimer C, Eliasson T, Andersson B, Bergh C-B, Augustinsson L-E, Emanuelsson H. Effects of spinal cord stimulation in angina pectoris induced by pacing and possible mechanism of action. *BMJ* 1993; **307**: 477–80.

Marchand S, Li JX, Charest J. Effects of caffeine on analgesia from transcutaneous electrical nerve stimulation. *NEJM* 1995; **333**: 325–6.

Maruta T, Swanson DW, McHardy MJ. Three year follow-up of patients with chronic pain who were treated in a multidisciplinary pain management center. *Pain* 1990; **41**: 47–53.

Masson EA, Hunt L, Gem JM, Boulton AJM. A novel approach to the diagnosis and assessment of symptomatic diabetic neuropathy. *Pain* 1989; **38**: 25–8.

Masur H, Papke K, Bongartz G, Vollbrecht K. The significance of 3-dimensional MR defined neurovascular compression for the pathogenesis of trigeminal neuralgia. *J. Neurol.* 1995; **242**: 93–8.

Max MB. Treatment of post-herpetic neuralgia: antidepressants. *Ann. Neurol.* 1994; **35**: S50–3.

Max MB, Culhane M, Schafer SC, Gracely RH, Walther DJ, Smoller B *et al.* Amitriptyline relieves diabetic neuropathy pain with normal or depressed mood. *Neurology* 1987; **37**: 589–96.

Max MB, Kishore-Kumar R, Schafer SC *et al.* Efficacy of desipramine in painful diabetic neuropathy: A placebo-controlled trial. *Pain* 1991; **54**: 3–9.

Max MB, Lynch SA, Muir JM, Shoaf SE, Smoller B, Dubner R. Effects of desipramine, amitriptyline and fluoxetine in diabetic neuropathy. *NEJM* 1992; **326**: 1250–6.

McGill JI, White JE. Acyclovir and post-herpetic neuralgia and ocular involvement. *BMJ* 1994; **309**: 1124.

McKendrick MW, McGill JI, Wood MJ. Lack of effect of acyclovir on post-herpetic neuralgia. *BMJ* 1989; **298**: 431.

McLachlan EM, Janig W, Devor M, Michaelis M. Peripheral nerve injury triggers noradrenergic sprouting within dorsal root ganglia. *Nature* 1993; **363**: 543–5.

McQuay HJ, Carroll D, Glynn CJ. Dose-response for analgesic effect of amitriptyline in chronic pain. *Anaesthesia* 1993; **48**: 281–5.

McQuay HJ, Carroll D, Jadad AR, Wiffen P, Moore RA. Anticonvulsant drugs for management of pain: a systematic review. *BMJ* 1995; **311**: 1047–52.

McQuay HJ, Jadad AR, Carroll D, Faura C, Glynn CJ, Moore RA *et al.* Opioid sensitivity of chronic pain: a patient-controlled analgesia method. *Anaesthesia* 1992; **47**: 757–67.

McQuay HJ, Tramer M, Nye BA, Carroll D, Wiffen PJ, Moore RA. A systematic review of antidepressants in neuropathic pain. *Pain* 1996; **68**: 217–27.

Meaney JFM, Miles JB, Nixon TE *et al.* Vascular contact with the 5th cranial nerve at the pons in patients with trigeminal neuralgia—detection with 3-D FISP imaging. *Am. J. Roent.* 1994; **163**: 1447–52.

Mellick LB, Mellick GA. Successful treatment of reflex sympathetic dystrophy with gabapentin. *Am. J. Emergency Med.* 1995; **13**:96.

Melzack R, Stillwell DM, Fox EJ. Trigger points and acupuncture points for pain: correlations and implications. *Pain* 1977; **3**: 2–23.

Mendoza N, Illingworth RD. Trigeminal neuralgia treated by microvascular decompression—A long term follow-up study. *Brit. J. Neurosurg.* 1995; **9**: 13–19.

Miles J, Lipton S. Phantom limb pain treated by electrical stimulation. *Pain* 1987; **5**: 373–92.

Mittal B, Thomas DGT, Walton P, Calder I. Dorsal column stimulation (DCS) in chronic pain: report of 31 cases. *Ann. Roy. Coll. Surg. Eng.* 1987; **69**: 104–9.

Morris GC, Gibson SJ, Helme RD. Capsaicin-induced and vasodilatation in patients with post-herpetic neuralgia. *Pain* 1995; **63**: 93–101.

Nashold BS, Friedman H. Dorsal column stimulation for control of pain. Preliminary report in 30 patients, *J. Neurosurg.* 1972; **36**: 590–7.

Nathan PW. Chloroprothixene (Taractan) in post herpetic neuralgia and other severe chronic pain. *Pain* 1978a; **5**: 367–71.

Nathan PW. The gate control theory of pain. A critical review. *Brain* 1978b; **99**: 123–58.

Nathan PW. Effects on movement of surgical incisions into the human spinal cord. *Brain* 1994; **117**: 337–46.

Nathan PW, Wall PD. Treatment of post-herpetic neuralgia by prolonged electrical nerve stimulation. *BMJ* 1974; **3**: 645–7.

Neilson KD, Adams JE, Hosobuschi Y. Phantom limb pain. Treatment with dorsal column stimulation. *J. Neurosurg.* 1975; **42**: 301–7.

Nesheim BI. The use of transcutaneous nerve stimulation for pain relief during labour. *Acta Obst. Gyne. Scand.* 1981; **60**: 13–16.

Ochoa JL, Yarnitsky D. The triple cold syndrome. Cold hyperalgesia, cold hypoaesthesia and cold skin in peripheral nerve disease. *Brain* 1994; **117**: 185–97.

Ochoa JL. Pain mechanisms in neuropathy. *Curr. Neurol.* 1994; **7**: 407–14.

Onghena P, Houdenhove BV. Antidepressant-induced analgesia in chronic non-malignant pain: a meta-analysis of 39 placebo-controlled studies. *Pain* 1992; **49**: 205–19.

Pappagallo M, Campbell JN. Chronic opioid therapy as alternative treatment for post-herpetic neuralgia. *Ann. Neurol.* 1994; **35**: S54–6.

Pfeifer MA, Ross DR, Schrage JP, Gelber DA, Schumer MP, Crain GM *et al.* A highly successful and novel model for treatment of painful diabetic peripheral neuropathy. *Diabetes Care* 1993; **16**: 1103–15.

Pockett S., Spinal cord synaptic plasticity and chronic pain. *Anesth. Analg.* 1995; **80**: 173–9.

Portenoy RK. Pharmacologic management of chronic pain. In Fields HL ed. *Pain syndromes in neurology.* Butterworth-Heinemann, Oxford. 1990: 257–77.

Portenoy RK, Foley KM, Inturrisi CE. The nature of opioid responsiveness and its implications for neuropathic pain: new hypotheses derived from studies of opioid infusions. *Pain* 1990; **43**: 273–86.

Price DD, Bennet G, Rafii A. Psychophysical observations on patients with neuropathic pain relieved by sympathetic block. *Pain* 1989; **36**: 273–88.

Price DD, Mao J, Frenck H, Mayer DJ. The *N*-methyl-D-aspartate antagonist dextromethorphan selectively reduces temporal summation of second pain. *Pain* 1994; **59**: 165–74.

Price DD, Graceley RH, Bennett GJ. The challenge and the problem of placebo in assessment of sympathetically maintained pain. In Janig W, Stanton-Hicks in ed. *Progress in pain research and* management, Vol. 6. IASP Press, Seattle. 1996.

Rayner HC, Atkins RC, Westerman RA. Relief of local stump pain by capsaicin. *Lancet* 1989; **ii**: 1276–7.

Reder AT, *Arnasson* BGW. Trigeminal neuralgia in multiple sclerosis relieved by prostaglandin E analogue. *Neurology* 1995; **45**: 1097–1100.

Richardson J, Sabanathan S, Mearns AJ, Sides C, Goulden CP. Post-thoracotomy neuralgia. *The Pain Clinic* 1994; **7**: 87–97.

Richardson RR, Siquiera EB, Cerullo LJ. Spinal epidural neurostimulation for treatment of acute and chronic intractable pain: initial and long term results. *Neurosurgery* 1979; **5**: 344–8.

Rigge, M., Pain. *Which? Way to health* 1990; April: 66–8.

Rockliff BW, Davis EH. Controlled sequential trial of carbamezepine in trigeminal neuralgia. *Arch. Neurol.* 1968; **19**: 129–36.

Rosner H, Rubin L, Kestembaum A. Gabapentin Adjunctive therapy in neuropathic pain states. *Clin J. Pain*, 1996; **12**: 56–8.

Rowbotham MC. Managing post-herpetic neuralgia with opioids and local anaesthetics. *Ann. Neurol.* 1994; **35**: S46–9.

Rowbotham MC, Fields HL. Postherpetic neuralgia: the relation of pain compliant, sensory disturbance and skin temperature. *Pain* 1989; **39**: 129–44.

Rowbotham MC, Reisner-Keller LA, Fields HL. Both intravenous lidocaine and morphine reduce pain of post-herpetic neuralgia. *Neurology* 1991; **41**: 1024–8.

Rowbotham MC, Davies PS, Fields HL. Topical lidocaine gel relieves postherpetic neuralgia. *Ann. Neurol.* 1995; **37**: 246–53.

Rull J A, Quibrera R, Gonzalez-Millan H, and Lozano-Castadena O. Symptomatic treatment of peripheral diabetic neuropathy with carbamezepine: double-blind crossover study. *Diabetologica* 1969; **5**: 215.

Salorava P and Kunev K. The calcitonin treatment of patients with algodystrophy. *Vutreshni Bolesti* 1990; **29**: 102–5.

Schott GD. An unsympathetic view of pain. *Lancet* 1995; **345**: 634–6.

Schott JD. Visceral afferents: their contribution to 'sympathetic dependent' pain. *Brain* 1994; **117**: 397–413.

Segal AZ, Rordorf G. Gabapentin as a novel treatment for post-herpetic neuralgia. *Neurology* 1996; **46**: 1175–6.

Sicuteri F, Fusco BM, Marabini S, Campagnolo V, Maggi CA, Geppetti P *et al.* Beneficial effect of capsaicin application to the nasal mucosa in cluster headache. *Clin. J. Pain* 1989; **5**: 49–53.

Simon GS, Dewey WL. Narcotic and diabetes. The effect of streptozocin-induced diabetes on the antinociceptive potency of morphine. *J. Pharm. Exp. Therap.* 1981; **218**: 318–23.

Simpson B A. Spinal stimulation in 60 cases of intractable pain. *JNNP* 1991; **52**: 196–9.

Sindrup SH, Gram LF, Brosen K, Esh j O, Mogensen EF. The selective serotonin reuptake blocker paroxetine is effective in the treatment of diabetic neuropathy symptoms. *Pain* 1992; **40**: 135–44.

Sinoff SE, Hart MB. Topical capsaicin and burning pain. *Clin. J. Pain* 1993; **9**: 70–3.

Solarova P, Kunev K. The calcitonin treatment of patients with algodystrophy. *Vutreshni Bolesti* 1990; **29**: 102–5.

Solomon RA, Vierstein MC, Long DM. Reduction of postoperative pain and narcotic use by transcutaneous electrical nerve stimulation. *Surgery* 1980; **87**: 142–6.

Stanton-Hicks M, J nig W, Hassenbusch S, Haddox JD, Boas R, Wilson P. Reflex sympathetic dystrophy: changing concepts and taxonomy. *Pain* 1995; **63**: 127–33.

Stow P J, Glynn C J, and Minor B. EMLA cream in the treatment of post-herpetic neuralgia: efficacy and pharmacokinetic profile. *Pain* 1989; **39**: 301–5.

Stracke H, Meyer UE, Schumacher HE, Federlin K. Mexiletene in the treatment of diabetic neuropathy. *Diabetes Care* 1992; **15**: 1550–5.

Tallis RC, Illis LS, Sedgwick EM, Hardwidge C, Garfield JS. Spinal cord stimulation in peripheral vascular disease. *J. Neurol. Neurosurg. Psychiatr.* 1983; **46**: 478–84.

Tan LKS, Robinson SN, Chartterjee S. Glycerol versus radiofrequency rhizotomy—A comparison of their efficacy in the treatment of trigeminal neuralgia. *Brit. J. Neurosurg.* 1995; **9**: 165–9.

Taylor P, Hallet M, Flaherty L. Treatment of osteoarthritis of the knee with transcutaneous electrical nerve stimulation. *Pain* 1981; **11**: 233–46.

Thomas DG, Kitchen ND. Long term follow-up of dorsal root entry zone lesions in brachial plexus avulsion. *J. Neuro. Neurosurg. Psych.* 1994; **57**: 737–8.

Thomas PK. The anatomical substratum of pain. *Can. J. Neurol. Sci.* 1974; **1**: 92.

Torebjörk E, Wahren L, Wallin G, Hallin R, Koltzenburg M. Noradrenaline-evoked pain in neuralgia. *Pain* 1995; **63**: 11–20.

Tourian AY. Narcotic responsive 'thalamic pain' treatment with propranolol and tricyclic antidepressants. *Pain* 1987(suppl. 4): 411.

Treede R-D, Davis KD, Campbell JN, Raja SN. The plasticity of cutaneous hyperalgesia during sympathetic ganglion blockade in patients with neuropathic pain. *Brain* 1992; **115**: 607–21.

Tsigos C, Gibson S, Crosby SR, White A, Young RJ. Cerebrospinal fluid levels of beta endorphin in painful and painless diabetic polyneuropathy. *J. Diabetes Complications* 1995; **9**: 92–6.

Tsubokawa T, Katayama Y, Yamammoto T, Hirayam, AT, Koyama S. Chronic motor cortex stimulation in patients with thalamic pain. *J. Neurosurg.* 1993; **78**: 393–401.

Tyrings S. Famciclovir for the treatment of acute herpes zoster: Effects on acute disease and post-herpetic neuralgia. *Ann. Int. Med.* 1995; **123**: 89–96.

Veldman PHJM, Reynen HM, Ivo EA, Goris RJA. Signs and symptoms of reflex sympathetic dystrophy: prospective study of 829 patients. *Lancet* 1993; **342**: 1012–15.

Verdugo RJ, Ochoa JL. 'Sympathetic maintained pain': I and II. *Neurology* 1994; **44**: 1003–14.

Wall P D and Sweet W H. Temporary abolition of pain in man. *Science* 1967; **155**: 108–9.

Watson CPN, Evans RJ, Reed K, Merskey H, Goldsmith L, Warsh J. Amitriptyline versus placebo in post-herpetic neuralgia. *Neurology* 1982: 671–3.

Watson CPN, Evans RJ, Watt VR. Post-herpetic neuralgia and capsaicin. *Pain* 1988a; **33**: 333–40.

Watson CPN, Evans RJ, Watt VR. Post-herpetic neuralgia: 208 cases. *Pain* 1988b; **35**: 289–97.

Watson CPN, Evans RJ, Watt VR. The post-mastectomy pain syndrome and the effect of topical capsaicin. *Pain* 1989; **38**: 177–86.

Watson CPN, Deck JH, Morshead C, Van der Koog D, Evans RJ. Post-herpetic neuralgia: further post-mortem studies of cases with and without pain. *Pain* 1991; **44**: 105–17.

Wells J C and Miles J B. Pain clinics and pain treat. *British Medical Bulletin.* 1991; **47**: 762–85

Wilder RT, Berde CB, Wolohan M, Vieyra MA, Masek BJ, Micheli LJ. Reflex sympathetic dystrophy in children. Clinical characteristics and follow-up of seventy patients. *J. Bone Joint. Surg. (A)* 1992; **74**: 910–19.

Wilton TD. Tegretol in the treatment of diabetic neuropathy. *S. Afr. Med. J.* 1974; **48**: 869.

Woolf CJ. Somatic pain-pathogenesis and prevention. *Brit. J. Anaesth.* 1995; **75**: 169–76.

Woolf CJ, Chong MS. Pre-emptive analgesia-treating postoperative pain by preventing the establishment of central sensitisation. *Anesth. Analg.* 1993; **77**: 1–18.

Woolf CJ, Shortland P, Coggeshall RE. Peripheral nerve injury triggers sprouting of myelinated afferents. *Nature* 1992; **355**: 75–7.

Wynn Parry CB. Pain in avulsion lesions of the brachial plexus. *Pain* 1980; **9**: 41–53.

Young RF. Evaluation of dorsal column stimulator for the treatment of chronic pain. *Neurosurgery* 1978; **3**: 370–3.

4 | *Epilepsy and blackouts*

Nick Davies

Epilepsy is the most common of chronic neurological disorders and it imposes the biggest burden on health care systems. It is a disorder that varies greatly in its clinical features, aetiology, severity, and prognosis and its association with other neurological disability. For this reason, many different disciplines may be responsible for supplying care, including neurologists, paediatricians, geriatricians, psychiatrists, and specialists in mental handicap; and in all spheres, the professions allied to medicine will have an important input.

Unfortunately, services for people with epilepsy in the United Kingdom are poorly developed, varying considerably from region to region. The quality of care they offer is varied but often quite poor. A number of reasons are apparent for this. The primary one is that British neurology has remained a small speciality and relatively few British neurologists would express any major interest or expertise in epilepsy in particular, or the management of chronic neurological disease in general. This has meant that many patients with epilepsy are seen and managed by clinicians without significant neurological training. Furthermore, the epilepsy patient associations have remained small, poorly financed and without a major political voice.

However, this situation is beginning to change driven by rapid advances in the ability to diagnose and classify the epilepsies, and to offer newer more specific and effective pharmacological and surgical treatment. These changes will be more demanding on clinical skills and should provide a stimulus to the development of neurological specialist epilepsy services that, on one level will need to offer highly specialized diagnostic and management services, on the other to interact with community and primary care services in an effective way. Meeting these needs will require a significant expansion in the number of neurological posts available and an increase in specific training programmes in epilepsy.

THE DEFINITION OF EPILEPSY

Epilepsy is most easily defined in physiological terms, being 'the name for occasional sudden, excessive, rapid and local discharges of grey matter' (1). It is more difficult to offer a comprehensive ***clinical*** definition of epileptic seizures and epilepsy because of the varied clinical manifestations produced by cerebral neuronal discharge. However, an epileptic seizure can be defined as an intermittent, stereotyped, disturbance of consciousness, behaviour, emotion, motor function, or sensation that on clinical grounds is believed to result from cortical neuronal discharge. Epilepsy can thus be defined as a condition in which seizures recur, usually spontaneously.

The complexity of organization of the cerebral hemispheres means that epileptic seizures can result in a great diversity of clinical phenomena. Two major types are recognized, focal (partial) and generalized seizures.

Focal seizures and epilepsies are characterized by a localized onset in one part of one hemisphere. The initial electrical discharge and usually interictal electroencephalogram (EEG) abnormalities are localized and consciousness is usually maintained at the onset of the seizure. The patient, therefore, frequently has recall for the first parts of the seizure—the aura. Focal seizures, however, characteristically spread from the site of onset and consciousness may often be impaired as part of a complex partial or secondarily generalized tonic-clonic seizure.

In contrast, generalized seizures and epilepsies are characterized by synchronous discharge affecting both hemispheres early in the seizure. Such seizures start suddenly without an aura. The interictal EEG usually shows generalized spike wave abnormalities.

The international classification of epileptic seizures (ICES) was proposed in 1981 and is summarized in Table 4.1 (2). It makes use of both clinical and EEG information. Similar seizures may occur at different ages with very different implications. Conversely, however, a patient may experience differing seizures during the course of his/her life so that a classification of the different epileptic syndromes based on seizure types occurring within the syndrome, age of onset, and aetiology will also be of vital importance in the management of patients with epilepsy. A proposed classification of epilepsy syndromes is presented in Table 4.2 (3).

Epilepsy must be regarded as a symptom complex rather than a disease entity. The causes for epilepsy are many and varied and include purely genetic epilepsies (see later), as well as epilepsies that are solely the result of acquired cerebral insult. Virtually any disease process affecting the cortex of the cerebral hemispheres can result in seizures or epilepsy.

Table 4.1 International classification of epileptic seizures (ICES)

Partial seizures (seizures beginning locally):
Simple (consciousness not impaired)
• With motor symptoms
• With somatosensory or special sensory symptoms
• With autonomic symptoms
• With psychic symptoms

Complex (with impairment of consciousness):
• Beginning as simple partial seizures (progressing to complex seizure)
• Impairment of consciousness at onset
Partial seizures becoming secondarily generalized

Generalized seizures:
Absence seizures
• Typical (petit mal)
• Atypical
Myoclonic seizures
Clonic seizures
Tonic seizures
Tonic–clonic seizures
Atonic seizures

Reproduced with permission from the commission on the International League Against Epilepsy (1981). (see Ref. 2.)

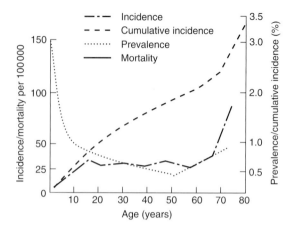

Fig. 4.1 Incidence, prevalence, and cumulative incidence rates for epilepsy in Rochester, Minnesota (1935–74). (Reproduced with permission from Anderson, V. E. *et al.* (1986). *Advances in neurology*, Vol. 44. Raven Press, New York.)

EPIDEMIOLOGY

Incidence rates vary in an age-specific way between approximately 20 and 70 per 100000 per year, whereas the prevalence for active epilepsy is in the range of 4–10 per 1000. Age-specific incidence, prevalence and cumulative incidence are given in Fig. 4.1 for a population in Rochester, Minnesota. It can be seen that the incidence of epilepsy is highest at the extremes of life but that there are significant differences between the cumulative incidence and prevalence of epilepsy, indicating that most patients who develop epilepsy do not suffer from a chronic disorder. The cumulative incidence of epilepsy by the age of 70 may be as high as 2–3% of the population. There is some evidence that incidental rates are declining in childhood (4) but the increasing numbers of elderly in the community mean that the size of the problem is unlikely to change.

The great majority of seizures and epilepsies developing in adult life will be regarded as symptomatic (i.e. associated with an underlying lesion). However, significant numbers of patients may be investigated without a cause becoming apparent. In the National General Practice Study of Epilepsy, 60% of all patients had no identifiable cause of epilepsy, although a proportion of these will have had a specific (genetically determined) epilepsy syndrome (5).

It may be useful to differentiate causes of seizures and epilepsy into acute symptomatic seizures occurring acutely in response to metabolic or cerebral insult, and remote symptomatic epilepsies in which epilepsy develops in relationship to a persisting cerebral lesion or damage. Some aetiologies, (e.g. head injuries, stroke, intracranial infections) may cause both acute symptomatic seizures and remote symptomatic epilepsy. The presence of the first does not necessarily result in the latter.

Sander *et al* (5) found that the commonest remote symptomatic causes of epilepsy were vascular disease (15%) and tumour (6%). Remote symptomatic epilepsy was commonest in the elderly, where vascular disease accounted for 49% of cases. Tumour was a rare cause of epilepsy below the age of 30 years (1%), but accounted for 19% of cases between 50 and 59 years. Trauma caused 3% of cases: infection 2%. Acute symptomatic seizures occurred in 15%, and alcohol was the commonest single cause (6%), its incidence being highest between 30 and 39 years of age.

Duncan and Hart (6) have estimated from a variety of sources the number of people with epilepsy in a hypothetical UK population of 1 million people (Table 4.3). In a survey of 1347 patients from 31 practices in the Mersey Region, northern England, the overall prevalence for active epilepsy was 0.8% (13% of whom were children) of the population, of whom approximately a third of adults and 85% of children had attended hospital services on at least one occasion within the previous 12 months. Fifty per cent of adults and 29% of children had been seizure-free since the previous year and 24% of adults and 39% of children had more than one seizure per month. Twenty per cent of adults and 40% of children had some additional neurological, mental, or psychiatric handicaps. Over 90% were receiving at least one antiepileptic drug. The costs to the UK health service are therefore significant and have been estimated at approximately £110m (7). Total costs (both direct and indirect) have been estimated at £1930 million (8).

DIAGNOSIS

The diagnosis of epilepsy is clinical and is based on a detailed description of events experienced by the patient before, dur-

Table 4.2 International classification of epilepsies, epileptic syndromes, and related seizure disorders

Localization-related (focal, local, partial)	Generalized
Idiopathic (primary)	
Benign childhood epilepsy with centrotemporal spike	Benign neonatal familial convulsions
Childhood epilepsy with occipital paroxysms	Benign neonatal convulsions
Primary reading epilepsy	Benign myoclonic epilepsy in infancy
	Childhood absence epilepsy (pyknolepsy)
	Juvenile absence epilepsy
	Juvenile myoclonic epilepsy (impulsive petit mal)
	Epilepsies with grand mal seizures on awakening
	Other generalized idiopathic epilepsies
	• Epilepsies with seizures precipitated by specific modes of activation
Cryptogenic	*Cryptogenic or symptomatic*
Defined by:	West's syndrome (infantile spasms, Blitz–Nick–Salaam–Krämpfe)
• Seizure type (see Table 4.1, ICES)	Lennox-Gastaut syndrome
• Clinical features	Epilepsy with myoclonic-astatic seizures
• Aetiology	Epilepsy with myoclonic absences
• Anatomical localization	
Symptomatic (secondary)	*Non-specific aetiology*
Temporal lobe epilepsies	Early myoclonic encephalopathy
Frontal lobe epilepsies	Early infantile epileptic encephalopathy with suppression bursts
Parietal lobe epilepsies	Other symptomatic generalized epilepsies
Occipital lobe epilepsies	*Specific syndromes*
Chronic progressive epilepsia partialis continua of childhood syndromes characterized by seizures with specific modes of precipitation	Epileptic seizures may complicate many disease states
Undetermined epilepsies	
With both generalized and focal seizures	*Special syndromes*
Neonatal seizures	Situation-related seizures
Severe myoclonic epilepsy in infancy	• Febrile convulsions
Epilepsy with continuous spike wave during slow-wave sleep	• Isolated seizures or isolated status epilepticus
	• Seizures occurring only when there is an acute or toxic event due to factors such as alcohol, drugs eclampsia, non-ketotic hyperglycaemia
Acquired epileptic aphasia (Landau–Kleffner syndrome)	
Other undetermined epilepsies	
Without unequivocal generalised or focal features	

Adapted with permission from the commission on classification and Terminology of the International League Against Epilepsy (1989). (See Ref. 3.)

Table 4.3 The epidemiology of epilepsy in a hypothetical UK population of 1 million persons

Prevalence and incidence	No. of cases
Annual incidence of febrile seizures (50/100 000)	500
Annual incidence of single seizures (20/100 000)	200
Annual incidence of new cases of epilepsy (50/100 000)	500
Prevalence of active epilepsy (500/100 000)	5000
Cumulative lifetime incidence of a seizure (2000/100 000)	20 000
Requirements for medical care	
Institutions	400
Residential care	300
Need for continuing medical attention	3300
Need for occasional medical attention	2600

Reproduced with permission from Duncan, J. and Hart, Y. M. (1991). *Epilepsy towards tomorrow.* Office of Health Economics, London.

ing, and after a seizure and, more importantly, on an eye witness account. In view of the social and economic implications, diagnostic errors need to be avoided at all costs. Thus, the first basic rule about diagnosing epilepsy is never to make the diagnosis without incontrovertible clinical evidence. If there is any doubt, the clinician should resist the temptation to attach a label and should rely on the passage of time and the further description of symptomatic events to reach a firm conclusion. Hardly anyone with epilepsy will come to any harm from a delay in diagnosis, whereas a false-positive diagnosis is gravely damaging. It seems essential that the diagnosis is made by someone with expertise in the area. While the diagnosis may be straightforward in some cases, in many it may be difficult. Referral to general physicians and other non-neurological specialists is inappropriate.

The events at the start of attacks must be determined. Do they occur without warning or are they preceded by symptoms of an epileptic aura (see below)? Are they preceded by faintness or syncope? Specifically epileptic symptoms include involuntary tonic or clonic movements lateralized to one side of the body, olfactory or gustatory hallucinations, and the complex perceptual changes associated with temporal lobe seizures—'it is indescribable'. Symptoms recorded by the patient after recovery of consciousness are also important. The presumptive diagnosis of a seizure may be secure when an individual wakes in a wet bed with a bitten tongue and complains of a headache and muscular aches and pains.

Most eye witnesses will be able to give a reasonable description of a tonic-clonic (grand mal) seizure. However, it may be harder to get a satisfactory description of more minor seizures. Here, direct questioning is often important, especially to elicit the characteristic features often associated with complex partial seizures—a fixed, motionless stare with subsequent automatisms that may include fidgeting, repetitive movements with the hands, or chewing or swallowing movements. Documentation of post-ictal confusion by an eye witness may be very important.

When the doctor has acquired as much clinical information as possible, he/she may be able to make certain judgements.

IS IT EPILEPSY?

Other causes of the events need to be considered. Syncope and pseudoseizures are most frequently mistaken for epilepsy (Table 4.4). Video-telemetry EEG (+/− ECG) monitoring has certainly allowed more definitive diagnoses to be made and help characterize the different causes more fully (9–12).

Syncope

Is defined by loss of consciousness and postural tone secondary to acute cerebral hypoxia (13). There are often obvious precipitants (e.g. emotional upset) but in other cases it remains unclear as to the trigger factor. Certain other features may assist in making the diagnosis: premonitory symptoms, such as nausea, sweating, lightheadedness, blurred/tunnel/greying vision, feeling distant; incontinence and tongue biting are extremely uncommon; duration is short (i.e. <25 seconds); recovery is rapid; post-ictal confusion is unusual; EEG during an episode often shows slowing, attenuating to a flat trace (14); prolactin levels are not usually increased (see below).

In an excellent study by Lempert *et al.* (12), video analysis of 56 induced syncopes demonstrated that myoclonic jerks were commonly associated (90%). They were usually multifocal or generalized and never preceded the fall. Forty-eight per cent fell flaccidly whereas the remainder fell stiffly with their legs

Table 4.4 Differential diagnosis of epilepsy

Syncope
Reflex syncope:
• Postural
• Psychogenic
• Carotid sinus syncope
• Micturition syncope
• Valsalva
Cardiac syncope:
• Dysrhythmias (heart block, tachycardias, etc.)
• Valvular disease (especially aortic stenosis)
• Cardiomyopathies
• Shunts
Perfusion failure:
• Hypovolaemia
• Syndrome of autonomic failure

Psychogenic attacks:
• Pseudoseizures
• Panic attacks
• Hyperventilation
• Night terrors
• Breath-holding

Transient ischaemic attacks
Migraine
Narcolepsy
Hypoglycaemia

Reproduced with permission from Appleton R. E. *et al* (1994). In *Epilepsy*. 3rd edn, p. 24. Martin Dunitz Ltd., London.

extended. Auditory and visual hallucinations occurred in 60% of cases but no olfactory phenomena were reported.

Cardiac syncope must not be missed and a search for an underlying arrhythmia should be made. Particularly important in this group is the prolonged QT syndrome. Although this condition was originally described in 1957 (15) it has only been recognized as an imitator of epilepsy since the 1980s (16–21). It may be hereditary or acquired. The misinterpretation as epilepsy has only been described with the hereditary causes. These include two eponymous syndromes: Jervell and Lange–Neilsen syndrome which is inherited in an autosomal recessive manner with nerve deafness; Romano–Ward syndrome with no accompanying deafness and autosomal dominant inheritance. These eponyms will no doubt be superseded as the ion channels (and the genes responsible for them) have recently been discovered (22,23).

The incidence is approximately 1 in 10 000. Mortality rate (from ventricular arrhythmias) for untreated patients may be as high as 71% in 15 years (24). In a review of 10 patients, Pacia *et al.* (21) found that the mean age at the time of first convulsion was 4.7 years. The age range for onset was 6 months to 16 years. The main reasons cited for misdiagnosis were: (1) patient was too young at onset to describe premonitory symptoms (dizziness, etc.); and (2) insufficient direct questioning of the witness (19). Singh *et al.* (19) recommended asking the witness whether the patient became still, 'like a dead body' prior to the convulsion. They suggested five points in the history which would strongly suggest long QT syndrome in young children:

1. Episodes of loss of consciousness preceding convulsions.
2. Episodes of loss of consciousness alternating with episodes of loss of consciousness and convulsions.
3. Patients whose convulsions respond to anticonvulsants but who continue to have episodes of loss of consciousness.
4. Family history of sudden and unexplained death.
5. History of deafness in the patient or other family member.

The presence of any of the above features should lead the physician to first check a number of baseline ECGs, as a single trace may be normal (25). A prolonged QT interval is usually taken as a QTc (i.e. QT/square root of R-R interval) of >0.44 but genetic studies have suggested that this is not always the case (26). An exercise ECG should be performed if there is any doubt.

Beta-blockers are the treatment of choice with excellent results. Other therapies may become available now that the ion channels responsible for three of the heritable conditions have been elucidated. Families of affected individuals should be screened for the genetic markers known to occur as well as having cardiological investigations.

Drop attacks are usually associated with already apparent symptomatic generalized epilepsy or partial seizures. The distinction is normally obvious but occasionally syncopal episodes can mimic complex partial seizures.

Cataplectic attacks are nearly always brought on by emotion e.g. laughter or anger and in 90–94% of cases are associated with narcolepsy (for a comprehensive review see Ref.27), so diagnosis should not be difficult. Having said this, many of these patients remain undiagnosed or misdiagnosed for several years.

Pseudoseizures

These are otherwise known as psychogenic seizures or non-epileptic seizures. They are events that may resemble epileptic seizures (and importantly may coexist) but are not accompanied by an underlying electrical disturbance. However, these patients often harbour underlying psychopathology (28). A common presentation is 'uncontrollable seizures' despite reasonable doses of anticonvulsants. In a series reported by Leis et al. (29), 13% had been treated as for status epilepticus. In pseudoseizures (PS), emphasis should be put on:

(1) Early recognition; and
(2) a secure diagnosis, made on the basis of a combination rather than any single 'test'.

Early recognition and treatment, as with other psychogenic disorders, seems to confer a better outcome long term (30). As discussed above, an incorrect diagnosis can lead to adverse psychosocial and economic effects.

Diagnosis is a minefield. History and an eye witness account are still extremely important. If a diagnosis of PS is thought likely, a full psychiatric history should be obtained (31).

Several papers (10,32,33) have been written on clinical features that aid differential diagnosis but none are good enough alone. The advent of video-telemetry EEG has probably been the greatest step forward but this too cannot be taken in isolation (29,33–41).

The main differential diagnoses to exclude are simple and complex partial seizures (especially frontal), as these may cause bizarre behavioural/motor manifestations and may have a normal ictal scalp EEG (42,43). Frontal complex partial seizures can, of course, be associated with psychiatric disturbance from the underlying pathology. The following features would point towards a diagnosis of PS: lack of stereotypies; asynchronous movements of extremities; longer duration (often with consciousness maintained) (10); lack of cyanosis or tongue biting; forced eye closure (44) and resistance to passive limb movements; do not occur during EEG confirmed sleep and may be preceded by a period of pseudo-sleep (36,45,46); patient does not turn to prone during episode (41); the patient may weep (47). Unlike Boon and Williamson (10), Saygi et al. found that history of psychiatric illness, body rocking, pelvic thrusting, pedalling, and rapid post-event recovery were as common in PS as in patients with proven frontal seizures (41). However, the latter often had magnetic resonance imaging (MRI) abnormalities. Incontinence has been reported in PS and can therefore not be relied on.

Most patients need no further investigation than that described above, to confirm or refute a diagnosis of pseudoseizures. In a small minority, seizure induction, post-event plasma prolactin levels, and more extensive neuroimaging may be helpful (the latter will be discussed in the section on neurological imaging below).

If handled sensitively and openly, seizure induction is ethically acceptable. The patient often has their medication reduced and under video-telemetry EEG is given a stimulus (e.g. intravenous normal saline), with the suggestion that it is likely to provoke a seizure. Several investigators have reported good results, interpreted with an element of caution (48–50). Slater et al. found that none of their 41 patients with a final diagnosis of epilepsy were inducible. Twenty-nine patients out of 32 with a final diagnosis of PS were inducible (50). As a single test it cannot, however, be depended on. This was well demonstrated by the fact that 2 out of 20 confirmed epileptic patients in the study by Walczak et al. had inducible episodes (49).

Despite the fact that plasma prolactin levels have been shown to rise after seizures (51), there are a number of pitfalls in using them to discern between PS, syncope, and bone fide fits: prolactin levels exhibit both diurnal and interindividual variation (52); the rise and fall of the plasma concentration is rapid (peak within 30 minutes of the attack, returning to basal levels after approximately 1 hour), leaving only a narrow window of opportunity for testing (53); drugs may alter prolactin levels (incl. psychotropics); prolactin levels may not rise following simple partial and complex partial seizures (54); some episodes of syncope can give rise to significant elevation of prolactin (55,56); the rise in prolactin level attenuates after multiple, sequential fits.

The best advice would appear to be that in the presence of a suggestive history, etc., a 3 to 4-fold increase in plasma prolactin (taken within 30 minutes of the first event) would be further evidence that the episode was epileptic.

Treatment of PS should involve a multidisciplinary approach, including psychiatric input (28,57). Prognosis, although variable, seems to be better in those who receive some sort of treatment and whose episodes and psychiatric disturbance come under control at an early stage (30).

WHAT KIND OF EPILEPSY?

The classification of seizures has important implications in terms of need to search for an underlying pathology, treatment, and prognosis. An acute symptomatic cause for a single seizure needs to be excluded in the first instance (e.g. alcohol, fever, drugs, metabolic disturbance). These are usually associated with confusional states or systemic disturbance that often outlast the seizures themselves. If no such abnormalities are found, a spontaneous epileptic disorder is probable. The question now is whether the episodes are partial or generalized (see Table 4.1). This may not always be as straightforward as it sounds. Ictal and interictal EEG can assist in this distinction. The second step is to see if the clinical scenario corresponds to any of the more specific epilepsy syndromes (see Table 4.2). Again, certain direct questions may need to be asked during history taking (e.g. morning myoclonus, automatisms) and correlated with EEG findings. The terms *idiopathic*, *symptomatic*, and *cryptogenic* need to be understood to follow the classification: *idiopathic* suggests no underlying cause other than a possible genetic predisposition; *symptomatic* relates to a probable underlying central nervous system disorder or lesion; *cryptogenic* are cases presumed to be symptomatic but the underlying cause is not known. In paediatric neurology an approach using both the above steps together with age of onset seems to aid diagnosis (58). It is important to note that more than one seizure type can occur in an epilepsy syndrome and that not all seizures will conform to a particular category.

PARTIAL SEIZURES (LOCALIZATION-RELATED)

Simple partial seizures alone are not accompanied by loss of consciousness. Most commonly they involve motor or sensory symptoms. Psychic and autonomic symptoms occur less frequently. They result from a localized aberrant neuronal discharge ordinarily from a single hemisphere. These phenomena often constitute the aura of a complex partial or secondary generalized seizure. The event may be followed by a period of paralysis of the affected limb—Todd's palsy. This may only persist for a few hours but may last up to several days. Jacksonian seizures (or march) involve a spread of neuronal hyperactivity across the motor homunculus of the cortex, sometimes leading to secondary generalization.

Complex partial seizures are associated with loss or impairment of consciousness. The onset may or may not be heralded by a simple partial seizure and automatisms may be apparent during the ictal or post-ictal phase. The presence or absence of the latter two phenomena forms the basis for classification (see Table 4.1). The episodes are due to localized neuronal discharge that swiftly spreads to the other cerebral hemisphere.

The category of partial seizures becoming secondarily generalized is fairly self-explanatory.

Simple and complex partial seizures (especially of frontal origin) are notoriously difficult to pick up on inter-ictal and even ictal scalp EEG (42,59). Sleep (non-REM) and sleep deprivation act as strong activators of seizures, so that EEGs performed under these conditions may increase their yield without having to resort to more invasive monitoring.

LOCALIZATION-RELATED (PARTIAL) EPILEPSY SYNDROMES

IDIOPATHIC

Benign childhood epilepsy with centrotemporal spikes (rolandic epilepsy)

This is the second most common childhood epilepsy syndrome behind febrile seizures. It accounts for 15–20% of children with epilepsy. It has a male predominance and shows a complex mode of inheritance in contrast to the original idea that it was an autosomal dominant condition (61). Onset is between 4 and 10 years with spontaneous remission at puberty. Seizures begin as partial sensory or motor disturbance involving the face, pharynx, and larynx on one side often going on to involve the arm.

Consciousness is usually preserved unless the episode becomes secondarily generalized, which most commonly happens at night. The seizure frequency is low in most cases but if treatment is required, carbamazepine is probably the drug of choice. Electroencephalography (EEG) demonstrates spikes and spike waves in the centrotemporal region. These may be seen in unaffected relatives.

Childhood epilepsy with occipital paroxysms

Sometimes confused with migrainous episodes (62,63). They start with visual symptoms such as amaurosis or hallucinations. A unilateral clonic seizure may follow, with or without automatisms. The episode is often followed by a migrainous headache, hence the confusion. These seizures are much less common than rolandic epilepsy but otherwise have a similar age of onset and prognosis.

SYMPTOMATIC

Temporal lobe seizures

In the days of MRI, SPECT, and PET scanners it may seem a bit pointless in trying to localize the source of a seizure by the clinical features. This has recently been highlighted in a partly prospective study comparing clinical features with localization by EEG and neuroimaging (70). Certain characteristics still may assist in directing further investigation (64).

Temporal lobe epilepsy (TLE) accounts for more than 50% of partial seizures. In contrast to frontal lobe epilepsy, complex partial temporal lobe seizures more commonly: involve an aura, which may be of localizing value; last longer (1–2 minutes); start with a stare and oroalimentary automatisms (e.g. swallowing); include other, more simple automatisms (e.g. picking at clothes); are accompanied by simple vocalization; are followed by confusion, drowsiness, and a longer post-ictal phase (30 min or more). Secondary generalization is less common with temporal lobe epilepsy.

Manford *et al.* (70) found that seizures arising from the temporal lobes were more often characterized by absences and an onset of fear, experiential (e.g. déjà vu, etc.), or sensory phenomena. There were however a significant number of extratemporal lesions that were associated with the same elements and duration was a poor predictor of site. They did agree that oroalimentary automatisms were predictive of a temporal focus. Where onset was followed by an absence phase prior to motor activity, a temporal lesion was more likely.

Mesial temporal sclerosis is the most common underlying finding in temporal lobe seizures. There is usually a history of febrile seizures followed by a latent period running into the second decade. The onset of these episodes is often different to that of lateral temporal lobe seizures. The former classically begin with a rising epigastric sensation; emotions; fear; déjà/jamais vu; olfactory hallucinations; and occasionally autonomic symptoms/signs. Lateral temporal lobe seizures tend to be heralded by simple auditory or gustatory hallucinations, receptive aphasia, or partial sensorimotor phenomena.

Auras, as mentioned above, may take the form of psychic, amnesic, emotional, dysphasic, hallucinatory, or autonomic phenomena. Psychic phenomena include depersonalization (feeling detached from the body or actions) and derealization (feeling detached from the outside world). As well as disturbance of memory—which is frequently associated with TLE—the occurrence of déjà/jamais vu is probably due to interruption of the interface between the right and left temporal lobes and consequently memory sequencing. Although pleasurable ictal emotions have been described (65), they are most commonly unpleasant. Fear seems to be the most frequent emotion and certainly experimentally arises from the amygdala (66). Anger and violence are not so prevalent. Directed violence rarely, if ever occurs in the setting of TLE (67), which may become relevant in medicolegal manoeuvrings. A distinction needs to be made between dysphasia at the onset of a seizure and ictal or post-ictal dysphasia. In practical terms this is not always easy, but the latter would suggest a dominant temporal lobe focus (68).

Visual hallucinations, of a complex nature are the prevailing type in TLE. They may involve perversion of shape,

colour, distance or size (macropsia/micropsia). It has been suggested that most of these arise from the right hemisphere (64). Simple visual hallucinations tend to accompany occipital lobe episodes. Simple auditory phenomena arise from the lateral temporal lobe. Noxious olfactory auras originate in the anteromesial temporal lobe but may be associated with basal frontal foci. Gustatory auras seem to suggest foci in the parietal opercular region. Rising epigastric sensations are autonomic phenomena most frequently experienced with mesial temporal lobe events. They have, however been reported in mesial/orbital frontal seizures. Nausea, piloerection, palpitations, pupillary changes, and respiratory disturbance are also seen.

Auras do not always precede the onset of a complex partial temporal lobe seizure. Staring or arrest of previous action occurring at the beginning may cause confusion with absence seizures. The subsequent ictal and post-ictal automatisms suggest TLE but they are not constantly associated. As with auras, automatisms may take several forms. Swallowing, lip-smacking, and chewing (oroalimentary automatisms) are most common with mesial TLE (69,70). Simple rather than complex (e.g. cursing) vocalization would suggest a temporal lobe focus, the latter more indicative of a frontal seizure. Picking at clothing and fidgeting are simple repetitive actions typical of temporal lobe phenomena. When these actions are unilateral they are often ipsilateral to the focus and are associated with dystonic posturing of the contralateral upper limb. This is most frequently seen in TLE but may be seen with extratemporal foci (70–72). Contraversive (i.e. away from side of focus) movements of the eyes and head are of localizing value only if they are forced and tonic or clonic. Equally, extratemporal foci can give rise to these phenomena.

Although actions may arrest during the seizure, for example walking, they may persist as part of the automatic behaviour. Cursive (running) seizures, although rare, do occur.

Emotional outbursts are seen as automatisms. These are not unique to TLE. Dacrystic (crying) and gelastic (laughing) seizures can be localized to frontal or temporal foci (73). Gelastic seizures have also been reported in association with hypothalamic hamartomata (74). The seizures begin in early childhood and are associated with complex partial and generalized seizures with progressive cognitive decline.

Autonomic phenomena, such as those already described above may present as ictal events. Respiratory arrest, tachycardia, and vomiting have all been described.

Frontal lobe seizures

The frontal lobe is the second commonest site for partial seizures. In comparison to complex partial seizures arising from the temporal lobe, frontal complex seizures have: a less specific, non-localizing aura; a shorter duration (<60 s); more complex associated vocalizations; more complex, semi-purposeful automatisms; a greater propensity to secondarily generalize; an absent or very transient period of post-ictal confusion (75). These are by no means hard and fast criteria to define a frontal seizure. Somatosensory and Jacksonian motor seizures seem to allow a prediction of a frontal (peri-rolandic) lesion in most cases. Other characteristics outlined above could equally be observed in a temporal lobe event. Manford *et al.* (70) found that version and posturing, if occurring early in the seizure, may suggest a frontal focus. Interestingly, but perhaps not surprisingly, a few patients with frontal lesions experienced epigastric and olfactory phenomena which in the past would have been thought typical of TLE.

Because of their bizarre manifestations, frontal lobe seizures are often mistaken for pseudoseizures. This is further compounded by the fact that even ictal scalp EEG recordings may be normal (some characteristics which can help distinguish pseudoseizures are outlined above). The other catch is that rapid spread to the opposite hemisphere is common, leading to the erroneous diagnosis of primary generalized epilepsy.

Auras tend to be non-specific and auditory and visual hallucinations are sparse. Olfactory phenomena, fear, and autonomic disturbance do occur at onset. The automatisms can involve complex motor phenomena (e.g. pedalling, boxing, and pelvic thrusting). Seizures arising from the primary and supplementary motor regions are associated with a longer initial period of retained consciousness as opposed to almost immediate loss of consciousness with foci in other frontal areas (76). A brief description of seizures characteristic of these regions follows. There is obviously overlap between the regions as there is, on occasion, spread of seizure activity into the temporal lobes.

Primary motor area (rolandic) seizures tend to manifest as tonic-clonic motor phenomena affecting the face and arm with retained consciousness. Jacksonian march and Todd's palsy may follow.

Supplementary motor area (SMA) seizures seem to be more frequent during sleep which may prove useful in differentiating them from pseudoseizures. Bilateral bizarre motor activity can occur but usually the seizure starts with dystonic posturing of the contralateral arm and contraversion of the head and eyes (72). In the past, confusion also arose in distinguishing SMA phenomena from paroxysmal nocturnal dystonia. The latter is now recognized as a form a frontal seizure. Consciousness is usually retained with SMA seizures and speech arrest has been described.

Anterior (polar) frontal seizures are characterized by early loss of consciousness, contralateral tonic activity, contraversive head and eye movements, followed by secondary generalization. Pseudoabsences occur. Autonomic disturbance may be apparent.

Dorsolateral frontal seizures involve contraversive head and eye deviation with or without impaired consciousness, speech arrest, and occasionally forced thoughts. They may rapidly generalize but they can also become complex partial seizures with automatisms.

Cingulate gyrus seizures are often misdiagnosed and may mimic absence seizures. Scalp electrodes may not be sensitive enough to pick up the initial activity of the event. Simple seizures arising from this region often start with profound fear. Autonomic changes are common and sexual automatisms may occur.

Orbitofrontal seizures may include olfactory and gustatory phenomena with prominent autonomic features. The 'typical' clustered, short duration, rapid recovery, nocturnal episodes are more likely to emanate from here. Bipedal and bimanual motor manifestations and sexual automatisms are seen.

Occipital lobe seizures

Similar episodes to those described in childhood (see above) occur in adults with an occipital focus. Simple visual hallucinations, amaurosis, and head and eye deviation are typical. The important point is to appreciate this onset, as the seizures frequently spread to the temporal lobe, clouding the issue, leading to incorrect localization and treatment (77). The episodes can mimic classical migraine. An interesting association has been discovered between occipital lobe epilepsy, occipital lobe calcifications, and coeliac disease (78,79). Sturge–Weber syndrome may give a similar appearance.

Parietal lobe seizures

The regions with the largest cortical representation are most commonly involved. Sensory disturbance may therefore affect the face (even bilaterally), arm, or hand. This can spread like the motor seizures of a Jacksonian march. Strange abdominal sensations occur but visual hallucinations are uncommon. Vertigo has been described, possibly in association with lesions of the suprasilvian parietal lobe. Non-dominant parietal lobe lesions may lead to *episodic anosognosia*. This term was first coined by Babinski, describing a lack of awareness of a limb/ weakness of a limb. *Asomatognosia* is used interchangeably with this term. Paracentral lobule involvement can rarely lead to sensory phenomena in the lower limbs.

Epilepsia partialis continua (EPC)

This was first described in patients with encephalitis by Kojewnikow (80). It is basically a form of focal motor status epilepticus. The face, arm, or leg exhibit repeated clonic movements (distal muscles of the limbs most commonly) which may only persist for hours but can last months (81). The seizures do not generalize. Diffuse myoclonic jerks do, however, occur and some patients with EPC have been incorrectly diagnosed as having an extrapyramidal syndrome. An EEG will usually help in showing focal slowing or spike waves. This type of seizure disorder is often refractory to conventional anticonvulsant therapy.

GENERALIZED SEIZURES

These constitute the majority of epileptic disorders. Of them, tonic-clonic (grand mal) seizures are the commonest and probably the most straightforward to diagnose. The clinical picture and EEG appearance would suggest simultaneous activity in both cerebral hemispheres. An underlying structural lesion is unlikely but inherited metabolic disorders often give rise to this seizure type. In recent times most of the genetically determined epilepsies have also been found to be of generalized type.

Tonic–clonic seizures

Without warning, loss of consciousness is followed by the tonic phase with flexion of the limbs (mostly the arms) which then abduct, elevate, and externally rotate. The eyes are open and often deviate upwards. The tonic phase continues with extension of the back and neck followed by the limbs. The respiratory muscles are involved in this phase and the patient becomes apnoeic. There is cyanosis and dilatation of the pupils which are unreactive. This all lasts about 10–20 seconds.

The transition phase—between tonic and clonic components—is heralded by a mild generalized tremor which coarsens before leading on to powerful, rhythmic flexor spasms. Respiration does not return until this phase has come to an end. Autonomic disturbance is marked during this stage.

Once the clonic phase has died down, the patient is initially comatose and flaccid. In the recovery stage there is confusion, headache, and myalgia. This can last for several hours but most often is masked by the fact that the patient falls into an exhausted sleep.

Absence (petit mal) seizures

These are characterized by the sudden onset of a blank stare without warning. The patient is usually unresponsive during the episode which commonly lasts 5–15 seconds. There is little or no post-ictal period. Peak age at onset is 4–8 years (82,83). Onset does not occur in adulthood and the seizures rarely persist into adult life. The episodes are sometimes accompanied by mild clonic features (e.g. flickering of the eyelids), autonomic disturbance, and automatisms. In reference to the latter, chewing and lip-smacking may cause confusion with TLE. However, absence seizures are not preceded by an aura, are not usually followed by a post-ictal phase and have a typical EEG.

The characteristic ictal EEG shows generalized 3 per second spike wave complexes which are symmetrical (hyperventilation can provoke this response in inter-ictal recordings). The seizures are usually easily controlled with anticonvulsants. About half of the cases go on to develop other seizure types (often grand mal) which tends to be a bad prognostic indicator. Onset of seizures after age 9 does not bode well either. Actual intelligence does not seem to be impaired but psychosocial difficulties may arise later.

Atypical absences can involve impaired rather than absent responsiveness with atonic elements and automatisms. Tonic phenomena (including deviation of the eyes) with impaired consciousness can also occur. Patients with these seizures are more likely to have impaired intellect and do not have the distinctive EEG changes of typical absences. Atypical absences are part of the Lennox–Gastaut syndrome which is described below.

Myoclonic seizures

Myoclonus is a brief, shock-like jolt in a muscle giving rise to a sudden jerky movement. This can occur in healthy individuals (e.g. when just going off to sleep) but also occurs in myoclonic epilepsy. Patients with this, may only admit to morning myoclonus if directly asked about the phenomenon. They sometimes notice themselves that a generalized seizure only occurs on a day when they get the morning jerking. The usual story is that they spill their breakfast, etc. because of the movements. Myoclonus can occur with other seizure types (e.g. absences) and may be associated with rare progressive neurodegenerative conditions (e.g. Lafora body disease, Unverricht–Lundborg disease).

Identifying a person as suffering from myoclonic epilepsy is important in terms of prognosis and treatment (see below).

Clonic seizures

These are rare and may be most easily described as generalized tonic-clonic seizures without the tonic phase.

Tonic seizures

This type of seizure is more common during non-REM (rapid eye movement) sleep. They may initially be misconstrued as a normal stretching action. Ocular deviation, eyelid retraction, and dilatation of the pupils may occur together with more widespread autonomic disturbance. Axorhizomelic (from the Greek *rhiza* root, *melos* limb) tonic seizures cause axial muscle hypertonicity together with proximal limb muscle involvement leading to elevation of the shoulders and abduction of the arms.

GENERALIZED EPILEPSY SYNDROMES

IDIOPATHIC

These are best discussed in the order of age that they tend to occur.

Neonatal

Benign familial neonatal seizures

These are associated with an autosomal dominant pattern of inheritance (see below) and a good prognosis. They tend to start on the second or third day, leading to clonic seizures occurring many times a day. They will often remit before the age of six months. A few patients do, however, go on to develop epilepsy.

Benign neonatal convulsions

Otherwise known as 'fifth day fits', they rather unsurprisingly occur on day five of life. A familial link has not been demonstrated and there are no long-term sequelae. They are often clonic and can result in apnoea.

Infancy

Myoclonic epilepsy of infancy

This can be of severe or benign type. The severe form is similar to the syndrome of early myoclonic encephalopathy. Presentation occurs in the first few months, often in the presence of fever, with unilateral or bilateral clonic seizures. There is usually evidence of photosensitivity. Focal phenomena may develop including automatisms and autonomic disturbance. Developmental delay is frequently seen and the seizures are often refractory to treatment.

The benign form is characterized by episodes of repetitive jerks starting in the first or second year of life. Control is easily attained and development is not affected. Generalized seizures may occasionally follow in adolescence.

Childhood

Childhood absence seizures

As described above.

Adolescence

Juvenile absence epilepsy

This tends to be more associated with generalized tonic-clonic seizures and onset is around puberty. Seizures are less frequent than in the childhood variant and the EEG spike wave discharge may be faster (3.5–4 Hz).

Juvenile myoclonic epilepsy (JME)

This is also known as Janz syndrome following its first description in 1957 (84). It is quite common (about 5% of all epilepsy) and usually starts around puberty. On direct questioning, the patient describes myoclonic jerks that occur in the morning. In 90% of patients these will be followed by a tonic-clonic seizure on that day, before midday. Absence seizures may be present but not so frequently. Photosensitivity is common and other provoking factors are sleep deprivation and alcohol. EEG performed after sleep deprivation and during the morning may be characteristic with paroxysmal polyspike wave (85).

Distinction from generalised tonic-clonic seizures is important for two reasons. First, phenytoin and carbamazepine may have no effect on the seizures but the latter may also exacerbate them. Second, despite being adequately controlled with treatment, recurrence is common on withdrawal of medication. Therefore a more prolonged period of treatment is required.

This syndrome seems to have a strong hereditary element and studies have suggested that the gene may lie on chromosome 6p. However, some have found linkage (86) while others have not (87).

Epilepsy with generalized tonic–clonic seizures on awakening

This syndrome has its onset in late teens with seizures occurring predominantly on waking (88). There seems to be genetic predisposition. Other types of seizure coexisting are unusual. Photosensitivity is common, as is exacerbation by sleep deprivation. Most anticonvulsants will prove effective.

CRYPTOGENIC OR SYMPTOMATIC

These will be described in the age order in which they occur.

Infantile spasms

The main seizure type consists of spasms of flexion, extension, or a mixture of the two (89). They are often multiple and show high amplitude slow wave on EEG. The onset is usually between 3 and 12 months. Other seizure types can occur depending on the underlying cause (focal, tonic–clonic, and myoclonic).

West syndrome (90) is defined as the triad of infantile spasms, mental retardation and hypsarrhythmia (from Greek *hypsi* high) on the EEG. An underlying cause is found in 70–80% of cases. The most common are perinatal anoxia, trauma, or infection; cerebral malformations (e.g. tuberose sclerosis, lissencephaly); and metabolic disorders (e.g. phenylketonuria). Prognosis often depends on the aetiology but the seizures are frequently resistant to treatment. Severe intellectual disturbance is common. Occasionally, the syndrome leads on to more generalized seizures and to Lennox–Gastaut syndrome.

Although the mechanism is not clear, ACTH (adrenocorticotropic hormone) or prednisolone may be effective in treating West syndrome. Other possible useful therapies include sodium valproate, vigabatrin, and benzodiazepines. A thorough search for underlying focal abnormalities has been suggested by a number of investigators (91). Surgical intervention, in some highly selected cases identified with PET or SPECT, may lead to improvement in seizures.

Lennox–Gastaut syndrome

This may occur as a sequel to West syndrome and has similar aetiologies. It begins between the ages of 1 and 5 years. The patients exhibit a number of different generalized seizures. Most often axial tonic, atypical absence, atonic, and tonic-clonic seizures (92). Myoclonic seizures are less common and if prominent other syndromes should be considered. Up to 90% are significantly mentally retarded. The interictal EEG shows 1.5–2.5 Hz spike waves and generalized 10 Hz rhythms when asleep.

Prognosis is poor and treatment difficult. A compromise has to be found between seizure control and unacceptable side-effects of polypharmacy. Sodium valproate, lamotrigine, and benzodiazepines seem to be of benefit but phenobarbitone, phenytoin, carbamazepine, and steroids have all been used with an occasional favourable response. Anterior corpus callosotomy has been shown to ameliorate the atonic seizures.

Epilepsy with myoclonic-astatic seizures

These were first described by Doose *et al.* (93). Onset tends to be between 2 and 5 years of age. The main seizure type is myoclonic or myoclonic-astatic but generalized tonic-clonic seizures are the first manifestation. Atypical absences may also occur. There may be a period of remission but the outcome is variable. Prognosis is not as poor as for Lennox–Gastaut syndrome. Status epilepticus is quite common. The EEG shows 2–3 Hz spike waves that are bilaterally synchronous superimposed on a background of 4–7 Hz rhythms.

Epilepsy with myoclonic absences

This is characterized by absences with bilateral rhythmic myoclonus (94). Onset is between 5 and 8 years of age. They are frequently refractory to treatment and may evolve into other syndromes, including Lennox–Gastaut syndrome. Mental retardation is common. Ictal EEG demonstrates 3 Hz spike waves.

UNDETERMINED EPILEPSIES

Landau–Kleffner syndrome (acquired epileptic aphasia)

This was first recognized in 1957 (95). Onset is between 3 and 10 years, initially with loss of acquired language (receptive or expressive or both). Overt epileptic seizures may not occur but in 75% partial motor or generalized tonic-clonic seizures develop. The EEG shows focal or generalized epileptiform features that are more prominent during non-REM sleep. An underlying aetiology has not been discovered. SPECT studies have particularly pointed to the perisylvian cortex as a site of origin of both the seizures and the language deficit (96).

Despite the fact that the seizures are not difficult to control the language deficit rarely improves. Behavioural disturbance often develops later.

SPECIAL SYNDROMES

Febrile seizures

These are most common between the ages of 6 months and 5 years. In this range they may affect 3–5% of children (97). By definition, the episodes are associated with fever but not intracranial infection or underlying chronic central nervous system (CNS) disorders. Seventy-five per cent of the episodes are generalized, short-lived (<15 min), with no sequelae. Complicated febrile seizures may involve focal, prolonged events, status epilepticus, and even Todd's palsy.

The uncomplicated events lead to a small increase (2–5%) in the risk of epilepsy in later life. Thirty per cent of patients will have a further seizure associated with fever. Prophylactic therapy is not generally recommended but diazepam may be given for prolonged episodes.

There does seem to be a genetic element to febrile seizures (98). Those with a positive family history should be educated about the possibilities of seizures and their management. Patients with complicated febrile seizures seem to be at greater risk of developing mesial temporal sclerosis and the accompanying seizure disorder (99).

Reflex epilepsies

A detailed description of these phenomena is beyond the scope of this chapter but may be found in Ritaccio (100).

Since the majority of patients have spontaneous seizures as well as stimulus induced episodes, an alternative term that is used is 'epilepsy with reflex seizures'. These may be further divided into those associated with generalized seizures and those associated with partial seizures.

Reflex seizures characterized by generalized events include those precipitated by light and those provoked by thinking and decision making.

Partial seizure-associated reflex epilepsies include those induced by: reading; startle; somatosensory stimuli; proprioception; sound (including certain types of music); eating; immersion in hot water; and vestibular stimulation.

Seizures precipitated by light are the most common in this classification. A suggestive history and photoparoxysmal response to intermittent photic stimulation on EEG are the diagnostic criteria. (A photoparoxysmal response consists of generalized spike waves, not necessarily accompanied by convulsion.) The EEG response can, however, be seen in patients who do not develop epilepsy. In pure photosensitive epilepsy no spontaneous seizures occur. That is, all episodes are set off by light stimuli including television, reflected sunlight, and disco lights. Juvenile myoclonic epilepsy is the syndrome most commonly associated with a strong photosensitive element.

Scoto-sensitive (associated with eye closure) epilepsy is less common. The provoked seizures may be tonic-clonic, absence, or myoclonic (101).

Treatment of epilepsy with reflex seizures first consists of trying to avoid the precipitant. In the case of light-induced seizures, other manoeuvres involve placing oneself more than 2.5 metres from the television set, monocular shielding, and the use of blue sunglasses (102). Conventional anticonvulsants are added if these measures do not suffice. It is important to realize that photosensitivity tends to continue into early adult life, but remission rates of 74% have been reported in the third decade, that is, withdrawal of therapy should not be considered too early in this condition.

Rasmussen's syndrome

This was first reported in 1958 (103). The peak age of onset is 3–6 years (range 1–15). The child usually has no significant past medical history but develops increasingly frequent simple partial motor seizures. Initially, there is no obvious structural abnormality on imaging. Epilepsia partialis continua (EPC) develops in 50% of cases. An inexorable neurological deterioration follows with severe impairment of cognition and hemiplegia together with focal cortical atrophy centred around the perisylvian region.

The aetiology of the condition still remains unclear. An autoimmune mechanism has been suggested and is supported by some of the neuropathological findings; the fact that approximately 50% of cases have cerebrospinal fluid (CSF) oligoclonal bands; the partial response to different immunomodulatory therapy; and the possible association with antibodies to the glutamate receptor GluR3 (104). Other reports would suggest a direct effect of viral infections. Ctyomegalovirus (CMV) and other herpes viruses have been detected in the brain biopsies of several cases. This prompted a non-controlled trial of ganciclovir with limited success (105).

It would, therefore, seem reasonable, in the early stages to try steroids, immunoglobulin, plasmapheresis, or ganciclovir. Subpial cortical transection may be a useful procedure in patients who have not yet developed a hemiplegia. If hemiplegia has already developed the best long-term results are gained with hemispherectomy (either disconnection or removal).

WHAT IS THE AETIOLOGY OF EPILEPSY?

No specific cause is found in about 60–70% of epileptics. Clues may be gained from the history by directly asking about perinatal events and development, severe head injury, CNS infection and family history. Virtually any cerebral pathology can give rise to seizures. Systemic disturbance (e.g. hypoxia, electrolyte imbalance, hypoglycaemia) can provoke seizures. The age of onset of the seizures may also give a hint towards the aetiology (e.g. in those over 60 years of age, cerebrovascular disease is a common cause).

Some important causes of epilepsy are outlined below.

Pyridoxine-dependent seizures

This is thought to be inherited in an autosomal recessive manner. Seizures start within the first 24 hours of life. Generalized seizures predominate and are refractory to all anticonvulsants. Intravenous pyridoxine (up to 100 mg) will lead to an immediate clinical response but the EEG may take a few weeks to settle. Unfortunately, most infants will show intellectual impairment despite treatment.

Genetic epilepsies

Conditions where both a genetic and environmental element contrive together to cause epilepsy (e.g. febrile seizures) will not be discussed. Likewise, hereditary structural abnormalities of the brain (e.g. periventricular heterotopia) are not outlined (for a review see Ref. 106).

Benign familial neonatal convulsions (as discussed above) are inherited in an autosomal dominant fashion and show genetic heterogeneity with loci on chromosome 20q (EBN1 locus, about 80% of cases) and 8q (EBN2 locus, about 20% of cases) (107,108).

Benign familial infantile convulsions (also as above) are also inherited in an autosomal dominant manner but have not shown linkage to either of the EBN loci.

Autosomal dominant nocturnal frontal lobe epilepsy was first differentiated by Scheffer *et al.* (109). Because of variable severity within families and 70% penetrance, the familial nature is not always appreciated. The seizures may be misconstrued as night terrors or psychiatric disturbances as they are brief, may be accompanied by retained awareness, and involve hyperkinetic motor seizures. The syndrome of paroxysmal nocturnal dystonia includes frontal lobe seizures of this type. Ictal EEG may help localize the seizures. Conventional anticonvulsants are usually effective (110). Linkage to chromosome 20q13.2 was found in one family and further investigation suggested that the defect was in the alpha4 subunit of the neuronal nicotinic acetylcholine receptor. This would raise the question as to whether disruption of the ion channel receptor is responsible, in some way, for seizure production (111,112).

Familial temporal lobe epilepsy, like nocturnal frontal lobe seizures above, is often missed. Penetrance is about 60% and it appears to an autosomal dominant disorder. The episodes are often typical of mesial temporal seizures. However, interictal EEG is frequently normal and MRI scans show no hippocampal atrophy or disturbed relaxometry. Treatment is usually straightforward (113,114). A single family with seizures more typical of lateral temporal lobe phenomena showed autosomal dominant inheritance and linkage to chromosome 10q (115).

Juvenile myoclonic epilepsy and its genetic links are discussed above.

There are numerous causes of progressive myoclonic epilepsy (116). Recently, the gene for Unverricht–Lundborg disease was cloned (117). The EPM 1 gene, on chromosome 21q, encodes cystatin B. This intracellular protein inhibits cathepsins (intralysosomal proteases). How this leads to the clinical picture of myoclonic epilepsy and neurological deterioration is as yet unknown.

Post-traumatic seizures

About 4% of epilepsy is caused by head trauma. Post-traumatic seizures can be immediate (at the time of the injury or within a few hours of it), early (within the first week), or late (beyond 5 years post-trauma). Immediate seizures do not predispose to epilepsy at a later date.

Overall, approximately 5% of non-missile head injuries (admitted to hospital) will develop late post-traumatic seizures. The main factors which increase this risk are a depressed skull fracture (31% increase); the presence of early post-traumatic seizures (25% increase); and the presence of an intracranial haematoma (15% increase) (118). Other contributory factors are post-traumatic amnesia (PTA), of more than 24 hours duration and in children, age under 2 years (119,120).

There is no evidence that prophylactic anticonvulsant therapy reduces the risk of late post-traumatic seizures (121). Therapy should be reserved for uncontrolled seizures that may otherwise hinder the patients recovery. Even in this situation, it has been argued that conventional anticonvulsants may have an adverse effect on functional recovery (122–124). Further studies on the newer anticonvulsants may lead to safer alternatives.

The risk from non-trauma-related neurosurgical lesions depends on the site and underlying pathology. For instance, clipping of an anterior cerebral artery aneurysm is more risky than a middle cerebral artery aneurysm in terms of increased incidence of late post-traumatic epilepsy (38% vs. 21%). Craniotomy for cerebral abscess carries the highest risk at 92% increased incidence.

INVESTIGATING EPILEPSY

Except in the acute situation, screening for biochemical or haematological abnormalities is rarely fruitful unless the history suggests otherwise (e.g. inborn errors of metabolism). The usual tests performed are, therefore, some form of neurophysiological investigation and neuroimaging.

OF WHAT VALUE IS THE EEG?

The electroencephalogram is used to record spontaneous electrical activity arising from the cerebral cortex. The 'normal' awake EEG varies with age but generally consists of mainly alpha and some beta rhythm (125). The alpha rhythm (8–12 Hz) may be rather asymmetrical and more prominent in the parieto-occipital regions. This rhythm is attenuated by eye opening and mental activity. Beta rhythm is a little faster (>12 Hz) but of lower amplitude and can be seen mainly over the frontal regions. Theta and delta are the slow waves and tend to be of greater amplitude than alpha and beta. Theta activity (4–7 Hz) can occur in normality, especially over the temporal regions and more so in patients over 60 years old. Delta waves (1–3 Hz) are not present in the normal awake adult. Spikes are high-voltage, peaked wave forms. If present on an inter-ictal recording of an epileptic patient they are referred to as epileptiform discharges.

Activating procedures are used to try to increase the yield of the resting EEG. As mentioned above sleep acts as a powerful activator (e.g. in temporal lobe seizures) but other manoeuvres include hyperventilation and photic stimulation (with a stroboscope). Reaction to these stimuli is age-dependent with children being far more sensitive.

The quality of neurophysiology services in the United Kingdom varies greatly. EEGs are often requested by clinicians who have little understanding of its sensitivity or specificity and reported by neurophysiologists or other specialists who have little or no clinical exposure to epilepsy. Rectifying these two failings would be a major step in improving epilepsy services.

The EEG provides valuable information that may: (1) add weight to the clinical diagnosis; (2) aid the classification of the epilepsy; and (3) show changes that may increase the suspicion of an underlying structural lesion.

As a diagnostic aid, the routine inter-ictal EEG is one of the most abused investigations in clinical medicine and is unquestionably responsible for great human suffering. The diagnostic value of an inter-ictal EEG is widely misunderstood. EEGs are often requested either to exclude or confirm a diagnosis of epilepsy—something that can seldom, if ever, be done. Between 10% and 15% of the population may have what may be construed as an 'abnormal' EEG; most such abnormalities are mild and of no diagnostic importance. By use of more rigid definitions of focal or generalized spike or polyspike and slow wave abnormality in the EEG, probably only 1% of a non-epileptic population have such abnormalities [this figure may be higher in children (126)]. A single waking inter-ictal EEG will show an epileptiform abnormality in about 50% of patients with epilepsy. This figure increases slightly with a second and third recording.

Scalp recording is influenced by intervening soft tissue and bone and particularly with deeply placed structures (mesial temporal lobe and orbitofrontal region) epileptic discharges can be difficult to detect. Special electrode placements (sphenoidal, foramen ovale) can be helpful in these situations. Video-telemetry EEG has been a major step forward in correlating the clinical picture with the underlying neurophysiological disturbance and is discussed further in the section on epilepsy surgery. The EEG is important as an aid to the diagnosis of pseudoseizures and particularly in reducing the morbidity associated with sedating and ventilating patients in pseudo-status epilepticus.

In terms of classifying epilepsy, the EEG is especially important in two clinical settings. In patients with seizures occurring without an aura that are characterized by a brief period of absence with or without automatism, it may be difficult to differentiate typical absence seizures from complex partial seizures. The finding of generalized spike wave or focal spike activity, respectively, will clarify the diagnosis. The distinction has important implications for the treatment and prognosis. In patients with tonic-clonic seizures without an aura, especially when these occur during sleep, the EEG can again differentiate between primary generalized epilepsies characterized by generalized spike wave and seizures with a focal onset in which there may be a localized disturbance.

Focal neuroimaging abnormalities are found in 70% of patients with focal slow wave activity on the EEG. It can therefore be used as aid to diagnosis of an underlying structural abnormality but not as the sole investigation.

WHAT NEUROIMAGING SHOULD BE PERFORMED?

It would seem reasonable that most adult patients with focal seizures should at least have a computerized tomographic (CT) scan of their head. Surveys of a somewhat selected population (epilepsy centres) with established epilepsy have shown that 60–80% may have an abnormal scan. These abnormalities were, however, mostly atrophic. Tumours were picked up in about 10%. Patients who present with a first seizure or early epilepsy have a much lower frequency (<20%) of anomalies which are again atrophic. As suggested above, the pick-up rate is much higher if there is a history of focal seizures and a focal EEG abnormality.

Magnetic resonance (MR) imaging should probably be restricted to patients with focal seizures and what are thought to be generalised seizures that prove to be refractory to anticonvulsant therapy. It is particularly useful in detecting hippocampal and mesial temporal atrophy and more recently for demonstrating neuronal migration disorders.

Further discussion of magnetic resonance imaging (MRI), single photon emission computerized tomography (SPECT), and positrm emission tomography (PET) techniques can be found in the section on epilepsy surgery.

COMMUNICATION AND COUNSELLING

1. DIAGNOSIS

The diagnosis of epilepsy is often frightening and disconcerting for patients and their families. There remains a considerable misunderstanding of the nature of the condition and it is one of the few organic neurological diagnoses still associated with considerable stigmatisation. For this reason patients need a careful explanation of the basis of epilepsy, an emphasis that it is an organic disorder and that it has no major associations with psychiatric disorder or stroke. Patients and their families need time to assimilate this information and to ask any relevant questions. Supplementary written information is extremely valuable and the various epilepsy associations are good sources of this. Very often, doctors are poor information-givers and patients may feel unable to ask the questions that they want answered. As clinical time is often limited, intervention by knowledgeable counsellors or a specialist nurse probably represent a better way of addressing these issues. As yet this support is not widely available.

2. EFFECTS OF PROGNOSIS AND TREATMENT

At the time of diagnosis, patients do need to be given a clear indication of the likely outcome of their epilepsy and in particular whether treatment with antiepileptic drugs is necessary, and if so, for how long will they need to be maintained. Failure to provide satisfactory information is bound to complicate the problems of poor compliance in a chronic condition.

3. IMPLICATIONS OF EPILEPSY AND LIMITATION OF SOCIAL DISADVANTAGE

The unpredictable nature of epileptic seizures and the stigmatization and concealment that often comes with the diagnosis creates particular problems that must be addressed at an early stage. There can be a very considerable fear of accidental injury and indeed death. Any counselling about these risks needs to be put clearly in context. While sensible avoidance of higher risk situations needs to be emphasized, overprotection should be guarded against except in the most severe of epilepsies.

It is clear (see below) that patients can be identified who are at particular risk. For others, reassurance about the low risks of serious accidental injury appears appropriate, perhaps with advice to avoid climbing to significant heights, to use microwave cooking rather than gas or electric hobs, and to ensure fires are adequately guarded. Showers are preferred to baths and swimming in open water or unsupervised is best avoided. For most people, a full range of leisure activities should otherwise be possible with supervision if appropriate (e.g. cycling on a busy road).

For patients with frequent seizures complicated by falls, a greater level of supervision is required.

For children, satisfactory liaison with schools concerning the diagnosis of epilepsy is important and in particular teaching staff need to be reassured and advised about the child being able to fulfil as complete a range of school activity as possible. Epilepsy itself is rarely a reason for special education and most children will be in main stream schooling. Special education is usually necessary for those with associated mental or neurological handicap.

In the adult population the most important implications involve driving, pregnancy, and employment.

Driving and epilepsy

Losing their driving licence has a profound effect on most adults in terms of independence and employment. Not surprisingly, this leads to a lot of concealment. In a study of 2000 police reported accidents due to drivers collapsing at the wheel but surviving (127), the largest number were due to epileptic seizures. Of those with established epilepsy, 71% had failed to declare their condition to the UK DVLA (Driver and Vehicle Licensing Agency).

During counselling, it should be made clear that a diagnosis of epilepsy will prohibit the patient from driving and that it is his/her responsibility to inform the DVLA (this advice should also be recorded in the notes). It should be stressed that driving under these circumstances is illegal and will invalidate insurance cover. To maintain the doctor–patient relationship, it needs to made clear that the doctor has no legal responsibility to inform the DVLA. If, however, every effort to gain patient compliance has failed and it is judged to be in the best interests of the patient or public, confidential information may then be disclosed to the licensing authority.

The current regulations (128) for patients with epilepsy allow a licence to be granted if:

(1) the patient has been seizure free for one year (with or without treatment); *or*
(2) the patient has had seizures *only* while asleep, and this pattern has persisted for 3 years; *and*
(3) allowing the patient to drive is not likely to be a danger to the public.

The patient must be made aware that the regulations do not just relate to tonic-clonic episodes but also include simple partial seizures and brief absences.

In the case of an isolated seizure without an obvious precipitant the one-year seizure-free period will still apply before a licence is granted (depending on the study, between 30% and 80% of patients with a first seizure will have another in the following two years). Acute symptomatic seizures (i.e. with a clear provoking factor) still need to be reported but the patient may be allowed back to driving at an earlier date. Obviously, a single seizure accompanied by an EEG showing a generalized 3 Hz spike wave will be accompanied by the full regulation period.

Seizures occurring while the patient is asleep are not the same as nocturnal seizures. Not all nocturnal seizures occur during sleep and attacks while asleep can occur during the day.

Withdrawal of anticonvulsant therapy is discussed in detail later but patients in remission, who have had there licence returned, may request that they come off medication. The risk of a seizure in the two years following withdrawal is about 40–50%. Most of this risk occurs in the period of dose reduction and within six months of stopping therapy. Therefore, patients wishing to cut down and stop their medication should be advised not to drive for six months *after discontinuation* of the treatment.

Pregnancy and epilepsy

Women of childbearing age do not necessarily plan to get pregnant. The first advice, therefore, should be about contraception. In choosing an anticonvulsant in this age group, if possible, anticonvulsants that are not inducers of the cytochrome p450 system are preferable: that is, phenytoin, phenobarbitone, carbamazepine, and more recently, oxcarbazepine and topiramate will all increase the metabolism of oestrogen hence increasing the likelihood of contraceptive failure. Sodium valproate, gabapentin, and lamotrigine do not induce the p450 system and therefore do not reduce the efficacy of the oral contraceptive pill (OCP). Vigabatrin probably does not interfere either (129). If an enzyme inducer cannot be avoided then the patient should be advised to take an OCP with at least 50 µg (microgram) of oestrogen (regular OCP has 35 µg) or another form of contraception suggested (eg barrier method).

PRIOR TO CONCEPTION

Ideally, the patient should be counselled well before the stage that she wishes to get pregnant. This is unfortunately not always possible. If control is good, one could argue that there is no good reason to change to a drug of perceived lower risk, unless perhaps the patient has a family history of neural tube defect, when valproate and carbamazepine may not be advisable. It is a decision between the physician and the patient, on an individual basis as to whether the newer antiepileptic drugs are continued, as not enough experience has been gained with these medications to assess their safety (see section on Treatment below). The patient should preferably be on monotherapy with the lowest dose possible that best controls the seizures. Preconception seizure frequency predicts the likely control during pregnancy (130). Folate supplementation (4 mg daily) is recommended *before* becoming pregnant, to decrease the frequency of neural tube defects particularly (131–133).

The risks associated with pregnancy should be fully explained and information given so that the patients feel that they are actively involved in minimizing these. It should be stressed that although there is an increased risk of major congenital malformations (4–6% as opposed to 2–3% in non-epileptic mothers) that more than 90% of women with epilepsy will have normal babies. More minor abnormalities, comprising the fetal anticonvulsant syndrome (134) may occur in <10% of cases.

PREGNANCY

Seizure frequency has been reported to increase in about 20% of pregnancies (135) and the main contributory factors are noncompliance, sleep deprivation, and pharmacokinetic changes of pregnancy.

Unfortunately, the view that any medication taken during pregnancy is harmful is taken a little too far and the risks to the mother and fetus of seizures are not emphasized. The patient should be reassured that on one drug, at a low dose the chances of fetal abnormality are small and the benefits of compliance spelled out (i.e. to prevent seizures causing miscarriage, haemorrhage, eclampsia, etc.). As with epilepsy in the general population, sleep deprivation can lead to deterioration in seizure control and the patients should try to modify their lifestyle accordingly.

Physicians are not always aware of the pharmacokinetic changes in pregnancy. Although total plasma levels of anticonvulsants decline during the course of pregnancy, the free drug levels (i.e. active) do not drop so markedly and in fact may increase (valproate). The main mechanisms for the fall in total levels are decreased plasma protein binding, reduced albumin concentration, and increased drug clearance (135). Dosage alterations should be made primarily if the patients clinical condition changes, that is, although drug levels should be monitored they should not be acted on unless seizure control or side-effects are unsatisfactory. In refractory cases free drug levels should be used. Devinsky and Yerby (135), however, advocate maintenance of drug levels within the therapeutic range during the last trimester, when the medication will have less of an effect on the fetus. The rationale being that this is when the fetus is at greatest risk of trauma from a generalized seizure and that it may prevent some of the 1–2% of seizures that occur during labour.

In view of the risks of cardiac, neural tube, and limb defects associated with anticonvulsant medication, most women will have an ultrasound examination at around 18 weeks. If this is equivocal amniocentesis may be advised.

Vitamin K supplements (20 mg/day) should be administered in the 3–4 weeks up to the presumed date of delivery. This will prevent neonatal haemorrhage and is given in addition to the vitamin K administered to the neonate.

Throughout the pregnancy it is imperative that the obstetric and neurology team co-operate and communicate regularly.

LABOUR AND THE POST-PARTUM PERIOD

If seizures do occur during labour or the immediate post-partum period, benzodiazepines are the drug of choice. Drug levels should be monitored up to eight weeks post-partum as they often rise and may lead to toxicity, which is particularly important if the patient is breast feeding. Nearly all the anti-convulsants are excreted in the breast milk. The drugs that are highly protein bound tend to be present in lower concentrations. Breast feeding is not recommended while being treated with phenytoin, vigabatrin, gabapentin, or topiramate. Infants can become sedated when being breast fed by a mother on phenobarbitone and this needs to be carefully monitored.

Employment and epilepsy

Even in these days of equal opportunities people with epilepsy still experience an unwarranted amount of discrimination when applying for jobs. Counselling should involve advice about how and when to disclose a history of epilepsy to a prospective employer. Certain types of employment are off limits because of statutory limitations—driving of public service and heavy goods vehicles, airline pilot, train driver, armed forces—but other employers dismiss epileptics with few sound reasons. The employers need educating about the relatively few situations when epileptic staff can be put at risk. Working at heights and close to large expanses of water should be avoided. The perceived danger of working with machinery demands individual evaluation, as most such machinery should, in this day and age, be adequately protected.

4. COMPLICATIONS OF EPILEPSY

Patients' concerns regarding the possibility of premature death and the risk of injury secondary to epilepsy are often not addressed. Reassurance about the low risk of either in a person with well-controlled seizures should be given along with advice about how to minimize the likelihood of injury.

Accidental injury

Injuries due to falling are not uncommon in people with epilepsy but most are not severe. Intuitively, these are more likely to occur in patients whose epilepsy involves frequent loss of consciousness with or without falls. Unfortunately, very few systematic analyses have been performed and indeed, no prospective study of incidence of these events has been undertaken.

Hauser *et al.* (136) showed that patients with epilepsy were over-represented in a study of non-fatal head trauma. These patients accounted for 7.4% of admissions to five New York hospitals, which was three times the expected incidence for a population of similar age distribution. In another study, 2.7% of seizures resulted in a clinically significant head injury although only 1 in over 9000 seizures resulted in skull fracture or intracranial haematoma (137).

A number of investigators have reported the high incidence of burns in epileptic patients (138–141). Hampton *et al.* (139) reported that of a population of patients with epilepsy, 38% had a history of burns with 13% seeking hospital treatment. Of the latter, 4% required admission and 1% skin grafting. Those who sustained burns were older, had a longer history of epilepsy and were more likely to have complex partial seizures. Spitz *et al.* (141) surveyed 244 patients with epilepsy. Ten per cent had burns significant enough to warrant medical attention and half of these required admission. The risk factors appeared to be high seizure frequency, inter-ictal neurological impairment, and female sex. The latter was explained by cooking-related injuries.

From the above, as with other epilepsy-related complications, it can be seen that reducing seizure frequency is important in minimizing the risks of injury. Simple advice about kitchen appliances (e.g. using a microwave oven as opposed to hob cooking) and perhaps occupational therapy input is just as important.

Mortality in epilepsy

Although most patients with a new diagnosis of epilepsy will have a favourable outcome, they do have a significantly higher mortality rate than the general population. The prospective, community based study by Cockerell *et al.* (142) put the overall standardized mortality ratio (SMR) for patients with definite epilepsy at 3. This value included patients with symptomatic (e.g. underlying tumours) as well as idiopathic epilepsy. Consequently, the SMR was highest in the first year of diagnosis (5.1) and thereafter declined. For remote symptomatic epilepsy alone, the SMR was 4.3. The SMR for idiopathic epilepsy alone was 1.6.

Deaths in epilepsy can be considered as unrelated to the epilepsy, related to the underlying disease causing the seizures or related to the epilepsy. Unrelated deaths would include conditions that lead to death in the general population (e.g. myocardial infarction or cancer). Underlying conditions that may cause seizures and lead to death would include cerebrovascular disease, cerebral tumours, and CNS infection.

Several causes of epilepsy-related deaths are avoidable. Drowning is a common cause usually relating to a fit while having a bath or swimming unsupervised. Status epilepticus has an associated mortality of about 18% (143). Suicide incidence is greater in the epileptic population and in some cases may be unavoidable (144). However, early signs and symptoms of depression should be acted on urgently and a psychiatric opinion sought. Preventing asphyxiation and aspiration as a direct effect of a fit depends greatly on when and where it occurs.

A lot of interest in recent years has centred on the phenomenon of sudden unexpected death in epilepsy (SUDEP). Jay and Leestma (145) defined SUDEP as 'non-traumatic death occurring in an individual within minutes or hours of the onset of the final illness or ictus, the individual having been previously relatively healthy, or suffering from a disease which would not ordinarily be expected to produce immediate or sudden death'. Cockerell (146) added that no cause can be found at autopsy and deaths immediately after a seizure are excluded. It tends to occur in younger age groups and other risks factors for SUDEP include uncontrolled seizures, long-term institutionalization, polytherapy (which is obviously linked to refractory seizures), psychotropic therapy, male sex, and alcohol abuse. Unfortunately, the studies on the subject are difficult to compare because of lack of agreement in terms of definition and they mostly look at highly selected groups (147). Consequently, the estimates of incidence vary but a figure of 1 in 200 deaths per epilepsy patient per year has been suggested by Nashef *et al.* (148).

The underlying mechanism has not been categorically proven but is thought most likely to be secondary to an un-witnessed seizure. Although several studies have shown that sinus tachycardia is the only arrhythmia associated with seizures a number of case reports (149, 150) have documented significant bradycardia or asystole with seizures. Nashef *et al.* (151) took the investigation one step further by demonstrating episodes of centrally mediated apnoea preceding bradyarrhythmias. The suggestion being that cardiorespiratory reflexes (triggered by apnoea) mediate the disturbance.

Whatever the cause for SUDEP it seems obvious that the known risk factors should be minimized in the individual, including tight control of seizures and more vigilant supervision in long-term care facilities.

Psychosocial handicap in epilepsy

The social, psychological, and emotional problems encountered with epilepsy have been extensively reviewed in terms of the severity of epilepsy, the additional effects of associated neurological handicaps including the effects of anti-convulsant therapy and the societal attitudes towards people with epilepsy (152, 153). High rates of psychosocial problems among individuals with epilepsy have been reported and these may be the result of the unpredictability and the severity of the seizures, rather than their frequency. No matter how well-controlled a person's seizures are, the fear of seizures may always be present, for epilepsy is as often a threat as an active condition (154). The fear evoked by the unpredictable nature of the seizures may lead to social withdrawal, with loss of existing friendships and an inability to form new relationships. Loss of employment or inability to compete in the job market may lead to loss of self-esteem and financial hardship. These factors not infrequently result in anxiety, depression, and a loss of sense of control (153, 155). The patient should receive adequate counselling and advice regarding gaining employment (e.g. retraining schemes) and benefits available.

Psychiatric disorders and epilepsy

The relationship between epilepsy and psychiatric disorders has evoked much discussion. A number of studies on unselected populations of patients have demonstrated an increased incidence of psychiatric illness in patients with epilepsy (156, 157). These studies provide evidence that the increased incidence occurs in both adults and children and that having epilepsy rather than other chronic conditions is associated with increased psychopathology. A general practice survey (158), using an accurate measure of psychiatric disorder and a detailed examination of the seizure type, has shown that psychiatric morbidity (especially anxiety and non-psychotic depression) occurs more commonly in people with epilepsy than would be expected by chance and is particularly common in patients with focal as opposed to primarily generalised epilepsy.

There have been a number of conflicting studies investigating the incidence and prevalence of psychosis in patients with epilepsy. Pond and Bidwell (156) in a study of 14 general practices found 29% of their sample had a history of psychiatric illness but none had been, or were, psychotic. In contrast, a number of hospital outpatient studies (159, 160) have reported an incidence of between 2% and 5%. In an earlier study of 69 patients with schizophrenia-like psychosis, 80% were found to have focal temporal lobe EEG abnormalities (161), leading the authors to conclude that the characteristics of the psychoses accompanying epilepsy were distinct from functional psychosis. This finding has not, however, been confirmed in subsequent prospective studies (162).

As already stated, suicide and self-harm are more common in patients with epilepsy in comparison to the general population. Exact figures are difficult to acquire but Barraclough (144) estimated that the incidence in people with temporal lobe epilepsy was five times that of the general population.

If seizures can be controlled by medication and if patients are provided with adequate information about the extent to which their lives may or may not be restricted, then they may be capable of developing effective coping strategies and avoid such extreme measures as suicide. Early recognition of and intervention for depression must be stressed.

5. SHARING CARE

Because of the variable nature and severity of the epilepsy, no single system of care is appropriate for all patients and many different agencies may become involved. For this reason, effective liaison should occur between these agencies, with the primary aim of offering continuity of care with a single clearly identified clinician having the prime responsibility for the medical management of the individual patient.

The diagnosis and initiation of treatment of epilepsy will usually require specialist skills. However, the majority of patients with newly diagnosed epilepsy quickly enter a remission and at this stage the patient's general practitioner can usually assume responsibility. Re-referral to specialist services may be required after two to three years remission for counselling about drug withdrawal. Patients with poorly controlled seizures may also benefit from specialist referral for reconsideration of the diagnosis, second line or newer drug therapy, or where appropriate, surgical treatment. There is no doubt that standards of care could frequently be improved by better liaison between primary care and specialist services. The use of liaison cards for epilepsy is poorly developed and would seem highly appropriate. Shared care systems for people with diabetes have made extensive use of nurse practitioners as 'key workers'. Gradually, we are seeing the introduction of similar nurses in epilepsy services but their provision is still too patchy. These nurses help to improve communication between the specialist services and the general practitioners together with other agencies (e.g. learning disability team, psychiatric services).

One area where communications frequently breakdown is in the transfer of care of people with epilepsy from paediatric to adult care. This is a particularly traumatic time, in that the state guarantees the individual a place in society with his/her peer group up until the age of 16 but after leaving school no such guarantee is extended to further education, training, or employment. At the same time, the young person is often discharged from the well-integrated paediatric services and has to cope with forming relationships with a new adult clinician who is less well equipped to provide a comprehensive system of clinical and social support. Here, there seems to be a clear role for joint specialist clinics run by paediatricians and adult neurologists to facilitate the process of handover of care.

6. PROGNOSIS

Most patients when told that they have epilepsy will want to the know whether their condition will remit and when. The data available on this subject are improving but suffer from variable periods defined as a remission and variable follow-up

duration. Many of the studies have been hospital-based and therefore probably underestimate favourable outcome.

Two studies of importance, were community-based. Annegers *et al.* (163) studied 457 patients in Rochester, USA, with a history of two or more non-febrile seizures, with follow-up for at least 5 years and in 141 for 20 years. The probability of being in a remission lasting 5 years or more was 61% at 10 years and as high as 70% at 20 years (Fig. 4.2). Cockerell *et al.* (164), in their update of the initial results of the BNGPSE study, reported their findings of a 9-year follow-up period. They reported on the original cohort of 564 patients with definite epilepsy and 228 with possible/probable epilepsy. From the index seizure (the seizure that registered the patient) 96% achieved a 1-year remission, 93% achieved a 2-year remission, 87% a 3-year remission, and 71% achieved a 5-year remission by 9 years follow-up (obviously, the figures represent patients who initially went into remission but subsequently relapsed). Looking at the underlying aetiology, those achieving a 5-year remission by 9 years was 69% for idiopathic seizures and 61% for remote symptomatic epilepsy.

Several factors are known to affect prognosis including age of onset, early course, and response to treatment, whether partial or primary generalized, particular epilepsy syndromes and whether the seizures are symptomatic (i.e. with an underlying lesion).

There is general agreement that the commencement of seizures within the first year of life (when it is usually sympto-

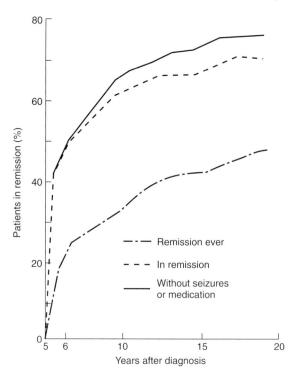

Fig. 4.2 Actuarial percentage of patients in remission after a diagnosis of epilepsy. (Reproduced with permission from Annegers, J. F. *et al.* (1979). *Epilepsia*, **20**, p729–37.)

matic of cerebral pathology), carries an adverse prognosis (165, 166).

The possible importance of the early course and treatment of epilepsy in its long-term outcome has been discussed in detail elsewhere (167). In this paper, data was analysed from a number of sources which showed that the frequency of both partial and primarily generalized seizures prior to treatment had an adverse effect on outcome and also that intervals between seizures may decrease progressively. Hauser *et al.* (168) showed that the risk of subsequent seizures increases from the first to the second and third seizures. The BNGPSE (164) reinforced these earlier findings.

Partial seizures have been thought to be more resistant to treatment than primarily generalized seizures. The 3-year remission rates at 9 years follow-up were 80% with partial onset and 91% with generalized onset (164).

Some of the outcomes from the different epilepsy syndromes have been discussed above. Between 70% and 80% of patients with simple absences are likely to enter remission (165, 169). Complex absences show a lesser remission rate of about 35–65% and in patients with the West or Lennox–Gastaut syndromes lower rates again can be expected.

Epilepsy of unknown aetiology has a better prognosis than symptomatic epilepsy (163, 170). In keeping with this, epilepsy complicated by an associated neurological or psychiatric deficit carries an adverse prognosis (165).

An attempt to quantify the weight that prognostic factors carry was made by Shaffer *et al* (171). The group examined the prognosis of 306 patients diagnosed between 1935 and 1978 and used Cox's proportional hazards model to investigate those factors determining the likelihood of achieving a 5-year seizure-free period and a 5-year seizure-free period off drugs. They calculated the relative risks and confidence intervals for a number of factors. Those of importance are presented in Table 4.5. It can be seen that no individual factor is very strongly predictive of remission but those that are include, the absence of generalized spike wave activity from a number of EEGs, the absence of brain damage, and never having had a tonic clonic seizure.

Table 4.5 Factors affecting prognosis of epilepsy

Factor	Five years seizure-free Relative risk (95% CL)*	Five years seizure-free and off medication Relative risk (95% CL)
Age < 16 at first fit	1.09 (0.82–1.44)	1.88 (1.23–2.8)
No early brain damage	2.15 (1.22–3.78)	4.27 (1.35–13.47)
No known aetiology	1.50 (1.05–2.13)	2.64 (1.45–2.84)
Never had a tonic-clonic fit	1.37 (1.03–1.82)	2.19 (1.48–3.24)
No generalized spike wave in third year EEG	3.47 (1.37–8.8)	2.36 (0.56–10.16)

* Univariate Cox regression estimate of relative risk from 298 patients. CL confidence limits. Reproduced with permission from Shaffer, S. Q. *et al.* (1988). *Epilepsia*, **29**, p590–600 (see Ref. 171.)

TREATMENT OF EPILEPSY: DRUG THERAPY

STARTING THERAPY

Antiepileptic treatment has, in the past, been advocated before seizures occur. Such prophylactic treatment has been undertaken in patients with a high prospective risk of epilepsy after head injury and craniotomy for various neurosurgical conditions (172). Because no clear evidence exists that antiepileptic treatment is effective in preventing late epilepsy (121,173), it seems better to delay treatment until seizures have occurred rather than to adopt a policy of treatment of all potentially epileptic patients—particularly as there may be a relatively high incidence of side-effects with prophylactic treatment (174) and relatively poor compliance (175).

Most neurologists do not treat a single seizure. The risk of recurrence varies in studies from 27% to 80%. The exceptions to this are if the patient's EEG is clearly abnormal or there is other evidence of a progressive cerebral disorder.

When two or more seizures have occurred within a short interval, antiepileptic therapy is usually indicated. Problems do, however, arise in defining a short interval. Most clinicians would include periods of six months to one year within the definition but difficulties arise in knowing whether seizures more widely separated in time require therapy. Even where seizures occur in a close temporal relationship, the identification of specific precipitating factors may make it more important to counsel patients than to commence therapy. The most common examples are febrile convulsions in children and alcohol withdrawal seizures in adults. Less commonly, seizures may be precipitated in photosensitive subjects by television, visual display units, or other photic stimuli (see above).

There is now considerable evidence (176) that patients with newly diagnosed epilepsy should be treated with a single drug. Up to 70–80% of patients rapidly enter a prolonged remission of their seizures (163,177). This raises the question as to which of the available antiepileptic agents should be used as drugs of first choice for which patients. The major factors that influence choice of drug are comparative efficacy and toxicity.

In practice, assumptions made about the comparative efficacy of the antiepileptic drugs have been of major importance. While many clinicians have been persuaded that one is likely to be the most effective against particular seizure types and epileptic syndromes, it is difficult to identify satisfactory clinical trials that support this contention (178). In children, the differences in the efficacy between sodium valproate and ethosuximide on the one hand, and phenytoin and carbamazepine on the other, in the treatment of absence seizures seem too obvious to demand confirmation in a prospective clinical study. Studies do not, however, differentiate between the efficacy of sodium valproate and ethosuximide in absence epilepsy (179). Similarly, the preferential response of juvenile myoclonic epilepsy to sodium valproate seems to identify this as the drug of choice in this syndrome (180). It is much more doubtful whether there are major differences in efficacy between carbamazepine, phenytoin, barbiturates, and sodium valproate in the treatment of partial epilepsies (178, 181–183).

The newer anticonvulsants are currently only licensed as add-on therapy in partial seizures with the exception of lamotrigine (licensed as monotherapy and for primary generalized seizures). Although no head-to-head trials of these drugs have been performed, a meta-analysis of several randomized controlled trials, did not show any major differences in efficacy when comparing gabapentin, lamotrigine, tiagabine, topiramate, vigabatrin, or zonisamide (184). Table 4.6 outlines suggested therapies in the different epilepsies.

Where differences in efficacy are marginal, the importance of comparative drug toxicity becomes a major consideration in the choice of antiepileptic agent. Antiepileptic drugs have four distinct types of toxicity: acute dose-related toxicity, acute idiosyncratic toxicity, chronic toxicity, and teratogenicity.

Acute dose-related toxicity

Most anticonvulsants including phenytoin, carbamazepine, barbiturates, and benzodiazepines, give rise to a non-specific encephalopathy associated with high blood concentrations. Patients exhibit sedation and nystagmus and with increasing blood levels, ataxia, dysarthria, and ultimately confusion and drowsiness (185). In some instances seizure frequency may increase with high blood levels and occasionally involuntary movements are seen particularly with phenytoin (186), but also with carbamazepine (187) and gabapentin (188). Phenytoin is especially likely to result in dose-related toxicity because of its unusual pharmacokinetics (see below). Sodium valproate does not appear to be associated with this typical syndrome of neurotoxicity but patients with high blood levels may exhibit restlessness, irritability, and occasionally confusion. Postural tremor is a common accompaniment (189).

Undoubtedly, important criteria influencing the choice of drug are the potential effects on cognitive function and behaviour. All antiepileptic drugs have adverse effects that can be detected at therapeutic concentrations and which become more apparent both with polytherapy and with increasing

Table 4.6 Choice of antiepileptic drugs

	First line drugs	Second line drugs
Generalized epilepsy		
Idiopathic		
• Simple absence	VPA, ESM	LTG
• Juvenile myoclonic	VPA, LTG	CNZ, TPM
• Awakening tonic-clonic	VPA, LTG	CBZ, PHT
Symptomatic	VPA, LTG	CBZ, PHT, TPM
Partial epilepsy	CBZ, VPA, LTG	PHT, GBP, TPM, VGB
Unclassified epilepsy	VPA	LTG

VPA, sodium valproate, ESM, ethosuximide, LTG, lamotrigine, CNZ, clonazepam; TPM, topiramate, CBZ, carbamazepine, PHT, phenytoin; GBP, gabapentin; VGB, vigabatrin. Adapted with permission from Chadwick, D. W. and Turnbull, E. H. (1985). *JNNP*, **48**, p1073–7 (see Ref. 178.)

blood levels of individual drugs (190). The fact that agents, such as carbamazepine and sodium valproate, have fewer adverse effects on cognitive function and behaviour is perhaps one of the most powerful arguments for preferring these agents to longer-established drugs (e.g. phenobarbitone). The newer antiepileptic drugs, in general, promise less adverse effects on cognitive function.

Acute idiosyncratic toxicity

Most antiepileptic drugs, particularly phenytoin and carbamazepine, may cause a maculopapular, erythematous eruption which, in more severe cases, may be associated with fever, lymphadenopathy, and hepatitis (185). The incidence of allergic skin reaction with phenytoin may be as high as 5–10% and with carbamazepine up to 15% (174). Lamotrigine may be associated with rash in up to 5–10% of patients (191). It is severe (e.g. Stevens–Johnson syndrome) in about 0.1% of patients overall but may be as high as 1% in patients less than 12 years old and with concomitant sodium valproate therapy (figures from Glaxo Wellcome UK Ltd). It may be possible to avoid these reactions with a cautious build-up of initial doses. Rarer but potentially more serious idiosyncratic reactions can occur, although these are unpredictable and less likely to influence the choice of drug. Marrow aplasia seems to be extremely rare and fears concerning carbamazepine appear largely unfounded. Concern has arisen because of reports of fatal cases of liver failure in association with sodium valproate therapy. These largely involved children under the age of 2 years who are often multiply handicapped, and receiving many different antiepileptic drugs. It may be that they have an underlying inborn error of metabolism that predisposes them to liver failure (192). Vigabatrin, although an effective new anticonvulsant, has been associated with confusion and psychosis, particularly in patients with a previous psychiatric history.

Chronic toxicity

Antiepileptic drugs are unusual in that they may be administered to patients over a long period as treatment for chronic epilepsy. This may lead to the development of a wide range of syndromes of chronic toxicity (Table 4.7). A number of factors seem to predispose to the development of these disorders (i.e. the use of polypharmacy, the dosage, and the length of therapy). Although it appears that sodium valproate and carbamazepine may have fewer chronic toxic effects than barbiturates and phenytoin, the length of time that elapsed before quite common chronic toxic effects were recognized with the older agents should warn us that continued vigilance is needed in the use of any antiepileptic drugs (193).

Teratogenicity

All antiepileptic drugs should be regarded as potentially teratogenic. This has been discussed in the section above on

Table 4.7 Chronic toxicity of anticonvulsant drugs

Nervous system
Memory and cognitive impairment
Hyperactivity and behavioural disturbance
Pseudodementia
Cerebellar atrophy
Peripheral neuropathy

Skin
Acne
Hirsutism
Alopecia
Chloasma

Liver
Enzyme induction

Blood
Megaloblastic anaemia
Thrombocytopenia
Lymphoma

Immune system
IgA deficiency
Drug-induced systemic lupus crythematosus (SLE)

Endocrine system
Decreased thyroxine concentrations
Increased cortisol and sex hormone metabolism

Bone
Osteomalacia

Connective tissue
Gum hypertrophy
Coarsened facial features
Dupuytren's contracture

Pregnancy
Obstetric complications
Teratogenicity
Fetal hydantoin syndrome

Adapted from Reynolds, E. H. (1975). Chronic Antiepleptic Toxicity: A Review. *Epilepsia* **16**: p319–52.

prescribing in pregnancy. There is still not enough information available to comment on the safety of the newer anticonvulsants in pregnancy. Pharmaceutical companies hold registers of pregnancies occurring while on their drug and a recent review describes the outcome of some of these pregnancies (129).

MONITORING THERAPY

The great majority of patients developing epilepsy achieve a long-lasting remission that begins very soon after the start of therapy. For these patients, drug withdrawal may be considered after two, three, or more years (see below). Unfortunately, some 20% of patients developing epilepsy have a chronic disorder, uncontrolled by drugs.

Patients with chronic epilepsy have often been exposed to increasing doses of multiple drugs with frequent changes of drugs and dosages. Such a policy needs to be questioned. In patients receiving, and complying with, optimal doses of a

single antiepileptic drug, the addition of further agents is likely to result in a significant (> 75%) improvement in seizure control in only approximately 10% of patients (194). Such a policy, however, inevitably increases the risks of dose-related, idiosyncratic and chronic toxicity. In essence, a law of diminishing returns applies. Thus, for this group of patients an appropriate aim may not be complete remission of seizures but a compromise of reduced seizure frequency with less severe seizures, to be achieved with one or at most two drugs. The concept of assessment of the patient's quality of life is an important one in this situation. Studies have shown that not only does the diagnosis of epilepsy and the severity and frequency of seizures have a great impact on their quality of life but also the adverse effects of medication (195).

Patients who continue to be disabled by the occurrence of seizures despite treatment with a single drug at optimal dosage demand further careful consideration. In particular, it is important to consider whether there are factors that would explain an unsatisfactory response to therapy (e.g. unidentified structural pathology, the presence of complex partial seizures, or poor compliance). If this is not the case, then it is important to review the diagnosis. A common reason for failure of therapy is that the patient does not have epilepsy. Furthermore, it must be remembered that some patients have both true epileptic seizures and pseudoseizures (see above). Has the appropriate drug been used? In particular, it is important to differentiate clearly between generalized absence seizures and partial seizures, which may in some instances be similar in their symptomatology.

Where none of these conditions apply, it may be reasonable to try alternative drugs as monotherapy and in some instances to undertake a trial of the addition of a second drug. However, this demands careful discussion with the patient and the understanding that the second drug will be withdrawn in the absence of a satisfactory sustained response. Finally, patients with intractable partial seizures despite adequate drug therapy, may benefit from surgical treatment (see below).

In monitoring drug therapy, it is important to have a clear understanding of the pharmacokinetics of antiepileptic agents. Pharmacokinetics defines drug absorption, distribution, metabolism, and elimination and while having an important influence on drug effects it does not describe the mode of action of the drugs in the CNS. When measuring serum levels of drugs it must therefore be remembered that the samples are taken from a physiological pool that can be remote from the site of the drug action.

Monitoring serum or plasma concentrations of antiepileptic drugs has become routine in the United Kingdom and Europe for largely historical reasons: phenytoin has a non-linear relation between the dose and the serum concentration (196) and a dose-related neurotoxicity. This results in a narrow therapeutic window, and monitoring is necessary to avoid toxicity in patients who continue to have seizures. The concept of the therapeutic or optimal range for phenytoin has been extended to other antiepileptic drugs, and many laboratories now routinely estimate serum concentrations of drugs other than phenytoin. This is seen as an increasingly questionable practice.

A single measurement will give a good approximation of the steady state for drugs with long half-lives (phenytoin and phenobarbitone) but not for drugs with short half-lives. Measurements of the sodium valproate concentrations from specimens taken at random during the day are virtually uninterpretable.

It is important to be aware of what is measured during routine estimations of blood concentrations of antiepileptic drugs and perhaps what is not measured. Some drugs have metabolites that seem to contribute to the therapeutic effect but which are not routinely assayed. These include the 10,11-epoxide of carbamazepine. Most UK laboratories determine the drug concentration in whole plasma or serum. Phenytoin, carbamazepine, and sodium valproate are heavily protein-bound but only the free drug fraction is in equilibrium with the brain and pharmacologically active.

Even when concentrations of free drugs and their metabolites in the blood are known, important pharmacodynamic considerations may alter the relationship between the blood concentration and the therapeutic effect. Thus, for sodium valproate the onset of action is slower and longer lasting than can be explained by the pharmacokinetics of the drug (197). Similarly, tolerance to the neurotoxicity and therapeutic effects of benzodiazepines and barbiturate drugs is not explained by pharmacokinetic changes and must be due to drug–receptor interaction.

There are further fundamental biological reasons for doubting the value of routine monitoring of blood concentrations of antiepileptic drugs. The upper limit of a therapeutic range may be defined as the concentration of the drug at which toxic effects are likely to appear. The most consistent relationship between the serum concentration and toxic effect is for phenytoin but even with this drug, some patients may tolerate and indeed require serum concentrations above 20 μg/ml (198). At the other end of the spectrum, patients with satisfactory control of seizures and low blood concentrations may have their doses needlessly increased. From this it is clear that treating the patient is much more important than treating the blood results.

Routine monitoring should increasingly be restricted to certain categories of patients: first, those receiving phenytoin or multiple drug treatment in whom dosage adjustment is necessary because of dose-related toxicity and poor seizure control; second, mentally retarded patients in whom the assessment of toxicity may be difficult; third, patients with renal or hepatic disease, and perhaps pregnant patients (as outlined above); and finally, patients who may not be complying with treatment.

WITHDRAWING THERAPY

Most patients who have been seizure-free for two or more years should be considered for withdrawal of therapy. The decision has to be a joint one between the patient and the clinician. It is not just about the statistical risk of recurrence or long-term effects of medication. The patient's age and circumstance will affect the impact that seizure recurrence will have. Patients should be counselled in detail prior to drug withdrawal (199). The regulations as regards driving, and reducing and stopping therapy need to be made clear (see above).

Overall, the risk of relapse is 25% at 1 year and about 29% at 2 years. Relapse after this is not common but possible (200). The main predictors of relapse include age of onset, aetiology, epileptic syndrome, and possibly EEG. Adolescent onset predisposes to a greater likelihood of relapse followed by adult onset with childhood onset being the least likely to relapse (200,201). Patients with remote symptomatic epilepsy are more at risk of relapse (200). The presence of mental retardation does not seem to bode well for drug withdrawal (201).

As already mentioned, some of the epileptic syndromes have a very good outlook (e.g. benign rolandic epilepsy) whereas others (juvenile myoclonic epilepsy) have a high relapse rate.

The EEG may be of some help in predicting relapse in certain situations. Inter-ictal epileptiform activity prior to drug withdrawal does not seem to affect relapse rate. The presence of slow wave abnormalities, however, does predict a poorer outcome, especially if it is seen when not previously present (201).

The period over which the medication is withdrawn depends partly on which drug is involved. Barbiturates and benzodiazepines need to be withdrawn very slowly (perhaps 12 months for phenobarbitone). Importantly, a prospective study on withdrawal of therapy in children did not show any significant increase in recurrence risk if drugs were tapered over 6 weeks as opposed to 9 months (202).

MORE ABOUT THE DRUGS . . .

A brief description of each of the anticonvulsant drugs follows, dosages are not included and can be found in the BNF (British National Formulary):

Carbamazepine is used for simple and complex partial seizures and primary generalized seizures. The dose and frequency are started low then increased as the drug exhibits autoinduction of its metabolism. A slow release (twice daily) version is available which may improve compliance and control. It may exacerbate juvenile myoclonic epilepsy. Carbamazepine reduces the efficacy of the oral contraceptive pill (OCP) and may enhance clearance of concomitant anticonvulsant medication. Dose-related side-effects include dizziness, diplopia, unsteadiness, nausea, and vomiting. Rashes occur in about 15% of patients. Monitoring of white blood count is not required unless patient develops sore throat or fever. Hyponatraemia as a consequence of carbamazepine needs to be remembered.

Clobazam is used in generalized and partial seizures but continuous treatment is not recommended. As with the other benzodiazepines it exhibits tachyphylaxis. It is most useful in patients with a clear catamenial clustering of their seizures as intermittent therapy on the days when seizure occurrence is deemed to be most likely. Drowsiness and sedation are its main drawbacks.

Clonazepam is most helpful in absence and myoclonic epilepsies. It can be useful as an infusion in partial status epilepticus. As a regular oral dose it unfortunately exhibits tachyphylaxis. Sedation is a common side-effect and the intravenous infusion can lead to respiratory depression.

Diazepam is really only used in the management of status epilepticus. The main advantages are that it is available in parenteral forms (iv, im, or pr; intravenous, intramuscular, per rectum). It causes sedation and repeated dosage is associated with respiratory depression.

Ethosuximide is used in simple absences. It causes a dose-related syndrome of nausea, dizziness, drowsiness, and unsteadiness. It may worsen tonic-clonic seizures.

Gabapentin (203,204) is licensed for add-on therapy in partial seizures and appears not to have an effect on generalized seizures. Increased anticonvulsant effect has been seen up to a dose of 7200 mg a day. Cognitive impairment is not common but dizziness, fatigue, somnolence, and ataxia have been reported. The incidence of these can be minimized by slow dose increase (i.e. slower than that outlined in the BNF). It does not affect the metabolism of the OCP. It does not interact with other anticonvulsant drugs. Because of relatively infrequent side-effects it has been suggested that it may be especially useful in the elderly.

Lamotrigine (205–207) is licensed for monotherapy or add-on therapy in partial or primary generalized seizures. Recent studies have shown it to be of value in the Lennox–Gastaut syndrome. It is necessary to initiate therapy slowly, especially with concomitant sodium valproate therapy to avoid a high risk of rash. The maximum dose is also lower in combination with sodium valproate. As discussed above, rash occurs in 5–10% but may be severe in 1%. Other reported side-effects include ataxia, diplopia, dizziness headache, and nausea. It has no effect on the OCP. Enzyme inducing anticonvulsants can decrease lamotrigine's half-life by as much as 50%, necessitating dose increase.

Oxcarbazepine (208, 209) is licensed for the treatment of generalized tonic-clonic and partial seizures. It has a keto substitution at the 10 position of the dibenzazepine nucleus which differentiates it from carbamazepine and is thought to be responsible for its better tolerability. It has similar efficacy to carbamazepine and may exacerbate juvenile myoclonic seizures. Oxcarbazepine seems to have a lower tendency to produce idiosyncratic reactions and drug interactions but it has the same effect on the OCP as carbamazepine. Side-effects include dizziness, drowsiness, diplopia, nausea, and vomiting.

Phenobarbitone is effective in tonic-clonic and partial seizures. It is also used in refractory epilepsy (including West syndrome). Because of its effects on cognitive function and marked sedation it is not used as widely as in the past. As with other barbiturates, it causes habituation and drug withdrawal has to be undertaken cautiously. As an enzyme inducer it lowers the plasma concentrations of several of the anticonvulsant drugs and the OCP.

Phenytoin is used in partial and tonic-clonic seizures. It has the advantage of once-daily dosing and can be given intravenously in the presence of status epilepticus or in postneurosurgical seizures. Unfortunately, it exhibits zero-order kinetics which may cause large increases in plasma concentration with only small increments in dosage. It has dose-related side-effects such as drowsiness, unsteadiness, and movement disorders and may impair cognition. Idiosyncratic reactions are mainly seen as a rash. The chronic side-effects are often more of concern in female patients (i.e. hirsutism, coarsening of facial features, and gum hypertrophy). It is an enzyme inducer and therefore interacts with other anticonvulsants and reduces the efficacy of the OCP.

Sodium valproate is effective in partial, tonic-clonic, and absence seizures. Because of its broad spectrum of action, some would recommend it as the drug of choice in new onset seizures. Its use in women may be limited by its propensity to cause weight gain. It can be given intravenously in acute situations. A slow release preparation is available which may help with compliance (it can be given once daily) and control. Dose-related side-effects include tremor, irritability, and occasionally confusion. Idiosyncratic reactions include hepatotoxicity (rare, except in paediatric cases). Alopecia can complicate more chronic therapy. Care needs to be taken with co-administration of lamotrigine. Sodium valproate does not reduce the efficacy of the OCP.

Tiagabine (210, 211) is useful in partial seizures as add-on therapy but may exacerbate absence seizures. Dose-related side-effects include ataxia, dizziness, fatigue, somnolence, and tremor. It does not affect the OCP metabolism. Trials are currently being undertaken to compare tiagabine with carbamazepine in partial seizures and sodium valproate in primary generalized seizures.

Topiramate (212–214) is licensed for partial seizures as add-on therapy. As well as ataxia, dizziness, fatigue, and somnolence, problems with concentration, anorexia, and weight loss have been reported. If profound, therapy should be discontinued. There is a 1.5% incidence of renal calculi with this therapy which requires monitoring. Topiramate reduces the efficacy of the OCP.

Vigabatrin (215–219) is licensed for add-on therapy in partial seizures and has shown promise in the treatment of West syndrome (particularly in association with tuberose sclerosis). It may worsen myoclonic seizures. As well as similar dose-related side-effects as other anticonvulsants, weight gain can be a problem. Psychiatric disturbance (including psychosis) has been reported and it should be used with caution if there is a past medical history of depression. Recent reports have described visual field constriction in patients on long-term vigabatrin (> 2 years). It is as yet unclear whether it is a direct effect of vigabatrin as most patients were on polytherapy. It should, however, prompt visual field assessment and consideration of therapy withdrawal if a patient complains of such visual disturbance. It does not seem to interfere with the metabolism of the OCP but it may decrease the plasma level of phenytoin by 20%.

Zonisamide (220–222) is licensed for the treatment of partial seizures as add-on therapy. Apart from the usual dose-related side-effects as noted above, initial studies showed an excess occurrence of renal calculi. This seemed to be associated with the European and American patients and not the Japanese. If therapy with this agent is initiated then monitoring for nephrolithiasis should be undertaken. It seems to cause quite marked sedation and interacts with several other anticonvulsants.

EMERGENCY TREATMENT SITUATIONS

STATUS EPILEPTICUS

The management of tonic-clonic status epilepticus has been extensively reviewed by Shorvon (223). It is defined as prolonged or recurrent tonic-clonic seizures lasting 30 minutes or more. It is not the only form of status epilepticus (i.e. complex and simple partial status epilepticus, absence status epilepticus) but it tends to require more urgent treatment. Most cases occur in children (224) and greater than 30% of all cases have no history of epilepsy (225). In the latter cases, acute cerebral disturbances are responsible (e.g. CNS infection, tumour, trauma), and it tends to be this that actually causes death. The mortality rate from tonic-clonic status epilepticus is approximately 5–10% and morbidity is associated with duration of the status (223).

It must be remembered that a significant proportion of patients thought to be in tonic-clonic status epilepticus turn out to have pseudoseizures (see above). Caution should be exercised in starting the following cascade of treatment, if there are atypical features to the seizures or an EEG is entirely normal. Admittedly, some forms of frontal lobe seizures may also fall into this category.

Initially, the patient may just exhibit an increased frequency of seizures which, if left unchecked, will deteriorate in to convulsions without inter-ictal recovery, and then coma. Treatment is therefore most useful in this prodromal period. At the onset of status epilepticus there is a marked increase in cerebral metabolism which is mostly compensated for. However, as the seizures continue cerebral autoregulation fails, leaving the cerebral circulation reliant on systemic blood pressure. The vicious circle then takes over of hypotension (secondary to drug therapy and autonomic disturbance), leading to cerebral hypoxia and central respiratory depression further worsening this hypoxia. The cerebral ischaemia may cause oedema leading to raised intracranial pressure (ICP) further

reducing tissue perfusion. All of this may occur over a matter of hours and obviously requires the patient to be in an intensive care facility.

Treatment prior to this catastrophic decline starts simply. The prodromal period should be recognized if possible and the seizures treated with diazepam or paraldehyde while the patient's regular therapy (if they are known to be epileptic) is adjusted. If the patient has entered a phase of recurrent seizures without inter-ictal recovery, hospital admission will have frequently been arranged where the usual assessment of cardiorespiratory function should be undertaken, with the airway secured, supplemental oxygen, and adequate output.

If the patient has been fitting for more than 10 minutes, full blood screen (biochemical, haematological, and blood gases) should be performed to rule out hypoglycaemia, etc., thiamine deficiency thought about, and emergency anticonvulsant therapy started. The usual choice would be: **lorazepam** (this is probably preferable to diazepam at this stage), as it has a longer duration of action (12 h) and lack of accumulation in lipid stores. It is given as a slow intravenous injection. In adults, 0.07 mg/kg (max. of 4 mg). A further single dose can be given after 20 min. **OR: diazepam** can be used, but repeated doses may be required as it is rapidly redistributed. Repeated doses may however cause sudden CNS depression and cardiorespiratory collapse. It can be given rectally or intravenously. The adult dose is 10–20 mg intravenously, with further doses given at 15-minute intervals to a maximum of 40 mg.

If seizures continue or return after this, an attempt to further establish an aetiology should be made. That is, an EEG should be performed to demonstrate the neurophysiological disturbance, possible focus and help to rule out pseudo-status epilepticus. A CT scan and lumbar puncture (if safe) will assist diagnosis if an infective aetiology is thought likely.

While these investigations are being arranged, the next level of anticonvulsant therapy should be started: **phenytoin**: this is usually given as a loading dose and should be administered with ECG monitoring. The adult loading dose is 15–18 mg/kg which often works out as 1000 mg which should be given over 20–30 min. Daily maintenance doses of 5–6 mg/kg are then started. There is little associated respiratory depression but hypotension can be problematic. Levels can be checked to attain optimal dose. **OR: phenobarbitone**: may not be used as frequently as phenytoin probably because of its greater propensity to cause respiratory depression and hypotension. It is a highly effective treatment, with long duration of action and possible cerebral protective action. It can accumulate and shows strong autoinduction. In adults, an intravenous loading dose of 10 mg/kg is suggested (max. rate 100 mg/min). Maintenance dose is 1–4 mg/kg per day. Prolonged therapy should be accompanied with drug level monitoring if toxicity or poor response occurs.

Patients continuing to fit (clinically or neurophysiologically) despite the above management strategy should be transferred to an intensive care facility and arrangements made for general anaesthesia, ventilation, and EEG monitoring (+/− inotrope support, central venous pressure, and intracranial pressure measurements, etc.). The two agents commonly in use for this are: **thiopentone**: apart from requiring ventilation when this agent is used, its profound hypotensive effect often needs counterbalancing with plasma expanders and inotrope support. This drug has the propensity to accumulate, and despite stopping therapy, it may take several days for it to have cleared sufficiently to assess the patient. Prolonged therapy can cause pancreatitis and hepatic disturbance. The usual adult regimen involves a 100–250 mg intravenous bolus over 20 s, with further 50 mg boluses every 2–3 min, until the seizures stop or burst suppression is attained on the EEG (interburst gaps of 2–30 s are acceptable). A maintenance infusion of 3–5 mg/kg/h is then usually sufficient adjusted according to the EEG and blood pressure. It is suggested that thiopentone is continued for at least 12 h after seizure activity has ceased before tapering. **OR: propofol**: oddly, this is known to cause seizures in general anaesthetic practice but seems to be an effective treatment for refractory status epilepticus. Like thiopentone it causes profound respiratory depression but dose not have such a marked hypotensive effect and despite high lipid solubility once discontinued its action diminishes quickly. In adults, an intravenous 2 mg/kg bolus is given and is repeated if seizures continue. An infusion is then set up of 5–10 mg/kg/h according to the EEG. Discontinuing therapy should be done as for thiopentone but obviously occurs more quickly and allows sooner assessment of the patient. During the patient's stay in the intensive care unit, a decision should be made about longer-term anticonvulsant medication based on the underlying aetiology or previous drug regimens.

The above is not meant to be an all-encompassing list and other therapies have their supporters. A more extensive list can be found in Shorvon (226).

ECLAMPSIA

Two large studies have proven that magnesium sulphate is more effective in preventing eclamptic seizures in pre-eclamptic women than phenytoin (227) and that it is more effective in treating established eclampsia than phenytoin or diazepam (228). Magnesium sulphate treatment was associated with decreased maternal and neonatal morbidity.

SURGICAL TREATMENT OF EPILEPSY

Although the surgical treatment of epilepsy was pioneered in the United Kingdom over 100 years ago, it has never been made widely available to patients with epilepsy. The increasing sophistication of the EEG investigation, neurological imaging, and neuropsychology, however, means that this form of treatment can be highly successful in large numbers of patients. It has been estimated that at least 75 000 patients in the United States may be suitable for surgical treatment (229) and in the United Kingdom there may be well over 12 000 patients who would benefit. There is an urgent need to expand the number of regional and supraregional centres able to offer adequate pre-surgical evaluation and surgical treatment.

The philosophy of surgical treatment requires either the accurate identification of the localized site of seizure onset (by a neurophysiological method, with or without neuroradiological techniques) or the disconnection of epileptogenic zones, so as to interrupt seizure spread in a palliative procedure (callosotomy or multiple subpial transections). Inevitably, excisions of epileptogenic lesions and zones will also involve interruption of their connections to some degree.

In a recent report of the varying procedures undertaken worldwide (230), 73% of operations involved some form of temporal lobe surgery, while extratemporal cortical excisions accounted for 15% of operations and 9% corpus callosotomy. To be considered for any of these procedures, patients will need to demonstrate a history of medically refractory epilepsy. There may be some controversy about a precise definition of refractory epilepsy but this will usually be established within two years of onset, if appropriate antiepileptic drugs have been administered singly or in combination in optimal doses. Thereafter, there can be little optimism that further manipulation of drug therapy is likely to alter radically the outcome of epilepsy in such a patient. Patients will be sufficiently disabled by their epilepsy to warrant the risks of surgical treatment and the necessary pre-surgical evaluation. There should be a high probability that an improvement in seizure control will lead to a significant improvement in the individual's quality of life. This concept and the modalities used to assess quality of life has been addressed in a number of studies and is well demonstrated in the paper by Kellett *et al.* (231). Other factors determining suitability of treatment will relate to the type of procedure to be performed but the above criteria may be relaxed when neuroimaging shows the presence of a lesion, possibly a low grade tumour, that would demand surgical treatment in its own right. Factors that may mitigate against a surgical option are: IQ less than 70; age over 50 years; disabilities other than epilepsy being predominant; lesions in areas where resection would lead to unacceptable deficit.

It is important that patients are referred earlier in the course of their epilepsy than previously so that the psychological consequences of prolonged disability do not hamper the rehabilitation of a patient whose seizures are halted.

SURGICAL PROCEDURE

Temporal lobe surgery

There is no doubt that patients with mesial temporal lesions experience the best results of epilepsy surgery (approximately 60% seizure-free, Ref. 230). The ideal candidate for temporal lobe surgery will have a history of seizures typical of a medial temporal onset, an initial epigastric aura being the most common mode of onset (232). The two pathologies with the best outcomes are those of mesial temporal sclerosis (MTS) or an indolent glioma of the medial temporal region (233). In the former, a history of a prolonged/complicated febrile seizure before the age of 4 or 5 years is a particularly strong clinical indicator. A more extensive list of clinical, neurophysiological, and neuroimaging features of mesial temporal lobe epilepsy can be found elsewhere (232).

If a patient has a history very suggestive of MTS, an EEG with a unilateral, inter-ictal anterior temporal spike, suggestive psychometry and evidence of hippocampal sclerosis on MRI there is usually no need for further, more invasive investigation to consider surgery. Obviously, when the situation is not so clear-cut, other tests may be required (see below).

Surgery may consist of anterior temporal lobectomy or selective amygdalohippocampectomy. The seizure control is similar for both but reoperation may be needed more often in the less complete resections (234). Amygdalohippocampectomy may be indicated in patients shown to have only borderline memory function on the contralateral side (235).

Overall, surgical procedures seem to carry a risk of transient neurological deficit of 0–1.5%, permanent neurological deficit of 0-3.9%, and death of 0.3-3.6% (230).

Extratemporal surgery

Frontal lobectomy is the next commonest focal resection. Care has to be taken to avoid involvement of the primary motor area (mapping is usually performed). The outcome in terms of percentage seizure-free is about 40% (230), but may be higher in those with a structural lesion (236). Parietal lobe and occipital lobe resections are performed less frequently but also seem to have a success rate of 40–45% of patients becoming seizure-free (230).

Callosotomy

Section of the corpus callosum and hippocampal commissure is an accepted palliative procedure for uncontrolled secondary generalized seizures (237, 238). The procedure seeks to prevent the generalization of seizures, particularly those that generalize rapidly, resulting in falls (tonic and atonic seizures). Early operations were often complicated by ventriculitis, meningitis, and hydrocephalus and by more severe and frequent focal seizures immediately post-operatively and by a characteristic disconnection syndrome of mutism, apraxia of the non-dominant limbs, agnosia, apathy, confusion, and infantile behaviour. Refinements of the procedure and the introduction of anterior and two-stage operations have reduced morbidity (239). In some series, up to 80% of patients have had a complete cessation of generalized seizures with falls, although about 25% may have more intense partial seizures than previously (only 5–6% became seizure-free, Ref. 230). It also seems that a callosotomy may reduce the incidence of status epilepticus.

The selection criteria for corpus callosotomy are more poorly defined than for other surgical procedures. The operation will be most commonly considered in children and adolescents with very severe epilepsy, with a multifocal origin of seizures or with seizures of sudden onset resulting in falls (e.g. Lennox–Gastaut syndrome).

Hemispherectomy

This procedure may be suitable for patients with intractable epilepsy and an infantile hemiplegia with a useless hand (e.g. Rasmussen's syndrome, see above). From a recent study (230), 60% of patients become seizure-free following this operation and behavioural abnormalities can also improve. However, the operation fell into disrepute as up to 25% of those undergoing hemispherectomy developed delayed complications (240). Most suffered from recurrent subdural haemorrhage from the subdural membrane lining in the hemispherectomy cavity. Adams (241) modified the procedure to eliminate the large extradural space and to insulate the ventricular system from the subdural cavity. Hemispherectomy should probably now be restored to its previous position in children with infantile hemipegia and epilepsy and also in those rare children with chronic progressive focal encephalitis (Rasmussen's syndrome). Functional hemispherectomy (removal of central and temporal areas and only disconnection of the anterior and posterior poles of the hemisphere) is the most commonly performed procedure of this type (242).

Multiple subpial transections

This operation seems to be a reasonable alternative to hemispherectomy in Rasmussen's syndrome prior to the patient becoming hemiplegic (243). Other intractable seizures arising from the primary cortices may benefit similarly.

PRE-SURGICAL EVALUATION

A detailed clinical history is essential to describe the features of seizures and past medical history. Development and educational histories are particularly important.

It must be stressed that no single test can be relied upon to localize seizure onset and be used as a guide for surgery. Non-invasive techniques are generally employed first and if doubts still arise, more invasive techniques are used to try to localize a focus.

It has already been mentioned that in certain straightforward cases (e.g. typical mesial temporal sclerosis, MTS) only a few investigations are required.

Inter-ictal scalp EEG remains a useful investigation but can be misleading, occasionally being falsely localizing. Ictal EEG (especially video-telemetry EEG) in combination with other information (psychometric testing and MRI) can be of significant localising value.

The psychological evaluation involves assessment of verbal IQ and memory (left hemisphere) and performance IQ and visual memory (right hemisphere). Major discrepancies suggest temporal lobe dysfunction. This is often followed by a

WADA (intra-carotid amytal) test in the case of temporal lobe seizures (244). This has two functions: first, it demonstrates whether the temporal lobe contralateral to that to be resected can sustain memory; second, memory impairment on the side of the suggested focus strongly supports this localization and good outcome post-operatively.

MRI (magnetic resonance imaging) scanning has been of significant benefit in terms of the non-invasive investigation prior to surgery. Hippocampal atrophy identified either by inspection or by volumetric analysis together with T2 relaxometry is particularly sensitive in cases of MTS (245). FLAIR (fluid attenuated inversion recovery) sequences increase this sensitivity (246). Three dimensional MRI reconstruction can demonstrate neuronal migration disorders that were previously missed (247).

SPECT (single photon emission computerized tomography) seems to be most reliable when performed during a fit. It has some drawbacks, for instance, variability depending on the timing of the isotope injection, and is still not widely available. Ictal Tc-HMPAO SPECT is most useful in localizing temporal lobe seizures (248). Ictal hyperperfusion is demonstrated and localizes correctly to the side of the seizure in about 97% of cases (248). Ictal SPECT may be more useful than inter-ictal PET (positron emission tomography) in localizing extratemporal foci.

Inter-ictal fluorodeoxyglucose (FDG)-PET demonstrates alterations in glucose metabolism in the brain. It can help localize the side of a lesion/focus but needs to be correlated with EEG abnormalities (249, 250). The major drawback of this investigation is the cost and lack of availability of the equipment necessary to perform a scan.

Major steps forward in MRI technology may well make PET redundant as a practical clinical investigation. MR spectroscopy, functional MRI, and diffusion-weighted imaging (DWI) are all being developed with a view to assisting non-invasive seizure localization (251).

Invasive investigations are resorted to if initial tests fail to prove a single epileptogenic focus or in those where the focus may partly involve important functional areas. Sphenoidal and foramen ovale electrodes can be used, especially when a temporal lobe focus is suspected.

Subdural grids and depth electrodes are predominantly used for extratemporal foci. Electrocorticography is used intra-operatively to try to define an epiletpogenic focus (although its use to predict outcome is controversial). Functional mapping is employed to avoid resection of eloquent areas.

VAGAL STIMULATION

This involves the implantation of a subcutaneous stimulator with electrodes attached to the left vagus nerve. About 130 patients have undergone this treatment but no truly blinded study has been possible and no substantial long-term data are available. The mode of action is not known (which could also

be said of a number of the newer antiepileptic drugs), but it may cause a reduction in seizures of over 50% in 39% of patients with partial seizures (252). This is comparable to the add-on effects of the newer anticonvulsant medications.

In view of cost and possible complications, it seems reasonable for further studies to be performed with longer follow-up to assess the usefulness, safety, and precise clinical application before widespread use is recommended.

CONCLUSION

It is generally recognized that services to people with epilepsy in the United Kingdom are poor, except for a few widely separated centres. How then can facilities be improved and what should be the form and content of epilepsy services?

It should be apparent from the this chapter that any comprehensive service must have a clear diagnostic capability and precision. Every person diagnosed as having epilepsy should have that diagnosis confirmed by an appropriate specialist with a specific interest and expertise in epilepsy. The specialist service should have access to all necessary investigations, including high quality neurophysiology as well as CT and MRI scanning. An adequate diagnosis implies not only differentiating seizures from non-epileptic events but also requires appropriate classification of seizures and epilepsy syndromes and an identification of any underlying cause. Diagnostic services need to be backed up by adequate information provision from people with genuine experience who may not, however, necessarily be medically qualified. Written information on the treatment for epilepsy and its implications should be provided.

People with chronic epilepsy, particularly those in the first two or three decades of life should be regularly reviewed. Here, the major aims are again diagnostic, to differentiate epilepsy from pseudoseizures and also therapeutic, so as to ensure optimal pharmacological treatment and the evaluation and the ability to evaluate for and provide surgical procedures to treat epilepsy. Once again, counselling and adequate information needs to be provided to reduce the psychosocial consequences of chronic epilepsy.

These requirements demand multidisciplinary skills of neurologists, neurophysiologists, neuroradiologists, neurosurgeons, psychologists, and psychiatrists. A specialist nurse may have a particularly important role to play in the liaison with primary care services. It is evident that the rapid advances in both the pharmacological and surgical treatment of epilepsy mean that the needs for specialist services are increasing all the while and that effective implementation of advances will be dependent on the development of adequate systems of care for people with epilepsy. While in the past excellent epilepsy services have been developed and run by non-neurological specialists, particularly neuropsychiatrists and clinical pharmacologists, it seems highly unlikely that these very small specialities can train clinicians swiftly enough to meet the demand. The only specialities capable of doing this would appear to be paediatric and adult neurology. The authors believe that each regional neuroscience centre in the United Kingdom should, by the start of the next millennium, have appointed a neurologist and paediatric neurologist with a specific interest and expertise in epilepsy. Their major responsibility should be the provision of specialist services for people with epilepsy that have direct links to primary care services. This goal should be achievable provided British neurology's neglect of epilepsy does not continue. Indeed, providing adequate services for people with epilepsy must be a major factor in favour of a rapid expansion in training posts and consultant appointments in epilepsy and neurology.

REFERENCES

1. Jackson JH. On the anatomical, physiological and pathological investigation of epilepsies. West Riding Lunatic Asylum Medical Reports **3**: 3.5. Reprinted in Taylor J. (ed) *Selected writings of John Hughlings Jackson.* Hodder and Stroughton, London. 90–111. 1873.
2. Commission on the International League Against Epilepsy. Proposal for revised clinical and electroencephalographic classification of epileptic seizures. *Epilepsia* **22**: 489–501. 1981.
3. Commission on Classification and Terminology of the International League Against Epilepsy. Proposal for revised classification of epilepsies and epileptic syndromes. *Epilepsia* **30**: 389–99. 1989.
4. Hauser WA, Annegers JF, Kurland LT. Incidence of epilepsy and unprovoked seizures in Rochester, Minnesota: 1935–1984. *Epilepsia* **34**: 453–68. 1993.
5. Sander JWA, Hart YM, Johnson AL, Shorvon SD. National general practice study of epilepsy: newly diagnosed epileptic seizures in a general population. *Lancet* **336**: 1267–71. 1990.
6. Duncan J, Hart YM. In *Textbook of epilepsy*, 4th (edn) (ed.) Laidlaw J, Richens A, Chadwick D. Churchill Livingstone, Edinburgh. 705–22. 1992.
7. Griffin J and Wiles M. *Epilepsy towards tomorrow.* Office of Health Economics London. 1991.
8. Cockerell OC, Hart YM, Sander JWAS, Shorvon SD. The cost of epilepsy in the United Kingdom: An estimation based on the results of two population-based studies. *Epilepsy Res.* **18**: 249–60. 1994.
9. Fisher RS, ed. *Imitators of epilepsy.* Demos, New York. 1994.
10. Boon PA, Williamson PD. The diagnosis of pseudoseizures. *Clin. Neurol. Neurosurg.* **95**: 1–8. 1993.
11. Hoefnagels WAJ, Padberg GW, Overweg J, Roos RAC *et al.* Syncope or seizure? The diagnostic value of the EEG and hyperventilation test in transient loss of consciousness. *JNNP* **54**: 953–6. 1991.
12. Lempert T, Bauer M, Schmidt D. Syncope: a videometric analysis of 56 episodes of transient cerebral hypoxia. *Ann. Neurol.* **36**: 233–7. 1994.
13. Kapoor WN. Diagnostic evaluation of syncope. *Am. J. Med.* **90**: 91–106. 1991.
14. Aminoff MJ, Scheinman MM, Griffin JC, Herre JM. Electrocerebral accompaniments of syncope associated with malignant ventricular arrhythmias. *Ann. Int. Med.* **108**: 791–6. 1988.
15. Jervell A, Lange-Nielsen F. Congenital deaf-mutism, functional heart disease with prolongation of the Q-T interval and sudden death. *Am. Heart J.* **54**: 59–68. 1957.
16. Ballardie FW, Murphy RP, Davis J. Epilepsy: a presentation of the Romano–Ward syndrome. *BMJ* **287**: 896–7. 1983.
17. Sundaram MBM, McMeekin JD, Gulamhusein S. Cardiac tachyarrhythmias in hereditary long Q-T syndromes presenting as a seizure disorder. *Can. J. Neurolog. Sci.* **13**: 262–3. 1986.
18. O'Callaghan CA, Trump D. Prolonged Q-T syndrome presenting as epilepsy. *Lancet* **341**: 759–60. 1993.
19. Singh B, Al Shawan SA, Habbab MA. *et al.* Idiopathic long Q-T syndrome: asking the right question. *Lancet* **341**: 741–2. 1993.
20. Gatto EM, Fernandez Pardal MM, Micheli F, Gonzalez MA, Daru VD. The long Q-T syndrome: Epilepsy as the form of presentation. *Rev. Clin. Esp.* **192**: 380–2. 1993.
21. Pacia SV, Devinsky O, Luciano DJ, Vazquez B. The prolonged Q-T syndrome presenting as epilepsy. A report of two cases and literature review. *Neurology* **44**: 1408–10. 1994.
22. Splawski I, Timothy KW, Vincent GM, Atkinson DL *et al.* Molecular basis of the long Q-T syndrome associated with deafness. *N. Engl. J. Med.* **336**: 1562–7. 1997.
23. Ackerman MJ, Clapham DE. Ion channels—basic science and clinical disease. *N. Engl. J. Med.* **336**: 1575–86. 1997.
24. Schwartz PJ. Idiopathic long Q-T syndrome: progress and questions. *Am. Heart J.* **109**: 399–411. 1985.
25. Chaudron JM, Heller F, Van den Berghe *et al.* Attacks of ventricular fibrillation and unconsciousness in a patient with prolonged Q-T interval: a family study. *Am. Heart J.* **91**: 783–91. 1976.
26. Vincent GM, Timothy KW, Leppert M, Keating M. The spectrum of symptoms and Q-T intervals in carriers of the gene for the long Q-T syndrome. *N. Engl. J. Med.* **327**: 846–52. 1992.
27. Bassetti C, Aldrich MS. Narcolepsy. *Neurologic Clinics* **14**: 545–71. 1996.
28. Bowman ES. Aetiology and clinical course of pseudoseizures: relationship to trauma, depression and dissociation. *Psychosomatics* **34**: 333–42. 1993.
29. Leis AA, Ross MA, Summers AK. Psychogenic seizures: Ictal characteristics and diagnostic pitfalls. *Neurology* **42**: 95–9. 1992.
30. Lempert T, Schmidt D. Natural history and outcome of psychogenic seizures: A clinical study in 50 patients. *J. Neurol.* **237**: 35–8. 1990.
31. Kristensen O, Alving J. Pseudoseizures—risk factors and prognosis: a case control study. *Acta Neurol. Scand.* **85**: 177–80. 1992.
32. Gates JR, Ramani V, Whalen S, Lowenson R. Ictal characteristics of pseudoseizures. *Arch. Neurol.* **42**: 1183–7. 1985.
33. Gulick TA, Spinks IP, King DW. Pseudoseizures: ictal phenomena. *Neurology* **32**: 24–30. 1982.
34. Holmes GL, Sackellares JC, McKiernan J, Ragland M *et al.* Evaluation of childhood pseudoseizures using EEG telemetry and video tape monitoring. *J. Pediatr.* **97**: 554–8. 1980.
35. Luther JS, McNamara JO, Carwile S *et al.* Pseudoepileptic seizures: methods and video analysis to aid diagnosis. *Ann. Neurol.* **12**: 458–62. 1982.
36. Desai BT, Porter RJ, Penry JK. Psychogenic seizures: a study of 42 attacks in six patients, with intensive monitoring. *Arch. Neurol.* **39**: 202–9. 1982.
37. King DW, Gallagher BB, Murvin AJ *et al.* Pseudoseizures: diagnostic evaluation. *Neurology* **32**: 18–23. 1982.
38. Krumholz A, Niedermeyer E. Psychogenic seizures: a clinical study with follow up data. *Neurology* **33**: 498–502. 1983.
39. Gumnit RJ, Gates JR. Psychogenic seizures. *Epilepsia* **27**(**suppl.** 2): S124–9. 1986.
40. Mattson RH. Electroencephalographic (polygraphic) studies in the diagnosis of non-epileptic seizures. In *Non-epileptic seizures*, (ed.) Rowan AJ, Gates JR. Butterworth, New York. 85–92. 1993.
41. Saygi S, Katz A, Marks DA, Spencer SS. Frontal lobe partial

seizures and psychogenic seizures: comparison of clinical and ictal characteristics. *Neurology* **42**: 1274–7. 1992.

42. Devinsky O, Kelley K, Porter RJ, Theodore WR. Clinical and electrographic features of simple partial seizures. *Neurology* **18**: 1347–52. 1988.

43. Ramsey RE, Cohen A, Brown MC. Coexisting epilepsy and non-epileptic seizures. In *Non-epileptic seizures*, (ed.) Rowan AJ, Gates JR. Butterworth, New York. 47–54. 1993.

44. Alhalabi M, Verma NP. Closure of eyes is a frequent and reliable sign of pseudoepileptic seizures (abstract). *Epilepsia* **35(suppl. 8)**: S15.

45. Benbadis SR, Lancman ME, King LM, Swanson SJ. Preictal pseudosleep: A new finding in psychogenic seizures. *Neurology* **47**: 63–7. 1996.

46. Bazil CW, Walczak TS. Effects of sleep and sleep stage on epileptic and non-epileptic seizures. *Epilepsia* **38**: 56–62. 1997.

47. Bergen D, Ristanovic R. Weeping as a common element of pseudoseizures. *Arch. Neurol.* **50**: 1059–60. 1993.

48. Lancman ME, Asconape JJ, Craven WJ *et al*. Predictive value of induction of psychogenic seizures by suggestion. *Ann. Neurol.* **35**: 359–61. 1994.

49. Walczak TS, Williams DT, Berten W. Utility and reliability of placebo infusion in the evaluation of patients with seizures. *Neurology* **44**: 394–9. 1994.

50. Slater JD, Brown MC, Jacobs W, Ramsey RE. Induction of pseudoseizures with intravenous saline placebo. *Epilepsia* **36**: 580–5. 1995.

51. Trimble MR. Serum prolactin in epilepsy and hysteria. *BMJ* **2**: 1682. 1978.

52. Yerby MS, van Belle G, Friel PN, Wilensky SJ. Serum prolactins in the diagnosis of epilepsy: sensitivity, specificity and predictive value. *Neurology* **37**: 1224–6. 1987.

53. Collins WCJ, Lanigan O, Callaghan N. Plasma prolactin concentration following epileptic and pseudoseizures. *JNNP* **46**: 505–8. 1983.

54. Sperling MR, Prichard PB III, Engel J, Jr *et al*. Prolactin in partial epilepsy: an indicator of limbic seizures. *Ann. Neurol.* **20**: 716–22. 1986.

55. Anzola GP. Predictivity of plasma prolactin levels in differentiating epilepsy from pseudoseizures: a prospective study. *Epilepsia* **34**: 1044–8. 1993.

56. Oribe E, Amini R, Nissenbaum E, Boal B. Serum prolactin concentrations are elevated in syncope. *Neurology* **47**: 60–2. 1996.

57. Rosenbaum DS, Snyder S, Rowan AJ *et al*. Outpatient multidisciplinary management of non-epileptic seizures. In *Non-epileptic seizures*, (ed.) Rowan AJ, Gates JR. Butterworth, New York. 275–83. 1993.

58. Wallace SJ. Childhood epileptic seizures. *Lancet* **336**: 486–8. 1990.

59. Sharborough F. Scalp-recorded ictal patterns in focal epilepsy. *J. Clin. Neurophysiol.* **10**: 262–7. 1993.

60. Doose H, Baier WK. Benign partial epilepsy and related conditions: multifactorial pathogenesis with hereditary impairment of brain maturation. *Eur. J. Pediatr.* **149**: 152–8. 1989.

61. Loiseau P, Beaussart M. The seizures of benign childhood epilepsy with rolandic paroxysmal spikes. *Epilepsia* **14**: 381–99. 1973.

62. Gastaut H. A new type of epilepsy: benign partial epilepsy of childhood with occipital spike waves. Clin. Electroencephalogr. **13**: 13–22. 1982.

63. Duchowny M, Harvey AS. Paediatric epilepsy syndromes: an update and critical review. *Epilepsia* **37(suppl. 1)**: S26–40. 1996.

64. Palmini A, Gloor P. The localising value of auras in partial

65. Currier RD, Little SC, Suess JF, Andy OJ. Sexual seizures. Arch. Neurol. **25**: 260–4. 1971.

66. Gloor P, Olivier A, Quesney LF *et al*. The role of the limbic system in experiential phenomena of temporal lobe epilepsy. *Ann. Neurol.* **12**: 129–44. 1982.

67. Delgado-Escueta AV, Mattson RH, King L *et al*. The nature of aggression during epileptic seizures. *N. Engl. J. Med.* **305**: 711. 1981.

68. Gabr M, Luders H, Dinner D *et al*. Speech manifestations in lateralisation of temporal lobe seizures. *Ann. Neurol.* **25**: 82–7. 1989.

69. Kotagal P. Seizure symptomatology of temporal lobe epilepsy. In Epilepsy surgery, (ed.) Luders H. Raven, New York. 143–56. 1991.

70. Manford M, Fish DR, Shorvon SD. An analysis of clinical seizure patterns and their localising value in frontal and temporal lobe epilepsies. *Brain* **119**: 17–40. 1996.

71. Kotagal P, Luders H, Morris H. Dystonic posturing in complex partial seizures of temporal lobe onset: a new lateralising sign. *Neurology* **39**: 196–201. 1989.

72. Bleasel A, Kotagal P, Kankirawatana P, Rybicki L. Lateralising value and semiology of ictal limb posturing and version in temporal lobe and extratemporal epilepsy. *Epilepsia* **38**: 168–74. 1997.

73. Sackeim HA, Greenberg MS, Weiman AL *et al*. Hemispheric asymmetry in the expression of positive and negative emotions. Neurologic evidence. *Arch. Neurol.* **39**: 210–18. 1982.

74. Berkovic SF, Kuzniecky RI, Andermann F. Human epileptogenesis and hypothalmic hamartomas: New lessons from an experiment of nature (editorial). *Epilepsia* **38**: 1–3. 1997.

75. Chauvel P, Delgado-Escueta AV, Halgren E, Bancaud J. (ed.). Advances in neurology: Frontal lobe seizures and epilepsies. Raven, New York. 1992.

76. Morris HH. Frontal lobe epilepsies. In Epilepsy surgery, (ed.) Luders H. Raven, New York. 157–65. 1991.

77. Williamson PD, Thadani VM, Darcey TM *et al*. Occipital lobe epilepsy: clinical characteristics, seizure spread patterns and results of surgery. *Ann. Neurol.* **31**: 3–13. 1992.

78. Ambrosetto G, Antonini L, Tassinari CA. Occipital lobe seizures related to clinically asymptomatic coeliac disease in adulthood. *Epilepsia* **33**: 476–81. 1992.

79. Gobbi G, Bouquet F, Greco L *et al*. Coeliac disease, epilepsy and cerebral calcifications. *Lancet* **340**: 439–43. 1992.

80. Bancaud J. Kojewnikow's syndrome (epilepsia partialis continua) in children. In *Epileptic syndromes in infancy, childhood and adolescence*, (ed.) Roger J, Draver C, Bureau M *et al*. John Libbey Eurotext, London. 286–98. 1985.

81. Thomas JE, Regan TJ, Klass DW. Epilepsia partialis continua: a review of 32 cases. *Arch. Neurol.* **34**: 266. 1977.

82. Loiseau P. Childhood absence epilepsy. In *Epileptic syndromes in infancy, childhood and adolescence*, (ed.) Roger J, Dravet C, Bureau M *et al*. John Libbey Eurotext, London. 106–20. 1985.

83. Porter RJ. The absence epilepsies. *Epilepsia* **34(suppl. 3)**: S42–8.

84. Janz D, Christian W. Impulsiv-petit mal. *Dtsch. Z. Nervenheilk* **176**: 346–86. 1957.

85. Enrile-Bascal FE, Delgado-Escueta AV. Myoclonic, tonic-clonic seizures of adolescence. The syndrome of Janz. *Neurology* **31**: 113. 1981.

86. Delgado-Escueta AV, Serratosa JM, Liu AW *et al*. A juvenile myoclonic epilepsy locus proximal to HLA: the value of studying a large family. *Epilepsia* **35(suppl. 7)**: 8. 1994.

87. Whitehouse WP, Rees M, Curtis D *et al.* Linkage analysis of idiopathic generalised epilepsy and marker loci on chromosome 6p in families of patients with juvenile myoclonic epilepsy: no evidence for an epilepsy locus in the HLA region. *Am. J. Hum. Genet.* **53**: 652–62. 1993.

88. Wolf P. Epilepsy with grand mal on awakening. In *Epileptic syndromes in infancy, childhood and adolescence*, (ed.) Roger J, Dravet C, Bureau M. *et al.* John Libbey Eurotext, London. 259–70. 1985.

89. Kellaway P, Hrachovy R, Frost JD, Zion T. Precise characterisation and quantification of infantile spasms. *Ann. Neurol.* **6**: 214–18. 1979.

90. West WJ. On a peculiar form of infantile convulsions. *Lancet* **i**: 724–5. 1841.

91. Shields D, Sherman A, Chugani HT *et al.* Treatment of infantile spasms: Medical or surgical? *Epilepsia* **33**: S26–31. 1992.

92. Aicardi J. The Lennox–Gastaut syndrome. *Intl. Pediatr.* **3**: 152–6. 1988.

93. Doose H, Gerken H, Leonhardt R *et al.* Centrencephalic myoclonic-astatic petit mal. *Neuropediatrie* **2**: 59–78. 1970.

94. Tassinari CA, Bureau M. Epilepsy with myoclonic absences. In *Epileptic syndromes in infancy, childhood and adolescence*, (ed.) Roger J, Dravet C, Bureau M *et al.* John Libbey Eurotext, London. 121–9. 1985.

95. Landau WM, Kleffner FR. Syndrome of acquired aphasia with convulsive disorder in children. *Neurology* **7**: 523–30. 1957.

96. O'Tuama LA, Urion DK, Janicek MJ *et al.* Regional cerebral perfusion in Landau–Kleffner syndrome and related childhood aphasias. *J. Nucl. Med.* **33**: 1758–65. 1992.

97. Nelson KB, Ellenborg JH. *Febrile seizures.* Raven, New York. 1981.

98. Wallace RH, Brekovic SF, Howell RA *et al.* Suggestion of a major gene for familial febrile convulsions mapping to 6q 13–21. *J. Med. Genet.* **33**; 308–12. 1996.

99. Maher J, McLachlan RS. Febrile convulsions: is seizure duration the most important predictor of temporal lobe epilepsy? *Brain* **118**: 1521–8. 1995.

100. Ritaccio AL. Reflex seizures. *Neurologic Clinics* **12**: 57–83. 1994.

101. Barclay CL, Murphy WF, Lee MA, Darwish HZ. Unusual form of seizures induced by eye closure. *Epilepsia* **34**: 289–93. 1993.

102. Takahashi T, Tsukahara Y. Usefulness of blue sunglasses in photosensitive epilepsy. *Epilepsia* **33**: 517–21. 1992.

103. Rasmussen T, Olsezewski J, Lloyd-Smith D. Focal seizures due to chronic localised encephalitis. *Neurology* **8**: 435–45. 1958.

104. Rogers SW, Andrews PI, Gahring LC *et al.* Autoantibodies to glutamate receptor GluR3 in Rasmussen's encephalitis. *Science* **265**: 648–51. 1994.

105. McLachlan RS, Levin S, Blume WT. Treatment of Rasmussen's syndrome with Ganciclovir. *Neurology* **47**: 925–8. 1996.

106. Flint AC, Kriegstein AR. Mechanisms underlying neuronal migration disorders and epilepsy. *Current Opinion in Neurology* **10**: 92–7. 1997.

107. Leppert M, Anderson VE, Quattlebaum TG *et al.* Benign familial neonatal convulsions linked to genetic markers on chromosome 20. *Nature* **337**: 647–8. 1989.

108. Lewis TB, Leach RJ, Ward K *et al.* Genetic heterogeneity in benign familial neonatal convulsions: identification of a new locus on chromosome 8q. *Am. J. Hum. Genet.* **53**: 670–6. 1993.

109. Scheffer IE, Bhatia KP, Lopes-Cendes I *et al.* Autosomal dominant frontal epilepsy misdiagnosed as sleep disorder. *Lancet* **343**: 515–17. 1994.

110. Scheffer IE, Bhatia KP, Lopes-Cendes I *et al.* Autosomal dominant nocturnal frontal epilepsy: a distinctive clinical disorder. *Brain* **118**: 61–73. 1995.

111. Phillips HA, Scheffer IE, Berkovic SF *et al.* Localisation of a gene for autosomal dominant nocturnal frontal lobe epilepsy to chromosome 20q 13.2. *Nature Genet.* **10**: 117–18. 1995.

112. Steinlein OK, Mulley JC, Propping P *et al.* A missense mutation in the neuronal nicotinic acetylcholine receptor alpha 4 subunit is associated with autosomal dominant nocturnal frontal lobe epilepsy. *Nature Genet.* **11**: 201–3. 1995.

113. Berkovic SF, Howell RA, Hopper JL. Familial temporal lobe epilepsy: a new syndrome with adolescent/adult onset and a benign course. In *Epileptic seizures and syndromes*, (ed.) Wolf P. John Libbey, London. 257–63. 1994.

114. Berkovic SF, McIntosh AM, Howell RA *et al.* Familial temporal lobe epilepsy: a common disorder identified in twins. *Ann. Neurol.* **40**: 227–35. 1996.

115. Ottman R, Risch N, Hauser WA *et al.* Localisation of a gene for partial epilepsy to chromosome 10q. *Nature Genet.* **10**: 56–60. 1995.

116. Berkovic SF, Cochius J, Andermann E, Andermann F. Progressive myoclonus epilepsies: clinical and genetic aspects. *Epilepsia* **34(suppl. 3)**: S19–30. 1993.

117. Pennacchio LA, Lehesjoki AE, Stone NE *et al.* Mutations in the gene encoding cystatin B in progressive myoclonus epilepsy (EPM 1). *Science* **271**: 1731–4. 1996.

118. Jennett B. *Epilepsy after non-missile head injuries*, (2nd edn). Heinemann, London. 1975.

119. Annegers JF, Grabow JD, Groover RV *et al.* Seizures after head trauma: a population study. *Neurology* **30**: 683–9. 1980.

120. Kieslich M, Jacobi G. Incidence and risk factors of post-traumatic epilepsy in childhood (letter). *Lancet* **345**: 187. 1995.

121. Temkin NR, Dikmen SS, Wilensky AJ *et al.* A randomised, double blind study of phenytoin for the prevention of post-traumatic seizures. *N. Engl. J. Med.* **323**: 487–502. 1990.

122. Dikmen SS, Temkin NR, Miller B *et al.* Neurobehavioural effects of phenytoin prophylaxis of post-traumatic seizures. *JAMA* **265**: 1271–7. 1991.

123. Smith KR, Goulding PM, Wilderman D *et al.* Neurobehavioural effects of phenytoin and carbamazepine in patients recovering from brain trauma: a comparative study. *Arch. Neurol.* **51**: 653–60. 1994.

124. Goldstein LB. Prescribing of potentially harmful drugs to patients admitted to hospital after head injury. *JNNP* **58**: 753–5. 195.

125. Kellaway P. An orderly approach to visual analysis: characteristics of the normal EEG of adults and children. In *Current practice of clinical electroencephalography*, (ed.) Daly DD, Pedley TA. Raven, New York. 139–99. 1990.

126. Mizrahi EM. Avoiding the pitfalls of EEG interpretation in childhood epilepsy. *Epilepsia* **37(suppl. 1)**: S41–51. 1996.

127. Taylor JF. Driving and epilepsy. In *Fourth International Symposium on sodium valproate and epilepsy*, (ed.) Chadwick David. Royal Society of Medicine, International Congress of symposium series no. 152, London and New York: 270–3. 1989.

128. Chadwick D. Epilepsy. In *Medical aspects of fitness to drive*, (5th edn). Medical Commission of Accident Prevention. 61–77. 1994.

129. Morrell MJ. The new antiepileptic drugs and women: efficacy, reproductive health, pregnancy and foetal outcome. *Epilepsia* **37(suppl. 6)**: S34–44. 1996.

130. Knight AH, Rhind EG. Epilepsy and pregnancy: A study of 153 pregnancies in 59 patients. *Epilepsia* **16**: 99–110. 1975.

131. Dansky LV, Andermann E, Rosenblatt D *et al.* Anticonvulsants, folate levels and pregnancy outcome: a prospective study. *Ann. Neurol.* **21**: 176–82. 1987.

132. Ogawa Y, Kaneko S, Otani K, Fukushima Y. Serum folic acid levels in epileptic mothers and their relationship to congenital malformations. *Epilepsy Res.* **8**: 75–8. 1991.

133. Medical Research Council Vitamin Research Group. Prevention of neural tube defects: results of the Medical Research Council Vitamin Study. *Lancet* **338**: 131–7. 1991.

134. Yerby MS. Pregnancy, teratogenesis and epilepsy. *Neurologic Clinics* **12**: 749–71. 1994.

135. Devinsky OD, Yerby MS. Women with epilepsy. *Neurologic Clinics* **12**: 479–95. 1994.

136. Hauser WA, Rich SS, Jacobs MP, Anderson VE. Patterns of seizure occurrence and recurrent risks in patients with newly diagnosed epilepsy. *Abstracts* of the 15th *Epilepsy International Symposium*. Hartford, Connecticut. American Epilepsy Society, 16. 1983.

137. Russell-Jones DL, Shorvon SD. The frequency and consequences of head injury in epileptic seizures. *JNNP* **52**: 659–62. 1989.

138. Tempest MN. Burns in epileptic patients: a survey of admissions to a regional burns centre over a period of 20 years. In Malles P, Barclay L, Konckova Z (ed.). *Research in burns. Transactions of the 3rd international conference on research in burns.* Hans Huber, Berne. 1970.

139. Hampton KK, Peatfield RC, Pullar T *et al.* Burns because of epilepsy. *BMJ* **296**: 1659–60. 1988.

140. Spitz MC. Severe burns as a consequence of seizures in patients with epilepsy. *Epilepsia* **33**: 103–7. 1992.

141. Spitz MC, Towbin JA, Shantz D, Adler LE. Risk factors for burns as a consequence of seizures in persons with epilepsy. *Epilepsia* **35**: 764–7. 1995.

142. Cockerell OC, Johnson AJ, Goodridge DMG *et al.* The mortality of epilepsy: results from the National General Practice Study of Epilepsy. *Lancet* **344**: 918–21. 1994.

143. Shorvon SD. *Status Epilepticus: its clinical features and treatment in children and adults.* Cambridge University Press. 1994.

144. Barraclough B. Suicide and epilepsy. In *Epilepsy and psychiatry*, (ed.) Reynolds E, Trimble M. Churchill Livingstone, Edinburgh: 72–6. 1980.

145. Jay GW, Leestma JE. Sudden death in epilepsy. A comprehensive view of the literature and proposed mechanisms. *Acta Neurol. Scand. Suppl.* **82**: 1–66. 1981.

146. Cockerell OC. The mortality of epilepsy. *Current Opinion in Neurology* **9**: 93–6. 1996.

147. Leestma JE, Annegers JF, Brodie MJ *et al.* Sudden unexplained death in epilepsy: observations from a large clinical development program. *Epilepsia* **38**: 47–55. 1997.

148. Nashef L, Fish DR, Sander JWAS, Shorvon SD. Incidence of sudden unexpected death in an adult outpatient cohort at a tertiary referral centre. *JNNP* **58**: 462–4. 1995.

149. Gilchrist JM. Arrhythmogenic seizures: diagnosis by simultaneous EEG/ECG recording. *Neurology* **35**: 1503–6. 1985.

150. Wilder-Smith E. Complete atrio-ventricular conduction block during complex partial seizures. *JNNP* **55**: 734–6. 1992.

151. Nashef L, Walker F, Allen P *et al.* Apnoea and bradycardia during epileptic seizures: relation to sudden death in epilepsy. *JNNP* **60**: 297–300. 1996.

152. Dodrill CB, Batzel L, Queisser HR, Temkin NR. An objective method for the assessment of psychological and social problems among epileptics. *Epilepsia* **21**: 123–35. 1980.

153. Betts TA. Depression, anxiety and epilepsy. In *Epilepsy and psychiatry*, (ed.) Reynolds EH, Trimble MR. Churchill Livingstone, Edinburgh. 1981.

154. Lechtenberg R. *Epilepsy and the family.* Harvard University Press, Cambridge, MA. 1984.

155. Garber J, Seligman M (ed.). *Human helplessness: Theory and application.* Academic Press, New York. 1980.

156. Pond A, Bidwell BH. A survey of epilepsy in fourteen general practices. *Epilepsia* **1**: 285–99. 1959.

157. Gudmundsson G. Epilepsy in Iceland. *Acta Neurol. Scand.* **43(suppl. 25)**: 1–124. 1966.

158. Edeh J, Toone B. Relationship between interictal psychopathology and type of epilepsy: results of a survey in general practice. *Br. J. Psychiat.* **151**: 95–101. 1987.

159. Currie S, Heathfield KWG, Henson RA, Scott DF. Clinical course and prognosis of temporal lobe epilepsy: a survey of 666 patients. *Brain* **94**: 173–90. 1971.

160. Bruens JH. Psychoses in epilepsy. In *handbook of clinical neurology*, (ed.) Vinkin PL, Bruyn LW. Amsterdam, North Holland. Vol. 15, 593–610. 1974.

161. Slater E, Beard AW, Glithero E. The schizophrenia-like psychoses of epilepsy. *Br. J. Psychiat.* **109**: 5–150. 1963.

162. Perez MM, Trimble MR. Epileptic psychosis—diagnostic comparison with schizophrenia. *Br. J. Psychiat.* **146**: 155–64. 1980.

163. Annegers JF, Hauser WA, Elverback LR. Remission of seizures and relapse in patients with epilepsy. *Epilepsia* **20**: 729–37. 1979.

164. Cockerell OC, Johnson AL, Sander JWAS, Shorvon SD. Prognosis of epilepsy: A review and further analysis of the first nine years of the British National General Practice Study of Epilepsy, a prospective population based study. *Epilepsia* **38**: 31–46. 1997.

165. Sofijanov NG. Clinical evolution and prognosis of childhood epilepsies. *Epilepsia* **23**: 61–9. 1982.

166. Kiorboe E. The prognosis of epilepsy. *Acta Psychiat. Scand.* **36(suppl. 150)**: 166–78. 1961.

167. Reynolds EH. Early treatment and prognosis of epilepsy. *Epilepsia* **28**: 97–106. 1987.

168. Hauser WA, Anderson VE, Loewenston RB, McRoberts SM. Seizure recurrence after a first unprovoked seizure. *N. Engl. J. Med.* **307**: 522–8. 1982.

169. Group for the study of the prognosis of epilepsy in Japan. Natural history and prognosis of epilepsy: report of a multi-institutional study in Japan. *Epilepsia* **22**: 35–53. 1981.

170. Juul-Jensen P. Epilepsy: a clinical and social analysis of 1020 adult patients with epileptic seizures. *Acta Neurol. Scand.* **40(suppl. 5)**: 1–285. 1964.

171. Shaffer SQ, Hauser WA, Annegers JF, Klass DW. EEG and other early predictors of epilepsy remission: a community study. *Epilepsia* **29**: 590–600. 1988.

172. Foy PM, Copeland GP, Shaw MDM. The incidence of post-operative seizures. *Acta Neurochir.* **55**: 253–64. 1981.

173. Foy PM, Chadwick DW, Rajgopalan N *et al.* Do prophylactic anticonvulsant drugs alter the pattern of seizures following craniotomy? *JNNP* **55**: 753–7. 1992.

174. Chadwick DW, Shaw MDM, Foy PM *et al.* Serum anticonvulsant concentrations and the risk of drug-induced skin eruptions. *JNNP* **47**: 642–4. 1984.

175. McQueen JK, Blackwood DH, Harris P *et al.* Low risk of late post-traumatic seizures following severe head injury: implications for clinical trials of prophylaxis. *JNNP* **46**: 899–904. 1983.

176. Reynolds EH, Shorvon SD, Galbraith AW *et al.* Phenytoin monotherapy for epilepsy: a long term prospective study, assisted by serum level monitoring, in previously untreated patients. *Epilepsia* **22**: 475–88. 1981.

177. Turnbull DM, Howell D, Rawlins MD, Chadwick DW. Which drug for the adult epileptic patient: phenytoin or valproate? *BMJ* **290**: 815–19. 1985.

178. Chadwick DW, Turnbull EH. The comparative efficacy of

antiepileptic drugs for partial and tonic-clonic seizures. *JNNP* **48**: 1073–7. 1985.

179. Callaghan N, O'Hare J, O'Driscoll D *et al.* Comparative study of ethosuximide and sodium valproate in the treatment of typical absence seizures (petit mal). *Develop. Med. Child. Neurol.* **24**: 830–6. 1982.

180. Delgado-Escueta AV, Enrile-Bascal F. Juvenile myoclonic epilepsy of Janz. *Neurology* **34**: 285–94. 1984.

181. Mattson RH, Cramer JA, Collins JF *et al.* A comparison of valproate with carbamazepine for the treatment of complex partial seizures with secondarily generalised tonic-clonic seizures in adults. *N. Engl. J. Med.* **327**: 765–71. 1992.

182. Heller AJ, Chesterman P, Elwes RDC *et al.* Phenobarbitone, phenytoin, carbamazepine or sodium valproate for newly diagnosed adult epilepsy. *JNNP* **58**: 44–50. 1995.

183. Richens A, Davidson DLW, Cartlidge NEF *et al.* on behalf of the adult EPITEG Collaborative Group. A multicentre comparative trial of sodium valproate and carbamazepine in adult onset epilepsy. *JNNP* **57**: 682–7. 1994.

184. Marson AG, Kadir ZA, Chadwick DW. Efficacy and safety of the new antiepileptic drugs. *BMJ* **313**: 1169–74. 1996.

185. Schmidt D. *Adverse effects of antiepileptic drugs.* Raven, New York. 1982.

186. Chadwick DW, Reynolds EH, Marsden CD. Anticonvulsant induced dyskinesias: a comparison with dyskinesias induced by neuroleptics. *JNNP* **39**: 1210–18. 1976.

187. Labar DR. Antiepileptic drug toxic emergencies. In *The medical treatment of epilepsy* (ed.) Rosor S, Kutt H. Marcel Dekker, New York. 573–88. 1992.

188. Reeves A *et al.* Movement disorders associated with the use of gabapentin. *Epilepsia* **37**: 988–90. 1996.

189. Turnbull DM, Rawlins MD, Weightman D, Chadwick DW. Plasma concentrations of sodium valproate: their clinical value. *Ann. Neurol.* **14**: 38–42. 1983.

190. Reynolds EH. Mental effects of antiepileptic medication: a review. *Epilepsia* **24**(**suppl. 2**): S85–9. 1983.

191. Richens A. Lamotrigine. In *Recent advances in epilepsy*, (ed.) Pedley TA, Meldrum BS. Churchill Livingstone, Edinburgh. Vol. 5, 197–210. 1992.

192. Dreifuss FE, Santilli N, Langer DH *et al.* Valproic acid fatalities: a retrospective review. *Neurology* **37**: 379–85. 1987.

193. Reynolds EH. Chronic antiepileptic toxicity: a review. *Epilepsia* **16**: 319–52. 1975.

194. Schmidt D. Two antiepileptic drugs for intractable epilepsy with complex partial seizures. *JNNP* **45**: 1119–29. 1982.

195. Baker GA, Jacoby A, Buck D *et al.* Quality of life of people with epilepsy: A European Study. *Epilepsia* **38**: 353–62. 1997.

196. Richens A, Dunlop A. Serum phenytoin levels in the management of epilepsy. *Lancet* **ii**: 247–9. 1975.

197. Gannaway DJ, Mawer GE. Serum phenytoin concentrations and clinical response in patients with epilepsy. *Br. J. Clin. Pharmacol.* **12**: 833–9. 1981.

198. Rowan AJ, Binnie CD, Warfield CA *et al.* The delayed effect of sodium valproate on the photoconvulsive response in man. *Epilepsia* **20**: 61–8. 1979.

199. Jacoby A, Baker G, Chadwick D, Johnson A. The impact of counselling with a practical statistical model on patient's decision making about treatment for epilepsy: findings from a pilot study. *Epilepsy Res.* **16**: 207–14. 1993.

200. Berg AT, Shinnar S. Relapse following discontinuation of antiepileptic drugs: a meta-analysis. *Neurology* **44**: 601–8. 1994.

201. Shinnar S, Berg AT, Moshe S *et al.* Discontinuing antiepileptic drugs in children with epilepsy: a prospective study. *Ann. Neurol.* **35**: 534–45. 1994.

202. Tennison M, Greenwood R, Lewis D, Thorn M. Rate of taper of antiepileptic drugs and the risk of seizure recurrence in children. *N. Engl. J. Med.* **330**: 1407–10. 1994.

203. US Gabapentin Study Group. Gabapentin as add-on therapy in refractory epilepsy: a double-blind, placebo-controlled, parallel group study. *Neurology* **43**: 2292–8. 1993.

204. Anhut H, Ashman P, Feuerstein TJ *et al.* Gabapentin as add-on therapy in patients with partial seizures: a double-blind, placebo-controlled study. *Epilepsia* **35**: 795–801. 1994.

205. Risner M. The Lamictal Study Group: Multicentre, double-blind, placebo- controlled, add-on, crossover study of lamotrigine (Lamictal) in epileptic outpatients with partial seizures. *Epilepsia* **31**: 619–20. 1994.

206. Matsuo F, Bergen D, Faught E *et al.* placebo-controlled study on the efficacy and safety of lamotrigine in patients with partial seizures. US Lamotrigine Protocol 0.5 Clinical Trial Group. *Neurology* **43**: 2284–91. 1993.

207. Donaldson JA, Glauser TA, Oldberding LS. Lamotrigine adjunctive therapy in childhood epileptic encephalopathy (the Lennox–Gastaut syndrome). *Epilepsia* **38**: 68–73. 1997.

208. Oxcarbazepine (editorial). Lancet **11**: 196–8. 1989.

209. Dam M, Ekberg R, Loyning Y *et al.* A double-blind study comparing oxcarbazepine and carbamazepine in patients with newly diagnosed, previously untreated epilepsy. *Epilepsy Res.* **3**: 70–6. 1989.

210. Ben-Menachem E. International experience with tiagabine add-on therapy. *Epilepsia* **36**(**suppl. 6**): S14–21. 1995.

211. Leppik IE. Tiagabine: the safety landscape. *Epilepsia* **36**(**suppl. 6**): S10–13. 1995.

212. Faught E, Wilder BJ, Ramsay RE *et al.* Topiramate placebo-controlled dose ranging trial in refractory partial epilepsy using 200-, 400- and 600mg daily dosages. *Neurology* **46**: 1684–90. 1996.

213. Rosenfield WE, Doose DR, Walker SA, Nayak RK. Effect of topiramate on the pharmacokinetics of an oral contraceptive containing norethindrone and ethinyl oestradiol in patients with epilepsy. *Epilepsia* **38**: 317–23. 1997.

214. Shorvon S. Safety of topiramate: adverse events and relationships to dosing. *Epilepsia* **37**(**suppl. 2**): S18–22. 1996.

215. French J, Mosier M, Walker S *et al.* and the Vigabatrin Protocol 024 Investigative Cohort; A double-blind, placebo-controlled study of vigabatrin 3g/day in patients with uncontrolled partial seizures. *Neurology* **46**: 54–61. 1996.

216. Sander JW, Hart YM, Trimble MR, Shorvon SD. Vigabatrin and psychosis. *JNNP* **54**: 435–9. 1991.

217. Chiron C, Dumas C, Dulac O *et al.* Vigabatrin versus hydrocortisone as first-line monotherapy in infantile spasms due to tuberose sclerosis. *Epilepsia* **36**(**suppl. 3**): S265. 1995.

218. Eke T, Talbot JF, Lawden MC. Severe persistent visual field constriction associated with vigabatrin. *BMJ* **314**: 180–1. 1997.

219. Backstrom JT, Hinkle RL, Flicker MR (comment on ref. 218). *BMJ* **314**: 1694–5. 1997.

220. Leppik IE, Willmore LJ, Homan RW *et al.* Efficacy and safety of zonisamide: results of a multicentre study. *Epilepsy Res.* **14**: 165–73. 1993.

221. Schmidt D, Jacob R, Loiseau P *et al.* Zonisamide for add-on treatment of refractory partial epilepsy: a European double-blind trial. *Epilepsy Res.* **15**: 67–73. 1993.

222. Berent S, Sackellares JC, Giordani B *et al.* Zonisamide (CI-912) and cognition: results from preliminary study. *Epilepsia* **28**: 61–7. 1987.

223. Shorvon SD. Tonic-clonic Status Epilepticus. *JNNP* **56**: 125–34. 1993.

224. Gross-Tsur V, Shinnar S. Convulsive status epilepticus in children. *Epilepsia* **34**(**suppl. 1**): S12–20. 1993.

225. Runge JW, Allen FH. Emergency treatment of status epilepticus. *Neurology* **46**(**suppl. 1**): S20–3. 1996.

226. Shorvon SD. Status epilepticus: its clinical features and treatment in children and adults. Cambridge University Press. 1993.

227. Lucas MJ, Leveno KJ, Cunningham FG. A comparison of magnesium sulfate with phenytoin for the prevention of eclampsia. *N. Engl. J. Med.* **333**: 201–5. 1995.

228. The Eclampsia Trial Collaborative Group. Which anticonvulsant for women with eclampsia? Evidence from the Collaborative Eclampsia Trial. *Lancet* **345**; 1455–63. 1995.

229. Dreifuss FE. Goals of surgery for epilepsy. In *Surgical treatment of the epilepsies*, (ed.) Engel J. Raven, New York. 31–50. 1987.

230. ILEA Commission Report. A global survey on epilepsy 1980–1990: A report by the Commission on neurosurgery of epilepsy. *Epilepsia* **38**: 249–55. 1997.

231. Kellett MW, Smith DF, Baker GA, Chadwick DW. Quality of life after epilepsy surgery. *JNNP* **63**: 52–8. 1997.

232. Engel J Jr Update on surgical treatment of the epilepsies. *Neurology* **43**: 1612–17. 1993.

233. Oxbury JM, Adams CBT. Neurosurgery for epilepsy. *Br. J. Hosp. Med.* **41**: 372–7. 1989.

234. Germano IM, Poulin N, Olivier A. Re-operation for recurrent temporal lobe epilepsy. *J. Neurosurg.* **81**: 3–36. 1994.

235. Yasargil MG, Wieser HG. Selective amygdalohippocampectomy at the University Hospital, Zurich. In *Surgical treatment of the epilepsies*, (ed.) Engel J. Raven, New York. 652–8. 1987.

236. Salanova V, Quesney LF, Rasmussen T *et al.* Re-evaluation of surgical failures and the role of re-operation in 39 patients with frontal lobe epilepsy. *Epilepsia* **35**: 70–80. 1994.

237. Spencer SS, Gates JR, Reeves AR *et al.* Corpus callosum section. In *Surgical treatment of the epilepsies*, (ed.) Engel J. Raven, New York. 425–44. 1987.

238. Black PM, Holmes G, Lombroso C. Corpus callosum section for intractable epilepsy in children. *Pediatr. Neurosurg.* **18**: 298–304. 1992.

239. Spencer SS, Spencer DD, Sass K *et al.* Anterior, total and two-stage corpus callosum section: differential and incremental seizure responses. *Epilepsia* **34**: 561–7. 1993.

240. Oppenheimer DR, Griffith HB. Persistent intracranial bleeding as a complication of hemispherectomy. *JNNP* **29**: 229–40. 1966.

241. Adams CBT. Hemispherectomy—a modification. *JNNP* **46**: 617–19. 1983.

242. Villemure J-G, Adams CBT, Hoffman HJ, Peacock WJ. Hemispherectomy. In *Surgical treatment of the epilepsies*, (ed.) Engel J. Raven, New York. 511–18. 1993.

243. Fisher RS, Uthman BM, Ramsay RE *et al.* Alternative surgical techniques for epilepsy. In *Surgical treatment of the epilepsies*, (ed.) Engel J. Raven, New York. 549–64. 1993.

244. Loring DW, Murro AM, Meador KJ *et al.* Wada memory testing and hippocampal volume measurements in the evaluation for temporal lobectomy. *Neurology* **43**: 1789–93. 1993.

245. Jack CR. Epilepsy: surgery and imaging. *Radiology* **189**: 635–46. 1993.

246. Jack CR, Rydberg CN, Krecke K *et al.* Mesial temporal sclerosis: diagnosis with FLAIR versus spin-echo MR imaging. *Radiology* **199**: 367–73. 1996.

247. Sisodiya S, Stevens J, Fish D *et al.* The demonstration of gyral abnormalities in patients with cryptogenic partial epilepsy using three-dimensional MRI. *Arch. Neurol.* **53**: 28–34. 1996.

248. Newton MR, Berkovic SF, Austin MC *et al.* SPECT in the localisation of extratemporal and temporal seizure foci. *JNNP* **59**: 26–30. 1995.

249. Spencer SS. The relative contributions of MRI, SPECT and PET imaging in epilepsy. *Epilepsia* **35**(**suppl. 6**): S72–89. 1994.

250. Sperling MR, Alavi A, Reivich M *et al.* False lateralisation of temporal lobe epilepsy with FDG positron emission tomography. *Epilepsia* **36**: 722–7. 1995.

251. Prichard JW. New nuclear magnetic resonance data in epilepsy. *Current Opinion in Neurology* **10**: 98–102. 1997.

252. Fisher RS, Krauss GL, Ramsay E *et al.* Assessment of vagus nerve stimulation for epilepsy: report of the Therapeutics and Technology Assessment Subcommittee of the American Academy of Neurology. *Neurology* **49**: 293–7. 1997.

5 | Headache

Richard Peatfield

Large-scale epidemiological surveys of the general population, such as that undertaken by Waters in South Wales in 1968, have established that up to 92% of all women aged 21–34 have had at least one headache in the previous year. This prevalence falls with age and is consistently a little lower in men, but remains 22% even in men over the age of 75. Although only a small minority of these patients seek medical advice, headache is by far the commonest single symptom in patients attending neurological clinics (Table 5.1). Structural causes of headaches requiring specific diagnosis and medical or surgical treatment are important but unusual in patients complaining of headache as a whole, and the majority of these have migraine, variants of migraine such as cluster headache, or the so called 'tension type headache', which have to be seen as non-structural 'functional' disorders. It is important that neurologists assess and reassure all these patients, particularly now that there is such a wide variety of effective therapies. Mere reassurance that there is no evidence of a 'brain tumour' is no longer sufficient.

Table 5.1 Prevalence of neurological diseases

	Point prevalence per 100 000[a]	No. needing neurological attention[a]	Percentage of neurological patients[b]
Migraine	10 000	2000	8.3%
Other severe headache	15 000	1500	9.0%
Epilepsy	650	650	12.6%
Stroke	600	600	6.7%
Lumbar pain syndrome	500	50	
Parkinson's disease	200	200	
Multiple sclerosis	60	60	3.2%
Subarachnoid haemorrhage	50	50	
Motor neurone disease	6	6	
Malignant primary brain tumour	5	5	
Meningitis	5	5	

[a] From Kurtzke (1992).
[b] From the Association of British Neurologists, Audit (1992).

DIFFERENTIAL DIAGNOSIS

This chapter will be concerned very largely with patients whose principal complaint is of headache. If a patient with headache also has fixed focal symptoms or signs, such as a hemiparesis or papilloedema one is much better advised to establish the cause of these other clinical features, as the cause of the headache will then usually become evident. While patients with migrainous auras do have intermittent focal symptoms, however, the vast majority of patients seeking help for headaches have few if any physical abnormalities to provide clinical clues, and much of the assessment has to be done from the clinical history. One will seldom gain much from physical examination, and only rarely are special investigations of any value. One should record the duration of the headache history and the pattern of attacks, with their duration, severity, and frequency as well as other clinical symptoms such as nausea, vomiting, and visual, limb, or speech disturbances. The relationship of headache to coughing, foodstuffs, exercise, neck, and jaw movements may also be significant.

The proportion with different diagnoses in a series of headache patients varies enormously depending on the source of these patients. For example, intracranial tumours requiring neurosurgical treatment constitutes no more than 1 in 1000 patients attending a specialist migraine clinic and slightly more in a general neurological clinic in a district general hospital, but up to 3% in patients attending a casualty department with 'the worst headache in my life' (Fodden *et al.* 1989). Conditions such as meningitis and subarachnoid haemorrhage, where a prompt and accurate diagnosis can be genuinely life-saving, are very rare in outpatients at all, but are much more common (up to 10%) in such casualty series and should always be borne in mind in an acute general practice setting.

Before this chapter goes on to discuss the assessment, pathogenesis, and management of 'functional' headache syndromes, such as migraine, the important alternatives that may require specific therapies will be discussed.

MASS LESIONS

Headache is very seldom the earliest symptom of a mass lesion within the cranium—only the meninges and basal blood vessels are pain-sensitive and there has to be very considerable anatomical distortion before these pain receptors are stimulated, either directly due to the tumour mass or to obstruction of cerebrospinal fund (CSF) pathways. While most patients with cerebral tumours will have headache among their symptoms at the time of diagnosis, and may well have sought medical attention largely because of this, virtually all these patients will have additional symptoms or physical signs that provide the clue that a thorough investigation is necessary. These include, for example, hemipareses, personality change, sensory or speech disturbances, and visual field defects with or without papilloedema. Seizures, or a progressive history over only a matter of weeks are further features justifying structural investigations. Many surveys of patients with tumours seeking advice about headache have supported the view that the proportion with clinically relevant structural abnormalities without atypical features or physical signs is so small that routine scanning cannot be considered economical. In most cases arranging to review a patient after about three months will establish that the headache pattern is indeed benign.

Potentially relevant mass lesions include not only malignant gliomas and benign tumours, such as meningiomas, pituitary adenomas, and posterior fossa haemangioblastomas, but also cerebral abcesses and intracranial haematomas, especially when subdural. Once diagnosed by appropriate scanning, advice should be sought from a neurosurgeon. It must be appreciated that routine computerized tomographic (CT) scanning will miss many patients with Arnold–Chiari malformations and a substantial proportion of those with subdural haematomas, meningitis or subarachnoid haemorrhage (see below), so a normal scan *per se* does not necessarily mean that the patient has a migraine like headache, if careful clinical assessment points elsewhere.

HYDROCEPHALUS

Most tumours obstructing the CSF pathways causing acquired hydrocephalus will lead to headache, most noticeably when the usual outflow pathway for cough-induced intracranial pressure waves is obstructed at the level of the foramen magnum by descent of the cerebellar tonsils (the Arnold–Chiari malformation) (See Fig. 5.1). While all headaches are liable to be increased by coughing, straining, sneezing, or bending over, any headache starting *de novo* after coughing warrants thorough investigation, as at least half will have the Arnold–Chiari malformation or some other major posterior fossa abnormality. The Arnold–Chiari malformation is most usually seen on a sagittal magnetic resonance imaging (MRI) scan—normal CSF pathways through the foramen magnum can be restored by surgical decompression, a procedure that is well justified if the history is typical.

Congenital hydrocephalus is a slower process, usually presenting with increasing head size, personality change, and optic atrophy rather than with headaches. Sixth nerve palsies are commonly seen. Colloid cysts of the third ventricle are

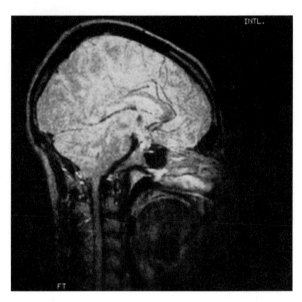

Fig. 5.1 Sagittal MRI scan of a 29-year-old man with attacks of headache triggered by lifting or straining, showing protrusion of the cerebellar tonsils through the foramen magnum (the Arnold–Chiari malformation). The headaches were relieved by posterior fossa decompression.

very rare but often present with headache, which may be positional, and the majority of patients have papilloedema or some other abnormality on clinical examination.

BENIGN INTRACRANIAL HYPERTENSION

Occasional patients presenting with new or worsening generalized headache, perhaps pulsatile, and sometimes associated with retro-ocular pain worsened by eye movements, are found to have papilloedema (Fig. 5.2), but CT scanning reveals normal or small ventricles without a mass lesion as a cause for the raised intracranial pressure. Unilateral VIth nerve palsies can be seen but other signs are unusual. Provided that the patient remains fully conscious it is considered safe to perform a lumbar puncture, when the pressure will be found to be raised, often above 200 mm of CSF, and the CSF itself is normal.

The cause of the raised intracranial pressure is often not clearly established. Patients with cerebral sinus thrombosis (e.g. following ear sepsis or associated with the contraceptive pill) can present with this clinical picture: usually this can be diagnosed on a CT or MRI scan, and confirmed angiographically. Blood clotting abnormalities (e.g. deficiencies of protein C or protein S) have been reported in many otherwise idiopathic patients, which would suggest that minor degrees of cerebral thrombosis are common in these patients, and routine angiograms with this in mind have been advocated by some authorities. Other cases are associated with head injuries, tetracyclines, and even corticosteroids. However, a substantial proportion of patients are significantly obese, which seems to be linked to a disturbance of brain water content.

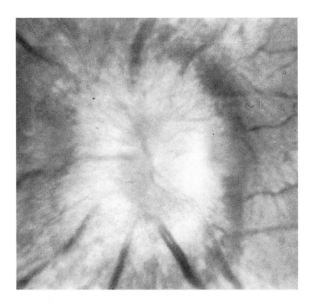

Fig. 5.2 The swollen optic disc of a patient with benign intracranial hypertension.

The headache is often relieved by removal of CSF at the original lumbar puncture, a procedure that can be repeated as necessary. Acetazolamide is used to reduce the excess production, and steroids have been used, although many feel their disadvantages outweigh the advantages. If the headaches persist they are often relieved by the insertion of a permanent lumboperitoneal shunt (Corbett and Thompson 1989).

The condition usually resolves spontaneously, but about 10% of patients suffer progressive visual loss—visual obscurations and an enlarged blind spot may be followed by peripheral field constriction or a central scotoma. Regular follow-up is therefore essential. The visual deterioration may respond to surgical decompression of one optic nerve by making a small hole in its covering meninges. (Fig. 5.3.)

ARTERIOVENOUS MALFORMATIONS

Knotted masses of distended blood vessels forming high flow fistulous communications between arteries and veins may occur in all parts of the brain, producing atypical enhancing area on a CT scan or angiography, usually without distortion of adjacent structures. Arteriovenous malformations (AVMs) should be distinguished from cavernous hemiangiomas which are seen on MRI scanning but are not demonstrable angiographically. Most AVMs come to medical attention by rupturing, either into the brain substance or the subarachnoid space, and they can also cause epilepsy. Headaches resembling migraine, sometimes with visual disturbances, can occur but are unusual, although there is a proven statistical association between arteriovenous malformation and migrainous symptoms. These malformations can be excised surgically, embolized via an intra-arterial catheter, or shrunk by radiation—all

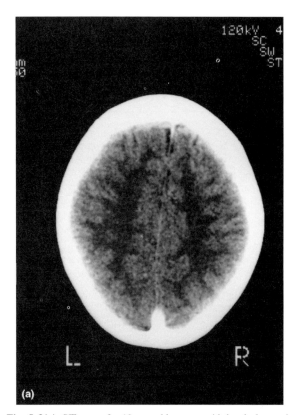

Fig. 5.3(a) CT scan of a 19-year-old woman with headaches and optic disc swelling; the third ventricle is effaced and there is midline opacity posteriorly suggesting sagittal and transverse sinus thrombosis.

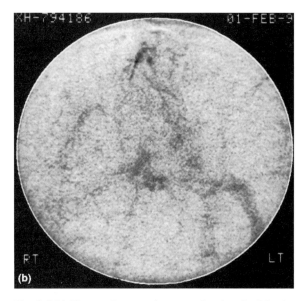

Fig. 5.3(b) Venous phase arteriogram undertaken the following day: only the distal left transverse sinus is opacified, with no contrast in the superior sagittal or right transverse sinus.

these procedures carry risks which may well be justified in a patient whose malformation has already bled but probably is not in most patients presenting only with headaches. AVMs are very rare among patients presenting with migrainous symptoms and scanning cannot be justified merely to detect such patients.

PAIN FROM THE NECK

There is an overlap of several segments in the lower brain-stem and cervical cord between the descending tract of the trigeminal nerve and the cervical nerve roots—thus, patients with cervical spondylosis can present with pain in the fore-head, although usually this is predominantly felt in the neck and is worsened by neck movements. Spondylitic pain is often associated with pain or paraesthesae in a root distribution in the arms. Radiological evidence of cervical spondylosis in older subjects is so common one has to be cautious in at-tributing headaches to the neck at least without excluding temporal arteritis. Most patients will respond to non-steroidal anti-inflammatory drugs (NSAIDs) in an appropriate dose.

The pain of acute disc prolapse and of other diseases of the cervical vertebrae is usually confined to the neck and is sel-dom a cause only of pain in the head.

SINUSITIS

A recent cold, pyrexia, or malaise are clues that a pain local-ized in the face originates in the sinuses—pain in the frontal sinus usually starts an hour or two after rising, clearing up in the afternoons, while that in the maxillary sinuses is worse on waking and is relieved by getting up. These patients often have a purulent nasal discharge. Sinusitic pain is very common in acute general practice or casualty department settings but is unusual in neurological clinics—the possibility that prolonged radiological opacification of the sinuses (Fig. 5.4) may in fact be malignant should always be borne in mind and an ENT (ear, nose, and throat) opinion sought in appropriate cases.

TEMPORAL ARTERITIS

Temporal or giant cell arteritis is a very common disease of the elderly—it is so easy to treat and has such devastating complications when untreated that one's index of suspicion must remain high. The pain may be frontal, occipital, or gen-eralized and is only rarely confined to the temple. All patients over the age of 55 with a recent history of headache should have their erythrocyte sedimentation rate (ESR) and/or C-reactive protein (CRP) checked and biopsy of the artery is advisable in all patients with an ESR above 2 standard devi-ations above the mean (which is often described as half the age in men and half the (age +10) in women) (Miller *et al.* 1983). Biopsy may be justified even if the ESR is within nor-mal limits in any patient with typical features such as scalp or

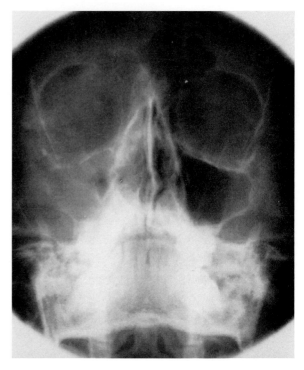

Fig. 5.4 Plain skull X-ray showing opacification in the right maxil-lary, ethmoid, and frontal sinuses. (Photo by courtesy of Dr Ian Colquhoun.)

muscle tenderness or tender arteries. High dose steroids (prednisolone 80 mg daily is advisable for at least the first 3 days) should be started as soon as the diagnosis is suspected, as they will not affect the biopsy changes for several days. The headache in typical patients resolves overnight. The CRP usually resolves more rapidly that the ESR, which will return to normal in two to four weeks. As long as it remains so, and the patient is asymptomatic it is usually possible to tail down the steroids over a period of one to two years, although in some cases the arteritic process continues for longer. Relapse is more likely in the first 18 months of treatment, and within 1 year of stopping steroids.

FACIAL AND DENTAL PAIN

Pain due to dental disease, and disease of the temporo-mandibular joint is usually easily distinguishable from con-ventional headaches and is best managed by appropriate specialists. There is no convincing evidence that temporo-mandibular joint disease can cause spontaneous migraine-type headaches. These patients' symptoms may be related to overclosure of the jaw, and they (but not those with straight-forward migraine) may be helped by the provision of a rear denture or bite-raising appliance.

Many patients seek advice for facial pain without a clear temporal pattern, precipitating causes, or even anatomical distribution, in that it may extend beyond the boundaries of the trigeminal nerve on the face, and a few are bilateral. Diseases of the teeth, ears, eyes, and related structures must be excluded but the majority of these are now classified as 'atypical facial pain'. A number of these patients are clearly depressed and in recent controlled trials they have been shown to improve with antidepressant drugs, independent of their prior psychiatric state.

MENINGITIS

That the consequences of missing bacterial or tuberculous meningitis can be disastrous hardly needs emphasis—meningitis is a rare but significant cause of headache presenting to accident and emergency departments and in general practice, although it is uncommon in outpatient clinics dealing with chronic or recurrent headache. Any patient with a pyrexia, neck stiffness, or positive Kernig's sign should be investigated thoroughly. It is often prudent to administer antibiotics, such as penicillin and chloramphenicol, once the diagnosis is suspected, after only blood cultures have been taken. No harm will have arisen if the headache turns out to be due to viral meningitis, a subarachnoid haemorrhage, or is even considered entirely benign after a CT scan and CSF examination. There is a wide variety of possible microorganisms in debilitated and immunosuppressed patients such as those with AIDS. Tuberculosis may present with a subacute lymphocytic meningitis and a low CSF glucose, and several CSF examinations may be needed to establish that the CSF glucose is falling and to culture the bacillus. Cryptococcal infection and granulomatous conditions such as sarcoidosis, Behçet's syndrome, and Lyme disease may occasionally present as meningitic headache. Broad-spectrum antibiotics should be begun urgently and the regime then modified after discussion with a microbiologist.

SUBARACHNOID HAEMORRHAGE (SAH)

This condition again is commonest in emergency situations, although occasional patients do present some time after their initial bleed. If this is recognized by careful history taking and confirmed by lumbar puncture, it will not have to be classified as a 'warning bleed' recognized only in retrospect after a more devastating major bleed. Suddenness of onset is the most important clue, particularly as the stiff neck may take up to three hours to develop, if at all. Any patient with a history even slightly reminiscent of a subarachnoid haemorrhage in the last two weeks should have a CT scan and lumbar puncture as a matter of urgency, and a case can be made for four vessel arteriography in patients whose major event occurred over two weeks before, if the history is sufficiently typical. Magnetic resonance angiography can sometimes be an appropriate compromise. About 30% of confirmed SAH patients have a normal initial CT scan, so both tests are necessary. In a substantial number of typical patients SAH cannot be confirmed; these are now labelled 'thunderclap headache' and usually develop migraine, cervical spondylosis, or anxiety symptoms during follow-up. Advice on the management of patients with proven subarachnoid haemorrhage should be sought from a neurosurgeon.

NEURALGIAS

This term is best applied to short-lived episodes of pain which may be very severe, and occur within the distribution of a sensory nerve. Individual episodes of, for example, trigeminal neuralgia usually last for a matter of seconds, which should be contrasted with the 20 minutes or longer of cluster headache. Trigeminal neuralgia usually affects the mandibular or maxillary divisions, and is often triggered by innocuous local stimuli such as eating, touching the face, or even just gusts of wind. In the majority of cases the pain is believed to be due to an aberrant artery in the posterior fossa impinging on the trigeminal nerve as it leaves the pons, although in about 2% of patients, often among the younger, it is a symptom of a plaque of multiple sclerosis within the brainstem. The mainstay of management is therapy with carbamazepine, which is usually well tolerated if the dose is increased slowly from 100 mg twice-daily: phenytoin, baclofen, and clonazepam are possible alternatives.

If the pain remains uncontrolled despite the maximal tolerated doses of anticonvulsants, surgical treatment should be considered—either percutaneous radiofrequency lesions of the trigeminal ganglion or a related procedure, or a direct surgical approach to the aberrant artery, placing a piece of sponge between it and the nerve. The former procedure is generally less hazardous, although it is not always effective and the pain can be expected to recur within one to three years. A minority will develop facial numbness with persisting pain, which can be particularly distressing. The posterior fossa procedure is more suited to younger patients once demyelinating disease has been excluded, as it carries a much better long-term prognosis.

Only a minority of zoster infections involve the neck or face, but post-herpetic neuralgia, which is much more common in older patients, can be particularly distressing. Management can prove very difficult, as the pain originates at the level of the dorsal root ganglion and is unresponsive to peripheral destructive procedures. Increasing the non-noxious sensory input to the segmental root entry zone by cold sprays, vibration, or percutaneous nerve stimulation may be of value, with pain relief lasting longer than the stimulus. Tricyclic antidepressants, such as amitriptyline, sometimes in conjunction with anticonvulsants (e.g. valproate), have also been shown to be of benefit.

BLOOD PRESSURE

Paroxysmal hypertension is a feature of phaeochromocytomas, raised intracranial pressure, renal failure, and vasculitis, and phaeochromocytoma is particularly commonly associated with paroxysmal headache. Vasodilator drugs given for the treatment of hypertension, such as nifedipine, hydralazine, and reserpine may also induce headaches, but of course beta-blockers may relieve it.

There is a definitely increased prevalence of headache in patients with hypertension exceeding 130 mm/Hg diastolic, a level that often produces hypertensive encephalopathy. The relationship of the blood pressure and headache is less clear at lower levels of hypertension, even though these may be within the range warranting antihypertensive treatment. It is certainly possible that the hypertension came to light when the patient sought advice about migrainous or other non-specific headaches and, of course, knowledge of the presence of hypertension can itself compound anxiety.

EPIDEMIOLOGY OF HEADACHE

The scale of headache as a public health problem is still best appreciated from the epidemiological studies of Waters, discussed briefly in the introduction—in his survey of 773 men and 945 women, taken from a voters' register in South Wales in 1968, 92% of the women aged 21–34 years said they had had a headache in the previous year. This figure declined to 55% of women over the age of 75 and the corresponding figures for men were 74% falling to 22% in those over 75. Waters drew attention to the inadequate definitions of 'migraine' at the time. A substantial proportion of patients experiencing headaches at all had had either an aura (visual or otherwise), nausea, or headache in a unilateral distribution and he found that approximately twice the number of patients he would expect by chance had all three of these symptoms. He put forward the view that all forms of headache, whether traditionally described as 'tension type' or 'migraine', lie on a continuum, rather than there being easily definable syndromes.

Until recently most epidemiological surveys were undertaken without using clear-cut diagnostic criteria at all, although some did use those used by Vahlquist in a study of Swedish schoolchildren in 1955. For a diagnosis of migraine to be made a patient has to have headaches in isolated attacks separated by headache-free intervals, with two of the following clinical features: (1) an aura to the attacks; (2) nausea or vomiting; (3) unilateral headache; (4) a positive family history. This last criterion was necessarily the least precise and has very properly been criticized by Waters. If a diagnosis of migraine is based on two of the three remaining criteria one-year prevalence figures of 30.9% in women and 17.2% in men can be derived from Waters' observations.

The diagnostic criteria of the International Headache Society (1988) (Table 5.2) championed by Professor Jes Olesen in Copenhagen, have transformed the clinical epidemiology of headaches, although it must be admitted that they have not as yet been validated against any measure of therapeutic responsiveness. An increasing number of epidemiological surveys have now been undertaken using these criteria

Table 5.2

1.1 Migraine without aura

A At least five attacks fulfilling B-D.

B Headache attacks lasting 4–72 hours (untreated or unsuccessfully treated).

C Headache has at least two of the following characteristics:
  1 Unilateral location.
  2 Pulsating quality.
  3 Moderate or severe intensity.
  4 Aggravation by walking stairs or similar routine physical activity.

D During headache at least one of the following:
  1 Nausea and/or vomiting.
  2 Photophobia and phonophobia.

1.2 Migraine with aura

A At least two attacks fulfilling B.

B At least three of the following four characteristics:
  1 One or more fully reversible aura symptoms indicating focal cerebral cortical—and/or brain stem dysfunction.
  2 At least one aura symptom develops gradually over more than four minutes or, two or more symptoms occur in succession.
  3 No aura symptom lasts more than 60 minutes. If more than one aura symptom is present, accepted duration is proportionally increased.
  4 Headache follows aura with a free interval of less than 60 minutes. (It may also begin before or simultaneously with the aura.)

International Headache Society diagnostic criteria for migraine. Reprinted from Cephalalgia 1988, 8 suppl. 7.

(Rasmussen *et al* 1993), however, many of these have confined themselves to specific age ranges, or have been undertaken in populations clearly different from those found in Britain or the United States. The ones most likely to prove representative of British practice include that undertaken by Stewart *et al.* (1992) using over 20000 subjects aged 12–80 taken from representative households throughout the United States. They reported their own symptoms on a questionnaire to which International Headache Society (IHS) criteria were applied, and it was established that 17.6% of the women and 5.7% of the men had had one or more migrainous headaches in the last year, and that about 40% of these were considered 'severe'. The Copenhagen group themselves (Rasmussen *et al.* 1991) have undertaken a random population sample in a suburb of their city—again using IHS criteria. They provide one year migraine prevalence figures of 15% in women and 6% in men. The lifetime prevalence figures are little higher, particularly in the women but there was no significant fall with age. The sex ratio was almost unity for migraine with aura but there were five times as many females as males with migraine without aura. In contrast the one year prevalence figures for 'tension type' headache, again diagnosed using IHS criteria were 86% for women and 63% for men. These figures are very comparable to those obtained by Waters and again were found to fall with age more convincingly.

It has long been recognized that patients with a long history of episodes of migraine can develop more chronic headache later in life—the Copenhagen study confirmed that tension type headache and migraine often coexist but did not find that tension type headaches were commoner in patients with migraine as well, whether or not this was accompanied by aura.

Migraine is as common in prepubertal boys as girls, but then there is a much higher incidence of new cases at the time of puberty in girls. The cumulative prevalence figures published by Dalsgaard Nielsen (1970) established that most patients who are likely to develop migraine during their lifetime would have done so by the age of 32 in men and 42 in women —these figures provide a useful indication as to the age at which more thorough investigation of newly developed headache may be justified.

The long-term prognosis of headache has not yet received much attention. The majority of these epidemiological studies, of course, are cross-sectional but do suggest that many patients will resolve as they grow older. One very small longitudinal study (Whitty and Hockaday 1968) did confirm that many patients' attacks became less frequent or less severe, although a minority were worse. They studied 28 female patients who had passed through the menopause, finding that 18 were unchanged, 6 were worse (1 starting at the menopause), 2 were improved and in only 2 had the attacks ceased.

Only a minority of headache patients will seek medical advice, for example, in one study of civil servants (Espir *et al.* 1988), 578 of 747 subjects responding to the questionnaire said they had had a headache in the previous year. Thirty-four per cent of these said that headache had interfered with their work, and 14% had had to take one or more days off work because of headache, but only 11% had contacted even their general practitioner about headache. One suspects that recent pharmacological advances may have increased this proportion somewhat, particularly now that publicity is indirectly reaching the general public.

Death during a wholly convincing migraine attack is exceptionally rare but there is a substantial morbidity associated with chronic or episodic headache in the community. There have been several recent attempts to assess the economic cost of migraine, in terms both in the number of days completely missed from work and by decreased productivity in subjects remaining at work despite their headache. In one British study (Cull *et al.* 1992) for example, drawn from a representative population sample of migraine sufferers, the men were absent from work for an average of 1.5 days a year with reduced effectiveness contributing the equivalent of a further 4.1 days a year.

Equivalent figures for women were 2.1 days absent, and the equivalent of 4.6 days lost due to reduced effectiveness. The economic cost of this was calculated at £611 million per annum. In a recent survey in the United States (Stewart *et al.* 1996) 51% of female and 38% of male migraine patients experienced 6 or more lost work day equivalents per year, a figure combining both absences and reduced effectiveness at work. An earlier study in the United States, based on the experience of 648 severe migraine patients recruited into a drug trial, provided an annual cost there of these patients alone of between 5.6 and 17.2 million dollars, corresponding to at least 5 billion dollars for the entire US population (Osterhaus *et al.* 1992)

When seen from an epidemiological perspective, therefore, the management of recurrent headache has to be a balance between seeking out the genuinely disabled, particularly those who do not realize how much help is now available, and overloading an already overstretched health service both in terms of manpower resources for the necessary clinical assessment, and indeed, the cost of more expensive therapies.

MECHANISMS OF HEADACHE

An understanding of the mechanism of headache is still of limited relevance in clinical diagnosis, or in establishing optimal drug therapy in an individual patient. Indeed, we can still assert that more pharmacological information has been derived from the study of drugs found effective in migraine on an empirical basis, than has been used to develop new drugs.

Even though serotonin does seem to be released from platelets and/or nerve terminals at the time of the attacks, it has been known for 30 years that the intravenous administration of serotonin will ameliorate headache, albeit with intolerable side-effects. Headache is definitely associated with vasodilatation of scalp and meningeal vessels, although this is probably initiated via brainstem nuclei and possibly perpetuated by a feedback loop involving both the trigeminal and facial nerves. There is release of calcitonin gene related peptide, but not substance P or vasoactive intestinal polypeptides into the jugular venous blood during attacks of headache (Edvinsson and Goadsby 1994).

The mechanism of the aura phase of the classical attack remains controversial—isotopic studies of cerebral blood flow have shown no significant changes in patients experiencing headaches without aura, but some reduction in the areas affected by aura symptoms in those with, for example, visual or sensory disturbances. In most cases cortical blood flow falls to levels consistent with reduced neuronal function, although in occasional patients the blood flow is indeed low enough to cause reversible or even permanent cortical ischaemia and therefore even infarction. Some authorities feel that scattered radiation from adjacent brain with normal blood flow leads to an overestimation of the flow in affected areas, and therefore that ischaemia is much commoner if not universal. The finding that the hypoperfusion may start before the aura symptoms and often extends well into the headache phase after the resolution of the aura, however, lends support to the notion that the aura symptoms are themselves due to a phenomenon akin to the 'spreading depression of Leao'. However, it has to be admitted that no direct evidence in support of this hypothesis is as yet available (Olesen *et al.* 1990). This controversy is so far of little relevance to practising neurologists. The observation that rebreathing may abort migrainous attacks is as easily explained by the effect of carbon dioxide on spreading depression in experimental animals as it is on vaso-constriction as the supposed mechanism of the aura symp-toms. The serotonin agonist sumatriptan is considered to be a vasoconstrictor of large diameter vessels sensitive to pain—it has no demonstrable effect on cerebral blood flow in man, and extensive studies of the drug administered during migrainous auras has not shown any undue prolongation of them.

THE ROLE OF SEROTONIN

It is now clear that ergotamine is effective by stimulating one subtype of serotonin receptor, which is a vasoconstrictor in certain cerebral arteries, although its side-effects may be due to effects of other serotonin receptors at marginally higher concentrations. The new agent, sumatriptan, which promises to be the first of a new pharmacological class, was specifically developed to be a selective agonist of this type of serotonin re-ceptor. While undoubtedly a constrictor of inflamed dilated arteries sumatriptan may also have a presynaptic inhibiting effect on the neurogenic inflammatory pathways within the vessel wall (Moskowitz 1992).

The role of other serotonin receptors in the pathogenesis and treatment of migraine is even less clearly understood. The principal metabolite of methysergide (methyl ergo-metrine) is known to have an effect on 5-HT_1 receptors akin to sumatriptan, and the finding that *m*-chlorophenylpiper-azine (which is a metabolite of the antidepressant trazadone) can induce migraine-like headaches, particularly in patients with a personal or family history of migraine, probably by stimulating some subtypes of 5-HT_2 receptors, has yet to be fully exploited (Fozard and Kalkman 1994). Although 5-HT_3 receptor antagonists were originally developed in the hope that they would prove useful in migraine they are now mar-keted for the suppression of chemotherapy-induced vomiting, and seem to have little, if any, effect in headache patients. The mechanism of action of the prophylactic agents, pizotifen and propranolol, are very poorly understood—the former has a wide variety of pharmacological properties including sero-tonin re-uptake inhibition, and an antagonistic effect on 5-HT_2 receptors, and the latter is probably acting as a vasoconstric-tor, as beta-blockers with intrinsic sympathomimetic activity seems less effective as migraine prophylactics (Peatfield 1986).

MANAGEMENT

The first duty of a clinician assessing and treating a patient complaining of headache is to exclude specific structural dis-eases, as has been outlined earlier in this chapter. Many of these will need specific neurosurgical or drug therapy such as the administration of antibiotics or corticosteroids.

CLUSTER HEADACHE

There is no doubt that cluster headache is a separate identifiable syndrome which responds best to a range of drug treatment different from those used in migraine (Krabbe 1986). Patients are predominantly male and experience at-tacks of pain of extreme severity that are usually situated in, behind or around one eye, although they can be felt elsewhere in the face or even in the neck. The pain is always unilateral and is usually on the consistent side of the head—the patients can have between one and six attacks of pain daily often at fixed times of day, and they commonly wake the patient from sleep about one hour after retiring. Episodes usually last for between 20 minutes and 3 hours and the patient is usually quite unable to lie still during the bout, getting out of bed and even considering hitting their head against a wall. The eye may water and become bloodshot with a ptosis and occasional patients experience congestion of the nostril on the same side. About 90% of the patients experience bouts of such attacks lasting for between 6 and 16 weeks with headache-free inter-vals for between 6 months and 5 years, although 10% of the patients have unremittent daily attacks for periods exceeding 3 months and sometimes for many years. The condition is seen in women, although sometimes it is atypical, the com-monest pattern being regular but infrequent attacks following a similar format. The vast majority of cluster headache pa-tients smoke regularly but unfortunately there is no evidence that stopping smoking has any effect on the natural history of the disease. Many patients find that alcoholic drinks of all kinds will trigger attacks during the 'bouts' of pain.

Patients with a wholly typical history of cluster headache do not warrant extensive investigation, although the pain can sometimes be simulated by pituitary tumours and other cav-ernous sinus abnormalities. Few simple analgesics can be ad-ministered fast enough to affect an individual episode of pain but there is now considerable evidence that breathing 100% oxygen will abort an attack, and more recently, subcutaneous sumatriptan has been shown to be extremely effective. How-ever, the financial viability of daily administration of this drug has to be questioned. Many patients gain relief from ergo-tamine taken at bedtime in anticipation of attacks.

For many years, the mainstay of medical management has been drug prophylaxis (Solomon *et al.* 1991). There is some evidence that the migraine prophylactic agents, pizotifen and methysergide, are of modest benefit in cluster headache, but propranolol seems ineffective. There is now good evidence to support the use of corticosteroids, verapamil and lithium in the management of cluster headache patients. A reasonable working policy is to use corticosteroids (prednisolone 40 mg daily for a week, declining to zero over the second week), in patients with episodic cluster headache presenting in the middle of their bouts and therefore likely to settle down spon-taneously within two or three weeks, using verapamil (120 mg 3 times daily in the beginning) for most other patients and re-serving lithium (Priadel 800 mg or more, dependent on blood levels) for patients with chronic cluster headache that has proved unresponsive to verapamil. It is, of course, essential to monitor lithium levels in patients given Priadel and this usu-ally requires weekly attendances until the level is stabilized—

it should certainly be above 1 mmol/litre before alternative therapies are tried. Intranasal capsaicin has also proved effective and percutaneous thermocoagulation of the Gasserian ganglion has been advocated in otherwise intractable patients.

Once patients with specific structural diseases and with cluster headaches have been excluded the practising neurologist is left with a large number of patients complaining of constant or episodic headache without any abnormalities on clinical examination. The epidemiological evidence reviewed earlier would suggest these patients lie on a continuum and there is certainly no convincing evidence to support the view that it is valid to distinguish between, for example, 'migraine', and 'tension headache', before deciding what form of therapy to offer. With a few exceptions, therefore, most of the therapeutic suggestions in this chapter can be applied to all these patients irrespective of their place within the continuum.

It remains essential to take the patient's problems seriously—they have, after all, selected themselves by seeking advice about their headaches and it is no longer sufficient to reassure the patient that they do not have a structural disease, leaving them to depend on over-the-counter analgesics. This reassurance is essential and certainly may interrupt a vicious circle in which a patient worries so much about their headache that the headache itself is worsened.

There is very little acceptable evidence to support the view that dietary measures are of value in the management of patients with headache. About 20% of migraine patients attending a tertiary referral clinic say that they have noticed an association with cheese, chocolate, and citrus fruit and many of these have also implicated alcoholic drinks of various types. However, they have usually already eliminated these from their diet and are actually seeking advice about spontaneous attacks. There is no acceptable evidence to support the view that the elimination of fresh dairy products, wheat or any other major dietary constituents have had anything more than a placebo effect in suggestible patients.

The contraceptive pill in contrast, does often initiate or exacerbate migraine, often after a delay of several months and it is often worth advising patients to discontinue the pill for a minimum of six months before considering any other form of regular medication. This effect may be less pronounced with the progesterone only contraceptive pill when compared to the conventional combined type, though there is no systematic evidence to confirm this.

The role of chronic analgesic administration in the perpetuation of headache remains contentious. This certainly applies to ergotamine, which is a vasoconstrictor with a very long functional half-life. Many patients will develop a further headache as the vasoconstrictor effect wears off one or two days after each dose, which they can easily treat with further doses of ergotamine thus perpetuating the headache. These patients are undoubtedly improved by discontinuing ergotamine completely, once the initial withdrawal headache (which usually lasts less than a week) has passed (Tfelt-Hansen and Krabbe 1981). Most patients taking large doses of analgesics

are taking preparations containing codeine and/or caffeine rather than pure aspiring or paracetamol and it seems very likely that both these agents are addictive and that patients may improve by discontinuing these as well. Excessive consumption of pure aspirin or paracetamol is seen very rarely and there is no evidence to support the view that this is anything other than a reflection of the severity of the patients' headaches. There is considerable clinical evidence to support the view that the regular administration of non-steroidal anti-inflammatory drugs, such as ibuprofen or naproxen, may actually be helpful in the management of headache patients and it is often prudent to suggest that patients taking large doses of compound analgesics convert to the use of these as an alternative.

A wide variety of non-drug measures have been advocated in headache patients, including psychological assessment and treatment, neck physiotherapy, biofeedback of various kinds, dental treatment, including the adjustment of the bite, and acupuncture. Acupuncture certainly has an effect on circulating endogenous opioids and has a role in the management of patients experiencing chronic pain, but there is as yet no evidence to support the use of any of these other treatments in headache patients.

ANALGESICS

Patients experiencing relatively mild attacks and those experiencing severe attacks at intervals of, for example, a month or more are best managed with analgesics taken when needed. Most patients will have already tried paracetamol, aspirin, and low dose codeine preparations before seeking advice even from their general practitioners, although sometimes these may be sufficient taken in conjunction with an antiemetic such as metoclopromide. This drug accelerates gastric emptying and the absorption of analgesics taken simultaneously by mouth, and is to be preferred to phenothiazines as antiemetics in headache patients. NSAIDs are particularly effective in the management of severe headaches, although the doses have to be reasonably large and some patients are unable to tolerate the gastric side-effects—ibuprofen 600 mg or naproxen 750 mg at a time have been shown to be effective in clinical trials. In general, ergotamine preparations have now been superseded by sumatriptan but there may be a place for administering these either as a suppository or inhaler in patients with infrequent but disabling attacks. It is safe to administer 3–4 mg of ergotamine during an attack, but is essential that the patient does not take any further ergotamine for at least a week and preferably for four weeks.

Sumatriptan (Imigran) now has a well-established place in the clinical repertoire (Dechant and Clissold 1992). Clinical trials have shown that it is undoubtedly more effective than conventional analgesics and has many fewer side-effects than ergotamine. In one large series (Visser *et al.* 1996), 89% of migraine patients responded consistently to the subcutaneous form within two hours, and 75% to the tablets; in contrast 9%

and 19%, respectively, responded well in less than one-third of attacks. Sumatriptan has substantial antiemetic properties in its own right and, of course, the subcutaneous auto-injector form is particularly useful in patients who vomit early in their attacks. It appears to be potent enough to enable many patients to remain at work during attacks, and to treat patients with attacks so severe that they have hitherto had to call out their general practitioner to administer intramuscular analgesic—benefits which should be offset against the undoubtedly high cost of the drug, both as tablets and the auto-injector. Sumatriptan is probably best reserved for patients with infrequent severe attacks that have failed to respond to high doses of NSAIDs agents and it should not be seen as a substitute for adequate prophylaxis in patients experiencing two or more attacks each month.

Transient side-effects, including paraesthesae and muscle aching are very common. The drug can cause coronary ischaemia, and should not be used in patients with ischaemic heart disease. It does not affect short-lived visual or sensory auras, but should not be used if these symptoms have previously persisted for more than about 2 hours. The relatively short duration of action of sumatriptan results in recurrent headache after about 12 hours in at least 5% of the patients; the best treatment for this is yet to be established.

Two new related compounds were marketed in 1997, in tablet form only, and several others are undergoing clinical trials. Zolmitriptan is more lipid-soluble than sumatriptan, with greater bioavailability and a slightly longer half-life. Clinical trial results are essentially similar, although a smaller proportion of patients relapse and the tablets are a little cheaper (Ferrari 1997). Naratriptan is absorbed even better, with a much lower relapse rate and many fewer side effects, but the onset of the clinical response is rather slower (Elkind *et al.* 1997).

PROPHYLACTIC MEDICATION

The mainstay of headache management for many years has been the administration of drugs to attempt to suppress the pain, particularly in those experiencing two or more attacks monthly. There is a lot of evidence that the pathophysiological processes that initiate the migraine attack start perhaps 48 hours before the onset of the pain and even parenteral sumatriptan only ameliorates the attack after about 30 minutes, leaving the patient in considerable distress for this time.

The drugs of first choice remain pizotifen and non-selective beta-blockers such as propranolol, atenolol, nadolol, or metoprolol (Lance 1992). As discussed above, beta-blocking drugs with intrinsic sympathomimetic activity (most notably oxprenolol and acebutalol) do not seem to be so effective in migraine, and benefit in headache does seem to correlate with the side-effect of peripheral vasoconstriction. Relatively large doses of beta-blockers may be required—it is conventional to start with propranolol 40 mg twice-daily and many patients gain relief only when the daily dose is increased from 160 to 320 mg daily. Side-effects are unusual—peripheral vasocon-

striction is best managed by appropriate insulation (gloves, socks, etc.), and bad dreams by changing from propranolol to the more water-soluble atenolol, but postural hypotension occasionally proves to be a dose-limiting side-effect. Beta-blocking drugs, of course, should not be used in asthmatic patients.

Pizotifen is the other front-line prophylactic drug—it has a variety of actions on serotonin receptors, as well as antidepressant and antihistamine effects, but its mode of action remains poorly understood. It is perhaps a little more sedative than propranolol, and it has the problem of stimulating the appetite, although weight gain can usually be pre-empted if the patient is warned in advance of this and told not to increase his/her food intake. Patients usually respond to 1.5 or 3 mg daily and the side-effect seems to become more troublesome at higher doses without a commensurate improvement in the headache.

About 70% of patients respond to propranolol and 70% to pizotifen, responses that are probably independent. A small minority of patients, therefore, are unresponsive to both. In these, methysergide should be tried, building up from 1 mg three times daily to 2 mg three times daily. If the dose does not exceed 6 mg daily and the drug is stopped for one month in every six the risk of retroperitoneal fibrosis appears to be negligible. The drug is usually well tolerated although a minority of patients have an ill-defined malaise which may prove doselimiting.

There is no convincing evidence to support the view that clonidine is effective in migraine prophylaxis and this drug can no longer be recommended. There have been extensive trials of a variety of calcium antagonists in migraine—verapamil is, of course, highly effective in cluster headache but the trials in migraine are as yet very small. Nimodipine has not been shown to be effective and flunarizine (which is very fat-soluble and sedative) is only available in some other European countries.

Tricyclic antidepressants such as amitriptyline or prothiaden have a well-established role in headache patients—they are certainly of value in patients with undoubted migraine but are, perhaps, more used in those with tension type headaches, or chronic daily headache. However, there have been no systematic clinical trials exploring which clinical features are particularly likely to predict responsiveness to tricyclic antidepressants. Many patients respond well to small doses of amitriptyline, but it may be necessary to increase the dose to 75 or even 100 mg daily. The role of the newer serotonin reuptake inhibitors, such as fluoxetine, is less well understood—they may be of more value in chronic daily headache than in migraine, as there are some published reports of migrainous headaches being exacerbated at least in the first few weeks of therapy. Recent trials have shown that the anticonvulsant, sodium valproate, is also effective in migraine.

FUTURE DEVELOPMENTS

It is only in recent years that the potential market for antimigraine therapies has been evident to drug companies, with the resultant rise in interest in the pharmacology of potential migraine mediators, and of drugs used both as analgesics and for prophylaxis. Sumatriptan is proving very successful, and a number of other drug companies are known to be developing alternative agents acting on the same receptor, perhaps with slightly different pharmacokinetic properties.

The role of the 5-HT$_{2b}$ and 5-HT$_{2c}$ receptors remain to be evaluated and it is certainly possible that antagonists of these receptors will prove of value in migraine patients. The increasing evidence that inflammatory peptides, such as CGRP, are released during migrainous attacks certainly suggests that antagonists of these agents, if they can be developed for clinical use, may be much more effective than any existing therapy. We can expect many more developments of this kind in the future.

REFERENCES

Corbett, J. J. and Thompson, H. S. (1989). The rational management of idiopathic intracranial hypertension. *Archives of Neorology*, **46**, 1049–51.

Cull, R. E., Wells, N. E. J., and Miocevich, M. L. (1992). The economic cost of migraine. *British Journal of Medical Economics*, **2**, 103–15.

Dalsgaard-Nielsen, T. (1970). Some aspects of the epidemiology of migraine in Denmark. *Headache*, **10** 14–23.

Dechant, K. L. and Clissold, S. P. (1992). Sumatriptan. *Drugs*, **43**, 776–98.

Edvinsson, L. and Goadsby, P. J. (1994). Neuropeptides in migraine and cluster headache. *Cephalagia*, **14**, 320–7.

Espir, M. L. E., Thomason, J., Blau, J. N. and Kurtz, Z (1988). Headache in civil servants; effect on work and leisure. *British Journal of Industrial Medicine*, **45**, 336–40.

Elkind, A., Webster, C., Laurenza, A. *et al.* (1997). Efficacy and tolerability of naratriptan tablets in the treatment of migraine: results of a double-blind, placebo-controlled, parallel-group trial. Poster presented at the 8th Congress of the International Headache Society, Amsterdam.

Ferrari, M. D. (1997). 311C90: increasing the options for therapy with effective acute antimigraine 5HT$_{1B/1D}$ receptor agonists. *Neurology*, **48**(suppl. 3), S21–4.

Fodden, D. I., Peatfield, R. C., and Milsom, P. L. (1989). Beware the patient with a headache in the Accident and Emergency Department. *Archives of Emergency Medicine*, **6**, 7–12.

Fozard, J. R. and Kalkman, H. O. (1994). 5-HT and the initiation of migraine: new perspectives. *Naunyn–Schmeideberg's Archives of Pharmacology*, **350**, 225–9.

International Headache Society (1988). Classification and diagnostic criteria for headache disorders, cranial neuralgia and facial pain. *Cephalalgia*, **8** (suppl. 7), 1–96.

Krabbe, A. A. (1986). Cluster headache, a review. *Acta Neurologica Scandinavica*, **74** 1–9.

Kutzke, J. F. (1992). The current neurologic burden of illness and injury in the United States. *Neurology*, **32**, 1207–14.

Lance, J. W. (1992). Treatment of migraine. *Lancet*, **339**, 1207–9.

Miller, A., Green, M., and Robinson, D. (1983). Simple rule for calculating normal erythrocyte sedimentation rate. *British Medical Journal*, **286**, 266.

Moskowitz, M. A. (1992). Neurogenic versus vascular mechanisms of Sumatriptan and ergot alkaloids in Migraine. *Trends in Pharmacological Sciences*, **13**, 307–10.

Olesen, J., Froberg, L., Skyhoj Olesen, T., Iversen, H. K. Lassen, N. A., Andersen, A. R. *et al.* (1990). Timing and topography of cerebral blood flow, aura and headache during migraine attacks. *Annals of Neurology*, **28**, 91–8.

Osterhaus, J. T., Gutterman, D. L., and Plachetka, J. R. (1992). Healthcare resource and lost labour costs of migraine headache in the US. *PharmacoEconomics*, **2**, 67–76.

Peatfield, R. C. (1986). *Headache*. Springer, Berlin.

Rasmussen, B. K., Jensen, R., Schroll, M., and Olesen, J. (1991). Epidemiology of headache in a general population—a prevalence study. *Journal of Clinical Epidemiology*, **44** 1147–57.

Rasmussen, B. K., and Breslau, N. (1993). Epidemiology. In *The Headaches*, (ed. J. Olesen, P. Tfelt-Hansen, and K. M. A. Welch.), pp. 169–73. New York, Raven.

Solomon, S. S., Lipton, R. B., and Newman, L. C. (1991). Prophylactic therapy of cluster headache. *Clinical Neuropharmocology*, **14**, 116–30.

Stewart, W. F., Lipton, R. B., Celantano, D. D., and Reed, M. L. (1992). Prevalence of headache in the United States. *JAMA*, **267**, 64–9.

Stewart, W. F., Lipton, R. B., and Simon, D. (1996). Work-related disability: results from the American migraine study. *Cephalalgia*, **16**, 231–8.

Tfelt-Hansen, P. and Krabbe, A. A. (1981). Ergotamine abuse, do patients benefit from withdrawal? *Cephalagia*, **1**, 29–32.

Vahlquist, B. (1955). Migraine in children. *International Archives of Allergy*, **7**, 348–55.

Visser, W. H., de Vrien, R. H. M., Jaspers, N. M. W. H., and Ferrari, N. D. (1996). Sumatriptan in clinical practice: a 2 year review of 453 migraine patients. *Neurology*, **47**, 46–51.

Waters, W. E. (1986). *Headache*. Croom Helm, London & Sydney.

Whitty, C. W. M. and Hockaday, J. M. (1968). Migraine: a follow up study of 92 patients. *British Medical Journal*, **1**, 735–6.

6 | *Neuromuscular disease*

John Winer

The management of patients with neuromuscular disease occupies a fairly large part of the general neurologist's outpatient and inpatient workload. Accurate figures for the prevalence of neuromuscular disease are difficult to obtain but peripheral neuropathies alone have an incidence twice that of Parkinson's disease (1). It is impossible to cover the management of all types of neuromuscular disease within the scope of a short chapter such as this and I shall not attempt to be comprehensive in choice of topic. Management or care of patients with neuromuscular disease falls into two main categories. The first category of patients are those in whom it is possible to reverse or ameliorate the disease process with active measures using drugs or other procedures which can alter the pathophysiology of the disease. This usually involves altering the immune response in the treatment of immune-mediated disorders. The second method of management involves the overall care of patients with chronic disease in maintaining maximum function despite a continuing disease process. This is a very extensive area requiring considerable skill and expertise and involves many disciplines not only neurological. I will deal, in this chapter, with three diseases that typify the first category of management in which it is possible to alter the disease process by the use of immunosuppression. Lastly, I will deal with a disease of a chronic nature in which it is possible to improve the quality of life of patients to a considerable extent although at the moment it is not possible to alter the pathophysiology of the disease process. I take the view that the provision of care to patients with neuromuscular disease is best carried out in a specialist neuromuscular clinic. Without these specialist clinics it is very difficult to coordinate the many disciplines required in the delivery of care. A centralized clinic also makes it easier to carry out patient education and to put patients in touch with the various self-help groups which carry out an important job in providing information on disease and educating patients and their relatives. Centralization of neuromuscular care in a single clinic also has the advantage of ensuring better continuity of care than is possible in busy general neurology clinics, which frequently have junior neurological staff who rotate fairly rapidly and are only seeing patients for perhaps one visit before they move on to another discipline or post. Continuity of neurological care is clearly very important for the management of patients with chronic diseases of this type. There is frequently an important balance between providing easy access to a centralized clinic of this sort and not taking over the role of a patient's general practitioner. Each neurologist will find his balance in this area. This often involves educating the patient's GP who may not be used to dealing with relatively rare neuromuscular disease, so that they can still become the first line for management problems. Centralized neuromuscular clinics also have the advantage of being able to update patients on the latest advances within the specialty, which is particularly important, bearing in mind the tremendous changes that have taken place recently in the genetics of neuromuscular disease. The management of patients with chronic neuromuscular disease is a multidisciplinary process and involves frequent liaison with colleagues, such as occupational therapists, physiotherapists, and speech therapists, and again this more easily delivered where there is good communication between these groups and a centralized neuromuscular clinic provides a good opportunity for this communication to take place. Many chronic neurological diseases render patients incapable of full-time employment and this in itself raises many financial difficulties and an attached social worker is very important in good provision of overall care, together with good liaison with the local occupational health departments so that if employment is possible the optimal job can be arranged for the disabled patient.

I intend to consider two diseases that fall into the category of neuropathies, Guillain–Barré syndrome (GBS) and hereditary motor and sensory neuropathy (HMSN). These two diseases have very different management problems requiring different expertise. I then consider the management of polymyositis as a typical example of a common myopathic disorder and then finally the management of myasthenia gravis as an example of a disorder at the neuromuscular junction.

NEUROPATHIES

GUILLAIN–BARRÉ SYNDROME (GBS)

Guillain, Barre, and Strohl described their now well-known syndrome in 1916 in two new recruits seen at an army neurological centre (2). The disease they described was a rapidly progressive paralysis with sensory symptoms, but predominantly motor signs. They described absent reflexes as a key feature of the disease and also noticed that the cerebrospinal fluid (CSF) showed a high protein content without an increase in CSF cell count. The diagnosis of GBS is usually relatively straightforward based on progressive weakness of more than one limb over a period of up to four weeks. Electrophysiological tests are very helpful in confirming that diagnosis and exclude central causes of progressive paralysis which can occasionally cause diagnostic difficulties. Recent trials of treatment in GBS included one or two cases of botulism which can closely mimic the syndrome. Patients with demyelination of the central nervous system can sometimes cause diagnostic confusion as can acute myopathies particularly associated with hypokalaemia. Even examples of patients with brainstem strokes can be misdiagnosed as GBS. Although the diagnosis of GBS is usually relatively straightforward the management is not. The disease is usually typically a monophasic illness with progression over three or four weeks followed by a plateau phase of five or six weeks and then a gradual improvement. Sixty-five per cent of patients will return to all normal activities within one year (3), even without treatment. Patients are frequently very disturbed by the rapidity of their illness and frightened not only by the hospital environment, but also by the fear of being permanently disabled. In the first instance, management frequently involves detailed discussion with patients about the likely outcome and the methods of treatment available. The relatives need to be included in these discussions and frequently patients and relatives will be considerably relieved to hear that the condition usually resolves completely with appropriate management.

Management of Guillain–Barré syndrome falls into two categories. Supportive management is vital to reduce complications and a number of treatments are available in order to try and modify the disease process. Supportive treatment involves careful monitoring of respiratory function with a view to instigating assisted ventilation if and when this becomes necessary. Vital capacity is the most appropriate measure of lung function in this disease and this should be carried out at least daily and sometimes three or four times daily in a patient confined to bed with progressive motor weakness. A vital capacity approaching one litre should be an indication to consider assisted ventilation, although it is the rate of fall of vital capacity that is more important than the absolute value. It is much better to instigate elective ventilation before respiratory reserve is exhausted, because emergency intubation is fraught with difficulty and leads to considerable morbidity. I prefer, if at all possible, to monitor patients with rapidly falling vital capacities in the intensive care unit so that ventilation can be carried out electively in the most atraumatic manner. Once ventilation has become necessary patients should be managed with the minimum use of sedative drugs, unlike many other intensive care conditions. Although Guillain–Barré syndrome may be a painful condition pain can usually be controlled with non-narcotic agents so that patients can cooperate as much as possible with passive and later active physiotherapy. Chest physiotherapy is very important to prevent

chest infections which is one of the main causes of the rare event of death in this disease. Frequent movement of the legs together with the use of support stockings and subcutaneous heparin can reduce the complication of pulmonary emboli. The use of end expiratory pressure during ventilation helps to protect against closure of terminal airways and chest infection. Autonomic disturbance is extremely worrying in this condition. Patients that are tetraplegic and ventilated have a relatively high incidence of autonomic disturbance. Bradycardias appear to be particularly worrying and the literature contains reports (4) of patients who have died following tracheal suction-induced cardiac asystole. My own practice is to insert a temporary prophylactic cardiac pacing wires in patients that show episodic bradycardia. Communication with paralysed patients in intensive care units is extremely difficult.

Active treatment of GBS is limited to the use of plasma exchange or intravenous gamma globulin. Five controlled trials (5–9) have been carried out to investigate the efficacy of exchange in GBS and the two largest have shown a highly significant benefit. Plasma exchange appears to reduce the time spent in intensive care units by about half and considerably reduces the time taken for patients to regain the ability to walk. The maximum benefit from plasma exchange appears to be largely confined to the first two weeks after onset of the neuropathy. This would be in keeping with the theory that myelin damage occurs early in the evolution of the symptoms of GBS and that persistent deficit relates to established neuropathy and not to continuing inflammation. A Dutch controlled trial (10) suggested that intravenous gamma globulin is as effective as plasma exchange in accelerating recovery in GBS and this finding has recently been confirmed by a multicentre international study (11).

HEREDITARY MOTOR AND SENSORY NEUROPATHY (HMSN)

The diagnosis of the classical case of HMSN or Charcot–Marie–Tooth disease is usually straightforward especially in the presence of a clear family history, pes cavus, and classic peroneal wasting, likened to an inverted champagne cork. In patients without a clear family history the diagnosis is often more difficult but will be suggested by a longstanding neuropathy with electrophysiological evidence of demyelination on nerve conduction studies. Axonal forms of HMSN may be very difficult to distinguish from other acquired neuropathies. Careful examination of family members will often provide the clue and several clinical studies suggest that genetically inherited neuropathies represent the largest group of so-called idiopathic neuropathies on initial screening (12). Recent recognition of the chromosome 17 duplication associated with demyelinating autosomal forms of HMSN (CMT1a) (13), together with other rapidly advancing genetic tests, will soon provide readily available blood tests of considerable diagnostic usefulness. Nerve biopsy may become unnecessary in the future but at the moment is still sometimes useful in patients without a family history and with no recognizable DNA mutation.

At least seven varieties of HMSN are described and advancing genetic understanding will almost certainly increase the subgroups of this neuropathy.

Currently, there is no prospect of active treatment for these inherited neuropathies, and management consists of patients education, genetic counselling, physical strategies to maximize function, and advice on social aspects of the illness, particularly in relation to the provision of disability benefit together with informed advice in relation to coping with disability.

Patient education

Patients need to be informed about the nature of the disease and the presumed pathogenesis. They frequently have anxieties about the progression of the disease and the chances of significant handicap in the future. Such discussions are dependent on the nature of the individual case together with the type of HMSN, age of presentation, etc. In general, patients can be reassured that the disease is only slowly progressive and produces only relatively mild handicap in the majority of afflicted individuals. The CMT Society* produces regular patient education leaflets and organizes local meetings to discuss advances in understanding of the disease.

Genetic counselling

Many concerns about HMSN will centre around the possible future chances of asymptomatic family members being affected and the risks to offspring. The increasing understanding of the genetic predisposition to the disease makes such genetic counselling more accurate although more complicated. Most genetic departments offer a counselling service to deal with these sorts of problems. Most patients with HMSN will benefit from a formal genetic appointment to discuss the implications of their diagnosis and to store DNA for future diagnostic tests that may be relevant to subsequent generations.

Occupational therapy and physiotherapy

Many patients with HMSN develop foot drop which can be helped by the provision of ankle–foot orthoses via the local orthotic department. More specialized orthoses may be required in individual cases and multidisciplinary assessments may be helpful in designing these. Weakness of the hands may require the provision of eating utensils with large handles, etc. If necessary, the provision of wheelchairs and the appropriate selection needs to be discussed.

Social support

In keeping with all chronic disease a proportion of the most severely affected individuals need ongoing support from social

* Charcot–Marie–Tooth Society, CMT International UK, 121 Lavernock Road, Penarth, South Glamorgan, CFG 2QG

workers. This may involve advice in relation to claiming appropriate benefits, disabled driving permits, etc. Retraining for more appropriate employment may be necessary for those with a physically demanding job and a realistic chance of an alternative sedentary or clerical occupation.

Complications

As the disease progresses foot deformity together with achilles tendon shortening may require surgical correction and referral to an appropriately experienced orthopaedic surgeon is important. Arthrodesis, tendon transfers, and lengthening, all have their part to play in maintaining maximum function. Scoliosis is recognized association of some varieties of HMSN and requires joint orthopaedic management and careful monitoring of vital capacity and lung function. Very rare cases of HMSN have developed nocturnal hypoventilation requiring consideration of external respiratory support such as a curasse or nasal positive pressure ventilation through a face mask. Such cases are fortunately rare and raise difficult ethical considerations in relation to the question of providing permanent respiratory support in patients with progressive neuromuscular disorders.

MUSCLE DISEASES

POLYMYOSITIS

Inflammatory muscle disease may occur with or without associated connective disease. Patients with myositis as part of connective disease (e.g. dermatomyositis) are usually referred directly to rheumatologists, whereas patients with muscle weakness and or pain usually arrive directly in the neurologist's clinic. A proportion of these patients were considered to develop their neurological symptoms in association with systemic malignancy but the frequency of this association appears to be low 14.

Patients with polymyositis usually present with a subacute history of muscle weakness and tenderness over weeks to months. The weakness is classically of the shoulder girdle or hips leading to difficulties with climbing stairs or holding the arms up. Swallowing may be affected and neck and trunk weakness usually exists. Reflexes and sensation remain normal.

The diagnosis is confirmed by a rise in the creatinine kinase enzyme level together with electromyography (EMG) findings of inappropriately full interference patterns, with small polyphasic motor units. Muscle biopsy typically reveals inflammatory infitrates consisting of predominantly CD8-positive lymphocytes. The disease process may be patchy so that biopsy findings may be normal in unaffected muscles. A small group of patients may have biopsy findings consistent with inclusion body myositis where the inclusion bodies have been shown to contain prion protein (15). The differential diagnosis also involves late onset muscular dystrophy, mitochondrial myopathies, and some rare metabolic myopathies.

The muscle damage that occurs in polymyositis is generally thought to be mediated by cytotoxic T cells and therefore treatment is aimed at reducing cell-mediated immunity. Steroids are the mainstay of treatment and are frequently given with other immunosupressants in an effort to reduce the steroid dose required. Azathioprine was the favoured drug for some time but methotrexate has become popular in recent years because of its fewer side-effects. Unfortunately, no controlled trials of any size have adressed the optimal treatment probably because of the lack of sufficient patients in any single centre.

My practice is to give 60 mg prednisolone a day at diagnosis accompanied with 7.5 mg of methotrexate once a week, increasing to 15–20 mg each week over a few months if the drug is well tolerated. Folic acid is usually given as a supplement. I perform liver function tests and a full blood count every two weeks for six weeks and then every month. The dose of steroids can be reduced over a few weeks to a maintenance dose of about 20 mg a day and then more slowly reduced over the next year.

Progress is predominantly judged by improvement in symptoms and return of muscle strength. Myometry may be helpful in measuring increasing strength and the serum creatine phosphokinase (CPK) gives a measure of persisting muscle damage. The level of the CPK may fall if the volume of muscle tissue becomes very reduced even in the presence of active inflammation so that care has to be exercised in the interpretation of CPK levels. It is frequently possible to withdraw steroids altogether and maintain normal muscle activity with an immunosupressant alone. Occasional patients can be managed without any treatment if they remain in remission for some years. However, such patients can relapse even after being off treatment for many years.

High dose steroid treatment for some years can lead to a steroid myopathy which may be mistaken for persistent activity of the inflammatory process. Reducing steroid treatment will lead to increase in strength in these patients. Treatment with cyclophosphamide has its advocates but is usually associated with increased morbidity and there are a few reports of success with plasma exchange for polymyositis although the logic of such treatment seems shaky. Long-term steroid treatment will exacerbate osteoporosis and hormone replacement therapy should be considered in post-menopausal women (16). The use of biphosphonates may confer some benefit as a prophylactic agent in preventing severe osteoporosis (17), but in view of the complications of these drugs (18) I would not wish to use agents such as Fosamax outside a trial situation at the present time.

MYASTHENIA GRAVIS

Myasthenia gravis is but one of a number of clinical disorders of the neuromuscular junction and is the most common. The disease is characterized by symptoms and signs of variable weakness of eyelids, extraocular muscles, or limbs. Edrophonium given intravenously will briefly reverse clinical weakness and forms the basis of the most useful confirmatory test of the diagnosis. Antibodies to the acetylcholine receptor are found in the serum of 85–90% of patients with generalized disease and show correlation with weakness within a given individual when measured longitudinally. Antibodies against striated muscle are detectable in about 30% of patients but much more frequently in individuals with a thymoma. EMG studies are useful in confirming the diagnosis with a decrement in muscle action potential on repetitive stimulation especially in proximal muscles in a proportion of patients. An increase in electrophysiological finding of jitter (the variation in time interval between action potentials of adjacent muscle fibres supplied by the same motor unit) is much more sensitive as a diagnostic test but less specific.

Treatment of myasthenia was revolutionized by Mary Walker's report (19) of the effect of anticholinesterases in temporarily reversing the defect in neuromuscular transmission. These agents are still very extensively used for the treatment of mild to moderate disease. Prostigmine and pyridostigmine are the two agents used most commonly and given every three or four hours if possible. I usually commence pyridostigmine at a dose of 30 mg 4 times daily and increase the dose as required. Very high doses of anticholinesterases often predispose to cholinergic crises and are theoretically undesirable because of concern that they may cause a reduction in the number of functional post-synaptic receptors.

Thymomas are best detected by computerized tomography (CT) scanning of the thorax and may be suggested by the presence of antistriated muscle antibodies. Removal of such tumours is required and may, if incomplete, require radiotherapy or chemotherapy. Young patients (under 40 years) appear to benefit from thymectomy in the absence of a thymoma and I advise thymectomy in such patients not completely controlled on anticholinesterases. Patients still symptomatic on anticholinesterases require immunosupression and a combination of steroids and azathioprine is conventional. A controlled trial comparing steroids alone with steroids and azathioprine has recently finished recruiting patients and further information on any advantage of combined therapy should become available.

The risk of patients with generalized myasthenia deteriorating initially on commencing steroids is well recognized and is greater in patients with bulbar symptoms. A suitable starting steroid dose of 10 mg on alternate days has been recommended with increases in 10 mg increments every second dose. Doses of 100–120 mg on alternate days may be needed. Patients with severe disease may require plasma exchange as a holding measure, but antibody synthesis is stimulated following exchange soon returning the antibody titire to the previous level making a definitive decision about future immunosupression essential. Plasma exchange is very useful in the acute treatment of a myasthenic crisis while waiting for the longer-acting drugs, such as azathioprine, to start to exert effect. Plasma exchange can also be a useful diagnostic test in the selection of patients without detectable antibodies but likely to respond to manipulations of the immune response with azathioprine or other immunosupressants.

Very rare cases of congenital myasthenia are encountered with a history of fatigable weakness of eye movements with ptosis and limb weakness. A series of enzyme defects has been described at every stage in the function of the neuromuscular junction. Diagnosis is based on electrophysiological studies *in vivo* and *in vitro* and an intercostal muscle biopsy may allow examination of the motor end plate to determine the abnormality in individual cases. Such patients may respond to anticholinesterases or to 3,4-diaminopyridine, depending on the nature of the abnormality in individual cases.

The early recognition of acute respiratory difficulties in myasthenia still represents the most effective way to prevent death and morbidity and the management of patients with acute respiratory failure is difficult. Intravenous edrophonium is recommended to distinguish between cholinergic and myasthenic crises but such patients may be very sensitive to small doses of edrophonium and can develop asystole and respiratory arrest acutely during the diagnostic test. I generally give only 5 mg of edrophonium slowly by intravenous infusion in the context of a sick patient in intensive care, ensuring that resuscitative equipment is readily available. It is frequently safer to ventilate patients with respiratory difficulties stopping all medication and then reintroduce the anticholinesterases slowly. Plasma exchange is frequently invaluable in the management of such patients.

Intravenous immunoglobulin (IVIG) has been shown to be an alternative treatment option for the acute management of myasthenia although clinical experience of IVIG in myasthenia is limited (20, 21). Autoimmune myasthenia may become inactive and patients who remain asymptomatic for many years should have their treatment slowly withdrawn. It is my practice to stop symptomatic treatment with anticholinesterases first, then tail down the steroid dose before finally considering stopping azathioprine. Some of these patients will relapse many years later but I do not feel justified in subjecting asymptomatic patients to the risks of long-term immunosupression if they have been totally well for several years. Azathioprine is known to increase the risk of certain malignancies particularly of the lymphoid system when continued for many years (22).

CONCLUSION

Recent advances in our understanding of the pathophysiology of neuromuscular disease together with advances in immuno-suppressive drugs makes the management of neuromuscular disease one of the most difficult but yet exciting areas in neurology. Clinical expertise is needed across several disciplines to cope with the unique challenge of reducing symptoms and preventing secondary deterioration in the more chronic conditions while on the other hand managing acute life threatening disorders requiring intensive care and complex immuno-suppressive therapy.

REFERENCES

1. Wade DT, Langton-Hewer R. Epidemiology of some neurological diseases. *Int Rehab Med.* 1987; **18**: 129–37.
2. Guillain G, Barré JA, Strohl A. Sur un syndrome de radiculonevrite avec hyperalbuminose du liquide cephalorachidien sans reaction cellulaire. Remarques sur les caracteres cliniques et graphiques des reflexes tendineux. *Bull Soc Med Hop Paris* 1916; **40**: 1462–70.
3. Winer JB, Hughes RAC, Osmond C. Aprospective study of acute idiopathic neuropathy: 1. Clinical features and their prognostic value. *J Neurol Neurosurg Psychiat* 1988; **51**: 605–12.
4. Winer JB, Hughes RAC. Identification of patients at risk of arrhythmia in the Guillain–Barré syndrome. *Q J Med* 1988; **68**: 735–9.
5. Osterman PO, Lundemo G, Pirskanen R *et al.* Beneficial effects of plasma exchange in acute inflammatory polyradiculoneuropathy. *Lancet* 1984; **ii**: 1296–9.
6. Mendell JR, Kissel JT, Kennedy MS *et al.* Plasma exchange and prednisone in Guillain–Barré syndrome. A controlled randomised trial. *Neurology* 1985; **35**: 1551–5.
7. Guillain–Barré Syndrome Study Group. Plasmapherisis for acute Guillain–Barré syndrome. *Neurology* 1985; **35**: 1096–104.
8. French Cooperative Group in plasma exchange in Guillain–Barré syndrome. Efficiency of plasma exchange in Guillain–Barré syndrome: role of replacement fluids. *Ann Neurol* 1987; **22**: 753–61.
9. Greenwood RJ, Newsom Davis JM, Hughes RAC *et al.* Controlled trial of plasma exchange in acute inflammatory polyradiculoneuropathy. *Lancet* 1984; **i**: 877–9.
10. Van der Meche FGA, Schmidz PIM, and the Dutch Guillain–Barré Study Group. A randomized trial comparing intravenous gammaglobulin and plasma exchange. *N Eng J Med* 1992; **326**: 1123–9.
11. Plasma exchange/sandoglobulin Guillain–Barré Syndrome Trial Group. Randomised trial of plasma exchange, intravenous immunoglobulin and combined treatments in Guillain–Barré syndrome. *Lancet* 1997; **349**: 225–30.
12. Dyck PJ, Oviatt KF, Lambert EH. Intensive evaluation of referred undiagnosed neuropathies yields improved diagnosis. *Ann Neurol* 1981; **10**: 222–6.
13. Vance J, Barker DF, Yamaoka LH *et al.* Localisation of Charcot–Marie–Tooth disease type 1A (CMT1A) to chromosome 17. p 11.2 *Genomics* 1991; **9**: 623–
14. Sigurgeirsson B., Lindelof B, Edhag O., Allander E. Risk of cancer in patients with dermatomyositis or polymyositis. A population based study. *New England Journal of Medicine* 1992; **326** (6) 363–7.
15. Mendell JR, Sahenk Z, Gales T, Paul L. Amyloid filaments in Inclusion Body Myositis. *Arch Neurol* 1991; **48**: 1229–34.
16. Anonymous. Managing osteoporosis. *Drug Therapeut Bull.* 1996; **34**: 45–8.
17. Diamond T, McGuigan L, Barbagallo S, Bryant C. Cyclical etidronate plus ergocalciferol prevents glucocorticoid-induce bone loss in post menapausal women. *Am J Med* 1995; **98**: 459–63.

18. Committee on Safety of Medicines. Oesophageal reactions with alendronate sodium (Fosamax). *Curr Prob Pharmacovig* 1966; **22**: 5.

19. Walker MB. Treatment of myasthenia gravis with physostigmine. *Lancet* 1934; **i**: 1200.

20. Annane D. *IVIG in myasthenia gravis.* Fourth International Congess on IVIG. *Interlaken.* 1996.

21. Edan G, Landgraf F. Experience with intravenous immunoglobulin in myasthenia gravis: a review. *Neurol Psychiat* 1994; **57**: 55–6.

22. Kinlet LJ. Incidence of cancer in rheumatoid arthritis and other diseases after immunosuppressive treatment. *Am J Med* 1985; **78**: 44–9.

7 | *Multiple sclerosis*

David A. Francis

Multiple sclerosis (MS) remains the commonest reason for chronic disability in young adults today with an estimated 80 000 sufferers in the United Kingdom alone. Comprehensive pathological accounts of the central nervous system (CNS) lesions responsible for symptoms, dating back to the beginning of the century (Dawson 1916), have failed to elucidate the underlying cause. Current evidence points to a combined aetiological role for both environmental and genetic factors. For many decades, treatment strategies have revolved around the use of immunosuppressant agents often with disappointing results. However, at no other time in the history of MS research has the future potential for understanding and controlling the disease looked more promising.

The well-recognized geographical prevalence gradient of MS first raised the possibility of an environmental influence on disease causation. It is predominantly a disorder of northern temperate climates. Prevalence rates reach their highest (>50 per 100 000 population) above a latitude of 40° North and decline towards the equatorial regions (Kurtzke 1980). The Southern Hemisphere shows a similar, although less impressive, frequency gradient with increasing latitude. Prevalence rates in Australia and New Zealand are approximately half those reported in Northern Europe suggesting a protective element, or perhaps a weakening of some predisposing factor, in the Antipodean environment (Miller *et al.* 1992). Further evidence stems from studies looking at migration from 'high-risk' to 'low-risk' regions. In a study of British migrants to South Africa 'age at migration' was a crucial factor. Emigrants taking up residence in early childhood adopted the low risk of their new home whereas adolescents and adults conveyed the higher risk of their parent country (Kurtzke *et al.* 1970). This data suggests that whatever environmental factor is implicated its maximum influence occurs before adolescence. Although this 'factor' is unknown popular theory believes it to be viral. Compston *et al.* (1986) have demonstrated an increased risk for the development of MS in individuals who experience a variety of common viral illnesses in late childhood although no specific agent has been implicated. Early viral exposure might explain the increased susceptibility to MS observed in the offspring of first-generation immigrants from Africa, the Indian subcontinent and the Caribbean to the United Kingdom. The UK-born children of these normally resistant racial groups show prevalence rates almost identical to their Caucasian counterparts (Elian *et al.* 1990).

Not all races succumb to these postulated environmental influences; the Oriental races, despite living at 'high-risk' latitudes, show an inherent resistance to MS and prevalence rates rarely rise above 5 per 100 000. (Kuroiwa *et al.* 1975). These with other important observations lend credence to a genetic influence. A positive family history is recorded in 15% of patients and the clinical concordance amongst monozygotic twin-pairs approaches a highly significant 30% in recent analyses (Ebers *et al.* 1986; Kinnunen *et al.* 1988; Mumford *et al.* 1994). The empirical risks for other family members, adjusted for age, have been calculated from extensive familial date (Sadovnick *et al.* 1988). The offspring of an affected patient has a 5% risk of developing MS, siblings between 3% and 5% and the parents a risk in the order of 2–4% dependent on the sex of the index case. These risks are not inconsiderable when compared to a background population point prevalence of 0.1% More specific genetic associations linking disease susceptibility to certain genes within the major histocompatibility complex (MHC) and at other loci involved in immune regulation (Spurkland *et al.* 1991) have added important therapeutic implications which will be discussed later.

NATURAL HISTORY

Attempts to predict the prognosis for any given individual are confounded by the disease's clinical heterogeneity. Eighty per cent of patients will follow a typical relapsing–remitting course from onset, the majority accruing disability with each relapse; but up to 20% will have many years of unrestricted activity punctuated only by short-lived visual or sensory disturbances which resolve completely. Relapses involving the motor system, especially in association with disturbances of brainstem function, co-ordination and/or balance, carry a less favourable prognosis. Other adverse prognostic signs are the development of the disease after the age of 40 years, particularly in males, and a short interval between the initial period and first relapse (Weinshenker *et al.* 1991). A large proportion of individuals will ultimately convert from the remittent form to a secondary stage of progressive disability and in

20% of all patients this unrelenting progressive course occurs from onset, maximum disability ensuing either within a few months or over several years.

MS and pregnancy

MS is more frequent in women than in men. Prior to 1950 most investigators felt that pregnancy had an adverse effect on the disease and should be avoided. Several large studies performed subsequently have shown either no effect of pregnancy on the condition or improvement during the antepartum period, followed by a small increased risk for exacerbation post-partum. Taken overall, there was no net effect, adverse or otherwise, on disease progression (Duquette and Girard 1993; Stenager *et al.* 1994). These recent clarifications of the effects of pregnancy and inheritability of MS has made it easier to counsel patients who wish to start a family.

MS at the extremes of life

The occurrence of MS in childhood is now well established. Earlier this century, when diagnosis relied heavily on dogmatic clinical criteria, the true incidence in children was underestimated. The largest register to date reports an incidence of 2.7% with onset before 16 years of age; confirmed by modern imaging techniques most individuals followed a relapsing/remitting course (Duquette *et al.* 1987). Only 25 patients with onset of MS before the age of 5 years have been reported in the literature (Harefield *et al.* 1991). Brainstem and cerebellar involvement seems to be more frequent in children than in adults and monosymptomatic onset often delays the correct diagnosis. In a proportion of children (22%) the disease is rapidly progressive heightening the need for early diagnosis and effective interventional treatment.

Patients with onset after the age of 50 years also suffer from the rigid age guidelines of most current diagnostic criteria. Increased recognition of this group of individuals have shown them to have a monosymptomatic slowly progressive onset affecting predominantly the motor system producing a spastic paraparesis. Fortunately, they show a high frequency of cerebrospinal fluid (CSF) oligoclonal IgG banding which, with the characteristic features of demyelination on magnetic resonance imaging (MRI) usually confirms the diagnosis (Fig. 7.1).

The assessment of MS in treatment trials has, in the past, relied on the repeated clinical examination of matched groups of patients over prolonged periods of time using established, but subjective, disability scoring systems (Kurtzke 1965). These are prone to both inter- and intra-observer error (Francis *et al.* 1991). Furthermore, the use of serial MRI in patients with 'clinically quiescent' disease has revealed ongoing disease activity occurring in the absence of symptoms. Patients with 'benign' disease accumulated MRI-detected lesions as quickly as patients following a more aggressive course (Thompson *et al.* 1990). MRI scanning methods are now being developed to monitor the disease process more directly by determining the initial extent and subsequent development of 'active' lesions within the central nervous system (CNS)

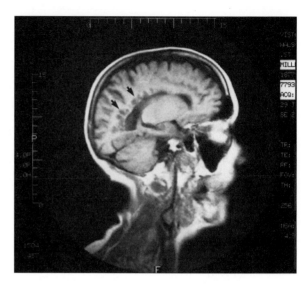

Fig. 7.1 Sagittal (TR500, TE20) MRI of a 70-year-old woman with a 20-year history of slowly evolving spastic paraparesis showing typical periventricular plaques of demyelination. (black arrowheads). Her cerebrospinal fluid also contained oligoclonal IgG bands.

during and after treatment (Miller *et al.* 1991). It is hoped that these disease parameters will provide more objective treatment end-points in future studies.

DIAGNOSIS

Currently, the definitive diagnosis of MS relies heavily on historical evidence of at least two distinct attacks of neurological disturbance and clinical evidence of two separate CNS lesions at the time of examination (Poser *et al.* 1983). In established disease this is rarely difficult; although patients with a steadily progressive non-compressive myelopathy may require long periods of observation. Certain laboratory investigations; for example cerebrospinal fluid immunoglobulin electrophoresis (Fig. 7.2) and/or evoked potential studies are used as 'paraclinical' evidence of a subclinical lesion or a lesion which may have caused symptoms in the past. Neither test is particularly sensitive nor specific for MS but they can be incorporated into the diagnostic criteria when any clinical doubt remains.

MRI is currently the most sensitive means available for detecting cerebral lesions in MS, Characteristic periventricular and discrete white matter abnormalities are seen in over 95% of patients with clinically definite MS (Fig. 7.3). Even these changes are not specific; similar abnormalities are documented in a wide variety of neurological conditions, for example; as an incidental finding in cerebrovascular disease (Fig. 7.4) neurodegenerative disorders, granulomatous conditions and occult infective processes of the CNS. With our increasing knowledge, subtle differences in form and distribution of these lesions strongly favour one diagnosis more than another,

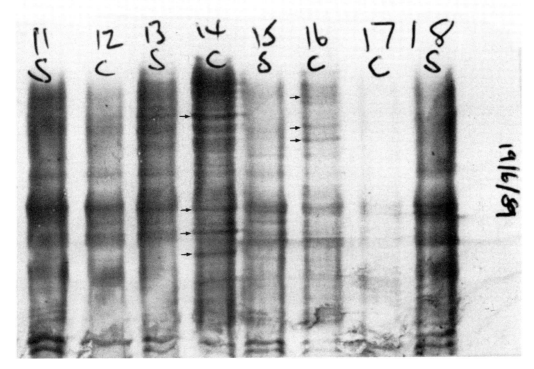

Fig. 7.2 Isoelectric focusing on agarose of paired unconcentrated cerebrospinal fluid (C) and serum (S) blotted on to nitrocellulose and stained using a double antibody peroxidase technique specific for human IgG. Arrows denote the oligoclonal IgG bands which when absent in the serum denotes the presence of increased intrathecal IgG synthesis; typical of, but not specific for, MS. Columns 13 + 14 and 15 + 16 represent two patients with MS bordered by two normal controls. (Courtesy of Dr P. Giles, Edinburgh Medical School.)

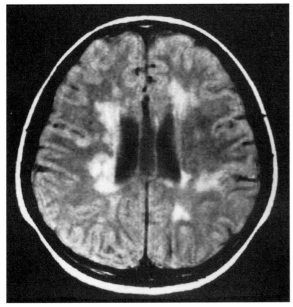

Fig. 7.3 MRI scan (TR2300, TE14) of a patient with clinically definite MS showing discrete white matter lesions and more confluent periventricular abnormalities.

and the appearances can usually be interpreted correctly in the light of the clinical picture. The realization that MRI is a profoundly sensitive method of detecting subclinical abnormalities in the brain of patients with multiple sclerosis will ultimately change our approach to diagnosis and render many of the less objective investigations obsolete.

Once the diagnosis is established there is no good reason to withhold this information from the patient. Failure to do so commonly produces life-long resentment and conspiratorial accusations directed towards the medical profession which jeopardizes trust at future consultations. The patient's fears should be freely discussed at an early stage of their disease particularly when it becomes obvious that the illness is continuing or new symptoms are developing. Open discussion at this stage can be used to dispel the common perceptions of us that are read in the lay-press and utilized by the Multiple Sclerosis Society in its successful 'shock tactics' advertising campaign. It is often the first job of the specialist to put these elements into context.

The Multiple Sclerosis Society of Great Britain and Northern Ireland has adopted a dual role in not only promoting and funding clinical and scientific research into MS through advertising but also provides much needed welfare and support services for MS sufferers and their families. Over 350 branches

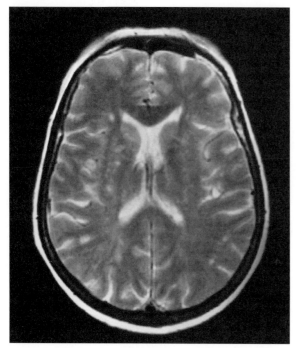

Fig. 7.4 MRI scan (TR2300, TE85) of a hypertensive 53-year-old woman with vertigo who had a cerebellopontine angle tumour. This image reveals the coincidental asymptomatic discrete white matter lesions of small vessel vascular disease which can be indistinguishable from MS.

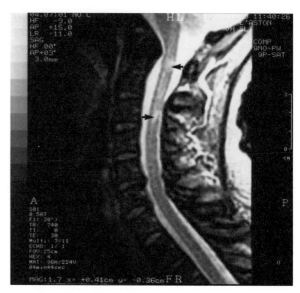

Fig. 7.5 Sagittal (TR740, TE30) MRI of the cervical cord of a 44-year-old woman with a partial Brown–Sequard sensory disturbance and mild spastic paraparesis. In addition to cervical spondylitic degeneration are the more notable areas of increased signal intensity denoting demyelination (arrows).

in the United Kingdom, run primarily by volunteers, provide an opportunity for patients and their carers to discuss problems and exchange ideas with others in a similar situation. Practical assistance is given in the form of advice on welfare, financial assistance, holidays, or contact with other voluntary organizations. Regular publications (*MS Matters*) keep individuals abreast of latest treatments and research in addition to advice on the more practical aspects of daily living. Short-stay and holiday centres are provided, many offering nursing care for the more disabled, giving well-deserved respite for carers and a sense of independence for sufferers. (Further information can be obtained from the Multiple Sclerosis Society of Great Britain and Northern Ireland, 25 Effie Road, Fulham, London, WS6 1EE.)

The dilemma that remains is whether to investigate a patient following an isolated clinical episode which is suspected as being due to demyelination but not proven. Long-term follow-up studies suggest that over 70% of adults will develop multiple sclerosis following isolated optic neuritis (Francis *et al.* 1987). The conversion rate for isolated brainstem lesions and spinal cord syndromes approaches 50% (Miller *et al.* 1989). The clinical presentation of such syndromes is of limited value in predicting future outcome. In transverse myelitis, for example, the more acute and complete lesions, often associated with a high CSF pleocystosis, tend not to progress to MS, particularly in older patients (aged 50 years or more), whereas

those of a partial or remitting nature, in young individuals with little or no CSF cellular response, often herald further attacks. MRI scanning of the spinal cord can be a sensitive means of detection (Fig. 7.5) and has shown widespread asymptomatic cerebral white matter abnormalities in up to two-thirds of patients with clinically isolated syndromes. While these appearances have been shown to be a powerful predictor of subsequent clinical progression to MS not all individuals will inevitably follow this course (Morrissey *et al.* 1993). The clinician who refers his patients for early MRI scanning is often left with the problem of discussing a strongly positive MRI scan with a patient who has little or no current disability. Such investigations are best avoided and discussion of the likely diagnosis is more sensibly deferred in these patients unless they themselves raise the possibility of MS.

TREATMENT

Many patients when diagnosed are returned prematurely to the care of their general practitioner. The developing role of the hospital-based but community-orientated 'nurse practitioner' will hopefully soften this often resented transference. In such situations a nurse with specialized training fills the void that follows discharge from the hospital or outpatient clinic and continues to provide educational and emotional support, listening and responding to feelings and concerns in the more comfortable environment of the individual's own home. He or she will be able to give general guidance on diet, hygiene, and exercise and provide an important link between the patient and other paramedical workers, the general practitioner or hospital specialist to maintain regular and effective interdisciplinary communication. The more disabled patient will require the combined help of the physiotherapist, occupational therapist, speech therapist, and social worker. These services may be easier to liaise through a hospital clinic and the additional support from a hospital specialist at this time is often welcome.

The time will also come in most patients when some form of active intervention is required. The decision to actively treat a patient with MS will revolve around three major strategies:

1. Treatment of the acute exacerbation.
2. Prevention of disease progression.
3. Symptomatic treatment.

I. TREATMENT OF THE ACUTE EXACERBATION

Most patients with MS will, at some stage during their disease, experience a period of acute worsening of their current symptoms or develop a new neurological disturbance. Its severity will depend on the site and size of the responsible plaques. Comparatively small lesions occurring at functionally important sites within the brainstem or spinal cord may produce severe neurological deficit, whereas larger plaques deep within the cerebral white matter may be clinically silent. Spontaneous recovery, following resolution of the acute inflammatory changes seen in and around new lesions, is usual but varies considerably between individuals. Thus, attempts to alleviate, and possibly reduce, the duration and extent of neurological damage, resulting from such exacerbations, are frequently made.

Corticosteroids

Adrenocorticotrophic hormone (ACTH) has been the principal agent in use for several decades. Early studies demonstrated a shortening in duration of attacks of around 10–15% after a 10-day course of daily intramuscular injections (Rose *et al.* 1970). Although the synthetic glucocorticoids have now largely superseded ACTH there is no strong clinical evidence they are superior. Theoretically, the glucocorticoids are more potent, cause less sodium retention, less potassium loss, and have a longer duration of action than ACTH. Small trials comparing the efficacy of bolus methylprednisolone to ACTH have demonstrated that the former is at least as effective with fewer side-effects (Abbruzzese *et al.* 1983; Milligan *et al.* 1987). ACTH may also be less reliable because adrenal cortisone secretion in response to ACTH infusion has been shown to be reduced in MS sufferers compared to control subjects (Maida and Summer 1979). Intravenous methylprednisolone therapy (1000 mg daily for three days or 500 mg daily for five days) has demonstrable benefit in reducing disability during the immediate post-relapse period (Milligan *et al.* 1987), but MRI studies have shown that it appears to have little effect on disease course. High dose methylprednisolone, by improving the integrity of the blood–brain barrier, was shown by sequential MRI scanning to reduce inflammatory oedema around active plaques but it did not prevent the development of new lesions during, or immediately after, the treatment period (Kesselring *et al.* 1989). This finding also supports the clinical impression of many that the use of long-term ACTH or synthetic steroid administration does not alter the frequency of exacerbations or limit progression of the disease. Furthermore, prolonged therapy has been associated with a high complication rate (Rose *et al.* 1970; Hughes 1983).

Intravenous steroids would seem to induce remissions more quickly but whether they are superior to oral corticosteroids is less clear. No controlled trial has tested the use of conventional prednisolone regimes. Oral prednisolone, in daily or alternate day regimes, at moderate to high dosages is occasionally used as a tapering supplement in patients with advanced disease, or those who relapse shortly after intravenous bolus therapy. More recent evidence suggests that high dose methylprednisolone is tolerated by the oral route and is no less effective (Alam *et al.* 1993). A multicentre randomized trial comparing oral with intravenous methylprednisolone has been completed in the United Kingdom. Their findings support those of the earlier study (Barnes *et al.* 1997).

Other treatments for acute relapse

Plasma exchange (PE) and intravenous gamma globulin (IVIG) have both been evaluated for the treatment of exacerbations. In the former, benefits were observed, but these were minimal and did not justify the cost or confer superiority over steroids (Weiner *et al.* 1989). A more recent study of 11 patients with secondary progressive disease failed to demonstrate a reduction in gadolinium-enhancing MRI lesions following treatment with PE and azathioprine (Sorenson *et al.* 1995).

IVIG used alone as a short course (400 mg/kg body weight, daily for 5 days) followed by a single 2 monthly maintenance booster produced fewer relapses in a small group of treatment patients over a 12-month follow-up period. The expense of this agent again militated against any significant benefit over conventional steroid therapy (Achiron *et al.* 1992). A trial involving IVIG (500 mg mg/kg) in conjunction with intravenous methylprednisolone in chronic progressive MS was not shown to have any stabilizing effect on clinical symptoms (Cook *et al.* 1992). Nevertheless, following a number of subsequent studies which held promise of a more favourable response a multicentre European trial of 300 patients with secondary progressive MS is currently being planned.

Overview of acute treatments

The general view is that steroid therapy, in whatever form, will hasten recovery from a clinically significant relapse. The high incidence of side-effects lead most neurologists to reserve its use for serious or disabling exacerbations and restrict pulse therapy to no more than two treatments within a 12 month period.

2. PREVENTION OF DISEASE PROGRESSION

Immunosuppression

The generally agreed consensus that MS is a disorder resulting from aberrant immune function, supported by the occasionally dramatic remission of an acute exacerbation in response to corticosteroids, prompted an exhaustive evaluation of the major immunosuppressive agents from the early 1960s onwards.

Azathioprine. (Imuran–Wellcome), is a readily absorbed nitroimidazole-substituted form of 6-mercaptopurine, and as the least toxic of the immunosuppressants, has been the most popular agent used in the treatment of this condition. The size and construction of initial studies produced conflicting results and prevented firm conclusions from being made about its efficacy. Larger, properly controlled, trials showed beneficial, but non-significant, trends favouring prolonged azathioprine treatment (Swinburn and Liversedge 1973; Mertin *et al.* 1982; Goodkin *et al.* 1990). These findings have been repeated in the largest multicentre trial of azathioprine in MS to date. After three years the treated group showed small improvements in overall disability, ambulation, and relapse rate but none of these parameters reached statistical significance (British and Dutch Multiple Sclerosis Azathioprine Trial Group 1988). Combination therapy has not clarified the issue. A placebo controlled, double-blind, randomized trial of azathioprine, with and without methylprednisolone, in 98 chronic progressive MS patients found those receiving active treatment did significantly better than placebo-treated patients on some, but not all, clinical measures (Ellison *et al.* 1989).

A recent meta-analysis of all published, controlled studies of azathioprine treatment in MS has concluded that the drug appears to reduce the annual relapse rate during each year of treatment and that progression of the disease was slowed after three years (Yudkin *et al.* 1991). This effect was most evident in the first few years of treatment. Reservations about the potential for inducing cancer following the prolonged use of azathioprine have been highlighted by the study of Amato and colleagues who found an increased malignancy rate in patients on regular azathioprine compared to untreated individuals (Amato *et al.* 1990).

Cyclophosphamide (Endoxana–Asta Medica) is a more powerful, and hence more toxic, immunosuppressant and appears to be better tolerated when given in short bursts of intravenous therapy spread over several weeks. Data from early uncontrolled studies of this alkylating agent suggested a modest benefit similar to that of azathioprine. In one study, 21 patients with chronic progressive MS were treated with low dose cyclophosphamide and only one had worsened, using stand-

ard clinical scoring, a year later compared to 14 out of 24 patients who worsened after standard corticosteroid therapy (Mauch *et al.* 1989). The interim results from a North American multicentre trial of intravenous cyclophosphamide/ACTH, with or without two-monthly cyclophosphamide maintenance boosters, in a five-year, randomized, single-blinded study showed a positive effect on the rate of disease progression in favour of booster therapy (Northeast Co-operative Multiple Sclerosis Treatment Group 1990). Conflicting evidence from a well-conducted Canadian multicentre trial showed no difference in outcome between untreated patients and those treated with either oral or intravenous cyclophosphamide, even when this was combined with oral prednisolone (Canadian Co-operative Multiple Sclerosis Study Group 1991). The final verdict of the Northeast Co-operative Multiple Sclerosis Treatment Group was that progression could be slowed by the use of two-monthly cyclophosphamide maintenance boosters and that this occurred particularly in younger patients. (Weiner *et al.* 1993b). These opposing views stimulated a wealth of correspondence between the proponents of the two main study groups and will require several more years of careful evaluation before a consensus of agreement, similar to that for azathioprine, can be reached on the place of cyclophosphamide in MS therapy. A not inconsiderable factor will be its greater toxicity in long-term treatment regimes.

Cyclosporin A (Sandimmun–Sandoz), is a simple peptide molecule of fungal extraction, and has theoretical advantages in that it has more selective suppressor activity on T lymphocyte function. All studies to date have shown a modest effect by slowing disease progression but only at dosages which have produced unacceptable side-effects. In a multicentre, double-blind, placebo controlled randomized trial of cyclosporin A in chronic progressive MS, by the American MS Study Group, initially 6 mg/kg/day was used (Multiple Sclerosis Study Group 1990). European investigators have used 5 mg and 7 mg/kg/day, respectively (Rudge *et al.* 1989; Steck *et al.* 1990). Significantly reduced disability scores were produced after two years with the higher dosages but these had correspondingly high drop-out rates owing to treatment side-effects, including hypertension and impaired renal function. The lower doses were better tolerated but the therapeutic benefit was correspondingly reduced.

Mitoxantrone, which has a non-specific white cell suppressor effect, plays a primary role in the treatment of leukaemia. Its efficacy has been assessed in the rapidly progressive form of MS using the more objective method of lesion enhancement seen on MRI scan at entry and follow-up as an outcome criterion. Its clinical effect was only modest with potent side-effects, of which cardiotoxicity was of the most concern, but a significant reduction in the number of enhancing lesions was observed over six months of therapy (Kappos *et al.* 1990). This study was an important forerunner of others using MRI scanning to measure disease activity during treatment protocols, the latest of which have again confirmed a notable effect on MRI disease activity (Krapfo *et al.* 1995; Edan *et al.* 1997).

Total lymphoid irradiation

This has a similar 'blanket-suppression' of the white blood cell population although targeted primarily at lymphocytes. As a consequence the side-effects, and infection rate in particular, can be troublesome. Women of child-bearing age are rendered permanently infertile and have to be counselled appropriately. The early optimism that this treatment slowed disease in those individuals with rapidly progressive MS has not been repeated in a recently published trial (Wiles *et al.* 1994).

Immunostimulation

The majority of investigators accept that the most plausible explanation for the demyelinating lesion in MS is the triggering of an inflammatory response directed against a component of myelin in response to a preceding, or previous, viral infection. The proponents of immunostimulation therapy argue that it results primarily from an inadequate immune response to this inciting agent. This has led to the paradoxical situation of attempting to *boost* the patients immunoresponsiveness.

Transfer factor

The earliest studies of immunostimulation involved the use of transfer factor a crude extract of disrupted human leucocytes. This was thought to confer to the recipient cell-mediated immunity against viruses and other indeterminate antigens to which the donor has acquired immunity. A large open study in New South Wales, Australia suggested transfer factor slowed deterioration in MS over an 18-month period, as measured by the Kurtzke disability scale (Frith *et al.* 1986). The results of a more meticulously conducted Belgian trial did not confirm this trend after a longer follow-up period (Van Haver *et al.* 1986) with the result that this treatment has largely fallen out of favour.

Interferons

Current interest has focused on the use of interferons (IFNs) to treat MS. These glycoproteins have a wide biological activity which include the activation of macrophages, enhancement of natural killer cells, and inhibition of virus replication, hence their theoretical use as 'antiviral' agents. IFNs may also produce relative immunosuppression and thus be of value in the control of abnormal immunological responses in MS. All three major forms; alpha, beta, and gamma interferons have now been evaluated in this condition.

Alpha-interferon produced by lymphocytes and macrophages, has an antiviral effect which has been used successfully to treat viral hepatitis and a variety of virus-induced tumours. No significant benefit has been demonstrated in MS, to date, at doses tolerated by the patient. Fever, fatigue,

and neutropenia were commonly encountered side-effects (Austims Research Group 1989).

The most encouraging data have come from the use of beta-IFN. Originally harvested from fibroblast cultures and given intrathecally, to bypass the blood–brain barrier, a small cohort of patients with remittent disease experienced significantly lower exacerbation rates than a similar number of placebo-treatment patients (Jacobs *et al.* 1987). Not all subsequent studies were as promising and dose-related side-effects via this route were troublesome (Milanese *et al.* 1990). This method of administration has been superseded by the production of recombinant beta-IFN which is stable via the subcutaneous route. This has enabled longer and more powerful studies to be performed the results of which hold promise for the most effective form of treatment for MS to emerge in recent years. The major finding of a double-blind randomized study of 372 patients with remittent disease, given alternate day subcutaneous injections of recombinant beta-IFN, was the reduction in frequency of clinical relapses by up to one third. In addition, the accumulation of brain lesions, as judged from serial MRI scanning throughout the treatment period, was significantly less in the treatment groups when compared to untreated patients. (IFNB Multiple Sclerosis Study Group 1995.)

The success of this study has been tempered by the high incidence of local inflammation at the injection site (60% of the beta-IFN patients; 6% of placebo patients) although this appears to be transient. Two other concerns of this trial persist. Despite the impressive reduction in MRI lesion load noted throughout the three-year trial, and its two-year extension for patients receiving 8 MIU (Million International Units) of *beta 1b-interferon*, there remains important limitations in the ability of MRI change to predict a treatment effect on disease progression. Secondly, a significant number of treated patients (39% at 3 years) developed neutralizing antibodies which appeared to correlate with reduced clinical benefit. What effect these two observations may have on the long-term course of MS is presently unknown. Not withstanding these reservations this agent has been licensed for use in remittent MS in North America for several years (Beneseron) and in 1995 was given its UK and European Licence (Betaferon–Schering) for ambulatory MS patients who had experienced at least two significant attacks in the previous two years.

A second major trial of 301 patients supports the use of beta-IFN. Avonex-Interferon-beta1a (Biogen) differs from Betaferon (Schering) by virtue of is manufacture and the resultant requirement for only once-weekly intramuscular injections. This study demonstrated a similar decrease in the annual exacerbation rate (32%) over a two-year period with a significant reduction in the number of active lesions (defined by the use of gadolinium-DTPA) seen on serial MRI scanning. The primary end-point for this study, however, was time to sustained disability progression of at least 1.0 point on the Kurtzke expanded disability status scale (EDSS). Treatment with interferon-beta1a was associated with a slower rate of disease progression (3.1 years to advance 1 EDSS point in placebo-treated patients compared with 5.4 years in patients on active treatment). The major criticism of this study has been the variable length of follow-up for patients before the study was prematurely closed for final analysis. This left incomplete two-years' data on 129 patients (43%) (Jacobs *et al.* 1996)

For the reasons stated above some European neurologists and most UK neurologists have been reluctant to prescribe Betaferon until further evaluation has been undertaken. Trials are underway world-wide to confirm and extend the role of beta-IFN in the treatment of MS. Many hundreds of patients, not only those with a relapsing–remittent course but also those currently in a secondary progressive phase and individuals presenting with their first demyelinating episode, are undergoing evaluation with the three proprietary forms of beta-IFN in the expectation that its influence on disease progression and/or development will be unequivocally defined.

One potential benefit of beta-IFN may be the down-regulation of antigen recognition by major histocompatibility complex (MHC) molecules. In contrast, gamma-IFN is a potent stimulator of MHC class II expression on cell surfaces, including endothelium. The up-regulation of antigen presentation, on this vulnerable interface, to circulating cytotoxic T cells promotes tissue damage. This theoretical danger was realized with gamma-IFN in a small pilot study involving 18 patients with relapsing–remitting disease, who experienced a disproportionate increase in the number of relapses during 'active' treatment (Panitch *et al.* 1987).

Other therapies.

Copolymer 1

Experimental allergic encephalomyelitis (EAE), the closest animal model to MS, can be induced by the repeated injection of extracts of myelin basic protein (MBP) a major constituent of CNS myelin (Zamvil and Steinman 1990). Although confirmatory evidence is lacking, MBP has long been suspected as the target antigen which provokes the inflammatory response in MS. Copolymer 1 (COP-1) is a short synthetic polypeptide of four amino acids which, by pre-inoculation, has been shown to suppress the subsequent development of EAE in several species of laboratory animal (Arnon and Teitelbaum 1980). Early uncontrolled studies involving daily subcutaneous injections of COP-1 in patients with MS were favourable and stimulated formal controlled trials in both progressive and relapsing–remitting disease. These studies noted modest, but non-significant, benefits in slowing disease progression (Bornstein et al. 1987, 1991). The results of a Phase III study of this agent have been reported (Johnson *et al.* 1995). This randomized, double-blind, placebo controlled trial involved 251 patients in 11 US Centres (125 receiving the active drug) over a two-year period. The authors reported a 29% mean reduction in relapse rate over placebo treated patients. A beneficial effect on disability was also

noted in several, but not all, the scales utilized in this study, suggesting some influence on disease progression.

The adverse effects with COP-1 were not severe, the main complication being that of transient localized injection site reactions. An as yet poorly understood systemic reaction was seen at least once in 15% of patients. This occurred within moments of injection of COP-1 and consisted of chest pain, palpitations, and/or dyspnoea lasting up to 30 minutes. Antibodies reactive to COP-1 were detected in many patients on active treatment but did not appear to have any neutralizing effect and had no influence on clinical outcome.

Although this agent has been granted an FDA licence in the US (December 1996: Copaxone TEVA-HMR) and a UK licence has been applied for, further trials are planned in Europe and Canada to obtain more comprehensive MRI data. Copolymer-1 represents a novel approach to treatment by 'desensitization' of the host to a potential immunogenic trigger. It is hoped that this further evaluation will establish its efficacy.

Hyperbaric oxygen

The reasoning behind the use of hyperbaric oxygen (HBO) in MS stems from the clinical similarity, albeit superficial, of the symptoms of MS with those of decompression sickness; and the, now outdated, suggestion that microthrombi or fat emboli in the capillaries of the CNS initiated the destructive process which led to demyelination. More recent claims point to benefit through influences on immune function (Hansbrough *et al.* 1990). A number of uncontrolled anecdotal reports purporting the effectiveness of this relatively harmless treatment falsely raised public expectations; and demand, fuelled largely by self-referral, soon outstripped the availability of hyperbaric chambers. A number of national registries of HBO treatment were set up to evaluate these therapeutic claims on a larger scale. It soon became clear from this data that there was continuation or worsening of symptoms despite treatment and that no useful effect was discernible on any objective parameter of the disease process (Kindwall *et al.* 1991). In 1995, Kleijen and Knipschild evaluated 14 published controlled trials of which only one found that HBO had a useful effect in MS. The authors concluded that HBO could not be recommended and few neurologists now support this treatment.

Overview of preventative treatments

In practice, few patients in the United Kingdom receive therapy aimed at slowing progression of the disease. Azathioprine has been more widely adopted in Europe and cyclophosphamide tends to be favoured in the United States. There is general agreement among all neurologists that the beneficial effects of current immunotherapy are at best modest and may not outweigh the risks of treatment in all but those patients with the most severe forms of the disease. It is hoped that the emergent treatments still under evaluation (linomide, cladribine, and sulphasalazine) will provide us with more effective alternatives which carry no greater risk to the individual.

3. SYMPTOMATIC TREATMENT

In the absence of effective therapy to halt progression of the disease many patients will require relief from those paroxysmal or persistent symptoms which are sufficient to interfere with the quality of their daily life. The amelioration of these can be considered under two broad headings: general symptomatic treatment and specific symptomatic treatment.

General symptomatic treatment

Treatments under this category are designed either to re-establish conduction through demyelinated nerve fibres in an attempt to restore function; or to inhibit ephaptic transmission between adjacent nerve tracts involved in larger areas of demyelination. The latter mechanism is thought to underlie the well recognized paroxysmal symptomatology of MS.

Restoration of conduction

The potassium channel-blocking agent, 4-aminopyridine, has been the most comprehensively assessed agent in this category. It acts by prolongation of the nerve action potentials; thereby enhancing conduction across demyelinated segments. Preliminary studies demonstrated neurological improvement in temperature-sensitive patients (Jones *et al.* 1983) and more recently its long-term efficacy has been evaluated. Patients who initially responded to treatment were reported to have persisting benefits in ambulation, fatigue, and visual function for periods of up to 32 months on dosages ranging from 15 mg to 40 mg daily (Polman *et al.* 1994). Paraesthesia and dizziness are common but well-tolerated side-effects; although its potential for triggering generalized epileptic seizures is of more concern. These and other encouraging results have prompted the development of a slow-release formulation which is hoped to reduce toxicity.

Inhibition of paroxysmal symptoms

Tonic seizures, trigeminal neuralgia, and paroxysmal dysarthria–ataxia are well-recognized symptoms which by definition are of short duration (i.e. less than 2 minutes) (Espir and Millac 1970). Carbamazepine, often in relatively small dosage, 100–200 mg daily, has proved the most useful treatment for paroxysmal disturbances of neurological function. Its beneficial effect may be related to its inhibitory action on voltage-sensitive sodium channels (Willow *et al.* 1985). Unfortunately, carbamazepine may aggravate fatigue and increase existing neurological deficits through its inhibitory influences, thereby limiting its dose range. Phenytoin is an alternative which has been shown to ameliorate these symptoms (Mathews 1958) and acetazolamide can be used in patients intolerant of either (Voiculescu *et al.* 1975). A recent preliminary study by Reder and Arnason (1995) has also sug-

gested a potential role for the long-acting prostaglandin E_1 analogue, misoprostol (Cytotec–Searle) in patients who fail to respond to conventional therapy.

Diet

Polyunsaturated fatty acids. Dietary supplementation with polyunsaturated fatty acids (PUFAs) and the avoidance of saturated animal fats, have their origins in epidemiological surveys of fish-eating communities which had a low incidence of MS. They may have other genuine therapeutic benefits; PUFAs exert an immunosuppressant effect (Mertin 1980) and linolenic acid and linolenic acids, as essential fatty acids are major constituents of myelin. Many early studies were disappointing but an analysis of the results of three controlled trials of supplementation with linolenic acid (around 20 g/day) concluded that in treated patients progression of disability was retarded and the severity and duration of relapses was reduced (Dworkin *et al.* 1984).

Gluten-free diet. The rationale for using a gluten-free diet in MS is more anecdotal and based on self-reported dramatic clinical recoveries in a few individuals (Matheson 1974). The possibility that MS stemmed from an intestinal disorder resulting in malabsorption of fatty acids and other vital nutrients has never been proven. In the largest open trial of gluten exclusion undertaken, Liversedge (1975) studied 42 patients, five of whom had to be withdrawn through intolerance of the dietary restriction. The relapse rate and accumulated disability in the remainder over a mean follow-up of almost two years was no different to that of patients on unrestricted diets.

Most neurologists will give general dietary advice aimed at avoiding obesity particularly when mobility is impaired. Although favoured by many, the cost of PUFA supplements is a major drawback. Sunflower seed oil and evening primrose oil are not yet licensed for use in multiple sclerosis. The introduction of a gluten-free diet has no theoretical basis and is not to be recommended

Specific symptomatic treatment

Treatments in this category target specific neuronal pathways and involve the combined approach of physical therapy, pharmacological intervention, and patient education.

Spasticity

Spasticity is by far the commonest symptom encountered in MS. Sustained muscle hypertonicity causes difficulties in maintaining posture, thereby impairing mobility in the ambulant patient; in the bedridden patient it is a major predisposing factor in the development of pressure sores. In addition, some patients experience painful flexor/extensor spasms, affecting predominantly the lower limbs, occurring spontaneously, particularly at night, or in response to passive movement. The effective treatment of spasticity needs to be balanced against the relative benefit of maintaining a 'rigid frame' for walking or transferring and requires not only the collaboration of doctors, nurses, and physiotherapists but also of the patient and their immediate carers. Many factors exacerbate spasticity by increasing afferent input; comfortable loose clothing, appropriate seating or positioning, and attention to skin and bladder hygiene are as important as more conventional therapies.

Physiotherapy. The mobile patient with mild to moderate spasticity, causing for example gait impairment, will often respond to well-directed physiotherapy alone. Observation of the individual and re-education of the muscles used in posture and gait may be sufficient. Heat treatments either in the form of ultrasound or local compresses are commonly used preparatory adjuncts to relax spastic muscles before active stretching to minimize the risk of muscle injury. Joint contractures can occur in untreated or badly treated patients with spasticity. All joints should be put through a full range of movement for 2 hours in every 24-hour period. Achieving this through direct electrical stimulation or by the use of 'toning beds' does not confer any specific advantage. Simple positioning prevents the patient from becoming fixed in a position favoured by the pull of spastic muscles. Prone positioning avoids marked flexor spasticity; side-lying and standing also produces stretch on spastic muscles by utilizing antagonistic muscle groups. If a limb has become contracted, its range may be improved by serial splinting. New casts being applied every week as the range of movement increases. Once the desired position has been achieved permanent splinting may be required to maintain an optimum posture or restore mobility.

Driving and employment. Patients with chronic spasticity often seek advice on the regulations for driving. There are three main groups of physical impairment which may influence their ability to drive or require vehicle modifications: limb (upper or lower) and spinal disability, which produces deformity or joint restriction, and the more general impairment of ability produced by associated muscular weakness. Driving assessment centres exist to offer advice on all aspects of transport. For a reasonable fee they provide assessments for driving ability and advice on car adaptations. The Motability organization, a registered charity (MOTABILITY, 2nd Floor, Gate House, Westgate, Harlow, Essex, CM20 1HR) provides helpful information about financial aspects of purchasing or adapting vehicles for the disabled. As soon as the individual is diagnosed as having MS, they must inform the DVLA (Driver and Vehicle Licensing Authority), and their own insurance company. This does not mean that the licence is automatically revoked but it may be subject to an approach to that person's medical attendant for further clinical information. Anyone who has difficulties obtaining motor insurance as a result of MS can approach the MS Society who hold information about sensitive insurance companies. If a patient's condition is likely to progress, short-term licenses of one to three years may be issued and are subject to renewal. In addition, it is important that vision, co-ordination and reaction time, memory, or concentration are not sufficiently impaired to render the potential driver at increased risk of an accident.

It is equally important that newly diagnosed patients with fixed disability are put in touch with the various government and charitable agencies whose aim is to advise, find work, or teach new skills to disabled people. The decision to inform current employers, mention their condition on applying for new jobs, or to seek a reduction in working hours has to be made on an individual basis and not influenced by the unjustified pessimistic expectation of unrelenting disease progression.

Oral medication Drug therapy is not to be regarded as an alternative to physiotherapy or other physical treatments and should be carefully titrated to provide relief of spasticity without producing or exacerbating muscle weakness.

Benzodiazepines. The effect of benzodiazepines in spasticity is mediated by their ability to enhance the action of the inhibitory neurotransmitter gamma-aminobutyric acid (GABA) on spinal stretch reflexes. Diazepam is an effective antispastic agent lasting 6–8 hours after an oral dose. Clonazepam is a suitable alternative, as a single bedtime dose, to prevent nocturnal muscle spasms. Adverse effects such as drowsiness, aggression, depression, and enhancement of weakness often prove unacceptable. There are also problems with drug dependence and withdrawal.

Baclofen (Lioresal–CIBA) has GABA agonist properties which act at the spinal cord level by inhibition of polysynaptic spinal reflexes. This gives it theoretical advantage in 'spinal cord' spasticity, as seen in MS, and is therefore the most commonly used preparation. The effects of each dose last 3–5 hours and side-effects of drowsiness, fatigue, and muscle weakness tend to be dose-dependent. The optimal dose in most patients averages 60 mg daily in divided doses. Abrupt withdrawal should be avoided as confusional states, hallucinosis, and convulsions have been recorded.

Dantrolene sodium (Dantrium–Procter and Gamble). This agent has a peripheral mode of action on skeletal muscle. Contraction is inhibited by suppressing the release of calcium ions from the sarcoplasmic reticulum within muscle fibres. Drowsiness, dizziness, weakness, and fatigue are again commonly reported side-effects and hepatotoxicity may occur in the long-term on high dosage regimes. Liver function should be monitored and the drug avoided in anyone with known liver dysfunction. A slow incremental regime is used to effect tolerance as dosages of up to 400 mg daily (100 mg 4 times a day, in divided doses) may be required.

Tizanidine (Sirdalud-Sanofi-Withrop). This recently evaluated antispastic agent, which has a similar action to baclofen on excitatory spinal pathways, appears to be a valid alternative. It compared favourably against baclofen in a number of double-blind trials in MS (Hoogstraten *et al.* 1988), and has just been licensed in the United Kingdom. Sedation, weakness, and dry mouth were noted side-effects.

Intrathecal medications. Historically, the use of intrathecal phenol, glycerine or alcohol to alleviate severe spasticity in patients with late-stage MS was first described over 30 years ago (Kelly and Gautier-Smith 1959). These techniques were reserved for patients already rendered paraplegic and incontinent; intrathecal phenol, in particular, was non-selective, damaging adjacent lumbosacral nerve roots. Painful lower limb spasms were abolished but often at the expense of reduced skin and bladder sensitivity, increasing the frequency of pressure sores. Recent experiences in the use of intrathecal baclofen for spasticity have made these irreversible procedures unnecessary. Following its introduction in 1984 (Penn and Kroin 1984) the application of baclofen, via the intrathecal route, has become increasingly popular. By circumventing the blood–brain barrier extremely low concentrations of baclofen are proving to be as effective as large oral dosages with fewer side-effects (Ochs *et al.* 1989). Most patients selected for this procedure have severe and disabling spasticity resistant to oral antispastic agents. A prerequisite is a positive response to an intrathecal test-bolus of either 25, 50, or 100 micrograms (μg). The beneficial effects of this should last for 6–8 hours and any potential side-effects or unwanted muscle relaxation can be noted.

An implantable drug administration device for long-term usage avoids the potential infection risk of repeated injections. The drug is applied at lumbar level producing maximal beneficial effect on the lower limbs thus preserving upper limb strength and preventing the central side-effects which would result from high brainstem concentrations. Following implantation, the pump can be programmed and the dosage titrated to the individuals requirements, a usual starting dose would be about 60 μg per day eventually averaging about 200 μg per day. Patients and their primary carers must be conversant with the systemic side-effects which may occur even on stable low concentration regimes. The judicious use of intrathecal baclofen today looks set to replace the many surgical procedures and nerve ablations performed for intractable spasticity over previous decades.

Ataxia

Ataxia and limb tremor remain one of the most disabling and difficult symptoms to treat. Although many strategies have been employed to alleviate this distressing problem their true efficacy remains uncertain largely because there are few objective methods of assessment. Reliability is further compromised by the effect of fatigue and emotional stress on performance. It has been suggested that the repeated practice of exercises of increasing complexity not only helps reinforce the experience-dependent plasticity of cerebellar neuronal networks but also redevelops self-confidence (Hardie 1989). The involvement of occupational therapists is important; even simple devices such as special hand grips on pens and cutlery, non-slip mats, and corrected seating positions can be beneficial for patients with ataxia. Mechanical loading, by weighting a patients wrists, for example, can reduce the amplitude of moderately severe tremor but has no observable benefit in patients at either the mild or very severe ends of the tremor spectrum (Michaelis 1993). It is also important to realize that the proportion of weighting bears no relationship to the amelioration of tremor and that arm function may be worsened if the increased inertia produced compromises underlying muscle weakness. An increasingly employed solution is to directly dampen the tool the patient is trying to manoeuvre (i.e. a feeding spoon rather than the limb itself). The increasing complexity of such devices bears testimony to the ingenuity of engineers in hospital medical physics departments.

The specific management of disabling tremor remains largely pharmacological (see Table 7.1). Most drugs employed to date have no more than a dampening effect on incapacitating tremor with the likelihood of tolerance developing or the production of unacceptable side-effects. On theoretical grounds, a number of investigators have advocated the use of isoniazid, an inhibitor of GABA-aminotransferase, in an attempt to increase intracerebral GABA which has been shown to be reduced in patients with advanced cerebellar disease (Kuroda *et al.* 1982). Both subjective and objective improvement in tremor have been recorded but the high doses required (up to 1200 mg) produce limiting side-effects and the benefits appear greater for postural cerebellar tremor than intention tremor (Sabra *et al.* 1982; Francis *et al.* 1986). Isoniazid has also been used to reduce oscillopsia due to acquired pendular nystagmus in MS (Traccis *et al.* 1990). A possible role for gabapentin (Neurontin–Parke-Davis) in the treatment of nystagmus has also been reported (Averbuch-Heller *et al.* 1995). The more recent results of a single-blind, crossover, trial encourages the use of carbamazepine for both postural and intention tremor (Sechi *et al.* 1989); the latter more typically associated with MS. While intravenous ondansetron (Zofran–Glaxo) may be useful in severe cerebellar outflow tremor.

Fatigue

This is an underrated symptom which many MS sufferers have to bear; often occurring early in the course of the disease and out of proportion to the patients' objective disability. Both physiological and psychological components are implic-

Table 7.1 Pharmacological treatment of tremor in multiple sclerosis

Beta-adrenergic blockers
Propranolol

Anticholinergics
Benzhexol
Orphenadrine

Anticonvulsants
Carbamazepine
Primidone

'Antibiotics'
Isoniazid

Benzodiazepines
Diazepam
Clonazepam

ated, the latter responding to standard antidepressant drugs and counselling. The recently introduced antidepressants (e.g. fluoxetine) have been shown to be especially beneficial. Several other drugs have been reported to help with this symptom. In two well-conducted studies approximately 60% of patients found that amantadine (Symmetrel, Mantidine, 100 mg twice-daily) lessened their fatigue (Rosenberg and Appenzeller 1988; Cohen and Fisher 1989); although the subsequent widespread use of this drug has been disappointing. Pemoline (Volital–LAB) has a CNS stimulant action and was promising in preliminary trials (Bass *et al.* 1990). In a more recent study, although 46.3% of patients reported good relief of fatigue, 25% were intolerant of its side-effects: anorexia, irritability, and insomnia (Weinshenker *et al.* 1992).

Urinary symptoms

Urinary frequency and urgency often leading to incontinence are common and distressing. Formal urodynamic assessment and a multidisciplinary approach between neurologist, urologist, and a continence nurse may be required to determine which neurogenic pathway is predominately disturbed and hence the most appropriate therapy. One should also remain alert to the possibility of an underlying urinary tract infection producing, or exacerbating, symptoms of bladder dysfunction. Prompt antibiotic treatment may be all that is required to return continence and peace of mind to a distraught patient. Recurrent infection may require low dose prophylactic antibiotics but this is best avoided in patients who are permanently catheterized unless systemic symptoms supervene.

Symptoms due to an unstable detruser muscle can be alleviated by anticholinergic agents, such as propantheline bromide (15 mg 2–4 times a day). Oxybutinin (Cystrin, Ditropan), now licensed in the United Kingdom, has similar properties to propantheline and confers no particular advantage. Many clinicians will utilize the anticholinergic properties of a tricyclic antidepressant (e.g. amitriptyline, imipramine) combating depression or neuralgic pain at the same time. Paradoxically, the major unwanted effect of treatment with these agents is dry mouth which can result in increased fluid intake thereby aggravating the original symptoms. The value of desmopressin in controlling nocturia is now well established; a recent study gave 20 μg as the optimal dose for effectiveness and preventing clinically significant hyponatraemia (Eckford *et al.* 1995). Temporary alleviation of bladder frequency; for example, in anticipation of a social event or a long car journey during waking hours can alternatively be achieved from simple 'cold cures' (e.g. Eskornade) which incorporate phenylpropranolamine, an antihistamine, which 'clamps' the bladder neck sphincter for short periods.

Symptoms due to intermittent bladder neck obstruction often respond to alpha adrenergic blockade with prasozin (Hypovase: 1 mg 3 times a day) or phenoxybenzamine (Dibenyline: 10 mg twice-daily). Where this fails intermittent self-catheterization should be considered as an adjunct to oral medication. Advancing physical disability is no bar to efficient and hygienic bladder catheterization provided initial tuition, preferably from a contenence adviser, is adequate or a close relative is fully instructed. An increasing range of disposable, individually sealed, and self-lubricated catheters has rendered this technique fault-free and patients who catheterize themselves up to four times daily have not experienced higher rates of infection. The principle objective of this technique is to prevent chronic urinary retention and consequent renal damage, secondary to reflux, which in the pre-antibiotic era was a major contributor to mortality.

FUTURE PROSPECTS

A major aim for the treatment of MS in the future will be the development of target-specific immunotherapy, with little or no systemic toxicity, which halts the progression of the disease. Such treatment would be effective early in its course before disability becomes established. The successful application of potential therapies is dependent upon our increased understanding of the immunological triggers responsible for MS and their interaction with the prime effectors of damage, T lymphocytes. For example, if MS is initiated by pathogenic T cells; manufactured monoclonal antibodies, directed against them, present a potentially ideal reagent either for their destruction or alternatively blockade at the MHC–T cell receptor site. A recent double-blind, placebo controlled trial to assess the effect of infusions of a monoclonal antibody to inducer T lymphocytes (anti-CD4 antibodies), which block the destructive autoimmune activity of the CD4 white cell has been reported. It had been suggested that this may lead to a reduction in the incidence of new CNS lesions thereby slowing disease progression. Unfortunately, using MRI activity as the primary end-point, no reduction of new lesions was seen in the treated group over an 18-month follow-up period (Miller *et al.* 1995).

Alternative strategies have employed either the parenteral inoculation of attenuated T cells which recognize the inciting agent (Hafler *et al.* 1992) or the oral ingestion of myelin constituents, akin to COP-1, leading to their subsequent toleration by the host (Weiner *et al.* 1993a); both manoeuvres theoretically remove the factors which may be responsible for the induction of the disease process. Attention is also being drawn to the potential of suppressing cytokines, particularly TNFα (tumour necrosis factor alpha) and blocking the binding of certain 'adhesion' molecules which may be implicated in the pathogenesis of MS. A number of clinical trials are underway.

Finally, one has to consider the future role of nerve cell implantation. Techniques are being developed in which the autoimplantation of either astrocytes or oligodendrocyte progenitors into lesions at sites of eloquent CNS function, possibly stimulated by specific nerve cell growth factors, may stimulate oligodendrocyte remyelination (Franklin *et al.* 1991). These exciting possibilities are currently under evaluation and will, it is hoped, open new, and effective methods of either preventing disability or restoring neuronal function in this enigmatic disease.

REFERENCES

1. Abbruzzese, G. Gandolfo, C., and Loeb, C. (1983). 'Bolus' methylprednisolone versus ACTH in the treatment of multiple sclerosis. *Italian Journal of Neurological Sciences*, **4**, 169–72.

2. Achiron, A., Pras, E., Gilad, R., Ziv, I., Mandel, M., Gordon, C. R., *et al.* (1992). Open controlled therapeutic trial of intravenous immune globulin in relapsing-remitting multiple sclerosis. *Archives of Neurology*, **49**, 1233–6.

3. Alam, S. M., Kyriakides, T., Lawden, M., and Newman, P. K. (1993). Methylprednisolone in multiple sclerosis: a comparison of oral with intravenous therapy at equivalent high dose. *Journal of Neurology, Neurosurgery and Psychiatry*, **56**, 1219–20.

4. Amato, M. P., Siracusa, G., Fratiglioni, L., and Amaducci, L. (1990). Azathioprine therapy and cancer risk in multiple sclerosis: a prospective long-term study. *Annals of Neurology*, **28**, 282.

5. Arnon, R. and Teitelbaum, D. (1980). Densitization of experimental allergic encephalomyelitis with synthetic peptide analogues. In *The suppression of experimental allergic encephalomyelitis and multiple sclerosis*, (ed. A. N. Davis and M. L. Cuzner), pp. 105–17. Academic Press, New York.

6. Austims Research Group (1989). Interferon-a and transfer factor in the treatment of multiple sclerosis: a double blind, placebo-controlled trial. *Journal of Neurology, Neurosurgery and Psychiatry*, **52**, 566–74.

7. Averbuch-Heller, L., Stahl, J. S., Rottach, K. G., and Leigh, R. J. (1995). Gabapentin as treatment for nystagmus (Abstract). *Annals of Neurology*, **38**, 972.

8. Bass, B., Weinshenker, B. G., Penman, M., Ebers, G. C., and Rice, G. P. A. (1990). A double-blind, placebo-controlled randomised trial to compare the efficacy of Cylert (pemoline) and placebo in the control of fatigue in multiple sclerosis. *Neurology*, **40** (suppl. 1), 261.

9. Bornstein, M. B., Miller, A., Slagle, S., Weitzman, M., Crystal, H., Drexler, E. *et al.* (1987). A pilot trial of Cop 1 in exacerbating-remitting multiple sclerosis. *New England Journal of Medicine*, **317**, 408–14.

10. Bornstein, M. B., Miller, A., Slagle, S., Weitzman, M., Drexler, E., Keilson, M. *et al.* (1991). A placebo-controlled, double-blind, randomised, two centre, pilot trial of Cop 1 in chronic progressive multiple sclerosis. *Neurology*, **41**, 533–9.

11. British and Dutch Multiple Sclerosis Azathioprine trial group (1988). Double-masked trial of azathioprine in multiple sclerosis. *Lancet*, **2**, 179–83.

12. Canadian Co-operative Multiple Sclerosis Study Group (1991). The Canadian Co-operative Trial of cyclophosphamide and plasma exchange in progressive multiple sclerosis. *Lancet*, **337**, 441–6.

13. Cohen, R. A. and Fisher, M. (1989) Amantadine treatment of fatigue with multiple sclerosis. *Archives of Neurology*, **46**, 676–80.

14. Compston, D. A. S., Vakarelis, B. N., Paul, E., McDonald, W. I., Batchelor, J. R., and Mims, C. A. (1986). Viral infection in patients with multiple sclerosis and HLA-DR matched controls. *Brain*, **109**, 325–44.

15. Cook, S. D., Troiano, R., Rohowsky-Kochan, C., Jotkowitz, A., Bielory, L., Mehta, P., *et al.* (1992). Intravenous gamma globulin in progressive MS. *Acta Neurologica Scandinavica*, **86**, 171–5.

16. Dawson, J. W. (1916). Disseminated sclerosis. *Edinburgh Medical Journal*, **17**, 311–77.

17. Duquette, P. and Girard, M. (1993). Hormonal factors in susceptibility to multiple sclerosis. *Current Opinion in Neurology and Neurosurgery*, **6**, 195–201.

18. Duquette, P., Murray, T. J., Pleines, J., Ebers, G. C., Sadovnick, D., Weldon, P. *et al.* (1987). Multiple sclerosis in childhood: Clinical profile in 125 patients. *Journal of Paediatrics*, **111**, 359–63.

19. Dworkin, R. A., Bates, D., Millar, J. H. D., and Paty, D. W. (1984). Linoleic acid and multiple sclerosis. *Neurology*, **34**, 1441–5.

20. Ebers, G. C., Bulman, D. E., Sadovnick, A. D., Paty, D. W., Warren, S., Hader, W. *et al.* (1986). A population-based twin study in multiple sclerosis. *New England Journal of Medicine*, **315**, 1638–42.

21. Eckford, S. D., Carter, P. G., Jackson, S. R., Penney, M. D., and Abrams, P. (1995). An open in-patient incremental safety efficacy study of desmopressin in women with multiple sclerosis and nocturia. *British Journal of Urology*, **74**, 459–63.

22. Edan, G., Miller, D., Clanet, M., Confavreux, C., Lyon-Caen, O., Lubetzki, C. *et al.* (1997). Therapeutic effect of mitoxantrone combined with methylprednisolone in multiple sclerosis: a randomised multicentre study of active disease using MRI and clinical criteria. *Journal of Neurology, Neurosurgery and Psychiatry*, **62**, 112–18.

23. Ellison, G. W., Myers, L. W., Mickey, M. R., Graves, M. C., Tourtellotte, W. W., Syndulko, K. *et al.* (1989). A placebo-controlled, randomized double-masked variable dosage, clinical trial of azathioprine with and without methylprednisolone in multiple sclerosis. *Neurology*, **39**, 1018–26.

24. Espir, M. L. E. and Millac, P. (1970). Treatment of paroxysmal disorders in multiple sclerosis with carbamazepine (Tegretol). *Journal of Neurology, Neurosurgery and Psychiatry*, **33**, 528–31.

25. Francis, D. A., Grundy, D., and Heron, J. R. (1986). The response to isoniazid of action tremor in multiple sclerosis and its assessment using polarised light goniometry. *Journal of Neurology, Neurosurgery and Psychiatry*, **49**, 87–9.

26. Francis, D. A., Compston, D. A. S., Batchelor, J. R., and McDonald, W. I. (1987). A reassessment of the risk of multiple sclerosis developing in patients with optic neuritis after extended follow-up. *Journal of Neurology, Neurosurgery and Psychiatry*, **50**, 758–65.

27. Francis, D. A., Bain, P., Swan, A. V., and Hughes, R. A. C. (1991). An assessment of disability rating scales used in multiple sclerosis. *Archives of Neurology*, **48**, 299–301.

28. Franklin, R. J. M., Crang, A. J., and Blakemore, W. B. (1991). Transplanted type-1 astrocytes facilitate repair of demyelinating lesions by host oligodendrocytes in adult rat spinal cord. *Journal of Neurocytology*, **20**, 420–30.

29. Frith, J. A., McLeod, J. G., Basten, A., Pollard, J. D., Hammond, S. R., Williams, D. B. *et al.* (1986). Transfer factor as a therapy for multiple sclerosis: a follow-up study. *Clinical and Experimental Neurology*, **22**, 149–54.

30. Goodkin, D. E., Bailly, R., Teetzen, M., and Hertsgaard, D. (1990). Azathioprine in relapsing-remitting multiple sclerosis: 2 year follow-up results of a randomized double-masked placebo-controlled trial. *Neurology*, **40**(suppl. 1), 284.

31. Hafler, D. A., Cohen, I., Benjamin, D. S., and Weiner, H. L. (1992). T cell vaccination in multiple sclerosis: a preliminary report. *Clinical Immunology and Immunopathology*, **62**, 307–13.

32. Hanefeld, F., Bauer, H. J., Christen, H. J., Kruse, B., Bruhn, H., and Frahm, J. (1991). Multiple sclerosis in childhood: Report of 15 cases. *Brain Development*, **13**, 410–16.

33. Hansbrough, J. F., Piacentine, J. G., and Eiseman, B. (1990). Immunosuppresion by hyperbaric oxygen. *Surgery*, **87**, 662–7

34. Hardie, R. J. (1989). Principles of management of neurological disability. In *Neurology in clinical practice*, Vol. 1, (ed. W. G. Bradley,

R. B. Daroff, G. M. Fenichel, and C. D. Marsden), pp. 749–87. Butterworth-Heinemann, Boston.

35. Hoogstraten, M. C., van der Ploeg, R. J. O., Vreeling, A., van der Burg, W., van Marle, S., and Minderhoud, J. M. (1988). Tizanidine versus baclofen in the treatment of spasticity of multiple sclerosis patients. *Acta Neurologica Scandinavica*, **77**, 224–30.

36. Hughes, R. A. C. (1983). Immunological treatment of multiple sclerosis. *Journal of Neurology*, **230**, 73–80.

37. IFNB Multiple Sclerosis Study Group (1995). Interferon beta-1b in the treatment of MS: final outcome of the randomised, controlled trial. *Neurology*, **45**, 1277–85.

38. Jacobs, L., Salazar, A. M., Herndon, R., Reese, P. A., Freeman, A., Jozafowicz, R., *et al.* (1987). Intrathecally administered natural human fibroblast interferon reduces exacerbations of multiple sclerosis: results of a multi-centre double-blinded study. *Archives of Neurology*, **44**, 589–95.

39. Jacobs, L. D. (The Multiple Sclerosis Collaborative Research Group) (1996). Intramuscular Interferon beta-1a for disease progression in relapsing multiple sclerosis. *Annals of Neurology*, **39**, 285–94.

40. Johnson, K. P. (Copolymer 1 Multiple Sclerosis Study Group) (1995). Copolymer 1 reduces relapse rate and improves disability in relapsing-remitting multiple sclerosis: results of a phase III multicentre, double-blind, placebo-controlled trial. *Neurology*, **45**, 1268–76.

41. Jones, R. E., Heron, J. R., Foster, D. H., Snelgar, R. S., and Mason, R. J. (1983). Effects of 4-aminopyridine in patients with multiple sclerosis. *Journal of the Neurological Sciences*, **60**, 353–62.

42. Kappos, L., Gold, R., Künstler, E., Rohrbach, E., Heun, R., Städt, D. *et al.* (1990). Mitoxantrone (MX) in the treatment of rapidly progressive MS: a pilot study with serial gadolinium (Gd)-enhanced MRI. *Neurology*, **40**(suppl. 1), 261.

43. Kelly, R. E. and Gautier-Smith, P. C. (1959). Intrathecal phenol in the treatment of reflex spasms and spasticity. *Lancet*, **2**, 1102–5.

44. Kesselring, J. Miller, D. H., MacManus, D. G., Johnson, G., Milligan, N. M., Scolding, N. *et al.* (1989). Quantitative magnetic resonance imaging in multiple sclerosis: the effect of high dose intravenous methylprednisolone. *Journal of Neurology, Neurosurgery and Psychiatry*, **52**, 14–17.

45. Kindwall, E. P., McQuillen, M. P., Khatri, B. O., Gruchow, H. W., and Kindwall, M. L. (1991). Treatment of multiple sclerosis with hyperbaric oxygen. Results of a national registry. *Archives of Neurology*, **48**, 195–9.

46. Kinnunen, E., Juntunen, J., Ketonen, L., Koskimies, S., Konttinen, Y. T., Salmi, T. *et al.* (1988). Genetic susceptibility to multiple sclerosis: a co-twin study of a nation-wide series. *Archives of Neurology*, **45**, 1108–11.

47. Kleijnen, J. and Knipschild, P. (1995). Hyperbaric oxygen for multiple sclerosis: review of controlled trials. *Acta Neurologica Scandinavica*, **91**, 330–4.

48. Krapf, H., Mauch, E., Fetzer, U., Laufen, H., and Kornhuber, H. H. (1995). Serial Gadolinium-enhanced magnetic resonance imaging in patients with multiple sclerosis treated with mitoxantrone. *Neuroradiology*, **37**, 113–19.

49. Kuroda, H., Ogawa, N., Yamawaki, Y., Nukina, I., Ofuji, T., Yamamoto, M. *et al.* (1982). Cerebrospinal fluid GABA levels in various neurological and psychiatric diseases. *Journal of Neurology, Neurosurgery and Psychiatry*, **45**, 257–60.

50. Kuroiwa, Y., Igata, A., and Itahara, K. (1975). Nationwide survey of multiple sclerosis in Japan. Clinical analysis of 1084 cases. *Neurology*, **25**, 845–51.

51. Kurtzke, J. F. (1965). Further notes on disability evaluation in multiple sclerosis, with scale modifications. *Neurology*, **15**, 654–61.

52. Kurtzke, J. F. (1980). Geographic distribution of multiple sclerosis: an update with special reference to Europe and the Mediterranean region. *Acta Neurologica Scandinavica*, **62**, 65–80.

53. Kurtzke, J. F., Dean, G., and Botha, D. P. J. (1970). A method for estimating the age of immigration of white immigrants to South Africa with an example of MS importance. *South African Medical Journal*, **44**, 663–9.

54. Liversedge, L. A. (1975). In *Multiple sclerosis research*, (ed. A. N. Davison, J. H. Humphrey, L. A. Liversedge, W. I. McDonald, and J. S. Porterfield), pp. 236–7. HMSO, London.

55. Maida, E. and Summer, K. (1979). Serum cortisol levels of multiple sclerosis patients during ACTH treatment. *Journal of Neurology*, **229**, 143–8.

56. Matheson, N. (1974). Multiple sclerosis and diet. *Lancet*, **2**, 831.

57. Matthews, W. B. (1958). Tonic seizures in disseminated sclerosis. *Brain*, **81**, 193–206.

58. Mauch, E., Kornhuber, H. H., Pfrommer, U., Hähnel, A., Laufen, H., and Krapf, H. (1989). Effective treatment of chronically progressive multiple sclerosis with low dose cyclophosphamide with minor side effects. *European Archives of Psychiatry and the Neurological Sciences*, **238**, 115–17.

59. Mertin, J. (1980). Essential fatty acids and immunity. In *Progress in multiple sclerosis research* (ed. H. J. Bauer, S. Poser, and G. Ritter), pp. 436–41 Springer, Berlin.

60. Mertin, J., Rudge, P., Kremer, M., Healey, M. J. R., Knight, S. C., Compston, A. *et al.* (1982). Double-blind controlled trial of immunosuppression in the treatment of multiple sclerosis: Final report. *Lancet*, **2**, 351–4.

61. Michaelis, J. (1993). Mechanical methods of controlling ataxia. In *Clinical neurology: international practice and research*, Vol. 2, (ed. C. D. Ward) pp. 121–39. Baillière Tindell, London.

62. Miller, D. H., Ormerod, I. E. C., Rudge, P., Kendall, B. E., Moseley, I. F., and McDonald, W. I. (1989). The early risk of multiple sclerosis following isolated acute syndromes of the brain-stem and spinal cord. *Annals of Neurology*, **26**, 635–9.

63. Milanese, C., Salmaggi, A., La Mantia, L., Campi, A., Eoli, M., Savoiardo, M. *et al.* (1990). Double-blind study of intrathecal beta-interferon in multiple sclerosis: Clinical and laboratory results. *Journal of Neurology, Neurosurgery and Psychiatry*, **53**, 554–7.

64. Miller, D. H., Barkhof, F., Berry, I., Kappos, L., Scotti, G., and Thompson, A. J. (1991). Magnetic resonance imaging in monitoring the treatment of multiple sclerosis: concerted action guidelines. *Journal of Neurology, Neurosurgery and Psychiatry*, **54**, 683–8.

65. Miller, D. H., Hornabrook, R. W., and Purdie, G (1992), The natural history of multiple sclerosis: a regional study with some longitudinal data. *Journal of Neurology, Neurosurgery and Psychiatry*, **55**, 341–6.

66. Miller, D. H., Lai, H. M., Lewellyn-Smith, N., Cuzner, L., and McDonald, W. I. (1995). Phase 2 trial of anti-CD4 antibodies in the treatment of multiple sclerosis. *Journal of Neurology*, **242** (suppl. 2), S23.

67. Milligan, N. M., Newcombe, R., and Compston, D. A. S. (1987). A double-blind controlled trial of high dose methylprednisolone in patients with multiple sclerosis. 1. Clinical effects. *Journal of Neurology, Neurosurgery and Psychiatry*, **50**, 511–16.

68. Morrissey, S. P., Miller, D. H., Kendall, B. E., Kingsley, D. P. E., Kelly, M. A., Francis, D. A. *et al.* (1993). The significance of brain magnetic resonance imaging abnormalities at presentation with clinically isolated syndromes suggestive of multiple sclerosis. A 5-year follow-up study. *Brain*, **116**, 135–46.

69. Multiple Sclerosis Study Group (1990). Efficacy and toxicity of cyclosporine in chronic progressive multiple sclerosis: a ran-

domised, double-blind placebo-controlled clinical trial. *Annals of Neurology*, **27**, 591–605.

70. Mumford, C. J., Wood, N. W., Kellar-Wood, H., Thorpe, J. W., Miller, D. H., and Compston, D. A. S. (1994). The British Isles survey of multiple sclerosis in twins. *Neurology*, **44**, 11–15.

71. Northeast Co-operative Multiple Sclerosis Treatment Group (1990). IV cyclophosphamide/ACTH plus maintenance cyclophosphamide boosters in progressive MS: Interim report of the Northeast Co-operative MS Treatment Group *Neurology*, **40** (suppl. 1), 260.

72. Ochs, G., Struppler, A., Meyerson, B. A., Linderoth, B., Gybels, J., Gardner, B. P. *et al.* (1989). Intrathecal baclofen for long-term treatment of spasticity: a multi-centre study. *Journal of Neurology, Neurosurgery and Psychiatry*, **52**, 933–9.

73. Panitch, H. S., Hirsch, R. L., Schindler, J., and Johnson, K. P. (1987). Treatment of multiple sclerosis with gamma interferon—exacerbations associated with activation of the immune system. *Neurology*, **37**, 1097–102.

74. Penn, R. D. and Kroin, J. S. (1984). Intrathecal baclofen alleviates spinal cord spasticity. *Lancet*, **1**, 1078.

75. Poser, C. M., Paty, D. W., Scheinberg, L., McDonald, W. I., Davis, F. A., Ebers, G. C. *et al.* (1983). New diagnostic criteria for multiple sclerosis: guidelines for research protocols. *Annals of Neurology*, **13**, 227–31.

76. Reder, A. T. and Arnason, B. G. W. (1995). Trigeminal neuralgia relieved by a prostaglandin E analogue. *Neurology*, **45**, 1097–100.

77. Rose, A. S., Kuzma, J. W., Kurtzke, J. F., Namerow, N. S., Sibley, W. A., and Tourtellotte, W. W. (1970). Co-operative study in the evaluation of therapy in multiple sclerosis: ACTH vs placebo. Final report. *Neurology*, **20**, 1–59.

78. Rosenberg, G. A. and Appenzeller, O. (1988). Amantadine, fatigue and multiple sclerosis. *Archives of Neurology*, **45**, 1104–6.

79. Rudge, P., Koetsier, J. C., Mertin, J., Mispelblom Beyer, J. O., Van Walbeek, H. K., Clifford-Jones, R. *et al.* (1989). Randomised double-blind controlled trial of cyclophosphamide in multiple sclerosis. *Journal of Neurology, Neurosurgery and Psychiatry*, **52**, 559–65.

80. Sabra, A. F., Hallet, M., Sudarsky, L., and Mullally, W. (1982). Treatment of action tremor with isoniazid. *Neurology (NY)*, **32**, 912–13.

81. Sadovnick, A. D., Baird, P. A., and Ward, R. H. (1988). Multiple sclerosis: updated risks for relatives. *American Journal of Medical Genetics*, **29**, 533–41.

82. Sechi, G. P., Zuddas, M., Piredda, M., Agnetti, V., Sau, G., Piras, M. L. *et al.* (1989). Treatment of cerebellar tremors with carbamazepine: a controlled trial with long-term follow-up. *Neurology*, **39**, 1113–15.

83. Sorenson, P. S., Wanscher, B., Szpirt, W., Jensen, C. V., Ravnborg, M., Christianson, P. *et al.* (1995). A controlled trial of plasma exchange in multiple sclerosis using serial MRI and multimodal evoked potentials as efficacy parameters. *Journal of Neuroimmunology*, (suppl. 1), 74.

84. Spurkland, A., Ronningen, K. S., Vandvik, B., Thorsby, E., and Vartdal, F. (1991). HLA-DQA1 and HLA-DQB1 genes may jointly determine susceptibility to develop multiple sclerosis. *Human Immunology*, **30**, 69–75.

85. Steck, A. J., Regli, F., Ochsner, F., and Gauthier, G. (1990). Cyclosporine versus azathioprine in the treatment of multiple sclerosis: 12 month clinical and immunological evaluation. *European Neurology*, **30**, 224–8.

86. Stenager, E., Stenager, E. N., and Jensen, K. (1994). Effect of pregnancy on the prognosis for multiple sclerosis. A 5-year follow-up investigation. *Acta Neurologica Scandinavica*, **90**, 305–8.

87. Swinburn, W. R. and Liversedge, L. A. (1973). Azathioprine and multiple sclerosis. *Journal of Neurology, Neurosurgery and Psychiatry*, **36**, 16–9.

88. Thompson, A. J., Kermode, A. G., MacManus, D. G., Kendall, B. E., Kingsley, D. P., Moseley, I. F., *et al.* (1990). Patterns of disease activity in multiple sclerosis: Clinical and magnetic resonance imaging study. *British Medical Journal*, **300**, 631–4.

89. Van haver, H., Lissoir, F., Droissart, C., Ketelaer, P., Van Hees, J., Theys, P. *et al.* (1986). Transfer factor therapy in multiple sclerosis: a 3 year prospective double-blind clinical trial. *Neurology*, **36**, 1399–401.

90. Voiculescu, V., Pruskauer-Apostol, B., and Alecu, C. (1975). Treatment with acetazolamide of brain-stem and spinal paroxysmal disturbances in multiple sclerosis. *Journal of Neurology, Neurosurgery and Psychiatry*, **38**, 191–3.

91. Weiner, H. L., Dau, P. C., Khatri, B. O., Petajan, J. H., Birnbaum, G., McQuillen, M. P. *et al.* (1989). Double-blind study of true vs sham plasma exchange in patients treated with immunosuppression for acute attacks of multiple sclerosis. *Neurology*, **39**, 1143–9.

92. Weiner, H. L., Mackin, G. A., Matsui, M., Orav, E. J., Khoury, S. J., Dawson, D. M. *et al.* (1993a). Double-blind pilot trial of oral tolerization with myelin antigens in multiple sclerosis. *Science*, **259**, 1321–4.

93. Weiner, H. L., Mackin, G. A., Orav, E. J., Hafler, D. A., Dawson, D. M., La Pierre, Y. *et al.* (1993b). Intermittent cyclophosphamide pulse therapy in progressive multiple sclerosis: Final report of the Northeast Co-operative Multiple Sclerosis Treatment Group. *Neurology*, **43**, 910–18.

94. Weinshenker, B. G., Rice, G. P. A., Noseworthy, J., Carriere, W., Baskerville, J., and Ebers, G. C. (1991). The natural history of multiple sclerosis: a geographical based study: 3. Multivariate analysis of predictive factors and models of outcome. *Brain*, **114**, 1057–67.

95. Weinshenker, B. G., Penman, M., Bass, B., Ebers, G. C., and Rice, G. P. A. (1992). A double-blind randomised crossover trial of pemoline in fatigue associated with multiple sclerosis. *Neurology*, **42**, 1468–71.

96. Wiles, C. M., Omar, L., Swan, A. V., Sawle, G., Frankel, J., Grunewald, R. *et al.* (1994). Total lymphoid irradiation in multiple sclerosis. *Journal of Neurology, Neurosurgery and Psychiatry*, **57**, 154–63.

97. Willow, M., Gonoi, T., and Catterall, W. A. (1985). Voltage clamp analysis of the inhibitory actions of diphenylhydantoin and carbamazepine on voltage-sensitive sodium channels in neuroblastoma cells. *Molecular Pharmacology*, **27**, 549–58.

98. Yudkin, P. L., Ellison, G. W., Ghezzi, A., Goodkin, D. E., Hughes, R. A. C., McPherson, K. *et al.* (1991). Overview of azathioprine treatment in multiple sclerosis. *Lancet*, **338**, 1051–5.

99. Zamvil, S. S. and Steinman, L. (1990). The T lymphocyte in experimental allergic encephalomyelitis. *Annual Review of Immunology*, **8**, 579–621.

Disorders in which there is either an excess of involuntary movements (hyperkinesias) or a paucity of normal movements (hypokinesias) are among the most dramatic in neurology. The hypokinesias including Parkinson's disease are discussed elsewhere. Patients with involuntary movements have their distress particularly accentuated by the overt and immediately visible nature of their disorder. Quite apart from drug treatments, strategies, and support, either physical or psychological, that help patients cope with this distress are especially valuable in the management of involuntary movements. In this chapter I have deliberately underplayed the use of laboratory and radiological investigations. This is to emphasize the clinical features that allow rational classification of the hyperkinetic movement disorders. Judicious use of appropriate radiological magnetic resonance imaging techniques can be helpful in certain situations but in general, these are less useful in the clinical management of hyperkinetic movement disorders than in many other areas of neurological practice.

Hyperkinesias can be divided into: tremor, dystonia, chorea, athetosis, ballism, myoclonus, tics, stereotypies, and akathisia. These are considered below.

TREMOR

Although there are numerous causes of tremor, adult patients who present with tremor are most frequently worried about having Parkinson's disease. The characteristics of a tremor generally enable an accurate clinical diagnosis to be made and allow a rational attempt at treatment. Tremor can affect any part of the body but most frequently is seen in the limbs. It can be present at rest, with posture testing, or with action, or to varying degrees with all of these. It may be a fast tremor as in thyrotoxicosis or a slow one as in hepatic encephalopathy. Normal muscle physiology dictates that fast tremors are necessarily fine, low amplitude tremors and that slow ones are more likely be coarser ones. All tremor is exacerbated by stress, for instance, while waiting to see the doctor in the outpatient's clinic or attending a job interview. Most tremors disappear during sleep. Some of the commoner causes of tremor presenting in neurological practice are discussed below.

PHYSIOLOGICAL TREMOR

Using accelerometric techniques it can be seen that everyone has a low amplitude, high frequency tremor. This physiological tremor is usually unnoticeable in day-to-day life but in situations of stress, it can become unmasked and is sometimes labelled an 'exaggerated physiological tremor'. Anxiety is a strong precipitant of a fine and high frequency tremor not unlike thyrotoxic tremor. In its mildest form it affects the hands, but can be manifest in the trunk and lips and face. Anxiolytic strategies are often all that is required in this situation. Occasionally, the source of anxiety is a self-limiting one such as an impending examination or a job interview. Sometimes anxiety starts off in relation to a single impending event but the superimposed anxiety about the cause of the tremor then perpetuates the shakiness. Relaxation exercises and other stress management strategies can help. Anxiolytic medication may also help but, particularly when benzodiazepines are used, the duration of pharmacological treatment needs to be regulated and kept brief. Beta adrenoceptor blocking agents can relieve the distress of and the intensity of physiological tremor. Alcohol too can alleviate this discomfort—a point of importance in the assessment of possible essential tremor—but usually not to the degree with which essential tremor is sometimes alleviated. Physiological tremor is probably under hormonal control as shown by its exacerbation during pregnancy. The relationship of this tremor to anxiety, fear and anger and its response to treatment with beta-blockers indicates a catecholaminergic mechanism in its causation. This is further supported by similarities between this tremor and that caused by beta agonist drugs such as salbutamol, used, for instance, in asthma treatment. An obvious but sometimes perilously overlooked point is the need to avoid using beta-blocking agents in treating salbutamol-induced tremor, as this is very likely to exacerbate the asthma. Xanthines, such as in tea and coffee, or in bronchodilators, such as theophylline, also exaggerate this tremor. These are important considerations in advising non-pharmacological strategies for improvement in various tremors. Hypoglycaemia is another cause of an exaggerated physiological tremor. This is usually seen in patients with diabetes treated with oral hypoglycaemic drugs or with insulin, although it can also occur in the rare but important condition, insulinoma.

THYROTOXIC TREMOR

Excess of thyroxine action causes a tremor similar to physiological tremor. Its prompt recognition is frequently what leads to a diagnosis of previously unrecognized thyrotoxicosis—a potentially hazardous condition to leave untreated. Treatment of the thyrotoxic state cures the tremor, and temporary respite can be obtained by using beta-blockers while definitive treatment is awaited. Sometimes, this is seen in patients receiving thyroxine as replacement therapy for hypothyroidism. The tremor in this situation should lead to a review of the dose of thyroxine as it may be too high or the patient may be taking more than the prescribed dose.

ESSENTIAL TREMOR

This is characterized by a tremor that is either absent or is considerably subdued at rest, is severe on posture testing (e.g. with the arms outstretched) and although present on intention or action testing (e.g. finger nose test) is less marked with posture than with action testing. The tremor persists throughout the range of movement without the terminal exacerbation seen in cerebellar tremors. It commonly affects the arms and the head (so called 'no-no' or 'yes-yes' tremors). It is uncommon for the tremor to affect the trunk or lower limbs with any severity but occasionally a postural trunk and leg tremor is precipitated by standing up—so-called orthostatic tremor. When it affects the hands, the movements are usually a flexion–extension of the fingers or adduction–abduction but not usually a pronation–supination movement as is the case in a parkinsonian tremor. Also, unlike parkinsonian tremor, essential tremor (ET) is bilateral and fairly symmetrical in the majority of cases. The task-specific, primary writing tremor also has some features in common with essential tremor and others linking it to writer's cramp. These similarities have led to the search for a common causative gene for both ET and dystonia. ET is not linked to the DYT1 mutation seen in idiopathic torsion dystonia. Often there is a family history (in about 50%) and the same tremor may be called 'benign familial tremor'. Sometimes, there is a history of a dramatic response to alcohol, exemplified by the patient who says that the first pint of beer shakes all over the place but the second goes down smoothly! This tremor is seen at all ages including rarely in paediatric practice. When seen in the elderly it is sadly still sometimes labelled a 'senile tremor'. Although labelled 'benign' this condition can be incapacitating owing to the exacerbation of the tremor during voluntary movement.

Beta adrenoceptor blockers have a more marked beneficial effect on ET than on physiological tremor. Doses of propranolol as high as 320 mg per day have been used and frequently 120–160 mg per day is tried. In my experience, lower doses are often just as effective with some patients showing satisfactory response at 20–40 mg per day. The response, however, is rarely complete and marked improvement is only seen in about half the patients. When propranolol has failed to give adequate relief or when its use is contraindicated, for instance, by cardiac or respiratory considerations, primidone can be effective in this disorder but some patients show a marked sensitivity to the sedative effects of primidone. Doses of 50–100 mg of primidone per day (as the syrup) may alleviate the tremor. Combinations of propranolol and primidone have also been used with a suggestion of an additive beneficial effect. Benzodiazepines and barbiturates can alleviate the distress caused by ET, sometimes by attenuating the tremor and occasionally by blocking the psychological consequences of having an embarrassing tremor. The benzodiazepine, clonazepam, is the drug of choice for the rare condition of orthostatic tremor. There are some reports of benefit from amantadine in ET. Drug treatment of essential tremor works best on postural arm tremor with head tremors being more resistant to therapy. Local injections of botulinum toxin have been used in ET; and as one would expect there is an increase in weakness of the injected muscles with a corresponding decrease in tremor severity. Recently, a number of investigations have been carried out looking at the response of ET to carbonic anhydrase inhibitors and to the anticonvulsant, gabapentin. No conclusions can yet be drawn on the effectiveness of these therapies. For severe, drug-unresponsive ET, contralateral ventrolateral thalamotomy is sometimes helpful, but as with all surgical procedures its safety and efficacy are closely linked with the surgeon's experience. There is a real risk of speech defect arising as a result of such stereotactic procedures and in a minority of those undergoing bilateral operations there may be total anarthria. Thalamic electrode implantation with variable frequency thalamic stimulation have also been reported helpful in essential tremor and although this procedure has the advantage of not making a deliberate lesion in the thalamus it has the disadvantage of predisposing to cerebral infection by virtue of a foreign body implanted into the brain. This procedure, like thalamotomy, is clearly best reserved for patients with severe, drug-unresponsive, incapacitating tremor.

PARKINSONIAN TREMOR

The typical tremor of Parkinson's disease (PD) is an asymmetric rest tremor of the arms, most severe in a hand, attenuated by posture testing or by action. When the thumb and first finger are affected a 'pill-rolling' label is applied. Some patients develop an additional action tremor, resulting in debates about whether this is a feature of the PD or whether it represents coexistent essential tremor. The occurrence of other cardinal features of PD (discussed elsewhere) fortunately makes the diagnosis of PD relatively easy even in cases where the tremor is atypical but in cases where there is no akinesia or rigidity at presentation, prolonged follow-up may prove the only practical and widely available means of determining whether an individual has PD or essential tremor. In common with other tremors, patients with PD develop ways of disguising their involuntary movements, for instance, by sitting on their hands to hide a rest tremor or by keeping their hands in their pockets or hidden behind a handbag. The tremor of PD occasionally shows a very good response to treatment with levodopa but usually the response is much less impressive than that for the bradykinetic and rigidity related symptoms. In patients who have sufficient symptoms arising from bradykinesia and rigidity to warrant treatment with levodopa it makes good sense to check whether the tremor also responds to levodopa before contemplating further therapy. When levodopa therapy is not indicated and when the tremor shows a marked situational exacerbation, a lipid-soluble beta-blocker such as propranolol may be helpful. The anxiolytic effect of beta-blockade may also improve the patient's feeling of well-being. In some patients with tremor that is unresponsive to levodopa but other symptoms that require levodopa, combinations of levodopa with either propranolol or an anticholinergic drug, such as benzhexol, procyclidine, or orphenadrine, may be needed. In addition to the usual precautions in using beta blockers it is important to remember that patients with PD may experience nocturnal hallucinations and vivid dreams, both of which are exacerbated by propranolol, especially when taken late in the day. I advise either a long-acting preparation as a single daily dose in the morning or a low dose twice-daily regime with the second dose taken no later than 2 p.m. Anticholinergic drugs can ameliorate PD tremor but their other effects such as on accommodation or sphincter function, or on memory and cognitive function limit their usefulness. Depression is common in PD. Some of the newer antidepressant drugs can either worsen PD or can interact with other anti-PD drugs (e.g. fluoxetine and selegiline). I therefore still use the older tricyclic antidepressant drugs such as imipramine, amitriptyline, or dothiepin. The anticholinergic side-effects of these can be put to good use to try to help PD tremor and the excessive salivation that is sometimes so troublesome in PD. Drug-resistant PD tremors can be treated surgically. In experienced hands the risks of procedures such as thalamotomy, pallidotomy, and subthalamic stimulation are low and beneficial results reported. Thalamotomy and thalamic stimulation have both been reported to alleviate PD tremor but are not free of risk as discussed in the section on essential tremor.

Tremor is seen less commonly in the parkinsonism induced by phenothiazines and other dopamine receptor blocking agents. When it occurs, it is usually more symmetrical than in PD but it may be indistinguishable from that of PD. It can respond dramatically to treatment with anticholinergics but on occasion the parkinsonism induced by these drugs may take over a year to resolve. It is tragic that this avoidable form of parkinsonism still occurs, frequently in patients receiving phenothiazines or butyrophenones for dubious indications or for inappropriate duration, and that it often escapes early recognition resulting in considerable disability. Such drug-induced parkinsonism, which is at least as common as idiopathic PD can also sometimes respond to levodopa but, as in PD, levodopa is only worth trying in cases where there is associated bradykinesia and rigidity.

ESSENTIAL TREMOR OR BENIGN TREMULOUS PARKINSON'S DISEASE?

In the early stages of PD it can be difficult to distinguish between essential tremor and PD tremor; this is particularly so if bradykinesia and rigidity are absent. Usually, follow-up over a year or two will clarify whether there is progressive neurological disability as in PD or whether the tremor remains the only substantial source of disability as in essential tremor. In a few cases, however, the patient remains tremulous without developing any of the other features of PD for several years. This tremor has all the characteristics of PD tremor and unlike a typical essential tremor, may be unilateral. There may be an associated action component. The condition is often termed 'benign tremulous Parkinsonism'. It may be difficult to distinguish between this disorder and so-called rubral tremors, believed to arise from defects in the dentato–rubro–thalamic pathway. Unlike rubral tremor which is often unilateral, essential tremor is usually bilateral. The response to levodopa, propranolol, or anticholinergic drugs in these disorders is variable, suggesting the possibility that this symptom collection may represent more than one disease. Rubral-type tremors have been linked with trauma. The injury can be either peripheral or central. For instance, there is a growing literature on the occurrence of tremor in a limb that has been injured, even in the absence of any obvious deafferentation. Similarly, closed head injury, including injuries that are regarded as mild have been linked with tremor. Such tremors pose not only a diagnostic and management challenge but a legal one as well, as there is frequently some litigation pending with the inevitable issue of whether the tremor is an organic one or a functional disturbance.

The issue of whether essential tremor occurs more frequently in individuals who suffer from PD and vice versa remains undecided but the lack of features of PD on autopsy in eight patients with ET suggests that if there is an increased risk of co-occurrence of PD and ET, that risk is not enormous.

CEREBELLAR TREMOR

Unlike PD and essential tremor, the tremor of cerebellar disease is not present at rest and is only mildly present on posture testing with marked exaggeration on action testing such as with the finger–nose or heel–shin tests. Its increase with action makes it disabling. Typically, there is a terminal exacerbation so that a hand may be relatively steady in its approach to a plateful of food but as it nears the food the amplitude of the tremor increases. Excluding drug intoxication, system degenerations such as the spinocerebellar syndromes, and inflammatory disturbances such as multiple sclerosis are the most commonly seen causes of severe, unremitting, and protracted cerebellar tremor. When cerebellar tremor is severe and possibly only when the adjacent brainstem is affected as well there is a rest component to the tremor. Tremulous movements also affect the articulation apparatus causing dysarthria. Propranolol sometimes lessens the tremor but not usually enough to make a difference to limb function. Isoniazid in high doses (up to 10 mg per kg of body weight) has also been shown to decrease tremor amplitude but again it only helps a small minority to a degree where they are able to feed, wash, or dress themselves. High dose isoniazid causes a number of side-effects including the potential for causing severe irreversible hepatic failure and must therefore be used with caution. Other techniques such as mechanical devices designed to decrease the amplitude of oscillations (both of the hand and of the head) may restore sufficient hand-mouth coordination to allow self-feeding. When the cause of the cerebellar disturbance is treatable, this offers the best prospect of relief from the cerebellar tremor. For instance, treatment of unrecognized hypothyroidism can eliminate cerebellar tremor in some patients. Chronic ingestion of certain drugs including the anticonvulsant, phenytoin, can cause a severe cerebellar syndrome, which can sometimes persist despite withdrawal of the drug.

NEUROPATHIC TREMOR

In some of the inherited neuropathies of the Charcot–Marie–Tooth type there is probably co-inheritance of essential tremor rather than occurrence of tremor as a consequence of deafferentation. In other neuropathies, the latter situation applies with a coarse and irregular tremor of variable frequency arising from the effects on sensory fibres of the neuropathy. Patients with paraproteinaemic polyneuropathies can also rarely present with a tremor that has features similar to those of a cerebellar tremor. The management of these tremors is essentially the treatment of the underlying neuropathy or its cause.

HYSTERICAL TREMOR

As a rule, most movement disorders are physical conditions rather than functional, non-organic ones. The finding of a peculiar tremor which is beyond one's normal experience is not, in itself sufficient to make a diagnosis of a hysterical tremor. A particular difficulty in evaluation of hysterical tremors is the question of definition. There is no gold standard so that an empirical attempt must be made at definition with the hope that patients defined in this way will be successfully treated with psychotherapy or pharmacotherapy including possibly using placebo treatments. In many areas of medicine it is no longer considered important to make a distinction between physical and psychological disorders; the emphasis being on symptom treatment if an underlying aetiology is not readily apparent. However, in the assessment of tremor there is merit in deciding whether a tremor is a hysterical one, as this avoids the use of potentially toxic agents or other potentially hazardous interventions, such as the ones discussed above. Features that help in diagnosing a tremor as being a hysterical conversion symptom include variability in time, frequency, and amplitude including distractibility, spontaneous remissions and, importantly, features that do not fit into recognized, alternative physical disorder. Hysterical tremors fatigue more often. Some patients with hysterical tremor may have other hysterical conversion symptoms such as hemiparesis or sensory deficit. In addition to these features that suggest the absence of physical disease it is helpful to have positive evidence of psychiatric disease (e.g. a previous history of hysterical conversion symptoms or of other psychiatric disease associated with hysteria, such as deliberate self-harm). Looking for personal secondary gain arising from the conversion symptom is generally unhelpful unless there is an obvious gain such as pending litigation or an insurance claim. Entrainment of a hysterical tremor may be another useful sign (i.e. speeding up of a tremor with increased frequency of voluntary repetitive action).

Treatment of hysterical tremors is not an easy task. Confrontation of the patient with the diagnosis is even less helpful in hysteria than it is in frank malingering. If a physical cause has not been found for the tremor it is advisable to avoid medications that are effective in physical disorders. In some cases, hysterical tremors may respond to supportive psychotherapy but the number of such cases is not large. Other non-pharmacological interventions such as behavioural psychotherapy, physiotherapy, hypnosis, and acupuncture have been successful in anecdotal cases but the majority fail to respond to these as well. Placebo treatments have been used with successful outcome in some patients but the ethics of using a treatment that may amount to deception are questionable. Any treatment that works in alleviating this hysterical symptom must allow the patient a face-saving and 'respectable' way out of a complex situation that he/she has got into. Attempting to abreact the patient with methohexitone will sometimes reveal an underlying psychological conflict that requires addressing and, more importantly, in the recovery phase from the barbiturate the patient may note that the tremor is better/gone and this may make the foundation for recovery. As with other patients with hysteria, it is almost inevitable that the patient will develop other hysterical symptoms in the future—cure is rare.

TASK-SPECIFIC TREMORS

Any skilled manual task can be associated with a specific tremor but in practice the one complained of most often is that which occurs while writing. This is termed 'primary writing tremor' (PWT). PWT has similarities with both essential tremor and the task-specific focal dystonia, writer's cramp. In many cases of writer's cramp there are tremulous movements as indeed there are in many of the dystonias. This has suggested that PWT is no different to writer's cramp except in the prominence of the tremor in relation to the dystonia. The debate is unresolved. Some authors have reported success with treatment with propranolol whereas others have treated this condition as a dystonia with anticholinergic drugs with some success. Propranolol seems to result in short-lived improvement (months) of the tremor without sustained long-term improvement. Contralateral ventralis intermedius thalamotomy is reported to be effective in PWT.

WILSON S DISEASE TREMOR

Wilson's disease (WD) is an autosomal recessively inherited defect of copper metabolism, characterized by increases in tissue copper concentrations and a decrease in the rate of incorporation of copper into cuproproteins such as caeruloplasmin and superoxide dismutase. The gene for WD codes for a copper-binding ATPase and is located on chromosome 13. A search for flanking linked markers can help identify presymptomatic individuals in a family known to have WD—particularly useful only in those individuals with equivocal blood and urine copper studies. Although WD has been reported to express first symptoms at age 50 in rare cases, the vast majority of patients are under 30 years old and frequently under 15 years old. Before adolescence, the presentation is nearly always non-neurological, with hepatic or haematological difficulties. In WD with neurological symptoms and signs, Kayser–Fleischer rings can be found in the eyes using slit lamp examination. When this examination is performed by an experienced ophthalmologist, KF rings are found in nearly all cases of neurological WD.

The tremor of WD can mimic most tremors but classically is a flapping one usually termed a 'bat's wing tremor'. A rough rule that can be applied to young patients with a tremor is that the occurrence of two or more movement disorders in one individual should activate a search for WD. Thus, a patient in his/her teens presenting with akinesia and a tremor should be regarded as having WD unless this is excluded by appropriate copper studies and slit lamp examination. A low threshold to considering the possibility of WD needs to be maintained. Other clues to the diagnosis can include psychiatric symptoms with the movement disorder preceding any antipsychotic medication, unexplained episodes of haemolytic anaemia, renal tubular damage, and most significantly, hepatic dysfunction in a patient before any medication. Serum copper and serum caeruloplasmin are good initial screening tests for WD. A low serum caeruloplasmin in an individual with a movement disorder is suggestive of WD but a normal serum copper or caeruloplasmin does not exclude the disease. Caeruloplasmin is an acute phase protein which is also under hormonal control, so that its concentrations increase with acute bacterial infections and may also rise with viral illness— these rises can bring the caeruloplasmin concentration into the normal range. Women have higher caeruloplasmin concentrations and these are further increased by the oral contraceptive pill. Twenty-four-hour urinary copper excretion measurement can be a useful adjunct to the diagnosis provided care is taken to avoid cross-contamination of the urine bottle with extraneous copper.

Treatment

The tremor and many of the other neurological manifestations of WD can be successfully treated by copper chelation therapy provided treatment is instituted early. In some instances, patients can be rendered asymptomatic. Early recognition and prompt treatment are essential. *d*-Penicillamine remains the mainstay of copper chelation therapy in WD, although its position is being challenged strongly by zinc. *d*-Penicillamine mobilizes stored copper from liver and other tissues and the penicillamine–copper ligates are excreted in the urine. The rate of copper excretion depends on the total body copper load, the dose of penicillamine used, the extent of renal impairment, and possibly the biochemical form in which the copper is stored. There is a well-described syndrome of exacerbation of WD following commencement of penicillamine therapy that may result from a shift in copper ions between different intracellular, intercellular, or intertissue compartments. Anecdotal reports indicate that this exacerbation can be avoided by slow introduction of the chelating agent and by regulation of the rate of excretion of copper. My practice is to aim at a four- to fivefold increase compared with the basal rate of copper excretion. The normal 24-h urine copper excretion is less than 1.5 micromoles or approximately 100 microgrammes. In WD, the basal excretion is increased and following start of penicillamine can increase to several milligrams per day. The dose of penicillamine is gradually increased to maintain a cupriuresis—sometimes requiring doses of 2 grams per day or more. Penicillamine causes significant side-effects in a number of patients. They include pyrexia, rashes, a systemic lupus erythematosus-like condition, and haematologic abnormalities, most notably, thrombocytopenia. A clinical response is seen in two to three weeks, with the first effect sometimes a worsening in neurological symptoms and signs. Tremor and the dystonia of WD frequently improve quickly but psychiatric disorders may take longer. Even prolonged and severe disability can improve dramatically with treatment. Treatment with penicillamine needs to be lifelong as patients who have discontinued therapy in a stable state are reported to have a very high rate of early relapse with severe and often irreversible liver failure. Penicillamine is best given in three or four divided doses with an inevitable effect on compliance. Constant education of the patient is required to ensure that the drug is not stopped. Metal chelates excreted via the kidney can result in renal tubular damage and cause proteinuria and a tubular acidosis. This should be avoidable with slow introduction of the drug and with vigilant monitoring of the urine for proteinuria. Patients on penicillamine also need to have their blood white cell counts and platelet counts monitored. Monitoring the platelet count is particularly important in those patients who already have a thrombocytopenia secondary to hypersplenism. In the maintenance phase of penicillamine therapy (i.e. after initial decoppering) I start patients on pyridoxine supplements as well, to avoid neurological complications arising from deficiency of this vitamin. I avoid using it in the initial phases in patients with a reasonable dietary intake, in the belief that compliance with one drug is easier to ensure than with two and clearly the penicillamine is the more important one.

Patients who cannot tolerate penicillamine or who fail to respond satisfactorily to this drug require other or adjunctive treatment. There are reports of the successful use of zinc salts as adequate therapy for decoppering in WD with claims that zinc may be as effective as penicillamine. Zinc appears to work via reduction in the absorption of copper from the gut by increasing the production of a copper-binding metallothionein. Zinc is certainly useful adjunct to penicillamine where the chelator has failed as single agent therapy. The toxicity of zinc salts is low and this increases their attractiveness as treatment in WD; there are, for instance, suggestions that zinc therapy may be safer in pregnancy than penicillamine therapy. Trientine (triethylene tetramine dihydrochloride) at a dose of 750–2000 mg per day in divided doses is another metal chelating agent that is reportedly effective in WD. Its use is best reserved for those patients failing to respond to the above measures or more importantly, those unable to tolerate the other drugs. Older chelators such as British antiLewisite (BAL) are outdated and their use is hardly ever necessary in WD. Sodium dimercaptopropane sulphonate has been successfully used in resistant cases. There is renewed interest in an old chelator, ammonium tetrathiomolybdate, which has the potential for decreasing the absorption of copper from the gastrointestinal tract and also for binding to low molecular weight copper ion complexes in plasma and removing them from the toxic copper pool. Although this drug has been reported beneficial in a small number of patients with no major adverse effects, it still remains an investigationed drug but nevertheless a promising agent. As a temporary measure, albumin infusions and plasma exchange have been used to reduce the toxic copper pool while waiting for more definitive decoppering therapy to work. This is only needed in the rarely seen patient with severe, fulminant neurological disease who cannot wait 2–4 months for the effects of penicillamine. Haemodialysis should not be used as this has been associated with death probably via increases in the free-copper pool in plasma. Liver transplantation is reserved for the Wilson's disease patient with liver failure. The wisdom of using it in severe, unresponsive neurological Wilson's disease without major liver malfunction is questionable.

Whatever decoppering treatment is used in WD there is need for reduction in the amount of copper ingested. A low copper diet should be instituted. In practice, this limits the amount of liver, nuts, seafood, and lentils eaten but does not make the diet too restrictive.

During treatment, monitoring of and encouraging good compliance are vital. Intermittent checking by measurement of urinary copper excretion rates helps in this regard; for instance, a sudden increase in the urine copper may indicate intermittent use of penicillamine. Measurement of tissue copper concentrations is particularly important in ensuring continued adequate decoppering. This effectively means measurement of liver copper concentrations by liver biopsy. On arbitrary grounds, my practice is to recommend liver biopsy for this purpose every two to five years, depending on the clinical state, the likelihood of compliance and the ease with which the clinical features responded to initial decoppering treatment.

DYSTONIA

Dystonia is a sustained abnormal involuntary posturing of any part of the body. It may be generalized or focal and may be either idiopathic or symptomatic. Childhood onset dystonia often progresses to become generalized, whereas adult onset symptoms usually remain confined to the area where they first manifest themselves. The most common focal dystonias include blepharospasm, writer's cramp, oromandibular dystonia, spasmodic dysphonia, and spasmodic torticollis. The abnormal posturing may be accompanied by rapid movements variably regarded as either a tremor, as in writer's cramp, or as myoclonic as in some of the jerky dystonias. The dystonia can be present either at rest or with action or both. In the early stages of idiopathic torsion dystonia, where typically, onset is in one lower limb in a child, the dystonia is present only on action. In contrast, dystonia as a feature of inherited metabolic disease or structural brain injury is typically present at rest. Tremor is a frequent accompaniment of dystonia. Sometimes, the tremor is coarse and irregular, leading to the description of jerky dystonia. In rare familial cases, usually in the first two decades of life, the dystonia may be combined with rapid, lightning-like movements. These families have usually worked out for themselves that the involuntary movements respond to treatment with alcohol! This condition is termed 'myoclonic dystonia'. In recent years, the development of botulinum toxin as a treatment for movement disorders and clearer definition of its clinical indications has made a major difference to the treatment of dystonia.

IDOPATHIC TORSION DYSTONIA

Diagnosis of this condition requires a high index of suspicion. Its clinical manifestations can be very diverse making the diagnosis difficult especially in the early stages. Typically, the childhood and adolescent forms begin with leg dystonia and frequently spread to a more generalized state. Adult-onset idiopathic torsion dystonia (ITD) is often focal at onset and remains so after several years of follow-up. It is possible that as our diagnostic techniques improve, many focal and task-specific dystonias currently classified as ITD may require reclassification to other disorders.

ITD is an autosomal dominant condition with variable penetrance (overall penetrance estimated at 30%). The gene for this disorder has been localized to chromosome 9 (9q34) and has been called the DYT1 gene. ITD in Ashkenazi jews, previously regarded as autosomal recessive is now believed to also be a dominant condition with relatively low penetrance being responsible for the apparent generation skipping found in some families. Another, genetically distinct familial form of torsion dystonia, Segawa disease, is a condition characterized by diurnal fluctuation and marked levodopa responsiveness. It was predicted from the sustained good response to treatment with levodopa that the gene defect lay in the dopamine synthesis pathway proximal to dopa decarboxylation. This proved to be correct and the genetic defect in this disorder has recently been identified as an abnormality of GTP cyclohydrolase 1. This enzyme is involved in the production of tetrahydrobiopterin, a cofactor necessary for tyrosine hydroxylation, the rate limiting step in dopamine biosynthesis. In one sibship, dopa-responsive dystonia was reported to be caused by an inherited defect in tyrosine hydroxylase. This defect is not found in the majority of patients with Segawa disease. It is now known that whereas marked diurnal fluctuation appears to predict dopa responsiveness there are well-documented cases of dopa responsiveness in patients with little or no diurnal variation in symptoms. This has lowered the threshold for attempting treatment of dystonias with levodopa. Another genetically distinct syndrome comprising dystonia and parkinsonism has been described in the Philippines (Lubag). This is an X-linked condition. Diagnosis of ITD is currently dependent on detection of clinical dystonia in an affected individual, there being no laboratory or genetic test currently available. As in other inherited neurological conditions it is important to offer the patient access to an established neurogenetic counselling service. For ITD, the risk of a sibling or child being affected, when there are at least two affected family members one of whom has the generalized type, is estimated at 20%.

Mild action dystonia in its early stages may not require pharmacotherapy. At this stage, physiotherapy may help by teaching the patient simple tricks that result in changes in posture. Some patients learn techniques to disguise their involuntary movements. For instance, a patient with spasmodic torticollis may use a *geste antagonistique* to keep his head from turning and a patient with writer's cramp may hold the pen differently to avoid dystonia. When pharmacotherapy becomes necessary, focal dystonias can often be adequately treated with botulinum toxin injections (e.g. as in blepharospasm, torticollis, and to a degree in writer's cramp). In generalized dystonia, however, botulinum toxin has little to offer except where one part of the body is very severely affected with other areas only mildly affected. In generalized dystonia a trial of treatment with levodopa should be attempted. Gradually increasing doses of levodopa as sinemet or madopar are given up to the equivalent of sinemet-275 four times a day. In cases that show a response to levodopa but are unable to tolerate the drug owing to adverse effects, other dopaminergic drugs, such as bromocriptine, may be helpful. Many of the adverse effects of levodopa are dopaminergic effects and are therefore similar to those of bromocriptine and the other dopamine agonists. I have successfully used a test of

subcutaneous apomorphine injection to predict levodopa responsiveness in dystonia—a situation analogous to apomorphine tests in Parkinson's disease. When there is no response to levodopa, benzhexol is the drug of choice. Often, high doses are required to see useful improvement which is seen in about half of all patients—more often in children than in adults. I have used doses of up to 80 mg per day and others have reported a requirement for doses as high as 160 mg per day. These high doses are better tolerated by children than by adults and side-effects are decreased by gradual dose escalation. Peripherally acting anticholinesterases, such as pyridostigmine, may be required in a small number of patients to counteract anticholinergic side-effects (blurred vision, dry mouth, constipation, and bladder disturbance) that may occur at high doses of benzhexol or related drugs. Between a third and a half of all patients fail to get satisfactory relief from either levodopa or benzhexol. These patients may show response to baclofen, benzodiazepines, such as clonazepam, or to carbamazepine. Occasionally, patients with refractory dystonia show response to dopamine-depleting agents, such as reserpine or tetrabenazine, or to dopamine receptor blocking agents, such as sulpiride. The use of neuroleptic medications has to take careful account of their risks including that of inducing tardive dyskinesias to add to the patient's dystonia. Some patients who fail to respond to medication as single agents may show a fair response to combinations, for instance, of baclofen and benzhexol. When these medical measures have failed, stereotactic thalamic surgery can afford relief but with a significant risk of increasing the overall disability. In addition to drug treatment a rehabilitation-type approach may enhance the patient's quality of life. This can vary from, for example, advice on obtaining a disabled person's car parking permit to providing total 'environment control systems'. School-going children require adequate explanation of their condition to their teachers; firstly to emphasize that the disorder is a physical one and not just the child 'playing up' and secondly to allow the disability to be taken into account in assessing the child's educational needs (e.g. provision of extra time in examinations for a child with writer's cramp).

As emphasized elsewhere, there is a need for giving the patient and their families/carers appropriate information promptly but in fractionated doses so that they are not overwhelmed by too much too soon. The role of a trained (nurse) counsellor in aiding this process can be invaluable as seen in other neurological disorders. Patient support organizations also play a useful role by providing information to patients on specific disability needs and by educating health care personnel in the management of this disorder that may be reasonably common in neurological practice but is rarely seen by general practitioners or by non-neurological specialists.

SYMPTOMATIC DYSTONIA

This is seen more often than idiopathic dystonia. The most common causes are drug-induced acute dystonic reactions, tardive dystonia, and levodopa-induced dystonia in Parkinson's disease. Dystonia as a feature of metabolic disease is relatively rare but as some of these conditions are effectively treatable if recognized early (such as Wilson's disease), their prompt identification cannot be emphasized strongly enough. Some of the other metabolic conditions that cause dystonia (e.g. glutaric aciduria) are even less common. Their investigation requires the support of a specialist laboratory dealing with inherited metabolic disorders. However, further discussion of the investigation of and management of the rare metabolic causes of dystonia is beyond the scope of this chapter. Dystonia can be a presentation of a hysterical disorder. Usually other non-dystonic symptoms are also present and these may guide the diagnosis of hysteria but sometimes no other helpful clinical features are found, making the distinction between organic and hysteric dystonia difficult. It should be emphasized here (as above in the section on hysterical tremor) that more patients with organic dystonia have been harmed by being labelled as having a hysterical disorder than vice versa.

Phenothiazines, butyrophenones, and metoclopramide can cause an acute dystonic reaction minutes to hours after ingestion of the drug. The dystonia typically affects the head and neck and results in an oculogyric crisis. In neurological practice, dystonia is seen most commonly in association with parkinsonism usually in the setting of dopa-induced dystonia after a period of drug treatment of idiopathic PD, but in some cases as a feature of the PD (e.g. early morning foot dystonia), and in rare cases as a part of uncommon parkinsonian syndromes such as juvenile PD, Lubag, etc. Dopa dyskinesias including dystonia, their relation to timing of dopa doses and their treatment are discussed elsewhere in this book. Tardive dystonia (TD) is defined as dystonia caused by three months or longer treatment with a neuroleptic drug. Retrocollis and torticollis are common in TD, as are orofacial dyskinetic movements frequently involving the tongue. Other choreiform movements of the type seen in other tardive dyskinesias are also common in dystonia-prevalent tardive syndromes (i.e. the conditions often overlap). Similar movement disorder are sometimes seen after shorter exposure (of only a few days) and a semantic debate continues over whether this can also be labelled tardive: 10–20% of neuroleptic-exposed patients develop this. It is seen more often in the elderly (40%) and especially in post-menopausal women who are less likely to remit spontaneously. The risk of tardive dyskinesia and dystonia is increased in diabetics. It is unclear whether this results from diabetic microangiopathy. Only about 30% remit completely. It frequently coexists with drug-induced parkinsonism. The severity of TD does not correlate with duration of neuroleptic exposure. There are some reports of TD-like movement disorder occurring in schizophrenic patients prior to treatment with neuroleptic medication suggesting that these patients have a particular predisposition to these involuntary movements; a predisposition that becomes unmasked by neuroleptics. On some occasions TD can develop after withdrawal of the offending drug. This usually occurs within six weeks of drug withdrawal.

Treatment

Management of TD and of other tardive disorders has got to start with adequate counselling of patients about to start protracted phenothiazine or butyrophenone medication. It is tragic enough when TD develops as a complication of the necessary use of neuroleptics for the treatment of major psychosis, but the avoidable occurrence of these side-effects in patients given these drugs for dubious indications or for inappropriate duration is a cause for greater lament. It is worth thinking whether using prochlorperazine for six months to treat mild non-specific dizziness is justified in view of the risk of extrapyramidal reactions, some of which may not resolve even with subsequent drug withdrawal. Phenothiazines should never be used as hypnotic agents, their use in treating vertigo should be restricted to short duration of no more than a few weeks and combination therapies, such as mixed preparations containing an antidepressant and a phenothiazine, should be avoided. Newer antipsychotic agents are being developed with lower risks of all tardive dyskinesias but many have other limitations to their use. Clozapine is one such drug which can cause agranulocytosis and therefore requires close haematological monitoring during use. The treatment of TD and other tardive problems with neuroleptic withdrawal has to recognize the observation that 50% of patients with schizophrenia (a major indication for long-term neuroleptic use) relapse within one year of stopping neuroleptics when the patient has had at least two psychotic episodes.

Considerable morbidity, both physical and psychological, arises from tardive movement disorders. In some cases the morbidity is severe enough to result in suicide. The cosmetic effects of abnormal orofacial movements can result in social and occupational isolation. The physical consequences of tardive oral movements (e.g. loosening teeth, impairing swallowing, muffling speech due to abnormal tongue movements) need attention, for instance with, dental or speech and language therapy referral. Treatment may also be needed for respiratory dyskinesias and for the consequences of dyskinesia on gastrointestinal motility causing dysphagia that is marked enough to cause weight loss. GABA (gamma-aminobutyric acid) agonists have been used to help, but they do not. TD can be worsened in the short term by stopping neuroleptics. Slow stopping is desirable for other reasons but does not protect against the risk of TD. There is some research data implicating free radicals in the pathophysiology of TD and some limited trial data that vitamin E supplements can improve TD. On the basis that if one antioxidant helps then others should be tried—lazaroids and ceruletide may also eventually be shown to help. Diltiazem, a calcium channel antagonist is reported helpful in some severe cases.

Withdrawal emergent dyskinesias are similar to TD but only start following stopping neuroleptics. They can take up to five weeks to begin, especially after depot injections and generally improve over weeks although they can go on for months. These are more likely to occur with oral medication particularly in older patients who have taken neuroleptics for prolonged periods. Acquired immunodeficiency syndrome (AIDS) can present with this type of movement disorder.

Tardive myoclonus may occur as a separate entity. It seems to be more common in men. Tardive tremor is probably a form of drug-induced parkinsonism although the features are sometimes those of essential tremor rather than parkinsonism (without a pre-existing history of either condition). A 'rabbity' chin tremor is seen along with drug-induced parkinsonism. Tics and obsession–compulsion without diagnostic features of Gilles de la Tourette syndrome are sometimes seen. This raises concern about unnecessary use of neuroleptic drugs in Tourette's (discussed later in this chapter). Various other disorders have been described to occur as tardive phenomena (e.g. tardive pain and tardive akathisia).

DRUG-INDUCED PARKINSONISM

In a large survey, 90% of the patients who developed parkinsonism following exposure to phenothiazines developed it in the first 72 days. Approximately 10–15% of neuroleptic exposed patients developed this complication. Women are more commonly affected than men and the elderly seem particularly prone in the same way as they seem at increased risk of tardive dyskinesia. Other risk factors include hyperthyroidism, concomitant therapy with fluoxetine, family history of PD, and a history of affective disorder. As a result of the occurrence of fairly acute parkinsonism, disability such as capacity to stand is more severely affected than in ordinary PD. Tremor is less common, bradykinesia more marked, and the features more symmetrical than for PD. However, the tremor can be asymmetric affecting extremities, fingers, jaw, mouth, tongue, and lips and can closely mimic that seen in PD. Prompt recognition requires keeping a low threshold to thinking of this complication. There have been numerous cases of failure to recognize drug-induced parkinsonism resulting in inappropriate treatment with dopaminergic medication while continuing on antidopaminergic neuroleptics. Withdrawal of the offending drug usually allows these symptoms to resolve, although such resolution can take up to 18 months. Approximately 10% of those recovering from drug-induced parkinsonism have later developed idiopathic PD. In Ayd's large survey of drug-induced parkinsonism 3% went on to develop PD in the five years after phenothiazine withdrawal. Two patients who recovered from drug-induced parkinsonism and later died of unrelated cause were found at autopsy to have Lewy bodies within the substantia nigra, indicating that the occurrence of drug-induced parkinsonism may be predictive of the predisposition to idiopathic PD. Sometimes the patient's psychiatric state does not allow drug withdrawal as discussed in the section on tardive dyskinesia. In this situation treatment with anticholinergic drugs such as procyclidine, orphenadrine

or benzhexol may be helpful. However, it is worth noting that prolonged concomitant use of neuroleptics and anticholinergics is regarded as a risk factor for the emergence of tardive dyskinesia. Paradoxically, sometimes increasing the dose of the neuroleptic agent (for psychiatric indications) improves the parkinsonism. This happens infrequently and unreliably and must, therefore, be regarded as an interesting observation but must not result in indiscriminate increase in neuroleptic doses in patients with drug-induced parkinsonism. When continuing with a neuroleptic is mandatory, switching to one of the newer agents with a low risk of extrapyramidal side-effects is worthwhile. Risperidone and clozapine are two such drugs. Clozapine has been used longer. It is clear that extrapyramidal problems are less marked with clozapine but there is a serious risk of agranulocytosis which requires frequent monitoring of blood tests. In the past, electroconvulsive therapy (ECT) was noted to have an incidental beneficial effect on the severity of drug-induced parkinsonism but given the concerns about ECT it is unlikely that anyone would use it specifically to alleviate drug-induced parkinsonism.

ACUTE DYSTONIA

In contrast to tardive dyskinesia, which occurs more often in elderly patients, acute dystonic reactions are seen more commonly in children or younger adults following short exposure to a phenothiazine, butyrophenone, or to metoclopramide. Typically, within an hour of taking a tablet or receiving an injection of one of these drugs the patient experiences retrocollis or torticollis with oculogyric movements, sometimes associated with blepharospasm. When this occurs without prior warning it is a frightening experience for both the sufferer and the clinician. Reassurance and a mild sedative, such as a benzodiazepine, may be all that is necessary in mild cases but where the anxiety is greater or where the attack is more severe, treatment with an anticholinergic drug such as intravenous benztropine may be needed. Intravenous anticholinergic drugs are highly effective in this setting. Failure to get prompt relief after intravenous benztropine injection should prompt a search for other causes of dystonia.

Botulinum toxin in movement disorders

Among the first therapeutic uses of botulinum toxin were in the focal dystonias, particularly in the treatment of blepharospasm. Subsequently, use spread to include hemifacial spasm and strabismus, and now the ever increasing list of its uses includes other focal dystonias such as torticollis, spasmodic dysphonia (laryngeal dystonia), oromandibular dystonia, and the focal limb dystonias such as writer's cramp; the treatment of spasticity in such diverse conditions as cerebral palsy, spinal trauma, and multiple sclerosis and in the treatment of an assortment of other movement disorders including essential tremor. A discussion of the management of movement disorders in current day practice would be incomplete without specific mention of this important treatment advance.

Botulinum toxin is derived from *Clostridium botulinum*. There are seven different subtypes of the toxin. Type A is the most widely used but as antibodies to it have emerged types B and F are also being investigated. All subtypes act presynaptically at the neuromuscular junction to prevent acetylcholine release. Immunoresistance to the blocking properties of botulinum toxin A appears in about 5% of all patients during chronic use.

Blepharospasm

Within a few days of botulinum toxin A injection into the orbicularis oculi of patients with blepharospasm, an improvement is seen in the majority of patients. This improvement may last 15 weeks or even longer in some individuals but generally the duration of benefit is shorter and most patients will need repeat injection in less than 15 weeks. Ptosis, blurred vision, diplopia, precipitation of acute glaucoma, excessive lacrimation, facial weakness are all seen to some degree but as techniques of injection have improved and as experience of use of the drug has increased these adverse effects have become less common and less troublesome. Detailed description of injection doses and sites is beyond the scope of this chapter. Botulinum toxin A can be helpful in treating symptomatic blepharospasm seen in other diseases, for instance in Parkinson's disease and can be useful in treating disabling blepharospasm tics (blinking tics) in Tourette's syndrome.

Cervical dystonia

Botulinum toxin is undoubtedly effective at relieving torticollis and other cervical dystonias. It does not have a licence for this indication in the United Kingdom. Pain and movement improve in over 90% of cases treated by injection into the appropriate sternocleidomastoid, scalene, or trapezius muscles. Some practitioners base their decision as to which muscles are most likely to be involved on purely clinical observation and palpation whereas others prefer electromyographic (EMG) control. No clear advantage can be demonstrated for the use of EMG guidance. Apart from an excess of neck muscle weakness there is a risk of dysphagia which can rarely be severe enough to lead to aspiration pneumonitis. The risk of this is low and, as with the treatment of blepharospasm, the incidence of adverse events has fallen with increasing use and experience. Respiratory difficulties arising from an effect of the injection on laryngeal structures is less common than the effect on swallowing but is potentially more worrying.

Laryngeal dystonia

Over the years, a number of patients with disorders of the voice have been regarded as having a non-organic or functional speech problem. Some of these have now come to be regarded as having a focal dystonia of laryngeal structures resulting in either an adduction type of laryngeal dystonia characterized by a strained, hoarse voice or an abduction type with a 'breathy' type of speech. EMG-guided injection of botulinum toxin A into either the adductors or abductors (de-

pending on the type of dystonia) can result in significant improvement of voice quality. Treatment of both types carry a risk of excessive laryngeal weakness but clearly the risk of excessive weakening the abductors is far greater. As a result, the patients with the abductor type of laryngeal dystonia require even more care than usual. These injections should ideally be done in a dedicated voice clinic.

Oromandibular dystonia

The jaw closure type of oromandibular dystonia can be eased by botulinum toxin A injection into the masseter muscles with a low but significant risk of dysphagia. The jaw opening type of dystonia requires injection into pterygoid muscles and this has a much higher risk of inducing dysphagia, even in experienced hands. Apart from the cosmetic and psychosocial advantages of improving a facial dystonia, treatment of oromandibular dystonia reduces the long-term effects on diet, dentition, and on temporomandibular joint stability and function.

Hemifacial spasm

Although hemifacial spasm is not a focal dystonia, it is included here in view of the dramatic effect that treatment with botulinum toxin A can have on this condition. Features of hemifacial spasm can resemble those of blepharospasm. Hemifacial spasm is always unilateral, unlike blepharospasm. The patient complains of twitching movements usually starting over the cheek or around the eye. They commonly affect the angle of the mouth as well. Botulinum toxin A injection into the muscles of facial expression improves the symptoms reliably and consistently albeit incompletely. Pharmacological treatment of this movement disorder other than with botulinum toxin, is inadequate. Clonazepam is frequently used but is not very effective even when the doses are pushed to highly sedating levels. Some of these patients can be demonstrated to have a aberrant blood vessel traversing the cerebellopontine angle and abutting onto the trigeminal and/or facial nerves. Microvascular decompression of this aberrant blood vessel has been advocated for hemifacial spasm as it has for trigeminal neuralgia and even for vertigo. Undoubtedly, some patients appear to benefit dramatically from such surgery and the benefit can be a lasting one. In the responders, the benefit is better than in the patients treated with botulinum toxin injections but in view of the operative risks, including the risk of death, it would seem prudent to reserve posterior fossa surgery for those patients who have failed to show a response to botulinum toxin or those who are intolerant of the injections.

CHOREA

Chorea describes involuntary movements that are fairly rapid, irregular, and often result in dystonic postures. Patients with mild chorea may just appear fidgety and nervous and given that anxiety is a common accompaniment of several chorea syndromes, the fidgety movements may remain undiagnosed or just attributed to anxiety. Chorea can be mistaken for myoclonus, particularly when multiple myoclonic movements occur. In theory, the distinction between myoclonus and chorea should be straightforward. Myoclonus is faster, more regular, and does not result in abnormal posturing. Chorea generally shows flowing involuntary movements drifting from one part of the body to another giving them a dance-like rhythmic appearance. Other clinical features can allow the diagnosis to be made with greater certainty. For instance, involuntary movements occurring in an individual who has recently suffered diffuse cerebral hypoxia may be post-anoxic action myoclonus.

Chorea is seen in Huntington's disease, in Sydenham's chorea, sometimes in pregnancy or during oral contraceptive use, in cerebral systemic lupus erythematosus (SLE), in other anticardiolipin antibody syndromes, and as a reaction to levodopa use in Parkinson's disease. There are numerous other causes including drug-induced chorea but these will not be discussed here.

HUNTINGTON'S DISEASE

Genetic advances

This is an autosomal dominant, inherited condition with high penetrance, low new mutation rate, and shows the phenomenon of anticipation (i.e. inheritance through the paternal line results in an earlier age of onset of symptoms). Early onset cases have more dystonia and more severe dementia and epilepsy but less chorea. Akinetic rigid syndromes are also seen in younger patients. The gene responsible for this disease is located on the short arm of chromosome 4 and contains an expanded CAG trinucleotide-repeat sequence—the normal length of this sequence is 11–34 trinucleotides but in HD this is expanded to between 37 and more than 80 repeats. It is unknown whether these CAG repeats which code for the amino acid, glutamine, are present in the final gene product. Patients with early onset disease (namely, those who have inherited the faulty gene from the paternal line) have very long trinucleotide repeat sequences but the correlation of repeat length with age of onset is not sufficiently accurate to enable prediction of the age of onset in an at-risk individual.

The availability of a good genetic test is likely to help establish a clear diagnosis of Huntington's disease (HD) in cases where the clinical diagnosis was uncertain. Misdiagnoses will also be clarified, including some in cases with a known family history. These may include examples of neuroacanthocytosis or another, genetically distinct disorder of an unstable trinucleotide repeat expansion called dentato-rubro-pallido-luysian atrophy (DRPLA). Epilepsy and myoclonus are more prominent in DRPLA. When the genetic defect of HD has been found in a family with a clinical history of HD, the test can be offered to at-risk family members. Numerous ethical problems have already arisen due to this, and others are likely to follow. Some of these have come relatively unanticipated. Among the expected ethical difficulties is the conflict between an individual's right to know whether they have the gene defect when their at-risk parent has no wish to have the diagnosis confirmed. A positive test in the former, of course, necessarily means a positive test in the latter. Careful thought needs to go into genetic testing and requires professional counselling preferably by a clinical geneticist within a neurogenetics clinic. Post-test counselling is required not only for those testing positive but equally so for those with negative tests as there can be considerable feelings of guilt in 'survivors' who know that other family members have a positive result. So far, the risk of suicide in those tested positive has been no higher than that of the disease in pre-gene test days but this may be an artefact of inadequate length of post-testing follow-up for what is a relatively new test.

Dramatic advances are taking place in the molecular understanding of HD including insights into the function of huntingtin, the protein that the HD gene locus codes for including its interaction with important enzymes involved in energy metabolism. It is known, both by inference from the nature of autosomal dominant disorders and from animal experiments, that HD results from the effects of the abnormal huntingtin protein rather than a deficiency of the normal protein. However, a number of issues remain unresolved, including whether the polyglutamine encoded by the CAG repeats remains in the functioning protein and how it effects cell damage in the basal ganglia. Understanding the interrelation between huntingtin, polyglutamine and excitatory amino acid-mediated damage sets the scene for considering anti-excitotoxic treatment in HD.

Drug treatment

Mild chorea can be treated with low dose benzodiazepines or even a beta-blocker (using its anxiolytic properties). A combination of a barbiturate and low dose benzodiazepines can also be successful and may pose less of a threat to the patient's well-being than do the phenothiazines. Butyrophenones and phenothiazines suppress chorea and can be remarkably effective in the short term. However, as discussed in the sections above, the risk of drug-induced movement disorders is appreciable. Tetrabenazine is also effective and has a different spectrum of adverse effects but depression, tiredness, and drug-induced parkinsonism may also limit its use. The newer antipsychotic drugs, which also have a dopamine receptor blocking action, such as sulpiride and clozapine, may be more useful. Sulpiride seems to cause fewer extrapyramidal side-effects although there are well-described cases of tardive dyskinesia when taking it. Clozapine is newer still and probably causes even fewer extrapyramidal reactions but its usefulness is limited by its haematological side-effects.

Dopamine receptor blocking drugs can, by their major tranquillizer actions, help the behaviour disturbance that can be a troublesome feature of the disease and the more sedative ones like thioridazine can help the sleep disturbance that families find difficult to manage.

As there is GABA cell loss in the brain in HD, attempts have been made to increase brain GABA concentrations using isoniazid, baclofen, and valproate; without any success. Similarly disappointing results are obtained with cholinergic manipulation. The increased understanding of serotonin receptor subtypes and the development of new agonists and antagonists of these receptors bodes well for the development of more successful therapies for movement disorders but has not achieved this at present.

Pharmacological treatment is sometimes required for the psychiatric manifestations of HD. Dementia with severe behavioural disturbance can often require major tranquillizers; anxiety may need treatment with benzodiazepines. As in other disabling conditions, the presence of depression must be looked for in both, the patient and in their carers. Prompt treatment of depression may improve the families' well-being to a greater extent than the treatment of chorea.

Other treatments

Apart from dementia and chorea, there are numerous symptoms of HD requiring drug treatment. For instance, in the latter stages of disease pain can be a major problem. Awareness of this problem allows rational prescribing of suitable analgesia. Communication and nutrition can be compromised by the chorea and can cause much distress, especially in patients who have good cognitive function. Access to speech therapy and a good dietician can be invaluable. Progressive physical disability that proves unresponsive to dopamine receptor blockade may require attention from a physiotherapist or occupational therapist. The needs may vary from one individual needing a foot-drop splint to another needing a complete environment control system. The network of care advisers run, for instance, by the UK patient support organization, COMBAT, can help to channel patients into receiving assistance appropriate to their current needs.

Looking after the carers is an important aspect of the management of all chronic disabling disorders. However, in HD this is even more important than in most other conditions as the carers are often other individuals at risk of the disease and therefore all too acutely aware that their parent's or their sibling's condition is what could happen to them in years to come. Counselling by trained staff can be invaluable.

OTHER CHOREAS

When chorea occurs as a familial disorder with autosomal dominant pattern of inheritance the usual explanation is HD and in a small number of cases it represents a syndrome incorporating chorea and acanthocytosis on a peripheral blood film. Increasing numbers of patients thought to have HD are now being recognized as having the rare condition, dentato-rubro-pallido-luysian atrophy (DRPLA). This distinction has

been made possible by the recent identification of a trinucleotide expansion in the DRPLA gene. Seizures occur frequently in the early stages of both chorea-acanthocytosis syndrome and DRPLA, whereas fits are rare in the early stages of adult onset HD. A few families have been reported to show chorea without cognitive deterioration and without acanthocytes. In these cases, the chorea is generally nonprogressive and may begin in early childhood.

Non-familial causes of chorea outnumber the familial ones, with drug-induced chorea being the commonest. The most frequent offenders are antiparkinsonian medications causing choreiform dyskinesias and the phenothiazines and butyrophenones causing tardive chorea. The oral contraceptive pill is another important cause of chorea which is of the same type as chorea gravidarum—underlining the influence of hormones on chorea. The link, if any, between these and Sydenham's chorea or post-streptococcal chorea or rheumatic chorea needs to be clarified. The incidence of Sydenham's chorea is increasing again, after a lull of over two decades. It is not clear whether this represents an increase in the virulence of present-day streptococci. The principles of management of the chorea remain as described above, bearing in mind the self-limiting nature of the chorea in these cases. The streptococcal infection is also treated with antibiotics, and associated manifestations of rheumatic fever, including particularly cardiac ones, require attention. Thyrotoxicosis, although more commonly associated with a tremor, can cause chorea which improves with treatment of the thyrotoxic state. However, like any chorea, the movement disorder can respond to treatment with butyrophenones even in the thyrotoxic state. Two other important general medical conditions linked with chorea are systemic lupus erythematosus (SLE) and polycythemia rubra vera. In general, other clinical features are sufficiently prominent to make these diagnoses relatively obvious and the treatment is that of the underlying condition. Electrolyte imbalance such as in renal failure and other metabolic problems such as hypoglycemia can induce chorea.

PAROXYSMAL CHOREA

A disorder that is frequently autosomal dominant in inheritance, causes intermittent choreas that is induced by movement and lasts a few seconds and occurs many times a day. This is termed, paroxysmal kinesigenic choreoathetosis (PKC) and can occasionally respond dramatically to treatment with anticonvulsants such as phenytoin or carbamazepine. A longstanding debate over whether PKC is an epileptic phenomenon or just a focal dystonia remains unresolved; an academic distinction in most clinicians' view as the treatments of choice are the anticonvulsants listed above. A less common disorder is paroxysmal dystonic choreoathetosis (PDC)—this is also often familial but the paroxysmal events can last minutes or hours and may only occur a few times each week. Some of the movements seen in these conditions are bizarre in appearance and are frequently mistakenly labelled hysterical. The paroxysmal disorders seen in multiple sclerosis—tonic spasms—can resemble those seen in PKC and PDC.

BALLISM

Large amplitude proximal movements usually affecting one limb are seen in hemiballismus, a disorder that may be regarded as a severe form of a hemichorea. It is characteristically associated with a lesion in the contralateral subthalamic nucleus but a variety of lesions in the basal ganglia can produce this abnormality. The most common pathology producing this condition is a vascular event in the subthalamic nucleus but it can be caused by a metastatic tumour deposit. Studies in experimental animals show that the pathways predominantly affected are the subthalamopallidal (a glutamatergic pathway) and the pallidothalamic ones with relative preservation of the subthalamonigral pathway. The principles of treatment are as those for chorea. Hemiballismus is generally more distressing than chorea, in part because of its sudden onset in a vascular event and partly by the very disabling and dramatic nature of the involuntary movements; so that, whereas many cases of chorea can be treated without resorting to drug therapy, hemiballismus usually requires pharmacotherapy, with haloperidol or tetrabenazine.

ATHETOSIS

Confusion over the term 'athetosis' helps to exemplify the arbitrary nature of some of the currently used classification of movement disorders. Athetosis is generally used to label a particular type of perinatal injury called athetoid cerebral palsy. The slow, writhing limb movements result in abnormal posturing of the affected limbs and may therefore quite reasonably be called dystonic; furthermore some of the movements are quick enough to be called chorea or even myoclonus and others are of large enough amplitude to be labelled ballistic.

In conditions where slow, writhing movements are seen it would seem important to determine whether the main problem is one of dystonia or whether it falls into the chorea–ballism group. This distinction is of practical importance as the treatment of these two broad categories is different (as discussed above). The term 'pseudoathetosis' still retains usefulness. This is used to describe involuntary twitching movements usually of an outstretched hand in patients with a deafferented limb. This can occur with a large fibre peripheral neuropathy, with spinal cord (dorsal column) disease, or even with parietal lobe lesions.

MYOCLONUS

This refers to rapid, brief lightning-like movements which may be segmental, focal, or generalized and can be either single movements or repetitive to the point of seeming like a tremor. They may involve an active muscle contraction termed 'positive myoclonus' or there may be a transient loss of muscle contraction called 'asterixis' or 'negative myoclonus'. Myoclonic movements can be physiological, as seen with the repetitive movements of hiccups or the single movement of a sneeze. Even when non-physiological, myoclonic movement disorder may be a static and exaggerated physiologic response to external stimuli such as a severe startle response in a nervous individual—myoclonus therefore does not necessarily imply underlying progressive neurological disease. In a hospital setting the most common cause of myoclonus is metabolic encephalopathy associated with renal or hepatic disease, electrolyte imbalance or hypoglycaemia, and occasionally as an adverse effect of medication. Some myoclonus is seen as a part of epileptic disorders. Epileptic myoclonus, whether 'spontaneous' or reflex represents one type of cortical myoclonus. On physiological grounds it is possible to distinguish between myoclonus of cortical origin or that arising from subcortical structures probably within the brainstem, and possibly the nucleus reticularis gigantocellularis. In some instances, myoclonus that arises as a cortical phenomenon may spread via subcortical structures. Most cases of symptomatic myoclonus probably arise from brainstem structures or their connections.

PHYSIOLOGICAL MYOCLONUS

This is more common during sleep. It includes the sudden, startling hypnic jerk which most individuals have encountered, and periodic movements of sleep (PMS), which are seen as a part of the spectrum of the restless legs syndrome (RLS). Hypnic jerks rarely warrant any pharmacological treatment. PMS, however, can be troublesome and may require treatment of both this and other aspects of RLS. Treatment of predisposing disorders such as anaemia offers the best prospect of early relief but such reversible factors are only found in a small minority of patients. Some require treatment with clonazepam, opiates, or dopamine agonists. Hiccups may also be thought of as a myoclonic disorder which, when protracted, can be treated with metoclopramide—a dopamine receptor blocker but one that stimulates gastric motility; this latter action may be important in its anti-hiccup action.

METABOLIC MYOCLONUS

The myoclonus of metabolic disorders is commonly encountered in general hospitals. Acute deterioration in renal function commonly causes myoclonus as a part of uraemic encephalopathy but the other features such as the delirium may overshadow the movement disorder. Similar movements can be seen in patients with acute or rapidly deteriorating liver function. Even patients with chronic hepatic encephalopathy can present with asterixis or liver flap, a form of myoclonus. Patients with respiratory failure with carbon dioxide retention often show a similar flapping tremor. Changes in electrolyte concentrations including hyponatraemia and hypocalcaemia cause myoclonus. Other metabolic upsets including hypoglycaemia and hyperglycaemia, particularly with hyperosmolarity, can cause myoclonus. Symptomatic treatment of the myoclonus in these cases is usually futile as the outcome is clearly related to the diagnosis and treatment of the underlying condition.

POST-HYPOXIC MYOCLONUS

In the recovery phase from the effects of acute cerebral hypoxia (such as during transient cardiac arrest) some individuals develop a combination of cortical and subcortical myoclonus that is precipitated particularly by action and is called post-hypoxic action myoclonus (PHAM). These patients may have additional signs of hypoxic injury including hemiparesis. Cerebellar signs are reported in some patients but these may represent myoclonic movements interfering with action. The occurrence of myoclonus in an appropriate clinical setting helps to establish the diagnosis. Rehabilitation of these patients is frequently seriously hampered by the PHAM. In recent years, some dramatic responses have been obtained by treatment with piracetam. When the response to piracetam is unsatisfactory, clonazepam, valproate, or a combination of 5-hydroxytryptophan, and carbidopa can be used. It is reported that patients with spike wave discharges on electroencephalogram (EEG) are more likely to show a favourable response to pharmacotherapy.

EPILEPTIC MYOCLONUS

This requires early recognition as certain anticonvulsants are more likely to be effective in epilepsy with myoclonus, and more importantly, some anticonvulsants such as carbamazepine may be contraindicated in these conditions owing to the risk of exacerbating the epilepsy. A few children with myoclonic epilepsy may have rare inherited progressive neurodegenerative disorders, early recognition of which is important for both prognostic reasons and for genetic counselling. These include Lafora body disease and the lipid storage diseases. A mixed bag of disorders has been labelled the Ramsay–Hunt syndrome comprising a combination of ataxia, dysarthria, and myoclonus. Some of the patients given this label have subsequently been found to have a mitochondrial cytopathy and others to have a multisystem degeneration called dentato-rubro-pallido-luysian atrophy (DRPLA), recognition of which has been facilitated by the finding of a trinucleotide repeat expansion in the gene defective in this disease. A few have a prion disease, Gerstmann–Straussler syndrome. Nevertheless, the term 'Ramsay–Hunt syndrome' retains a clinical usefulness so long as the descriptive and syndromic nature of the symptom complex is remembered. Stimulus-sensitive startle myoclonus, starting asymmetrically and progressing to cognitive impairment is known to occur in the rare disorder, corticobasal degeneration. This condition is an inexorably progressive condition, leading to severe disability and death.

INFECTIONS AND MYOCLONUS

Prion diseases such as Creutzfelt–Jakob disease (CJD) commonly cause myoclonus, often of a severity greater than that seen in other dementing disorders such as Alzheimer's disease. The occurrence of a rapidly progressive dementia with myoclonus in an adult should initiate a search for CJD including an EEG, which frequently shows repetitive and periodic complexes. The identification of prion protein mutations in this disease has made the diagnosis easier. The myoclonus is generally a minor symptom in this rapidly fatal condition. The progressive degenerative condition, subacute sclerosing panencephalitis (SSPE) seen as a rare sequel to measles in adolescents also results in myoclonus. Periodic complexes are also seen on the EEG in this disease, in which both serum and cerebrospinal fluid have high titres of antimeasles antibodies. In the cerebrospinal fluid (CSF) these may be present as an oligoclonal band identifiable on electrophoresis with isoelectric focusing. More acute viral encephalitides, such as herpes simplex encephalitis, are another infective cause of myoclonus. This is characterized by a short history (a few days) of encephalopathy with confusion, seizures that may be focal in onset and other lateralizing signs sometimes in the setting of evidence of herpes simplex infection or activation (e.g. cold sores on the lips). Early recognition and prompt start of appropriate antiviral medication with acyclovir are required to improve the eventual outcome. The syndrome of dancing eyes and dancing feet (opsoclonus–myoclonus syndrome) occurs with equal frequency as either a post-infectious condition (following rubella, mumps, infectious mononucleosis, and other infections) or as a feature of underlying neuroblastoma. The combination of opsoclonus and myoclonus sometimes combined with eyelid flutter and dysarthria is unmistakable. Whether paraneoplastic or post-infectious the condition responds to treatment with oral steroids in many cases. There are reports of improvement on propranolol in a few steroid-unresponsive cases.

Prion disorders with some similarity to CJD have recently caused great public interest in the United Kingdom. This arises from the observation that there have been rather more cases of a CJD-like disorder in younger patients than would have been expected in the UK population. Some of these younger patients have been associated with the meat industry and have presented with an anxiety state with emergence of dementia and myoclonus later in the course of the disease. This disorder has come to be linked with bovine spongiform encephalopathy (BSE) although the scientific evidence establishing this link is far from conclusive.

MYOCLONUS AS A FEATURE OF EXTRAPYRAMIDAL
DISEASES

Patients with Parkinson's disease sometimes show myoclonic movements usually attributed to their treatment with levodopa. Myoclonus also occurs as a feature of other basal ganglia disorders such as Huntington's disease (HD), DRPLA, Hallervorden–Spatz disease, Wilson's disease, and even (rarely) in Steele–Richardson–Olszewski syndrome. Corticobasal degeneration is a disorder comprising apraxia, dementia, and among numerous movement disturbances, a stimulus-sensitive myoclonus. The pattern of reflex myoclonus seen in corticobasal degeneration has recently been likened to that seen in some cases of HD. A few patients with dystonia show jerky myoclonic movements which can be very strikingly alcohol-responsive.

SPINAL MYOCLONUS

Segmental myoclonus of spinal origin sometimes follows structural spinal injury or occurs in association with identifiable structural pathology on imaging studies. However, it can also arise from what seems to be a structurally sound spinal cord. Structural disturbances linked with this are vascular events affecting the cord, demyelination, syringomyelia, and tumours, both intra- and extramedullary. In para-infectious causes and in para-neoplastic disorders, aetiological factors may be difficult to identify. As in other para-neoplastic conditions the spinal myoclonus may precede the declaration of the neoplasm. In general, the myoclonus is confined to a small number of spinal myotomes. Axial flexion or rarely, extension myoclonic spasms are seen in the recently described propriospinal myoclonus that has been linked with trauma to the cervical spinal cord. The principles of drug treatment of spinal myoclonus are the same as those of other myoclonus syndromes. Clonazepam is occasionally very successful. In resistant cases tetrabenazine, levodopa, and piracetam have been tried.

NON-SPINAL SEGMENTAL MYOCLONUS

Palatal myoclonus also called palatal nystagmus is a repetitive movement of the soft palate which can interfere with speech and with swallowing and occasionally causes an irritating tinnitus, which unlike most tinnitus, can also be heard by the doctor! The movements of the soft palate can be extremely rapid (up to 8–10 Hz) and although these are temporarily suppressed by talking and swallowing, the movement disorder can cause dysphagia and dysarthria. Most often, patients present in middle to late years of life, sometimes with features of a posterior fossa stroke in addition to the myoclonus. Other structural abnormalities in the vicinity of the inferior olivary nucleus can also cause palatal myoclonus. Imaging studies can show hypertrophy of the contralateral inferior olivary nucleus. A few cases are associated with other involuntary movements such as blepharospasm or oromandibular dyskinesia and, in the rare condition of Whipple's disease, with facial myorhythmia. In view of the association with dystonia a few cases have been treated with benzhexol with some success. Others have tried more conventional treatments with antimyoclonus agents with only limited success. The place, if any, of piracetam in palatal myoclonus remains to be determined.

Opsoclonus which is associated with myoclonus in the limbs as a post-infective or a para-neoplastic disorder may also be regarded as a form of non-spinal segmental myoclonus. Both the main features of the syndrome sometimes respond well to treatment with oral glucocorticosteroids.

TICS

Tics are rapid movements, motor or vocal that are of short duration and often repetitive but usually of random, non-rhythmic timing. There is partial control over these semi-involuntary movements. For example, patients can sometimes suppress tics while involved in absorbing activity or when in a situation that may cause embarrassment. Frequently, there is some gratification obtained from carrying out these movements and patients may be able to draw the distinction between 'it happens' and 'I have to make it happen'. Tics are very common: 8–12% of all children have at least one tic which in most cases is dismissed as a mannerism; usually not causing any disruption to the child's day-to-day functioning. Multiple tics are less frequently. When a child presents with multiple vocal (coughing, sniffing, grunting, throat clearing, animal sounds, etc.) and motor tics (blinking, head nodding, shoulder shrugging, touching, etc.) a diagnosis of Gilles de la Tourette syndrome is entertained. This disorder, which may be inherited as an autosomal dominant condition with variable penetrance, has attracted a lot of attention owing to one rather uncommon feature. Coprolalia or involuntary swearing is dramatic but infrequent and is not required to make the diagnosis. Tics can be suppressed partially during intense concentration, such as during examinations, and their occurrence does not *per se* usually pose a hindrance to the child's education. However, the social morbidity from the tics including teasing by schoolmates and adverse comments from ill-informed teachers can be considerable. Multiple motor and vocal tics can require pharmacological treatment for these reasons, particularly where behavioural approaches have failed to give relief and where follow-up over a year has failed to show spontaneous resolution. The drugs that are most effective at suppressing tics are the butyrophenones and the phenothiazines. Haloperidol is the most frequently used of these drugs in this context. These drugs have potentially serious side-effects including the possibility of tardive dyskinesia and other drug-induced movement disorders, as discussed above. Tardive dyskinesia is seen more commonly in the elderly but children are not exempt from such adverse effects and the dyskinesia may not be reversible. It is therefore imperative that the lowest dose required to alleviate symptoms sufficiently to allow social functioning is used. It is also advisable to withdraw the medication at intervals to determine if it is still required. Mild tics that are nevertheless incapacitating are sometimes treated with benzodiazepines such as clonazepam. Both butyrophenones and benzodiazepines have a sedating action and can affect a child's learning. Clonidine and tetrabenazine have also been used for tic suppression. I have not found clonidine helpful and tetrabenazine has extrapyramidal side-effects which limit its usefulness.

Multiple tic syndrome (Gilles de la Tourette) is frequently accompanied by attention deficit hyperactivity disorder (ADHD) and by a combination of obsessions and compulsions. The obsessive–compulsive disorder can involve complicated rituals of washing, dressing, etc., and can become more disabling than the tics. Treatment with the newer serotonin reuptake inhibitors, such as fluoxetine, or with the older tricyclic drug, clomipramine, can be effective at alleviating these symptoms. A few individuals will exhibit obsessive compulsions leading to potential serious self-harm. When these obsessions fail to respond to pharmacological manipulation and carry a serious risk of, for instance, blinding oneself, stereotactic cingulotomy has been used successfully. Pharmacological treatment of ADHD is probably best avoided as it is not very effective, it can exacerbate tics, and the very long-term effects of drugs such as methylphenidate and pemoline are unknown. Selegiline has been used to treat the ADHD in Tourette's syndrome and some limited success reported. However, with the recently reported findings of increased death rates in patients with Parkinson's disease treated with selegiline, it would seem sensible to avoid using selegiline until the exact significance of the Parkinson's disease findings is clarified.

STEREOTYPIES

No entirely satisfactory definition exists for stereotypies. The term is often used for ritualized movements carried out by mentally handicapped children in whom the issue of whether these movements are under voluntary control or under semivoluntary control cannot be readily established. They probably differ from true obsessive–compulsive behaviour, in that obsessive compulsions are usually under a fair degree of voluntary thought and possibly voluntary control. In obsessive–compulsion an individual may experience either an overwhelming desire to carry out an activity or may be terrified of disastrous consequences of avoiding carrying out that activity. Stereotypies are generally not thought to involve complex thoughts about the consequences or otherwise of carrying out an action, suggesting that they are not under full voluntary control and possibly are completely involuntary. Habit spasms occurring in normal individuals (e.g. leg-shaking while seated or foot-tapping) may be thought of as stereotypies which, in this setting, are under partial voluntary control (i.e. they can

be voluntarily suppressed but their restarting occurs without active thought). Boredom may be a driving force for these movements in some cases and in others, a more diffuse lack of sensory stimulation may be relevant. In addition to sensory deprivation, abnormal sensation may drive some of these movements as in akathisia where an inner restlessness impels the patient into carrying out a ritualized action. This may also occur in Ekbom's syndrome although in that condition relief from restlessness is obtained by any movement rather than one specific activity. Unlike these conditions, in which the movements are carried out to make up for a lack of stimulation or to counter an abnormal sensation, stereotypic actions can be involved in complex partial epileptic seizures in which they are totally involuntary. In a number of mental handicap syndromes, particularly in the more severely affected individuals, stereotypic behaviour and action is frequently seen. In autism, rocking movements of the whole body, flapping of arms, and flicking fingers before the eyes can be troublesome. Some children will concentrate intensely and apparently endlessly on rocking toys or revolving tops. On rare occasions, stereotypic behaviour becomes more serious with a potential for deliberate self-harm. Stereotypic behaviour also forms a part of the obsessive–compulsive disorder seen in Gilles de la Tourette syndrome although, as discussed above, the degree of voluntary control over obsessive compulsions may preclude considering them as a stereotypic action. In Rett syndrome, a disorder that affects girls from infancy onwards with a normal peri-natal period, hand-wringing stereotypies are prominent and heavily relied on in making the diagnosis. These girls lose communication skills and also lose purposeful hand use. However, their condition can stabilize and sometimes even improve. This disorder has been regarded as a defect of the X chromosome but the lack of affected boys and the absence of a history of male fetus abortions is not easy to reconcile with that view. Mitochondrial abnormalities have also been considered especially as a few of these patents have suffered sudden cardiac death. The aetiology is unknown but the marked reduction of pigment in the substantia nigra indicates a primary disorder of the extrapyramidal system.

On the basis that there may be a mitochondrial abnormality underlying the aetiopathogenesis of Rett syndrome, an attempt at treatment was made using l-carnitine. This was an isolated report of benefit. Seizures can occur in this condition but there is no evidence that the hand-wringing is an epileptic phenomenon. When stereotypies are seen as a part of mental handicap syndromes the other features of the syndrome usually overshadow the movement disorder. Symptomatic treatment with medication is rarely necessary. Behavioural approaches including the recognition that some of the movements may result from boredom, frustration, or some sensory deprivation may help with management. When the movements are socially incapacitating or when they pose a danger to the patient, treatment on empirical grounds with haloperidol or other major tranquillizers may be tried. The risks in using such medications have been referred to above.

FURTHER READING

Joseph, A. B. and Young, R. R. (ed.) (1992). *Movement disorders in neurology and neuropsychiatry*. Blackwell, Oxford

Kurlan, R. (ed.) (1995). *Treatment of movement disorders*. Lippincott, Philadelphia.

Marsden, C. D. and Fahn, S. (ed.) (1994). *Movement disorders*, Vol. 3. Butterworth–Heinemann, Oxford.

Werner, W. and Lang, A. E. (1989). *Movement disorders. A comprehensive survey*. Futura, New York.

9 | *Parkinson's disease*

Christopher Ward and Piers Newman

Parkinson's disease (PD) is the commonest cause of progressive neurological disability in later life with a prevalence of 1–2 per 1000. Many aspects of the management of PD are relevant to people with PD-like syndromes. PD 'look-alikes' constituted a further 1 per 1000 in one epidemiological study (1, 2). In this chapter the emphasis will be on rehabilitation rather than on purely medical aspects of management. The range of medical and surgical interventions is especially wide in PD, including symptomatic drug treatment, symptomatic neurosurgical procedures, and implantation surgery which aims to be restorative. In addition, several agents have been proposed on theoretical grounds to be neuroprotective, but there is as yet no firm evidence that the neurodegenerative process can be retarded or halted by drug treatment (3).

The exceptionally wide range of medical and surgical options has proved to be a disadvantage as well as an advantage for people with PD. In the first place, neurologists and others have often had excessively high expectations of such treatment, ignoring the fact that distressing symptoms and disabilities are experienced by most patients even when drugs are effective. Secondly, physicians have sometimes had a blinkered view of the purposes of treatment, emphasizing physical disabilities which are typically influenced by drugs while failing to take account of other less conspicuous problems which may be more important to the patient.

The first section of this chapter comments selectively on clinical issues which are most directly relevant to rehabilitative management. In the next section, the general principles of management and of non-medical and medical therapy are reviewed. The final two sections describe practical aspects of management most often encountered, respectively, in early and in late PD.

CLINICAL FEATURES IN A REHABILITATION CONTEXT

Multiple physical, cognitive, and psychiatric disorders combine to produce a wide spectrum of disabilities. These must be taken into account as the disease advances, if management is to be effective.

PHYSICAL IMPAIRMENTS AND DISABILITIES

The principal motor symptoms and disabilities need not be described here comprehensively since they are well documented in textbooks. They are clearly attributable to the classical parkinsonian triad of tremor, rigidity, and bradykinesia, together with the fourth cardinal motor feature, impaired postural reflexes (4). Other symptoms are less easily categorized. *Musculoskeletal* problems such as shoulder stiffness and pain are common, as are other less clearly defined aches and pains (5). Postural flexion can cause kyphosis and scoliosis.

Three distinct forms of *speech impairment* are dysphonia (reduction in volume), dysarthria (loss of articulatory clarity), and dysfluency (6). The term 'festinating speech'—an extreme form of dysfluency—draws an analogy with the gait disorder: despite the misleading term 'akinesia', both speech and gait are subject to rapid, irregular action, as well as to slowing. Speech dysfluency can additionally have a cognitive basis, since PD characteristically reduces the speed of production of lists of nouns.

Dysphagia is often due to poor bolus formation during the oral phase, leading to premature reflex swallowing (7, 8). *Autonomic* impairments are frequently described (9), including bladder symptoms, typically urinary frequency, sexual dysfunction, and constipation. The neurological basis of these problems is poorly understood. There is little evidence of a specific neurogenic bladder dysfunction (10). There is a strong clinical impression that PD causes erectile failure in the absence of factors such as mood disorder. Constipation as well as other autonomic symptoms can sometimes be attributed to drug treatment (11). Another inadequately documented problem is *sleep disturbance* (12). The cause may be depression, or the physical discomfort associated with bradykinesia and rigidity, but a specific abnormality of the sleep–wake cycle may occur. *Extraocular* disorders are another frequent source of symptoms (13). Reading difficulties can be caused by slow, jerky saccadic eye movements, or by impaired convergence (which is correctable with prisms).

PSYCHOLOGICAL FACTORS

In many ways PD is best viewed as a behavioural rather than as a physical disorder. The cognitive perspective helps us to understand how skilled motor performance breaks down in

PD. For example, the cognitive aspect of a task such as walking across a room is evident from the everyday observation that environmental stimuli such as obstacles or thresholds can cause akinetic freezing. Another example of the complexity of parkinsonian deficits is the finding that impaired communication has a receptive as well as an expressive component: patients have difficulty in perceiving and responding to prosodic (expressive) cues provided by other speakers (14). Similarly, dysphagia is not caused solely by a simple neuromuscular malfunction but can be due to a failure in higher-level oral control.

Selective cognitive deficits can be demonstrated psychometrically early in the course of PD (15). There is impairment in performing two tasks simultaneously, in switching tasks (16), and in processing complex sequences of tasks. There is also a specific deficit in verbal learning. Some studies suggest that PD impairs the learning of new motor skills (17) but patients can benefit from practice in a reaction time task (18). Many selective cognitive deficits reflect the role of the basal ganglia in information processing and can be regarded as an integral part of the parkinsonian syndrome. Selective deficits have not been shown to presage dementia although prospective studies may yet demonstrate a link.

Mood disorders affect most people with PD to some extent and are sometimes the critical determinants of overall disability and handicap. Controlled studies suggest that depression is a specific complication of PD, presumably as a neuropharmacological effect (19). Anxiety (often combined with depression) is also common although less well documented (19, 20). Dramatic changes in a mood state termed 'affect-arousal' occur in parallel with fluctuations in mobility as a result of response to L-dopa treatment (21). People with PD and their families often report that anxiety impairs motor tasks. Motor performance in PD is characteristically variable and affective tone undoubtedly affects the observed level of disability. Anxiety and depressive apathy contribute to social withdrawal, which is a major source of distress for spouses and other helpers of people with PD. Impaired communication leads to isolation not only from the outside world but also within the family home (22, 23).

Psychotic symptoms are not seen as a complication of PD but can be caused by all the drugs used for its treatment (24). Mild hallucinations are a common experience during L-dopa treatment. L-dopa is less likely than other agents to cause severe psychiatric reactions, which are more commonly associated with ergot drugs. Psychotic symptoms may also be provoked idiosyncratically in some people who are started on relatively small doses of anticholinergic drugs.

Dementia (i.e. progressive multimodality cognitive failure) affects 10–30% of patients with PD (25). Severe dementia never occurs as a presenting feature of PD but is liable to become clinically significant in parallel with severe physical disability.

DIAGNOSIS AND PROGNOSIS

How important is accurate diagnosis? There are some valid arguments in favour of a liberal approach to clinical diagnosis. From the point of view of drug treatment the penalty for misdiagnosis is not as high as for some conditions, since the effects of drug treatment can be tested empirically over a period of time. There is justification in the argument that all people with suspected PD and significant disability should be given a therapeutic trial of antiparkinsonian drug treatment, with the important proviso that clinical response must be monitored objectively so that ineffective treatment can be discontinued promptly. However, accurate diagnosis has purposes beyond that of determining decisions about treatment. Prognostic information, which depends critically on diagnosis, can be valuable in the planning of rehabilitation and care and is demanded by many patients. Some individuals find diagnostic uncertainty especially hard to bear, especially if they have preconceptions about prognosis. They are understandably unhappy with the neurologists's reassurance that 'time will tell'. Ideally, diagnosis should therefore be established rapidly, and also accurately.

This is difficult to achieve. The diagnosis of PD is more problematic than is often appreciated (26). Outside the neurologist's clinic the most likely misdiagnosis is essential tremor which is more than twice as prevalent as PD. No patient with monosymptomatic tremor can confidently be classified as PD. Other parkinsonian syndromes can closely mimic PD in the early stages although differing in their rate of progression and clinical features. Although neuroimaging techniques, such as single photon emission computerized tomography (SPECT), hold some future promise as objective markers of PD, the only generally available objective test is response to L-dopa or apomorphine. The apomorphine test is not widely used because, even with the largest doses of domperidone pre-treatment, some patients experience very unpleasant (although brief) side-effects. A single dose of oral L-dopa can be used in a similar way. Unequivocal, measurable improvement provides objective evidence against essential tremor but the test's usefulness is limited by the fact that some non-PD syndromes can respond to some extent to L-dopa. The test thus has limited negative predictive value. Its positive predictive value is also somewhat limited: a negative test—no observable response to a single L-dopa challenge—provides evidence against PD but a more extended therapeutic trial may be required.

Given the difficulties of diagnosis the patient should be seen at least once by a consultant who is capable of evaluating critically the clinical evidence, but even then the diagnostic error rate is likely to be at least 20% on a single assessment (26).

LAYING THE FOUNDATIONS FOR GOOD MANAGEMENT

Good management depends firstly, on the assessment and monitoring of problems; secondly, on the setting of appropriate short-term and long-term goals; and thirdly, on the provision of services which can meet identified needs.

METHODS OF ASSESSMENT

The World Health Organization (27) distinguishes impairments (deficits in anatomy or physiology), disabilities (failure to perform standard tasks to an agreed standard), and handicaps (disadvantages). Handicap is the level of assessment which is of most immediate importance to an individual but the idiosyncratic nature of handicap makes it especially difficult to assess. By contrast, impairments such as bradykinesia are often easy to measure. Measuring the time taken to move the finger 20 times between two marks 25-cm apart on a sheet of paper provides a useful index of response to anti-parkinsonian treatment and can be quickly assessed at every clinic visit, but does not in itself predict either disability (what the patient cannot do) or handicap (what the patient wishes to do but cannot do). The times taken to walk 10 metres and back, or to write a standard sentence three times have similar applications in the monitoring of response to drugs. They are also measures of disability but provide only limited information about a person's daily function, and little or none about handicap/disadvantage.

At least as much importance must be attached to assessment of handicap/disadvantage as to impairment or disability. Much of the assessment is necessarily subjective but can be recorded systematically. I use the mnemonic 'PILS' as a framework for this part of the assessment, to signify four different domains of potential disadvantage. The first of these, *P*revention, encompasses assessments of risks, including avoidable physical, psychological, and social complications. At each medical encounter a physician should rapidly consider the scale of risk of *future* physical complications such as accidents (notably falls and fractures; and road accidents) as well as future psychological and social problems, for example, stemming from social isolation and progressive dependency. The second assessment target, *I*ndependence, includes the assessment of all functional aspects of daily life, including indoor and outdoor mobility. Even the busiest of professionals has a duty to be aware of major obstacles to independence: screening questionnaires are time-saving tools for this purpose. Third, *L*ifestyle refers to the person's roles and aspirations. Early in PD, paid employment may be a central concern. However, 'lifestyle' issues must not be conflated with independence and physical function; for example, the parental role can be conserved despite a very high level of physical dependency. In considering the effect of PD on personal and social life it is easy to underestimate the stigmatizing effect of parkinsonism, especially tremor which has cultural connotations such as nervousness and alcoholism. Any visible neurological abnormality, however slight, is widely as regarded as a sign of incompetence if not of mental instability. Fourth, *S*ocial resources include the people (spouse, friends, carers) as well as the physical resources (money, housing, transport) which so largely reduce the level of handicap experienced by individuals with PD.

Many scales have been developed for the measurement of deficits in PD (28). The widely used Hoehn and Yahr Scale provides an indication of the stage of progression of motor impairment but is of little value in short-term monitoring of disease. The Webster Scale (29) has the advantage of brevity and ease of use. Because it measures motor impairments and disabilities, the aggregate score is of little value as a guide to management. The Unified PD Rating Scale (30) provides a tool for assessing physical and psychological function but is more suitable for research than for routine use. The PD39 provides a brief, validated overall measure of well-being and function (31).

SETTING SHORT- AND LONG-TERM GOALS

Goal-setting is not a traditional medical concept but is fundamental to good medical as well as non-medical management in PD. The existence of a remedy such as levodopa must not blind the physician to the practical purposes of treatment. The patient must be fully aware that drugs do not modify the course of disease and are justifiable only in so far as they control symptoms which contribute to disabilities or handicaps which are important to the patient, as revealed through the assessment process. Problems which are of central concern to the patient, but not amenable to medical treatment, must be the object of separate therapeutic goals. Such goals must be monitored so that treatment can be tailored to them.

Case report

A local government worker aged 59 was troubled by tremor in his left (non-dominant) hand. He had little or no physical disability. Even the smallest doses of a range of antiparkinsonian drugs caused severe side-effects. A major reason for his rejecting drugs was his anxiety and it became clear that anxiety was as much a cause as an effect of his disability. He was convinced that his colleagues regarded him as incompetent, and he was reluctant to mix socially because of his tremor. Over the next three years, during which he retired from work, it became clear that anxiety rather than tremor should have been the principal target for treatment. The two most effective interventions for him were not drugs, but forms of social support. First, he joined the local branch of the Parkinson's Disease Society and subsequently was helped by a specialist nurse in his locality to set and achieve some simple goals which increased his local mobility while reducing dependency on his wife.

From the moment when the diagnosis has been established the patient, the family, and their professional and non-professional helpers have opportunities to be positive rather than merely reacting to problems as they arise. These opportunities are rarely taken, partly because of a lack of awareness of what can be done. The tendency to 'live each day as it comes' is an essential coping mechanism for some individuals facing the prospect of progressive disability but is indefensible as a professional attitude. It is important that people with PD are aware of how they can, if they wish, modify future outcomes. In PILS terminology, social resources can be adjusted at the earliest stage in order to facilitate future prevention, independence, and lifestyle. For example, a person seeking a new home would be well advised to seek one without steps or stairs, and future transport needs could be taken into account. Similarly, sensible planning at an early stage may enable someone to remain employed as long as possible. At least some action can be taken to promote long-term physical and psychological well-being. For example, a patient can usefully monitor body weight as a future indicator of physical complications or depression. All the publicly available advice concerning healthy eating and physical activity can and should be adapted to people with PD.

SERVICES FOR PARKINSON S DISEASE

Even if drug treatment reverses all disabilities, the psychological fact of PD is immutable and requires a process of psychological adjustment. The most basic service need is for a well-informed professional person who can be a source of information, a contact point for resources, and a listening ear throughout the course of the disease. The general practitioner (GP), who seems a natural choice for this role, can only fulfil it partially. The first major obstacle to providing a comprehensive PD service in general practice is the lack of clinical experience. A group practice of 10000 will include less than 20 patients with PD and only half of these will be significantly disabled (2). A second barrier to broad-based management of PD in general practice is a bias towards purely medical aspects of the disease. GPs refer relatively few patients with PD to therapists (2, 32), partly because PD which is viewed as a 'treatable' (i.e. drug-responsive) disorder. Many individual GPs have demonstrated an ability to overcome these difficulties and to be effective advisers and advocates for people with PD, and more could be done to improve GP training in the management of neurological disorders.

Neurologists based at Regional centres tend to be relatively inaccessible, and could not offer even annual review to most patients with PD. Moreover, British neurologists lack the training to offer a comprehensive support service. Few have detailed knowledge of community health or social services and they rarely encounter patients who are too disabled to attend outpatient clinics. Geriatricians are often in a better position to provide rehabilitative support for all stages of disability (33). However, the extent of their training in the diagnosis and management of PD is variable.

Given current financial constraints, effective new services for people with PD are likely to be based on imaginative and flexible deployment of existing regional and local resources. Diagnosis and early post- diagnosis follow-up should be handled by a consultant geriatrician, neurologist, or general physician with a specific interest in movement disorders. A specialist PD clinic facilitates multidisciplinary support involving, for example, a specialist social worker or nurse (34, 35). The specialist PD clinic can maintain different levels of involvement depending on the requirements of different patients and the capabilities of different primary health care teams. The GP must be closely involved in post-diagnosis counselling and should be identified as the pivotal medical contact for subsequent care. A designated community nurse could potentially monitor the needs of chronically disabled people in a locality and liaise with more specialist services (36).

A specialist PD nurse adviser, ideally based in a specialist PD clinic, can greatly increase the quality of services both locally and centrally. With appropriate training and through the educational effect of clinical experience a nurse can equal and surpass medical trainees in the expert assessment and supervised medical management of PD. In order to acquire adequate clinical experience of complicated PD the nurse adviser must serve a large catchment population and cannot therefore be the mainstay of routine management. The nurse adviser can, however, be a valuable advisory and educational resource for less specialized nursing colleagues working in the community.

THERAPY IN PARKINSON'S DISEASE

There is a growing literature on physiotherapy in PD. There has been a tendency for physiotherapy to emphasize motor impairment rather than disability. Some impairment-orientated studies have shown small or no benefit (37), but several studies have demonstrated improvements in posture or mobility (38).

Much of this work is based on an outpatient model. The work of community physiotherapists in PD has been little studied but appears to be a useful way of assessing and facilitating mobility in the home. Since home mobility is strongly related to equipment and to environmental considerations community physiotherapists must work closely with their occupational therapy colleagues.

Home-based occupational therapy interventions can be of immense practical importance, These range from the supply of small items of equipment such as chair raises to the installation of major home adaptations. There has been lamentably little research on small or large environmental adaptations but they can decisively enhance independence and in many cases self-evidently reduce the risk of home accidents. Occupational therapists can provide more extended, goal-orientated treatment programmes often in a day hospital or outpatient setting with home visits as required. The Parkinson's Disease Society (215 Vauxhall Bridge Road, London SWIV IEJ; tel. 0171 931 8080) has recently produced helpful information packs for occupational therapists and physiotherapists.

In common with physiotherapy, much speech therapy research has been concerned to demonstrate beneficial effects on specific speech impairments in PD (e.g. voice production, articulation, and prosody) (39). Prosody, the patterning of pitch and stress in speech, is specifically impaired in PD. Prosody makes a large contribution to the intelligibility, communicative content, and interest of speech. There is also impairment in the perception of prosodic cues in the speech of others (14), and this receptive deficit also can respond to treatment (40).

One therapeutic technique used in the therapy of PD speech disorders is to provide augmented feedback information displayed graphically on a computer screen (e.g. Visispeech) (41). Voice amplifiers are helpful for severe dysphonia, especially if the spouse has impaired hearing. An important preliminary to any speech therapy is to assess the patient's and spouse's hearing. Therapy for dysfluent, 'festinating' speech includes pacing, teaching the patient to tap the finger slowly for each word, or providing a marked ruler along which the finger moves to signal each word in the phrase. A device to provide delayed auditory feedback increases intelligibility by slowing speech and improving voice volume (41). Dysfluency and festinating are exacerbated by anxiety which should be a specific target for counselling and therapy

Several forms of PD therapy can be effectively delivered in a group setting. One group occupational therapy study showing benefits for patients with PD included an element of physiotherapy, to enhance mobility, as well as inputs focused on self-care (42). Another example of an interprofessional approach was a study in which nurses implemented exercise programmes (43). Physiotherapy groups are popular with patients and are often set up by a local branch of the Parkinson's Disease Society (PDS). At the very least they can be expected to enhance physical and social confidence.

Speech therapy can also be enhanced by group work. Any successful group is likely to lessen the social impact of impaired communication. A swimming group is an example of an enjoyable setting for enhancing communication (41). Such activities help to restore a sense of control or self-efficacy. Day centres can potentially fulfil some of the same social functions, provided the client's communicative and other specific needs are understood and met. Another important setting for peer support is local branch meetings of the PDS. A link with the branch can often be set through a non-professional welfare worker employed by the PDS branch.

Drug therapy

L-dopa (levodopa). In the 1950s, PD was shown to be due to deficiency of dopamine in the striatum. Dopamine does not cross the blood–brain barrier but levo-dihydroxyphenylalanine (L-dopa) does. In the brain it is metabolized to dopamine and, in PD, stored and used by the surviving dopaminergic neurones. In the 1960s, L-dopa was introduced for the treatment of PD and produced dramatic symptomatic improvement, it has remained the mainstay of treatment ever since. Initially, large doses of L-dopa were given to compensate for metabolism to dopamine outside the brain by peripheral dopa decarboxylase. The peripherally produced dopamine caused severe side-effects such as vomiting, cardiac dysrhythmias, and hypotension. Later, L-dopa was combined with a peripherally acting dopa decarboxylase inhibitor (carbidopa in Sinemet and benserazide in Madopar) allowing the use of lower doses of L-dopa and reducing the incidence and severity of the peripheral side-effects. Most patients with early PD demonstrate a complete or good symptomatic improvement with L-dopa and failure to respond should prompt a reconsideration of the diagnosis.

The major problem in the treatment of PD is that the initial smooth response to L-dopa usually only lasts a few years, the 'honeymoon period'. After five years of treatment at least 50% of patients will be experiencing motor fluctuations and dyskinesias and this percentage increases with time. The motor fluctuations begin with a 'wearing off' of the effect of L-dopa as the time for the next dose approaches. Later, erratic and unpredictable fluctuations occur with a state of mobility switching to akinesia over minutes, the 'on-off' effect. Dyskinesias usually appear at about this time. These consist of involuntary choreoform or dystonic movements initially occurring at the time of peak action (peak dose dyskinesia) and later occurring as the plasma level of L-dopa is rising and falling (biphasic dyskinesia). The consistent long duration improvement seen with each dose early in the disease declines and eventually the patient is either 'on', but dyskinetic, or 'off'. These complications may be related to postsynaptic receptor changes or the continued depletion of dopaminergic neurons with a reduction in the dopamine storage capacity. L-dopa can also precipitate confusion and psychosis particularly in the elderly or demented patients, and despite the dopa decarboxylase inhibitor can cause nausea and hypotension.

It has been suggested that L-dopa, while providing symptomatic treatment, may increase the rate of dopaminergic neurone depletion and actually accelerate the disease process. The conversion of L-dopa to dopamine and the metabolism of dopamine produce free radicals that may induce damaging oxidative stress within dopaminergic neurones. L-dopa induces nigral cell loss in rodent models of PD (44), but not in normal rodents and causes apoptosis in cultured neuronal cells (45). However, there is no clinical evidence that treatment of PD with L-dopa accelerates the disease process.

Dopamine agonists exert their therapeutic effect by direct stimulation of postsynaptic dopamine receptors. There is no reliance on surviving dopaminergic neurones. Agonists can be divided into those derived from ergotamine (bromocriptine, cabergoline, and pergolide) and those not ergot-derived (apomorphine, ropinirole, and pramipexole). Both groups can produce confusion, hallucinations, nausea, and hypotension but only the ergot-derived have been associated with pulmonary and peritoneal fibrosis. Agonists rarely produce motor fluctuations and dyskinesia but have a greater tendency to produce psychosis in the elderly or demented and appear less therapeutically potent than L-dopa. In newly diagnosed PD patients, bromocriptine monotherapy was successful in 40% at one year and 6% at five years (46), although in a recent report (47) cabergoline monotherapy was as effective as L-dopa monotherapy (80% adequately treated) at one year. Pergolide is probably better tolerated and more effective than bromocriptine (48) but at present there appears to be little difference in efficacy between the newer agonists, ie pergolide, cabergoline, ropinirole and pramipexole. . Early combination of an agonist with L-dopa allows lower doses of L-dopa to be used with satisfactory response and may delay the onset of motor fluctuations and dyskynesias (46), although this has not been demonstrated in all studies.

There is speculation that agonists may be neuroprotective; stimulation of presynaptic D_2 autoreceptors reduces the firing rate of dopaminergic neurones, possibly reducing oxidative stress within those neurones. However, there is no evidence that agonists delay the progression of PD.

Selegiline (Deprenyl) inhibits monoamine oxidase B prolonging the half-life of dopamine. Laboratory experiments suggested it may be neuroprotective. The DATATOP study (49) reported that selegiline treatment delayed the need for L-dopa and suggested this may be due to neuroprotection. However, reassessment of the results of the DATATOP study concluded that all the benefit from selegiline could be due to mild improvement in symptoms and that there is no evidence of neuroprotection (3). The latest updates on the patients who participated in the DATATOP study found that selegiline treatment did not confer any lasting benefit (50, 51). Selegiline delays the need for L-dopa and lower doses of L-dopa can be used but it does not delay the onset of fluctuations nor dyskinesia 50. In 1995, it was reported that selegiline treatment was associated with a 60% increased mortality that had not been reported in previous studies (52). Selegiline's place in the treatment of PD continues to be debated, occasional patients derive good symptomatic improvement. Selegiline is generally well tolerated but can cause insomnia and hallucinations.

Antimuscarinic agents and amantadine. Antimuscarinic agents have little or no effect on bradykinesia but may reduce tremor. They are infrequently used because of side-effects including dry mouth, urinary retention and confusion, especially in the elderly. Amantadine was developed as an antiviral agent and fortuitously found to improve the symptoms of PD. This may be due to increasing dopamine release. However, few patients derive significant benefit and it can cause livedo reticularis, insomnia, and hallucinations.

Catechol-*O*-methyl transferase (COMT) inhibitors. COMT is an enzyme widely distributed in the central nervous system (CNS) and periphery. L-dopa is converted by COMT to a metabolite that competes with L-dopa for active transport across both the gut and the blood–brain barrier. Tolcapone, the first of the group, is due for release in late 1997. Tolcapone inhibits COMT peripherally and centrally prolonging the action of L-dopa and reducing L-dopa requirement (53), its main side-effect is diarrhoea which occurs in about 7%.

SOCIAL AND PSYCHOLOGICAL SUPPORT

The psychological and social effects of PD are often a significant source of disability and handicap (22, 23, 54). Referral to a social worker is a useful means of mobilizing practical resources including financial benefits, but a social worker's counselling skills can also be invaluable to individuals and families (55). Published descriptions of the experience of PD give valuable insight into the territory which supportive counselling may encounter (56).

At a national and regional level the Parkinson's Disease Society (PDS) provides peer support for different subgroups, including younger people with PD. Activists can find a useful social role within self-help groups such as the PDS or through other organizations campaigning on behalf of disabled people.

PHASES OF MANAGEMENT

For the patient, the family and the physician, the management of PD is a lifelong task which can be divided into a number of phases. The first phase is initiated by establishing the diagnosis and discussing its implications. One obvious task in this first phase is to establish a therapeutic plan to control presenting symptoms. There then often follows a period of successful response to treatment with few if any physical disabilities. This period provides an opportunity to lay the foundations for good management in succeeding phases. While some patients will opt to 'live each day as it comes', others will wish to plan actively for the future, taking whatever action is possible to prevent disabilities and complications.

A second phase is marked by the reassertion of impairments. A continuous process of therapeutic 'nipping and tucking' aims to keep pace with progressive disease and to accommodate more complex responses to treatment. In the third phase, often overlapping with the second phase, management of disability becomes the dominant issue.

PHASE 1: DIAGNOSIS AND EARLY TREATMENT

COMMUNICATING THE DIAGNOSIS AND PROGNOSIS

This is a skilled process. All too often this crucial task is delegated to a relatively inexperienced doctor—perhaps a junior trainee—who has limited understanding of the multiple manifestations of PD and little or no knowledge of the range and severity of disabilities experienced outside the confines of a hospital clinic.

Learning the diagnosis is a defining moment in the life—the 'career'—of someone with PD. For many people personal experience rather than general knowledge determines their concerns about the future. Their imagined identities as PD 'sufferers' are likely to be coloured by diverse images, for example of an elderly relative in a wheelchair, or of someone with severe Alzheimer's disease. On the other hand, they may have seen a television documentary in which someone with PD appears to be miraculously cured by neurosurgery. People with such variable preconceptions are ill-prepared for standardized information whether from a doctor or nurse, or from a book or leaflet. They need sources of advice and information which match their own requirements at different stages in a process of learning and adaptation which often continues for years after initial diagnosis.

Prognosis needs to be communicated first in terms of natural history and secondly in terms of response to treatment. The patient's initial questions about *natural history* of PD are likely to be confined to the rate of progression, which varies from one individual to another but does not vary dramatically for any one individual. Individuals differ greatly in their demand for details of impending disabilities. There may (or may not) be prejudices and fears concerning the nature of the disease process and the way in which it advances. Is it like a cancer? Does it cause pain? What kills you? The cause of death is often bronchopneumonia and it is reasonable to use the phrase 'you die *with* PD, not *of* PD'. To many, the concept of PD as a brain disorder immediately suggests the spectre of dementia and it is often important to draw a clear distinction between 'the brain' and 'the mind'. The possibility of future dementia cannot be denied but the risk of severe or early onset dementia is low.

Many people are given misleading information about prognosis for *response to treatment*. On the one hand, there are physicians who eulogize the effects of drugs, as though patients should be grateful to have the diagnosis of PD since it is 'treatable'. This approach ignores the considerable risk of misdiagnosis and therefore the possibility of disappointing response to treatment. Moreover, even when the diagnosis is correct the patient cannot expect all impairments to respond equally well to drugs. Bradykinesia, and all the motor disabilities stemming from slowness of movement, usually respond to drug treatment. The response of tremor is less predictable. Some other impairments, for example in speech, are much less responsive. Predicting response to treatment must also take account of the likelihood of future fluctuations in response to drugs. These can be a source of disability in their own right but their effects are sometimes exaggerated in the imaginations of patients who have never experienced them. They are experienced by the majority of those receiving effective treatment over a 3-to 5-year period but only a relatively few patients are severely disabled by them. Many people with PD are still gaining functional benefit from drug treatment throughout their lives.

After diagnosis the patient and family need time for reflection. The first interview will have raised new questions without necessarily answering all their original concerns. At least one follow-up interview is required even if subsequent care is to be co-ordinated elsewhere. An appropriately experienced professional such as a social worker, working closely with a consultant, can improve the quality of communication and can lay the foundations for effective subsequent support (54, 57). If the cost of such a service is prohibitive there is some benefit in a follow-up phone call by a nurse or doctor from the clinic, the day after an initial appointment.

SETTING GOALS FOR DRUG TREATMENT

As emphasized earlier, good management depends on establishing appropriate therapeutic goals. The therapeutic goals of drug treatment are not self-evident but need to be specified and agreed. Drugs represent just one of the modalities available within a management plan which must encompass issues,

such as prevention, independence, lifestyle, and social resources. The patient must understand that success is judged solely by the extent to which psychological and practical benefits are experienced in daily life, since drug treatment cannot arrest the disease process. Accordingly, patients should be encouraged to influence decisions about timing and dosage: compliance is usually good, and most patients err on the side of rigid adherence to drug regimes when a little flexibility would be more helpful to them.

Common sense dictates that drug dosage should be minimized and polypharmacy avoided. Controversy surrounds strategies to prevent later problems of dyskinesia and variable drug response. The early use of selegiline has a L-dopa-sparing effect. Alternatively, dopamine agonists used *de novo* are less likely to lead to such complications but are also less likely to be sufficiently effective to attain a specific functional goal. When such a goal is clearly in sight, it is sometimes hard to justify delaying the use of the most consistently effective drug, L-dopa, merely in order to delay the onset of later complications.

DRUG TREATMENT IN EARLY PARKINSON'S DISEASE

The major difficulties in the treatment of PD, (i.e. motor fluctuations and dyskinesia), are related to duration of dopamine replacement. L-dopa therapy is delayed at least until motor symptoms are having a significant impact on the patient's activities. There is a trend towards prescribing dopamine agonists earlier, rather than use them as L-dopa sparing agents when the complications of L-dopa therapy appear. This trend is justified by the findings in most of the relevant studies that patients treated with an agonist as monotherapy or in combination with low dose L-dopa have a lower incidence of fluctuations and dyskinesia than patients treated with L-dopa alone.

At the time of diagnosis many patients have minor symptoms which do not warrant symptomatic treatment. Some neurologists continue to recommend selegiline at this stage. When symptomatic treatment becomes necessary the choice is between L-dopa, an agonist, or both, except in a young otherwise healthy patient whose main symptom is tremor when an antimuscarinic agent may be tried first. Antimuscarinic agents and agonists are avoided in the elderly who are more prone to develop the psychiatric side-effects.

In the elderly (>70 years old) most agree that L-dopa monotherapy is the first line treatment. It is often started in two or three doses a day of 50 mg with 12.5 mg of dopa decarboxylase inhibitor. The dose is increased every two or three days until there is an adequate response or the side-effects develop. In younger patients there are three alternatives to this approach:

1. Start L-dopa monotherapy but if more than a moderate dose (300 mg a day) is necessary add an agonist rather than continue increasing the L-dopa dose.

2. Start agonist monotherapy and increase the dose until there is an adequate response or the dose is not tolerated in which case add low dose L-dopa (58).
3. Start low dose L-dopa and an agonist in combination (46).

Young patients, with onset at less than 40 years of age, are less likely to develop the psychiatric side-effects of agonists and may develop L-dopa-related fluctuations and dyskinesia earlier (59). The argument in favour of a trial of agonist monotherapy is most persuasive in this group of patients. However, against the possible advantages of agonist monotherapy one needs to balance the cost of the drug and the psychological setback incurred if the agonist fails to produce symptomatic improvement or the benefit is short lived. Nocturnal akinesia can interfere with sleep and may be improved by taking a controlled release (CR) preparation of L-dopa on retiring. Akinesia on waking may also improve with a late dose of a CR preparation, alternatively dispersible Madopar can be used as a 'kick-start' to the day.

The most common early side-effects of L-dopa and agonists are nausea, vomiting, and postural hypotension. Taking the L-dopa with food can prevent nausea. Domperidone, a dopamine antagonist that does not cross the blood–brain barrier so does not aggravate PD, can alleviate all three adverse effects. Fludrocortisone in a dose of 0.1 mg once or twice a day may correct the postural hypotension.

PREVENTIVE MEASURES

Individuals will vary in the extent to which they wish to take action in an attempt to anticipate and prevent future problems. Some general preventive issues (e.g. concerning housing) were discussed earlier in the section on goal-setting. Such considerations may come to the fore at the earliest stage of PD, or they may not seem relevant until a later stage, when disabilities become obvious. Many people will ask for advice on physical exercises designed to maintain mobility and fitness. A physiotherapist may provide such a programme following a single assessment, rather than engaging in an extended (and costly) series of repeated outpatient visits at a stage when physical disability is minimal. There is some support for the intuition that preventive exercises are helpful. An early study retrospectively compared the outcomes of 200 patients, half of whom received physiotherapy. After 10 years only 13 of the treated group had severe disability, compared with 55 in the untreated group (60). General physical fitness and healthy eating are important in PD as in the general population. Good dental care is especially important: later in the disease process dental problems may impair communication and swallowing.

An important aim of management of early PD is to prevent psychiatric complications. While there is no evidence that either anxiety or depression can be prevented, common sense suggests that at least some predisposing factors can be modified. The provision of effective support and adequate

information at the outset and at all subsequent stages of PD is likely to reduce the risk of anxiety. Relaxation routines are built into some physiotherapeutic regimes and may help the patient to retain some control over mood swings (61). Early advice, with insight into the progressive negative effects of anxiety, may help to prevent anxiety becoming amplified to the point that social life becomes severely restricted.

Depression in PD is at least partly situational and the most useful preventive interventions may be measures to reduce social isolation and to increase communication rather than drug treatment (62). Maintaining relationships and social roles depends to a great degree on effective communication (63). Patients and families may be better able to compensate for the negative social effects of impaired communication if a therapist is able to give them insight into present and potential problems at an early stage. Patients are insufficiently aware of the monotony and low volume of their speech and of its adverse social effects (64). It may help them to realize that reduced facial expression has an effect on the social impression which a person makes. With a soft voice and an undemonstrative body (65), the person with PD may find it difficult to gain entry into a group conversation. Because PD speech is slow and disjointed friends and family need to be reminded to allow time for the person with PD to contribute. These insights need to be established early, before bad communicative habits become established within the family unit.

Psychological support is often helpful in adjusting to loss of status, of competencies, and of independence. Withdrawn mood and impaired communication are among a number of factors which can lead to a shift in roles within and outside the home. As the person's physical dependency increases a spouse may adopt a dominant role so that the 'patient' is progressively excluded from an equal marital relationship or position in a family. Family and social relationships may suffer progressively from maladaptive processes which can be reversed or at least mitigated through skilled counselling by a social worker or other qualified and suitably experienced professional.

One relatively easily prevented psychiatric problem is acute drug-induced psychosis. This complication must be avoided if at all possible since it may trigger catastrophes such as premature loss of employment, irremediable marital breakdown, or institutional care. Predisposing factors include any previous episode of hallucination or confusion, any evidence of coexisting cerebral pathology, coexisting infection, high doses of any antiparkinsonian medication (especially in elderly people) (66), the use of ergot agonists (58) and other dopamine agonists, and polypharmacy. In one large series, 8% of hospital admissions for drug-induced delirium or psychosis were patients with PD.

INDEPENDENCE

Practical problems in washing, dressing, and eating are often due to bradykinesia, for example, manifesting in deficits in rapid repeated movements such as tooth brushing. These impairments often respond to levodopa and their associated disabilities often also benefit from occupational therapist (OT) advice (67). One of the simplest ideas is to use velcro fastenings for clothes and shoes. Patients will gain new practical ideas from exhibitions of equipment held in local equipment stores. Among many useful items are electric toothbrushes, adapted cutlery, non-slip plates, and other adaptations for crockery, and equipment such as trolleys to facilitate carrying (67).

General mobility including walking and transfers are also generally improved by dopaminomimetic drugs such as levodopa. Transfers are improved by raising the level of the bed, chairs, and toilet seat, and by installing grab rails. The OT will also help with access to the house and garden, and transfers into a car. Driving is an important consideration in early PD (68). The UK licensing authority must be informed by the licence holder following the diagnosis of PD. Competence depends less on physical than on cognitive factors. Simple reaction times—and therefore stopping times—are delayed in PD and cannot easily be predicted from other measures of bradykinesia (69). Impairments in performing dual tasks, and in shifting mental 'set' (16), raise questions about how the driver will respond to complex traffic situations. The presence of peripheral visual illusions, especially at night, presents a further potential hazard. When an individual with PD feels subjectively competent to drive and is legally permitted to do so, the best advice is to cease driving if passengers expresses anxieties about competence. If in doubt, driving should be restricted to familiar conditions in daylight. The physician should discourage driving if there is clinical evidence of perceptual or cognitive impairment. Difficulties can be resolved by obtaining a road assessment either in a driving assessment centre or with a qualified instructor.

LIFESTYLE: ROLES AND OCCUPATIONS

Steps taken in early PD can be helpful in conserving and developing social roles. The person with PD may wish for a social worker in collaboration with a doctor to negotiate with employers to maintain employment or to negotiate early retirement. The importance of other equally important roles must be understood and accommodated so far as possible. The sustaining of roles is often complicated by other life transitions occurring in parallel with the onset of disease: children may be leaving home, and retirement age may be approaching. Early advice and interventions can help to prevent the development of a sick role, and to protect symbolic as well as practical aspects of existing roles among family and friends.

Occupational therapy advice can be helpful, for example, in suggesting simple pieces of equipment which can facilitate role performance at home or in the workplace. These include, for example, thickened pens, computer keyboards, electronic notebooks, and alarm watches as memory aids at home or at work. For many, the scope for meaningful occupation is lim-

ited (70) but some people are able to continue unlikely hobbies such as painting and model-making. If there is diplopia for close work, as in reading, the problem may be impaired ocular convergence which is correctable with spectacle lens prisms.

SEXUAL FUNCTION, MENSTRUATION, AND CHILDBEARING

Sexual dysfunction is rarely discussed at any stage of PD but is a concern of many couples of all ages. Most are grateful for the opportunity of discussing their concerns even if there is no practical outcome. Sexual dysfunction has been increasingly documented in PD (71, 72). Physical factors include autonomic dysfunction due to PD itself or to drugs, lack of mobility, fatigue, and bladder dysfunction. Psychological factors include depression and depleted self-image associated with PD. Communicative difficulties were often identified as damaging the sexual relationship in 20 couples surveyed by Wilkinson and Ward (unpublished). Antiparkinsonian drugs can cause increase in sexual content of dreams and an increase in sexual behaviours which are not always welcomed by partners. A partner who is also a carer may withdraw from a sexual relationship. A trained sexual counsellor can help to unravel these complexities but will need to understand the special context of PD. Counselling can assist in increasing insight between partners, and in providing 'permission' for different expressions of physical affection. Strategies such as choosing different times of day for intercourse and altering drug schedules to increase mobility can be helpful for some. Practical measures include vaginal lubrication, and drugs to enhance erectile function.

Few women spontaneously report menstrual difficulties and the topic must be raised by the doctor as a routine enquiry. Nursing advice will often produce practical solutions to menstrual problems due to the difficulty of managing menstrual hygiene when disability is severe. Parkinsonian deficits can worsen during the menstrual period (73). Numerous women with PD have had successful pregnancies (74). Evidence is necessarily limited and manufacturers' advice is cautious, but there is no evidence that L-dopa and decarboxylase inhibitors are teratogenic even though, theoretically, L-dopa might be expected to affect etal dopaminergic cells.

MOOD DISTURBANCE

Preventive management of anxiety was discussed earlier. Psychological forms of anxiety management, supervised by a clinical psychologist, can be effective. Anxiolytic drugs have a limited role. Benzodiazepines are not often effective. For mild anxiety, especially when associated with sleep disturbance, amitriptyline is often useful. For more severe anxiety a neuroleptic such as flupenthixol may be unavoidable. The benefit of relieved anxiety often outweighs any extrapyramidal adverse effects. The non-drug management of depression was discussed earlier under the heading of prevention. Antidepressant drugs are often useful, as would be expected in view of evidence that depressive illness is specifically associated with PD and is not merely a reaction to chronic disability (75). Since depression in PD is often associated with sleep disorder and also with anxiety, a tricyclic such as amitriptyline is often the drug of choice. There is no evidence that newer antidepressant agents, such as selective serotonin re-uptake inhibitors, are as effective as amitriptyline, although there have unfortunately been no relevant trials as yet.

Drug-induced psychosis is difficult to manage (24). Withdrawal of medication does not necessarily resolve the episode. Clozapine is an effective antipsychotic agent with relatively mild extrapyramidal side-effects (76), but patients on clozapine must be monitored closely.

SLEEP

Sleep disturbance, which is a common complaint in PD, is distressing and places a large burden on carers when they are required to help in transferring out of bed many times during the night. Sleep disturbance also reduces the quality of life during the day. This is partly because motor impairment is worsened after a sleepless night. Dopamine receptors are more responsive after sleep (12), and the clinical phenomenon of 'sleep benefit' is well recognized. Disturbed nights are often caused by the sheer physical discomfort of rigidity and bradykinesia, compounded by difficulty in turning in bed. The first recourse should be to the usual range of 'sleep hygiene' measures which do not require specific medication. Secondly, the patient can be taught manoevres to make it possible to turn over in bed independently. These include (for some individuals) nylon sheets, bed socks, a rope attached to the side or end of the bed, a monkey pole above the bed, suitably placed rails, or methods of physical mobility learned from a physiotherapist. A third possibility is the addition of antiparkinsonian medication to reduce nocturnal bradykinesia. L-dopa at bedtime with repeated doses as necessary, usually in controlled release form, can be very effective provided they do not cause nightmares, confusion, or excessive involuntary movements. Benzodiazepines such as temazepam are often ineffective; chloral hydrate or its derivatives, or amitriptyline are preferable.

PAIN

Musculoskeletal aches and pains are a frequent presenting symptom in PD. Increasing the dose of L-dopa can be helpful when muscle rigidity is causing physical discomfort (5).

PHASE 2: PROGRESSIVE DISABILITY

Following the early phase of PD, during which response to treatment is often relatively uncomplicated, physical disabilities begin to reassert themselves. Response to drugs becomes less predictable and drug treatment becomes more complex.

Good management aims, as at all stages of PD, to focus on specific functional goals. Doses and dose schedules are determined empirically in close collaboration with the patient. Communication between the doctor and the patient must be clear: both must understand the goals of treatment and both must agree what constitute better and worse outcomes. Achieving such a consensus is difficult: for example, the doctor may be more alarmed by drug-induced dyskinesias than is the patient or the doctor, or the patient and the carer may have different views on the advisability of sacrificing mobility in order to reduce the incidence of hallucinations. A further potential source of confusion arises when the patient and the doctor do not have a common language to describe 'on' and 'off' states: this can be overcome by asking the patient to fill in a diary of mobility whilst under observation in the clinic.

During the second phase of PD the emphasis of care, and therefore of the preventive agenda, still encompasses psychosocial issues but is also increasingly concerned with critical physical factors such as safety (falls and fractures), skin care and positioning (seating, bedding), nutrition (dysphagia, loss of weight or, less commonly, obesity), and bladder and bowel management.

RECOGNIZING DISABILITY

At a certain stage, a person with PD begins to regard him or herself as 'disabled'. For many people this perception occurs some time after the fact of PD has been absorbed, because effective initial treatment often eliminates most disabilities. Disability will often not be acknowledged initially lest visible physical limitations be seen as a signal of defeat in the continuing struggle against disease. Recognizing disability therefore often entails a new phase of psychological and social adjustment, confronting some of the themes (notably of loss) covered at the time of diagnosis. Practical issues connected with employment, housing, finances, transport, and so on, may now be openly considered in a forward-looking strategy which seemed unthinkable in the first phase of the disease. Family and professional attitudes are also often transformed. A spouse or partner becomes labelled as a 'carer'. This is helpful in so far as it raises awareness of the psychological, social, and physical resources which can support the caring role. However, the 'patient' (as he or she is now openly called) is right to fear that the carer role can disastrously undermine pre-existing relationships. For GPs, acknowledgment of disability is usually helpful and sometimes long overdue. The horizons of management become wider when the GP realizes that drug treatment is not the sole or even necessarily the primary consideration.

POSTURE, MOBILITY, AND FALLING

Postural changes associated with PD cause many problems. Head flexion is socially stigmatizing, impairs communication (see above), and can contribute to dysphagia (see below).

Kyphoscoliosis is unsightly, is uncomfortable, and sometimes painful, and adds to the risk of falling. Moreover severe scoliosis, which develops in some patients with markedly asymmetrical parkinsonism, causes uneven weight distribution in the sitting position and is a risk factor for pressure sores. The preventive effects of good positioning and of orthoses are well recognized in spasticity but are uncertain in PD. Contractures of the extremities are rare in PD although they do occur (77) and require splinting in the hope of preventing further deformity and disability. It is uncertain whether postural correction in gait training is helpful but it can be recommended early in PD with the aim of reducing the likelihood of severe disability later on. Seating should be reviewed if kyphoscoliosis is developing. Good side support for the trunk is advisable for reasons of safety and comfort, and may reduce future deformity. A slight recline to the back of a chair is more likely than a collar to be helpful for dystonic neck flexion. side support, or in extreme cases strapping, is required for scoliosis.

As PD advances, mobility is characteristically erratic, despite optimal drug treatment. Freezing episodes are more likely at times when drug treatment is generally less effective and may be reduced by optimizing drug regimes, but are still liable to occur at any time. They can often be overcome by various manoeuvres. Many patients discover for themselves 'tricks' such as making a high stepping motion over a carer's shoe, or a real or imagined line on the floor (78). A similar cue can be provided by a short cross-piece attached to the lower end of a walking stick, and some patients walk with an inverted stick, using the handle to similar effect. (79). Sometimes, a helper can set off the gait pattern by gently grasping the person's shoulders and gently rocking motion the upper body from side to side. Relaxation techniques can reduce freezing episodes which are much more likely when there is a sense of urgency (e.g. in crossing a busy road or getting out of a taxi). When all else fails, akinesia can nearly always be reversed with a subcutaneous injection which can be administered, through clothing if necessary, to resolve a crisis. Most patients continue to require regular doses of oral domperidone (80). The availability of apomorphine is helpful in itself. The existence of a potential 'life-belt' relieves anxiety and makes possible a wider range of social activities by boosting confidence.

Walking aids have not been formally evaluated in PD. Walking sticks are of little mechanical value—the patient with PD often carries the stick rather than leaning on it. The stick acts as a signal to passers-by to keep their distance. Standard Zimmer frames are unsatisfactory because lifting the frame requires a ballistic truncal movement of a type which is impaired in PD. The most useful walking frames are those with wheels, especially if there is a braking mechanism as in the triangular Delta frame (67). Wheelchairs are not used solely for severe disability; a chair is very helpful for someone with well-preserved walking but unpredictable akinetic episodes.

Falling is common in PD (81) and there is a high risk of fractures. Many risk factors for falling are not specific to PD.

These include cognitive impairment, sedative drugs, environmental factors, and postural hypotension. The latter is specifically associated with multisystem atrophy of Shy–Drager type, but also seems to be more prevalent in PD (82), although postural hypotension did not account for the high frequency of falls in one survey (81). The postural hypotension sometimes associated with L-dopa treatment is partly due to peripheral effects of dopamine which can sometimes be alleviated by increasing the dose of decarboxylase inhibitor or by the addition of selegiline. The peripheral effects of dopaminergic agonists also cause postural hypotension which can often be corrected by the addition of domperidone as a peripherally acting dopamine antagonist. These manoeuvres fail when the cause of postural hypotension is central rather than peripheral. Amitriptyline is of special note among the many other drugs which cause postural hypotension, since it is often used and often helpful in PD (see above).

Several risk factors are specific to PD. Postural instability is a cardinal feature of parkinsonism. Patients often report that falls are entirely unpredictable, but turning and reaching are typical causes. The best advice is to walk through an arc rather than turning abruptly on the heel (doing a 'military wheel' rather than 'about turn') because in a sharp turn the pivotal heel tends to drag, producing instability (Ashburn, personal communication). However, it is impossible to avoid impulsive turns and the most useful interventions are home adaptations supervised by an OT, for example, removing the need to reach upwards (e.g. to fix curtains), lowering cupboards, and installing grab rails. Stooping is another risky manoeuvre, as is carrying, and a grab stick and a trolley are useful. A physiotherapist can teach the patient and carer techniques for getting up off the floor and a newly available inflatable device can enable a person to rise to the standing position independently. For those living alone an alarm system is required. Severe drug-induced truncal dyskinesia is likely to be implicated in some falls although not a major cause of falls in one study (81).

The risk of fractures, especially of the hip, is further increased by a reduction of bone density associated specifically with PD (83). Routine vitamin D supplements, and other measures to reduce the rate of decreasing bone density, should be considered.

FEEDING AND NUTRITION

PD raises numerous dietetic issues (84). These include the management of protein intake in order to manage erratic L-dopa treatment (85), obesity (which is uncommon, but adds to disability), and weight loss.

Recording of body weight is invaluable in the management of all stages of PD. Obesity is rare, but weight loss is common. The cause is sometimes mysterious but most weight loss is due to treatable (or at least manageable) factors. Drug-induced nausea is a common cause, often correctable with domperidone. Another important cause of weight loss is increased caloric demand caused by severe tremor, muscle rigidity, or drug-induced dyskinesia. Caloric supplements are required. Depression is a common and treatable cause of weight loss in PD.

Weight loss is one manifestation of feeding and swallowing problems. Very slow or inefficient feeding makes cooked food grow cold and unappetizing. The cause of slowness may be general bradykinesia or the problem may be impaired mastication and swallowing. Dental problems may contribute. Weight loss is sometimes the only clue to the presence of dysphagia. Dysphagia is relatively common in PD although only a minority of patients experience severe complications such as aspiration pneumonia (8). The patient will sometimes report difficulty in swallowing; significant aspiration is sometimes asymptomatic although there may be clues such as postprandial bronchospasm or recurrent episodes of pneumonia. Although dysphagia does partially respond to improved antiparkinsonian drug treatment (86) a speech/language therapist will often be required to advise on safe feeding techniques, postural problems such as excessive neck flexion, and food consistency. Indications for the use of a percutaneous endoscopic gastrostomy (PEG) feeding tube are controversial but a PEG is certainly justified if feeding is causing distress despite optimal management of dysphagia.

Drooling, reported by 40% of patients in one survey (32), is a distressing symptom which probably results from reduced automatic swallowing rather than from abnormal salivary secretion. Reducing salivary flow with anticholinergic drugs or by irradiating salivary glands does not always have sufficient cosmetic effect and may reduce the efficiency of swallowing. A less drastic measure is to improve head posture in the sitting position. If a bib is used, black towelling will make the patient look ecclesiastic rather than paediatric.

RESPIRATION

Bronchopneumonia is a common cause of death in PD. Mechanisms of respiratory dysfunction in PD are multifactorial (87). One potentially preventable factor is dystonic postural flexion leading to kyphosis. Respiratory exercises are of unproven value. Recurrent episodes of upper respiratory tract infection should suggest the presence of dysphagia and aspiration.

BLADDER AND BOWELS

There is evidence against the widely held belief that PD causes specific neurogenic bladder dysfunction. Nevertheless, urinary urgency and frequency are common complaints (88). Incontinence is often a secondary effect of motor slowing during the process of going to the lavatory and undressing. Velcro fastenings and other modifications to clothing are helpful. During the night, frequent visits to the lavatory are one of the major causes of carer stress. They are often caused more by nocturnal restlessness and anxiety than by urological prob-

lems and the solution may lie in improved sleep (see above). Nocturnal Desmopressin nasal spray occasionally helps by reducing night-time urinary secretion, but many patients have a subjective desire to pass urine even with small bladder volumes. Anticholinergic drugs, and constipation, are two other factors which commonly cause bladder problems. The many psychological and physical factors contributing to bladder problems should be thoroughly investigated, ideally by a trained continence advisor with experience of PD. Many men with PD are submitted to prostate operations, only to find that their symptoms are unchanged.

People with PD are often troubled by constipation. Specific PD-related causative factors include reduced fluid intake on account of dysphagia or bladder problems; anticholinergic drugs; and possibly intrinsic autonomic dysfunction. Pseudo-obstruction is an occasional complication of chronic constipation. Initial management includes a decisive increase in fluid intake, a modest increase in fibre intake, stool softeners, and stimulant laxatives. Large increases in fibre and agents which increase faecal bulk will be ineffective and potentially hazardous if bowel mobility is reduced either by drugs or by autonomic dysfunction.

DRUG TREATMENT OF LATE PARKINSON S DISEASE

As symptomatic control deteriorates the doses of L-dopa and the agonist are gradually increased. If fluctuations, dyskinesia, and psychiatric symptoms emerge the physician and patient need to find the most acceptable balance between the mobility gained and the side-effects induced by the treatment.

Motor fluctuations and dyskinesia may improve by giving less L-dopa more often, switching to CR preparations of L-dopa (18) or reducing the total dose of L-dopa, and if necessary increasing the dose of the agonist. Dietary amino acids compete with L-dopa for absorption and transport into the brain so taking L-dopa 30 minutes before food and avoiding high protein meals may help prevent large fluctuations in the plasma level of L-dopa and smoothen the response. Selegiline prolongs the action of L-dopa and can reduce the wearing-off effect. Cabergoline is a long-acting ergot agonist and may be more useful than other agonists in treating patients with motor fluctuations (90). Tolcapone may be also be beneficial producing a smoother response to L-dopa and allowing a reduction in the dose (53). Apomorphine can help selected patients severely handicapped by fluctuations and dyskinesia that have not responded to the above measures. It is given subcutaneously as bolus doses to treat severe, unpredictable periods of akinesia or as a continuous daytime infusion allowing large reductions in the doses of L-dopa. Pallidotomy can dramatically improve contralateral dyskinesia, this is discussed below.

Psychiatric symptoms usually consist of paranoia, hallucinations, or confusion. The hallucinations are usually visual and are generally non-threatening. The onset of psychiatric symptoms frequently lead to nursing home placement. The first step is to reduce the dose of the agonist and any antimuscarinic agents. It may be necessary to increase the dose of L-dopa to maintain mobility but this can cause a re-emergence of the psychiatric symptoms. The newer atypical neuroleptics, clozapine, risperidone, and olanzapine can help control the treatment related psychosis and are less likely than the older neuroleptics to aggravate the parkinsonian symptoms.

SURGICAL TREATMENT OF PARKINSON'S DISEASE

In 1817, James Parkinson noted that the tremor of one of his patients markedly improved following a stroke. In the 1950s, surgery aimed at several targets within the thalamus and globus pallidus was commonly performed but poorly reported. The introduction of L-dopa in the 1960s led to these procedures being virtually abandoned but recently there has been a resurgence of interest. The most popular techniques are stereotactic destructive surgery or deep brain stimulation (DBS) of the globus pallidus internus (GBi) or the ventral intermediate nucleus of the thalamus (Vim) (91). Interestingly, the effects of stimulation or destruction of a particular target appear to be the same. Vim surgery is usually performed to reduce contralateral tremor (92). GBi surgery can reduce contralateral bradykinesia and rigidity with improved gait and dexterity as well as reducing L-dopa-induced dyskinesia. Both types of surgery may result in hemiparesis due to haemorrhage in the internal capsule, this is more likely in thalamic surgery when it occurs in upto 5% (91). Bilateral destructive surgery is rarely performed because when the Vim is the target the incidence of dysarthria is about 35% and when the GBi is the target there is significant risk of cognitive damage. However, DBS contralateral to a destructive procedure may be less hazardous (91). Patients with disabling unilateral tremor that does not respond to drug treatment and patients whose tolerance of medication is limited by severe unilateral dyskinesia should be considered for surgery. Transplantation of embryonic mesencephalic tissue into the striatum has been shown to produce lasting improvement in symptoms (93).

LATE PARKINSON'S DISEASE AND PALLIATIVE CARE

People with Parkinson's disease constitute a disproportionately large minority of nursing home residents, probably because the physical and psychological manifestations of end-stage PD pose such severe challenges to community carers. It is necessary for professional and informal carers to recognize the increasing need for symptom control as opposed to active rehabilitation, although there is no sharp distinction between the two: in a sense, much of what has been described here as rehabilitation has a palliative aspect, and much of what is encompassed by modern palliative medicine has a rehabilitative dimension. Good nursing care is required to minimize the risk of complications such as pressure sores: although sensation is intact, the severe immobility of end-stage PD predisposes to pressure sores, as does undernutrition. Musculoskeletal pain must be controlled through correct positioning and handling, but also with adequate antiparkinsonian and analgesic drug treatment.

CONCLUSION

This chapter began with a comment on the tendency for neurologists and other physicians to regard Parkinson's disease as a solely medical condition in which their role is restricted to drug management. A less blinkered view can be achieved through direct observation of *all* stages of PD and also through working with other professionals: neurologists, general physicians, geriatricians, and family practitioners must be conversant with the principles of rehabilitation and must gain direct experience of skilled multidisciplinary management of progressive disabling disorders such as Parkinson's disease. Outcomes of a wide range of services—medical and surgical treatment, therapy, counselling, social services, and so on—are then much more likely to coincide with the aspirations of people with PD and of their families.

REFERENCES

1. Mutch WJ, Digwall-Fordyce I, Downie AW, Paterson JG, Roy SK. Parkinson's disease in a Scottish city. *Br Med J* 1986; **292**: 534–6.
2. Mutch WJ, Strudwick A, Roy SK, Downie AW. Parkinson's disease: disability, review and management. *Br Med J* 1986; **293**: 675–7.
3. Ward CD Does selegiline delay progression of Parkinson's disease? A critical re-evaluation of the DATATOP study. *J Neurology Neurosurgery and Psychiatry* 1994; **57**: 217–20.
4. Schieppati M, Nardone A. Free and supported stance in Parkinson's disease. The effect of posture and 'postural set' on leg muscle responses to perturbation, and its relation to severity of disease. *Brain* 1991; **114**: 1227–44.
5. Quinn NP, Koller WC, Lang AE, Marsden CD. Painful Parkinson's disease. *Lancet* 1984; **2**: 1366–9.
6. Critchley EMR. Speech disorders in parkinsonism: a review. *J Neurol Neurosurg Psychiatry* 1981; **46**: 140–4.
7. Johnston BT, Li Q, Castell JA, Castell DO. Swallowing and esophageal function in Parkinson's disease *Am J Gastroenterology* 1995; **90**: 1741–6.
8. Wintzen AR, Badrising UA, Roos RAC, Vielvoye J, Liauw L, Pauwels EKJ Dysphagia in ambulant patients with Parkinson's disease: common, not dangerous. *Can J Neurol Sci* 1994; **21**: 53–6.
9. Goetz C, Lutge W, Tanner CM. Autonomic dysfunction in Parkinson's disease. *Arch Neurol* 1986; **36**: 73–5.
10. Gray R, Stern G, Malone-Lee J. Lower urinary tract dysfunction in Parkinson's disease: changes relate to age and not disease *Age and Ageing* 1995; **24**: 499–504.
11. Jost WH. Gastrointestinal motility problems in patients with Parkinson's disease. Effects of antiparkinsonian treatment and guidelines for management *Drugs and Aging* 1997; **10**: 249–58.
12. Parkes JD. *Sleep and its disorders* WB Saunders, London. 1985: 413–14.

13. Shibasaki H, Sadatoshi T, Kuroiwa Y. Oculomotor abnormalities in Parkinson's disease. *Arch Neurol* 1979; **36**: 360–4.

14. Pell MD. On the receptive prosodic loss in Parkinson's disease *Cortex* 1996; **32**: 693–704.

15. Cooper JA, Sagar HJ, Jordan N, Harvey NS, Sullivan EV. Cognitive impairment in early, untreated Parkinson's disease and its relationship to motor disability. *Brain* 1991; **114**: 2095–122.

16. Brown RG, Marsden CD. Dual task performance and processing resources in normal subjects and in patients with Parkinson's disease. *Brain* 1991; **114**: 215–31.

17. Frith CD, Bloxham CA, Carpenter KN. Impairments in the learning and performance of a new manual skill in patients with Parkinson's disease. *J Neurol Neurosurg Psychiatry* 1986; **49**: 661–8.

18. Worringham CJ, Stelmach GE. Practice effects on the pre-programming of discrete movements in Parkinson's disease. *J Neurol Neurosurg Psychiatry* 1990; **53**: 702–4.

19. Schiffer RB, Kurlan R, Rubin A, Boer S. Evidence for atypical depression in Parkinson's disease. *Am J Psychiatry* 1988; **145**: 1020–2

20. Routh LC, Black JL, Ahlskog JE. Parkinson's disease complicated by anxiety. *Mayo Clin Proc* 1987; **62**: 733–5.

21. Brown RG, Marsden CD, Quinn NP, Wyke MA. Alterations in cognitive performance and affect-arousal state during fluctuations in motor function in Parkinson's disease. *J Neurol Neurosurg Psychiatry* 1984; **47**: 454–5.

22. Singer E. The social costs of Parkinson's disease. *J Chron Dis* 1973; **26**: 243.

23. McCarthy B, Brown R. Psychosocial factors in Parkinson's disease. *Br J. Clin Psychol* 1989; **28**: 41–52.

24. Saint Cyr JA, Taylor AE, Lang AE. Neuropsychological and psychiatric side effects in the treatment of Parkinson's disease. *Neurology* 1993; **43**: S47–52.

25. Brown RG, Marsden CD How common is dementia in Parkinson's disease? *Lancet* 1984; **2**: 1262–5.

26. Ward CD, Gibb WR. Research diagnostic criteria for Parkinson's disease. *Adv Neurol* 1990; **53**: 245–9.

27. World Health Organization. *The international classification of impairments, disabilities, and handicaps—a manual of classification relating to the consequences of disease* WHO Geneva. 1980.

28. Marsden CD, Schachter M. Assessment of extrapyramidal disorders. *Br J Clin Pharmacol* 1981; **11**: 129–51.

29. Webster DD. Critical analysis of the disability in Parkinson's disease. *Modern Treatment* 1968; **5**: 257–82.

30. Fahn S, Elton RL. *et al*. Unified Parkinson's disease rating scale. In *Recent developments in Parkinson's disease* (ed. S Fahn, CD Marsden, DB Calne, M Goldstein). Macmillan Healthcare Information, New Jersey. 1987.

31. Peto V, Jenkinson C, Fitzpatrick R, Greenhall R. The development and validation of a short measure of functioning and well being for individuals with Parkinson's disease *Quality of Life Res.* 1995; **4**: 241–8.

32. Oxtoby M. *Parkinson's disease patients and their social needs.* Parkinson's Disease Society, London. 1982.

33. Wilkinson DG The psychogeriatrician's view: management of chronic neurological disability in the community. *J Neurol Neurosurg Psychiatry* 1992; **55**(suppl.): 41–4.

34. Oxtoby M, Findley L, Kelson N. *et al. A strategy for the management of Parkinson's disease and the long-term support of patients and their carers.* Parkinson's Disease Society, London. 1988.

35. Mutch WJ. A better way to care? The role of specialist clinics. *J Neurol Neurosurg Psychiatry* 1992; **55**(suppl.): 36–40.

36. Vetter N, Jones D, Victor C. Health visiting with the elderly in general practice. In *Research in preventive community nursing care*, (ed. A While). Wiley, Chichester. 1986: Ch. 5.

37. Gibberd FB, Page NGR, Spencer KM, Kinnear B, Hawksworth JB. Controlled trial of physiotherapy and occupational therapy for Parkinson's disease. *Br Med J* 1981; **282**: 1196.

38. Comella CL, Stebbins GT, Brown-Toms N, Goetz CG. Physical therapy and Parkinson's disease: a controlled clinical trial *Neurology* 1994; **44**: 376–8.

39. Johnson JA, Pring TR. Speech therapy in Parkinson's disease: a review and further data. *Brit J Disord Commun* 1990; **25**: 183–94.

40. Scott S, Caird FI. The response of the apparent receptive speech disorder of Parkinson's disease to speech therapy. *J Neurol Neurosurg Psychiatry* 1984; **47**: 302–4.

41. Scott S. Speech therapy. In *Rehabilitation in Parkinson's disease*, (ed. FI Caird). Chapman & Hall, London. 1991.

42. Gauthier L, Dalziel S, Gauthier S. The benefits of group occupational therapy for patients with Parkinson's disease. *Am J Occup Ther* 1987; **41**: 360–5.

43. Hurwitz A. The benefit of a home exercise regimen for ambulatory Parkinson's disease patients. *J Neurosci Nurs* 1989; **21**: 180–4.

44. Blunt SB, Jenner P, Marsden CD. Suppressive effect of L-dopa on dopamine cells remaining in the ventral tegmental area of rats previously exposed to the neurotoxin 6-hydroxydopamine. *Mov Disord* 1993; **8**: 129–33.

45. Ziv I, Zilkha-Falb R, Offen D, Shirvan A, Barzilai A, Melamed E. Levodopa induces apoptosis in cultured neuronal cells—A possible accelerator of nigrostriatal degeneration in Parkinson's Disease? *Mov Disord* 1997; **12**: 17–23.

46. Rinne UK. Early combination of bromocriptine and levodopa in the treatment of Parkinson's disease: A 5 year follow-up. *Neurology* 1987; **37**: 826–8.

47. Rinne UK, Bracco F. *et al.* Cabergoline in the treatment of early Parkinson's disease: Results of the first year of treatment in a double-blind comparison of cabergoline and levodopa. *Neurology* 1997; **48**: 363–8.

48. Pezzoli G, Martignoni E, Pacchetti C, Angeleri V. *et al.* A crossover, controlled study comparing pergolide with bromocriptine as an adjunct to levodopa for the treatment of Parkinson's disease. *Neurology* 1995; **45**(suppl. 3): S22–7.

49. Parkinson Study Group. Effects of Tocopherol and Deprenyl on the progression of disability in early Parkinson's disease. *N Engl J Med* 1993; **328**: 176–83.

50. Parkinson Study Group. Impact of Deprenyl and Tocopherol treatment on Parkinson's Disease in DATATOP patients requiring levodopa. *Ann Neurol* 1996; **39**: 37–45.

51. Parkinson Study Group. Impact of Deprenyl and Tocopherol treatment on Parkinson's disease in DATATOP subjects not requiring levodopa. *Ann Neurol* 1996; **39**: 29–36.

52. Lees AJ on behalf of the Parkinson's Disease Research Group of the United Kingdom. Comparison of the therapeutic effects and mortality data of levodopa and levodopa combined with selegiline in patients with early, mild Parkinson's disease. *Br Med J* 1995; **311**: 1602–7.

53. Kurth MC, Adler CH, St Hilaire M. *et al.* Tolcapone improves motor function and reduces levodopa requirement in parients with Parkinson's disease experiencing motor fluctuations: A multicentre, double-blind, randomized, placebo-controlled trial. *Neurology* 1997; **48**: 81–7.

54. Nanton V. The consequences of Parkinson's disease—Needs, provisions and initiatives. *J Roy Soc Health* 1983; **105**: 52–4.

55. Baker M, Smith P. The social worker. In *Rehabilitation in Parkinson's disease*, (ed. FI Caird). Chapman & Hall, London. 1991.

56. Todes CJ. Inside parkinsonism: a psychiatrist's personal experience. *Lancet* 1983; **1**: 977–8.

57. The Neurological Alliance. *Living with a neurological condition: Standards of care*. London, 1996.

58. Montastruc JL, Rascol O, Senard JM, Rascol A. A randomised controlled study comparing bromocriptine to which levodopa was later added, with levodopa alone in previously untreated patients with Parkinson's disease: a five year follow up. *J Neurol Neurosurg Psychiatry* 1994; **57**: 1034–8.

59. Kostic V, Przedborski S, Flaster E, Sternic N. Early development of levodopa-induced dyskinesias and response fluctuations in young-onset Parkinson's disease. *Neurology* 1991; **41**: 202–5.

60. Doshay LJ. Method and value of physiotherapy in Parkinson's disease. *N Engl J Med* 1962; **266**: 878–80.

61. Banks MA. Physiotherapy. In *Rehabilitation in Parkinson's disease*, (ed. FI Caird). Chapman & Hall, London. 1991: Ch. 4.

62. Scott S. Parkinson's disease: treatment can reduce social isolation. *Speech Therapy in Practice* 1988; **4**: 21.

63. Scott S, Caird FI, Williams BO. *Communication in Parkinson's disease*. Croom Helm, Kent. 1984.

64. Pitcairn TK, Clemie S, Gray JM, Pentland B. Impressions of parkinsonian patients from their recorded voices *Br J Disord Commun* 1990; **25**: 85–92.

65. Pentland B, Pitcairn TK, Gray JM, Riddle WJR. The effects of reduced expression in Parkinson's disease on impression formation by health professionals. *Clin Rehabil* 1987; **1**: 307.

66. Wolf B, Grohmann R, Schmidt LG, Ruther E. Psychiatric admissions due to adverse drug reactions. *Compr Psychiatry* 1989; **30**: 534–45.

67. Beattie A. Occupational therapy. In *Rehabilitation in Parkinson's disease*, (ed. F. I. Caird). Chapman & Hall, London. 1991. Ch. 5.

68. Dubinsky RM, Gray C, Husted D, Busenback K, Vetere-Overfield B, Wiltfong D *et al*. Driving in Parkinson's disease. *Neurology* 1991; **41**: 517–20.

69. Evarts EV, Teravainen H, Calne DB. Reaction time in Parkinson's disease. *Brain* 1981; **104**: 167–86.

70. Manson L, Caird FI. Survey of hobbies and transport of patients with Parkinson's disease. *Br J Occup Ther* 1985; **48**: 199.

71. Brown RG, Jahanshahi M, Quinn NP, Marsden CD. Sexual function in patients with Parkinson's disease and their partners. *J Neurol Neurosurg Psychiatry* 1990; **53**: 480–6.

72. Koller WC, Vetere-Overfield B, Williamson A, Busenbark K, Nash J, Parrish D. Sexual dysfunction in Parkinson's disease. *Clinical Neuropharmacology* 1990; **13**: 461–3.

73. Quinn NP, Marsden CD. Menstrual-related fluctuations in Parkinson's disease *Movement Disorders* 1986; **1**: 85–7.

74. Allain H, Bentue-Ferrer D, Milon D, Moran P, Jacquemard F, Defawe G. Pregnancy and parkinsonism: a case report without problem. *Clin Neuropharm* 1989; **12**: 217–19.

75. Gotham A-M, Brown RG, Marsden CD. Depression in Parkinson's disease: a quantitative and qualitative analysis. *J Neurol Neurosurg Psychiatry* 1986; **49**: 381–9.

76. Friedman JH, Lannon MC. Clozapine in the treatment of psychosis in Parkinson's disease. *Neurology* 1989; **39**: 1219–21.

77. Kyriakides T, Langton Hewer R. Hand contractures in Parkinson's disease. *J Neurol Neurosurg Psychiatry* 1988; **51**: 1221–3.

78. Stern GM, Lander CM, Lees AJ. Akinetic freezing and trick movements in Parkinson's disease. *J Neural Transm* 1980(suppl. 16): 137–41.

79. Dietz MA, Goetz CG, Stebbins GT. Evaluation of a modified inverted walking stick as a treatment for parkinsonian freezing episodes. *Mov Disord* 1990; **5**: 243–7.

80. Frankel JP, Lees AJ, Kempster PA, Stern GM Subcutaneous apomorphine in the treatment of Parkinson's disease. *J Neurol Neurosurg Psychiatry* 1990; **53**: 96–101.

81. Koller WC, Glatt S, Vetere-Overfield B, Hassanein R. Falls and Parkinson's disease. *Clin Neuropharmacol* 1989; **12**: 98–105.

82. Camerlingo M, Ferraro B, Gazzaniga GC, Casto L, Cesana BM, Mamoli A. Cardiovascular reflexes in Parkinson's disease: long-term effects of levodopa treatment in *de novo* patients *Acta Neurol Scand* 1990; **81**: 346–8.

83. Taggart H, Crawford V Reduced bone density of the hip in elderly patients with Parkinson's disease *Age and Ageing* 1995; **24**: 326–8.

84. Kempster PA, Wahlqvist ML. Dietary factors in the management of Parkinson's disease. *Nutrition Reviews* 1994; **52**: 51–8.

85. Berry EM, Growdon JH, Wurtman JJ, Caballero B, Wurtman RJ. A balanced carbohydrate: protein diet in the management of Parkinson's disease. *Neurology* 1991; **41**: 1295–7.

86. Bushmann M, Dobmeyer SM, Leeker L, Perlmutter JS. Swallowing abnormalities and their response to treatment in Parkinson's disease. *Neurology* 1989; **39**: 1309–14.

87. Borwon LK. Respiratory dysfunction in Parkinson's disease. *Clin Chest Med* 1994; **15**: 715–27.

88. Blaivas JG. Urinary bladder problems in Parkinson's disease. *Current Opinion in Neurology and Neurosurgery* 1988; **1**: 284.

89. Hutton JT, Morris MA, Bush DF, Smith ME, Liss CL, Reines S. Multicentre controlled study of Sinemet CR vs Sinemet (25/100) in advanced Parkinson's disease. *Neurology* 1989; **39**(suppl. 2): 67–72.

90. Geminiani G, Fetoni V, Gentrini S. *et al*. Cabergoline in Parkinson's disease complicated by motor fluctuations. *Mov Disord* 1996; **11**: 495–500.

91. Tasker RR, Lang AE, Lozano AM. Pallidal and thalamic surgery for Parkinson's disease. *Experimental Neurology* 1997; **144**: 35–40.

92. Capparos-Lefebvre D, Blond S, Vermersch P, Pecheux N, Guieu J, Petit H. Chronic Thalamic stimulation improves tremor and levodopa induced dyskinesias in Parkinson's disease *J Neurol Neurosurg Psychiatry* 1993; **56**: 268–73.

93. Wenning GK, Odin P, Morrish P. *et al*. Short-and long-term survival and function of unilateral intrastriatal dopaminergic gafts in Parkinson's disease *Ann Neurol* 1997; **42**: 95–107.

10 | *Dementia and delerium*

Christopher McWilliam and Kenneth Barrett

The diagnosis and management of the interrelated states of dementia and delerium demonstrates a distinction between the acute, often emergency, medical intervention required in the case of delirium and confusional states and the chronic medicosocial problems found in dementia which require a multidisciplinary approach to their management.

Although there are marked similarities in differential diagnosis the contrasting management strategies are worthy of separate discussion and are elaborated below.

MANAGEMENT OF DELIRIUM

Delirium is the commonest neuropsychiatric disorder and can be caused by numerous clinical conditions. There are three main elements to its management:

1. Recognize the disorder.
2. Identify and, where possible, remove the cause.
3. Provide short-term measures to alleviate the symptoms.

This review will consider these elements separately.

RECOGNIZING DELIRIUM

The definition of delirium in the World Health Organization, tenth edition of the International classification of diseases (ICD-10) is as follows:

An aetiologically non-specific synarome characterized by concurrent disturbances of consciousness and attention, perception, thinking, memory, psychomotor behaviour, emotion, and the sleep–wake cycle. It may occur at any age but is most common after the age of 60 years. The delirious state is transient and of fluctuating intensity; most cases recover within 4 weeks or less. . . The distinction that is sometimes made between acute and sub-acute delirium is of little clinical relevance; the condition should be seen as a unitary syndrome of variable duration and severity ranging from mild to very severe. (WHO 1993)

ICD-10 requires symptoms in five areas for the diagnosis to be definite. Included are:

1. Impairment of consciousness and attention. The inability to focus attention and to ignore distraction is a key feature. This may be associated with drowsiness, but heightened arousal can also occur.

2. Global disturbance of cognition. This may include disturbance in the flow and coherence of thought, and impairment in any higher function. ICD-10 includes perceptual disorders in this category. Many forms of abnormal perceptual experience occur. The mildest is the illusion or misinterpretation. For example, a 70-year-old man with a drug-induced delirium believed that people who walked past his window were his dead wife. Hallucinations can occur in any combination of sensory modalities and can merge into dream-like states. Visual hallucinations are the commonest, particularly small animals or insects. In metabolic delirium and delirium following sudden withdrawal from alcohol or sedatives, the patient commonly plucks at their clothing, sheets, or the air about them, apparently trying to touch hallucinated objects.

3. Psychomotor disturbance can be either agitation or reduced activity. Agitation is most severe in delirium following the withdrawal of central nervous system (CNS) sedatives and tranquillizers, including alcohol. Reduced activity is common where delirium occurs in the presence of more chronic conditions such as progressive renal and liver failure, or following stroke. These are not unbreakable rules, however.

4. Disturbance of sleep–wake cycle. Most characteristic is inability to sleep and a worsening of symptoms at night. A dark or dimly lit environment particularly fuels perceptual disorders which in turn can increase fear and disorientation.

5. Emotional disturbance can vary from anxiety to extreme fear, from depression and tearfulness to elation and fatuousness. Fear is at its most severe in alcohol and minor tranquillizer withdrawal and is fuelled by or provokes disturbing perceptual disorder. A sense of being followed or stalked is common in this situation. Emotional blunting and apathy are particularly common in renal and liver failure, and hyperglycaemia- induced delirium, but again this is not invariable.

It can be deduced from the above that the presentation of delirium can vary widely and does not conform to a single stereotyped state such as the classical delirium tremens. Failure to diagnose the condition is most commonly due to failure to consider the possibility in the presence of a calm or emotionally blunted patient with no obvious perceptual disorder. The clinical feature of greatest importance diagnostically is the impairment of attention (Geschwind 1981). This encompasses the inability to focus attention and the automatic remembering of ongoing events. The latter ability is analogous to a security video camera in a bank. Failure to record automatically ongoing events leads to disorientation in time and place; we know where we are in time and place because we know where we where a moment ago. Hence, the most important element of the mental state evaluation is determining whether or not the individual is disoriented in time and place. Delirium may not be diagnosed in the absence of disorientation, although in the early stages orientation may fluctuate over time. Delirium is typically of very rapid onset but again this feature is not invariable.

A useful tool for single or day-to-day monitoring of delirium is the Galveston orientation and amnesia test (GOAT) (Levin *et al.* 1979). This includes a scoring system and is useful particularly in post-traumatic delirium.

While delirium is generally reversible there is evidence that in the elderly who have recovered from an episode some degree of persisting functional decline is not uncommon (Murray *et al.* 1993; Koponen *et al.* 1989).

The following case examples present the commoner clinical variants of delirium.

Case report 1

A 47-year-old man was taken to the accident and emergency department by the police. He was dishevelled, had multiple abrasions and bruises and had been picked up in the street where he was behaving in a bizarre manner. He was apparently afraid of passers by and running aimlessly from place to place. He appeared terrified and repeatedly pointed to things in the room saying 'take them away'. He was disoriented in time and place and gave only occasional appropriate and coherent answers. He was flushed, had a course tremor, tachycardia, hypertension, and was hyperventilating. Physical examination revealed an enlarged liver but no other stigmata of liver disease or other abnormality. A full blood count revealed a mean cell volume of 105 and liver function tests an elevated gamma GT and alkaline phosphatase. A diagnosis of delirium tremens was made and he was treated with diazepam, initially intramuscularly, and thiamine. He rapidly settled but remained disoriented for a further 48 hours. He was then able to give a history. He had a 3-year history of increasing alcohol ingestion and for three months had drunk two bottles of spirits and several pints of beer daily. Two days before admission he had decided to stop drinking. Over the next 24 hours he became increasingly distressed and experienced terrifying auditory, visual, and tactile hallucinations coupled with the belief that he was being pursued by people who were trying to kill him.

This is the picture of 'delirium tremens'. While the extreme anxiety and terror is more commonly seen following the abrupt withdrawal of sedative and tranquillizing substances (such as benzodiazepines and barbiturates) this can also occur in metabolic encephalopathies of rapid onset, and in systemic or cerebral infection. Visual misinterpretations or hallucinations of small animals or insects are surprisingly common but may only be indicated by a drowsy and incoherent patient plucking at the air or bedclothes.

Case report 2

A 59-year-old man presented with impaired attention and orientation which had developed over a period of 6 hours. There was no evidence of drowsiness, agitation, fearfulness, or hallucinations. Speech was incoherent and rambling. He was disoriented in time and space and believed he was at work rather than the hospital. Seeing a filing cabinet he went over to it and proceeded to take out files. There was no previous psychiatric history and no history of substance abuse. He was hypertensive but no other abnormality was found on physical examination. Metabolic and endocrine investigations were normal. Computerized tomography (CT) scan of his brain revealed bilateral medial thalamic abnormalities which were likely to be infarcts.

Although thalamic infarcts are an uncommon cause of delirium this type of presentation is not. Attention, orientation, and the ability to think and communicate coherently were impaired but there were no other mental state abnormalities. The causes can include right middle cerebral thrombotic stroke and a wide range of metabolic, endocrine, and nutritional causes such as vitamin B_{12} deficiency. Normal pressure hydrocephalus may also present in this way, the characteristic gait disturbance developing later. A similar picture is seen in post-ictal delirium, although is generally much more short-lived. There is some evidence that right hemisphere stroke more commonly results in delirium than left hemisphere stroke (Mesulam *et al.* 1976). This and the fact that neglect is also most enduring after right hemisphere stroke has led to speculation that the mechanisms subserving focused attention are right hemisphere-based.

Case report 3

A 59-year-old man admitted with sudden onset severe headache, agitation, and disorientation. Investigation confirmed a subarachnoid haemorrhage from an anterior communicating aneurysm. This was surgically clipped but he experienced severe vascular spasm and subsequently had low density areas on CT scan in both inferior frontal areas. He recovered consciousness within 24 hours but was very agitated, disoriented, and assaulted all who approached him. He became calmer on major tranquillizers but remained disoriented, restless, and unable to sustain concentration for more than a few seconds. His concentration span gradually improved over many months but he remained disoriented and was found to have a severe impairment of learning and memory.

Case report 4

A 24-year-old man sustained a head injury in a road traffic accident. He was admitted to hospital with a Glasgow coma score of 4 and was found to have suffered a right parietal fracture, parietal and frontal contusions. He was ventilated for 36 hours and regained consciousness 72 hours after the accident. He was restless, disinhibited, disoriented, and irritable for a further 5 days and was particularly difficult to manage at night when he required sedation. Ten days post-injury he was oriented, mildly elated, had a nominal aphasia and made paraphasic errors in speech.

The patient in Case 4 had 'post-traumatic amnesia' lasting approximately 10 days. This is a confusing term as the state referred to is actually post-traumatic delirium. It is a feature of delirium that the affected individual has little or no recollection of the period in which they were delirious. The ability to remember depends on the ability to focus attention and this, as has been stated above, is always impaired in delirium. Some individuals retain a patchy memory of the delirious state and sometimes these recollections are distressing, particularly if they were of prolonged nightmarish experiences that spilled into the waking state. The patient in Case 3 had post-operative delirium and when this resolved was left with a profound amnesic state. Hence, although his post-surgical/traumatic amnesic state did not resolve his post-traumatic delirium did.

Case report 5

An 85-year-old woman was seen at home in the early hours of a February morning. Her neighbours had alerted her general practitioner that she had behaved oddly for a day or so and had been muttering abuse. This was out of character. On the day she was seen she had not responded to knocks on the door. She was sitting in a cool room in night attire and was muttering to herself. She was disoriented in time and space and was drowsy, with a prolonged response time to questions. She pointed at nothing in particular around the room and plucked at her dressing gown. She was on no regular medication and had shown no evidence of cognitive decline other than on the day in question. Her axillary temperature was recorded as 36 °C centigrade by her general practitioner but on repeat with a low reading thermometer in hospital it was 30°C. She made a full recovery from her hypothermic episode.

THE DIFFERENTIAL DIAGNOSIS OF DELIRIUM

Dementia

Failure to diagnose delirium is common in the elderly where the time course of the mental decline may be unclear. Most of the features of delirium may occur in the late stages of dementia. Both involve global cognitive impairment. An onset over days rather than months of years is key but even when decline is gradual a metabolic, haematological, thyroid, and cardiovascular screen is essential to exclude and remedy factors that can further impair cognition (Kane *et al.* 1993).

Other psychiatric disorders

Acute schizophrenia can have a rapid onset, and include incoherent speech, disorientation, hallucinations, agitation, and sleep disorder. But hallucinations are more commonly auditory and complex, and associated with delusional explanatory beliefs. In addition, clouding of consciousness does not occur. Depressive and catatonic stupor generally have an onset over weeks or months and there is usually a previous history of affective disorder or schizophrenia.

Dissociative disorder (fugue states and dissociative confusional states) is the most difficult to distinguish. Although non-organic psychiatric causes of delirium should be considered as part of the overall assessment it is clearly important to fully exclude organic causes before settling on such a diagnosis, even when there is a previous history of severe psychiatric disorder. Where the diagnosis remains in doubt, and particularly where there is no previous history of psychiatric disorder, an electroencephalogram (EEG) can be valuable: the presence of widespread delta frequencies is against a functional cause. Dissociative and schizophreniform states are the most likely causes of non-organic delirium. Both can be triggered by frontal and temporal brain pathology, which can further complicate matters.

IDENTIFYING THE CAUSE

We are all susceptible to delirium but a number of factors appear to make us more vulnerable. The most important is age, or at least the loss of neurones with advancing age. In some cases no single factor is found to be causing delirium, particularly in people with degenerative brain disease and the elderly, but a series of minor disturbances appear to combine. For example, a mildly elevated serum urea, and a urinary tract infection produced delirium in a 45-year-old woman with advanced multiple sclerosis.

The causes of delirium are summarized in Table 10.1.

ALLEVIATING THE SYMPTOMS OF DELIRIUM

Once the cause of delirium is found it is often possible to remove that cause, or await spontaneous recovery. The delirious state is, however, potentially hazardous and additional measures often need to be taken while the cause is being removed.

The perceptual disorders experienced in the delirious state may be misinterpretations or hallucinations. Both are exacerbated by a dimly lit environment or an environment which is a welter of sound and activity. Hence nursing in a quiet but well- lit environment is preferable.

Delirium tremens and Wernicke's encephalopathy carry a significant mortality if not identified and treated promptly. Abrupt alcohol withdrawal is associated with a high risk of epileptic seizures so sedatives with anticonvulsant action are favoured. Diazepam at an initial dose of 30–60 mg per day in divided doses is required, the dose being titrated against the symptoms of withdrawal. Thiamine is given whether or not there are signs of Wernicke's encephalopathy.

Delirium as a consequence of abrupt sedative withdrawal is best treated by reinstating sedation and withdrawing less abruptly.

Agitation and fear are the commonest management problems in delirium. Sedation with chlormethiazole is effective but is only acceptable for a period of a few days because of the danger of dependency and related withdrawal problems. The drug has a short half-life, around 5 hours, and so should be given in at least four daily doses of 0.5–1.5 gm each. Alternatively, it can be given intravenously. This is an effective way of maintaining sedation where it is necessary to keep the patient very drowsy and horizontal for short periods but it requires great care and appropriate equipment to prevent oversedation and risk of aspiration.

Table 10.1 Causes of delirium

Metabolic
Liver failure
Kidney failure
Hypoglycaemia
Hyperglycaemia
Hypo- and hypernatraemia, kalaemia, calcaemia

peri-ictal:
Post-ictal
Complex partial and petit mal status

Vascular/hypoxic:
Cerebral hypoxia and hypercapnia
Severe anaemia
Impaired cerebral perfusion (as in heart failure)
Thrombotic and embolic stroke
Cerebral haemorrhage (intracerebral, sub- and extradural)
Cranial arteritis
Severe hypertension

Trauma
Head injury
Neurosurgical

Infection
Encephalitis
Meningitis
Systemic infection (including wound/pressure sore)

Neoplastic:
Carcinomatosis
Primary and secondary (intracranial neoplasm)

Nutritional:
Vitamin deficiency (B$_{12}$, folate, thiamine, nicotinic acid, etc.)
Severe malnutrition

Endocrine:
Hypo- and hyperthyroidism
Cushing's disease
Addison's disease
Hyperparathyroidism

Withdrawal states:
Alcohol
Benzodiazepines and other minor tranquillizers
Barbiturates
Chlormethiazole and other hypnotics

Toxic:
Drug-induced (L-dopa and dopamine agonists, anticholinergics, Antidepressants, and many others)
Neuroleptic malignant syndrome
Heavy metals (lead)
Solvents

Others:
Raised intracranial pressure/hydrocephalus

Assessment:
Key questions to answer by taking a history (from an informant):

Is there a history of past or recent serious illness? in particular:
Psychiatric (schizophrenia, major depression, or mania, dissociative states, substance abuse)

Neurological (epilepsy, demyelinating disease, Parkinson's disease, stroke, cerebral tumour, head trauma)
Systemic (neoplasm, collagen disease, renal, and hepatic impairment, endocrine disease, infection, immune disorder)

What regular medication are they or should they be taking?

Could there have been occupational or other exposure to toxins/solvents?

Key questions to answer by physical examination:
Is the patient cyanosed, pale/anaemic, jaundiced, dehydrated, ketotic, pyrexial?
Is there a source of infection (particularly chest, renal tract, wounds/pressure sores)?
Are there stigmata of systemic disease?
Are there localizing neurological signs or papilloedema?

Where more prolonged control of agitation is required the administration of major tranquillizers may be necessary and haloperidol is usually favoured. It can be given orally, intramuscularly and in extreme cases intravenously. It produces calming without marked sedation, is less epileptogenic, and less likely to produce hypotension than the phenothiazines. Unlike the phenothiazines it is not hepatotoxic and so can be given when there is impaired liver function. A wide dose range is used from a starting dose of 2–5 mg to 80 mg daily. Extrapyramidal side-effects are common even at small doses. Acute painful dystonia and occulogyric crises have a sudden onset and are distressing. Both can be effectively treated in most cases by administering anticholinergics intramuscularly (e.g. procyclidine, 10 mg or benztropine 4 mg). Parkinsonian side-effects are also common and can be treated by oral anticholinergics (e.g. procyclidine 5–10 mg 2–3 times daily). Elderly patients often suffer more severe parkinsonian side-effects on haloperidol. The phenothiazine, thioridazine, is much less likely to produce such effects but is more sedative and can be hypotensive. A dose of 10–50 mg every 6–8 hours is usually effective, the dose titrated against response.

MANAGEMENT OF DEMENTING ILLNESS

The care of dementing illness presents one of the biggest challenges facing the health service and will continue to do so well into the next century. Current sociomedical and political debate is becoming increasingly focused on the problems caused by the requirement to care for an increasing number of progressively ill patients with limited resources. Care is mostly provided by non-professional carers outside hospitals or other institutional settings (i.e. 'Care in the Community').

Demographic changes in most Western countries will produce a rapid rise in the elderly population in the next 50 years and more particularly in those in the 75–85 and 85+ age bands. It also appears that the survival rate for patients with dementia is increasing. In 1982, the average survival was estimated at 18 months but is now as much as 5 years even in patients over the age of 85. These factors combined give projections for an increase in the number of cases of dementia by the year 2000 of 16% in Great Britain, 40% in the United States, and 79% in Canada (Jorm 1990). It should also be noted that, as a consequence of the same demographic changes, the age and hence potential infirmity of carers is also increasing.

Social changes have resulted in the geographically closely centred extended family becoming less common and the old traditional expectations for women in Western society to automatically provide care for ageing relatives are rapidly disappearing.

Most patients with dementia suffer from either Alzheimer's disease, a condition of unknown aetiology (60–65%), a vascular type of dementia (20–25%), or a combination of the two (10–15%), none of which is as yet amenable to significant modification by pharmacological techniques.

Scientific progress with regard to elucidating the various aetiologies of the dementias in order to develop possible treatment strategies has been slow. Although treatments for some of the symptoms have recently become available, effective drug treatment or prevention of the underlying disease process seem far off.

The combination of social and medical problems in patients with dementia and their carers, and a lack of specific medical treatment has meant that care throughout the course of the illness has to be not only multiprofessional but also must involve contributions from non-professional support groups and from the carers themselves. Provision of dignified and humane care must also be examined in a social context (Post 1996). Care and treatment of dementia requires an eclectic and pragmatic approach with no single group of care providers having a monopoly on expertise.

Probably the most useful approach is to regard dementing illness, of whatever aetiology, as an ongoing process which will require constant review and modification of treatment of each individual patient and support for their carers as the illness and any complications progress.

DEFINITION, AETIOLOGY, AND CLASSIFICATION OF DEMENTIA

When the concept of dementia is considered it is important to remember that the term itself means different things to professionals and lay people and also has different implications for various professional groups. The word 'dementia' also carries the burden of pejorative connotation and carries considerable emotional weight. Public awareness of issues surrounding dementia and its management is also increasing thanks to media coverage of Creutzfeldt–Jacob disease and an increasing number of articles on dementia in popular magazines and media coverage. It should not, however, be assumed that this increase in publicity has greatly informed the general public and a large part of the management of a patient with dementia is taken up in explaining the nature of the illness, its prognosis, and their implications to patients and, more often, their carers.

Probably the best way to understand dementia is not as a specific disorder but as a variable and progressively changing symptom complex which may be the result of a wide variety of pathological processes involving the central nervous system, in general, and the cerebral cortex and subcortex, in particular.

Although most definitions stress the progressive and irreversible aspects of the disease it is important to be constantly aware of a number of cases, perhaps up to 20% of the total, which are potentially reversible especially if diagnosed early. It is for this reason that comprehensive early screening of confusional states for treatable causes is essential. A reasonable working definition of dementia has been provided by the World Health Organization:

Dementia is the global impairment of higher cortical functions, including memory, the capacity to solve problems of day to day living, the performance of learned perceptuo-motor skills, the correct use of social skills and control of emotional reactions in the absence of gross clouding of consciousness. The condition is often irreversible and progressive. (WHO 1986)

The often-used distinction between *senile* and *pre-senile dementias* does not contribute to understanding the concept of dementing illnesses and their management and will not be used here.

It must also be remembered that dementing illnesses are often accompanied by other pathological changes in the body especially in the cardiovascular and central nervous systems, and the interplay and progression of these various diseases with the dementing process will play a large part in determining the presentation and course of illness. This inherent complexity and tendency to complications makes classification of dementia difficult.

Classifications may be based on histopathology, neurology, or on clinical and behavioural features with various indicators used to measure deterioration over time. A classification scheme based on genetics or histopathology may communicate little about clinical presentation or management problems and vice versa and care must be used in communication to avoid confusion. For research purposes computerized schemes such as CAMDEX (Roth *et al.* 1986) and GMS\AGECAT (Copeland *et al.* 1986) have been developed and these can be used to provide standardized diagnoses in ICD or DSM (*Diagnostic and statistical manual of mental disorders* American Psychiatric Association) form. These schemes, however, give no guidance to prognosis, treatment, or management.

The most useful classification schemes for aiding the understanding of the aetiology and management of the dementing illnesses are those which attempt to correlate clinical neuropsychological findings with neuropathological ones. Once this is done the principles can be applied to the individual circumstances of a given patient.

At the risk of oversimplification a pragmatically useful classification with some relevance to management can be based on the psychological and clinical distinctions between 'cortical' dementias and 'subcortical' dementias. Although this gives no clues as to aetiology it does at least correlate with behavioural findings and gives some indication as to probable progression of the illness (Cummings 1986). Cortical dementias such as Alzheimer's, Pick's, and human prion disease are those affecting primarily the cerebral cortex and hence the higher instrumental functions of language, perception, memory, calculation, volition, social behaviour, and personality. Subcortical dementias, such as dementia secondary to Parkinson's disease, spinocerebellar degeneration, Wilson's disease, Huntington's disease, toxic and metabolic encephalopathies, and progressive supranuclear palsy, are usually due to microvascular degeneration in these areas of the brain. They affect the more basic fundamental functions of arousal, motivation, mood, and attention mediated in the basal ganglia, thalamus, and their connections with the limbic system and frontal lobes. Involvement of the subcortical nuclei usually produces some form of motor disorder in addition to the above changes and these may present as great a management problem as the psychological features.

It is important to remember, however, that in the advanced cases of dementia which often present to professional caregivers, features of both types of dementia are present and emphasis shifts to assessing possible progression and prognosis in a multidisciplinary context.

DIFFERENTIAL DIAGNOSIS IN DEMENTIA

Once delirium has been eliminated as detailed above the following important differential diagnoses remain:

Pseudodementia

This is a condition of impaired cognition, memory loss, and disorientation occurring in a non-organic psychosis.

Clinically, the state can resemble dementia but typically they have is a well defined onset and the course is short.

Depressive illness is by far the commonest cause although it can be found secondary to mania and schizophrenia.

A therapeutic trial of antidepressant medication is often effective, to such an extent that many call the condition 'depressive syndrome of dementia' and advocate routine prescription of antidepressants to all patients with suspected or established dementia.

Normal pressure hydrocephalus

Classically, this presents with the clinical triad of motor disturbance, especially of gait, memory deficit with slowing, and urinary incontinence. CT scan will show marked ventricular enlargement with relatively normal cortical sulci and isotope cisternography will reveal obstruction to the flow of cerebro spinal fluid (CSF) over the cortex. Although theoretically treatable by a ventricular shunting procedure to divert CSF, improvement cannot be expected in all cases.

Intracranial lesions

Dementia syndrome may be secondary to any form of intracranial space-occupying lesion. Careful history and a high index of suspicion may lead to the diagnosis of primary or secondary tumour, brain abscess, or intracranial bleed and CT scan will usually confirm the diagnosis.

PRESENTATION AND CLINICAL FEATURES OF DEMENTIA

Although these are well known to most clinicians it is worthwhile studying some features of typical dementias in some detail.

Early forms of dementia tend not to be seen by hospital specialists or even by general practitioners, as onset in the non-vascular dementias may be so insidious as to be indistinguishable from a general decline in health. Many sufferers from dementia live in the community throughout most of their illness with their gradual deterioration dealt with by increasing support from the family with the help of statutory and voluntary care. Changes may be attributed to 'just old age' and may present as slowness, apathy, poor adaptability to change, increasing irritability, forgetfulness and vagueness, poor decision-making ability, and a general falling of in interest and activity. These symptoms are also found in early depressive illness and failure of such patients to respond to antidepressant medication or psychotherapy may be an indicator of the onset early dementia.

It is also unusual for patients with dementing illnesses to present themselves for treatment, especially as insight tends to be lost early on. More commonly, it is a carer who complains about some change in cognitive function, mood or behaviour, or changes are picked up during examination for some other complaint.

Vascular dementia secondary to disease of the anterior, middle and posterior cerebral arteries may begin in a mild transient form and be masked by other manifestations of cerebrovascular and cardiovascular disease such as stroke. The subcortical types of dementia often present with mental slowness, inertia, loss of drive and initiative, and apathy, in addition to cognitive deficits. These may be missed as these psychological symptoms may be secondary to the motor symptoms or misdiagnosed as depression or fatigue.

As the dementia progresses the memory deficits become more marked, with memory for recent events usually much worse than distant memory. Disorientation in place may become apparent with the additional appearance of personality change and behavioural disturbance such as wandering, neglect of hygiene and incontinence. The patient may often present a risk to him/herself and to others by leaving gas unlit, boiling pans dry, insisting on driving the car, and so on; and it is at this stage that health and/or social service professionals may become involved in assessment and care provision.

In severe dementia, the patient is dependent on others for support and may present with marked behavioural disturbance, aggression, total short-term memory loss, involuntary movements, and personality change. If untreated, the course of a dementing illness can often be predicted from the underlying pathology whether cortical or subcortical, degenerative, or vascular. Clinical features will depend on the relative degree of involvement of various parts of the brain and will change as the disease progresses.

This concept of dementia as a continuously changing disease process is valuable when undertaking assessment and planning management.

Emergency presentations of dementia which present so many problems for support services are usually due to failure of care in patients with established dementia or sudden deterioration in patients with vascular dementia. Ideally, such emergency presentations can be prevented by proactive planning and co-ordinated medical and social monitoring of patients with dementia living in the community.

The contrasting features of cortical and subcortical dementias, independent of aetiology, have been well summarized (Cummings 1986) and are shown in Table 10.2.

PRINCIPLES OF ASSESSMENT AND MANAGEMENT

Assessment and management of dementia at whatever stage requires close co-operation between all existing and potential providers of care. Assessment of medical, psychiatric, psychological, environmental, and social factors is imperative with close involvement of the patient if appropriate and carers in any decisions regarding future management.

The multiple aetiology and presentation of dementia often results in patients being assessed by various professionals according to local variations in service provision and referring habits of general practitioners. Patients may be first seen by general psychiatrists, specialist psychogeriatricians, geriatricians, general physicians, or neurologists and many cases are missed or ignored. Dementia may also present following admission to hospital for any other cause such as fractured neck of femur. Others may be brought to casualty departments or to emergency social services provision after being found wandering in the street. No two cases of dementia are alike and specific individualized treatment plans covering as many possible outcomes as possible must be drawn up. This process requires time and application and may take place in the patient's home or in hospital. It should be undertaken by a full multidisciplinary team and the end result should be a comprehensive treatment plan, tailored to the individual patient and their carers with full consideration of present and future needs.

Emphasis of care provision may shift as the illness progresses and this may usefully be co-ordinated by a designated key worker who will co-ordinate the efforts of the various care agencies for both statutory and voluntary sectors and attempt to match changing care needs with available resources through the course of the illness. This may result in a given

Table 10.2 Contrasting features of cortical and subcortical dementia

Aspect	Cortical dementia	Subcortical dementia
Neuropsychological features		
Severity	More severe deficits earlier in the disease course	Mild to moderate throughout the course
Speed of cognition	Normal	Slowed
Memory short term	Encoding deficit, aided little by clues	Recall partially facilitated clues and recognition tasks
Remote recall	Normal in early stages temporal gradient	No temporal gradient
Language	Anomia, comprehension deficit, paraphasia	Normal or mild anomia
Visuospatial skill	Impaired, poor model copying	Impaired, poor manipulation of egocentric space (map reading, judgement of horizontal and vertical)
Cognition	Impaired early, late untestable	Poor abstraction and categorization
Neuropsychiatric features		
Personality	Indifference, occasional disinhibition	Apathy, irritability
Depression	Uncommon	Common
Mania	Absent	Infrequent
Psychosis	Common, simple delusions	Common in some disorders may have complex delusion
Motor system		
Speech	No dysarthria	Dysarthria
Posture	Normal (flexed late)	Flexed or extended
Gait	Normal (until late)	Hypo- or hyperkinetic
Speed	Normal (until late)	Slow
Adventitious movements	None or myoclonus	tremor, chorea, dystonia
Tone	Normal early, rigid in later stages	Abnormal (hypotonic in choreic disorders, hypertonia in parkinsonian conditions)

From Cummings, J. L. (1986).

patient receiving care in various locations including: their own home; day care units run by voluntary agencies, social services or health services; day hospitals; respite care in hospital, nursing, or residential home; supervised 'sheltered' accommodation, or permanent care in a residential or nursing home.

PHARMACOLOGICAL TREATMENT IN DEMENTIA

The last decade has seen a marked advance in understanding the pathological mechanisms underlying the development and clinical presentation of the illness. This increase in theoretical knowledge has lead to the recent appearance of drugs capable of symptomatic treatment of cognitive deficits. Most of the current research has been directed towards enhancing cognitive performance and has become inextricably linked with the search for designer 'smart drugs' which may or may not improve memory and IQ test results in non-demented people. It is probably true that, for the foreseeable future, the treatment of dementia will not be by drugs alone but will require other physical and psychological methods in addition.

It is useful to divide the drug treatment of the dementias into four separate but overlapping groups:

1. Drugs enhancing cognition and memory.
2. Drugs treating associated emotional changes.
3. Drugs treating behavioural problems.
4. Drugs aimed at prevention of cerebrovascular illness.

TREATMENT OF COGNITIVE AND MEMORY DEFICITS

Research in this area over the last 15 years has largely concentrated on neurotransmitter function in the brain with attention being focused particularly on the role of the cholinergic system. To date, the only class of drugs demonstrating any clinical effectiveness are acetyl cholinesterase inhibitors (Giacobini 1994). The first of these to be licensed for the treatment of dementia is tetrahydroaminoacridine (Tacrine). While this has been shown to improve the core deficits of Alzheimer's disease and reduce the rate of clinical deterioration (Wilcock 1995), experience in thousands of subjects has highlighted many problems. Clinical improvement in most cases is minimal and transitory and occurs in only up to 30% of cases. Side-effects have been severe and dose-limiting in most subjects. Nevertheless, the introduction of Tacrine has helped to clarify the criteria for a successful anticholinesterase drug. Such a drug must demonstrate:

(1) a selective effect on the CNS;
(2) improvements in activities of daily living;
(3) prolonged efficacy of years rather than months;
(4) an ability to prevent deterioration in cognitive function;
(5) a reduction in the need for institutional care; and
(6) a realistic price for the duration of treatment.

Trials of future drugs for dementia will also need to address the problems of appropriate patient selection, determination of optimum dosage and duration of treatment, avoidance of tolerance, long-term effects, management of termination of treatment, and effects on carers.

In March 1997 a new anticholinesterase drug, Donepezil, was licensed for use in the United Kingdom. To date, although any clinical benefits appear to be modest and short-acting (UK Drug Information Service 1997); it does appear to represent an advance on Tacrine in that it is simple to administer and has a much more favourable side-effect profile. (Rogers and Friedhoff 1996). Information as to patient selection, long-term use, patient selection, management of discontinuation, and effects on carers is, as yet absent.

The introduction of clinically effective drugs for Alzheimer's disease raises many medicopolitical and ethical issues and has serious implications for the provision of health care. More drugs for the treatment of Alzheimer's disease and other dementias will soon be on the market and the need for rational procedures for their introduction based on sound clinical evidence and careful consultation becomes increasingly urgent.

TREATMENT OF EMOTIONAL PROBLEMS

Patients with dementia often display affective symptoms of depression, anxiety, inappropriate mood, and emotional lability. This is particularly common in the early stages of Alzheimer's disease or following an acute vascular episode in multi-infarct dementia. It is impossible to determine whether these symptoms represent part of the dementing process itself or a reaction to the patient's own deterioration and no specific treatment exists.

Some of these symptoms can be alleviated with appropriate symptomatic treatment and it is probably worth a therapeutic trial of antidepressant drugs especially if, as mentioned above, they may have some positive effects on cognition. This, coupled with the fact that patients with dementia tend to suffer from multiple physical illnesses and are poor treatment compliers, indicates that choice of antidepressant should be one of the new non-tricyclic compounds such as a specific serotonin re-uptake inhibitor (SSRI) or monoamine oxidase-B (MAO-B) inhibitor which appear to lack the troublesome side-effects of tricyclic antidepressants.

Comprehensive treatment of emotional problems is not purely pharmacological and may also involve some social therapy, counselling, or other interventions determined by full assessment.

DRUG TREATMENT OF BEHAVIOUR DISORDERS

As with emotional disorders, the factors producing behavioural disorders in patients with dementia and hence their presentation varies between patients and also within a given patient as the disease progresses. Much can and should be done by appropriate levels of care before pharmacological intervention is considered. Indeed, many management problems with demented patients are caused by inappropriate medication given for behaviour disorders without full assessment of all the contributory factors. Severe behavioural disturbances may present as emergencies especially if they involve violent or aggressive behaviour and require appropriate and immediate treatment.

Sleep disturbance and mild behavioural disorders such as wandering usually respond to small doses of neuroleptic medication. The lack of controlled research data in this area has led most psychogeriatricians to develop their own treatment strategy based on experience, largely by trial and error.

Dosage should start at a much lower level than used for psychoses in non dementing adults. Typical dosage may be 1–1.5 mg of haloperidol or 50 mg sulpiride 2–3 times daily. It is vital to ensure careful monitoring for side-effects and dose modification according to response and deterioration. More severe cases may require depot neuroleptics to stabilize their behavioural disturbance. Typical dosage here may be 25 mg of depot haloperidol or of flupenthixol decanoate every 2–3 weeks.

Again, treatment is often determined by the experience of the clinician rather than by any hard research data into efficacy. Constant review is essential as behavioural disturbance is often transitory in many cases and high levels of medication may only be required for a short period of the illness. It is also becoming increasingly recognised that many cases of dementia display subcortical features of Lewy body dementia rather than uncomplicated Alzheimer dementia. These patients react badly to neuroleptics with increased behavioural and extrapyramidal movement disorders. Drug treatment should be discontinued if this occurs.

PREVENTION OF CEREBROVASCULAR ILLNESS

Recent work has proved unequivocally the beneficial effect of low dose aspirin in the prevention of cerebrovascular disease in at-risk patients. It is also likely that in future better understanding of the pathogenesis of cerebral arterial disease will result in improved prophylaxis and hence a reduction in the incidence of multi-infarct dementia.

NON-MEDICAL INTERVENTIONS

The lack of effective drug treatments for dementia and the wide variation in clinical presentation has led to development of many non-medical management strategies which can be used to help sufferers and their carers at various stages of the illness. Unless and until simple and cost effective drug treatments for dementing illnesses are developed these non-medical interventions provide the mainstay of therapy in dementia and can be applied to care in hospital and, perhaps to a lesser extent, care in the community.

Reality orientation (RO)

This is perhaps the best known non-medical intervention in dementia and has been subjected to considerable evaluation and research (Holden and Woods 1988). Unfortunately, there is a lack of consensus about what reality orientation actually involves and it has been appropriately stated that RO is 'all things to all people'. Perhaps it is best understood as a philosophy of care rather than a rigidly defined set of techniques for patient management. Its effect has been most apparent on the care environment provided in hospitals, nursing homes, and day care centres where aspects of RO are used on a day-to-day basis.

RO is usually hospital-based and two main approaches are described. RO group sessions involve small groups of selected patients meeting staff for up to an hour at least twice a week. Specific RO classrooms may be used but these tend to have been superseded by having RO aids throughout the ward. These may include, posters, orientation data such as day, date, weather, meals, news items, and so on. The emphasis is on enhancing orientation in a pressure-free environment where fear of failure is eliminated. The other approach, 24-hour RO, is a continuous form of interactive therapy involving the patient, staff, and relatives in encouraging orientation and discouraging disorientation at every interaction. Behavioural orientation such as finding one's way around and verbal orientation have been separately identified.

The benefits of RO probably derive from the maximizing of existing function rather than regaining orientation skills that have been lost. It also is a powerful aid in reversing the effects of institutionalization and in promoting positive approaches in carers. It should also be noted that RO is not a blanket treatment for all patients with dementia as there is evidence that it can contribute to emotional distress in patients with more advanced illness.

Reminiscence therapy (RT)

It was formerly believed that reminiscence, 'dwelling on the past', contributed to the progression of mental deterioration in dementia. This is now known not to be the case and it has been shown to aid in the retention of cognitive function. As well as enhancing cognitive performance RT has the added advantage of 'empowering' the patient in relation to the care staff as in a very real sense the patient becomes an expert on the subject of the past and can also be better understood in the context of their life history. RT sessions have also been shown to increase self-esteem and social interaction between patients themselves and between patients and carers.

As with reality orientation, RT has been incorporated into many care environments and aspects of it form part of the day-to-day care in many long stay and day care establishments. RT techniques used on a less formal basis may be useful in the patient's home.

Validation therapy (VT)

This has important similarities to and differences from both RO and RT. Like them it is an interactive technique used mostly in care environments for the demented and can be used in individual or group therapy.

The basic tenet of VT is that the patient is managed within their own 'reality' rather than that of the external world. The role of the therapist is to interact with the patient within this world and improve verbal communication and behaviour.

Perhaps because of its strong grounding in dynamic psychotherapy, expertise in VT developed in the United States and Canada before the United Kingdom.

Experience with VT has produced new insights into the progression and management of dementia and work is now being focused on refining the technique and identifying specific VT strategies for different behavioural problems.

NON-DRUG TREATMENT OF BEHAVIOURAL DISORDER

Patients with dementia are well known for exhibiting disturbed behaviours. These can often be extremely distressing both for the patient and their carers and it is often the onset of behavioural disturbance in dementia that triggers a referral to professional agencies.

Assessment of behavioural disturbance and development of strategies to manage it throughout the course of a dementing illness forms a large part of management. This is of paramount importance as the successful management of behavioural problems will often determine whether a patient can be managed in their existing setting, perhaps in their own home or in residential care, or will require admission to hospital or to a nursing home specializing in the care of dementia.

The most common behavioural problems in dementia are: wandering, incontinence, and 'aggressive', 'challenging', or sexually inappropriate behaviour. These tend to change in nature and intensity as the illness progresses and must be assessed in detail on an individual basis according to the context and setting in which they occur. Once this assessment is complete certain principles of management can be applied.

Assessment may be carried out in the patients home or may require hospital admission. Involvement of carers at all stages of the assessment is imperative as the interaction between the patient and carers may often contribute to the behavioural difficulty.

Management will depend on the outcome of the assessment and should depend on the outcome of a multidisciplinary assessment, with appointment of a key worker to liaise between the patient, carers, and professionals.

SENILE DEMENTIA AND HEALTH LEGISLATION

Although most patients with dementia receive their treatment on an informal basis, workers in hospital and the community may have to deal with some of the legal methods used in their management. Legal methods are also available to safeguard the financial affairs of the demented patient.

Most health professionals, especially those working in the community are aware of the provisions and usage of the Mental Health Act (1983) which can be used to detain the mentally ill in hospital for assessment and/or treatment. Somewhat surprisingly there is no specific mention of senile dementia in the Act and there is a lack of guidance as to how to deal with the demented in its code of practice. This has

resulted in inconsistent application of the Act in patients with dementia, and practice may vary widely according to local interpretation of the legislation.

This is especially true of Guardianship orders which were devised to provide a mechanism for the protection of people who are rendered vulnerable to exploitation, ill treatment, or neglect because of mental disorder, and to provide the means whereby a responsible carer can act on their behalf. There is no doubt that, when used appropriately, Guardianship orders provide an authoritative framework for working with a patient in the community with the minimum of constraints to achieve as independent a life as possible.

The workings of the Court of Protection which oversees the management of the financial affairs of those rendered incapable of doing so by mental illness are also defined by the Act. This exists 'for the protection and management of the affairs of a person under a disability'. The Court also exercises supervisory jurisdiction over Enduring Powers of Attorney. These enable a person to make advance provision for eventual loss of capacity and allows for the appointment of a chosen person to administer their affairs and give instructions on how this should be carried out.

Other patients with dementia may be admitted to hospital under Section 47 of the National Assistance Act (1948). This empowers community medical officers to apply to a magistrate for compulsory removal of persons who: (a) are suffering from grave chronic disease, or being aged, infirm, or physically incapacitated are living in insanitary conditions; and (b) are unable to devote to themselves or are not receiving from other persons proper care and attention. The rate of use of this Order is difficult to determine as admissions under the Act are not routinely monitored but it appears that, as with Guardianship orders, practice varies greatly between localities. In general it is felt that this Order is not appropriate for the demented patient and admission under the Mental Health Act is more appropriate in nearly all cases. This has the advantage of protecting the patient's right to appeal against detention which do not form part of the National Assistance Act legislation.

MANAGEMENT OF ABUSE

It is becoming increasingly recognized that the elderly, in general, and patients with dementia, in particular, are the targets of abuse (Glendenning 1993). This may be perpetrated by informal or professional carers or indeed by society in general and can take any of several forms.

Classifications of abuse vary but all include, verbal, physical, psychological, sexual, and financial abuse; misuse of drugs, deprivation of care, and neglect. Estimates of the size of the problem vary and the very nature of the problem renders investigation and accurate measurement difficult if not impossible. As far as the demented patient is concerned abuse can be avoided by early and appropriate intervention with the patient and their carers and recognition of potential areas of abuse should form part of any assessment and treatment plan.

It is probably true to say that the continuing revelation of the nature and extent of the abuse of elderly people, in general, and of sufferers from dementia, in particular, will have ongoing effects on the future roles of anyone involved in the care of these people in either a professional or voluntary capacity.

REFERENCES

Copeland, J. R. M., Dewey, M. E., and Griffiths-Jones, H. M. (1986). Computerised psychiatric diagnostic system and case nomenclature for elderly subjects: GMS and AGECAT. *Psychology and medicine*, **16**, 89–99.

Cummings, J. L. (1986). Subcortical dementia. Neuropsychology, neuropsychiatry, and pathophysiology. *British Journal of Psychiatry*, **149**, 682–97.

Geschwind, N. (1981). Disorders of attention: a frontier in neuropsychology. *Philosophical Transactions of the Royal Society, London*, **B298**, 173–89.

Giacobini E (1994). In *Recent advances in the treatment of neurodegenerative disorders and cognitive dysfunction*, (ed. G. Racagni, N. Brunello, and S. Z. Langer).

Glendenning, F. (1993). What is elder abuse and neglect? In *The mistreatment of elderly people*, (ed. P. Decalmer and F. Glendenning), Ch.1. Sage, London.

Holden, U. P. and Woods, R. T. (1988). *Reality Orientation: Psychological approaches to the confused elderly*. Churchill Livingstone, Edinburgh.

Jorm, A. F. (1990). *The epidemiology of Alzheimer's disease and related disorders*. Chapman and Hall, London.

Kane, F. J. Jr, Remmel, R., and Moody, S. (1993). Recognising and treating delirium in patients admitted to general hospitals. *Southern Medical Journal*, **86**, 985–8.

Koponen, H., Stenback, U., Mattila, E., Soininen, H., Reinikainen, K., and Riekkinen, P. J. (1989). Delirium among elderly persons admitted to a psychiatric hospital: clinical course during the acute stage and one-year follow-up. *Acta Psychiatrica Scandinavica*, **79**, 579–85.

Levin, H. S., O'Donnell, V. M., and Grossman, R. G. (1979). The Galveston Orientation and Amnesia Test: A practical scale to assess cognition after head injury. *Journal of Nervous and Mental Diseases*, **167**, 675–84.

Mesulam, M., Waxman, G., Geschwind, N., and Sabin, T. D. (1976). Acute confusional states with right middle cerebral infarction. *Journal of Neurology, Neurosurgery and Psychiatry*, **39**, 84–9.

Murray, A. M., Levkoff, S. E., Wetle, T. T., Beckett, L., Cleary, P. D., Schor, J. D. *et al.* (1993). Acute delirium and functional decline in the hospitalised elderly patient. *Journal of Gerontology*, **48**, M181–6.

Rogers, S. L. and Friedhoff, L. T. (1996). The efficacy and safety of Donezepil in patients with Alzheimer's disease. Results of a US multi-centre, randomised, placebo controlled trial. *Dementia*, **7**, 293–303.

Roth, M., Tym, E., Mountjoy, C. Q., Huppert, F. A., Hendrie, H., Verma, S. *et al.* (1986). CAMDEX: a standardised instrument for the diagnosis of mental disorder in the elderly with special reference to the early detection of dementia. *British Journal of Psychiatry*, **149**, 698–709.

UK Drug Information Services (1997). *Donezepil Monograph*, 4/97/12.

Wilcock, G. K. (1995). Pharmacological approaches to treating Alzheimer's disease. In *Neurobiology of Alzheimer's disease*, (ed. D. Dawbarn and S. J. Allen), pp. 298–304. BIOS Scientific Publishers, Oxford.

World Health Organization (1986). *WHO Technical Report Series 730*. WHO, Geneva.

World Health Organization (1992). Mental disorders. In *International classification of diseases*, (ICD-10).

11 | *Motor neurone disease*

Adrian Williams

The management of motor neurone disease raises many challenges for the neurologist who will diagnose and care for the majority of patients. However, in many areas this is becoming a multidisciplinary business with specialist clinics, sometimes with domiciliary arms. Unfortunately, management is variable and depends to an extent on local interest, priorities, and geographical region. In many districts there is an increasing involvement of hospices in this terminal illness preceded by several years of increasing disability when rehabilitation expertise can have a major part to play.

Communication issues have for many years been a criticism levelled against neurologists who, not that long ago, used to evade serious issues or only tell the partner. Fortunately, this situation is improving and the importance of staging information and having the support and follow up of a specialist nurse practitioner is increasingly appreciated. Perhaps in the past neurologists themselves have under-rated how much support patients can receive simply by showing concern and interest and imparting information honestly but kindly, with adequate follow-up appointments. Indeed, we should take these factors into consideration, and not just write a prescription for drugs that may not substantially affect the problems that our patients still have to face.

Management, of course, varies depending on whether a diagnosis has been made and patients and paramedical staff, who are later concerned that information was sparse, must realize that in at least half the patients the diagnosis is not obvious and may only be clarified with tests and time until a pattern is complete and no other realistic diagnosis is on the cards. It is not always appreciated that there is no specific diagnostic test, certainly not from electromyograms (EMGs) and NCSs. Until we are certain, most of us do not use the term 'motor neurone disease' even in our letter to the family doctor, in order to avoid inadvertent leaks. We would only rarely mention it, even if it were the top of a differential diagnosis, until any other reasonable possibility had been eliminated.

This chapter is a fairly personal view of early management through the initial diagnostic phase. However, I do not always follow this myself because under different circumstances or with a different rapport and assessment of the patients prior knowledge and expectations, major modifications may be perfectly acceptable. The principles are to make the correct diagnosis and then impart it in such a way as to reduce the shock as much as is possible and to not leave the patient or their family with the feeling that they have been diagnosed but then abandoned. I would venture to suggest that possibly with extremely rare exceptions (a neurologist and general practitioner with a lot of time) the latter is almost impossible to achieve if the physician is not working closely with a specialist nurse practitioner at the minimum.

DIAGNOSIS

Diagnosis obvious during the initial consultation or even from the referral letter, for example, a bulbar palsy with a probable or definite fasciculating tongue with or without fasciculation in the limbs.

In such a situation there are not too many diagnostic catches. Occasionally, tongue tremors can mislead the less experienced and best avoided by making sure fasciculation is definite with the tongue at rest. A slowly moving tongue without much apparent weakness can be misinterpreted as being upper motor neurone but can be seen with myasthenia. Diagnosis of other cases of bulbar palsy, such as multiple sclerosis or vascular disease, should not cause too much difficulty. However, I have seen a thoracic aneurysm cause a purely motor cord lesion plus a hoarse voice, and swallowing problems and severe anterior osteophytes with spondylosis does the same, as indeed in one patient diagnosed with dysphagia or dysarthria, with an unsuspected foreign body in his throat, who we cured! It is also worth recalling that dysphagia but probably never dysarthria can be seen with polymyositis and that myotonic dystrophy can present with marked bulbar problems. It is possible to overlook X-linked Kennedy's disease which should be remembered in young males with a LMN syndrome particularly if they have gynaecomastia. Even if the diagnosis seems immediately certain it is advisable to see the patient as a day case or an extended outpatient to do an EMG and NCS, and sometimes a tensilon test and antiacetylcholine receptor antibodies. These procedures are largely for the record and it is hard to expect patients to accept such a serious diagnosis without any tests at all. Only rarely would one tell the patient at the first meeting, but perhaps warn them that it could be serious with no easy treatment but that further tests are needed to be sure (however, do not then delay an obvious diagnosis just because the EMG proves typical or even normal). Once it has been decided to tell the patient and the family, it is better to see them with the nurse practitioner. However, if this is not possible, a contact number could be given and possibly the address and phone number of the Motor Neurone Disease Association. Certainly, offer to see them again soon. Patients usually later thank you for not hiding too much and for saying what motor neurone disease will nor cause (e.g. dementia, incontinence, bed sores).

Diagnosis likely but not obvious, for example, a bulbar palsy without fasciculation or a weak limb or limbs with obvious fasciculation.

I would normally admit the patient as a day case or for a short admission. Management is similar to the above, although the patient is more likely to require magnetic resonance imaging (MRI) scanning of spine, head, or both. Routine blood tests should include thyroid function and a calcium test to pick up exceedingly rare motor syndromes related to thyrotoxicosis and hyperparathyroidism. Again, stage information so that it does not come as a complete surprise and in circumstances that both doctor and patient have got to know each other. Try not to leave it to junior members of the firm and do not tell patients in a public place. Try and impart concern about the seriousness of the situation at the same time as demonstrating that you and your team have dealt with it many times before and give the patient the confidence that you will help them throughout the course of the disease.

Diagnosis possible, but possible neuropathy as all the signs are lower motor neurone and reflexes are depressed or absent?

A lot has been written about this group of patients who are clearly important as they may have a treatable illness. Unfortunately, however, it is relatively rare that they do, particularly if there is considerable fasciculation. Nerve conduction studies are usually crucial. Conduction block, if found, needs to be taken seriously but can turn out to be a 'red herring' even when found by excellent neurophysiologists. Clear signs of neuropathy with excessive slowing, especially if there are abnormalities on the sensory side always needs to be taken very seriously. Cerebrospinal fluid (CSF) examination may be of help as the protein is at best slightly raised with classic motor neurone disease (MND). Ganglioside antibodies and monoclonal bands are of some help in diagnosing an autoimmune neuropathy but there are numerous false negatives and a few false positives. It usually turns out to be a matter of clinical judgement, taking all the above into consideration, particularly the nerve conduction tests. Then, in a few selected patients, give a trial of treatment either with immunoglobulin in the first instance if there is multifocal neuropathy with conduction block or other forms of immunosuppression, such as steroids with azathioprine, for a more conventional neuropathy. If the nerve conduction studies suggest that an accessible nerve, such as the superficial radial or sural, might be

involved, then a nerve biopsy may be in order. In addition, if changes of demyelination are observed long-term treatment with steroids/azathiopine should be considered. If there is any hint of vasculitis, which I have seen on one occasion mimic MND, cyclophosphamide can be administered.

Diagnosis not obvious or difficult.

The usual problem here is telling the difference between degenerative spinal disease with a radicular problem in an arm or a leg and MND. Prominent fasciculation is not often seen with a foot drop, for example due to a disc, but in the arms a lot of fasciculation can be seen with spondylosis. Obviously, in the usual age group one is dealing with, MRI scans may show significant degenerative disease that could turn out to be irrelevant. Even in the best of hands, surgery can be carried out in good faith and yet the diagnosis later clearly becomes MND. When investigating a spastic paraparesis with no fasciculation, MND may not be considered in the initial differential diagnosis. However, when all the usual tests are negative, and with time, fasciculation spreads into the arms and perhaps bulbar muscles, then a diagnosis of primary lateral sclerosis or if lower motor neurone features have developed, classical MND may emerge. Such situations can be difficult diagnostically together with knowing what to tell the patient. Again, one might be accused of lack of communication although it may simply be that the diagnosis could not have been made at an earlier juncture. In cases where, in retrospect, unnecessary surgery might have been performed, one was at least trying to treat the treatable.

Other surprises are relatively rare. Post-polio syndromes should be obvious from the history. Focal forms of spinal muscular atrophy can be an impediment. Lead or mercury poisoning should not be totally forgotten. Compared with most other neurological diagnoses, the differential diagnosis is hardly ever versus a functional disorder. However, I once saw a patient who was convinced that she had motor neurone disease but with no physical signs or evident disability whatsoever, but who came back a year later with the disease. There was another patient with a progressive weakness together with breathlessness who seemed convincing and in whom I was almost certain had motor neurone disease. However there was normal neurophysiology, and we later thought the patient must have been a hysteric.

MANAGEMENT OF THE ESTABLISHED CASE

I find the nurse practitioner role essential and would have great difficulty managing a case humanely without such support. Experience suggests that interested neurologists working at a distance from a centre that offers a multidisciplinary approach are perfectly capable of managing patients' care well, but it takes a lot of effort and availability if certain important aspects of patient care are not going to get left out. At the other extreme, it is quite possible for a multidisciplinary approach to get out of control and risk overwhelming the patient by possibly giving them too much information too quickly; or by allowing them to see cases of more advanced MND and frightening them badly. It is therefore important that the consultant, in concert with a nurse practitioner, undertakes a form of triage so that patients do not see too many health care professionals or see any before they really need them. One should also curb any enthusiasm for inappropriate procedures, such as gastrostomy, respiratory support, videofluroscopy, or administration of a new drug.

The component elements of multidisciplinary clinics usually include the consultant, the nurse practitioner, speech and swallowing therapists with links with the communication aids centre, a dietician with close links with an endoscopy team, physiotherapists, occupational therapists, a social worker, respiratory advisers, and often the local care adviser from the Motor Neurone Disease Association. Rehabilitationists, palliative care teams, and the chaplain may also be involved. It is therefore clear that one needs to be selective and timely in using these resources. Such clinics work best when whatever is advised can be delivered (e.g. equipment or some other service), rather than relying on some other agency or simply sending a list of recommendations back to the hapless general practitioner or neurologist working at the periphery.

PROGNOSIS

It is well known that the prognosis in motor neurone disease is generally poor compared with other degenerative diseases. Early respiratory symptoms and bulbar dysfunction are poor signs. Rapid progression until the time of diagnosis is at least as important. Exceptions occur, for example, the traditionally held view that purely lower motor neurone involvement is a good sign, can prove to be very wrong, and an occasional patient with an onset with bulbar palsy lives for 10 years. On the whole, approximately 30% of patients live for 5 years, 10% for 10 years, and a few for up to 20 years. Although the progressive weakness causes major problems, the usual retention of intellect and personality and the relative rarity of major depression often means that these years are used in a positive manner.

DRUG TREATMENT

Most patients with motor neurone disease are not benefited by any form of medication. It is not common even when one is actively looking for anxiety and depression, for anxiolytics or antidepressants to be required or requested. Antispasticity agents, such as Lioresal, are also relatively rarely indicated as the degree of spasticity or at least spasticity enough to be causing a significant problem is relatively rare, presumably due to the lower motor neurone component in most patients. A controlled control of Riluzole, a drug that decreases glutamate released from nerve terminals, showed a 3-month longer average survival, and a higher proportion of survivors at 18 months compared with placebo. The effects on the degree of disability were less convincing. Nevertheless, a number of patients in areas where the financial implications have been absorbed are now taking this drug usually as part of a shared care protocol with general practitioners. This normally simply involves an information sheet for the GP and the patients being followed up in a multidisciplinary clinic at more regular intervals than occurred previously, and having their biochemical indices of hepatic and renal function monitored. The dose is 50 mg twice-daily. Nausea, fatigue, and somnolence are the main problems and hepatic function can be markedly affected but soon recovers. Not all patients think the drug worth taking and quite a high proportion who start taking it stop when they deteriorate or get side-effects.

A number of trials of neurotrophic factors have not as yet, despite some promising animal models, been successful. Nevertheless, neurotrophins are currently the main area of interest and myotrophin is being used in selected trials in the United States, and it is possible that one of these growth factors will prove to be of modest benefit.

It goes without saying that Riluzole, and perhaps the next generation of drugs, may only delay slightly and not avoid any of the complications of MND. Thus, all the efforts that have been made over the last few years to improve support for these patients, needs to be kept firmly in place and enhanced.

OTHER MEDICAL INTERVENTIONS

Cricopharyngeal myotomy surgery seems to have gone out of fashion which is appropriate given that it had never been shown to be of benefit. However, it is conceivable there is a very small subgroup where it may still be appropriate so is worthy of a mention.

Feeding gastrostomy rather than nasogastric feeding has been a significant advance particularly in patients who have presented with major bulbar problems with intact or reasonably intact limb function. It is easier to use and less embarrassing than a nasogastric tube and many patients with a feeding gastrostomy can get out into the world and often travel extensively, in a way that they would not have done otherwise. Nevertheless, nasogastric feeding as part of late-stage terminal care, may be more appropriate in some cases. If it is clear that nasogastric feeding is going to be necessary it is best to discuss it several months beforehand with the patient and not to wait too long, particularly if the patient is beginning to lose a significant amount of weight or running an obvious risk of aspiration pneumonia. Videofluroscopy is of some help, as is pulse oximetry, in detecting early aspiration, although a lot of coughing and clinical common sense is almost as good. It is better to work with gastroenterologists or interventional radiologists who have carried out gastrostomies before under these circumstances, and can work as part of the multidisciplinary team and with the dieticians, in particular.

In such circumstances the whole procedure generally goes without a hitch during a short two-day admission.

Feeding gastrostomy used to be controversial but this has, by and large, now ended except in cases where respiratory support is necessary. Clearly, active intervention is more of an issue if the patient has presented largely with respiratory problems but is otherwise relatively undisabled, whereas at a later stage it is more a matter of comfort and terminal care. Forced vital capacities, around a half of predicted, makes it likely that respiratory failure will ensue. Prevention of aspiration, suctioning of secretions, and prompt treatment of pneumonia and atelectasis can delay onset, as can vocal cord assessment as a few will have stridor that may be quiet if the respiratory muscles are weak, and a tracheostomy is worth considering. Although it is highly dependent on the centre, intermittent positive pressure breathing is increasingly being used, as is intermittent negative pressure ventilation helping, by resting fatigued muscles.

However, long-term assisted ventilation remains rare and in this centre we have neither advised nor encouraged nor had any pressure from the patients to instigate it in recent years. Other centres have different views on this. However, one suspects that, for a variety of reasons, having gone through enthusiastic phases, attitudes may well regress to the reaction of both doctors and patients that life on a ventilator with eventual complete paralysis does not have worthwhile quality, not with stand the harrowing situation of switching off ventilators when the patient expresses a desire for that to happen.

GENETIC TESTING/COUNSELLING

Familial ALS is rare. The commonest adult type is dominant. There is a rare recessive juvenile form mapped to chromosome 2. In the dominant form, several single site mutations have been found in all but 3 of the 5 exons of the gene coding for CU/ZN sod (SOD1) on chromosome 21q. About 20% of all ALS families have one of these mutations. To find a mutation in a sporadic case has been recorded but is exceptionally rare. On the rare occasion that one is dealing with a family, we would see them in the joint neurogenetics clinic with a geneticist and counsellor and offer to test any at-risk adults if, after careful consideration, they wish, in a virtually identical manner to the way we deal with Huntington's chorea.

Occasionally, testing for the CAG repeat mutations in the androgen receptor (less than 25 normally, greater than 40 with Kennedy's syndrome) should be carried out. In young people, many screen for hexosaminidase A deficiency.

INVOLVEMENT IN CLINICAL TRIALS, RESEARCH, AND BRAIN BANKING

The majority of patients will appreciate being invited to be part of research studies in motor neurone disease if required

and will be happy to enter clinical trials. As with all trials, there may be some reluctance to hear about the placebo arm but if the alternative is no active treatment then many patients will wish to enter. Similarly, for simple requests for blood or urine, few patients will mind, particularly if they are given an explanation for the sort of research that is designed and reassurance that it has been approved by an ethical committee. More invasive tests, such as CSF examination may encounter a little more resistance. There has been little pressure in obtaining consent for post-mortem examination in MND, unlike in conditions such as Parkinson's disease. However, if it ever became a priority for the research community, there is no reason to believe that, with the support of the Motor Neurone Disease Association, similar arrangements could not be made both for sufferers and for controls (often partners) as has been so successful with the Parkinson's Disease Bank.

TERMINAL CARE

This is a critical part of the management of motor neurone disease. Fortunately, the majority of hospices have now expressed an interest and it is relatively rare for the neurologists to be actively involved at this stage. MND has been one of those conditions that has been actively debated by the euthanasia lobby. Most neurologists in this country would consider that it is important that in the last two months of this illness, patients are kept as comfortable as possible and that any inappropriate treatment is avoided. It is therefore essential that many patients have infusions that contain drugs to control dyspnoea, pain, drooling, insomnia, and fear. Opioids, hyoscine, benzodiazepines, usually by subcutaneous infusion, are therefore required and the response of the symptoms rather than concerns about the dosage should be the order of the day.

CONCLUSION

We now return to the multidisciplinary approach. There has been an attempt to put together protocols but one needs to be careful that these are appropriate and tailored to the individual patient. There are some patients who even when they have been told they have MND, do not wish to go to clinics or even have the name of the disease mentioned in front of them ever again. Although this situation relatively rare, it is worth mentioning, because these views need to be respected and it is rather difficult to write fixed protocols when there is still going to be such variation in attitude towards the disease.

The important principles are: that patients feel they know where to go or to phone when they need help; some of problems are predicted and avoided; when they need equipment or supportive letters about housing, etc. that it happens quickly. If the disease progresses rapidly and there are long delays, appropriate actions are rendered useless. A helpline is also invaluable.

A further principle is that one person should remain in charge so that the process does not get out of hand and that rigid views (encouraged by protocols!) are discouraged, good humour maintained, and feedback from patients encouraged.

FURTHER READING

Bensimon, G., Lacomblez, L., Meininger, V. *et al.* (1994). A controlled trial of Riluzole in amyotrophic lateral sclerosis. *New England Journal of Medicine*, **330**, 585–91.

Lange, D. J., Trojaborg, W. T., Latov, N. *et al.* (1992). Multifocal motor neuropathy with conduction block: a distinct clinical entity? *Neurology*, **42**, 497–505.

Murray, N. M. F. (1994). Neurophysiology. In *Motor neuron disease*, (ed. A. C. William), pp. 171–90. Chapman and Hall, New York.

Oliver, D. (1994). Terminal care. In *Motor neuron disease*, (ed. A. C. Williams), pp. 281–96. Chapman and Hall, New York.

Pegg, R. (1994) A carer's perspective. In *Motor neuron disease*, (ed. A. C. Williams), pp. 203–12. Chapman and Hall, New York.

Pestronk, A., Chaudhry, V., Feldman, E. L. *et al.* (1990). Lower motor neuron syndromes defined by patterns of weakness, nerve conduction abnormalities, and high titers of antiglycolipid antibodies. *Annals of Neurology*, **27**, 316–28.

Rosen, D. R., Siddique, T., Patterson, D. *et al.* (1993). Mutations in Cu/Zn superoxide dismutase gene are associated with familial amyotrophic lateral sclerosis. *Nature*, **362**, 59–62.

Tandan, R. (1994). Clinical features and differential diagnosis of classical motor neuron disease. In *Motor neuron disease*, (ed. A. C. Williams), pp. 3–27. Chapman and Hall, New York.

Unsworth, J. (1994). Coping with the disability of established disease. In *Motor neuron disease*, (ed. A. C. Williams), pp. 213–38. Chapman and Hall, New York.

12 | *Stroke and subarachnoid haemorrhage*

Peter Humphrey

In the United Kingdom stroke is cared for by a large number of specialists. General practitioners, geriatricians, and general physicians will manage most people in the acute phase. Neurological or neurosurgical advice may be sought but few neurologists are actively involved in the day-to-day management of acute stroke. The long-term rehabilitation of stroke patients also involves young disabled units and rehabilitation teams.

Management of stroke is expensive and accounts for about 5% of the UK health service's hospital costs. Stroke is the commonest cause of severe physical disability. About 100 000 people suffer a first stroke each year in England and Wales. It is important to emphasize that approximately 25 000 occur in people under 65. The incidence of stroke is 2 per 1000 per year (Oxford Community Stroke Project 1983). Each year approximately 60 000 people are reported to die of stroke, this represents approximately 12% of all deaths; only ischaemic heart disease and cancer account for more deaths.

Transient ischaemic attacks (TIAs) are defined as acute focal neurological symptoms/signs resulting from vascular disease which resolve in less than 24 hours: most settle in less than 30 minutes. The incidence of first ever TIA is 0.35 per 1000.

Over the last 20 years the mortality from stroke has fallen both in the United Kingdom and United States by approximately 20–30% (Khaw 1996). There has also been a fall in the incidence of stroke. This is probably real but may partly be accounted for by the reclassification of disease, for example, most cases of dementia are now thought to be due to primary degenerative disease and not atherosclerosis, as previously thought. The more successful treatment of hypertension is likely to be another important factor in the declining incidence of cerebrovascular disease. It is unlikely that this explains the whole picture as this improvement is also seen over the period 1950–60 before the treatment of hypertension became widely practised.

All those interested in stroke will appreciate that stroke or TIA is not a diagnosis. It is merely a description of a symptom complex thought to have a vascular aetiology. The management of stroke or TIA is, therefore, not a single process but will vary according to the type of event. It is important to classify stroke according to the anatomy of the lesion, its timing, aetiology, and pathogenesis. This classification will help to decide the most appropriate management.

CLASSIFICATION OF STROKE

ANATOMICAL

Carotid vs. vertebrobasilar

Carotid

Classifying whether a stroke is carotid or vertebrobasilar in territory is important especially if the patient makes a good recovery. Carotid endarterectomy is of proven value only in those with carotid symptoms. Carotid stroke usually produces hemiparesis, hemisensory loss, or dysphasia if the dominant hemisphere is involved. Apraxia and visuospatial problems may also occur. If there is severe deficit there may also be a homonymous hemianopia.

From a management point of view it is important to include vascular events affecting the eyes because the ophthalmic artery is the first branch of the internal carotid artery. Episodes of amaurosis fugax or central retinal artery occlusion are, therefore, also carotid events.

A Horner's syndrome can occur due to damage to the sympathetic fibres in the carotid sheath; this may follow vascular events in the internal carotid artery especially carotid dissections. Many patients presenting with localized headache and a Horner's syndrome have in the past been diagnosed as having had a 'severe migraine'. In our experience, carotid dissection is often the correct diagnosis in these patients if ultrasound and magnetic resonance scanning are performed soon after the onset of symptoms.

After an internal carotid artery occlusion there may be exaggerated pulsation in the branches of the external carotid artery (particularly the superficial temporal artery). Increased collateral blood flow through this artery shunts blood via the orbital vessels into the ophthalmic artery and then into the circle of Willis in an attempt to compensate for the internal carotid occlusion, the patient thus performing his own extracranial–intracranial anastomosis. This is an almost universal finding on ultrasound in internal carotid artery occlusion. Sometimes, the increased collateral flow is so marked that the superficial temporal artery on the side of the occlusion becomes tender and painful. This can mimic temporal arteritis. It is particularly important in this situation that the temporal artery is *not* biopsied or a major collateral source of blood supply will be obliterated.

Vertebrobasilar

The terminal branches of this system are the posterior cerebral arteries. Field defects, usually unilateral, are the principle result of ischaemia. Lesions on both sides are not uncommon and produce complete blindness, bilateral visual hallucinations (e.g. impression of frosted glass or water running across the whole of the vision). Anton's syndrome consists of bilateral cortical blindness (with little insight), normal pupillary responses, and confabulation.

Sometimes, amnesic syndromes may be seen following ischaemia to the medial part of the temporal lobe. However, in most patients transient global amnesia is no longer thought to be a TIA affecting the vertebrobasilar system (Hodges and Warlow 1990).

The posterior cerebral artery also supplies part of the thalamus: infarction here produces sensory impairment over the contralateral side of the body which may be accompanied by a very unpleasant pain: this can be spontaneous or induced by light touch of the skin (thalamic syndrome) and often reaches its peak some months after the stroke.

The signs following vertebrobasilar ischaemia depend on the level of the lesion in the brainstem (Caplan 1981). Midbrain ischaemia may result in pupillary changes with impaired vertical gaze or oculomotor nerve dysfunction. Damage to the pons produces horizontal gaze palsy with facial weakness or sensory loss. In either case, a quadriparesis or hemiparesis may occur.

A wide range of other syndromes are reported to follow ischaemia of localized areas of the brainstem. The basic pattern is one of ipsilateral cranial nerve palsies combined with contralateral paresis or sensory loss which may affect face, arm and leg, or arm and leg depending on the level in the brainstem at which this occurs. There may be ipsilateral cerebellar signs and/or a Horner's syndrome. Thrombosis of the posterior inferior cerebellar artery serves as a useful example. This produces ischaemia of the dorsolateral medulla with cranial nerve palsies V, VI, VII, IX, and X, cerebellar ataxia, and a Horner's syndrome on the same side of the lesion with contralateral spinothalamic loss in the arm and leg. Pain and temperature loss may occur over the ipsilateral face due to damage to the descending tract and nucleus of V. Hemiplegia is rare because the pyramidal tracts lying ventrally are spared.

Occlusion of the basilar artery itself is often fatal producing flaccid tetraplegia and loss of brainstem reflexes. Coma often occurs. It is important to distinguish this from the rare 'locked-in' syndrome in which there is ventral ischaemia of the midbrain. The clinical picture is similar except that the patient is fully alert. He may appear to be unconscious because he is completely immobile apart from vertical movements of the eyes and occasionally the eyelids. It is good practice to introduce oneself to any patient who appears to be 'unconscious' and immediately ask the patient to move his eyes vertically before accepting that the patient is truly unconscious.

There is little to be gained by memorizing many of the names of the different brainstem vascular syndromes. One word of caution—carotid artery dissection is one of the common causes of young stroke. It commonly presents with an ipsilateral Horner's and contralateral hemiparesis: it has also been described with ipsilateral lower cranial nerve palsies (IX–XII) due to the expanded carotid artery damaging these nerves in the neck where they lie adjacent to the carotid artery (Sturzenegger and Huber 1993). Classical teaching would have mistakenly put this vascular syndrome in the vertebrobasilar territory (q.v. carotid dissection).

It is particularly important that postural vertigo in the elderly, whether on lateral rotation or extension of the neck, is *not* thought to be diagnostic of vertebrobasilar TIAs. Isolated vertigo unaccompanied by other brainstem symptoms or signs, within six weeks of onset is unlikely to occur on the basis of vertebrobasilar insufficiency (Fisher 1967).

Lacunar

These small deep microinfarcts described by Fisher are commonly seen in hypertensive and diabetic patients (Fisher 1982): they rarely occur in patients with carotid stenosis. It is important, if possible, to recognize these lacunar syndromes because of their good prognosis and different pathogenesis. Lacunar infarcts (LACI) commonly present as pure motor stroke, pure sensory stroke, sensorimotor stroke, or ataxic hemiparesis (Table 12.1). Patients are required to have either complete face, arm, and leg or major face and arm or leg involvement. Those with more restricted deficits (e.g. weak hand only, are not included)—these are considered to be partial anterior circulation infarcts in the cortex. Acute focal movement disorders may also be lacunar.

Sometimes multiple lacunar infarcts occur. In such cases, there is often, but by no means always, a history of preceding minor stroke. The resulting syndrome is of a pseudobulbar palsy with dementia, dysarthria, small stepping gait (marche a petits pas), unsteadiness, and incontinence.

Bamford and colleagues (1991) have used the Oxford Community Stroke Data to classify strokes clinically into:

(1) lacunar infarcts;
(2) total anterior circulation (Carotid artery) infarcts;
(3) partial anterior circulation (Carotid artery) infarcts; and
(4) posterior circulation infarcts (vertebrobasilar).

Table 12.1 Common lacunar infarcts

Clinical type	Site of lesion
Pure motor hemiplegia	Internal capsule, pons, cerebral peduncle
Pure hemi-anaesthesia	Thalamus
Ataxic hemiparesis	Pons, internal capsule
Dysarthria/clumsy hand syndrome	Pons, internal capsule

Total anterior circulation infarct (TACI) presents with a combination of higher cerebral dysfunction deficit (dysphasia, dyscalculia, visuospatial disorder), homonymous visual field defect, and ipsilateral motor and/or sensory deficit of at least *two* areas of the face, arm, and leg. Partial anterior circulation infarcts (PACI) present with only two of the three components of the TACI syndrome with higher cerebral function alone *or* with a motor/sensory deficit more restricted than those classified as LACI (e.g. confined to *one* limb, or to face and hand but *not* to the whole arm). In posterior circulation infarcts (POCI), patients present with any of the symptoms/signs described under the section on vertebrobasilar disease.

Using these simple clinical criteria, it proved possible to classify most strokes into one of these four different categories. This may be important as the prognosis, aetiology, and risk of recurrent strokes varies in the different groups. The TACI group had a very poor prognosis, high mortality, but low recurrence rate, presumably as most of the carotid territory has been destroyed by the infarct. The PACI group had a good prognosis but high early recurrence rate, as this type of stroke is frequently embolic probably from internal carotid artery atheroma. These patients have a lot to lose from a second stroke. The lacunar group had an intermediate prognosis but a low risk of recurrence. This type of stroke is rarely due to embolic disease but follows microvascular thrombosis or haemorrhage often as a result of hypertension and/or diabetes.

The POCI group had a good prognosis but high early recurrence rate. This Oxford Community-based stroke study dispels the notion that brainstem strokes in general have a poor prognosis in the acute phase: it also emphasizes the significant risk of recurrence and need to advise about risk factors and offer early medical treatment to those with posterior circulation infarcts.

Subclavian steal syndrome

This follows occlusion or stenosis of the subclavian artery, usually on the left. The affected artery then fills retrogradely from the opposite vertebral artery or the carotid artery via the circle of Willis. Because of the blocked subclavian, blood flow in the relevant arm is dependent on retrograde flow in the vertebral artery. Patients are usually asymptomatic but may develop symptoms of brainstem TIAs characteristically but rarely when the arm is exercised since blood is stolen from the brainstem by the arm as it is exercised. This syndrome is largely a curiosity: there is a very low risk of stroke (Hennerici *et al.* 1988) and it is not necessary to consider any form of surgical intervention unless there are intractable vertebrobasilar TIAs. It is often possible to diagnose this clinically by measuring the blood pressure (BP) in both arms, especially in patients with vertebrobasilar TIAs. A systolic difference of more than 15 mm Hg between two arms suggests significant subclavian disease. It is usually not necessary to act on this except to ensure that in hypertensive patients the BP is monitored in the arm unaffected by the subclavian stenosis. Angioplasty is a less invasive alternative to surgery.

Border zone infarcts

Sometimes, infarction follows a generalised reduction in cerebral blood flow. This is most commonly seen after cardiac arrest or hypoxic damage during cardiac surgery. Ischaemia is then especially marked in the border zone between the territory of individual arteries because here perfusion is least. The parieto-occipital zone is the area most often affected; here border zone infarcts produce visual field defects (often partial and easily missed on routine examination), reading difficulties, visual disorientation, and constructional apraxia (Ross Russell *et al.* 1978). In the frontal border zone, slowing up, pathological grasp reflexes, gait disturbances, and incontinence may occur.

It should now be apparent that the clinical description is helpful in formulating an opinion about the anatomical site, aetiology, prognosis, and risk of recurrence. This may well have management consequences.

TIMING/PATHOGENESIS

The timing of events is important in our understanding of pathogenesis. Most TIAs are embolic. Embolic TIAs usually arise from the major extracranial arteries or from the heart. A small percentage are haemodynamic—these usually occur when there is severe widespread occlusive disease.

Sometimes it is possible to identify patients with haemodynamic TIAs clinically. Embolic TIAs usually occur for no apparent cause. However, haemodynamic TIAs may have a trigger; for instance, standing, exercising, lowering BP, eating, and straining have all been described as precipitating events. Haemodynamic amaurosis fugax may be triggered by a bright light or sunlight. Unlike patients with embolic amaurosis fugax, who usually describe a shutter or black shadow descending across the visual field, those with haemodynamic attacks often initially describe increased contrast between black and white and then whiteness of vision before the vision darkens. Haemodynamic amaurosis fugax is often more gradual than embolic amaurosis. Sometimes, haemodynamic TIAs may be proceeded by symptoms of presyncope such as dizziness and faintness. Finally they may occur many times a day over a considerable period of time: this is unusual in embolic TIAs.

While haemodynamic TIAs are rare compared with embolic TIAs it is important to try and identify them as it is unlikely that antiplatelet therapy will help these symptoms: some type of reconstructive vascular surgery is more likely to be appropriate (Ross Russell *et al.* 1983).

The risk of stroke after a TIA is approximately 30% in five years (Dennis *et al.* 1990). Stroke is usually secondary to thromboembolic disease. About 15% of all strokes are haemorrhagic. Of these, 5% are secondary to subarachnoid haemorrhage and 10% to intracerebral haemorrhage (Table 12.2). Thromboembolic stroke accounts for 85% of all stroke (Sandercock *et al.* 1985). It is usually possible on clinical grounds to differentiate those with subarachnoid haemorrhage.

Table 12.2 Causes of cerebral haemorrhage

1. Hypertension
2. Aneurysm (berry)
3. Atherosclerotic aneurysm
4. Perimesencephalic haemorrhage
5. Arteriovenous malformation
6. Anticoagulants
7. Bleeding into tumour
8. Mycotic aneurysm
9. Coagulation disorders
10. Arteritis
11. Amyloid angiopathy
12. Drug abuse (e.g. cocaine)
13. Venous thrombosis
14. Leukaemia
15. Cavernous Angioma

Table 12.3 Cardiac sources of emboli

Left atrium
Thrombus (usually secondary to atrial fibrillation)
Myxoma
Atrial septal aneurysm

Mitral valve
Rheumatic endocarditis
Infective endocarditis
Marantic endocarditis
Prosthetic valve
Mitral valve prolapse
Mitral annulus calcification
Libman–Sacks endocarditis

Left ventricle
Thrombus: myocardial infarction, cardiomyopathy

Aortic valve
Rheumatic endocarditis
Infective endocarditis
Marantic endocarditis
Bicuspid valve
Aortic sclerosis and calcification
Prosthetic valve
Syphilitic aortitis

Congenital cardiac disorders

Cardiac surgery
Air embolism
Platelet/fibrin embolism

Right to left paradoxical shunts
Patent foramen ovale
ASD/VSD
Pulmonary arteriovenous malformation

The clinical differentiation of thromboembolic disease and intracerebral haemorrhage is difficult. Various authors have attempted to develop a clinical score (Weir *et al.* 1994). Early loss of consciousness, early vomiting, bilateral extensor plantars, marked elevation of BP, all suggest haemorrhage. TIAs, the presence of peripheral vascular disease, suggest thromboembolic disease. However, no clinical score is sufficiently accurate to allow reliable differentiation. Computerize tomographic (CT) scan (provided it is performed within two weeks of the first symptom) is the only reliable method; stroke patients should have a CT scan as, clearly, the proper assessment and treatment of thromboembolism and haemorrhage are different.

What percentage of stroke are thrombolic and what percentage embolic is far more difficult to ascertain. It depends mainly on the frequency of embolic sources in the population at large (e.g. rheumatic heart disease is becoming less frequent), and the intensity of investigation to look for an embolic source (e.g. echocardiography, doppler, or duplex examination of the carotid arteries), (Table 12.3). Unfortunately, this is made even more complicated by the fact that vascular disease is a diffuse illness. The detection of a cardiac source of emboli does not necessarily mean that embolization has occurred. All will have seen the patient who is in atrial fibrillation and has a small intracerebral haemorrhage on CT accounting for his/her stroke.

It is estimated that approximately half of all thromboembolic strokes are embolic and half thrombotic.

The percentage of all strokes due to other causes such as primary hypoperfusion (q.v. border zone infarcts), vasospasm, and arteritis is small: these are all discussed under the relevant sections.

ACCURACY OF DIAGNOSIS/DIFFERENTIAL DIAGNOSIS

Managing any condition requires knowledge of differential diagnosis and accuracy of diagnosis (Norris and Hackinski

1982). The differential diagnosis of TIA and stroke includes epilepsy, migraine, tumour, demyelination, syncope, subdural haematoma, malignant hypertension, hyperventilation, hypoglycaemia, and giant intracerebral aneurysm. Focal motor seizures may be mistaken for TIA, especially in patients with a very severe carotid stenosis in whom the jerking of the limbs occurs as part of the TIA. Focal sensory seizures are even more difficult to distinguish although the march of the sensory symptoms in a focal seizure may be helpful. Migraine occasionally presents diagnostic difficulties. The slow build-up of a migrainous aura which often lasts 20–30 minutes would be unusual in a TIA. Visual migraine is often made up of positive visual symptoms, (e.g. scintillating scotomas), unlike the blackness of amaurosis fugax. The presence of a typical migrainous headache would be unusual in a TIA. Headache occurs in 16% of TIA patients (Koudstall *et al.* 1991).

The UK transient ischaemic attack study group have presented their data on tumours mimicking TIAs. Patients who present with sensory TIAs, jerking TIAs, loss of consciousness, or speech arrest should all be suspected of having a tumour until proven otherwise (Coleman *et al.* 1993). Demyelination will usually be suspected on the basis of the age of the patients, past history of previous attacks and more gradual onset of hemiparesis compared to that seen in a vascular hemiparesis.

Subdural haematomas rarely present with vascular like symptoms. They do, however, present a particular diagnostic difficulty. The diagnosis of a carotid TIA is usually reasonably consistent (Kraaijeveld *et al.* 1984; Landi *et al.* 1992). However, vertebrobasiliar TIAs are more variable. It is important to be wary of labelling the following as TIAs— loss of consciousness, dizziness, mental confusion, incontinence of faeces or urine, and bilateral loss of vision with reduced level of consciousness—these are all often secondary to hypoperfusion. Isolated symptoms such as vertigo, diplopia, dysphagia, dysarthria, loss of balance, tinnitus, sensory symptoms confined to one part of one limb or face, amnesia, drop attacks, and scintillating scotomas, should always be interpreted cautiously when they occur in isolation: they may, however, be consistent with TIAs especially if they occur together or with other more definite symptoms of TIAs. The reliability of the diagnosis of TIA can be improved if clear-cut criteria in plain language are used before assessment of TIAs is made (Koudstaal *et al.* 1986).

In the diagnosis of stroke the false positive rate with no investigations is between 1% and 5% if a careful history is taken of the event (Sandercock *et al.* 1985). It is important to emphasize that CT is no more accurate than the clinical opinion (Norris and Hachinski 1982); this is probably because some events which are clinically strokes are mistakenly diagnosed on CT as tumours, a diagnosis which is not substantiated with time. The accuracy of diagnosis in TIAs is not so consistent particularly for vertebrobasilar disease mainly because of the difficulty in interpreting the isolated symptoms mentioned above (Ferro *et al.* 1996).

The tendency to diagnose vague transient episodes as TIAS should be resisted (Martin *et al*, 1997).

RISK FACTORS

Advice about risk factors is one of the most important aspects of managing cerebrovascular disease.

Age

This is the most important predictive factor of cerebrovascular disease. The incidence of stroke is low below 40. It rises from an annual incidence of less than 1 per 100 000 per year below 40 to more than 2000 per 100 000 per year by the age of 75 (Kannel and Wolf 1983).

Hypertension

This is the most powerful risk factor for both haemorrhagic and atherosclerotic cerebrovascular disease (Prospective Studies Collaboration 1995). Although most physicians pay more attention to diastolic blood pressure, systolic blood pressure more closely reflects the risk of further stroke. There is no clear cut-off at which the risk begins to rise. The risk of stroke rises exponentially as diastolic blood pressure increases in the range 70–110 mm Hg. A 7.5 mm Hg rise in the usual diastolic blood pressure, within the range 70–110 mm Hg is associated with a doubling in the risk of stroke.

Transient Ischaemic Attacks

The risk of a stroke after TIA is approximately 30% in 5 years (Dennis *et al.* 1990). It is highest in the first year. The carotid surgery trials suggest that in patients with carotid stenosis the risk of stroke is approximately 10% in the first year even with best medical treatment.

Cardiac Disease

Patients with coronary artery disease are at increased risk of stroke. Cardiac enlargement on the chest X-ray, congestive cardiac failure, ECG changes such as left ventricular enlargement, conduction block, and ST/T wave changes also increase the risk of stroke (Kannel and Wolf 1983). Atrial fibrillation substantially increases the risk of stroke. There is also a long list of potential cardiac sources of emboli (see Table 12.3).

Diabetes Mellitus

This is an independent risk factor according to the Framingham data.

Smoking

There is no doubt that smoking is an important risk factor for stroke. (Donnan et al. 1993).

Cholesterol

This is a very important risk factor for coronary artery disease and myocardial infarction. An overview of cholesterol data has shown that an elevated cholesterol increases the risk of stroke by about 30% (Qizilbash *et al.* 1992). However, as most TIA patients die a cardiac death and cholesterol is an important risk factor for cardiac disease, advice about cholesterol is mainly aimed at preventing coronary events (Sacco *et al.* 1982).

Other risk factors

Alcohol, in excess, is probably a risk factor for cerebrovascular disease, especially haemorrhage. Homocysteinuria and fibrinogen may be independent risk factors for vascular disease (Clarke *et al.* 1991; Qizilbash *et al.* 1991). It is not known if obesity, stress, physical activity, have any part to play in the aetiology of stroke—if they do, it is likely to be small. Not surprisingly peripheral vascular disease is also a risk factor for stroke.

INVESTIGATIONS

The routine investigation of TIA or stroke patients requires a few simple tests: full blood count, ESR (erythrocyte sedimentation rate), urea and electrolytes, glucose and cholesterol, along with a chest X-ray and ECG. It is important to remember that most patients with strokes and elevated ESR do not have an arteritis or subacute bacterial endocarditis; in fact, a high ESR in stroke patients usually remains unexplained and settles without treatment.

Carotid TIAs or stroke with recovery also need a doppler/duplex ultrasound to detect carotid stenosis—this is highly accurate but very operator-dependent (Hankey *et al.* 1990; Humphrey *et al.* 1990; Howard *et al.* 1991); our own experience has shown that most X-ray departments setting up doppler/ duplex ultrasound services are highly inaccurate and all such units should have their results substantiated either by angiography or a proven ultrasound service (Fig. 12.1).

Other tests to be considered include:

1. Thyroid function tests: especially when cholesterol is raised or patient is in atrial fibrillation.
2. CT scan is indicated if there is:
   (a) doubt about diagnosis especially if gradual onset or no clear history;
   (b) need to exclude cerebral haemorrhage: ideally all strokes;
   (c) cerebellar stroke with deteriorating level of consciousness.
3. Cerebral angiography (digital subtraction/magnetic resonance) may be indicated if the patients is a candidate for carotid endarterectomy:
   (a) to look for evidence of arteritis;
   (b) in cerebral haemorrhage.
4. Echocardiography is indicated if:-
   (a) Abnormal cardiac findings are present, suggestive of valvular heart disease or evidence of recent myocardial infarction or left ventricular aneurysm clinically or on chest X-ray and ECG.
   (b) All young stroke (<50 yrs): if no other clear-cut cause for stroke is found.
   (c) Multiple territory stroke for no clear cause.
   (d) Antiphospholipid syndrome or systemic lupus erythematosis: ?Libman–Sacks endocarditis.
   (e) Positive blood cultures.
5. Blood cultures: if febrile—subacute bacterial endocarditis.
6. Temporal artery biopsy: arteritis.
7. Twenty-four hour ECG: arrhythmia (very rarely necessary: grossly overused).
8. Young stroke work-up (q.v.).

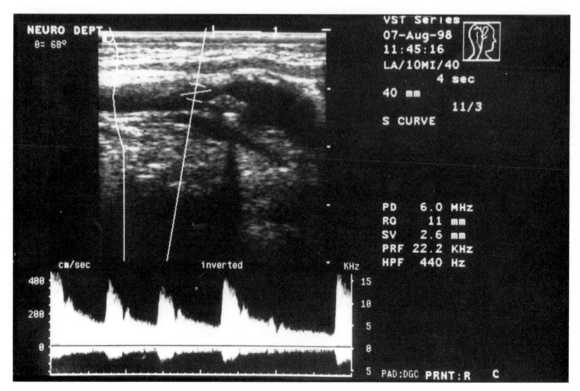

Fig. 12.1 The doppler trace shows a doppler shift of over 15 kHz and a peak systolic velocity (PSV) of over 400 cm/s (N< 120 cm/s) consistent with a tight stenosis: this is the most reliable ultrasound measurement for grading stenosis. A doppler shift of more than 4 kHz suggests a stenosis of more than 50%. Spending too much time assessing the ultrasound image and not enough assessing doppler changes is one of the most common sources of error. The image also demonstrates a tight stenosis at the origin of the internal carotid artery.

TREATMENT

MEDICAL

Vascular risk factors

Hypertension is the most important risk factor for stroke. As already stated, the risk of stroke rises exponentially as diastolic blood pressure increases in the range 70–100 mm Hg. A 7.5 mm Hg rise in diastolic BP within the range 70–110 mm Hg is associated with a doubling in the risk of stroke. This emphasizes the importance of blood pressure control including in the elderly. There is a risk of precipitating hypotension in a small number of patients, especially the elderly; this is often overstated as a reason for not being more aggressive about treating blood pressure, especially isolated systolic hypertension.

In the population at large, a modest fall of 5 mm Hg in mean population diastolic BP, achievable by modestly reducing the mean daily salt intake in the population by 50 mmol/l might reduce overall stroke mortality by 22% (Law *et al.* 1991). This would have a greater effect on the total number of strokes than just treating high blood pressure in people with diastolics of over 100 mm Hg.

Treating all hypertensives would reduce the mortality of stroke by 15%. This compares to aspirin which reduces the *overall* incidence of stroke by 1–2% and carotid endarterectomy which reduces the overall incidence by 0.5% (Dennis and Warlow 1991). Recent data suggest that inadequate treatment of high blood pressure is common and is the most important avoidable risk factor which is not being adequately monitored and treated (Payne *et al.* 1993).

Advice about smoking is clearly important. Good diabetic control is to be encouraged although there is limited data to prove that this reduces the risk of stroke.

There is no consensus about the value of cholesterol-lowering drugs. There is, however, no doubt that the lower the cholesterol the lower the chance of heart attack and I feel everyone under the age of 75 should be offered dietary advice. The average lifespan at 75 is approximately 10 years. Clearly at 75, many will choose not to change their lifestyle, but I think they should at least be offered a low cholesterol diet. In many this will not lower the cholesterol by a great deal. The West Coast of Scotland study (Shepherd *et al.* 1995) and the Scandinavian study (1994) strongly suggest that treating raised cholesterol reduces the risk of cardiac events.

A small number of patients have haematocrits over 50; these need assessment for polycythaemia followed by appropriate treatment if necessary.

Acute stroke/rehabilitation

In recent years there has been much debate over the value of stroke units. A recent overview leaves little doubt that patients treated in stroke units do better than those treated in general medical wards (Langhorne *et al.* 1993). There is no specific reason for this: it may just be an organizational matter rather than due to any one specific treatment. The major benefit from stroke units seems to come from rehabilitation. Rehabilitation should start immediately the stroke is diagnosed. The concept that acute care can be separated from rehabilitation does not seem sensible. There should be a seamless package with acute stroke care and rehabilitation under the direction of the same team; it is the emphasis of the care package which will vary at different moments. Pound *et al.* (1995) have also emphasized that important psychological needs during the acute stage of stroke were often better met by admission to hospital.

There is no proven medical treatment for acute stroke. Dextran has been shown not to be beneficial. The trials of calcium antagonists, steroids, and glycerol are inconclusive (Sandercock and Willems 1992); this is an area of active research.

High blood pressure after acute stroke is common and often settles spontaneously. In most people it does not require treatment. One should only start treatment if hypertensive encephalopathy is considered possible or the patient has had a proven cerebral haemorrhage and the blood pressure is markedly elevated (systolic >230 mm Hg: diastolic >130 mm Hg). It is also important to check the blood pressure in all strokes 1–2 months after discharge from hospital as a significant number will show a persistent rise in blood pressure after discharge which is severe enough to require treatment, even though that individual's blood pressure will have been satisfactory at the time of hospital discharge.

The International Stroke Trial (IST) suggests aspirin should be started immediately after stroke. Routine warfarin or thrombolysis are hazardous (Sandercock *et al.* 1993; Bogousslavsky 1996). Despite the lack of any proven treatment, except aspirin, it is one of the most exciting frontiers in acute neurology. There is no doubt that treatment will come: the increase in and interest created by large multicentre trials is rightly unstoppable. Stroke units makes these trials much easier to perform. We have only to see how the ISIS trials have transformed the care of myocardial infarction to know that we must encourage stroke units to investigate treatments for this most debilitating disease.

More difficult is the question of whether patients do better with rehabilitation at home or in hospital. The recent papers from Gladman *et al.* 1993 and Young and Foster 1992) have suggested home or day hospital care may be better. More work needs to be done on this. If the patient is kept at home, it is clearly important that he/she should still be investigated in the most appropriate manner. What is needed now are more trials comparing home with stroke units. We should not intrinsically assume that hospital is better. Motivation and 'do it yourself' physiotherapy are probably greatly enhanced by staying at home, provided adequate support from social services, paramedical teams, and the family are available.

Transient ischaemic attacks stroke with recovery

The treatment of TIAs has been transformed in the last 10 years with both medical and surgical trials. For the most part this is not because some new treatment has become available but old treatments have been property assessed. Clinicians owe a lot to the advice of good statisticians.

There is no doubt that aspirin reduces the risk of stroke and death in patients with TIAs by approximately 25% (Antiplatelet Trialist's Collaboration 1994). The exact dose is unclear. The evidence is best for doses of around 150–300 mg. Some believe smaller doses (37.5/75 mg) may be adequate but it is possible that the trials using these doses may be too small and that we may have missed a difference between 37.5 mg and larger doses due to a Type II error.

Ticlopidine is also an effective antiplatelet agent, it may be more effective than aspirin (*Lancet* 1991). It is available in the United States but not on general release in the United Kingdom. Unfortunately, it sometimes causes skin rash, diarrhoea, and reversible neutropenia—patients, therefore, need more careful monitoring. A sister to Ticlopidine, Clopidogrel, 75 mg once a day appears safe and may be more effective than aspirin (Caprie 1996). Dipyridamole may be helpful (Davis and Donnan 1998).

Warfarin is indicated for definite cardiac emboli. Lone atrial fibrillation has now been added to this list. The European atrial fibrillation study shows that warfarin reduces the risk of subsequent stroke by 60–70% compared to placebo in patients who have had an episode of cerebral ischaemia. The risk of serious bleeding was only 3% per annum with 0.2% intracranial bleeds (European Atrial Fibrillation study Group 1993).

I also use warfarin if a patient has had several TIAs not controlled by aspirin. I tend to give warfarin for 6–12 months and then switch back to aspirin provided no further ischaemic events occur. There is no good data to support this as yet.

A very common question is: when to start warfarin after a definite stroke? The risk of recurrent emboli is high after the first event but there is the danger of secondary haemorrhage into an infarct if warfarin/heparin is started too early. The Cardiac Embolism Study Group has shown that the risk of secondary haemorrhage is very low provided one is 14 days after the initial event. The risk is also very low in the first 14 days if the infarct is small or the deficit mild. Therefore, I start anticoagulants immediately if the deficit is mild but delay for 14 days if the deficit is severe (e.g. severe hemiparesis, hemisensory loss and dysphasia with a large infarct on CT: clearly, on day 1, CT may be negative and the decision then has to be made on the severity of the clinical deficit only). (Cardiac Embolism Study Group 1984.)

SURGICAL TREATMENT

In 1954, the first carotid endarterectomy (CEA) was performed. The risk of stroke in patients with a carotid stenosis who have had a TIA is approximately 10% per annum. The quoted surgical risk of carotid endarterectomy varies from 1% to 25%. It is not surprising, therefore, that for 37 years no one knew if this operation was worthwhile. It is only with the publication of the European Carotid Surgery Trial (ECST) and the North American Trial (NASCET) in 1991 that the true value of this surgery became known (Brown and Humphrey 1992).

The serious complication rate in ECST was 3.7% and in NASCET 2.1%. Patients were randomized to surgery and medical treatment or best medical treatment. In the group with 70–99% stenosis, there was a highly significant benefit from surgery—there were less than 75% strokes in those treated with carotid endarterectomy. Clearly, the lower the surgical complication rate the sooner the patient benefits from surgery. In the ECST trial the crossover was at approximately 5 months and in the NASCET 3 months. All fit patients with a tight symptomatic stenosis should therefore, be offered surgery—they should be given the natural history risk of stroke (i.e. 10% per annum), the local operation risk and advised that surgery reduce the risk of stroke to 2% per annum. Each patient can then make up his/her mind whether they wish to pursue this. If the surgical risk is over 10% then the benefit from this operation is lost: all units should aim for a surgical risk of under 5%.

There are a possible 5000 candidates for CEA in England and Wales: surgery to this group would prevent 500 strokes in the first year. It is not a cheap form of treatment but for the individual with a carotid TIA and a tight stenosis, surgery reduces the risk of a stroke by 75%. For patients with stenosis of less than 70%, surgery is of no benefit as the natural history risk is so small (European Carotid Surgery Trialists Collaborative Group 1996).

It is important to appreciate that this operation is only for patients with recent carotid symptoms (i.e. usually amaurosis fugax, hemiparesis, hemisensory loss, and dysphasia). Just how much this operation has been over used is emphasized by the report in 1988 (before the results of the ESCT and NASCET trials) which showed that only 35% of patients had this operation for appropriate reasons in a sample of 1302 patients in the United States (Winslow *et al.* 1988).

None of these surgical trials included the angiographic risk. While the risk of stroke after carotid angiography is generally quoted as 1%, it is almost certainly higher in patients with carotid stenosis, leaving approximately 2% with a permanent disability, (Davies and Humphrey 1993). Doppler/duplex ultrasound is undoubtedly the best screening test but it is very operator-dependent. Some units operate on ultrasound alone; unfortunately, obtaining information on the intracranial circulation is difficult with ultrasound. Ultrasound combined with magnetic resonance angiography (MRA) can give highly accurate information about both the carotid artery in the neck as well as an angiographic picture of the whole intracerebral circulation (Fig. 12.2). Our policy now is to operate on the basis of an entirely non-invasive work up with ultrasound and MRA if both tests agree (Young *et al.* 1994). In our hands,

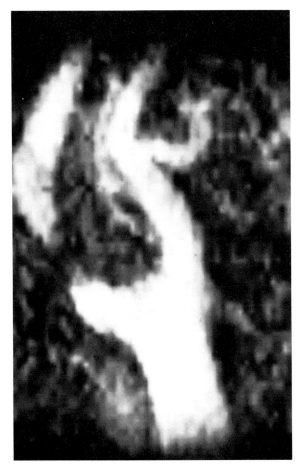

Fig. 12.2 Shows an MRA (Siemens 1.5T) with a tight stenosis at the origin of internal carotid artery. A gap on 3D TOF image signifies a stenosis of at least 80%.

in the 70–99% stenosis group the tests agree in 96% of cases: we only pursue digital subtraction angiography on the 4% in whom the non-invasive tests do not agree. If MRA proves to be less operator-dependent and becomes widely available it may replace the need for ultrasound; to do this would require an enormous expansion in MRA to all district general hospitals.

In expert hands a bruit is the best clinical guide to detect an underlying internal carotid stenosis (Harrison and Marshall 1975; Wilson and Ross Russell 1977). However, the bruit is lost in very tight stenoses (false negative): also, a false positive bruit is not infrequent in the presence of either a contralateral occlusion, external carotid stenosis, or just internal carotid atheroma. Furthermore, if the presence of a bruit is to be of value, it needs to be useful to those who are making the initial assessment. The presence or absence of a bruit in the referral letter to a cerebrovascular clinic showed a specificity of 70% and sensitivity of 57% for 70–99% stenosis (Davies and Humphrey 1994). On this basis, many patients with a carotid stenosis would be denied surgery if only those with a bruit were referred. All patients with carotid TIA or stroke with re-

covery should have carotid ultrasound in a department with a proven track record. I no longer listen for a bruit; if I wish to detect a carotid stenosis I perform an ultrasound examination.

My own personal work-up for carotid endarterectomy is, therefore, a careful history, simple examination of the cardio-vascular system (occasionally I examine the neurological system!), routine blood tests, chest X-ray and ECG. This combined with doppler/duplex ultrasound is all done at the first clinic visit. If a carotid stenosis is detected and the patient is symptomatic, fit, and agrees to the risk of surgery, then an urgent MRA as an outpatient is booked. The patient is then seen a few days after the MRA and referred for surgery if the MRA confirms the carotid stenosis detected by ultrasound.

I do not routinely perform CT or MRI scans on these patients: the value of CT scanning was evaluated in a prospective study of 469 patients being considered for carotid endarterectomy: the cost of CT in this study was considerable and the results did not alter management (Martin *et al.* 1991). In the increasingly cost-conscious health service, we need to look for value for money. Tumour 'TIAs' (Coleman *et al.* 1993) are rare and can often be suspected on clinical grounds—patients with speech arrest, pure sensory TIA, blackouts, and jerking in their TIAs should all raise the suspicion of alternative pathology. CT need only be performed in this group.

I remain convinced that a neurologist or physician with a major interest in vascular disease should perform the initial assessment. These are not patients who should be referred primarily to the vascular surgeons. In our cerebrovascular clinics we see 25 new patients each week, only 2–3, on average, meet all the criteria to be candidates for carotid endarterectomy. The differential diagnosis seen in our clinic includes, migraine, epilepsy, hyperventilation, tumours, Parkinson's disease, and motor neurone disease, to name but a few. In a population of 1 000 000 people, there are approximately 50–100 people who are candidates for carotid endarterectomy each year: this compares with approximately 15 000 people with asymptomatic carotid stenosis. The scope for inappropriate surgery is substantial.

Not all would agree with my own philosophy but the Editor of this book has encouraged us to be 'opinionated and controversial'. Like most unbiased observers (!!), I have no doubt that the above policy makes sure only appropriate patients come to surgery and that they are investigated at minimal risk. Our only problem is seeing the patients soon enough. There is little doubt that the risk of a stroke is highest in the first six months after the initial event and if the time from first symptom to assessment, investigation, and surgery, takes several months, then we are 'missing the boat' in significant numbers of patients. In the United Kingdom, we need to assess these patients within a few days of their symptoms and prepare patients for surgery if appropriate within 2 weeks after TIAs and 6–8 weeks after strokes with recovery. This will require changes in organization, more neurologists with an interest in vascular disease, and perhaps more vascular surgeons (Hankey and Warlow, 1990).

Asymptomatic bruits

These are common in the elderly population (approximately 5% over the age of 65). The risk of ipsilateral stroke is approximately 2% per annum. Surgery is of no proven value, although trials are in progress (Warlow 1995).

OTHER ASPECTS OF TREATMENT

Emotional aspects

These are very important; few doctors have sufficient time to address them fully. Depression and anxiety are common: with reassurance, especially about the risk of recurrence and advice about treatment to prevent further events, depression and anxiety often improves with time. Counselling the spouse and close family is also important (House 1987).

Emotionalism is also common: it is present in both bilateral and unilateral strokes. Often, it is sufficient to explain this is a physical symptom which improves with time: sometimes a small dose of amitriptyline (10–25 mg) may be highly beneficial (House *et al.* 1989).

Epilepsy

Early epilepsy occurs in approximately 10% of all stroke: it should be energetically treated (e.g. with iv phenytoin) as the cerebral metabolic rates doubles during a fit. Late epilepsy after a stroke is a common cause of epilepsy in the elderly population in general; however, it is rare in the individual stroke patient and should make one reassess the validity of the diagnosis of cerebrovascular disease.

Dysphagia

This is common even after unilateral strokes. It usually recovers but predisposes to aspiration, chest infection, dehydration, and death. It can be assessed by simply asking the patient to drink 50 ml of water and should be mandatory in all stroke patients (Gordon et al. 1987).

Thalamic pain

This is more common than is generally appreciated; it frequently starts weeks after the patient is discharged from hospital. It is a cause of great distress and may be helped by a variety of strategies (Bowsher 1993).

Other common problems

After acute stroke, deep vein thrombosis (DVT) occurs in more than 50% of paretic legs, although a relatively small number develop symptomatic pulmonary embolism. DVT can usually be managed with elasticated stockings. Pressure sores, septicaemia often secondary to urinary tract, or chest infection and hyperglycaemia should be watched for. Frozen shoulder is a common problem and can markedly slow the individual's recovery.

PROGNOSIS

The risk of a stroke after TIAs is approximately 30% in 5 years. It is highest in the first year: in patients with carotid stenosis it is approximately 10–12% in the first year after the TIA. The figures for stroke are similar: it is, therefore, important to reassure all stroke patients that the second stroke is not just around the corner. Even patients with bilateral internal carotid occlusions only have a recurrent stroke risk of 13% per year. Most TIA and stroke patients die of a cardiac death (Sacco *et al.* 1982).

Following an acute stroke 20–30% of patients die. A poor prognosis is associated with reduced consciousness, conjugate gaze palsy, signs of severe brainstem dysfunction, pupillary changes, and incontinence persisting beyond the first few days. Strokes resulting in cognitive impairment (e.g. apraxia, neglect) and visuospatial dysfunction also carry a poor prognosis for recovery.

One year after a stroke, 33% of patients will be dead, 22% dependent, and 45% independent. Most recovery occurs in the first few weeks: less recovery occurs in months 3–6 and even less, but still useful recovery occurs in months 6–12. It is known that some symptoms can show recovery over a long period of time (e.g. hemiplegic leg), while others often do not recover much unless they recover early (e.g. retinal infarction, homonymous hemianopia, and isolated spinothalamic sensory loss). For the hemiplegic hand, if there is no active hand grip by 3 weeks there is unlikely to be useful recovery. It is crucial to take the natural history of disability into account when planning rehabilitation.

Six months after a stroke half the patients will be physically independent, 15% will have speech problems, 11% will be incontinent of urine, and 7% incontinent of faeces, and 33% will still need assistance with feeding.

YOUNG STROKE/UNUSUAL CAUSES OF STROKE

Young stroke may be secondary to premature atherosclerosis. The investigation and treatment should initially exclude premature atherosclerosis. However, young stroke is more likely to be secondary to the more unusual causes of stroke (see Table 12.4) (Bogousslavsky and Pierre 1992; Martin *et al.* 1997).

Emboli from congenital heart disease or valvular disease are important. It is rare to find a potential cardiac source of emboli if the heart is clinically normal: however, I have seen two cases of mitral stenosis not detected clinically by myself or the physician looking after the patients. I tend to ask for echocardiography on all strokes under 50. Transoesophageal echo is more likely to pick up potential sources of emboli than the more usual transthoracic echo. Transthoracic echocardiography is reliable for imaging aortic and mitral stenosis and in the assessment of left ventricular wall movement, whereas

Table 12.4 Other causes of cerebral infarction

1. Arterial dissection
2. Cardiac embolism
3. Migraine
4. Haematological disorders
5. Inflammatory arterial disease
6. Antiphospholipid syndrome/Sneddon's syndrome
7. Venous thrombosis
8. Moya-Moya disease
9. Pregnancy
10. Metabolic disorders (e.g. homocysteinuria)
11. Fat embolism
12. Infection
13. Malignancy: neoplastic angioendotheliosis
14. Hypertensive encephalopathy
15. Cerebral arteriography
16. Subarachnoid haemorrhage
17. Post-therapeutic irradiation
18. Oral contraceptives
19. Fibromuscular dysphasia
20. Drug abuse
21. Fabry's disease
22. Hereditary collagen disorders, Ehlers–Danlos, Marfan's, pseudoxanthoma elasticum
23. Mitochondrial cytopathy
24. Syphilis
25. AIDS
26. Cadasil

Table 12.5 Additional tests to consider in young stroke

Carotid/vertebral ultrasound*
MRI/MRA*
Echocardiography*
Serology for syphilis*
Lupus anticoagulant, antinuclear factor*
Anticardiolipin antibody*
Conventional angiography
Haemoglobin electrophoresis
Haematological opinion: including protein S, C, and antithrombin III
24 Hour ECG
Screening tests for homocysteinuria
Lumbar puncture
Brain biopsy/meningeal biopsy
WBC alpha galactosiodase
Muscle biopsy
HIV screen
Drug screen
DNA analysis

* Should be performed in all young stroke.

transoesophageal echocardiography is the preferred modality for atrial thrombus, atrial septal defects, patent foramen ovale, valvular vegetations, and myxomas. (Table 12.3.)

The significance of mild valvular abnormalities, such as mitral valve prolapse, mitral annulus calcification, patent foramen ovale, remains controversial.

In many practitioner's experience, dissection of the carotid and vertebral arteries is the most commonest cause of young stroke (Humphrey 1996). There is frequently no history of trauma: even when there is a history of trauma, it is often very mild and easily missed. In carotid artery dissection there may be a Horner's syndrome. There is usually headache, often in the temples, sometimes in the neck itself, and symptoms of carotid or vertebrobasilar ischaemia. Most strokes or TIAs in dissection are secondary to emboli or lack of blood flow. Carotid artery dissection in the neck is the most common type. The artery does not rupture. There are no trials on which to base treatment but my policy is to anticoagulate for 6–12 months if the patient has a mild or moderate deficit and thus a lot to lose from a further attack. Doppler/duplex ultrasound and MRI/MRA are the investigations of choice (Fig. 12.3). Doppler/duplex shows a reduced flow or a to- and- fro flow in the internal carotid artery, and MRI of the neck through the carotid artery shows the blood in the wall of the artery (Eljamel *et al.* 1990; Mullges *et al.* 1992). Angiography may not be necessary. Some vertebral dissections can rupture and one has to be more cautious about anticoagulation in this group (Caplan and Tettenborn 1992).

The antiphospholipid syndrome with the presence of lupus anticoagulant and/or anticardiolipin antibody is being increasingly recognized (Hughes 1993). A history of miscarriage or previous thrombosis may be elicited, Livedo reticularis may be seen. These proteins predispose to thrombosis. Blood tests may also yield a positive VDRL and thrombocytopenia. Strokes in this setting (and in systemic lupus erythematosus) are usually thrombotic or embolic (Libman–Sacks endocarditis) and not arteritic. Therefore, if treatment is deemed necessary it is appropriate to use antithrombotic therapy rather than steroids. If there has only been one event I usually start aspirin unless the history or haematological investigation suggests the disease is very active. I usually use anticoagulants if recurrent events occur: I only use steroids in this setting for SLE if there is strong evidence of arteritis (Venables 1993).

There is a long list of arteritic causes of stroke (Hankey 1991; Caplan 1993). There is insufficient space to discuss the diagnosis and management of these conditions. Cerebral angiitis secondary to herpes zoster ophthalmicus is a poorly recognized condition and may respond to steroids and/or acyclovir. Granulomatous angittis is usually only diagnosed at post mortem. A meningeal/brain biopsy is necessary to make the diagnosis. This is clearly not undertaken lightly: if there is any suspicion of granulomatous angiitis a short course of high dose steroids sometimes results in striking clinical improvement, but this is not reliable.

Cerebral venous thrombosis may present in a vascular manner with TIA, stroke, or subarachnoid haemorrhage (Martin and Enevoldson 1996). It again will prove easier to recognize with the advent of MRI and MRA. The CT may be normal or just show a tight brain. However, in a small number of people the empty triangle sign (no contrast in the

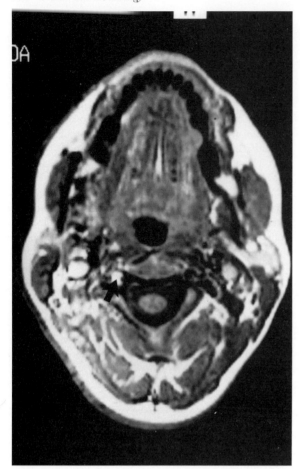

Fig. 12.3 The MRI scan is taken from a 30 year old lady with no vascular risk factors who developed a left homonymous hemianopia which lasted 1½ hours and was not associated with any other symptoms. The arrow shows the right vertebral dissection with blood (white) in the wall occluding almost the entire lumen (small black dot remaining). MRA confirmed the above findings, although it is not as useful in diagnosis as plain MRI taken through the *neck*.

sagittal sinus) or haemorrhagic infarcts in both cerebral hemispheres strongly suggests sagittal sinus thrombosis. It is important to recognize because a randomized trial suggests these patients benefit from anticoagulation even if there is a venous haemorrhagic infarct (Einhaupl *et al*. 1991). This trial has some flaws and is being repeated but it is particularly interesting to see how few patients were needed to demonstrate the benefit of anticoagulation over placebo. It is the first cause of young stroke in which treatment has been assessed by a randomized placebo controlled trial.

FIBROMUSCULAR DYSPLASIA

The significance of this rare condition has tended to be overemphasized in the past. It is often quoted as a reason for angiography. The risk of stroke in fibromuscular dysphasia is small. I manage it in the same way I do all TIAs. Angiography to detect this condition is usually an unnecessary hazard (Corrin *et al*. 1981).

CEREBRAL HAEMORRHAGE

Intracerebral haemorrhage accounts for 10% of all strokes and subarachnoid haemorrhage for 5%.

INTRACEREBRAL HAEMORRHAGE

Table 12.2 gives a list of the major causes. Most are secondary to hypertension, with lipohyalinosis of the small penetrating arteries and rupture of small microaneurysms.

Hypertensive haemorrhage particularly occurs in the internal capsule, putamen, caudate, thalamus, pons, lobar, or cerebellar hemispheres. Community-based studies suggest that intracerebral haemorrhage may be a more mild condition than appears from the many hospital-based studies (Boonyrakarnkulera *et al*. 1993). Surgical drainage for primary intracerebral haemorrhage is of unproven value. Most, however, would consider a surgical opinion in the presence of cerebellar haemorrhage and hydrocephalus if there is increasing drowsiness and neurological deficit.

Vascular malformations, particularly cavernous angiomas, are being recognized with increasing frequency with the advent of MR scanning. Amyloid angiopathy may account for up to a third of all haemorrhages in the elderly: it should be especially suspected if multiple haemorrhages occur sequentially or if there is an associated progressive underlying dementia.

SUBARACHNOID HAEMORRHAGE (SAH)

Surgery for SAH is one of the commonest neurosurgical operations. Despite the low morbidity and mortality attached to surgery, it makes only a small difference to the overall outcome.

Many patients (25–50%) are said to have premonitory headaches although it is very often difficult to identify this group. A CT scan and LP are needed in those with sudden onset of headache: there is often no neck stiffness or vomiting in these premonitory headaches. This emphasizes the diagnostic problem when less ominous headaches are so much more common: 95% of SAH cases will show blood on CT if performed within 24 hours: this falls to 50% after a week. LP is only needed if CT shows no blood or meningitis is a possible diagnosis. To detect xanthochromia the LP is best performed eight hours after the onset of headache.

Conventional contrast angiography is not indicated if CT and LP are negative and there is no focal neurological sign such as IIIrd nerve palsy. Angiography will show an aneurysm in about 80% of CT-positive cases. If the angiography is negative some surgeons undertake a second angiography a few days or weeks later—this is especially important if the site of bleeding on the initial CT suggests an underlying aneurysm. MRA has been helpful in some of these angiogram negative cases in our unit.

The importance of perimesencephalic haemorrhage as a non-aneurysmal cause of SAH has been emphasized by Van Gijn. This accounts for 10% of all SAH. The centre of bleeding is around the midbrain, most often in the interpeduncula fossa. These can be suspected from the initial CT. No aneurysm is usually found: the blood remains localized and does not spread into the ventricles or surrounding brain. The prognosis in this group is excellent (Van Gijn *et al.* 1985).

The risk of re-bleeding in aneurysmal SAH is 30% over the subsequent four weeks: this has resulted in early surgical intervention provided the patient is in good clinical condition. The immediate mortality of re-bleeding is 50%. Up to 25% of patients with aneurysmal SAH suffer delayed cerebral ischaemia usually 5–14 days after the bleed. The calcium antagonist, nimodipine, has been shown in a double-blind trial to significantly reduce the development of ischaemia: it is now routinely used by many neurosurgeons (Pickard *et al.* 1989). Hypertension is usually left untreated and circulating volume maintained. Epilepsy should be aggressively treated. Sudden deterioration in a patient with SAH is only due to re-bleeding in about 50% of cases. Hydrocephalus, ischaemia, epilepsy, and metabolic changes all need excluding.

Despite the improvement in care in SAH in recent years, there is still a high morbidity and mortality. Almost 50% die and 25% are left severely disabled (Van Gijn 1992).

CARE OF TRANSIENT ISCHAEMIC ATTACKS AND STROKE

In England and Wales there are approximately 100 000 first strokes each year and 25 000 initial TIAs.

TRANSIENT ISCHAEMIC ATTACKS

Most TIAs will be managed by general practitioners. A careful history, simple examination, some routine blood tests, chest X-ray, and ECG are all that is needed for the majority. All should be given advice about risk factors and started on aspirin 150–300 mg a day if at all possible. All reasonably fit patients with carotid events aged under 80 years should be referred to a neurologist or physician, with an interest in vascular disease, to investigate the possibility of carotid stenosis, provided the person is prepared to take the risk of surgery. The local surgical risk should be given to all patients. Ideally, investigation should be performed using carotid ultrasound of proven reliability and then MRA to confirm the ultrasound findings. There should be a small number of surgeons in each region performing the operation: each surgeon should do at least 25 carotid endarterectomies each year. The surgical res-

ults should be independently audited to ensure a low complication rate—preferably under 5% and definitely under 10%.

I do not think such patients should be referred to vascular surgeons for initial work-up. I run two cerebrovascular clinics each week seeing 25 new patients. Approximately 2–3 patients per week come to carotid endarterectomy. Thus, 22–23 patients either have alternative diagnoses, which is often not vascular, or have vascular disease for which endarterectomy is not appropriate. It is not reasonable to expect a vascular surgeon to perform this filtering. I investigate carotid stroke with recovery in the same manner. I think TIAs in patients under 50 years of age, whether carotid or vertebrobasilar, should be sent for specialist opinion—they are usually not due to atheromatous disease. Many are due to migraine, hyperventilation, and sometimes unusual causes of vascular disease. I spend a lot of my time reassuring and 'undiagnosing' vascular disease usually with enormous relief to the individual concerned. TIAs not controlled by aspirin or diagnostic difficulties should also be referred for specialist opinion.

STROKE

This is more difficult. The first question is whether the patient should be admitted to hospital. This is partly dependent on the severity of the deficit and age but more often on social factors such as the presence of carers and support services (Wade and Langton Hewer 1985). Whatever policy is followed, patients should be investigated appropriately and ideally all should have a CT scan.

I have no doubt that before long there will be treatment for acute stroke (as in myocardial infarction) and that acute stroke units will be needed to administer whatever treatment proves appropriate. The acute investigations will all be performed at the same time. After a short period in an acute stroke unit (perhaps just 24–72 hours), one could then consider what should happen to the patient. There are likely to be three options. First, the patient has a mild deficit and will do well whatever: he/she can go home needing only a small amount of domiciliary services. Second, there are the severely disabled who will not do well whatever is done: these patients may be managed at home or in nursing homes or other long-stay institutions. It is a waste of time and resources putting these people through a long and arduous rehabilitation programme which will do nothing except lead to frustration and disappointment for staff, patient, and family alike. These patients should still be assessed intermittently to check that the predicted prognosis is being followed. Realistic goals must be set at all times and the patient and carers understand what these are. Setting goals are, however, important.

Third, there are those presumably with disability between the first two options who need rehabilitation. Clinical criteria which identify these groups are slowly being identified. Where doubt exists the patient should be assumed to be able to benefit from rehabilitation: there is data now which is beginning to identify patients at an early stage who will not benefit from rehabilitation. One needs to decide whether rehabilitation is best delivered at home or in hospital. It is also necessary to ascertain what aspects of disability respond to physiotherapy, speech therapy, and occupational therapy. Could one type of generalized therapist delivery most of this type of care and advice, only calling on a more specialized service if necessary: this would certainly simplify a lot of domiciliary care if home care proves superior. Rehabilitation needs to answer simple questions in sufficient numbers to provide a useful long-term answer about the role of these therapists. Addressing simple questions in a simple manner, in a way in which many hospitals and general practitioners can participate, is enjoyable for both medical and paramedical staff. It helps to raise the interests in all and helps to encourage valuable discussion. It also helps to break down entrenched views which are usually not based on reliable facts. It might even be the attitude of the therapist which is most important aspect rather than anything he/she does. Wade (1993) is to be congratulated on his honesty—I quote:

Neurologic rehabilitation risks becoming a castle built on sand. The number of articles, books, journals, and conferences that relate to neurologic disability is growing rapidly, but much of the content is insubstantial, repetitive, or without evidence. The subject lacks a substantial agreed framework, and even the term 'rehabilitation' carries many meanings. More importantly, the subject lacks a firm scientific background of evidence to support many of its practices. Thus, although there is now more emphasis on the undoubted importance of the subject, there is a risk that resources may rapidly move away in the future when it is noticed that many of the rehabilitation emperors have no clothes.

As everyone must appreciate vascular disease followed this path in the past so that no useful therapy followed. In the last 10 years, however, enormous strides have been made with trials of aspirin, high blood pressure, and cholesterol, warfarin, and carotid endarterectomy. These studies will stand the test of time and cannot be ignored by clinicians—they serve as the benchmark from which to move forwards.

The next 10 years will be just as exciting. Rehabilitation has begun to follow this track. A simple relevant clinical end-point must be the yardstick for measurement. Multicentre trials with simple protocols are just as relevant to rehabilitation as drug trials.

I suspect that rehabilitation is best managed at home (Young and Forster 1992); one hour (if this is possible) inpatient physiotherapy a day will be trivial compared to the amount of 'physiotherapy' a motivated person will do in his/her own home. Clearly, it will be necessary to look after the carers and supply the appropriate aids and domiciliary therapists promptly but I would be surprised if this was more expensive than inpatient care. Care and rehabilitation at home should not be seen as a financially cheap political option which only requires partial funding. Social problems such as housing and finance need consideration. Routine follow-up every three to six months may help to reverse or slow down the late decline in mobility seen after stroke (Wade *et al.* 1992).

These services must be co-ordinated with a team leader. An integrated stroke service will be crucial. In hospital, this will be the consultant in charge of the stroke unit: in the community, the integrated stroke service liaising with the general practitioner will organize the necessary service. We do not want two completely separate services, one led by the hospital and one by the general practitioner. Large randomized trials are needed with detailed costings to see what is the most effective method of delivering optional care. All therapists must be aware of their role as counsellors (Forster and Young 1992). It is essential that we use the charities fully. The Stroke Association (CHSA House, Whitecross Street, London EC1Y 8JJ; Tel. 0171 566 0300) is becoming increasingly active. A whole host of support clubs are springing up in the United Kingdom; booklets about many aspects of stroke from TIAs to wheelchairs, and from epilepsy after stroke to young stroke are available.

Delivering stroke care is expensive: it uses a large percentage of the UK health budget and we need to deliver care in the most efficient and cost-effective manner. No view, however, stepped in tradition, should be exempt from proper clinical assessment with large properly conducted trials. The progress made in the last 10 years tells us this must be the way forward; it is exciting to answer questions which everyone involved in the care of patients faces daily. The ultimate beneficiary is the patient.

AUDIT

Properly carried out and reliable audit is difficult to do in clinical practice, particularly when most doctors individually see very few cases of even common conditions. The article by Hankey *et al.* (1993) which looks at the different outcomes in three large cohorts of patients with TIAs (1821, 469, and 184 patients), shows how misleading it can be analysing small groups of 'in-house' patients.

However, in cerebrovascular disease one could audit whether a diagnosis of carotid or vertebrobasilar ischaemic event has been considered. Checking for risk factors (q.v.) and advice about their management is also crucial, particularly with regard to good blood pressure control. Payne and colleagues (1993) have demonstrated that blood pressure control is far from good: this would probably make the greatest contribution to the future health of patients with cerebrovascular disease. Antiplatelet treatment is rarely overlooked but should be checked. The indications for anticoagulation should be considered.

It is very difficult to perform statistically robust audit in carotid endarterectomy. It is clearly important that patients are assessed by an 'independent' doctor after surgery. But reading too much into the initial successes or indeed failures will always be difficult when dealing with even moderately large numbers in operative terms but small numbers statistically. However, an operative complication rate of over 10% should merit a detailed assessment.

DRIVING

The rules about driving after a stroke have changed recently. Driving a car is allowed a month after a transient ischaemic attack.

After a stroke, the same rule applies provided clinical recovery is satisfactory. If epilepsy occurs in the first 24 hours, it can be ignored: thereafter, the normal epilepsy rules follow. HGV/PSV licences can be restored after five years provided a full and complete recovery has occurred.

It is sometimes difficult to know if partial visual field defects or impairment of cognitive function have not recovered sufficiently to allow driving to restart. Driving assessment centres are available throughout the United Kingdom. (The full list of centres is available in the September 1993 Guidelines on fitness to drive, issued by the Driver and Vehicle Licensing Agency (DVLA), Swansea. An information pack is available from MAVIS, Department of Transport, TRL Crowthorne, Berkshire, RG11 6AU; (Tel. 01344 661000.)

REFERENCES

Antiplatelets Trialists Collaboration Collaborative Overview of Randomized Trials of Antiplatelet Therapy. Prevention of death, myocardial infarction and stroke by prolonged antiplatelet therapy in various categories of patients. *BMJ*, 1994, **308**, 81–106.

Bamford, J., Sandercock, P., Dennis, M., Burn, J., and Warlow, C. Classification and natural history of clinically identifiable subtypes of cerebral infarction. *Lancet*, 1991, **337**, 1521–6.

Bogousslavsky, J. Thrombolysis in acute stroke. *BMJ*, 1996, **313**, 640–1.

Bogousslavsky, J. and Pierre, P. Ischaemic stroke in patients under the age of 45. *Neurologic. Clinics*, 1992, **10**, 113–24.

Boonyakarnkul, S., Dennis, M., Sandercock, P., Bamford, J., Burn, J., and Warlow, C. Primary intracerebral haemorrhage in the Oxfordshire Community Stroke Project. *Cerebrovascular Diseases*, 1993, **3**, 343–9.

Bowsher, D. Pain syndromes and their treatment. *Current Opinion in Neurology and Neurosurgery*, 1993, **6**, 257–63.

Brown, M. M., and Humphrey, P. R. D. on behalf of the Association of British Neurologists. Carotid endarterectomy: recommendations for management of transient ischaemic attack and ischaemic stroke. *BMJ*, 1992, **305**, 1071–4.

Caplan, L. R. Vertebrobasilar disease. *Stroke*, 1981, **12**, 111–4.

Caplan, L. R. Stroke in children and young adults. In *Stroke: a clinical approach*, pp. 469–85. 1993. Butterworth-Heinemann, Sevenoaks, Kent.

Caplan, L. R. Non-atherosclerotic ischaemia. In *Stroke: a clinical approach*, pp. 299–348. 1993. Butterworth-Heinemann, Sevenoaks, Kent.

Caplan, L. R. and Tettenborn, B. Vertebrobasilar occlusive disease: Spontaneous dissection of extracranial and intracranial posterior circulation. *Cerebrovascular Diseases*, 1992, **2**, 256–66.

Caprie Steering Committee. A randomized blinded trial of Clopidogrel versus Aspirin in patients at risk of ischaemic events (CAPRIE). *Lancet*, 1996, **348**, 1329–39.

Cardiac Embolism Study Group. Immediate anticoagulation of embolic stroke: Brain haemorrhage and management options. *Stroke*, 1984, **15**, 779–89.

Clarke, R., Daly, L., Robinson, K., Daughten, L., Cahalane, S. et al. Hyperhomocysteinaemia: an independent risk factor for vascular disease. *New. Engl. J. Med.* 1991, **324**, 1149–55.

Coleman, R. J., Bamford, J. M., and Warlow, C. P. for the UK TIA Study Group. Intracranial tumours that mimic transient cerebral ischaemia: lessons from a large multicentre trial. *J. Neurol. Neurosurg. Psychiatry*, 1993, **56**, 563–6.

Corrin, L. S., Sandok, B. A., and Houser, O. W. Cerebral ischaemic events in patients with carotid artery fibromuscular dysplasia. *Arch. Neurol.* 1981, **38**, 616–8.

Davies, K. N. and Humphrey, P. R. D. Complications of cerebral angiography in patients with symptomatic carotid territory ischaemia screened by carotid ultrasound. *J. Neurol. Neurosurg. Psychiatry*, 1993, **56**, 967–72.

Davies, K. N. and Humphrey, P. R. D. Do carotid bruits predict disease of the internal carotid artery. *Postgrad. Med. J.* 1994, **70**, 433–5.

Davis, S. M. and Donnan, G. A. Secondary Precrention for stroke after CARRIE and ESPS-2. *Cerebrovascular Diseases*, 1998, **8**, 73–7.

Dennis, M. and Warlow, C. Strategy for stroke. *BMJ*, 1991, **303**, 636–8.

Dennis, M., Bamford, J., Sandercock, P., and Warlow, C. Prognosis of transient ischaemic attacks in the Oxfordshire Community Stroke Project. *Stroke*, 1990, **21**, 848–53.

Donnan, G. A., You, R., Thrift, A., and McNeill, J. J. Smoking as a risk factor for stroke. *Cerebrovas. Dis.* 1993, **3**, 129–38.

Einhaupl, K. M., Villringer, A., Meister, W., Mehraein, S., Garner, C. et al. Heparin treatment in sinus venous thrombosis. *Lancet*, 1991, **338**, 597–600.

Eljamel, M. S. M., Humphrey, P. R. D., and Shaw, M. D. M. Dissection of the cervical internal carotid artery. The role of Doppler/ Duplex studies and conservative management. *J. Neurol. Neurosurg. Psychiatry*, 1990, **53**, 379–83.

European Atrial Fibrillation Study Group (EAFT). Secondary prevention in non rheumatic atrial fibrillation after transient ischaemic attack or minor stroke. *Lancet*, 1993, **342**, 1255–62.

European Carotid Surgery Trialists Collaborative Group. MRC European Carotid Surgery Trial: Interim results for symptomatic patients with severe (70–99%) or with mild (0–29%) carotid stenosis. *Lancet*, 1991, **337**, 1235–43.

European Carotid Surgery Trialists' Collaborative Group. Endarterectomy for moderate symptomatic carotid stenosis: interim results from MRC European Carotid Surgery Trial. *Lancet*, 1996, **343**, 1591–3.

Ferro, J. M., Falcao, I., Rodrigues, G., Canhao, P., Melo, T. P., Oliveira, V. et al. Diagnosis of transient ischaemic attack by the non-neurologist. *Stroke*, 1996, **27**, 2225–9.

Fisher, C. M. Vertigo and cerebrovascular disease. *Archs. Otolar.* 1967, **85**, 529–34.

Fisher, C. M. Lacunar strokes and infarcts: A review. *Neurology*, 1982, **32**, 871–6.

Forster, A. and Young, J. Stroke rehabilitation: Can we do better? Emphasizing physical recovery may be counterproductive. *BMJ*, 1992, **305**, 1446–7.

Gladman, J. R. F., Lincoln, N. B., and Barer, D. H. A randomised controlled trial of domiciliary and hospital-based rehabilitation for stroke patients after discharge from hospital. *J. Neurol. Neurosurg. Psychiatry*, 1993, **56**, 960–6.

Gordon, C., Langton Hewer, R., and Wade, D. T. Dysphagia in acute stroke. *BMJ*, 1987, **295**, 411–4.

Hankey, G. J., and Warlow, C. P. Symptomatic carotid ischaemic events: safest and most cost effective way of selecting patients for angiography, before carotid endarterectomy. *BMJ*, 1990, **300**, 1485–91.

Hankey, G. J. Isolated angiitis/angiopathy of the central nervous system. *Cerebrovascular Diseases*, 1991, **1**, 2–15.

Hankey, G. J., Warlow, C. P., and Sellar R. J. Cerebral Angiographic risk in mild cerebrovascular disease. *Stroke*, 1990, **21**, 209–22.

Hankey, G. J., Dennis, M. S., Slattery, J. M., and Warlow, C. P. Why is the outcome of transient ischaemic attacks different in different groups of patients? *BMJ*, 1993, **306**, 1107–11.

Harrison, M. J. G. and Marshall, J. Indications for angiography and surgery in carotid artery disease. *BMJ*, 1975, **1**, 616–18.

Hennerici, M., Klemm, C., and Rautenberg, W. The subclavian steal phenomenon: A common vascular disorder with rare neurologic deficits. *Neurology*, 1988, **36**, 669–73.

Hodges, J. R. and Warlow, C. P. The aetiology of transient global amnesia. *Brain*, 1990, **113**, 639–57.

House, A. Depression after stroke. *BMJ*, 1987, **294**, 76–8.

House, A., Dennis, M., Molyneux, A., Warlow, C. P., and Hawton, K. Emotionalism after stroke. *BMJ*, 1989, **298**, 991–4.

Howard, G., Cambless, L. E., Baker, W. H., Ricotta, J. J., Jones, A. M. *et al.* A multicentre validation study of Doppler ultrasound versus angiography. *J. Stroke Cerebrovasc. Dis.* 1991, **1**, 166–73.

Hughes, G. R. V. The antiphospholipid syndrome, ten years on. *Lancet*, 1993, **342**, 341–4.

Humphrey, P., Sandercock, P., and Slattery, J. A simple method to improve the accuracy of non-invasive ultrasound in selecting T.I.A. patients for cerebral angiography. *J. Neurol., Neurosurg. Psychiatry*, 1990, **53**, 966–71.

Humphrey, P. R. D. Dissection of carotid and vertebrobasilar arteries. Royal Society of Medicine: *Current Medical Literature, Neurology and Neurosurgery*, 1996, **12**, 31–6.

Kannel, W. B. and Wolf, P. A. Epidemiology of cerebrovascular disease. In Ross Russell (ed.), *Vascular disease of the central nervous system*, pp. 1–24. 1983, Churchill Livingstone, Edinburgh.

Khamasta, M. A., and Hughes, G. R. V. Antiphospholipid syndrome. *BMJ*, 1993, **307**, 883–4.

Khaw, K-T. Epidemiology of stroke. *J. Neurol. Neurosurg. Psychiatry*, 1996, **61**, 333–8.

Koudstaal, P. J., Van Gijn, J., and Kappelle, L. J. Headache in transient or permanent cerebral ischaemia. *Stroke*, 1991, **22**, 754–9.

Koudstaal, P. J., Van Gijn, J., Staal, H., Duivenvoorden, H. J., Gerritsma, J. G. M. *et al.* Diagnosis of transient ischaemia attacks: improvement of interobserver agreement by a check-list in ordinary language. *Stroke*, 1986, **17**, 723–8.

Kraaijeveld, C. L., Van Gijn, J., Schouten, H. J. A., and Staal, A. Interobserver agreement for the diagnosis of transient ischaemic attacks. *Stroke*, 1984, **15**, 723–5.

Lancet (1991). Ticlopidine (Editorial), **337**, 459–60.

Landi, G., Candelise, L., Cella, E., and Pinardi, G. Interobserver reliability of the diagnosis of lacunar transient ischaemic attack. *Cerebrovascular Disease*, 1992, **2**, 297–300.

Langhorne, P., Williams, B., Gilchrist, W., and Howie, K. Do stroke units save lives? *Lancet*, 1993, **342**, 395–8.

Law, M., Frost, C., and Wald, N. By how much does dietary salt reduction lower blood pressure: II. Analysis of data from trials of salt reduction. *BMJ*, 1991, **302**, 819–24.

Martin, J. D., Valentime, R. J., Myers, S. I., Rossi, M. B., Patterson, C. B., and Clagett, G. P. Is routine CT scanning necessary in the preoperative evaluation of patients undergoing carotid endarterectomy? *J. Vasc. Surg.* 1991, **14**, 267–70.

Martin, P. J. and Enevoldson, T. P. Classic diseases revisited. Cerebral venous thrombosis. *Postgrad. Med. J.* 1996, **72**, 72–6.

Martin, P. J., Enevoldson, T. P., and Humphrey, P. R. D. Causes of ischaemic stroke in the young. *Postgrad. Med. J.* 1997, **73**, 8–16.

Martin, P. J., Young, G., Enevoldson T. P., Humphrey, P. R. D. Overdiagnosis of TIA and minor stroke: experience at a regional Neurovascular Clinic. *Q. J. Med.* 1997, **90**, 759–63.

Mullges, W., Ringelstein, E. B., and Leibold, M. Non invasive diagnosis of internal carotid dissections. *J. Neurol. Neurosurg. Psychiatry*, 1992, **55**, 98–104.

Norris, J. W. and Hachinski, V. C. Misdiagnosis of stroke. *Lancet*, 1982, **i**, 328–31.

Oxfordshire Community Stroke Project. Incidence of stroke in Oxfordshire. First year's experience of a community stroke project. *BMJ*, 1983, **287**, 713–16.

Payne, J. N., Milner, P. C., Saul, C., Bowns, I. R., Hannay, D. R., and Ramsay, L. E. Local confidential injury into avoidable factors in deaths from stroke and hypertensive disease. *BMJ*, 1993, **307**, 1027–30.

Pickard, J. D., Murray, G. D., Illingworth, R., Shaw, M. D. M., Teasdale, G. M. *et al.* Effect of oral Nimopidine on cerebral infarction and outcome after subarachnoid haemorrhage; British Aneurysm Nimodipine Trial. *BMJ*, 1989, **298**, 636–42.

Pound, P., Bury, M., Gompertz, P., and Ebrahim, S. Stroke patients' view on their admission to hospital. *BMJ*, 1995, **311**, 18–22.

Prospective Studies Collaborative. Cholesterol, diastolic blood pressure and stroke: 13,000 strokes in 450,000 people in 45 prospective studies. *Lancet*, 1995, **346**, 1647–53.

Qizilbash, N., Jones, L., Warlow, C. P., and Mann, J. Fibrinogen and lipid concentrations as risk factors for transient ischaemic attacks and minor ischaemic strokes. *BMJ*, 1991, **303**, 605–9.

Qizilbash, N., Duffy, S. W., Warlow, C. P., and Mann, J. Lipids are risk factors for ischaemic stroke, overview and review. *Cerebrovascular Disease*, 1992, **2**, 127–36.

Ross Russell, R. W. and Bharucha, N. The recognition and prevention of border zone cerebral ischaemia during cardiac surgery. *Q. J. Med.* 1978, **47**, 303–23.

Ross Russell, R. W. and Page, N. G. R. Critical perfusion of brain and retina. *Brain*, 1983, **106**, 419–34.

Sacco, R. L., Wolf, P. A., Kannel, W. B., and McNamara, P. Survival and recurrence following stroke: the Framingham Study, *Stroke*, 1982, **13**, 290–5.

Sandercock, P., and Willems, H. Medical treatment of acute ischaemic stroke. *Lancet*, 1992, **339**, 537–9.

Sandercock, P., Molyneux, A., and Warlow, C. P. Value of computed tomography in patients with stroke: Oxfordshire Community Stroke Project. *BMJ*, 1985, **290**, 193–7.

Sandercock, P. A. G., Van der Belt, A. G., Lindley, R. J., and Slattery, J. Antithrombotic therapy in acute stroke: an overview of the completed randomized trials. *J. Neurol. Neurosurg. Psychiatry*, 1993, **56**, 17–25.

Scandinavian Simvastatin Survival Study Group. Randomized trial of cholesterol lowering in 4444 patients with coronary heart disease. The Scandinavian Simvastatin Survival Study (4S). *Lancet*, 1994, **344**, 1383–9.

Shepherd, J., Cobbe, S. M., Ford, I., Isles, C. G. *et al.*, for the West of Scotland Coronary Prevention Study Group. Prevention of coronary heart disease with Pravastatin in men with hypercholesterolaemia. *New Eng. J. Med.* 1995, **333**, 1301–7.

Sturzenegger, M. and Huber, P. Cranial nerve palsies in spontaneous carotid artery dissection. *J. Neurol. Neurosurg. Psychiatry*, 1993, **56**, 1191–9.

Van Gijn, J. Subarachnoid haemorrhage. *Lancet*, 1992, **339**, 653–5.

Van Gijn, J., Van Dongen, K. J., Vermeulen, M., and Hijdra, A. Perimesencephalic haemorrhage: a non-aneurysmal and benign form of subarachnoid haemorrhage. *Neurology*, 1985, **35**, 493–7.

Venables, P. J. W. Diagnosis and treatment of systemic lupus erythematosis. *BMJ*, 1993, **307**, 663–6.

Wade, D. T., Langton Hewer, R. Hospital Admission for Acute Stroke WHO: for How Long and To What Effect? *J. Epidemiol. Comm. Health*, 1985, **39**, 347–52.

Wade, D. T. Neurological rehabiliation (Editorial overview). *Current Opinion in Neurology*, 1993, **6**, 753–5.

Wade, D. T., Collen, F. M., Robb, G. F., and Warlow, C. P. Physiotherapy intervention late after stroke and mobility. *BMJ*, 1992, **304**, 609–13.

Warlow, C. P. Endarterectomy for asymptomatic carotid stenosis? *Lancet*, 1995, **345**, 1254–5.

Weir, C. J., Murray, G. D., Adams, F. E., Muir, K. W., Gossett, D. E., and Lees, K. R. Poor accuracy of stroke scoring systems for the differential clinical diagnosis of intracranial haemorrhage and infarction. *Lancet*, 1994, **344**, 999–1000.

Wilson, L. A. and Ross Russell, R. W. Amaurosis fugax and carotid artery disease: indications for angiography. *BMJ*, 1977, **ii**, 435–7.

Winslow, C. M., Solomon, D. H., Chassin, M. R., Kosecoff, J., Merrick, N. J., and Brook, R. H. The appropriateness of carotid endarterectomy. *New Engl. J. Med.*, 1988, **318**, 721–7.

Young, G., Humphrey, P. R. D., Shaw, M. D. M., Nixon, T. E., and Smith, E. T. S. A comparison of magnetic resonance angiography, Duplex ultrasound and digital subtraction angiography in the assesment of extracranial internal carotid artery stenosis. *J. Neurol. Neurosurg. Psychiatry*, 1994, **57**, 1466–78.

Young, J. B. and Forster, A. The Bradford Community Stroke Trial, results at six months. *BMJ*, 1992, **304**, 1085–9.

13 | *Spinal cord diseases*

Edmund M. R. Critchley

The vertebral column and its surrounding musculature provide the most effective protection afforded to any organ of the body. Not only are these structures a bulwark against trauma to the spinal cord but also render the cord relatively immune from infection and haemorrhage. The protective surround hides the spinal cord and its emerging nerve roots from direct examination hence diagnosis is correspondingly difficult and, in the light of the limited ability of the spinal cord to repair itself and recover from insult to its substance, an accurate diagnosis is always essential.

In early childhood, while the frame is still immature, the upper cervical spine is most susceptible to direct trauma and most developmental anomalies are seen at this site. In later life, injury and wear and tear particularly affect the lower cervical spine and lumbar region. In the adult the spinal cord ends at L1-2 and lesions below this level (e.g. disc disease) involve the cauda equina and the emergence of nerve roots through the exit formaina.

INDICATORS OF HIGH CERVICAL LESIONS

The signs and symptoms of high cervical and foramen magnum lesions are poorly taught and often imperfectly understood but advances in surgical techniques have led to dramatic changes in the management, for example, of rheumatic spines, and a careful examination of the symptomatology and investigation of lesions at this level is increasingly worthwhile. The spinal canal is widest at the first cervical vertebra and many anomalies at this site are asymptomatic. The rule of three can be applied: odontoid space; medullary space; and free posterior space. The main bony lesions seen are:

(1) occipitalization or assimilation of the atlas with partial fusion to the rim of the foramen magnum;
(2) basilar impression or invagination where the odontoid protrudes above Chamberlain's line (back of the palate to posterior rim of foramen magnum); and
(3) anomalies of the odontoid.

Laxity of the ligaments can occur with Down's syndrome and with hyperaemia during infections in childhood. Crowding of structures within the posterior fossa may be associated with Chiari type deformities (type I cerebellar tonsillar descent;

type II more severe herniation, medullary descent, and spina bifida) and these may be linked with syringomyelia, raised intracranial pressure, and lower cranial nerve dysfunction. Congenital lesions (such as atlanto-axial dislocation), trauma, rheumatoid arthritis with pannus formation, and benign tumours (predominantly meningiomas and neurofibromas), may occur at or below the foramen magnum.

SYMPTOMS AND SIGNS OF HIGH CERVICAL COMPRESSION

1. Localized neck pain often radiating to the vertex, increased by movement and associated with spasm and neck stiffness.
2. Wasting of suboccipital and paraspinal muscles, often unilaterally. Torticollis with wasting and weakness of sternomastoids and trapezii (from involvement of motor roots C2-4 and accessory nerves).
3. Uni- or bilateral wasting and paralysis of the tongue.
4. Spastic quadriparesis, sometimes with wasting of small muscles of the hands if the anterior spinal artery is involved.
5. Downbeat nystagmus, more prominent on lateral gaze.
6. Spinothalamic sensory loss (e.g. to pin-prick) over nape of neck and anywhere between C1-5 and, since the trigeminal sensory nucleus occupies the upper cervical cord, dissociated sensory loss may be present over the face.
7. Tingling and sensory loss in finger tips with loss of position sense and/or stereognosis (demonstrated by pseudotremor of outstretched hands).
8. Priapism.
9. Lhermitte's sign.
10. Loss of height.
11. Compression of the anterior part of the cord at C3/4 may give:
    (a) clumsy hands with occipital headache;
    (b) a progressive spastic quadriplegia; and
    (c) respiratory distress.

A number of conditions at the foramen magnum can give rise to very similar symptoms: namely, atlanto-axial dislocation which may be congenital, traumatic, or with rheumatoid arthritis or ankylosing spondylosis; fracture displacement or dislocation of the odontoid; exuberant pannus formation around the odontoid peg in rheumatoid arthritis.

Vertical or backward displacement of the odontoid into the foramen magnum can lead to intermittent or progressive compression of the brainstem and vertebrobasilar arteries with risk to life and the development of a myelopathy. Cervical pain and stiffness may occur as isolated symptoms with no immediate neurological deficits but 50% will progress. Ischaemia in vertebrobasilar territory may produce episodic loss of consciousness or blindness and sudden jolts result in transient paraesthesiae, pyramidal weakness, or tetraplegia. These episodes may last from minutes to hours but long tract signs can persist and the resulting incapacity become permanent at any time. Respiration may be embarrassed with the development of central sleep apnoea, and a delayed myelopathy follow after several years.

The diagnosis is apparent from plain lateral X-rays of the neck in flexion and extension. Magnetic resonance image (MRI) scanning has removed the risk inherent in other forms of radiography and provides a fuller picture. Emergency treatment by external fixation should be followed by surgical stabilization of the atlanto-axial joint.

EXTERNAL TRAUMA

The commonest sites of spinal injury in adult life are the lower cervical spine, thoracolumbar junction, and upper cervical segments—in that order. Fractures or dislocations of vertebral bodies or neural arches may be associated with discoligamentous injuries at other levels and with abnormalities of the prevertebral soft tissues due to haematoma. This in turn may produce constriction of the throat and trachea. Survival so often depends on the initial assessment, immobilisation of the affected area before any attempt is made to move the patient, and the care with which the patient is transported and examined.

If a spinal injury is suspected at the scene, the priorities of respiratory and cardiovascular stabilization are followed by immobilization of the spinal column in an anatomically neutral supine postion (Tucci *et al.* 1992). One should never attempt to free lift a potential spinal cord-injured patient. The log-rolling technique will minimize the chance of a secondary neurological injury. The patient should be prepared for transfer by being placed on a firm board with sandbags and adhesive tape securing the cervical area. Cervical collars are not recommended at this stage as they provide only limited immobilization and can act as a tourniquet if there is neck swelling from an associated vascular or other soft tissue injury and may hide tracheal deviation or subcutaneous emphysema from view (Green and Hall 1976). (Fig. 13.1)

The presence of skeletal instability may be suggested by torticollis with the assumption of a 'cock-robin' pose due to a

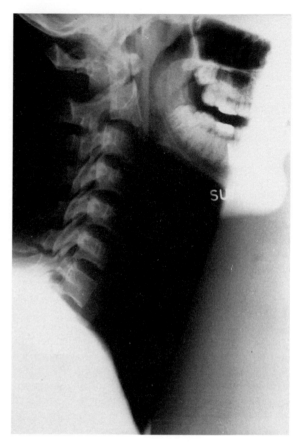

Fig. 13.1 X-ray and lateral view of fractures of the base of the odontoid peg and posterior elements of C1.

Jefferson fracture (i.e. fragmentation of the ring of the atlas caused by axial compression). Careful palpation of the spines may confirm any displacement. An ominous sign of cord involvement is paradoxical neurogenic ventilation whereby diaphragmatic breathing in the presence of intercostal paralysis results in abdominal distension with indrawing of the affected segments of the chest wall during inspiration. Respiratory support is a first priority. (Table 13.1.)

Early radiology is necessary to determine the stability of the spine. A Jefferson fracture and even a Hangman's fracture (fractures across the pedicles of C2 from a hyperextension injury) are not necessarily unstable but anterior subluxation is, as are fractures affecting both the vertebral body and neural arch. When in doubt, a useful system is to divide the spine into three columns, the first centred on the intralaminar line, the second on the posterior margin of the vertebral body, and the third on its anterior margin. If the injury has disrupted ligaments and/or bones of two of the three columns, the spine is considered acutely unstable and appropriate precautions taken (Denis 1983). A more chronic instability may occur if the posterior column is damaged.

Besides paradoxical neurogenic ventilation, impaired gaseous exchange may occur either from direct respiratory

Table 13.1 Recognition of cord trauma

Conscious patients	Unconscious patients
Local and radicular pains and tenderness	Absent tendon reflexes Except in deep coma,
Impaired limb movements	withdrawal from noxious
Spinal shock followed by paraplegia in flexion	stimuli above but not below lesion
Paradoxical neurogenic ventilation	Paradoxical neurogenic ventilation
Impaired movements of hands	Priapism
Post-traumatic torticollis	Post-traumatic torticollis

embarrassment or from cervical lesions. Ventilatory assistance is imperative with lesions above C4 and repeated examination is essential to detect any ascending abnormality with lesions involving segments just below C4.

Just occasionally, paraplegia may have a non-organic cause: 20 such patients out of a total of 7000 were seen at a spinal injuries centre over 40 years (Baker and Silver 1987). The physical findings were a disproportionate motor paralysis, non-anatomical sensory loss, the presence of down-going plantar resonses, normal tone, and reflexes. With recognition they made a rapid recovery. Notable features commonly included a high incidence of previous psychiatric illness, hospital-based employment, and an overwhelming desire for compensation.

SPINAL CORD LACERATION

Acute spinal cord laceration from birth injuries, gunshot wounds, road traffic accidents, etc. leads to immediate spinal shock with flaccid paralysis below the level of the lesion accompanied by, paralysis of bladder and rectum, paralysis of the sympathetic nervous system with impairment of peripheral blood vessels, faulty homeostasis, abolition of sweating, cessation of peristalsis, and loss of all sensation with arreflexia. Paralysis and sensory loss do not recover but after days or weeks, spinal shock is replaced by coarse reflex activity, spasms and paraplegia in flexion. Bilateral lesions above C5 cause respiratory paralysis and a complete quadriplegia.

Early management includes prevention of contractures and pressure sores and support to the shoulders to prevent painful frozen shoulders. The ambient temperature must be kept constant to maintain homeostasis. The bladder should be drained until automatic emptying is re-established. The bowels must be emptied by suppositories, a Ryles tube passed, and intravenous feeding continued until the bowel sounds return.

TRAUMATIC LESIONS WITHIN THE SPINAL CORD

'Spearing' or head-on tackling with forced hyperextension or hyperflexion of the neck can result in the temporary abolition of axonal function (neurapraxia) unaccompanied by neural degenerative changes with transient quadriparesis (Torg *et al.* 1986). Sensory changes include burning pain, numbness, tingling, and loss of sensation, while the motor changes range from weakness to complete paralysis. Complete recovery usually occurs in 10–15 minutes but can take up to 48 hours. Nearly all the athletes involved were found to have pre-existing cervical stenosis, congenital cervical fusion, cervical instability, or intervertebral disc herniation. In Torg's series of 117 American football players, none developed permanent paralysis. However, caution is advised and the prevalent opinion is that contact sports are better avoided after an episode of neurapraxia.

In an older age group, sudden compression resulting in hyperextension or flexion of the neck as may occur with a head injury can cause central contusion or haemorrhagic necrosis. The clinical manifestations are noticeably more severe in the upper than lower limbs, with flaccid paresis of the upper limbs, marked hyperpathia of arms and hands, retention of urine, a flaccid—followed by a spastic—paresis of the legs, and a variable impairment of sensation below the lesion. Atheroma, hypertension, and degenerative changes within narrow spinal canal influence the prognosis.

Post-traumatic syringomyelia may occur as a long-term complication of injury or operations on intrinsic tumours of the spinal cord (Anton and Schweigel 1986). Ascending cavitation of the cord, usually within the cervial region but sometimes bulbar, may present with pain, numbness, and intense hyperpathia meriting prompt action. The upward extension is accompanied by further signs of motor impairment and wasting and the risk of respiratory difficulties. The extent of cavitation can be clearly determined by MR scanning or by the presence of dye in the centre of the cord on computerized tomography (CT) myelography. Relief of hyperpathia in approximately 90% of cases can be obtained by decompression and shunting. There may also be some improvement in motor function but rarely in sensation.

SYRINGOMYELIA

This results from obstruction of cerebrospinal fluid (CSF) flow from the 4th ventricle with the subsequent development of a fluid-filled cavity (syrinx) in the substance of the spinal cord. There is usually a developmental Chiari type II malformation within the posterior fossa but a few cases are associated with intramedullary gliomas, spinal injury, basal arachnoiditis, or posterior fossa tumours. Downward extension of the syrinx damages anterior horn cells, spinothalamic, and corticospinal fibres, but seldom affects the posterior columns.

Clinical features usually develop at 10–30 years of age and many report an incidental 'crick in the neck' before the onset of dysaesthesiae. For others, the onset is more insidious with trophic ulceration following a burn, or weakness and wasting of a hand. A dissociated, and suspended, sensory loss to pain and temperature occurs in one or both arms, paradoxically with spontaneous burning shoulder pain, together with painless destruction of finger tips and joints of the hands and wrist. As the spinothalamic fibres ascend several segments within the cord before decussating the level of sensory loss on the skin does not indicate the level of an intrinsic lesions. Thus, ipsilateral spinothalamic loss due to compression of the lateral spinothalamic tracts may be associated with a segmental band of contralateral sensory loss from involvement of decussated fibres. The upper limbs are weak and arreflexic with atrophy of the small muscles of the hands. Leg involvement with spastic paraparesis is more insidious. Cervical lesions from C5 upwards may produce coarse rotatory nystagmus, vertigo, Horner's syndrome, and ataxia.

MR scanning, with gadolinium to define any tumour, has proved highly successful in demonstrating the pathological anatomy of syringomyelia, but CT myelography and vertebral angiography can also be helpful. Adequate surgical decompression of the craniocervical junction correcting hindbrain herniation or arachnoiditis is the most important aspect of treatment as tissue grafts or shunts may produce fibrosis if overenthusiastically applied. (Fig. 13.2)

BROWN–SEQUARD SYNDROME

Clinical hemisection of the cord, classically from trauma but mostly from a transverse plaque in multiple sclerosis or from transverse myelitis, results in ipsilateral spastic paralysis, loss of position sense, and contralateral loss of pain and temperature sensation. The complete syndrome is uncommon but elements of the syndrome are often suggested by finding a brisk extensor plantar response on one side and a sluggish response on the other.

THE VASCULAR SYSTEM

VASCULAR ANATOMY

The blood supply to the spinal cord is non-segmental. Most radicular arteries perfuse just the nerve roots within their territory. Radiculopial arteries also irrigate the pial-leptomeningeal arterial plexuses. Only at certain segmental levels do radiculomedullary arteries contribute to the blood supply of the cord; thus a longitudinal watershed area, liable to infarction, exists in the upper thoracic region around T4 between the downward flow of the anterior spinal artery (reinforced by a feeding vessel at C7) and the upward flow from the arteria magna of Adamkiewicz which arises between T9 and L2 on the left side. (Fig. 13.3)

VASCULAR DISORDERS

Occlusion of posterior spinal arteries seldom results in persistent sensory loss. These arteries, and circumferential arteries

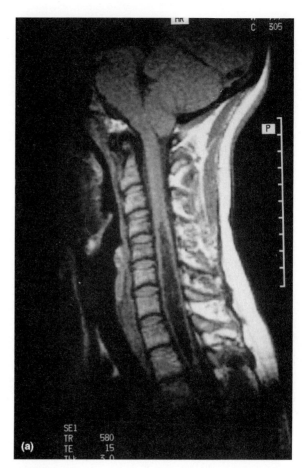

Fig. 13.2(a) Tonsillar herniation and syrinx. Sagittal MR scan of T1 weighted image.

arising from the anterior spinal artery, form a rich plexiform network perfusing the superficial areas of the cord. In addition, sulcal (central or sulcocommissural) arteries arise from the anterior spinal artery as asymmetric end-arteries to alternate sides supplying the innermost portion of white matter and the central grey matter apart from the posterior horns. Occlusion of a sulcal artery leads to a hemisectional deficit with central necrosis involving anterior horn cells, corticospinal tracts and, to a lesser extent, spinothalamic tracts. Venous occlusion of the same area produces a corresponding deficit, but with relative sparing of grey matter. (Table 13.2)

Thrombosis of the anterior spinal artery, or disease involving the aorta or heart, result in the most critical forms of ischaemic myelopathy with girdle pain (dependent on the level of involvement), flaccid paralysis, loss of sensation, and loss of sphincter control. Such events may follow cardiac arrest, surgery the heart or aorta, aortic aneurysmal rupture, blood loss, and angiography of the aorta, thyrocervical trunk, or radicular arteries. The pain and dysaesthesiae following anterior spinal artery thrombosis may prove refractory to

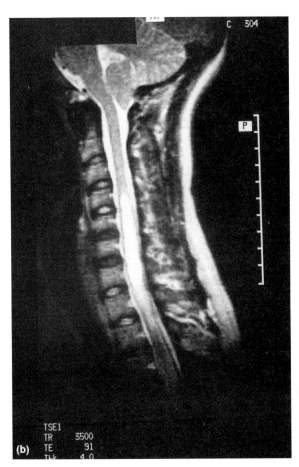

Fig. 13.2(b) T2 weighted image

Table 13.2 Vascular lesions

Ischaemic and watershed
myelopathies
Arterial disease
Venous Infarction
Embolism:
    Gas—decompression sickness
    Fat
    Atheromatous plaques
    Nucleus pulposus
    Parasites
    Bacterial
    Metastatic
Haemorrhage:
    Spinal subarachnoid
    Haematomyelia
Haematoma formation
ArterioVenous malformations
Neurogenic intermittent claudication:
    of spinal cord
    of cauda equina

However, in as many as 50% of patients (particularly in the older age group), no predisposing cause is determined other than widespread atheroma. Chronic ischaemic changes may produce a progressive flaccid paraparesis mimicking motor neurone disease.

Systemic diseases may occasionally affect the vasculature of the cord. Examples include polyarteritis nodosa, systemic lupus erythematosus, and giant cell arteritis. Vasculitic changes associated with osteitis as in brucellosis, abscess formation, or rheumatoid arthritis involving the spine may also cause inflammation within small- or medium-sized vessels in the vicinity. Vascular changes may accompany the meningitic reactions of sarcoidosis, tuberculosis or syphilis. Drug reactions to adulterated heroin or quinine can result in hypotension, embolism, or hypersensitivity reactions involving the cord.

Venous infarction of the cord is rare except in the context of an associated arteriovenous malformation. When it does occur, spinal venous stasis and thrombosis are usually associated with malignant disease, sepsis, vertebral disorders, or hyperviscosity. The differential diagnosis of infarction of the lower part of the cord and cauda equina includes occlusion of the aorta producing the Leriche syndrome of intermittent claudication with ischaemic changes in the legs and wasting. Recovery of sensation after infarction is usually good but that of power remains poor.

Septic emboli are relatively rare. Those from parasitic disease include malaria and schistosomiasis. Fat embolism may follow fractures of bones. Fragments of nucleus pulposus from lateral rupture of a degenerative disc can enter the arterial circulation under pressure through a tear in an adjacent radicular artery or vascular malformation with the rapid development of pain and paraparesis. In most cases, the diagnosis is established at autopsy. At altitude, hypobaric decompression

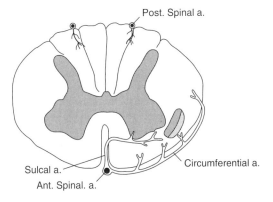

Fig. 13.3 Diagram of a transverse section of the spinal cord to show arterial supply.

opiate, anticonvulsant, or tricyclic antidepressant therapy (Triggs and Beric 1993). Less severe conditions such as hypotension, Stokes–Adams attacks, hyperviscosity syndromes, or blood dyscrasias may produce patchy or watershed infarction, perhaps mimicking the Brown–Sequard syndrome.

with multiple ischaemic foci can result in infarction of areas of the spinal cord.

There are no specific treatments for any of the above vascular changes other than to treat the underlying systemic condition. Except in the presence of embolic cardiac disease, anticoagulant therapy should be avoided. Antibiotics have been advocated in the presence of infarction, and control of hypertension should be achieved gradually to minimize the risk of a precipitous drop in pressure. High dose steroid therapy and even surgical decompression have been tried to prevent the development of a necrotizing myelopathy.

Diving and tunnelling, and recreational SCUBA diving, can lead to decompression sickness (Caisson's disease) with manifestations involving spinal cord and brain. Autochthonus bubbles of inert gas formed intra- or extravascularly within the nervous system as a result of rapid decompression can cause irreversible damage if recompression and slower decompression are not performed. Furthermore, gas emboli, formed as a result of pulmonary overinflation with alveolar rupture under pressure, circulating through the pulmonary venous system into the arterial system, may block small arteries causing an acute inflammatory response with ischaemia within the territory supplied by that artery, and may also produce the more severe forms of embolic paraplegia. However, it is not always possible to differentiate between arterial gas emboli and autochthonous gas bubbles.

Pearson (1992) cites the distribution and percentage incidence of presenting symptoms and signs in 935 patients with decompression sickness and central nervouse system (CNS) involvement: 21% had numbness and paraesthesia, 20% motor weakness, 6% paralysis, and 2.5% urinary symptoms. Treatment, as stated, depends on recompression and slow, often repeated, decompression. Prevention involves attention to rigid rules and training, limiting the time and depth of diving, the speed of ascent, and with very deep dives, the use of helium and oxygen mixtures.

HAEMORRHAGE

Bleeding into the substance of the cord (haematomyelia) tends to involve the cervical region. This uncommon condition may result from vascular anomalies, leukaemia, or indirect trauma, producing syringomyelia-like symptoms. The cord may appear swollen on MRI or myelography. Decompression is rarely required. In the acute stage, conservative treatment with a collar and bedrest is advised.

Spinal subarachnoid haemorrhage may present with back and girdle pain, followed later by pain at the base of the spine and a blood-stained CSF. No specific treatment is required except to confirm the bleeding site and where possible to operate to prevent further haemorrhage. Most spinal subarachnoid bleeds arise from arteriovenous malformations. Aneurysms can occur; as may aneurysmal dilatation of the anterior spinal artery.

SPINAL EPIDURAL AND SUBDURAL HAEMATOMATA

Haematomata can develop rapidly with sudden, severe back pain, constant over the site of haemorrhage. The pain may be enhanced by movement or manoeurves that increase the pressure on the vertebral venous plexus and by percussion over the affected area. Neural compression rapidly develops. Most haematomata result from trauma, particularly in neonates and older children, in whom the lower cervical spine is the most commonly affected site. In adults, haematomata usually occur in the thoracic or lumbar regions often as a result of minor injuries without accompanying fractures or dislocation, with vascular malformations, blood dyscrasias, or tumours, and can follow lumbar puncture or epidural anaesthesia with leakage of blood within the subdural space. Spinal haematomata are a potential hazard to anticoagulated patients.

Occasionally, a spinal haematoma may develop insidiously over days or weeks but more often the march of events is rapid, within hours, inevitably with cord compression—60% of those afflicted are left with a permanent paralysis. The diagnosis should be by MRI. If by myelography, a cisternal puncture is preferable, as a lumbar space is often the suspected site. Prompt surgical drainage is required with antibiotic cover and correction of any bleeding tendency. In patients on anticoagulant therapy, treatment should be stopped and vitamin K or fresh frozen plasma provided. Most of those who recover have been operated upon within 72 hours of the onset of symptoms. However, even with immediate palliative treatment, there still remains the hazard of early or delayed ischaemic necrosis of the cord.

SPINAL ARTERIOVENOUS MALFORMATIONS

These are often associated with other vascular anomalies in the central nervous system and elsewhere. Most are located below the T3 segment, are dural as well as intradural, and receive part of their blood supply from arteries that either do not supply the cord at all or only supply the posterior spinal circulation (Aminoff 1992). Symptoms may arise from subarachnoid bleeding (this is particularly true of those situated in the cervical region), or from infarction or ischaemia caused by shunting of blood away from the cord.

The myeloradiculopathy resulting from spinal arteriovenous malformations may have an insidious onset and follow a relapsing and remitting course. Symptoms include pain, dysaesthesia, limb weakness, or bladder dysfunction. Neurogenic claudication may be precipitated by changes of posture. Diagnostic difficulties often arise but recurrent myelopathic symptoms at the same spinal level, previously considered to be due to transverse myelitis or to multiple sclerosis, should always suggest the possibility of an arteriovenous malformation.

Spinal arteriovenous malformations may show as wormlike defects on myelography. They are less readily diagnosed by CT scanning or MRI. If the myelogram is sufficiently convincing selective angiography may not be required but can be helpful not only to confirm the presence, the level and extent of the vascular anomaly, but also to determine the presence of a fistula or shunt. Surgical excision using a dissecting microscope and cavitron probe, or embolic occlusion of the feeding vessels, may arrest the rapid progression of a myeloradiculopathy or prevent further bleeding. A symptomless malformation, discovered accidentally, is best left undisturbed.

NEUROGENIC CLAUDICATION

Intermittent claudication of the cauda equina (Blau–Logue syndrome) results from central disc compression with weakness in the legs with exertion, often associated with urinary retention or incontinence. Intermittent claudication of the spinal cord may arise from any vascular impairment such as atheroma or aortic steal syndromes affecting the anterior spinal artery, but the most common cause is vascular shunting due to a spinal arteriovenous malformation.

Claudication is also a symptom in 33% of patients with symptomatic lumbar stenosis. The majority of these patients complain of symptoms which appear during activity or with body postures that involve extension of the lumbar spine with mechanical compression of the nerve roots, as for example with hyperextension while receiving a general anaesthetic. Typically, patients attempt to ease their symptoms by adopting a stooping posture when walking. Both postural and exertional claudication result in transient root pains, paraesthesiae, weakness, and numbness. Reflex changes, sensory deficits, and impairment of straight leg raising may only become obvious after exertion. Conservative treatment with traction or lumbar supports may exacerbate the condition. The diagnosis should be clinical but confirmed by CT myelography, MRI, or electromyography. Increasingly, the preferred operative procedure is a partial undercutting facetectomy with decompression of the nerve root canal by removal of the hypertrophied bony foramina, ligamentum flavum, and sequestrated disc material. The operation has an added advantage in that it is possible to demonstrate the obstruction of the venous plexus and to observe the refilling of these vessels when surgical dissection has been completed.

MENINGITIS

Any inflammatory, irritative, or infiltrative disorder of the leptomeninges produces a meningitic reaction with exudation of cells and protein into the CSF of the subarachnoid space, involvement of the dura, and inflammatory and arteritic infiltration into the substance of the brain and spinal cord. Seen most acutely in bacterial meningitis, the cardinal symptoms are headache increasing in severity, fever, progressive drowsiness, and nuchal rigidity resulting from meningeal irritation. In a child too young or too ill to complain of headache, its presence may be confirmed by accompanying features such as photophobia, vomiting, or papilloedema.

All forms of meningitis are still associated with high morbidity and mortality. Thus, the emphasis must be on early treatment and avoidance of coning in the presence of cerebral oedema. Sir Charles Symonds wrote that the speciality of neurology was established through the use of the ophthalmoscope and lumbar puncture needle. Nowadays, the caution of prior ophthalmoscopy before lumbar puncture is more usually provided by CT or MR scanning and in the very young by ultrasound. Even so, the risks of coning from lumbar puncture in infants and preschool children are such that treatment should be started immediately and the diagnosis obtained by other means (blood cultures, culturing skin lesions in meningococcal meningitis, throat swabs).

At a later age, once the safety of lumbar puncture is established by scanning, and if necessary enhanced by the use of mannitol or dexamethasone, CSF should be withdrawn to enable an accurate diagnosis. (Tables 13.3 and 13.4) This may also be required in younger children if the meningitis fails to respond to broad-spectrum antibiotics. Repeated CSF examination may be needed in subacute or chronic meningitis, looking for tubercle bacilli, yeasts, fungi, or mitotic cells. If

Table 13.3 Examination of cerebrospinal fluid

1. Cell count + dark ground examination
2. Centrifuge + differential count (haemoglobin and erythrocytes)
3. Biochemical: protein and glucose
4. Gram stain (+ Indian ink for yeasts)
5. Culture on simple media
6. Enriched broth culture + carbon dioxide:
   for further subculture and antibiotic sensitivities
7. Centrifuge and store for:
   (a) viral culture
   (b) acid-fast ZN
   (c) inoculation
   (d) serology
   (e) rapid methods of diagnosis (see Table 13.4)

Table 13.4 Rapid methods of diagnosis

To determine specific bacterial capsular antigens:
  immunoelectrophoresis
  latex particle agglutination
  ELISA
Endotoxins of Gram-negative organisms:
  Limulus test
Bacterial aetiology for aseptic meningitis:
  C reactive protein >50 mg/l
  CSF lactate >2.2 mmol/l
  raised CSF lactic dehydrogenase

Pitfalls of diagnosis:
Absence of cells in CSF does not exclude a positive Gram
  stain for *Streptococcus pneumoniae*
Polymorph pleocytosis early in tuberculous (TBM) or viral meningitis
Lymphocytic meningitis with partially treated bacterial
  infection

there is still a risk of cerebral oedema, CSF may be withdrawn from a ventricular drain, permitting simultaneous measurement of intracerebral pressure. At the extremes of life, in the comatose, or in the immunocompromised, there may be a 'dearth' of symptoms—even nuchal rigidity may be absent—and survival depends on the clinician realizing that the CSF may be a locus of infection.

Viral encephalomeningitis is more common than a viral meningitis, limited largely to the meninges of the spinal cord. Meningitis may be the only feature of a viral illness or be associated with other neurologial manifestations such as shingles or paralysis (polio, echo, or Coxsackie infections) or with systemic diseases such as mumps, rubella, measles, or influenza. (Table 13.5.) Rashes may herald the infection and the CSF is characteristically lymphocytic (an aseptic meningitis). Viral meningitis must be differentiated from other forms of lymphocytic meningitis (Table 13.6). With a sterile CSF or where malignancy is a possibility (e.g. with malignant melanoma, lymphomas, leukaemia, or carcinoma of lung, breast, or gastrointestinal tract), the CSF should be examined for malignant cells. Unfortunately, conventional CSF cytological methods are frequently unsatisfactory with a reported rate of detection as low as 20% (Bigner and Johnston 1981). A frequent fault is to report malignant cells as lymphocytes. However, with the addition of monoclonal antibody immunocytology recognition is improved and the type of malignant cell may be detected (Moseley *et al.* 1989).

With recurrent attacks of bacterial meningitis (i.e. repeated after convalescence), investigation should include the possibility of head trauma, CSF leaks, congenital CSF fistulae, or dermal sinus tracts; other forms of dysraphism, parameningeal infections (see above), comprised or deficient immune conditions, or inadequacy of the initial treatment. CT scanning is of value, not only in the acute phase as indicated, but in the course of treatment of bacterial and other infec-

Table 13.5 Typical organisms causing meningitis

Neonatal	< 3 months	Children	Elderly
E. coli	Staphylococci	Neisseria meningitidis	E. coli
Streptobacillus	Pseudomonas	Strept pneumoniae	
Listeria	Klebsiella	Haemophilus influenzae	

Table 13.6 Pathological findings in cerebrospinal fluid in different types of meningitis

	Normal	Bacterial	Viral	TBM
Appearance	Clear	Cloudy	Clear/opalescent	
White blood cell count	<3/ml	>1000/ml	<200/ml	
Differential WBC	–	>60% poly-morphs	Lymphocytic	
Protein	20–40 g/1	>100 g/1	<100 g/1	>100 g/1
Glucose	2.2–4.5 mmol/1	<2.2	Normal	<2.2

Table 13.7 Non-viral causes of lymphocytic meningitis

Bacterial
Tuberculous meningitis
Partially treated bacterial meningitis,
Infection adjacent to the meninges:-
    osteitis, mastoiditis, abscess.
Uncommon organisms (e.g. brucellosis)

Other infections:
Leptospirosis
Neurosyphilis
Amoebae
Toxoplasmosis
Fungi, Yeasts

Neoplastic
Carcinomatous,
    leukaematous, lymphomatous,
    sarcoidosis

Toxins
Intrathecal chemotherapeutic agents
X-ray contrast media
Lead

Recurrent meningitis or encephalitis
Mollaret's benign recurrent meningitis
Behçet's disease
Reye's disease
Vogt–Koyangi–Harada syndrome

tions: to exclude abscesses and tuberculomas; if there is any suggestion of a skull fracture or penetrating injury; and to exclude the development of hydrocephalus.

TREATMENT

Supportive treatment for all forms of meningitis must not be neglected. This includes the monitoring of the conscious level, bedrest in a dimly lit or darkened room, reduction of temperature, treatment of rigors, analgesics (including opiates), antiemetics, and anticonvulsants as required. Cerebral oedema may have to be treated with dexamethasone or mannitol. Pressure monitoring may be needed and the early development of hydrocephalus require shunting. In epidemics, notification, warnings and prophylaxis for those at risk are also required.

For meningococcal infection where the sensitivities are already known penicillin may be effective (Klein *et al.* (1993). For most bacterial infections ampicillin is easiest to administer but rashes and sensitivity to beta-lactamase- producing *Haemophilus* can occur. Of the third generation antibiotics, given by injection, ceftriaxone is most effective with more rapid sterilization of CSF, and a milder risk of hearing impairment; but it does have the potential side-effects of diarrhoea and biliary pseudolithiasis. Tuberculosis is best treated with isoniazid 300–600 mg daily, rifampicin 600 mg daily, and ethambutol 1.5 mg daily, the regimen may be changed in the light of antibiotic sensitivities, but therapy is usually continued for at least 12 months. Cryptococcal meningitis is treated with amphotericin B and flucytosine. Other drugs for fungal infections include minocycline. Antimitotic agents and steroids may be given for malignant meningitis.

COMPLICATIONS

Residual defects affecting cranial nerves or extensively damaging the cord and nerve roots can occur, dependent on the organism, severity of infection, and adequacy of therapy. Obstruction can occur with basal meningitis or hydrocephalus. Localized infection may be associated with relapses or recurrent attacks, with abscesses or tuberculomas. (Fig. 13.4.) Where, for example, progressive paraplegia occurs in the presence of tuberculosis the differential diagnosis includes: vertebral collapse, cord compression related to arteritis, thrombophlebitis, and a granuloma or epidural abscess, from an expanding subdural empyema or from constrictive arachnoiditis.

ARACHNOIDITIS

Scarring of the leptomeninges with a constructive or adhesive fibroblastic proliferation is termed arachnoiditis. In developing countries it is often assumed to be associated with tuberculosis and manifests as the commonest cause of spinal compression (43 out of 123 operated cases in Madras; Ramamurthi 1961). In the West, the use of the oily contrast medium, Myodil as a cause of arachnoiditis has led to medicolegal controversy. The symptoms progression of developing over months or years are of spinal compression with pain, para-

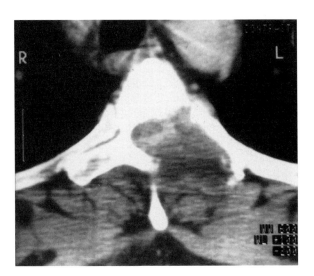

Fig. 13.4 Tuberculosis of the spine, showing destruction of posterior elements on the left with abscess formation (the spinal cord is on the right). CT, axial image.

lysis, wasting, paraesthesiae and sensory loss, and sphincter disturbances. A subacute ascending or transverse radiculopathy may occur at one or more levels. The CSF contains a raised protein and a few cells.

There are other causes of arachnoiditis. Trauma, disc disease, and cervical spondylosis may give a localized form. Contaminants in the CSF, toxic doses of drugs injected into the subarachnoid space, infections, and blood (e.g. after a subarachnoid haemorrhage) may result in localized or generalized arachnoiditis. It is also claimed to arise *de novo*. Other infections in addition to tuberculosis (e.g. syphilis, cryptococcus, cystercercosis, brucellosis, and fungi) may cause arachnoiditis but it does not appear to result from neoplasia, sarcoidosis, Behçet's syndrome, or Mollaret's meningitis. If from Myodil, locules may be seen on plain X-ray with the characteristics of fat on MRI, spinal arachnoid cysts may be present, neural compression and constriction may affect root sleeves or the spinal cord itself. Treatment is often ineffective but surgical decompression, steroids, and intrathecal streptokinase may be tried.

SPINAL EPIDURAL ABSCESSES

These are the result of pyogenic infections in the space between the dura mater and the surrounding vertebral bodies. In 1948, Heusner wrote that 'the decisive factor in the outcome . . . is the celerity with which the first physician suspects . . . and summons expert aid'. He defined three forms:-

1. Acute 'purulent' metastatic occurring over hours to days.
2. Subacute with a granular abscess cavity evolving over days to weeks, and, involving less than 10%.
3. Chronic (e.g. with osteomyelitis.

The history may be of a blunt injury usually to the thoracic or lumbar regions. The site of local bruising later becomes secondarily infected: in 50% from a blood-borne infection but sometimes spreading from contiguous structures. The most common organism is *Staphylococcus*. Other abscess forming-bacteria include streptococci, tuberculosis, *Brucella*, *E. coli*, *Proteus*, *Pseudomonas*, and increasingly uncommon organisms are seen among the immunocompromised and drug abusers.

Back pain is often dull at first and aggravated by movement. Rigidity of the paraspinal muscles then develops and the patient complains of radicular pains. Progression from the earliest symptoms of fever, backache, and local spinal tenderness to paralysis may be rapid. Diagnosis must be by MRI; other methods may become legally indefensible. Lumbar puncture may be difficult because of para-vertebral spasm and, although myelography will show the extent of the abscess, the introduction of contrast may increase the hazards of subsequent management. Without surgical intervention the mortality is 100%, and the longer the delay in evacuating the area of suppuration, the greater the morbidity and mortality (Galbraith and Barr 1974). Full bacteriology is imperative, and as the abscess lies anteriorly, extensive exposure is required. In children the prophylactic use of Harrison's rods may be needed to prevent subsequent scoliosis. Prolonged antibiotic therapy is essential, increasingly with broad-spectrum antibiotics, and many centres also employ hyperbaric oxygen therapy to the affected tissues (Ravicovitch and Spallone 1982).

WHIPLASH INJURY

The term 'whiplash' strictly refers to soft tissue injuries following rear end collisions but many of the details also apply to other neck sprains after accidents (Porter 1989). Symptoms may be minimal at first but develop over 24 hours with pain in the neck and lower back: 53% recover fully by 5 weeks (Gargan and Bannister 1992). A poor prognosis is associated with objective neurological signs, sharp reversal of the normal cervical lordosis on X-ray, and restricted movement at one level in flexion/extension. No patient with intrusive or disabling symptoms at three months went on to make a full recovery and a confident assessment of outcome can be given within nine months. The condition does not appear to be influenced by the pre-existing pscyhological personality or by litigation. Older patients, presumably because of pre-existing degenerative disease have the worst prognosis. Overall, there is a small but significantly increased ($P>0.01$) incidence of anterior cervical discectomy and fusion compared with the general population (Hamer *et al.* 1992) and radiographic evidence of degenerative changes in the spine occurs at an earlier age.

Treatment involves the use of a soft collar for up to 12 weeks, physiotherapy, and alleviation of symptoms by non-steroidal anti-inflammatory agents (NSAIDs) or by diazepam (5–10 mg o.n. to relieve muscle spasm).

TUMOURS

Treatment is essentially surgical but recognition clinical: with awareness of the importance of radicular symptoms before cord compression develops (see Table 13.8).

Byrne and Waxman (1990), emphasize the monitoring of early symptoms of back and radicular pain by MR scanning to exclude vertebral and intraspinal metastases well before the possibility of neural compression develops. Symptoms and signs can be grouped into four main categories: (1) a neuralgic stage of segmental and local pain; (2) impaired motor function leading to paralysis; (3) subjective and objective sensory signs; and (4) disturbances of sphincter and sexual function. The deleterious effects to neural function can arise as a result of any combination of mechanical compression, arterial occlusion leading to ischaemia, and venous occlusion with congestion and infarction. The signs of compression differ with the level involved, this, together with high cervical compression, has already been discussed.

Table 13.8 The frequency of intraspinal tumours in adults

Intramedullary (15% overall)
90% gliomas
65% ependymomas
30% other gliomas
5–10% dermoids, etc.

Intradural (55%)
30% neurofibromas
25% meningiomas, metastases, etc.

Extradural (30%)
Metastases
Myeloma
Bone tumours

The features of cervical impairment include:

1. Deep aching or burning pain affecting the neck, shoulders, and arms.
2. Segmental, radicular pain with reduced reflexes, wasting, and weakness; with radicular symptoms reflexes may be inverted.
3. Developing spastic paralysis below the level of the tumour.
4. A suspended, monkey-jacket, sensory loss; lateral spinothalamic compression may cause total loss below the lesion without sacral sparing.
5. Painless burns or atrophic injuries to the hands (intrinsic lesions).
6. Uni- or bilateral Horner's syndrome from sympathetic interruption either within the cord or involvement of the stellate ganglion.
7. Urgency or incontinence with intrinsic lesions.

The features of dorsal compression are similar: with an emphasis on girdle pains, the possibility of localized scoliosis from wasting, and weakness of paraspinal and intercostal muscles, and paralytic ileus from involvement of splanchnic nerves. (Fig. 13.6.) Compression below D11 to L1/2 can involve the conus and lower still the cauda equina. A pure conus syndrome will cause saddle anaesthesia, urinary retention or overflow incontinence, faecal incontinence, impotence, and absent anal reflexes. Cauda equina involvement will give lower motor neurone features as well as those of compression at other sites (Gurusinghe 1992).

ACUTE TRANSVERSE MYELOPATHY

Transverse myelitis, it is often classified as a demyelinative condition. It may be a secondary, non-specific hypersensitivity disorder involving the spinal cord and occurring in isolation or in combination with an acute polyneuritis and radiculopathy (as in the Guillain–Barré syndrome). The cord lesion is initially limited longitudinally to a few segments, but may spread as an ascending myelitis. A similar presentation

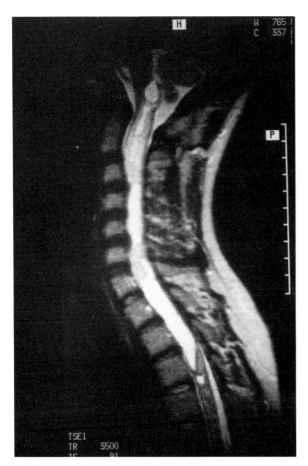

Fig. 13.5 Ependymoma and intramedullary cyst formation within the cervical cord. Sagittal MRI, T2 weighted images.

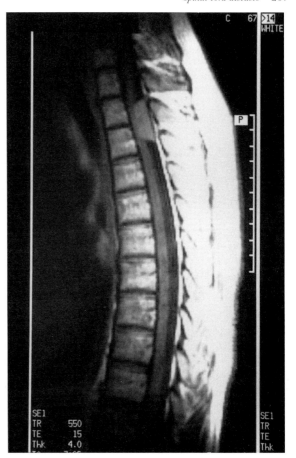

Fig. 13.6 Intradural, extramedullary meningioma compressing cord at T1-2, extending from craniocervical junction to T3-4. Sagittal MRI, T1 weighted images following gadolinium.

can occur with spinal multiple sclerosis. However, with myelopathy plaque formation is replaced by an inflammatory, allergic arteritis affecting the grey and white matter and meninges over several segments.

The mid or upper thoracic cord is commonly involved and the differential pathogenesis is set out in Table 13.9. A more chronic form may develop one to four years after spinal irradiation. Acute myelitis may develop over hours or days. The sequence of events is usually similar. An acute pyrexia with radiculopathy or back pain localized over a few spinal segments is followed by symptoms of spinal cord transection. There may be a persisting low grade pyrexia. Bilateral paraesthesiae start in the feet and ascend with numbness and sensory impairment giving rise to urinary retention and loss of bowel control. There follows a progressive flaccid weakness of the lower limbs and abdominal muscles. The paresis may remain flaccid if the spinal cord starts to necrose. More usually the initial flaccid weakness gives way to an increasingly spastic paraplegia. The CSF may contain up to 10 g/l of protein and up to 200 lymphocytes/ml. MR scans show high signal intensity on long TR sequences over several segments.

With milder degrees of myelopathy the full thickness of the cord need not be affected. Management depends on the underlying cause with additional use of corticosteroids, especially where there is a possibility of a collagen vascular or allergic reactive aetiology. The majority of patients pass from the initial stage to a stable plateau lasting days or weeks before a slow recovery over three or more months, often leaving a mild residual disability. Those who fail to recover may develop myelomalacia or necrosis (the Foix–Alajouanine syndrome). In a few instances, where recovery is slow, surgical decompression can help—although the mechanism of improvement is far from clear.

About a third of those with post-infective myelitis give a history of an antecedent viral infection. An acute onset with pain usually carries a poor prognosis, and the thoracic cord is affected in 90% of cases. There is evidence of primary demyelination with significant inflammation and a marked lymphocytic reaction in the CSF showing immune reactivity to myelin basic protein and P_2 proteins.

Myelopathies related to systemic lupus erythematosus (SLE) fall into two types. The acute type resembles post-

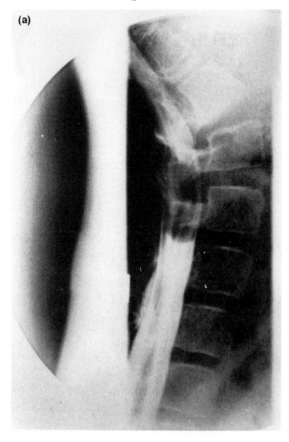

Fig. 13.7(a) Myelogram of a child. Implantation epidermoid lateral.

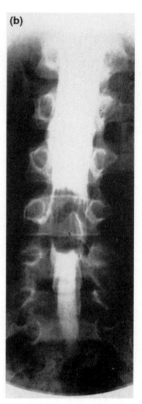

Fig. 13.7(b) anterior-posterior views. Water-soluble contrast medium.

infective myelitis. The CSF protein is raised with a pleocytosis and reduced CSF glusose to 50%. The cord may be oedematous and swollen with added infarction. Intense immunosuppression is required with high dose steroids, intravenous cyclophosphamide or short-term plasma exchange. The subacute form, which has also been called lupus sclerosis, may give a poorly defined sensory level and neurological signs elsewhere. The true nature of the illness is disputed (Dawson and Potts 1991).

Direct viral infection can occur with herpes zoster with dysfunction of the bladder and anus (Jellinek and Tulloch 1976). Recovery is usually complete and the segmental distribution of any rash does not necessarily coincide with the level of myelopathy. Herpes zoster infections can be unpredictable, remaining dormant until another viral infection reduces the body's resistance; and myelopathy can be a feature of symptomatic herpes zoster infections (e.g. developing at the site of trauma, a metastatic deposit, or disc prolapse). Immunosuppression in the recipients of renal transplants can set alight cytomegalovirus (CMV) infection with acute transverse myelopathy. A syndrome primarily involving the bladder with transient urinary retention may arise from myeloradiculitis of

Table 13.9 Causes of acute transverse myelopathy

Demyelinating:
Multiple sclerosis
Devic's d. neuromyelitis optica
Subacute myelo-optic neuropathy (SMON)
Guillain–Barré radiculomyelopathy

Virus-related
Post-infective, post-vaccination
Infections
AIDS-related

Non-viral infections
Spirochaetes: syphilis, Lyme disease
Parasites: schistosomiasis, larva migrans

Autoimmune
Collagen diseases
Stings, bites

Drugs
Heavy metals, arsphenamine,
intrathecal drugs, pamaquin,
orthocresyl phosphate

Physical agents
Burns, electric shock,
irradiation, heat stroke

Toxic and deficiency states
Lathyrism
Metabolic (e.g. calcium: remote effects)
Nutritional (e.g. Vitamin B_{12} deficiency)

the sacral segments as with anogenital herpes simplex infections, or with echo, CMV, and EBV (Epstein–Barr) infections. (Table 13.10.)

Lyme disease provides a good example of a radiculomyelopathy. In a Danish study (Hansen and Lebach 1992) 94 of 187 patients had Bannwarth's syndrome of painful lymphocytic meningoradiculits with paresis (61%) or with a radicular pain syndrome only (25%). Most responded to treatment with penicillin.

AIDS-related and ARDS (AIDs related disease states) myelopathies are fairly common. They tend to start insidiously and may remain asymptomatic for some time. Three types of primary myelopathy are recognized:

1. In children, bilateral corticospinal tract degeneration may occur with a distinct histopathology and the development of a progressive quadriparesis (Dickson *et al.* 1989).
2. A symptomatic transient myelopathy may develop at the time of seroconversion (Denning *et al.* 1987) and improve over 6 weeks apart from some residual signs.
3. A vacuolar myelopathy predominantly affecting the lateral and posterior columns in the thoracic region with histological features resembling vitamin B_{12} deficiency. As symptoms develop there is a progressive spastic paraparesis, incontinence, and ataxia. Position and vibration sensation may be affected. Accompanying features include chronic diarrhoea, wasting, and a peripheral neuropathy.

There is no specific treatment for these AIDS myelopathies which can occur during latent HIV infection.

In addition to these, zoster infection, normally dormant in the dorsal root ganglia may invade the cord. Kaposi sarcoma and lymphoma may compress the cord and a progressive ascending myelopathy occur due to either HSV-2 or cytomegaloviruses, the latter associated with a radiculopathy. Syphilitic meningovascular disease, mycobacterial meingomyelitis, and toxoplasmosis may also supervene. These myelopathies are more virulent and progressive than vacuolar myelopathy. Their presence may be determined by myelogaphy or MR scanning and herpetic infections may partially respond to acylovir.

RADICULOPATHIES

GUILLAIN–BARRÉ SYNDROME (GBS)

GBS can present as a peripheral neuropathy, myelopathy, or even encephalopathy and is generally described as an autoimmune disease, the basis of which is not precisely clear. In about 50% there is an antecedent viral infection but it may follow surgery, inoculation, mycoplasma infection, or be related to lymphoma, Hodgkin's disease, or systemic lupus erythematosus. A few cases may be drug-induced, as from gold. In its radicular-myelopathic form, such as with Landry's ascending paralysis, it may mimic acute transverse myelopathy.

Classically, there is proximal weakness with arreflexia in a limb spreading to other limbs in a cartwheel fashion over 4–6 weeks, associated with mild ataxia—which may be due to involvement of Clarke's column, sensory symptoms, a flaccid paralysis, and autonomic nervous system disturbance. Once the progressive phase arrests recovery starts after 2–4 weeks intermission and may continue over a period from 4 weeks to 3 years. Even so, residual signs may still persist at the end of that period. The CSF shows a raised protein with a cytoalbuminique dissociation and oligoclonal bands due to a rise in IgG. Other presentations not affecting the cranial nerves include sensory loss with arreflexia, pandysautonomia, and a chronic relapsing demyelinating neuropathy.

Steroids in various forms have not helped the prognosis except in the relapsing forms. Plasmaphoresis should be seriously considered for the more severe cases but the mildest do well with supportive and expectant treatment.

DIABETIC AMYOTROPHY (LOWER LIMB ASYMMETRIC MOTOR NEUROPATHY)

Develops as a painful polyradiculopathy prone to occur in elderly male diabetics and usually involving the musculature of the thigh with wasting and weakness. There is depression or loss of reflexes. Some sensory change does not exclude the diagnosis and the CSF protein is raised to about 100mg/l. The thoracic roots can be similarly affected with pain and dysaesthesia involving the chest wall and abdomen. Active denervation can be seen on electromyogram (EMG) in the paraspinal muscles.

Pain may respond to carbamazepine or valproic acid. The condition can recovery spontaneously or in response to

Table 13.10 Viral causes of acute transverse myelopathy

DNA viruses

Enveloped
Herpes: simplex, simiae, zoster,
    Epstein–Barr cytomegalovirus (CMV)
Pox viruses: vaccinia, variola

Non-enveloped
Hepatitis B

RNA viruses
Non-enveloped
Picorna viruses: polio, Coxsackie, echo
Other enteroviruses
Hepatitis A
Encephalomyocarditis virus

Enveloped
Togaviruses: arbovirus, tick-borne, rubella
Retroviruses: HIV
Orthomyxoviruses: influenza
Pavamyxoviruses: measles, mumps
Bunyaviruses: Californian encephalitis
Rhabdoviruses: rabies

careful diabetic control but may occasionally prove refractory. Myelopathic changes can occur with diabetes: as a pseudotabes involving the dorsal columns or the lateral columns as diabetic amyotrophic lateral sclerosis. In the more symmetric sensorimotor polyneuropathies loss of dorsal root ganglia can be a marked feature. Usually, these conditions occur in addition to a chronic peripheral neuropathy.

NEURALGIC AMYOTROPHY

The first symptom is a severe aching or burning pain across the shoulder, often radiating to an arm and aggravated by movement. Wasting may then occur affecting primarily the muscles of the shoulder girdle with neural involvement of the long nerve of Bell, the circumflex nerve and the phrenic to the ipsilateral hemidiaphragm. Sensory loss is particularly liable to be present over the deltoid, and slowing of nerve conduction found outside the area clinically affected (e.g. in the ulnar and median nerves). The pain may persist for 3 months and the syndrome develop over 4–6 months. Bilateral involvement can occur.

The aetiology is poorly understood. There may be an antecedent viral infection, or a history of immunizations, surgery, trauma, pregnancy, drug abuse, or collagen vascular disease, and there is a rare familial form. Recovery occurs in 80% within 2 years and 90% within 4 years. Steroids given early in the course of the illness ease pain and perhaps influence the degree of wasting. Analgesics may be needed and passive movements performed to prevent the development of a frozen shoulder.

THORACIC OUTLET SYNDROMES

A cervical rib can give rise to symptoms and result in arteriovascular changes in the hands, whereas neurogenic syndromes are more frequently associated with cervical bands. Neurogenic syndromes include the 'very rare true neurogenic syndrome' and the very common droopy shoulder syndrome (Swift and Nichols 1984). The nerve roots affected are C8 and T1. Plain X-rays of neck, CT, or MR scanning, and electrophysiological tests may define the syndrome which can vary from painless partial thenar wasting to paraesthesiae affecting the whole limb. Symptoms may be temporarily relieved by elevating the shoulder and permanently by surgical section of the band or by postural exercises.

SHINGLES

The zoster-varicella virus can be isolated from the vesicles of chicken pox or shingles; and may remain dormant in dorsal root ganglia for years after the primary infection. Varicella can involve the nervous system giving rise to a self-limiting cerebellar ataxic syndrome, encephalitis, aseptic meningitis, transverse myelitis, or Guillain–Barré-like syndromes, and is commonly accompanied by a mild lymphocytic pleocytosis and a raised protein in the CSF.

Shingles results from the reactivation of the dormant virus, affecting 1% of the general population and 25% of those with neoplasia, especially lymphomas. With shingles the thoracic and lumbar dermatomes are frequently afflicted but the virus may cause ophthalmic herpes or affect the motor system causing an internuclear ophthalmoplegia, geniculate herpes with otalgia and facial paresis, or sphincter disturbance. Anterior horn cell involvement is probably fairly common but frequently missed. Intercostal wasting may go unnoticed but C5 or C6 involvement produces weakness of shoulder blade abduction and flexion of the elbow with slow recovery.

Autonomic nervous system involvement may account for Horner's syndrome and some forms of bladder and bowel disturbance, but the commonest manifestation is a dermatomal sensory neuropathy with vesiculation. The eruption is best treated initially with boric powder or colloidon and kept dry. Vidarabine and acyclovir are indicated for the complications of *Herpes zoster* infection, both in normal individuals and in the immunosuppressed, but do not influence the development or severity of post-herpetic neuralgia. Simple analgesics are of temporary benefit if only to ensure an adequate night's rest. It is, however, a neuralgic pain and most painkillers do little more than sedate. Chlorpromazine, sparine, and antidepressants can help. Capsaicin cream or ethylchoride sprays applied topically are beneficial; as are Pifco vibrators or dorsal column stimulators.

TORTICOLLIS

Although spasmodic torticollis is moderately benign, the violent movements of torsion dystonia can lead through continuous wear and tear to degenerative changes including multiple subluxations between C5 and T1. Drugs, such as tetrabenazine, haloperidol, and benzhexol, can reduce the painful movements, but procedures such as anterior fixation are risky unless the movements can be stopped prior to operation and during convalescence.

The most effective treatment is the injection of botulinum toxin A (usually about 500 Units of Dysport at any one session) into the most active and the most painful muscles of the neck—usually the sternocleidomastoid, splenius capitis, and trapezius. The injections will weaken the muscles in spasm thus limiting the craniocervical dystonia. There is a delay of 7–10 days before the injections take effect and around that time swallowing difficulties can arise which are minimized if care is taken not to inject pairs of muscles. Rarely more than three muscles are injected at any time but after a week or so further muscles can be injected and the procedure repeated when the movements return. Some weakening of the neck muscles overall may occur occasionally necessitating the use of a supportive collar.

CERVICAL SPONDYLOSIS

Ageing, movement, and trauma involving the lower cervical spine result in degenerative changes which become radiologically apparent at around 50 years of age. The water content of the disc declines with age, the nucleus pulposus is replaced by fibrocartilage; spurs, osteophytes and ridges develop; changes occur in apophyseal joints; the ligamentum flavum thickens and loses elasticity; and blood vessels are constricted by atheroma. Especially if the spinal canal is already narrow (cervical stenosis), flattening of the cord occurs in the anterior-posterior direction and laterally the exit foramina of the spinal roots are encroached on. The brunt of these changes in cervical spondylosis (and with rheumatoid arthritis of the neck) falls between C5-6, and to a lesser extent at C6-7 and C7-8. Bulging or herniation of posterior discs with slippage and subluxation may occur, and, as the lower spaces become more rigid, spondylotic changes also impair movement of the spine at higher levels.

The first symptom is often a painful stiff neck. Rotation and flexion are reduced and the posture becomes fixed. A radiculopathy can develop with pain, paraesthesiae, muscle weakness, and fasciculations in the arms. Reflexes may be depressed, inverted or (below the level of the lesion) hyperactive. A myelopathy can occur due to compression of the cord with spasticity, weakness, even ataxia, sensory loss, and bladder and bowel impairment.

The first line of treatment is rest, local heat, muscle relaxants, and non-steroidal analgesics. Surgery—laminectomies and, increasingly, anterior fixation, taking care not to weaken the spine—is indicated to prevent progression of myelopathy. Just occasionally surgery is also indicated for unresponsive painful radiculopathies and to prevent further wasting or loss of function in the arms.

Similar ageing processes occur involving the lumbar spine which is less mobile but has a greater responsibility for weight bearing. If both cervical and lumbar spine are congenitally narrowed (tandem stenosis) anterior horn cell degeneration can occur at both levels with wasting, fasciculation, and lower limb spasticity mimicking motor neurone disease.

LHERMITTE'S PHENOMENON

Partial demyelination of the posterior columns in the cervical region may induce electric shock sensations which spread with lightening rapidity down the arms, back, or legs on flexion, or, occasionally hyperextension, of the neck. Although Lhermitte recognized its common occurrence in multiple sclerosis, it may also occur with cervical spondylosis, disc herniation, whiplash injury (where it develops over a latent period of 3 months and commonly remits spontaneously after 3 to 6 months), following irradiation, as a early sign of subacute combined degeneration (Vitamin B_{12} deficiency), with hypervitaminosis (e.g. pyridoxine excess), and with drugs which raise the CSF protein, such as cisplatin and perhexilene.

If the symptom occurs frequently or is painful it may be alleviated by the use of carbamazepine 100 mg twice-daily or sodium valproate 200 mg twice-daily. If still troublesome an MR scan of the neck is advisable to exclude cord compression.

DISC HERNIATIONS

CERVICAL

Most disc disease occurs at C5/6 or C6/7. Because of the lack of fat in the cervical spinal canal, diagnostic MR scanning is best performed using gadolinium. Acute cervical disc herniation is often associated with trauma. Lateral or posterolateral prolapse causes root compression with neck stiffness, pain, and radiculopathy. Symptoms may be delayed for some hours following the trauma and made worse with movement, straining, and coughing. Immobilization and traction are required. Cervical discs may also follow a chronic relapsing course or even, especially in the elderly, produce a sudden neurological deficit in an arm with little neck pain. Rest and traction are usually sufficient to produce a remission and surgery is best reserved for when these measures fail.

Central protrusion can cause acute cord compression with less dramatic subjective symptomatology. Again, immobilization with traction is usually sufficient to ameliorate most disc lesions but anterior discectomy is the operation of choice if the manifestations of cord dysfunction are severe and do not show some improvement within a few days.

THORACIC

In the thoracic region the lower discs are most at risk from straining injury. Lifting a heavy object may result in sudden back pain, radiating round the thorax or down to the buttocks. Root symptoms may be accompanied by weakness of the abdominal muscles and the pain mimic an acute abdomen. However, a central disc can be silent producing paraparesis immediately or insidiously. Calcification may be seen on plain X-ray but the myelographic appearances are often unspectacular with changes which do little to suggest the severity of the clinical signs.

LUMBAR

The history of an abrupt and painful experience when bending, lifting, and twisting with inability to straighten up immediately is often of greater help than the clinical examination. Root pain may be confirmed by an absent ankle jerk and occasional sensory loss. Straight leg raising may be impaired. A central disc can cause intermittent claudication of the cauda equina.

CT and MR scanning can be used to demonstrate types of disc herniation not visible on myelography. A far lateral or extreme lateral disc may compress the exiting nerve root in the intervertebral foramen distal to the nerve root sleeve. In the past this has been one explanation of the failed back syndrome. Free fragments (migratory disc material) may also show on CT or MR.

Relatively few patients with disc herniation require surgery but respond to bedrest, traction, or local analgesia. Recuperation should be linked with a course of exercises and active physiotherapy. If a sufficient trial of conservative management fails to relieve incapacitating pain, surgery is beneficial. Chemolysis and percutaneous lumbar discectomy have to some extent replaced open surgery but surgery is particularly required in the event of:

1. Acute cervical or thoracic disc herniation causing significant myelopathy.
2. Lumbar disc herniation causing cauda equina dysfunction such as impaired bowel or bladder control.
3. Wasting or foot drop that is severe or progresses.

REFERENCES

Aminoff, M. J. (1992). Spinal vascular disease In *Diseases of the spinal cord*, (ed. E. Critchley and A. Eisen), pp 281–300. Springer, London.

Anton, H. A. and Schweigel, J. F. (1986). Posttraumatic syringomyelia: the British Columbia experience. *Spine*, **11**, 85–8.

Baker, J. H. E. and Silver, J. R. (1987). Hysterical paraplegia. *Journal of Neurology, Neurosurgery and Psychiatry*, **50**, 375–82.

Bigner, S. H. and Johnston, W. N. (1981). Cytopathology of cerebrospinal fluid. *Acta Cytologica*, **25**, 461–79.

Byrne, T. N. and Waxman, S. G. (1990). *Spinal cord compression*. F. A. Davis, Philadelphia.

Dawson, D. M. and Potts, F. (1991). Acute nontraumatic myelopathies In *Disorders of the spinal cord*, (ed. R. M. Woolsey and R. R. Young), *Neurologic clinics*, Vol. 9, pp. 585–604. Saunders, Philadelphia.

Denis, F. (1983). The three column spine and its significance in the classification of acute thoracolumbar injuries. *Spine*, **8**, 817–31.

Denning, D. W., Anderson, J., Rudge, P., and Smith, H. (1987). Acute myelopathy associated with primary infection with human immunovirus. *British Medical Journal*, **294**, 143–4.

Dickson, D. W., Belman, A. L., Park, Y. D., *et al.* (1989). Central ner-vous system pathology in pediatric AIDS: an autopsy study. APMIS suppl. **8**: 40–57.

Galbraith, J. and Barr, V. (1974). Epidural abscess and subdural empyema. *Advances in Neurology*, **6**, 227–31.

Gargan, M. F. and Bannister, G. C. (1992). *The rate of recovery following soft tissue injury of the neck*. Paper read to the British Cervical Spine Society. See also *Journal of Bone and Joint Surgery* (1990), **72B**, 901–3.

Green, B. A. and Hall, W. J. (1976). Recognition and accident care for spinal cord injured patients. *Paraplegia Life*, **5**, 5–11.

Gurusinghe, N. T. (1992). Spinal cord compression and spinal cord tumours. In *Diseases of the spinal cord*, (ed. E. Critchley and A. Eisen), pp. 351–408. Springer, London.

Hamer, A. J. Prasad, R. Gargan, M. F. Bannister, G. C., and Nelson, R. J. (1992). *Whiplash injury and cervical disc surgery*. Paper read to the British Cervical Spine Society.

Hansen, K. and Lebach, A. M. (1992). The clinical and epidemiological profile of Lyme neuroborrelosis in Denmark, 1985–1990. *Brain*, **115**, 399–424.

Heusner, A. P. (1948), Nontuberculous spinal epidural infection. *New England Journal of Medicine*, **239**, 845–54.

Jellinek, E. H. and Tulloch, W. S. (1976) Herpes zoster with dysfunction of bladder and anus. *Lancet*, **2**, 1219–22.

Klein, N. J., Heyderman, R. S., and Levin, M. (1993). Management of meningococcal infection. *British Journal of Hospital Medicine*, **50**, 42–9.

Moseley, R. P., Davies, A. C., and Bourne, S. G. (1989). Neoplastic meningitis in malignant melanoma. *Journal of Neurology, Neurosurgery and Psychiatry*, **52**, 881–6.

Pearson, R. A. (1992). Decompression illness and the spinal cord. In *Diseases of the spinal cord*, (ed. E. Critchley and A. Eisen), pp. 301–18, Springer, London.

Porter, K. M. (1989). Neck sprains after car accidents. *British Medical Journal*, **298**, 973–4.

Ramamurthi, B. (1961). Intraspinal arachnoiditis. *Indian Journal of Medical Science*, **15**, 777–81.

Ravicovitch, M. A. and Spallone, A. (1982). Spinal epidural abscess. *European Neurology*, **21**, 347–57.

Swift, T. R. and Nichols, F. T. (1984). The droopy shoulder syndrome. *Neurology*, **34**, 212–13.

Torg, J. S., Pavlov, H., Genuario, S. E., Sennett, B., Wisneski, R. J., Robie, B. H. *et al.* (1986). Neurapraxia of the cervical spinal cord with transient quadriplegia. *Journal of Bone and Joint Surgery*, **66A**, 1354–74.

Triggs, W. J. and Beric, A. (1993). Sensory abnormalities and dysaesthesias in the anterior spinal artery syndrome. *Brain*, **115**, 189–98.

Tucci, K. A., Landy, H. J., Green, B. A., and Eismont, F. J. (1992). Trauma and paraplegia. In *Diseases of the spinal cord*, (ed. E. Critchley and A. Eisen), pp. 409–28. Springer, London.

14 | Controversies in the management of common tumours

Spiros Sgouros and A. Richard Walsh

The advent of computerized tomography (CT) and more recently magnetic resonance imaging (MRI) scanning has led to the earlier diagnosis on many intracranial neurological conditions requiring potential neurosurgical treatment (Helseth 1995). In addition to high quality imaging, a probable histological diagnosis can be made, although certain MRI appearances are more diagnostic than others. Classical mistakes in working diagnosis, such as misinterpreting multiple abscesses for multiple metastatic tumours or a multicentric low grade glioma for metastatic tumours, are well described and can only be differentiated by biopsy.

It is not the intention of this chapter to be a definitive text on all aspects of neurosurgery; the authors have been selective including areas where neurosurgical treatment is controversial. We begin the chapter with a brief overview of techniques that have developed over the last decade or are in extensive use at present.

OVERVIEW OF SURGICAL TECHNIQUES FOR INTRACRANIAL TUMOURS

STEREOTACTIC BIOPSY

Since the introduction of CT scanning in the early 1970s the potential of using this imaging modality in association with stereotactic frames for biopsy and ablative procedures has been realized (Kelly 1989). Existing stereotactic frames such as the Leksell frame were adapted for use with CT and later MRI, and new frames specifically for theses scanning modalities were also developed such as the BRW/CRW frame system.

Most stereotactic procedures use CT rather than MRI scan to select targets for biopsy because of the ease of use of this imaging modality and the inherent inhomogeneity of MRI scan, making it potentially non-linear.

Many reports in the literature have indicated achieving positive biopsies in at least 90% of cases, and the finding of an unexpected diagnosis leading to a modification of the proposed treatment in at least 12% of cases (Kratimenos 1993). Morbidity of between 0% and 10% has been reported, the most significant being an operative haematoma. Proximity to major blood vessels (e.g. adjacent to the sylvian fissure) increases the likelihood of this complication and may make the

surgeon either perform an open procedure or perform the biopsy using stereotactic angiography to avoid the major vessels (Kelly 1984). Stereotactic biopsy is most appropriate for small deep seated or diffuse lesions within the brain.

STEREOTACTIC CRANIOTOMY

The use of stereotactic localization to aid in the excision of small subcortical or deep lesions is well established (Hitchcock *et al.* 1989, Kelly 1989, 1992) although the authors' preference is to use per-operative ultrasound as a faster and less cumbersome technique.

PER-OPERATIVE ULTRASOUND

Once a craniotomy has been performed ultrasound is an excellent modality for identifying intracranial masses including haematomas, metastases, abscesses, and deep-seated intrinsic tumours (Hammoud *et al.* 1996). In addition, ultrasound with colour Doppler flow can identify the major blood vessels in relation to the lesion, aiding its safe removal.

IMAGE-GUIDED SURGERY

The development of computer assisted image-guided surgery came as an evolution of stereotactic principles, when computer technology advanced enough to allow processing and manipulation of images in real time. The whole concept of image-guided surgery relies on the co-registration of anatomical landmarks between preoperatively acquired images and the real patient in the operating theatre (Kelly *et al.* 1984). For accuracy, commonly preoperative MRI scans are performed with skin markers attached, acting as fiducials (Alexander *et al.* 1995; Ryan *et al.* 1996). Several systems have been developed, using as the guiding tool a mechanical arm, a locatable probe or the optical axis of the operating microscope which can be incorporated in the system. As with all technology, there is a learning curve, following which the surgeon can enjoy the full benefits of a system which can continuously inform him/her during the operation of his/her exact location in the intracranial cavity, in relation to pre-operative imaging (Alexander *et al.* 1995; Ryan *et al.* 1996; Weiner and Kelly 1996). Less invasive or traumatic surgery surgery is claimed by the advocates of this technology. It certainly seems that it offers an extra degree of confidence to the surgeon who is prepared to undertake surgery to poorly accessible parts of the brain (Weiner and Kelly 1996). Only time will show though whether surgical results are significantly better, to justify the expense of such systems. This technology is particularly useful for subcortical, deep-seated intracerebral or skull base tumours, where intraoperative navigation is needed most. The problem of peroperative shift of structures has not been solved yet but in practice does not really apply to deep seated tumours.

I. Intracranial Tumours

Common ways of presentation of intracranial tumours include symptoms of raised intracranial pressure acute or chronic, epilepsy and focal neurological disability relevant to the anatomic site of the lesion. Consequently, surgical management of these tumours is directed towards relieving, improving, or minimizing neurological disability as well as establishing diagnosis based on which appropriate treatment modalities can be employed to improve the prognosis of the patient.

At the time of first radiological diagnosis, a series of important questions need consideration, such as the confidence of diagnosis on radiological imaging alone, the natural history of the disease if left untreated, the likelihood of complete excision or substantial tumour mass reduction without incurring additional neurological disability, the benefits which such surgery can offer and whether indeed a major intracranial operation is necessary or is conservative expectant management more appropriate. In addition, the likely morbidity and mortality of any potential adjuvant treatment, such as radiotherapy and chemotherapy, need to be evaluated from the outset.

The preliminary radiological diagnosis in association with the age and the clinical condition of the patient will determine further management. The outcome of the proposed treatment will have to be judged against the natural history of the disease if left untreated. The expected benefit of the proposed treatment will have to be weighed against the likelihood of serious complications–temporary or permanent–resulting from it. This 'risk–benefit' approach to clinical management is becoming increasingly mandatory in an era of well-informed patients and increasing litigation.

Commonly, the first stage of management of intracranial tumours is some form of surgery. Although some procedures are initially performed to provide rapid relief of symptomatic raised intracranial pressure (e.g. temporary cerebrospinal fluid drainage in tumours that cause obstructive hydrocephalus), the majority of operations are aiming to provide histological diagnosis and if appropriate, effect reduction of tumour mass. The likelihood or feasibility of complete excision of a brain tumour will be determined by its nature and location. Anatomical relationship and infiltration of surrounding structures such as brainstem, motor cortex, speech areas, visual pathways, and hypothalamus are important. In general, operations for benign brain tumours are aiming at complete excision, whereas in malignant tumours such a goal is unrealistic as even total macroscopic excision of a tumour leaves behind macroscopically invisible tumour cells that have infiltrated the normal white matter and are responsible for recurrence. In such cases, the natural enthusiasm of the surgeon for complete excision should be moderated by the neurological deficit that such surgery may incur, compromising the quality of the remaining (short) life of the patient.

SUPRATENTORIAL TUMOURS

GLIOMAS

Although the term 'glioma' in its correct interpretation includes tumours of astrocytic, oligodendrocytic, and ependymal cell origin, in everyday clinical practice, is used as being synonymous to astrocytoma. This reflects the fact that astrocytomas are the commonest intrinsic brain tumours. Their biological behaviour varies depending on the cell of origin, the grade of malignancy, and the site of the tumour. Although a detailed analysis of the management of gliomas is beyond the scope of this account, several controversial issues deserve discussion as they affect both the neurosurgeon who is treating such patients and the physician who is involved in the overall care, whether that is the neurologist, the general physician, or the family doctor, depending on local circumstances.

Malignant gliomas of the cerebral hemispheres

Mainly affecting elderly individuals over the fifth to sixth decades of life, they are not uncommon in young adults in their second to third decades. Prognosis is dependent largely on age at presentation. It is clear now that younger patients have significantly better prognosis than older ones, although the dividing age varies between 50 and 60 years in different studies (Ayoubi *et al.* 1993; Devaux *et al.* 1993; Ganju *et al.* 1994; Helseth 1995; Kallio *et al.* 1991; Kleinberg *et al.* 1993; Peschel *et al.* 1993; Quigley and Maroon 1991; Sandeman *et al.* 1990; Ullen *et al.* 1990; Ushio 1991; Vertosick and Selker 1992; Whittle *et al.* 1991). There seems to be an underlying biological reason for this difference, mainly related to different chromosomal abnormalities seen in the two groups. In an oversimplified statement, young patients tend to have deletions of chromosomes 17 and 22 in contrast to deletion of chromosome 10 which is seen in older patients and is associated with poor outcome (Guha 1993). The detailed knowledge on biology of the involved tumour suppressor genes is rapidly expanding as research on immunotherapy of gliomas advances (Jen *et al.* 1994). Another prognostic factor is the severity of the pre-operative clinical disability: the better the pre-operative clinical condition, the better the quality of life post-operatively.

Both these factors (age and disability) weigh heavily on the decision for surgical treatment.

Malignant gliomas have usually characteristic radiological appearances both on CT and MRI scan (Fig. 14.1). On CT scans they present as mass lesions with mixed high density, irregular ill-defined margins, commonly low density necrotic centre and considerable associated surrounding white matter oedema, and shift of midline structures. Similarly, on MRI scan they present as mixed signal infiltrating mass lesions, causing significant oedema in the adjacent white matter. It is increasingly believed that this oedematous white matter does actually contain tumour cells (Jolesz *et al.* 1993), which would have surgical implications and bearing on recurrence potential.

The issue of the predictive value of the extent of surgical resection has not yet been resolved. It is now accepted that tumour cells are present beyond the macroscopically evident tumour. It has been observed that recurrence occurs in a zone of the first 3 centimetres from the resection margin, which makes total resection look almost a futile surgical exercise (Jolesz *et al.* 1993). Nevertheless, it seems that in young patients total macroscopic excision is offering an appreciable benefit in

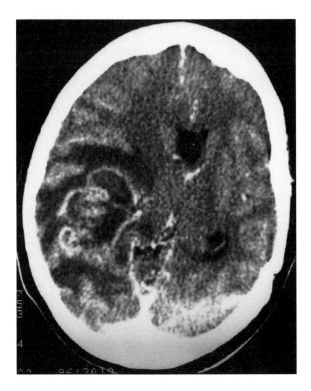

Fig. 14.1 Malignant glioma. Contrast-enhanced CT scan of a 60-year-old patient who presented with symptoms of raised intracranial pressure and left hemiparesis. A mixed density, contrast-enhancing right parietal lesion is seen. The mass has indistinct margins, spreading into the normal adjacent brain. There is considerable associated white matter oedema and significant midline shift. These are the typical appearances of a malignant glioma of the cerebral hemispheres.

long-term survival. In older patients, the benefit is less clear hence when the tumour is in a disadvantageous anatomical location or when the patient's disability is already advanced, surgical endeavours tend to be limited to modest debulking or just biopsy in cases of deep-seated tumours. Although blind radiotherapy based in radiological appearances has been advocated it is always worth considering at least a burr hole biopsy, to exclude an intracerebral abscess. Such a mistake in diagnosis would lead to embarrassing and disastrous complications.

Post-operative radiotherapy is proven to prolong survival appreciably, and various combinations with chemotherapy have been tried in an effort to maximize treatment potential (Arcicasa *et al.* 1994; Barker *et al.* 1996; Curran *et al.* 1993; Dinapoli *et al.* 1993; Feun *et al.* 1990; Hildebrand *et al.* 1994; Leibel *et al.* 1994; Mortimer *et al.* 1992; Rajan *et al.* 1994; Riese *et al.* 1994; Watne *et al.* 1991). This is administered commonly as conventional external beam whole brain radiotherapy, although both brachytherapy and stereotactic radiosurgery techniques have been exploited, with limited success so far (Chamberain *et al.* 1994; Coffey 1993, 1992; Florell *et al.* 1992; Hitchon *et al.* 1992; Kitchen *et al.* 1993; Loeffler *et al.* 1992; Masciopinto *et al.* 1995; Prados *et al.* 1992; Scerrati *et al.* 1993; Shrive *et al.* 1995; Sneed *et al.* 1992; Sofat *et al.* 1992).

In elderly patients, post-operative radiotherapy is likely to extend survival by two to three months and impacts the usual side-effects. This should always be borne in mind when counselling patients' families, who should be given a realistic interpretation of the situation from the outset, as the overall bad prognosis of these tumours does not allow room for wishful thinking. A mean survival of 6–9 months has been observed in elderly patients and 18–24 months in younger adults, following maximal surgery and radiotherapy (Aiken 1994; Ayoubi *et al.* 1993; Sandeman *et al.* 1990).

Management of recurrent malignant gliomas is largely a desperate situation as the prognosis is extremely poor, the treatment options very limited, and the emotional charge amplified by the rapid clinical deterioration. Chemotherapy and radiotherapy offer little practical benefit. Photodynamic therapy has been tried, with limited success. Poor availability and practical difficulties in administration have been prohibitive in its establishment as a valid treatment option. In young patients, there is limited scope for repeat cytoreductive surgery, followed by chemotherapy which has debatable benefit and is not free of side-effects. In older patients it is better to admit defeat as there is no treatment option which can offer any realistic benefit (Berger *et al.* 1992; Buckner *et al.* 1995; Lillehei *et al.* 1991; Merchant *et al.* 1992; Muller and Wilson 1995; Papanastasiou *et al.* 1993; Priestman *et al.* 1993; Strömblad *et al.* 1993).

It appears that the effect of surgery and radiotherapy has been exploited almost to its maximum, and that further radical improvements are likely to come from immunotherapy and genetic engineering (Barba *et al.* 1993; Bender *et al.* 1992; Buckner *et al.* 1995; Chatel *et al.* 1993; Holladay *et al.* 1992;

Jaeckle 1994; Merchant *et al.* 1992; Papanastasiou *et al.* 1993; Priestman *et al.* 1993; Riva *et al.* 1992; Saris *et al.* 1992; Takamiya *et al.* 1993; Yu *et al.* 1993; Watts and Merchant 1992).

Low grade gliomas of the cerebral hemispheres

Although these can present in the same manner as malignant gliomas they more commonly present with epilepsy with little or no additional symptoms. As they are slow growing tumours, symptoms tend to be present for a long time before diagnosis is made and is not uncommon for the patient to be treated by the family doctor alone for a while before appropriate referral is made.

The radiological appearance of low grade gliomas is distinctly different from that of the high grade ones. On CT scanning, they tend to have a diffuse low density appearance, commonly seen in the temporal or posterior frontal lobe. They tend to enhance poorly with intravenous contrast, and for this reason, CT scan is not offering accurate information on the extent of these tumours. In contrast, MRI scan offers more detailed anatomical information, as with T1 and T2 images differentiation can be made between tumour and surrounding white matter oedema (Fig. 14.2). As is evident, MRI scanning would be more appropriate in these tumours, in

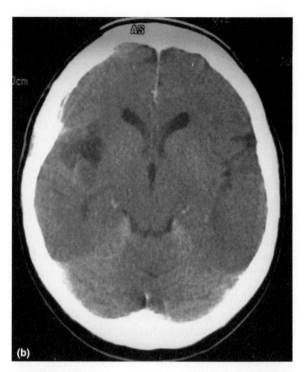

Fig. 14.2(b) Post-operative contrast-enhanced CT scan. Most of the tumour has been removed but there is an area of moderate enhancement in the posteromedial aspect of the resection, indicating possible tumour residuum.

comparison to high grade tumours that can be imaged well with CT scanning. This, in association with an overall better outcome of low grade gliomas, makes the use of costly resources justifiable. This is particularly relevant to hospitals where availability of MRI scanning is limited and priorities should be made.

Conclusive evidence on the best way to manage these tumours is not yet available. Most surgeons would accept, based on the management of low grade gliomas in children, that if total excision of the tumour is possible then it is likely to be curative (Berger *et al.* 1994; Pollack *et al.* 1995; Vecht 1993; Walsh *et al.* 1990; Whitton and Bloom 1990; Zentner *et al.* 1996). In the majority of cases where this is not possible because of unacceptable morbidity then radiotherapy with or without surgical debulking of the tumour has not been shown to be superior than expectant policy, although this mode of treatment is effective in arresting the progress of tumours both radiologically and clinically (Eyre *et al.* 1993; Miralbell *et al.* 1993; Recht *et al.* 1992; Shapiro 1992; Shaw 1990, 1992; Taphoorn *et al.* 1994).

Transformation from low to high grade tumour is well recognized and this should always be borne in mind during follow-up. The overall 5-year survival following total excision and radiotherapy is averaging 45%, falling to 30% after initial biopsy and radiotherapy (Pollack *et al.* 1995; Whitton and Bloom 1990).

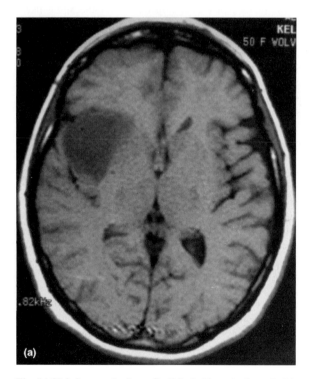

Fig. 14.2(a) Low grade glioma. Radiological investigations of a 51-year-old woman who presented with a 6-month history of complex partial seizures with predominant olfactory aura. (**a**) On T1 weighted MRI scan there is a well-defined low signal lesion in the the right insula and the adjacent opercula. The margins towards the deeply seated thalamus are indistinct.

CEREBRAL METASTASES

Clinical presentation of intracranial metastases is that of an expanding intracranial lesion, with symptoms of raised intracranial pressure, focal neurological deficits according to location, and occasionally fits. Although they usually present as solitary lesions (Fig. 14.3), it is not uncommon to encounter multiple metastases, on either side of the tentorium.

Where the overall condition of the patient is satisfactory to undergo intracranial surgery then resection of solitary intracranial metastases can provide excellent palliative symptom relief when used in conjunction with post-operative radiotherapy. Stereotactic radiosurgery has been tried as an alternative to surgery but has not been proven to be more effective (Bindall *et al.* 1996; Engenhart *et al.* 1993; Flickinger *et al.* 1994; French and Ansman 1977; Raskind *et al.* 1971; Simionescu 1960; Störtenbecker 1954; Veith and Odom 1965).

In cases of multiple cranial or systemic metastases, surgical excision is not considered appropriate. Radiotherapy is considered although the prospect for real benefit is rather poor.

Palliative treatment is adopted instead and in that context, shunting of any coexisting hydrocephalus often results in symptomatic improvement. The overall prognosis is usually determined by the primary tumour, with average survival around 18–24 months following excision of solitary metastases, the exception been metastatic oat cell carcinoma of the lung with a much worse outcome (Bindall *et al.* 1993; Davey *et al.* 1994; Kristensen *et al.* 1992; Wronski *et al.* 1995).

MENINGIOMAS

These represent about 10% of all intracranial tumours in most series. The diagnosis is best made by MRI scan without and with gadolinium enhancement. Characteristic position and morphology of a tumour arising from the meninges makes the diagnosis of meningioma very likely (Fig. 14.4), although they can be radiologically indistinguishable from dural metastases, intracranial haemangiopericytomas, and more rarely, primary cerebral lymphomas and plasmacytomas. In the suprasellar region they need to be distinguished from pituitary tumours and intracranial aneurysms and MRI scanning has made the latter differentiation much easier (Murtagh and Linden 1994; Wasenko *et al.* 1994).

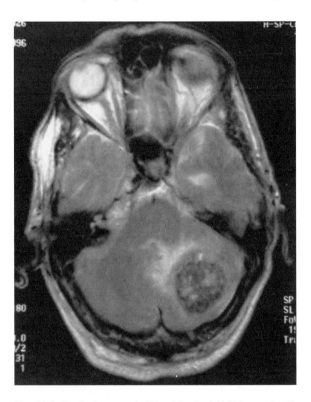

Fig. 14.3 Cerebral metastasis. T2 weighted axial MRI scan of a 69-year-old smoker who presented with a 3-week history of headaches, vomiting, and unsteady gait. On MRI scan there is a mixed density space-occupying lesion in the left cerebellar hemisphere. On his chest radiograph there was a distinct lesion on the base of the right lung. A pre-operative diagnosis of a lung primary tumour with cerebellar metastasis was made and confirmed after excision and histological examination of the posterior fossa lesion.

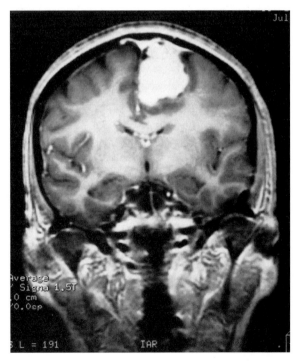

Fig. 14.4 Falx meningioma. Contrast-enhanced T1 weighted coronal MRI scan of a 52-year-old woman who presented with unsteady gait and left leg monoparesis. A brightly enhanced lesion is seen originating from the dura of the falx, growing towards the medial surface of the cerebral hemisphere and causing pressure. This is a typical appearance of a meningioma.

Most meningiomas are benign tumours although so-called atypical, and rarely malignant meningiomas do occur. Recurrence after surgical excision is dependent on the site of the meningioma, the degree of surgical excision, and the histological nature of the tumour. Cortical meningiomas have a lower incidence of recurrence less than 20% in most series compared to basal meningiomas with a recurrence rate of 40–50% (Black 1993; Cantore *et al.* 1994; De Monte 1995; Desai and Bruce 1994; Kinjo *et al.* 1995, Mahmood *et al.* 1994; Mastronardi *et al.* 1995; Miller 1994; Newman 1994; Ojeman 1993; Ransohoff 1994*a*, *b*; Risi *et al.* 1994; Rostomily *et al.* 1994; Rubin *et al.* 1994; Samii *et al.* 1996; Sekhar *et al.* 1994, *et al.* 1994*a*, *b*). Histological classification in benign and atypical or malignant meningiomas is usually made with atypical and malignant meningiomas recurring much more commonly than benign ones (Chamberlain 1996; De Jesús *et al.* 1995; Mahmood *et al.* 1993; Wilson 1994; Younis *et al.* 1995). Benign meningiomas have a recurrence-free rate of about 80% at 25 years in comparison to a recurrence-free rate of just over 50% at 10 years for atypical meningiomas, and a recurrence free-rate of just over 20% in malignant meningiomas at 5 years. Recent attempts to explore the value of radiotherapy and stereotactic radiosurgery in the management of aggressive meningeal tumours has been met so far with limited success (Ganz *et al.* 1993; Lunsford 1993, 1994; Maire *et al.* 1995).

Most meningiomas show slow growth on serial scanning but a small proportion, around 10%, appear to show no growth over many years. A decision to operate is therefore based on the position of the tumour and thus the ease of total excision, symptoms that it is causing, its size, and the general condition of the patient. It is reasonable to offer excision of a small cortical or parasagittal meningioma that is causing minimal symptoms in the expectation of achieving a total excision with low risk of morbidity, whereas a large basal meningioma causing few symptoms may be managed conservatively as total excision is not possible and surgical management would be entirely symptomatic (Gijtenbeek *et al.* 1993; Ide *et al.* 1995; McGrail and Ojemann 1994; Nishizaki *et al.* 1994).

Recent research has discovered that meningiomas exhibit a moderate degree of hormonal dependency owing to the presence of progestogen receptors which has been isolated in tumour tissue. Preliminary work has shown that antiprogestogen treatment may reduce tumour size, but no clinical application of this treatment has been established as yet (Grunberg 1994; Olsok 1994; Rubinstein *et al.* 1994).

PITUITARY TUMOURS

Although, as with all other intracranial tumours, the advent of CT and MRI scanning has substantially improved our ability to diagnose these tumours when they are still small (Grigsby 1993; Stadnik *et al.* 1994; Steiner *et al.* 1994; Wen and Loeffler 1995) the commonest mode of presentation to most neurosurgeons is with symptoms of chiasmal compression (Fig. 14.5) (Andrews 1994; Hennessy and Jackson 1995; Levy and

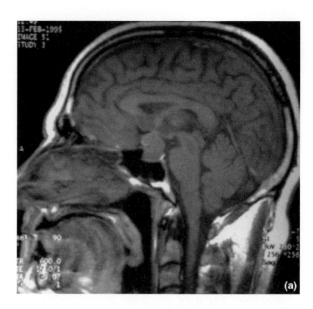

Fig. 14.5(a) Pituitary tumour. T1 weighted images of a patient who presented with a 5-month history of progressive bitemporal hemianopia. **(a)** Sagittal view: a pituitary tumour is seen, having grown outwith the pituitary fossa, towards the floor of the third ventricle. The contour of the tumour has an hourglass shape, the waist constriction been due to the diaphragm sellae.

Lightman 1994). The classical visual field deficit of bitemporal hemianopia occurs in about 60% of cases, but all visual field deficits are possible and homonymous hemianopia due to optic tract compression or monocular visual loss due to isol-

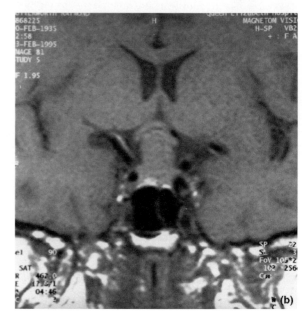

Fig. 14.5(b) Coronal view: the supracellar component has grown superiorly and is deforming the optic chiasm. It is easy to understand how this patient has developed bitemporal hemianopia.

ated optic nerve compression occur in a significant minority of cases (Jeffreys 1989; Laws *et al.* 1977).

Prolactinomas represent approximately 40% of pituitary tumours in most large series and so the syndrome of hyperprolactinaemia is by far the commonest endocrinological presentation. In women of childbearing age, commonly the only symptom is secondary amenorrhoea, but gynaecomastia or galactorrhoea can also occur. In males, hyperprolactinaemia leads to loss of libido and impotence due to suppression of production of testosterone, although this is rarely a presenting symptom. The first line of treatment for prolactinomas is dopamine agonist therapy, and complete resolution or dramatic reduction in the size of the tumour associated with normalization of prolactin levels can be expected in the majority of cases (Adams and Burke 1993; Barrow *et al.* 1984; Ferrari *et al.* 1992; Jaquet 1993; Jaspers *et al.* 1994; Jones 1995; Mbanya *et al.* 1993; McCutcheon 1994; Melis *et al.* 1989; Serri *et al.* 1994; Soule and Jacobs 1995). Elevated prolactin levels as a result of pituitary stalk compression by non-prolactinomas can lead to the elevation of prolactin levels to 5 times of the upper limit of normal, and values of up to 10 times the upper limit of normal are well described. The levels of prolactin will suppress with dopamine agonist therapy in these cases, but will not be associated with any reduction in tumour size. A small number of patients will not be able to tolerate dopamine agonist therapy and surgical removal of the tumour can be considered (Kovacs *et al.* 1995; Thomson *et al.* 1994). A small number of prolactinomas will be only partially responsive to dopamine agonist therapy and require surgical debulking (Soule *et al.* 1994, 1996), especially if there is a significant cystic component.

Growth hormone-secreting tumours represent about 10% of pituitary tumours. Those occurring before puberty and presenting with pituitary gigantism are rare, they usually present in middle decades of life although a small percentage can present in old age (Puchner *et al.* 1995). The clinical syndrome of acromegaly, with increase in the size of hands and feet, change in facial appearance, as well as hyperhydrosis, symptoms of carpal tunnel compression, and arthralgia (Yamada *et al.* 1993). Diabetes mellitus occurs in up to 30% of cases. Diagnosis is made by the failure of suppression of GH (growth hormone) levels in the blood across a glucose tolerance test. There is, however, no correlation between the degree of elevation of GH or insulin-like growth factor 1 (IGF1) and the clinical syndrome. Acromegaly leads to an approximate doubling in the risk of mortality (Bates *et al.* 1993) by increasing the risk of cardiovascular disease. Transphenoidal surgery will lead to endocrinological cure in almost all microadenomas (Davies *et al.* 1993; Laws and Thapar 1995; Long *et al.* 1996; Osman *et al.* 1994); Surgical cure is defined as a reduction in GH levels to less than 5 µg/1 although symptoms of acromegaly will often improve at higher levels than this. The higher the preoperative elevation of GH and the bigger the size of the tumour, the lower the chances of surgical cure. If GH levels remain elevated following surgery associated with

persisting symptoms of acromegaly, then the use of Octreotide can be considered. With the advent of a longer-acting formulation this therapy may become more widespread. Up to 30% of acromegalic patients have been reported to have a mixed prolactin and GH-secreting tumour (Nyquist *et al.* 1994). These tumours, 73% occurring in females whereas acromegaly overall has an equal occurrence by sex, can respond well to dopamine agonist therapy.

ACTH-secreting pituitary adenomas are rare and represent a progressively lethal disease. They frequently present as microadenomas, with high quality MRI scanning it is increasingly rare to have imaging-negative disease. A recent multicentre review of surgery for these tumours reported clinical and biochemical remission in 76% of cases (Bochicchio *et al.* 1995). Recurrence occurred in 13% of cases in remission, and low post-operative steroid levels and the need of long-term glucocorticoid substitution therapy were associated with a high probability of long-term cure. Similar results have also been reported by other studies (McCance *et al.* 1993; Post *et al.* 1995; Tyrrell and Wilson 1994).

Endocrinologically inactive tumours will present with pituitary failure, or more likely, chiasmal compression. The majority of these tumours are amenable to transphenoidal removal although lateral extension into the middle fossa, the occurrence of the so called 'cottage loaf' tumour and a suprasellar extension greater than 30 mm (Fig. 14.6) make total excision by transphenoidal root very unlikely (Adams and Burke 1993; Arafah *et al.* 1994; Bradley *et al.* 1994; Cooke and Jones 1994; Marazuela *et al.* 1994; Peter and Tribolet 1995; Petruson

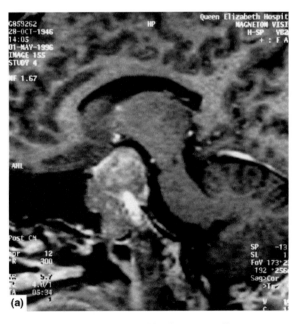

Fig. 14.6(a) Pituitary tumour with a large supracellar component. T1 weighted MRI images of a 49-year-old patient who in the course of 4 years became blind from his pituitary tumour, despite two surgical attempts and a course of radiotherapy: sagittal.

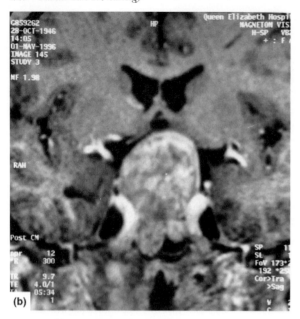

Fig. 14.6(b) coronal. A very large supracellar component of the pituitary tumour has displaced the optic chiasm superiorly, to an extreme.

et al. 1995; Sassolas *et al.* 1993; Vance 1994). The use of post-operative radiotherapy reduces the likelihood of further surgery from 30% to 3% in an unselected population of endocrinologically inactive tumours (Brada *et al.* 1993; Clarke *et al.* 1993; Fisher *et al.* 1993; Ganz *et al.* 1993; Jaffrain-Rea *et al.* 1993; Plowman 1995; Pollock *et al.* 1994; Zierhut *et al.* 1995).

INFRATENTORIAL TUMOURS

ACOUSTIC NEUROMAS

MRI scanning with gadolinium enhancement has revolutionized the diagnosis of small acoustic neuromas (Fig. 14.7). Most acoustic neuromas show progressive increase in size with serial scans but estimates range as high as 25% for those tumours that show no increase in size over many years. Morbidity for surgical excision of acoustic neurinomas relates to their size in terms of preservation of facial nerve function and more recently preservation for useful hearing (Fig. 14.8) (Arriaga *et al.* 1994; Black 1995; Black *et al.* 1995; Esses *et al.* 1994; Irving *et al.* 1995; Lalwani *et al.* 1995; Nutik 1994; Shelton *et al.* 1995; Telian 1994; Torrens *et al.* 1994; Wright and Bradford 1995). Haines and co-workers have reported preservation of useful hearing in 80% of intracanalicular tumours although results of this nature cannot be anticipated in most surgeons' hands (Haines and Levine 1993). Stereotactic radiosurgery has increasingly been advocated in the management of these tumours with stabilization or reduction in the size of tumours in all cases and preservation of hearing in

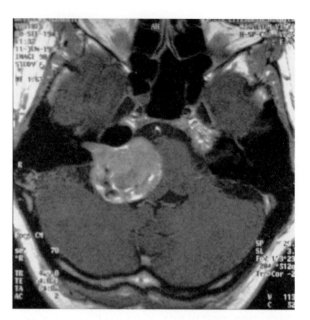

Fig. 14.7 Acoustic neuroma. T1 weighted contrast-enhanced MRI scan of a 53-year-old woman who presented with right-sided deafness and gait ataxia. A sizeable enhancing high signal tumour is seen on the VIIIth nerve complex, extending into the internal acoustic meatus.

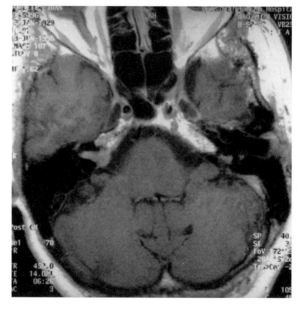

Fig. 14.8 Acoustic neuroma, intracanalicular. T1 weighted MRI scan of a 32-year-old woman who presented with a 4-month history of tinnitus and difficulty in understanding telephone communication, and she uses her right ear. A small lesion of 1-cm diameter is seen inside the dilated right internal accoustic meatus, on the VIIIth nerve complex. (Hearing preservation during surgery for a small intracanalicular acoustic neuroma has recently become an important issue.)

45% of tumours less than 3 cm in size at 2 years (Forster *et al.* 1996; Ogurinde *et al.* 1995).

BRAINSTEM GLIOMAS

Since the introduction of MRI scanning the knowledge on brainstem gliomas has improved dramatically. We now recognize certain discrete clinical patterns which have different biological profile and outcome: the diffuse tumours, the well-circumscribed tumours extending from the medulla to the pons, the dorsal exophytic medullary tumours, and the cervicomedullary tumours.

Patients with brainstem tumours present with lower cranial nerve sings, bulbar palsy, and long tract sings, these findings varying according to the exact location of the tumour. As for astrocytomas in other parts of the central nervous system, these tumours can be of low or high histological grade, the latter ones having very poor prognosis. The diffuse tumours have distinct radiological features. Diffuse mass usually in the centre of the brainstem, with indistinct margins, with variable contrast enhancement and occasionally areas of mixed density, indicating intratumoral necrosis (Fig. 14.9). They tend to be of high grade which makes the prognosis invariably poor, despite maximal treatment. Traditional management was that of biopsy, either open or commonly stereotactic, followed by radiotherapy. Commonly, radiotherapy is administered in the conventional overlapping-fields method, although stereotactic radiosurgery is claimed to offer similar good results (Guiney *et al.* 1993; Hirato *et al.* 1995; Linstadt *et al.* 1991; Packer *et al.* 1992; Shrieve *et al.* 1992). It is clear that surgery offers very little to these patients and in view of the characteristic radiological appearances, there has been a tendency in recent years to avoid biopsy and the associated morbidity, and offer radiotherapy relying on the radiological diagnosis (Albright *et al.* 1993; Epstein and McCleary 1986). Views differ on this issue as it is well documented that in up to 15% of the cases, biopsy of a brainstem lesion can produce an unexpected diagnosis, although this tends to apply to more circumscribed lesions (Kratimenos and Thomas 1993; Packer *et al.* 1991–2; Rajshekhar and Chandy 1995). An overall 5-year survival of 20% has been reported (Guiney *et al.* 1993; Packer *et al.* 1992).

The other varieties of brainstem tumours can be helped more by surgery. They are more often encountered in children and young adults and tend to be of low histological grade. With the help of the cavitron ultrasonic aspirator and the operating microscope, the dorsal exophytic tumours can be reduced in size substantially. The exophytic component can be resected safely, which improves both the symptoms and the overall outcome (Pollack *et al.* 1993; Takasato *et al.* 1993). In the case of pontomedullary and cervicomedullary tumours, surgical expectations tend to be modest. The tumour can be approached from an area where it comes close to the dorsal surface of the medulla and moderate reduction in size can be achieved (Langmoen *et al.* 1991; Packer *et al.* 1991–2, 1992; Robertson *et al.* 1994). Considerable morbidity can be

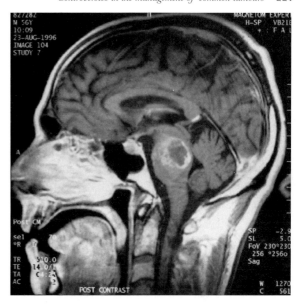

Fig. 14.9 Brainstem glioma, diffuse. Contrast-enhanced T1 weighted sagittal MRI scan of a 49-year-old man with a 3-week history of headaches and gait ataxia. A mixed density enhancing lesion is seen in the pons. Indistinct margins and infiltration of surrounding structures indicate the malignant nature of this tumour.

caused and this tends to moderate surgical enthusiasm. The presence of a tumour cyst (Fig. 14.10) occasionally facilitates surgical excision. Decompression of the cyst usually results in symptomatic improvement. The role of post-operative radiotherapy is controversial. In view of the low histological grade they are moderately responsive to radiotherapy. For this reason there has been a trend to reserve radiotherapy for later tumour progression following initial surgery (Hibi *et al.* 1992; Kretschmar *et al.* 1993; Packer *et al.* 1994; Wakabayashi *et al.* 1992). An overall 5-year survival of 40% has been reported (Hibi *et al.* 1992; Mulhern *et al.* 1994; Packer *et al.* 1992, 1994; Pollack *et al.* 1993).

EPENDYMOMAS

These are tumours arising from cells of the ependymal lining, found in the walls of the ventricular system. Commonly seen in the fourth ventricle (Fig. 14.11), are also seen less frequently in relation to the third and lateral ventricles. Less frequently they are found in the supratentorial compartment as well, usually in relation to the ventricular system, although they can present as lobar tumours (Furie and Provenzale 1995; Tortori-Donati *et al.* 1995). Infratentorial ependymomas are commoner in childhood whereas supratentorial ependymomas are commoner in adults. Mode of presentation is similar to any other mass lesion in similar location. In the posterior fossa in adult patients, there are commoner than other midline lesions. Surgical excision is mandatory, as the raised intracranial pressure and the obstructive hydrocephalus would

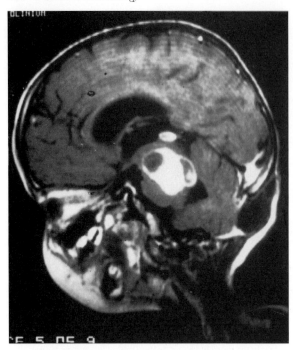

Fig. 14.10 Brainstem glioma, cystic. Contrast-enhanced T1 weighted sagittal MRI scan of a 3-year-old boy who presented with a 4-month history of gait unsteadiness. An enhancing lesion is seen at the pons. The margins are well demarcated and there is a cyst in the middle of the tumour. These are features of a low grade pontine glioma.

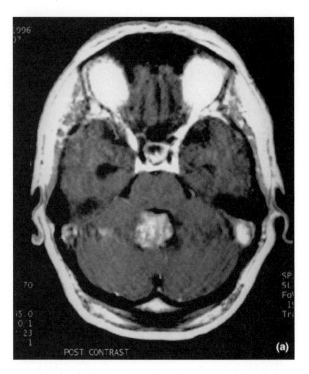

Fig. 14.11(a) Ependymoma of the fourth ventricle. T1 weighted axial MRI scans of a 49-year-old man who presented with a 3-week history of headaches, vomiting, and unsteady gait. Preoperative study. A mixed-density midline cerebellar lesion is seen, spreading into the fourth ventricle.

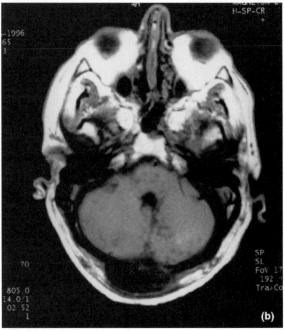

Fig. 14.11(b) Post-operative study. Through a posterior fossa craniectomy the lesion has been removed completely, and there is no evidence of residual tumour.

otherwise cause rapid clinical deterioration. In the posterior fossa it is common to achieve total macroscopic surgical removal, through a posterior fossa craniectomy, although adherence to the floor of the fourth ventricle is not uncommon and may result in subtotal removal. In the supratentorial compartment they tend to lie in relation to the lateral ventricles, which makes surgical removal feasible.

Ependymomas have a known tendency to spread through the subarachnoid pathways. During surgery, cerebrospinal fluid is obtained and examined for the presence of malignant cells. In the early post-operative period, whole neuraxis MRI scan is obtained, to detect the presence of satellite lesions in the spine. This will influence radiotherapy planning.

Following successful recovery from surgery, whole neuraxis irradiation is usually administered, with booster doses at the tumour site and at other possible sites of satellite lesions. In children younger than three years, where radiotherapy is contraindicated, there has been a tendency to consider aggressive chemotherapy, with modest results so far (Evans *et al.* 1996).

Outcome depends on age, site, and histological signs of malignancy. In adults, following surgery and radiotherapy a 5-year survival of 50% should be expected in the absence of malignant histological features, which falls to 20% in the presence of histological features, such as mitoses, endovascular proliferation, necrosis, and invasion of the surrounding brain. In infratentorial tumours of childhood a 40% 5-year survival should be expected in the absence of malignant features (Chiu *et al.* 1992; Ferrante *et al.* 1994; Jayawickreme *et al.* 1995; Kovalic *et al.* 1993; Palma *et al.* 1993; Pollack *et al.* 1995; Rousseau *et al.* 1994; Vanuytsel *et al.* 1992).

II. Spinal Tumours

SPINAL ASTROCYTOMAS

These are commonly seen in childhood, where they tend to be of low histological grade, in contrast to adults where high grade tumours are encountered more often. As with many other spinal space-occupying lesions, they present with spinal pain and progressive neurological deficit, relevant to the level of the lesion. In the pre-MRI era radiological diagnosis was often difficult and inconclusive as the sensitivity of CT myelography was poor. This had an inevitable negative influence on the surgical management of these tumours. The advent of MRI improved the diagnostic rate of intramedullary tumours and changed the previously negative attitude of neurosurgeons towards them. The typical MRI appearance is that of increased signal following gadolinium injection in a swollen enlarged spinal cord (Fig. 14.12). Good demarcation from the surrounding normal spinal cord tends to imply low histological grade. In contrast, radiological evidence of invasion and mixed signal indicating necrosis in the centre of the tumour, point towards a high grade lesion. Often in low grade gliomas there is a discrete cyst in the tumour centre, which proves helpful during surgery in locating the tumour with the help of per-operative ultrasound. Occasionally, syringomyelia cavities are seen on either side of the tumour (Samii and Klekamp 1994). These are not specific to astrocytomas, but are encountered in association to a variety of spinal tumours that cause obstruction of cerebrospinal fluid flow in the subarachnoid space.

Low grade lesions tend to be symptomatic for longer periods before diagnosis, with gradually evolving neurological deficits, due to the slow growth rate. In contrast, high grade tumours exhibit a more rapid evolution which results usually in severe neurological disabilities over shorter time periods. Their biological behaviour is not too different to cerebral gliomas, and similar considerations apply to management issues.

Commonly, the first treatment of a patient with a spinal intramedullary tumour is some form of surgery. The radiological appearance will heavily influence the surgeon's decision on the type of surgery. It is now well established that patients with high grade spinal astrocytomas do not benefit from radical aggressive surgical resection (Brotchi *et al.* 1992; Cristante and Herrmann 1994; Huddart *et al.* 1993). The outcome of these patients is invariably poor and aggressive surgery generates substantial morbidity without improving survival. For this reason there has been in recent years a move away from rad-

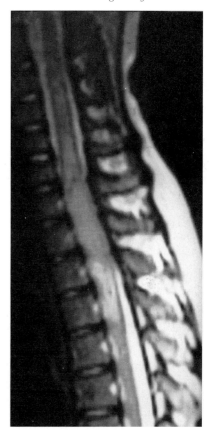

Fig. 14.12 Spinal astrocytoma. Contrast-enhanced T2 weighted sagittal MRI scan of a 23-year-old male who presented with a 4-month history of progressive leg weakness and muscle wasting. A high signal enhancing intramedullary lesion is seen in the upper thoracic region. At certain areas the transition between tumour and normal spinal cord become indistinct. Syringomyelic cavities are seen above and below the tumour.

ical excision of spinal tumours which radiologically and during operation have appearances of high grade astrocytoma. Following limited resective surgery, all these patients are receiving radiotherapy. A 5-year survival of 20% has been reported following this management (Epstein *et al.* 1992; Huddart *et al.* 1993; Hulshof *et al.* 1993; Minehan *et al.* 1995; Sandler *et al.* 1992; Shirato *et al.* 1995; Stein and McCormick 1992).

The situation is slightly different with low grade spinal astrocytomas. Tumours with typical radiological appearances of low grade glioma are favourable surgical propositions. A high rate of complete excision has been reported, and the use of the operative microscope and the ultrasonic surgical aspirator have substantially improved the chances of total macroscopic excision with little additional morbidity (Brotchi *et al.* 1992; Cristante and Herrmann 1994; Lunardi *et al.* 1993; Steinbok *et al.* 1992). The use of per-operative electrophysiological monitoring is said to minimize operative morbidity while offering to the surgeon a level of confidence, however, this is not a universally accepted view (Kearse *et al.* 1993; Koyanagi *et al.* 1993; Wagner *et al.* 1994).

The need for post-operative radiotherapy has not yet been resolved. Several studies have shown that the long-term outcome of completely excised low grade astrocytomas is very good and likely not to be improved any further with radiotherapy. A 5-year survival rate of 80% has been reported with surgery alone. In recent years there has been an increasing tendency to reserve radiotherapy for cases of recurrent tumour growth, following repeat surgical excision (Hulshof *et al.* 1993; Lunardi *et al.* 1993; O'Sullivan *et al.* 1994; Sandler *et al.* 1992; Shirato *et al.* 1995; Steinbok *et al.* 1992).

Special operative considerations apply to children with spinal tumours, relating to progressive spinal deformity following laminectomy. Laminotomy with replacement of the laminae at the end of the procedure tends to be associated with a smaller incidence of such problems (Abbott *et al.* 1992). The coexistence of neurological deficits inevitably tends to complicate spinal growth even further. A high rate of secondary scoliosis is observed in these children, imposing a further burden on their rehabilitation.

SPINAL EPENDYMOMAS

These are slow growing tumours and are considered of benign biological behaviour. They tend to be found in the third to fourth decade of life, and a common presenting symptom is that of chronic low back pain. There is a well-recognized clinical picture of a patient who has had orthopaedic treatment for chronic low back pain for years, and now is presenting with slowly progressing neurological deficit. In view of the chronicity of the symptoms, the new neurological deficits (e.g. loss of bladder control) occasionally are not appreciated properly, delaying diagnosis and adding more embarrassment to the whole situation. Neurological deficits will depend on the site of the tumour, as for any other spinal tumour. Cervical and upper thoracic lesions will cause spastic quadri- or paraparesis, respectively, to varying degrees. Cauda equina lesions will cause bladder, bowel, and sexual dysfunction and to variable degree loss of sensation in the distal leg dermatomes and distal leg weakness.

Radiologically, they appear as a well-defined contrast-enhancing high signal mass on MRI scanning (Fig. 14.13) (Fine *et al.* 1995). It is worth noting that in view of their slow growth they tend to cause changes in the vertebral bodies, usually appearing as scalloping of the posterior aspect, and clearly appreciated on plain spinal radiographs taken during investigation of chronic low back pain. There is a documented tendency for cerebrospinal fluid dissemination, but at much less frequency in comparison to intracranial ependymomas.

As with other spinal tumours, the introduction of the operating microscope and microinstruments, the use of the ultrasonic aspirator and better radiological imaging have

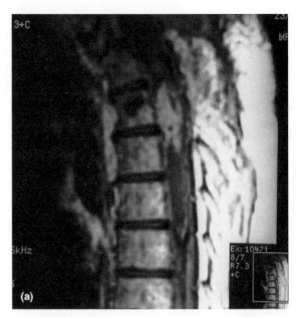

Fig. 14.13(a) Spinal ependymoma. Contrast-enhanced T1 weighted sagittal MRI scans of a 49-year-old man who presented with a 3-month history of progressive leg weakness. There is a well-defined high signal intramedullary lesion in the upper thoracic region of the spinal cord. The lesion is well demarcated from the surrounding normal spinal cord. (a) sagittal (b) axial

improved both functional outcome following surgery, as well as enhanced the likelihood of total or near total excision (Cooper 1985; Epstein *et al.* 1993; Fischer and Mansuy 1980; Garrido and Stein 1977; Guidetti *et al.* 1981; Sgouros *et al.* 1996).

Surgical excision is regarded as the primary treatment modality. Biopsy only, followed by radiotherapy is associated with very poor results. Today, it is very rare to declare a tumour inoperable.

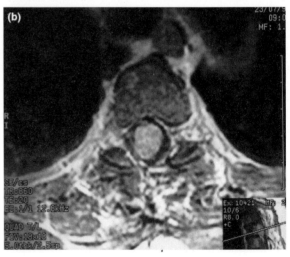

Fig. 14.13(b) axial.

An overall good long-term outcome is invariably reported, in contrast with its intracranial counterpart, which has much more aggressive biological behaviour. (Barone and Elvidge 1970; Mørk and Løken 1977; Rawlings *et al.* 1988). The cauda equina tumours have a better outcome than the intramedullary ones. An overall 5-year survival of over 80% should be expected following successful surgical excision. Subtotal excision carries only a slightly worse prognosis (Barone and Elvidge 1970; Epstein *et al.* 1993; Guidetti *et al.* 1981; Shaw *et al.* 1986; Shirato *et al.* 1995; Sgouros *et al.* 1996), and is associated with increased rate of disease progression (Cervoni *et al.* 1994; Clover *et al.* 1993; Linstadt *et al.* 1989; Sonneland *et al.* 1985; Waldron *et al.* 1993), but prolonged survival following treatment is well documented (Cooper 1989; Linstadt *et al.* 1989; Rawlings *et al.* 1988; Sgouros *et al.* 1996; Whitaker *et al.* 1991). In all circumstances age seems to have an effect, with patients under 40 years of age having a better outcome (Sgouros *et al.* 1996; Whitaker *et al.* 1991). It is of interest that histological features have little prognostic value in these tumours (Fokes and Earle 1969; Guidetti *et al.* 1981; Ross and Rubinstein 1989; Shaw *et al.* 1986; Sonneland *et al.* 1985).

Total excision is feasible for the well-circumscribed tumours (Cooper 1989; Cooper and Epstein 1985; Cristante and Hermann 1994; Fischer and Mansuy 1980; Garrido and Stein 1977; Morantz *et al.* 1979; Mørk and Løken 1977; Rawlings *et al.* 1988; Schweitzer and Batzdorf 1992; Sgouros *et al.* 1996). In the absence of disseminated tumour nodules in the central nervous system, following complete excision, the risk of recurrence is very low, obviating the need for additional irradiation (Cooper 1989; Schweitzer and Batzdorf 1992; Sgouros *et al.* 1996; Sonneland *et al.* 1985). There are situations where there is obvious macroscopic invasion of normal spinal cord, with indistinct transition margins, dictating subtotal excision. There is as yet no consensus on the management of such incompletely excised tumours (Cervoni *et al.* 1994; Cooper 1989; Cooper *et al.* 1985, Cristante and Hermann 1994; Di Marco *et al.* 1988; Fearnside and Adams 1978; Ferrante *et al.* 1992; Guidetti *et al.* 1981; Linstadt *et al.* 1989; Marks and Adles 1982; Mørk and Løken 1977; Peschel *et al.* 1983; Rawlings *et al.* 1988; Schweitzer and Batzdorg 1992; Sgouros *et al.* 1996; Shaw *et al.* 1986; Sonneland *et al.* 1985; Waldron *et al.* 1993; Whitaker *et al.* 1991). Traditionally, radiotherapy has been employed post-operatively for such tumours to discourage tumour progression (Barone and Elvidge 1970; Cervoni *et al.* 1994; Cooper 1989; Di Marco *et al.* 1988; Fearnside and Adams 1978; Linstadt *et al.* 1989; Marks and Adler 1982; Peschel *et al.* 1983; Schweitzer *et al.* 1992; Shaw *et al.* 1986; Sonneland *et al.* 1985; Waldron *et al.* 1993; Whitaker *et al.* 1991). However, in recent years this has been increasingly questioned. It has been argued that radiotherapy does increase the disease-free interval but without reducing the overall risk of disease progression and without improving the overall survival (Sgouros *et al.* 1996). Although many centres still administer radiotherapy routinely to such patients, a

conservative expectant approach with repeat MRI scanning, and consideration of further surgery in case of tumour progression would be justified. In case of recurrence following previous total excision, further surgery would be appropriate.

REFERENCES

Surgical techniques

Alexander E III, Kooy HM, van Herk M, Schwartz M, Barnes PD, Tarbell N. *et al.* Magnetic resonance image-directed stereotactic neurosurgery: use of image fusion with computerized tomography to enhance spatial accuracy. *J Neurosurg* **83**: 271–6, 1995.

Hammoud MA, Ligon BL, ElSouki R, Shi WM, Schomer DF, Sawaya R. Use of intraoperative ultrasound for localizing tumors and determining the extent of resection: a comparative study with magnetic resonance imaging. *J Neurosurg* **84**: 737–41, 1996.

Hitchcock ER, Issa AM, Sotelo MG. Stereotactic excision of deeply seated intracranial mass lesions. *Br J Neurosurg* **3**: 313–20, 1989.

Kelly PJ. Stereotactic biopsy and resection of thalamic astrocytomas. *Neurosurgery* **25**: 185–95, 1989.

Kelly PJ, Alker GJ Jr, Kall BA. *et al*: Method of computed tomography-based stereotactic biopsy with arteriographic control. *Neurosurgery* **14**: 172–7, 1984*a*.

Kelly PJ, Kall BA, Goerss S. Transposition of volumetric information derived from computed tomography scanning into stereotactic space. *Surg Neurol* **21**: 465–71, 1984*b*.

Ryan MJ, Erickson RK, Levin DN, Pelizzari CA, Macdonald RL, Dohrmann GJ. Frameless stereotaxy with real-time tracking of patient head movement and retrospective patient–image registration. *J Neurosurg* **85**: 287–92, 1996.

Weiner H, Kelly PJ. A novel computer-assisted volumatric stereotactic approach for resecting tumors of the posterior parahippocampal gyrus. *J Neurosurg* **85**: 272–7, 1996.

Malignant glioma

Aiken RD. Quality-of-life issues in patients with malignant gliomas. *Seminars in Oncology* **21**: 273–5, 1994.

Arcicasa M, Roncadin M, Bortolus R, Bassignano G, Boz G, Franchin G. *et al.* Results of three consecutive combined treatments for malignant gliomas. Ten-year experience at a single institution. *Am J Clin Oncol* **17**: 437–43, 1994.

Ayoubi S, Walter PH, Naik S, Sankaran M, Robinson D. Audit in the management of gliomas. *Br J Neurosurg* **7**: 61–9, 1993.

Barba D, Hardin J, Ray J, Gage FH. Thymidine kinase-mediated killing of rat brain tumors. *J Neurosurg* **79**: 729–35, 1993.

Barker II FG, Prados MD, Chang SM, Gutin PH, Lamborn KR, Larson DA. *et al.* Radiation response and survival time in patients with glioblastoma multiforme. *J Neurosurg* **84**: 442–8, 1996.

Bender H, Takahashi H, Adachi K, Belser P, Liang SH, Prewett M. *et al.* Immunotherapy of human glioma xenografts with unlabeled, 1311-, or 1251-labeled monoclonal antibody 425 to epidermal growth factor receptor. *Cancer Res* **52**: 121–6, 1992.

Berger MS, Tucker A, Spence A, Winn HR. Reoperation for glioma. *Clin Neurosurg* **39**: 172–86, 1992.

Buckner JC, Brown LD, Kugler JW, Cascino TL, Krook JE, Mailliard JA. Kardinal *et al.* Phase II evaluation of recombinant interferon alpha and BCNU in recurrent glioma. *J Neurosurg* **82**: 430–5, 1995.

Chamberlain MC, Barba D, Kormanik P, Shea WM. Stereotactic radiosurgery for recurrent gliomas. *Cancer* **74**: 1342–7, 1994.

Chatel M, Lebrun C, Frenay M. Chemotherapy and immunotherapy in adult malignant gliomas. *Curr Opin Oncol* **5**: 464–73, 1993.

Coffey RJ. Boost Gamma Knife radiosurgery in the treatment of primary glial tumors. *Stereotact Funct Neurosurg* **61**(suppl.): 59–64, 1993.

Coffey RJ, Lunsford LD, Flickinger JC. The role of radiosurgery in the treatment of malignant brain tumors. *Neurosurg Clin N Am* **3**: 231–44, 1992.

Curran WJ Jr, Scott CB, Weinstein AS, Martin LA, Nelson JS, Phillips TL, Murray K. *et al.* Survival comparison of radiosurgery—eligible and—ineligible malignant glioma patients treated with hyperfractionated radiation therapy and carmustine: a report of Radiation Therapy Oncology Group 83–92. *J Clin Oncol* **11**: 857–62, 1993.

Devaux BC, O'Fallon JR, Kelly PJ. Resection, biopsy, and survival in malignant glial neoplasms. A retrospective study of clinical parameters, therapy, and outcome. *J Neurosurg* **78**: 767–75, 1993.

Dinapoli RP, Brown LD, Arusell RM, Earle JD, O'Fallon JR, Buckner JC. *et al.* Phase III comparative evaluation of PCNU and carmustin combined with radiation therapy for high-grade glioma. *J Clin Oncol* **11**: 1316–21, 1993.

Feun LG, Maor M, Stewart DJ, Leavens ME, Savaraj N, Bodey GP. Pilot study of PCNU and cranial radiation therapy in the treatment of patients with malignant gliomas. *Oncology* **47**: 389–92, 1990.

Florell RC, Macdonald DR, Irish WD, Bernstein M, Leibel SA, Gutin PH. *et al.* Selection bias, survival, and brachytherapy for glioma. *J Neurosurg* **76**: 179–83, 1992.

Ganju V, Jenkins RB, O'Fallon JR, Scheithauer BW, Ransom DT, Katzmann JA. *et al.* Prognostic factors in gliomas. A multivariate analysis of clinical, pathologic, flow cytometric, cytogenetic, and molecular markers. *Cancer* **74**: 920–7, 1994.

Guha A. Tumor suppressor genes in human astrocytomas. In Black PMcL, Schoene WC, Lampson LA (ed.), *Astrocytomas: diagnosis, treatment, and biology.* Blackwell, Boston. pp. 228–40, 1993.

Helseth A. The incidence of primary central nervous system neoplasms before and after computerized tomography availability. *J Neurosurg* **83**: 999–1003, 1995.

Hildebrand J, Sahmoud T, Mignolet F, Brucher JM, Afra D. Adjuvant therapy with dibromodulcitol and BCNU increases survival of adults with malignant gliomas. EORTC Brain Tumor Group. *Neurology* **44**: 1479–83, 1994.

Hitchon PW, VanGilder JC, Wen BC, Jani S. Brachytherapy for malignant recurrent and untreated gliomas. *Stereotact Funct Neurosurg* **59**: 174–8, 1992.

Holladay FP, Heitz T, Chen YL, Chiga M, Wood GW. Successful treatment of a malignant rat glioma with cytotoxic T lymphocytes. *Neurosurgery* **31**: 528–33, 1992.

Jaeckle KA. Immunotherapy of malignant gliomas. *Seminars in Oncology* **21**: 249–59, 1994.

Jen J, Harper JW, Bigner SH, Bigner DD, Papadopoulos N, Markowitz S. *et al.* Deletion of p16 and p15 genes in brain tumors. *Cancer Research* **54**: 6353–8, 1994.

Jolesz FA, Schwartz RB, Guttmann CRG. Diagnostic imaging of intracranial gliomas. In Black PMcL, Schoene WC, Lampson LA (ed.), *Astrocytomas: diagnosis, treatment, and biology.* Blackwell, Boston. pp. 37–49. 1993.

Kallio M. Therapy and survival of adult patients with intracranial glioma in a defined population. *Acta Neurol Scand* **81**: 541–9, 1990.

Kallio M, Sankila R, Jaaskelainen J, Karjalainen S, Hakulinen T. A population-based study on the incidence and survival rates of 3857 glioma patients diagnosed from 1953 to 1984. *Cancer* **68**: 1394–400, 1991.

Kelly PJ. Stereotactic resection and its limitations in glial neoplasms. *Stereotact Funct Neurosurg* **59**: 84–91, 1992.

Kitchen ND, Hughes SW, Taub NA, Sofat A, Beaney RP, Thomas DG. Survival following interstitial brachytherapy for recurrent malignant glioma. *J Neuro-Oncology* **18**: 33–9, 1993.

Kleinberg L, Wallner K, Malkin MG. Good performance status of long-term disease-free survivors of intracranial gliomas. *Int J Radiat Oncol Biol Phys* **26**: 129–33, 1993.

Leibel SA, Scott CB, Loeffler JS. Contemporary approaches to the treatment of malignant gliomas with radiation therapy. *Seminars in Oncology* **21**: 198–219, 1994.

Lillehei KO, Mitchell DH, Johnson SD, McCleary EL, Kruse CA. Long-term follow-up of patients with recurrent malignant gliomas treated with adjuvant adoptive immunotherapy. *Neurosurgery* **28**: 16–23, 1991.

Loeffler JS, Alexander E III, Shea WM, Wen PY, Fine HA, Kooy HM. *et al.* Radiosurgery as part of the initial management of patients with malignant gliomas. *J Clin Oncol* **10**: 1379–85, 1992.

Masciopinto JE, Levin AB, Mehta MP, Rhode BS. Stereotactic radiosurgery for glioblastoma: a final report of 31 patients. *J Neurosurg* **82**: 530–5, 1995.

Merchant RE, McVicar DW, Merchant LH, Young HF. Treatment of recurrent malignant glioma by repeated intracerebral injections of human recombinant interleukin-2 alone or in combination with systemic interferon-alpha. Results of a phase I clinical trial. *J Neuro-Oncology* **12**: 75–83, 1992.

Mortimer JE, Crowley J, Eyre H, Weiden P, Eltringham J, Stuckey WJ. A phase II randomized study comparing sequential and combined intraarterial cisplatin and radiation therapy in primary brain tumors. A Southwest Oncology Group study. *Cancer* **69**: 1220–3, 1992.

Muller PJ, Wilson BC. Photodynamic therapy for recurrent supratentorial gliomas. *Seminars in Surgical Oncology* **11**: 346–54, 1995.

Papanastassiou V, Pizer BL, Coakham HB, Bullimore J, Zananiri T, Kemshead JT. Treatment of recurrent and cystic malignant gliomas by a single intracavity injection of 1311 monoclonal antibody: feasibility, pharmacokinetics and dosimetry. *Br J Cancer* **67**: 144–51, 1993.

Peschel RE, Wilson L, Haffty B, Papadopoulos D, Rosenzweig K, Feltes M. The effect of advanced age on the efficacy of radiation therapy for early breast cancer, local prostate cancer and grade III-IV gliomas. *Int J Radiat Oncol Biol Phys* **26**: 539–44, 1993.

Prados MD, Gutin PH, Phillips TL, Wara WM, Sneed PK, Larson DA. *et al.* Interstitial brachytherapy for newly diagnosed patients with malignant gliomas: the UCSF experience. *Int J Radiat Oncol Biol Phys* **24**: 593–7, 1992.

Priestman TJ, Bleehen NM, Rampling R, Stenning S, Nethersell AJ, Scott J. A phase II evaluation of human lymphoblastoid interferon (Wellferon) in relapsed high grade malignant glioma. Medical Research Council Brain Tumour Working Party. *Clin Oncol* **5**: 165–8, 1993.

Quigley MR, Maroon JC. The relationship between survival and the extent of the resection in patients with supratentorial malignant gliomas. *Neurosurgery* **29**: 385–8, 1991.

Rajan B, Pickuth D, Ashley S, Traish D, Monro P, Elyan S, Brada M. The management of histologically unverified presumed cerebral gliomas with radiotherapy. *Int J Radiat Oncol Biol Phys* **28**: 405–13, 1994.

Riese NE, Loeffler JS, Wen P, Alexander E III, Black PM, Coleman CN. A phase I study of etanidazole and radiotherapy in malignant glioma. *Int J Radiat Oncol Biol Phys* **29**: 617–20, 1994.

Riva P, Arista A, Sturiale C, Moscatelli G, Tison V, Mariani M. *et al.* Treatment of intracranial human glioblastoma by direct intratumoral administration of 131I-labelled anti-tenascin monoclonal antibody BC-2. *Int J Cancer* **51**: 7–13, 1992.

Sandeman DR, Sandeman AP, Buxton P, Hughes HH, Chadwick

DW, Williams IR. *et al.* The management of patients with an intrinsic supratentorial brain tumour. *Br J Neurosurg* **4**: 299–312, 1990.

Saris SC, Spiess P, Lieberman DM, Lin S, Walbridge S, Oldfield EH. Treatment of murine primary brain tumors with systemic interleukin-2 and tumor-infiltrating lymphocytes. *J Neurosurg* **76**: 513–19, 1992.

Scerrati M, Roselli R, Montemaggi P, Iacoangeli M, Prezioso A, Rossi GF. Interstitial irradiation for newly diagnosed or recurrent malignant gliomas: preliminary results. *Acta Neurochir* **58**(suppl.): 119–22, 1993.

Shrive DC, Alexander III E, Wen PY, Fine HA, Kooy HM, Black PM. *et al.* Comparison of stereotactic radiosurgery and brachytherapy in the treatment of recurrent glioblastoma multiforme. *Neurosurgery* **36**: 275–81, 1995.

Sneed PK, Gutin PH, Prados MD, Phillips TL, Weaver KA, Wara WM. *et al.* Brachytherapy of brain tumors. *Stereotact Funct Neurosurg* **59**: 157–65, 1992.

Sofat A, Hughes S, Briggs J, Beaney RP, Thomas DG. Stereotactic brachytherapy for malignant glioma using a relocatable frame. *Br J Neurosurg* **6**: 543–8, 1992.

Strömblad LG, Anderson H, Malmström P, Salford LG. Reoperation for malignant astrocytomas: personal experience and a review of the literature. *Br J Neurosurg* **7**: 623–33, 1993.

Takamiya Y, Short MP, Moolten FL, Fleet C, Mineta T, Breakefield XO. *et al.* An experimental model of retrovirus gene therapy for malignant brain tumors. *J Neurosurg* **79**: 104–10, 1993.

Yu JS, Wei MX, Chiocca EA, Martuza RL, Tepper RI.: Treatment of glioma by engineered interleukin 4-secreting cells. *Cancer Research* **53**: 3125–8, 1993.

Ullen H, Mattsson B, Collins VP. Long-term survival after malignant glioma. A clinical and histopathological study on the accuracy of the diagnosis in a population-based cancer register. *Acta Oncol* **29**: 875–8, 1990.

Ushio Y. Treatment of gliomas in adults. *Current Opin Oncol* **3**: 467–75, 1991.

Vertosick FT Jr, Selker RG. Long-term survival after the diagnosis of malignant glioma: a series of 22 patients surviving more than 4 years after diagnosis. *Surg Neurol* **38**: 359–63, 1992.

Watne K, Nome O, Hager B, Hirschberg H. Combined intra-arterial chemotherapy and irradiation of malignant gliomas. *Acta Oncol* **30**: 835–41, 1991.

Watts RG, Merchant RE. Cerebrovascular effects and tumor kinetics after a single intratumoral injection of human recombinant interleukin-2 alone or in combination with intravenous chemotherapy in a rat model of glioma. *Neurosurgery* **31**: 89–98, 1992.

Whittle IR, Denholm SW, Gregor A. Management of patients aged over 60 years with supratentorial glioma: lessons from an audit. *Surg Neurol* **36**: 106–11, 1991.

Low grade glioma

Berger MS, Deliganis AV, Dobbins J, Keles GE. The effect of extent of resection on recurrence in patients with low grade cerebral hemisphere gliomas. *Cancer* **74**: 1784–91, 1994.

Eyre HJ, Crowley JJ, Townsend JJ, Eltringham JR, Morantz RA, Schulman SF. *et al.* A randomized trial of radiotherapy versus radiotherapy plus CCNU for incompletely resected low-grade gliomas: a Southwest Oncology Group study. *J Neurosurg* **78**: 909–14, 1993.

Miralbell R, Balart J, Matias-Guiu X, Molet J, Ariza A, Craven-Bartle J. Radiotherapy for supratentorial low-grade gliomas: results and prognostic factors with special focus on tumour volume parameters. *Radiotherapy Oncol* **27**: 112–16, 1993.

Pollack IF, Claassen D, A1-Shboul Q, Janosky JE, Deutsch M. Low-

grade gliomas of the cerebral hemispheres in children: an analysis of 71 cases. *J Neurosurg* **82**: 536–47, 1995.

Recht LD, Lew R, Smith TW. Suspected low-grade glioma: is deferring treatment safe? *Ann Neurol* **31**: 431–6, 1992.

Shapiro WR. Low-grade gliomas: when to treat? *Ann Neurol* **31**: 437–8, 1992.

Shaw EG. Low-grade gliomas: to treat or not to treat? A radiation oncologist's viewpoint. *Arch Neurol* **47**: 1138–40, 1990.

Shaw EG. Role of radiation therapy in the management of low-grade gliomas *Ann Neurol* **32**: 835, 1992.

Taphoorn MJ, Schiphorst AK, Snoek FJ, Lindeboom J, Wolbers JG, Karim AB. *et al.* Cognitive functions and quality of life in patients with low-grade gliomas: the impact of radiotherapy. *Ann Neurol* **36**: 48–54, 1994.

Vecht CJ.: Effect of age on treatment decisions in low-grade glioma. *J Neurol Neurosurg Psychiatry* **56**: 1259–64, 1993.

Walsh AR, Schmidt RH, Marsh HT.: Cortical mapping and resection under local anaesthetic as an aid to surgery of low and intermediate grade gliomas. *Br J Neurosurg* **4**: 485–91, 1990.

Whitton AC, Bloom HJ.: Low grade glioma of the cerebral hemispheres in adults: a retrospective analysis of 88 cases. *Int J Radiat Oncol Biol Phys* **18**: 783–6, 1990.

Zentner J, Meyer B, Stangl A, Schramm J.: Intrinsic tumors of the insula: a prospective surgical study of 30 patients. *J Neurosurg* **85**: 263–271, 1996.

Cerebral metastases

Bindal RK, Sawaya R, Leavens ME, Lee JJ. Surgical treatment of multiple brain metastases. *J Neurosurg* **79**: 210–16, 1993.

Bindal AK, Bindal RK, Hess KR, Shiu A, Hassenbusch SJ, Shi WM. *et al.* Surgery versus radiotherapy in the treatment of brain metastasis. *J Neurosurg* **84**: 748–54, 1996.

Davey P, O'Brien PF, Schwartz ML, Cooper PW. A phase I/II study of salvage radiosurgery in the treatment of recurrent brain metastases. *Br J Neurosurg* **8**: 717–723, 1994.

Engenhart R, Kimmig N, Hover K-H. *et al.* Long-term follow-up for brain metastases treated by percutaneous stereotactic single high-dose irradiation. *Cancer* **71**: 1353–61, 1993.

Flickinger JC, Kondziolka D, Lunsford LD. *et al.* A multi-institutional experience with stereotactic radiosurgery for solitary brain metastasis. *Int J Radiat Oncol Biol Phys* **28**: 797–802, 1994.

French LA., Ausman JI. Metastatic neoplasms to the brain. *Clin Neurosurg* **24**: 41–46, 1977.

Kristensen CA, Kristjansen PEG, Hansen HH. Systemic chemotherapy of brain metastases from small cell lung cancer—a review. *J Clin Oncol* **10**: 1498–1502, 1992.

Raskind R, Weiss SR, Manning JJ, Wermuth RE. Survival after excision of single metastatic brain tumors. *AJR* **111**: 323–8, 1971.

Simionescu MD.: Metastatic tumors of the brain: a follow-up study of 195 patients with neurosurgical considerations. *J Neurosurg* **17**: 361–73, 1960.

Störtenbecker TP. Metastatic tumors of the brain from a neurosurgical point of view: a follow-up study of 158 cases. *J Neurosurg* **11**: 84–111, 1954.

Veith R. G, Odom GL. Intracranial metastases and their neurosurgical treatment. *J Neurosurg* **23**: 375–83, 1965.

Wronski M, Arbit E, Burt M, Galicich JH. Survival after surgical treatment of brain metastases from lung cancer: a follow-up study of 231 patients treated between 1976 and 1991. *J Neurosurg* **83**: 605–16, 1995.

Meningioma

Black PM. Meningiomas. *Neurosurgery* **32**: 643–57, 1993.

Cantore G, Delfini R, Ciappetta P. Surgical treatment of petroclival meningiomas: experience with 16 cases. *Surg Neurol* **42**: 105–11, 1994.

Chamberlain MC. Adjuvant combined modality therapy for malignant meningiomas. *J Neurosurg* **84**: 733–6, 1996.

De Jesús O, Rifkinson N, Negrón B. Cystic meningiomas: a review. *Neurosurgery* **36**: 489–92, 1995.

De Monte F. Current management of meningiomas. *Oncology* **9**: 83–91, **96**, 1995.

Desai R, Bruce J. Meningiomas of the cranial base. *J Neuro-Oncology* **20**: 255–79, 1994.

Ganz JC, Backlund EO, Thorsen FA. The results of Gamma Knife surgery of meningiomas, related to size of tumor and dose. *Stereotact Funct Neurosurg* **61**(suppl.): 23–9, 1993.

Gijtenbeek JM, Hop WC, Braakman R, Avezaat CJ.: Surgery for intracranial meningiomas in elderly patients. *Clin Neurol Neurosurg* **95**: 291–5, 1993.

Grunberg SM.: Role of antiprogestational therapy for meningiomas. *Human Reproduction* **9**(suppl.): 202–7, 1994.

Ide M, Jimbo M, Yamamoto M, Umebara Y, Hagiwara S, Kubo O. Growth rate of intracranial meningioma: tumor doubling time and proliferating cell nuclear antigen staining index. *Neurol Med Chir* **35**: 289–93, 1995.

Kinjo T, al-Mefty O, Ciric I. Diaphragma sellae meningiomas. *Neurosurgery* **36**: 1082–92, 1995.

Lunsford LD. Contemporary management of meningiomas: radiation therapy as an adjuvant and radiosurgery as an alternative to surgical removal? *J Neurosurg* **80**: 187–90, 1994.

Lunsford LD, Kondziolka D, Flickinger JC.: Stereotactic radiosurgery for benign intracranial tumors. *Clin Neurosurg* **40**: 475–97, 1993.

Maire JP, Caudry M, Guerin J, Celerier D, San Galli F, Causse N. *et al.* Fractionated radiation therapy in the treatment of intracranial meningiomas: local control, functional efficacy, and tolerance in 91 patients. *Int J Radiat Oncol Biol Phys* **33**: 315–21, 1995.

Mahmood A, Caccamo DV, Tomecek FJ, Malik GM. Atypical and malignant meningiomas: a clinicopathological review. *Neurosurgery* **33**: 955–63, 1993.

Mahmood A, Qureshi NH, Malik GM. Intracranial meningiomas: analysis of recurrence after surgical treatment. *Acta Neurochir* **126**: 53–8, 1994.

Mastronardi L, Ferrante L, Qasho R, Ferrari V, Tatarelli R, Fortuna A. Intracranial meningiomas in the 9th decade of life: a retrospective study of 17 surgical cases. *Neurosurgery* **36**: 270–4, 1995.

McGrail KM, Ojemann RG. The surgical management of benign intracranial meningiomas and acoustic neuromas in patients 70 years of age and older. *Surg Neurol* **42**: 2–7, 1994.

Miller DC. Predicting recurrence of intracranial meningiomas. A multivariate clinicopathologic model—interim report of the New York University Medical Center Meningioma Project. *Neurosurg Clin N Am* **5**: 193–200, 1994.

Murtagh R, Linden C. Neuroimaging of intracranial meningiomas. *Neurosurg Clin N Am* **5**: 217–33, 1994.

Newman SA. Meningiomas: a quest for the optimum therapy. *J Neurosurg* **80**: 191–4, 1994.

Nishizaki T, Kamiryo T, Fujisawa H, Ohshita N, Ishihara H, Ito H. *et al.* Prognostic implications of meningiomas in the elderly (over 70 years old) in the era of magnetic resonance imaging. *Acta Neurochir* **126**: 59–62, 1994.

Ojemann RG. Management of cranial and spinal meningiomas. *Clin Neurosurg* **40**: 321–83, 1993.

Olson JJ. Laboratory evidence for the hormonal dependency of meningiomas. *Human Reproduction* **9**(suppl.): 195–201, 1994.

Ransohoff J. Introduction to meningiomas. *Neurosurg Clin N Am* **5**: 191–2, 1994*a*.

Ransohoff J. Removal of convexity, parasagittal, and falcine meningiomas. *Neurosurg Clin N Am* **5**: 293–7, 1994*b*.

Rostomily RC, Eskridge JM, Winn HR. Tentorial meningiomas. *Neurosurg Clin N Am* **5**: 331–48, 1994.

Risi P, Uske A, de Tribolet N. Meningiomas involving the anterior clinoid process. *Br J Neurosurg* **8**: 295–305, 1994.

Rubin G, Ben David U, Gornish M, Rappaport ZH. Meningiomas of the anterior cranial fossa floor. Review of 67 cases. *Acta Neurochir* **129**: 26–30, 1994.

Rubinstein AB, Loven D, Geier A, Reichenthal E, Gadoth N. Hormone receptors in initially excised versus recurrent intracranial meningiomas. *J Neurosurg* **81**: 184–7, 1994.

Samii M, Carvalho GA, Tatagiba M, Matthies C, Vorkapic P. Meningiomas of the tentorial notch: surgical anatomy and management. *J Neurosurg* **84**: 375–81, 1996.

Sekhar LN, Babu RP, Wright DC. Surgical resection of cranial base meningiomas. *Neurosurg Clin N Am* **5**: 299–30, 1994*a*.

Sekhar LN, Swamy NK, Jaiswal V, Rubinstein E, Hirsch WE Jr, Wright DC. Surgical excision of meningiomas involving the clivus: preoperative and intraoperative features as predictors of postoperative functional deterioration. *J Neurosurg* **81**: 860–8, 1994*b*.

Younis GA, Sawaya R, DeMonte F, Hess KR, Albrecht S, Bruner JM. Aggressive meningeal tumors: review of a series. *J Neurosurg* **82**: 17–27, 1995.

Wasenko JJ, Hochhauser L, Stopa EG, Winfield JA. Cystic meningiomas: MR characteristics and surgical correlations. *Ajnr* **15**: 1959–65, 1994.

Wilson CB. Meningiomas: genetics, malignancy, and the role of radiation in induction and treatment. *J Neurosurg* **81**: 666–75, 1994.

Pituitary tumours

Adams CB, Burke CW. Current modes of treatment of pituitary tumours. *Br J Neurosurg* **7**: 123–7, 1993.

Andrews DW. Pituitary adenomas. *Curr Opin Oncol* **6**: 53–9, 1994.

Arafah BM, Kailani SH, Nekl KE, Gold RS, Selman WR. Immediate recovery of pituitary function after transsphenoidal resection of pituitary macroadenomas. *J Clin Endocrinol Metabol* **79**: 348–54, 1994.

Barrow DL, Tindall GT, Kovacs K, Thorner MO, Horvath E, Hoffman JC. Clinical and pathological effects of Bromocriptine on prolactin secreting and other pituitary tumors. *J Neurosurg* **60**: 1–27, 1984.

Bates AS, Van't Hoff W, Jones JM, Clayton RN. An audit of outcome of treatment of acromegaly. *Quarterly J. Med* **86**: 293–9, 1993.

Bochicchio D, Losa M, Buchfelder M. *et al.* Factors influencing the immediate and late outcome of Cushing's disease treated by transsphenoidal surgery. A retrospective Study by the European Cushing's Disease Survey Group. *J Clin Endocrinol Metabol* **80**: 3114–20, 1995.

Brada M, Rajan B, Traish D, Ashley S, Holmes-Sellors PJ, Nussey S. *et al.* The long-term efficacy of conservative surgery and radiotherapy in the control of pituitary adenomas. *Clin Endocrinol* **38**: 571–8, 1993.

Bradley KM, Adams CB, Potter CP, Wheeler DW, Anslow PJ, Burke CW. An audit of selected patients with non-functioning pituitary adenoma treated by transsphenoidal surgery without irradiation. *Clin Endocrinol* **41**: 655–9, 1994.

Clarke SD, Woo SY, Butler EB, Dennis WS, Lu H, Carpenter LS. *et al.* Treatment of secretory pituitary adenoma with radiation therapy. *Radiology* **188**: 759–63, 1993.

Cooke RS, Jones RA. Experience with the direct transnasal transsphenoidal approach to the pituitary fossa. *Br J Neurosurg* **8**: 193–6, 1994.

Davis DH, Laws ER Jr, Ilstrup DM, Speed JK, Caruso M, Shaw EG. *et al.* Results of surgical treatment for growth hormone-secreting pituitary adenomas. *J Neurosurg* **79**: 70–5, 1993.

Ferrari C, Paracchi A, Mattei AM, de Vincentiis S, D'Alberton A, Crosignani P. Cabergoline in the long-term therapy of hyperprolactinemic disorders. *Acta Endocrinol* **126**: 489–94, 1992.

Fisher BJ, Gaspar LE, Noone B. Radiation therapy of pituitary adenoma: delayed sequelae. *Radiology* **187**: 843–6, 1993.

Ganz JC, Backlund EO, Thorsen FA. The effects of Gamma Knife surgery of pituitary adenomas on tumor growth and endocrinopathies. *Stereotact Funct Neurosurg* **61**(suppl.): 30–7, 1993.

Grigsby PW. Pituitary adenomas: evolving diagnosis and management. *Int J Radiat Oncol Biol Phys* **27**: 1253–4, 1993.

Hennessey JV, Jackson IM. Clinical features and differential diagnosis of pituitary tumours with emphasis on acromegaly. *Baillière's Clinical Endocrinology and Metabolism* **9**: 271–14, 1995.

Jaffrain-Rea ML, Derome P, Bataini JP, Thomopoulos P, Bertagna X, Luton JP. Influence of radiotherapy on long-term relapse in clinically non-secreting pituitary adenomas. A retrospective study (1970–1988). *Eur J Med* **2**: 398–403, 1993.

Jaquet P. Medical therapy of prolactinomas. *Acta Endocrinol* **129**(suppl.): 31–3, 1993.

Jaspers C, Benker G, Reinwein D. Treatment of prolactinoma patients with the new non-ergot dopamine agonist roxindol: first results. *Clinical Investigator* **72**: 451–6, 1994.

Jeffreys R. Surgical treatment of large pituitary adenomas. *Br J Neurosurg* **3**: 147–52, 1989.

Jones TH. The management of hyperprolactinaemia. *Br J Hosp Med* **53**: 374–8, 1995.

Kovacs K, Stefaneanu L, Horvath E, Buchfelder M, Falhbuch R, Becker W. Prolactin-producing pituitary tumor: resistance to dopamine agonist therapy. *J Neurosurg* **82**: 886–90, 1995.

Laws ER Jr, Thapar K. Surgical management of pituitary adenomas. *Baillière's Clinical Endocrinology and Metabolism* **9**: 391–405, 1995.

Laws ER, Troutman JC, Hollenhorst RW Jr. Transphenoidal decompression of optic nerves and chiasm. *J Neurosurg* **46**: 717–22, 1977.

Levy A, Lightman SL. Diagnosis and management of pituitary tumours. *BMJ* **308**(6936): 1087–91, 1994.

Long H, Beauregard H, Somma M, Comtois R, Serri O, Hardy J. Surgical outcome after repeated transphenoidal surgery in acromegaly. *J Neurosurg* **85**: 239–47, 1996.

Lunsford LD, Kondziolka D, Flickinger JC. Stereotactic radiosurgery for benign intracranial tumors. *Clin Neurosurg* **40**: 475–97, 1993.

Marazuela M, Astigarraga B, Vicente A, Estrada J, Cuerda C, Garcia-Uria J. *et al.* Recovery of visual and endocrine function following transsphenoidal surgery of large nonfunctioning pituitary adenomas. *J Endocrinol Invest* **17**: 703–7, 1994.

Marks LB. Conventional fractionated radiation therapy vs. radiosurgery for selected benign intracranial lesions (arteriovenous malformations, pituitary adenomas, and acoustic neuromas). *J Neuro-Oncology* **17**: 223–30, 1993.

Mbanya JC, Mendelow AD, Crawford PJ, Hall K, Dewar JH, Kendall-Taylor P. Rapid resolution of visual abnormalities with medical therapy alone in patients with large prolactinomas. *Br J Neurosurg* **7**: 519–27, 1993.

McCance DR, Gordon DS, Fannin TF, Hadden DR, Kennedy L, Sheridan B *et al.* Assessment of endocrine function after transsphenoidal surgery for Cushing's disease. *Clin Endocrinol* **38**: 79–86, 1993.

McCutcheon IE. Management of individual tumor syndromes. Pituitary neoplasia. *Endocrinol Metabol Clin N Am* **23**: 37–51, 1994.

Melis GB, Gambacciani M, Paoletti AM, Mais V, Sghedoni D, Fioretti P. Reduction in the size of prolactin-producing pituitary tumor after Cabergoline administration. *Fertil Steril* **52**: 412–15, 1989.

Nyquist P, Laws ER Jr, Elliott E. Novel features of tumours that secrete both growth hormone and prolactin in acromegaly. *Neurosurgery* **35**: 179–83, 1994.

Osman IA, James RA, Chatterjee S, Mathias D, Kendall-Taylor P. Factors determining the long-term outcome of surgery for acromegaly. *Quarterly J Med* **87**: 617–23, 1994.

Peter M, De Tribolet N. Visual outcome after transphenoidal surgery for pituitary adenomas. *Br J Neurosurg* **9**: 151–7, 1995.

Petruson B, Jakobsson KE, Elfverson J, Bengtsson BA. Five-year follow-up of nonsecreting pituitary adenomas. *Arch Otolaryngol—Head Neck Surg* **121**: 317–22, 1995.

Plowman PN. Radiotherapy for pituitary tumours. *Baillière's Clinical Endocrinology and Metabolism* **9**: 407–20, 1995.

Pollock BE, Kondziolka D, Lunsford LD, Flickinger JC. Stereotactic radiosurgery for pituitary adenomas: imaging, visual and endocrine results. *Acta Neurochir* **62**(suppl.): 33–8, 1994.

Post FA, Soule SG, De Villiers JC, Levitt NS. Pituitary function after selective adenomectomy for Cushing's disease. *Br J Neurosurg* **9**: 41–6, 1995.

Puchner MJA, Knappe UJ, Lüdecke DK. Pituitary surgery in elderly patients with acromegaly. *Neurosurgery* **36**: 677–83, 1995.

Samuels MH. Gonadotroph adenomas. *Curr Ther Endocrinol Metabol* **5**: 52–6, 1994.

Sassolas G, Trouillas J, Treluyer C, Perrin G. Management of nonfunctioning pituitary adenomas. *Acta Endocrinol* **129**(suppl.): 21–6, 1993.

Serri O, Beauregard H, Somma M. Prolactinoma. *Curr Ther Endocrinol Metabol* **5**: 41–3, 1994.

Snyder PJ. Extensive personal experience: gonadotroph adenomas. *J Clin Endocrinol Metabol* **80**: 1059–61, 1995.

Soule SG, Powell M, Jacobs HS. Prolactinomas resistant to dopamine agonists: insights into pathogenesis and therapy. *Current Opin Obstet Gynecol.* **6**: 393–7, 1994.

Soule SG, Jacobs HS. Prolactinomas: present day management. *Br J Obstet Gynecol* **102**: 178–81, 1995.

Soule SG, Farhi J, Conway SG. *et al.* The outcome of hypophysectomy for prolactinomas in the era of dopamine agonist therapy. *Clin Endocrinol* **44**: 711–16, 1996.

Stadnik T, Spruyt D, van Binst A, Luypaert R, d'Haens J, Osteaux M. Pituitary microadenomas: diagnosis with dynamic serial CT, conventional CT and T1-weighted MR imaging before and after injection of gadolinium. *Eur J Radiol* **18**: 191–8, 1994.

Steiner E, Math G, Knosp E, Mostbeck G, Kramer J, Herold CJ. MR-appearance of the pituitary gland before and after resection of pituitary macroadenomas. *Clin Radiol* **49**: 524–30, 1994.

Thomson JA, Davies DL, McLaren EH, Teasdale GM. Ten year follow up of microprolactinoma treated by transsphenoidal surgery. *BMJ* **309**(6966): 1409–10, 1994.

Tyrrell JB, Wilson CB. Cushing's disease. Therapy of pituitary adenomas. *Endocrinol Metabol Clin N Am* **23**: 925–38, 1994.

Vance ML. Nonfunctioning pituitary adenoma. *Curr Ther Endocrinol Metabol* **5**: 31–3, 1994.

Yamada S, Aiba T, Sano T, Kovacs K, Shishiba Y, Sawano S. *et al.* Growth hormone-producing pituitary adenomas: correlations between clinical characteristics and morphology. *Neurosurgery* **33**: 20–7, 1993.

Wen PY, Loeffler JS.: Advances in the diagnosis and management of pituitary tumors. *Curr Opin Oncol* **7**: 56–62, 1995.

Zierhut D, Flentje M, Adolph J, Erdmann J, Raue F, Wannenmacher M. External radiotherapy of pituitary adenomas. *Int J Radiat Oncol Biol Phys* **33**: 307–14, 1995.

Acoustic neuroma

Arriaga MA, Luxford WM, Berliner KI. Facial nerve function following middle fossa and translabyrinthine acoustic tumor surgery: a comparison. *Am J Otol* **15**: 620–4, 1994.

Black FO, Brackmann DE, Hitselberger WE, Purdy J. Preservation of auditory and vestibular function after surgical removal of bilateral vestibular schwannomas in a patient with neurofibromatosis type 2. *Am J Otol* **16**: 431–43, 1995.

Black PM. Benign brain tumors. Meningiomas, pituitary tumors, and acoustic neuromas. *Neurol Clin* **13**: 927–52, 1995.

Esses BA, LaRouere MJ, Graham MD. Facial nerve outcome in acoustic tumor surgery. *Am J Otol* **15**: 810–2, 1994.

Forster DMC, Kemeny AA, Pathak A, Walton L. Radiosurgery: a minimally interventional alternative to microsurgery in the management of acoustic neuroma. *Br J Neurosurg* **10**: 169–74, 1996.

Haines SJ, Levine SC. Intracanalicular acoustic neuroma: early surgery for preservation of hearing. *J Neurosurg* **79**: 515–20, 1993.

Irving RM, Beynon GJ, Viani L, Hardy DG, Baguley DM, Moffat DA. The patient's perspective after vestibular schwannoma removal: quality of life and implications for management. *Am J Otol* **16**: 331–7, 1995.

Lalwani AK, Butt FY, Jackler RK, Pitts LH, Yingling CD. Delayed onset facial nerve dysfunction following acoustic neuroma surgery. *Am J Otol* **16**: 758–64, 1995.

Nutik SL. Facial nerve outcome after acoustic neuroma surgery. *Surg Neurol* **41**: 28–33, 1994.

Ogunrinde OK, Lunsford DL, Kondziolka DS, Bissonette DJ, Flickinger JC. Cranial nerve preservation after stereotactic radiosurgery of intracanalicular acoustic tumors. *Stereotact Funct Neurosurg* **64**(suppl.): 87–97, 1995.

Shelton C, Alavi S, Li JC, Hitselberger WE. Modified retrosigmoid approach: use for selected acoustic tumor removal. *Am J Otol* **16**: 664–8, 1995.

Telian SA. Management of the small acoustic neuroma: a decision analysis. *Am J Otol* **15**: 358–65, 1994.

Torrens M, Maw R, Coakham H, Butler S. Facial and acoustic nerve preservation during excision of extracranalicular acoustic neuromas using the suboccipital approach. *Br J Neurosurg* **8**: 655–65, 1994.

Wright A, Bradford R. Management of acoustic neuroma. *BMJ* **311**(7013): 1141–4, 1995.

Brainstem glioma

Albright AL, Packer RJ, Zimmerman R, Rorke LB, Boyett J, Hammond GD. Magnetic resonance scans should replace biopsies for the diagnosis of diffuse brain stem gliomas: a report from the Children's Cancer Group. *Neurosurgery* **33**: 1026–9, 1993.

Epstein F, McCleary EL. Intrinsic brain stem tumours: surgical indications. *J Neurosurg* **64**: 11–15, 1986.

Guiney MJ, Smith JG, Hughes P, Yang C, Narayan K. Contemporary management of adult and pediatric brain stem gliomas. *Int J Radiat Oncol Biol Phys* **25**: 235–41, 1993.

Hibi T, Shitara N, Genka S, Fuchinoue T, Hayakawa I, Tsuchida T. *et al*. Radiotherapy for pediatric brain stem glioma: radiation dose, response, and survival. *Neurosurgery* **31**: 643–50, 1992.

Hirato M, Nakamura M, Inoue HK, Ohye C, Hirato J, Shibazaki T. *et al*. Gamma Knife radiosurgery for the treatment of brainstem tumors. *Stereotact Funct Neurosurg* **64**(suppl.): 32–41, 1995.

Kratimenos GP, Thomas DGT. The role of image-directed biopsy in the diagnosis of brainstem lesions. *Br J Neurosurg* **7**: 155–64, 1993.

Kretschmar CS, Tarbell NJ, Barnes PD, Krischer JP, Burger PC, Kun L. Pre-irradiation chemotherapy and hyperfractionated radiation therapy 66 Gy for children with brain stem tumors. A phase II

study of the Pediatric Oncology Group, Protocol 8833. *Cancer* **72**: 1404–13, 1993.

Langmoen IA, Lundar T, Storm-Mathisen I, Lie SO, Hovind KH. Management of pediatric pontine gliomas. *Childs Nerv Syst* **7**: 13–15, 1991.

Linstadt DE, Edwards MS, Prados M, Larson DA, Wara WM. Hyperfractionated irradiation for adults with brainstem gliomas. *Int J Radiat Oncol Biol Phys* **20**: 757–60, 1991.

Mulhern RK, Heideman RL, Khatib ZA, Kovnar EH, Sanford RA, Kun LE. Quality of survival among children treated for brain stem glioma. *Pediat Neurosurg* **20**: 226–32, 1994.

Packer RJ, Nicholson HS, Johnson DL, Vezina LG. Dilemmas in the management of childhood brain tumors: brainstem gliomas. *Pediat Neurosurg* **17**: 37–43, 1991–92.

Packer RJ, Nicholson HS, Vezina LG, Johnson DL. Brainstem gliomas. *Neurosurg Clin N Am* **3**: 863–79, 1992.

Pollack IF, Hoffman HJ, Humphreys RP, Becker L. The long-term outcome after surgical treatment of dorsally exophytic brain-stem gliomas. *J Neurosurg* **78**: 859–63, 1993.

Packer RJ, Boyett JM, Zimmerman RA, Albright AL, Kaplan AM, Rorke LB. *et al*. Outcome of children with brain stem gliomas after treatment with 7800 cGy of hyperfractionated radiotherapy. A Childrens Cancer Group Phase I/II Trial. *Cancer* **74**: 1827–34, 1994.

Rajshekhar V, Chandy MJ. Computerized tomography-guided stereotactic surgery for brainstem masses: a risk–benefit analysis in 71 patients. *J Neurosurg* **82**: 976–81, 1995.

Robertson PL, Allen JC, Abbott IR, Miller DC, Fidel J, Epstein FJ. Cervicomedullary tumors in children: a distinct subset of brainstem gliomas. *Neurology* **44**: 1798–803, 1994.

Shrieve DC, *Wara WM*, Edwards MS, Sneed PK, Prados MD, Cogen PH *et al*. Hyperfractionated radiation therapy for gliomas of the brainstem in children and in adults. *Int J Radiat Oncol Biol Phys* **24**: 599–610, 1992.

Takasato Y, Arai T, Ohta Y, Yamada K. Gross total removal of adult brainstem glioma—two case reports. *Neurol Med Chir* **33**: 625–9, 1993.

Wakabayashi T, Yoshida J, Mizuno M, Kito A, Sugita K. Effectiveness of interferon-beta, ACNU, and radiation therapy in pediatric patients with brainstem glioma. *Neurol Med Chir* **32**: 942–6, 1992.

Ependymoma

Chiu JK, Woo SY, Ater J, Connelly J, Bruner JM, Maor MH. *et al*. Intracranial ependymoma in children: analysis of prognostic factors. *J Neuro-Oncology* **13**: 283–90, 1992.

Evans AE, Anderson JR, Lefkowitz-Boudreaux IB, Finlay JL. Adjuvant chemotherapy of childhood posterior fossa ependymoma: cranio-spinal irradiation with or without adjuvant CCNU, vincristine, and prednisone: a Childrens Cancer Group study. *Med Pediat Oncol* **27**: 8–14, 1996.

Ferrante L, Mastronardi L, Schettini G, Lunardi P, Fortuna A. Fourth ventricle ependymomas. A study of 20 cases with survival analysis. *Acta Neurochir* **131**: 67–74, 1994.

Furie DM, Provenzale JM. Supratentorial ependymomas and subependymomas: CT and MR appearance. *J Computer Assisted Tomography* **19**: 518–26, 1995.

Jayawickreme DP, Hayward RD, Harkness WF. Intracranial ependymomas in childhood: a report of 24 cases followed for 5 years. *Childs Nerv Sys* **11**: 409–13, 1995.

Kovalic JJ, Flaris N, Grigsby PW, Pirkowski M, Simpson JR, Roth KA. Intracranial ependymoma long term outcome, patterns of failure. *J Neuro-Oncology* **15**: 125–31, 1993.

Palma L, Celli P, Cantore G. Supratentorial ependymomas of the first two decades of life. Long-term follow-up of 20 cases (including two subependymomas). *Neurosurgery* **32**: 169–75, 1993.

Pollack IF, Gerszten PC, Martinez AJ, Lo KH, Shultz B, Albright AL. *et al.* Intracranial ependymomas of childhood: long-term outcome and prognostic factors. *Neurosurgery* **37**: 655–66, 1995.

Rousseau P, Habrand JL, Sarrazin D, Kalifa C, Terrier-Lacombe MJ, Rekacewicz C. *et al.* Treatment of intracranial ependymomas of children: review of a 15-year experience. *Int J Radiat Oncol Biol Phys* **28**: 381–6, 1994.

Tortori-Donati P, Fondelli MP, Cama A, Garre ML, Rossi A, Andreussi L. Ependymomas of the posterior cranial fossa: CT and MRI findings. *Neuroradiology*. **37**: 238–43, 1995.

Vanuytsel LJ, Bessell EM, Ashley SE, Bloom HJ, Brada M. Intracranial ependymoma: long-term results of a policy of surgery and radiotherapy. *Int J Radiat Oncol Biol Phys* **23**: 313–19, 1992.

Spinal astrocytoma

Abbott R, Feldstein N, Wisoff JH, Epstein FJ. Osteoplastic laminotomy in children. *Pediat Neurosurg* **18**: 153–6, 1992.

Brotchi J, Noterman J, Baleriaux D. Surgery of intramedullary spinal cord tumours. *Acta Neurochir* **116**: 176–8, 1992.

Cristante L, Herrmann HD. Surgical management of intramedullary spinal cord tumors: functional outcome and sources of morbidity. *Neurosurgery* **35**: 69–74, 1994.

Epstein FJ, Farmer JP, Freed D. Adult intramedullary astrocytomas of the spinal cord. *J Neurosurg* **77**: 355–9, 1992.

Huddart R, Traish D, Ashley S, Moore A, Brada M. Management of spinal astrocytoma with conservative surgery and radiotherapy. *Br J Neurosurg* **7**: 473–81, 1993.

Hulshof MC, Menten J, Dito JJ, Dreissen JJ, van den Bergh R, Gonzalez D. Treatment results in primary intraspinal gliomas. *Radiotherapy Oncol* **29**: 294–300, 1993.

Kearse LA Jr, Lopez-Bresnahan M, McPeck K, Tambe V. Loss of somatosensory evoked potentials during intramedullary spinal cord surgery predicts postoperative neurologic deficits in motor function. *J Clin Anesth* **5**: 392–8, 1993.

Koyanagi I, Iwasaki Y, Isu T, Abe H, Akino M, Kuroda S. Spinal cord evoked potential monitoring after spinal cord stimulation during surgery of spinal cord tumors. *Neurosurgery* **33**: 451–9, 1993.

Lunardi P, Licastro G, Missori P, Ferrante L, Fortuna A. Management of intramedullary tumours in children. *Acta Neurochir* **120**: 59–65, 1993.

Minehan KJ, Shaw EG, Scheithauer BW, Davis DL, Onofrio BM. Spinal cord astrocytoma: pathological and treatment considerations. *J Neurosurg* **83**: 590–5, 1995.

O'Sullivan C, Jenkin RD, Doherty MA, Hoffman HJ, Greenberg ML. Spinal cord tumors in children: long-term results of combined surgical and radiation treatment. *J Neurosurg* **81**: 507–12, 1994.

Samii M, Klekamp J. Surgical results of 100 intramedullary tumors in relation to accompanying syringomyelia. *Neurosurgery* **35**: 865–73, 1994.

Sandler HM, Papadopoulos SM, Thornton AF Jr, Ross DA. Spinal cord astrocytomas: results of therapy. *Neurosurgery* **30**: 490–3, 1992.

Shirato H, Kamada T, Hida K, Koyanagi I, Iwasaki Y, Miyasaka K. *et al.* The role of radiotherapy in the management of spinal cord glioma. *Int J Radiat Oncol Biol Phys* **33**: 323–8, 1995.

Stein BM, McCormick PC. Intramedullary neoplasms and vascular malformations. *Clin Neurosurg* **39**: 361–87, 1992.

Steinbok P, Cochrane DD, Poskitt K. Intramedullary spinal cord tumors in children. *Neurosurg Clin N Am* **3**: 931–45, 1992.

Wagner W, Peghini-Halbig L, Maurer JC, Perneczky A. Intraoperative SEP monitoring in neurosurgery around the brain stem and cervical spinal cord: differential recording of subcortical components. *J Neurosurg* **81**: 213–20, 1994.

Spinal ependymoma

Barone BM, Elvidge AR. Ependymomas. A clinical survey. *J Neurosurg* **33**: 428–38, 1970.

Cervoni L, Celli P, Fortuna A, Cantore G. Recurrence of spinal ependymoma. Risk factors and long-term survival. *Spine* **19**: 2838–41, 1994.

Clover LL, Hazuka MB, Kinzie JJ. Spinal cord ependymomas treated with surgery and radiation therapy. A review of 11 cases. *Am J Clin Oncol* **16**: 350–3, 1993.

Cooper PR. Outcome after operative treatment of intramedullary spinal cord tumors in adults: Intermediate and long-term results in 51 patients. *Neurosurgery* **25**: 855–9, 1989.

Cooper PR, Epstein F. Radical resection of intramedullary spinal cord tumors in adults. *J Neurosurg* **63**: 492–9, 1985.

Di Marco A, Griso C, Pradella R, Campostrini, Garusi GF. Postoperative management of primary spinal cord ependymomas. *Acta Oncol* **27**: 371–5, 1988.

Epstein FJ, Farmer JP, Freed D. Adult intramedullary spinal cord ependymomas: the result of surgery in 38 patients. *J Neurosurg* **79**: 204–9, 1993.

Fearnside MR, Adams CBT.: Tumours of the cauda equina. *J Neurol Neurosurg Psychiatry* **41**: 24–31, 1978.

Ferrante L, Mastronardi L, Celli P, Lunardi P, Acqui M, Fortuna A. Intramedullary spinal cord ependymomas—a study of 45 cases with long-term follow-up. *Acta Neurochir* **119**: 74–9, 1992.

Fine MJ, Kricheff II, Freed D, Epstein FJ. Spinal cord ependymomas: MR imaging features. *Radiology* **197**: 655–8, 1995.

Fischer G, Mansuy L. Total removal of intramedullary ependymomas: Follow-up study of 16 cases. *Surg Neurol* **14**: 243–9, 1980.

Fokes EC Jr, Earle KM. Ependymomas: Clinical and pathological aspects. *J Neurosurg* **30**: 585–94, 1969.

Garrido E, Stein BM. Microsurgical removal of intramedullary spinal cord tumors. *Surg Neurol* **7**: 215–19, 1977.

Guidetti B, Mercuri S, Vagnozzi R. Long-term result of the surgical treatment of 129 intramedullary spinal gliomas. *J Neurosurg* **54**: 323–30, 1981.

Linstadt DE, Wara WM, Leibel SA, Gutin PH, Wilson CB, Sheline GE. Postoperative radiotherapy of primary spinal cord tumours. *Int J Radiat Oncol Biol Phys* **16**: 1397–403, 1989.

Marks JE, Adler SJ. A comparative study of ependymomas by site of origin. *Int J Radiat Oncol Biol Phys* **8**: 37–43, 1982.

Morantz RA, Kepes JJ, Batnitzky S, Masterson BJ. Extraspinal ependymomas. *J Neurosurg* **51**: 383–91, 1979.

Mork SJ, Løken AC. Ependymoma. A follow-up study of 101 cases. *Cancer* **40**: 907–15, 1977.

Peschel RE, Kapp DS, Cardinale F, Manuelidis EE. Ependymomas of the spinal cord. *Int J Radiat Oncol Biol Phys* **9**: 1093–6, 1983.

Rawlings CE, Giangaspero F, Burger PC, Bullard DE. Ependymomas: A clinicopathologic study. *Surg Neurol* **29**: 271–81, 1988.

Ross GW, Rubinstein LJ. Lack of histopathological correlation of malignant ependymomas with postoperative survival. *J Neurosurg* **70**: 31–6, 1989.

Schweitzer JS, Batzdorf U. Ependymoma of the cauda equina region: Diagnosis, treatment and outcome in 15 patients. *Neurosurgery* **30**: 202–7, 1992.

Sgouros S, Malluci C, Jackowski A. Spinal ependymomas—The value of postoperative radiotherapy for residual disease control. *Br J Neurosurg* **10**: 559–66, 1996.

Shaw EG, Evans RG, Scheithauer BW, Ilstrup DM, Earle JD.

Radiotherapeutic management of adult intraspinal ependymomas. *Int J Radia Onco Biol Phys* **12**: 323–7, 1986.

Sonneland PRL, Scheithauer BW, Onofrio BM. Myxopapillary ependymoma. A clinicopathologic and immunocytochemical study of 77 cases. *Cancer* **56**: 883–93, 1985.

Waldron JN, Laperriere NJ, Jaakkimainen L, Simpson WJ, Payne D,

Milosevic M. *et al.* Spinal cord ependymomas: a retrospective analysis of 59 cases. *Int J Radiat Oncol Biol Phys* **27**: 223–9, 1993.

Whitaker SJ, Bessell EM, Ashley SE, Bloom HJG, Bell BA, Brada M. Postoperative radiotherapy in the management of spinal cord ependymoma. *J Neurosurg* **74**: 720–8, 1991.

15 | Infectious diseases

Milne Anderson

Successful management of a case of infection involving the central nervous system (CNS) requires that the diagnosis be made as early as possible and treatment instituted without delay. The two main factors which adversely affect the outcome of any form of CNS infection are the state of consciousness of the patient when the diagnosis is made, and any delay in treatment. To a large extent the state of consciousness of the patient prior to admission is beyond the control of the admitting doctor, yet it should be possible by education and exhortation to persuade family doctors to refer potential cases earlier. Media interest in, and in some cases hysterical reporting of, cases of meningitis have served to focus public interest on the subject, and the profession should capitalize on this to spread awareness of the early symptoms and signs of brain infection. Unfortunately, attendance at hospital does not guarantee rapid diagnosis and treatment. Delays occur in busy accident and emergency departments and time is sometimes wasted carrying out inappropriate investigations which might have been avoided had a proper history been obtained at the outset. This point is worthy of emphasis. It is not possible to glean much reliable information from a confused, distressed, or unconscious patient but a few minutes spent at the very beginning talking to relatives, friends, and ambulance attendants will usually provide sufficient information to indicate the likely problem. In this context it is particularly important to enquire if there has been recent travel abroad—cheap air travel has reduced the size of the world, with the result that infections which were previously regarded as exotic and rare may turn up in your own practice. Two or three times each year reports appear in the popular press of people dying of cerebral malaria which had not been recognized in time. Rabies cannot be contracted in Britain but people who have been bitten by a rabid animal abroad can travel to Britain while incubating the disease. Backpackers trekking in distant jungles may return with infestations, such as cysticercosis, which manifests months later.

Neurological infections most commonly affect the brain and its surroundings, less frequently the spinal cord, and uncommonly, peripheral nerve and muscle. Intracranial infection is conventionally described under three symptom-complex headings: (1) meningitis; (2) encephalitis; and (3) focal suppuration. These may be of acute, subacute, or chronic onset and evolution and this may have aetiological significance. Unfortunately, the presence of one of these clinical syndromes does not exclude the others and they commonly coexist, usually meningitis with encephalitis. Brain abscess may complicate meningitis or an abscess may rupture into the cerebrospinal fluid (CSF) and cause meningitis. Consequently, some signs and symptoms are common to all three syndromes. It is important to recognize that the usual signs of infection, including pyrexia, may be absent, and more often than not there is no obvious infection elsewhere in the body. This is particularly so in the early stages of disease, in the very young, the very old, and the immune compromised, and it behoves the physician to have a particularly high index of suspicion of infection when dealing with such patients. It is also important when infection is suspected to seek out any primary locus—such as heart and lung, ear, paranasal sinuses, kidney and gut, not forgetting teeth and genital tract—and to eradicate it.

Symptoms and signs which point to neurological infection are pyrexia, headache, and alteration of consciousness. Focal signs may also coexist. It is important to understand that most patients with meningitis and encephalitis, and a substantial number of those who develop intracranial suppuration, do not have any focal signs on first examination, and if such are found they imply abscess or granuloma formation, brain infarction from arterial or venous inflammation, or the development of necrotizing encephalitis. Focal epileptic seizures carry the same significance. With meningitis, photophobia, vomiting, neck stiffness, and variable degrees of altered consciousness are found. Encephalitis occurs when there is more involvement of brain parenchyma manifest by earlier and more marked reduction in conscious level, perhaps with focal signs and epileptic seizures. Epileptic seizures can be more easily provoked in an immature brain, as in febrile convulsions of childhood or in a brain already compromised by pre-existing disease, and their occurrence then has less clinical significance. Signs of raised intracranial pressure are common with all three syndromes. It cannot be stressed enough that alteration of conscious level is the commonest sign of raised intracranial pressure (ICP), and neck stiffness may be caused by the cerebellar tonsils herniating through the foramen magnum. Therefore, all cases who exhibit these signs—and this applies to most cases with suspected meningitis, encephalitis, and focal suppuration—*should be assumed to have significantly raised ICP and be managed accordingly*. Papilloedema takes time to develop. Its presence confirms the existence of raised ICP but its absence must not be taken to mean that ICP is normal, and it is therefore safe to examine the CSF by lumbar puncture. The same comments may be made about other signs classically associated with intracranial hypertension—VIth and IIIrd nerve palsies and variations in pulse and blood pressure. It is my belief that much of the morbidity and mortality associated with intracranial infection results from the failure of many clinicians to appreciate the significance of raised ICP in the evolution of these diseases. The subject is dealt with later in more detail.

The same neurological syndrome may be caused by many different organisms. For example, meningitis may be due to infection by viruses, bacteria, fungi, and protozoa. Meningism, that is the presence of photophobia, neck stiffness, headache, and sometimes pyrexia may occur from non-infectious causes such as subarachnoid haemorrhage. The temporal profile of the onset, evolution, progression, resolution, and response to intervention provide important clues to the likely aetiology. So too does information about pre-existing disease states and medication, occupation, or recreational pastimes which may expose the subject to particular pathogens, and a knowledge of the state of health of family, friends, and colleagues in his/her immediate environment.

Recognizing that the clinical syndromes may overlap and evolve, it remains useful to describe them under the headings of meningitis, encephalitis, and intracranial suppuration, and this convention will be followed here.

MENINGITIS

The patient with acute meningitis presents within a few hours or at most two to three days. The usual cause is viral, or less commonly, bacterial infection. Rarely, it may be caused by fungi or protozoa which in common with bacteria like tuberculosis and brucellosis, usually cause a subacute or chronic meningitic syndrome which may take weeks to evolve.

'Acute aseptic meningitis' is the term given by Wallgren to a syndrome of acute onset with meningeal irritation associated with CSF pleocytosis, lymphocytes predominating, no bacteria or fungi on culture, a short benign and self-limiting course, and complete recovery. It is now recognized that more than 70% of such cases are due to viral infection and the viruses that are responsible are listed in Table 15.1.

Children and young adults are most frequently affected. In temperate climates most cases occur in summer and autumn but may be seen at any time and in any age group. The onset is acute, even abrupt, with pyrexia, headache, malaise, myalgia, photophobia, irritability, and neck stiffness. Barring complications, the patient remains conscious and coherent; if drowsy he/she can be roused easily. There may have been a preceding influenza-like illness or gastrointestinal disturbance. Physical examination reveals neck stiffness and little else neurologically. If the conscious level deteriorates or focal signs

Table 15.1 Causes of viral meningitis

Enteroviruses
Echo
Polio
Coxsackie
Varicella zoster
Mumps
Herpes simplex
Lymphocytic choriomeningitis
HIV

are found, then encephalitis or bacterial infection is more likely. In a minority of patients abnormalities may be found on systemic examination, which may have aetiological significance. Parotitis and orchitis suggests mumps; myocarditis and myalgia may be found with Coxsackie; arthralgia and lymphadenopathy with HIV; and rashes may occur with enteroviral infections. The clinical course is short, spontaneous improvement taking place within days and resolution within two weeks. Myalgia, lassitude, and headache may continue longer and eventually settle. Epileptic seizures are not part of the syndrome unless there is an underlying predisposition to epilepsy, or complications ensue.

In order to confirm the diagnosis it is necessary to examine the CSF by lumbar puncture (LP). While the clinical syndrome is easy to recognize, similar findings may be seen in the early stages of bacterial meningitis, in partially treated meningitis, after subarachnoid haemorrhage, with parameningeal infection, inflammation or neoplasia, and collagen diseases. Although not necessary in every case, particularly if the signs are mild, cranial imaging with computerized tomography (CT) will be carried out in most cases to determine if there is evidence of these other pathologies. The CSF pressure may be raised and the fluid is usually clear in appearance. The white cell count is raised, commonly in the range of 100–$1000/mm^3$ and these are mainly lymphocytes. Sometimes, polymorphs may predominate causing confusion with early bacterial meningitis. In such cases, provided no organisms are seen on the Gram stain and the clinical state of the patient does not deteriorate, it may be prudent to re-examine the CSF some 12–24 hours later (Feigin and Shackelford 1973). If there is doubt it is best to treat for bacterial meningitis on a 'best guess' basis after samples have been sent for culture. The protein content may be raised but not much, and the glucose should be normal or only slightly reduced. None of the many other tests which have been applied to CSF is sufficiently specific to differentiate viral from other forms of meningitis. My own experience of PCR (polymerase chain reaction) is not yet sufficient to express a useful opinion. It is not necessary to establish an exact aetiology in most cases since the syndrome is benign and self-limiting. If considered necessary, the organism may be identified following culture, by the demonstration of IgM antibody or of antigen in CSF or blood or by the demonstration of a significant rise in antibody titre in samples of blood or CSF taken 14 days apart. Haematological and biochemical tests are seldom helpful, neither is the EEG (electroencephalogram).

The main part of the management of a case of viral meningitis revolves around reassuring the patient and relatives that the course of the disease is benign and that recovery without physical or mental deficit is the norm. Meningitis has received a bad press particularly in the popular tabloid newspapers, and the public are not able to discriminate between different forms. This is not made easier by the reporting of organisms like the *meningococcus* as a 'killer virus'. There is therefore an understandable desire by relatives for antibiotics to be given and this can usually be allayed by explanation. If it cannot, I am prepared to give a short course of penicillin provided there are no contraindications. If antibiotics have been administered prior to admission I usually complete the course. Headache should be relieved by adequate analgesia and attendants should have no scruples about giving medication by injection, and regularly. Experience suggests that this is the most efficacious route and this way the drug cannot be vomited back. Because of the anxieties engendered by a diagnosis of 'meningitis' it is prudent to review patients once after discharge in order to reassure them that any lingering symptoms will resolve. Just occasionally it is necessary to arrange for a 'therapeutic' scan or EEG to reinforce this and to confirm to them that no brain damage has occurred.

The epidemiology and pathogenesis of bacterial meningitis is complex. Any organism may cause meningitis given circumstances favourable to its proliferation such as immune suppression or direct access to CSF via a fracture of the skull. In practice, over 70% of cases beyond the neonatal period are caused by three organisms, each of which has virulent properties which allow colonization of the neuraxis: *Haemophilus influenzae*, *Neisseriae meningitidis*, and *Streptococcus pneumoniae*, most of these cases occur in children and young adults and a list of the common causal organisms is given in Table 15.2.

Certain disease states predispose the patient to infection by particular groups of organisms, and these are shown in Table 15.3

Clinical features

The clinical features of a straightforward case of meningitis are easy to recognize. The onset is quick, within hours or at

Table 15.2 Causes of bacterial meningitis

Children
Haemophilus
Meningococcus
Pneumococcus

Adults
Pneumococcus
Meningococcus
Staphylococcus
Streptococcus
Listeria

Tuberculosis may affect any age group

Table 15.3 Bacteria* and predisposing cause

Skull fracture
Staphylococci
Gram-negative bacilli
Multiple organisms

CSF leak
Pneumococci
Gram-negative bacilli
Multiple organisms

CNS shunt
Staphylococcus epidermidis

Alcohol
Pneumococcus

Sickle-cell disease
Pneumococcus

Diabetes
Pneumococcus
Staphylococcus
Gram-negative bacilli

Pregnancy / Peri-natal
Listeria
Streptococci

Neutropaenia
Pseudomonas

Immune defect: cells
Listeria

Immune defect: humoral
Pneumococci
Meningococci
Haemophilus
Multiple organisms

* Of these the meningococcus is the only organism to cause significant epidemics. Infection acquired in hospital is becoming increasingly frequent.

the most a couple of days. Fulminant cases may be dead within 24 hours so there is always pressure to diagnose and treat early. Fever, headache, nuchal rigidity, irritability, photophobia, confusion, and alteration of consciousness are characteristic. By comparison with the viral form, bacterial meningitis is more severe and becomes so more quickly. Unfortunately, a significant minority have atypical features, perhaps as many as 20% of cases and this can make diagnosis difficult. Neck stiffness and fever may be absent. Young children may present with a syndrome which mimics an upper respiratory or gastrointestinal infection or just a non-specific malaise. The very old may not have many signs and show little in the way of neck stiffness. Conversely, I have been referred elderly patients with pyrexia and marked neck stiffness who have turned out to have a urinary infection and neck stiffness caused by cervical spondylosis. Those who are immunocompromised may easily become very ill with little objective to show for it. Epilepsy may occur at any age, is common in young children and may be the presenting feature of meningitis (Hambleton and Davies 1975). Every child who presents with a 'febrile convulsion' is a potential case of meningitis so should every one have a lumbar puncture carried out? Two studies suggest that this is not necessary if the convulsion is of short duration and the child regains consciousness rapidly, has no neurological deficit or focal component to the seizure, or signs of meningitis (Lorber and Sunderland 1980; Rutter and Smales 1977). Then it is reasonable to observe the child recover over the next few hours and this must be done in hospital. Seizures occur in about 35% of cases in children and a lesser proportion in adults and should be treated aggressively because increased requirements for energy from firing neurones may exceed the capacity of cerebral perfusion to supply it and ischaemic damage may ensue (Kaplan and Fishman 1987).

In approximately 15% of cases focal neurological signs may be found due to inflammation of arteries or veins causing infarction, or rarely because a brain abscess is forming. Cranial nerve palsies affecting chiefly the IIIrd and VIth cranial nerves result from inflammation and exudate affecting the meninges at the base of the brain. Papilloedema usually indicates raised ICP but in some cases a swollen optic disc may be caused by septic optic neuritis in which case the visual acuity is severely disturbed.

Non-neurological signs which may be helpful include skin rashes which are evident in about a third of cases. Meningococcal infection is accompanied by a diffuse maculopapular rash in two-thirds of cases and this may become petechial and then frankly purpuric and be accompanied by shock. Other bacteria which may induce skin rashes are staphylococci, pneumococci, listeria, and haemophilus. Rashes caused by sensitivity reactions to antibiotics are unlikely to occur in the earliest stages of meningitis. Pneumonia frequently accompanies pneumococcal meningitis. It is important to search for any contemporaneous illness or focus of infection and obtain material for laboratory culture.

It has already been mentioned that the conscious level is of paramount importance in determining prognosis. It must be assessed and monitored closely. Unfortunately, our ability to influence it by treatment remains rather limited, not least because we do not fully understand the pathophysiological processes which cause deterioration. The present position may be briefly summarized thus. Bacteria which possess neurotropic properties penetrate the blood–brain barrier from the bloodstream in which they are protected from circulating complement by their polysaccharide capsule. In the CSF a neutrophil response is induced. Bacterial cell wall components are released into CSF where they stimulate the production of inflammatory cytokines including interleukins 1 and 6, tumour necrosis factor, and prostaglandins. Inflammation and further blood–brain barrier disruption ensue. Cerebral blood flow increases and vasogenic cerebral oedema pushes up ICP. The inflammatory products induce cytotoxic oedema which in turn cause interstitial oedema by limiting the flow of CSF from subarachnoid space to the bloodstream. ICP rises further, cerebral blood flow drops, vasculitis, and inflammation spread more widely, cerebral autoregulation is compromised and cerebral over-or underperfusion cause further brain damage (Quagliarello and Scheld 1992; Tunkel and Scheld 1993). Experimental studies of several agents capable of modifying or inhibiting some of these reactions are underway.

Management

From a clinical management perspective, whatever the mechanism, ICP is raised in bacterial meningitis. Experience suggests that this factor is frequently neglected and it is my belief that this neglect contributes considerably to the morbidity and mortality associated with the condition. Lumbar puncture in such circumstances is clearly hazardous and this has been confirmed by several studies (Horwitz *et al.* 1980; Minns *et al.* 1989; Rennick *et al.* 1993). The last of these studies shows, and experience confirms, that even after apparently normal brain imaging with CT or MR (magnetic resonance), CSF pressure may be dangerously high. At present, the best and not infallible parameters of when to carry out a lumbar puncture are clinical, reinforced by experience. If there are focal signs, if the patient cannot be readily roused, if neck stiffness is very marked, or if papilloedema or IIIrd or VIth nerve palsies are present it is best not to do a lumbar puncture, and to treat the patient on a 'best guess' basis guided by clinical circumstances. If brain imaging is normal I prefer to give such patients mannitol and dexamethasone before LP. In any event, the decision to examine the CSF in such a situation should be referred by junior medical staff to a senior colleague. CSF may be examined later when deemed safe and evidence of bacterial infection can be demonstrated by PCR or other molecular or immunological techniques (Desforges 1992).

When CSF has safely been obtained, the findings which confirm bacterial meningitis are a raised cell count with polymorphs predominating by 60%, elevation of the protein content, and reduction in glucose, which should be compared with a sample of venous blood taken simultaneously. A CSF : blood ratio of less than 0.3 is abnormal and is found in about 75% of cases, but is not a specific finding. Fresh CSF should be examined under the microscope after appropriate staining, by an experienced bacteriologist and cultures set up, and here a phone call to the laboratory to explain the circumstances of the case beforehand can pay immediate dividends. There are few situations which are more irritating than to get a report from the laboratory that Gram-positive cocci have been demonstrated on the film in the middle of the night, which is then contradicted in the morning by a senior colleague reporting the presence of appropriately staining debris which has been mistakenly reported as bacteria. Given adequate warning and full details of the case, most laboratories will provide a positive identification of the organism in over 80% of cases, but they do need clinical information to provide the best service. Many tests have been used over the years to try to separate bacterial from other forms of meningitis but none has been sufficiently specific to be consistently useful. Whether newer molecular biological methods are better remains to be proved.

Imaging of the intracranial contents should be carried out in cases of meningitis prior to lumbar puncture if there are focal signs or anxieties about raised intracranial pressure. It is best to ask for neuroradiological help if it is available, for some of the changes may be subtle, particularly in the early stages. MRI scans reveal more than CT but they are not so available in emergency and are not always appropriate to a very ill patient. For MR imaging the patient must be capable of lying still within a claustrophobic tunnel for 30 minutes or longer. It is possible to carry out MR imaging on seriously ill patients who require assisted ventilation but the anaesthetic equipment must be free from magnetic influence, and few centres are able to provide this facility. Early in the course of meningitis the CT scan is likely to be normal. Paranasal sinuses, including sphenoidal and ethmoid, should be inspected for fluid levels and evidence of chronic infection, similarly the mastoid air cells. Skull bone should be interrogated for fractures. Meningeal enhancement around the base of the skull, and enhancement of ventricular ependyma indicate meningitis. Small ventricles and effacement of cortical sulci indicate cerebral oedema, and enlarged ventricles point to hydrocephalus from obstruction. It may be possible to determine if there is evidence of uncal herniation and to see the position of the cerebellar tonsils in relation to foramen magnum. Infarction, subdural collections, and space occupation from abscess formation are detectable (Cabral *et al.* 1987; Sze and Zimmerman 1988).

Blood cultures should be set up and samples obtained from any obvious foci of infection. Blood electrolytes, osmolality, and gases should be monitored closely because inappropriate secretion of antidiuretic hormone can cause a potentially catastrophic fall in sodium level. Particularly with meningococcal infection, blood clotting factors and platelets need to be watched closely because of the danger of disseminated intravascular coagulation. Other tests are carried out according to clinical need.

Drug treatment

Treatment must be started immediately the diagnosis is established. It is prudent to discuss antibiotic choices with a bacteriologist or with a colleague specializing in infectious diseases who will have knowledge of local and nosocomial patterns of infection. Once decided, the antibiotic should be given parenterally at a rate and in a dose sufficient to achieve and maintain bactericidal levels in CSF 20 times higher than the minimal bactericidal concentration *in vitro*. *There is no place for the use of intrathecal antibiotics.* Every three or four years I am called on to see a patient who has been given penicillin intrathecally in grossly excessive dose and the outcome is usually fatal. Bacteriologists sometimes have a touching faith in

the literature concerning the dosage schedules of the latest antibiotics and may seek to persuade you that oral administration twice a day is adequate. Such advice should be resisted. While I do not suggest that antibiotics should be prescribed in a cavalier fashion, with meningitis there may be only one chance and in my view it is better to err on the side of antibiotic overkill. Potential adverse effects from such a course of action are substantially less disabling than those seen following inadequate treatment of meningitis. For *Haemophilus influenzae* type B meningitis a third-generation cephalosporin is recommended because an increasing number of beta-lactamase-producing strains are resistant to ampicillin and a small number now produce chloramphenicol acetyl transferase. Meningococcal and pneumococcal meningitis are best treated with penicillin. There is increasing evidence that mortality figures can be reduced in children if the doctor who sees the patient at home gives an injection of penicillin immediately before sending the child to hospital, provided there are no contraindications to the use of penicillin. Some pneumococcal strains and a few meningococci have been reported to be resistant to penicillin, and for these and for people with penicillin allergy, a third-generation cephalosporin or vancomycin can be given (Kaplan and Fishman 1988; Klein *et al.* 1992). Gram-negative bacillary meningitis should be given a third-generation cephalosporin, group B streptococci a combination of penicillin and ampicillin to cover those rare strains which are penicillin-resistant, *Staph. aureus* flucloxacillin in high dose with vancomycin for penicillin allergy, and *Listeria* ampicillin with co-trimaxazole for penicillin allergies. Anaerobic infections are best managed with a combination of penicillin, chloramphenicol, and metronidazole. When no organism can be identified children and adults can be given a third-generation cephalosporin, and the elderly a combination of a third-generation cephalosporin and ampicillin. For the immuno compromised if the defect is cellular, ampicillin will cover *Listeria*; humoral is treated with penicillin and a third-generation cephalosporin and neutropaenia with a third-generation cephalosporin and an aminoglycoside to cover *Pseudomonas*.

Adequate cardiorespiratory function, oxygenation, and tissue perfusion must be maintained. Intracranial pressure rises maximally in the first 48 hours and should be treated with a combination of dexamethasone and mannitol. If the patient's conscious level deteriorates, intracranial pressure monitoring should be used and if the pressure rises above 15 mmHg the head of the bed should be raised and hyperventilation induced (Pickard and Czosnyka 1993).

Several anti-inflammatory agents are being evaluated to determine if they will inhibit the various stages of inflammation and the release of bacterial cell wall products, and clinical results are awaited (Townsend and Scheld 1993). Dexamethasone has been used in this context and preliminary results with children have been encouraging (Lebel *et al.* 1988; Odio *et al.* 1991). Unfortunately, it does not look as though this is the case with adults and further results are awaited. My practice at present is to give dexamethasone in a dose of 0.15 mg/kg body weight 6-hourly for 4 days, starting as soon as possible and preferably before antibiotics are given.

Communication

Once a diagnosis of meningitis has been established, communication should be facilitated between the medical team, the patient, if in a state to understand, and the relatives. There is much misunderstanding about meningitis in the populace (from which nurses, paramedics, and doctors are not exempt). Realistic reassurance about the course of the disease should be given together with an explanation of the treatments being used. Relatives find it helpful to have explained to them what all the tubes going into and coming from the patient are for. If any form of operative intervention is likely to be required, such as tracheostomy or burr holes, it should be anticipated by the medical team and explanations given well beforehand. Once the causal organism is identified, community and public health physicians can be alerted if appropriate. In the case of children and students, experience suggests that no matter which organism is implicated, it is prudent to discuss the case with the local medical officer because he/she will learn of it from the educational institute in any event. A diagnosis of meningococcal meningitis means that 'kissing contacts', household contacts, and classmates need to be identified and offered prophylaxis, usually with rifampicin but it should be noted that resistant strains are emerging and alternatives may be necessary (Cuevas and Hart 1993). This is best dealt with by a consultant in infectious diseases. If the organism is *Haemophilus*, infant household contacts and perhaps others should be offered similar prophylaxis. Permission should be obtained to permit discussion with colleagues in the patient's workplace, who are often alarmed at the prospect that they may contract the disease. In these times, it is well to anticipate that when a diagnosis of meningitis is made in a schoolchild the press and broadcasting media are likely to become involved. However distasteful the prospect, it is better that they have informed comment to report, and co-operation with their requests for information and interviews should be complied with. A sympathetic commentator can often help to allay public fears, a hostile one can compound them. Clinicians should be prepared to make themselves available for these purposes and not leave the communication of medical details to lay administrators.

Prevention of bacterial meningitis is now a viable proposition with immunization. Encouraging results have been obtained against *Haemophilus* and against meningococcal and pneumococcal infection.

OTHER FORMS OF BACTERIAL MENINGITIS

Less common forms of bacterial meningitis also have to be considered. Tuberculosis (TB) has never disappeared from the scene and there is some evidence that it is becoming more of a problem in the general population, and mycobacterial infection is being recognized with increasing frequency amongst the AIDS population. Tuberculous meningitis accounts for between 5% and 10% of all cases of TB seen in Britain. At present it is very much a disease of immigrant groups, but not exclusive to them. Central nervous system TB is always a complication of TB elsewhere in the body but this may not be clinically evident. In children, TB may be brought to light by an acute infectious disease such as pertussis or measles. Rarely, the onset may be acute or even fulminant, in which case it is indistinguishable from other bacterial meningitides and the diagnosis may be missed unless there is evidence of TB elsewhere, or acid and alcohol-fast bacilli (AAFB) are seen on the microscopic preparation. The usual history is less acute, with a prodrome which may take 2–3 weeks of lethargy, irritability, anorexia, depression, confusion, and abnormal behaviour which is not uncommonly misinterpreted as being of psychiatric origin. Meningeal symptoms and signs follow with signs of raised intracranial pressure and cranial nerve palsies caused by basal exudation and arteritis. Rarely, choroidal tubercles may be seen on fundoscopy. CSF examination (with appropriate precautions) yields a fluid which may be slightly turbid or yellow and has a mononuclear pleocytosis, high protein content and reduced glucose. AAFB may be seen on the smear and the detection rate is in proportion to the experience of the observer. Unfortunately, it takes many weeks to culture the organism in the laboratory.

As with other forms of meningitis the application of the newer immunological and molecular biological techniques has not been as sensitive as we would like, and at the time of writing there is no test which can be done on CSF that will provide an instant answer. PCR is perhaps the most promising. It is therefore frequently necessary to commence treatment for TB without bacterial confirmation of the diagnosis. If there is evidence of TB elsewhere in the body the decision is made easier. If not, other causes of more chronic, lymphocytic meningitides need to be considered before anti-TB chemotherapy is started. These include brucella, fungi and parasites, sarcoidosis, and malignant meningitis.

There are no specific findings on brain imaging. Hydrocephalus is common the longer the disease persists and may require surgical treatment. Basal meningeal enhancement and areas of infarction are also seen. Some cases go on to develop tuberculomas, even after apparently adequate treatment. (Fig. 15.1). When the diagnosis has been decided and a treatment regime is required, it is my practice to consult a specialist in tuberculosis because patterns of drug resistance are developing world-wide and are subject to change. It is not uncommon for the recommendation to be to treat with as many as five front-line drugs in the first instance—streptomycin, rifampicin, pyrazinamide, ethambutol, and isoniazid—and modify the regime subsequently in the light of sensitivity reports. I never use second-line drugs without such expert advice. On such treatment, the patient must be monitored closely for side-effects, and blood and CSF levels are estim-

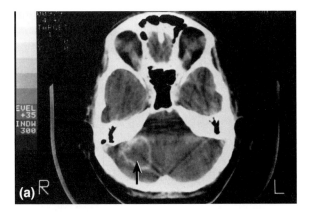
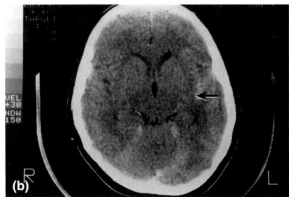
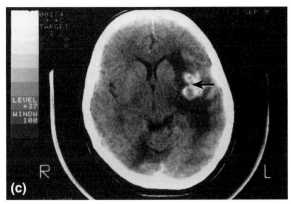
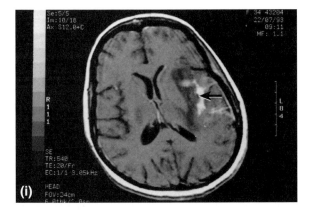
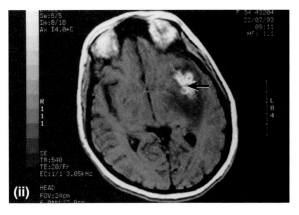

Fig. 15.1 Serial CT and MRI brain scans of an Indian woman with TB meningitis who, during a course of anti-TB chemotherapy, developed a right cerebellar tuberculoma [CT scan (a)], while meningeal enhancement of meningitis was evident in the left Sylvian fissure [CT scan (b)]. Following surgical excision of the cerebellar lesion, a further tuberculoma continued to develop in the left Sylvian fissure [MRI scans (i) and (ii), and CT scan (c)] after many months of anti-TB chemotherapy. Following the original surgical excision of the cerebellar lesion the patient has remained clinically well.

ated frequently. Despite such precautions it has been my unhappy experience to have treated two patients who died, in each of whom the diagnosis was expeditiously and accurately made, appropriate drugs, confirmed by subsequent sensitivity

reports, were given in adequate dosage confirmed by CSF drug levels. The first developed a hypothalamic tuberculoma and the second, upper spinal cord and brainstem adhesions. There is no evidence that intrathecal steroids have a beneficial effect, nor that dexamethasone used systemically is helpful, although we all use it if there is evidence of raised ICP. The length of time for which anti-TB chemotherapy should be given has not been established with certainty. Most give it for a year and some have reported success with a 9-month or even 6-month regime.

The same considerations should be extended to the families of patients with tubercular meningitis (TBM) as has been described above. I give a more guarded prognosis because the outcome is even more difficult to predict and the evolution of the illness is longer. The incidence of sequelae is also higher. Family and workplace contacts may need to be seen and followed up, so liaison with TB and public health doctors is important.

Infection with spirochaetes can rarely cause meningitis which if recognized quickly can be treated successfully. Syphilis causes an acute form of meningitis indistinguishable clinically from other forms of bacterial meningitis. This occurs within two years of the original infection. The CSF findings are of a mononuclear pleocytosis and raised protein and positive VDRL test with confirmation by a positive FTA-Abs test. Such cases are being recognized more frequently in association with AIDS when the disease may be rather more aggressive and behave in an atypical fashion (Katz *et al.* 1993). Treatment is with parenteral penicillin for 10 days with steroid cover for the first 24 hours to counter the effects of a Jarisch–Herxheimer reaction to the products of treponemal disintegration. All such cases should have repeat CSF examinations to ensure that treatment has been effective and reinfection has not occurred. It is important that contacts be traced and treated, frequently a difficult and delicate task which is best done by professional contact tracers who are attached to GUM (genitourinary medicine) or AIDS clinics. The other spirochaete which may cause acute meningitis is *Borrelia burgdorferi*, the agent of Lyme disease. Although rare in Britain, Lyme disease should be considered in the differential diagnosis of meningitis for which no cause can be found, and the diagnosis is confirmed by immunological examination of blood and CSF for raised titres to the organism. Treatment is with third-generation cephalosporins given parenterally for two weeks.

Rickettsial infection is rarely evident in Britain but must be considered if the patient has been abroad within the last month. The incubation period of most forms is two to three weeks, and the organisms, which are inoculated into humans by the bite of a mite or tick, produce their effects by invading small blood vessels where they induce endothelial and perivascular inflammation and thrombosis which results in meningoencephalitis if the brain is affected. Q fever (*Coxiella burnetti*) and typhus (*Rickettsia prowazekii*) are found world-wide, Rocky mountain spotted fever (*R. rickettsii*) in the Americas, Mediterranean spotted fever (*R. conorii*) in the Mediterranean basin, Africa and Asia, and scrub typhus (*R. tsutsugamushi*) in the Pacific, Australia, and Asia. The individual syndromes vary in detail but all share the clinical features of high fever, headache, and skin rashes, and meningoencepahalitis which develops in the second week. Sometimes, the rash may not be evident. Confusion, convulsions, and coma ensue in severe cases. There are no diagnostic features on scan or CSF examination and treatment with tetracycline for 10 days should be given if rickettsial infection is suspected and confirmed serologically later (Shaked 1991).

Such cases are best discussed with a consultant in infectious diseases.

ENCEPHALITIS

When pathogenic organisms invade brain tissue directly, the resultant inflammatory reaction together with the neurotropism of the organism, cause dysfunction of neurones and results clinically in encephalitis. The pathogen in the vast majority of cases is a virus and in certain locations malaria, rickettsiae, and fungi are important causes. A similar syndrome may be caused by an allergic or immunological reaction to a viral trigger producing peri-venous demyelination and after a latent period, post-infectious encephalitis. The usual route of entry of virus to the brain is haematogenous. A few, such as herpes simplex and rabies, ascend to the brain centripetally along axons from the periphery.

Viral encephalitis is fairly common. Because cases are not notified in Britain it is difficult to know the true incidence. It is said that 20 000 cases occur annually in the United States (almost certainly an underestimate). In Europe, cases occur sporadically and accompany infections such as mumps, measles, chicken pox, and rarely cytomegalovirus and Epstein–Barr virus infection. Elsewhere, in the United States and Asia, cases occur sporadically and in epidemic form, the latter due to arboviruses.

Clinical features

Certain clinical features are shared by all cases of encephalitis. There is an overlap with the meningitic syndromes in that neck stiffness and photophobia may be encountered. Similarly, there is often a prodrome of malaise, non-specific upper respiratory symptoms, myalgia, arthralgia, fever, parotitis, or skin rash. Because encephalitis implies parenchymal brain disease, disturbance of consciousness and epileptic seizures are more common than with meningitis. Headache, confusion, disorientation, speech upset and drowsiness occur. Progression to coma may follow and accompany signs of raised ICP. Focal signs of hemiparesis, spasticity, sensory loss, dysphasia, ataxia, incoordination, hallucinations, and memory upset serve to indicate that part of the brain which is bearing the brunt of the infection. Some viruses demonstrate tropism to particular parts of the brain. Herpes simplex virus (HSV) colonizes the temporal lobes, rabies the limbic system, and the resultant clinical manifestations have diagnostic significance. Evidence of infection elsewhere should be sought—the rash of measles, parotitis of mumps. Has there been a recent insect bite? Has there been travel abroad to areas with known vectors of arbovirus disease, and has the patient undertaken activities which may render him liable to the bite of ticks? (Although rare in Britain I have seen Central European encephalitis in Birmingham.)

Herpes simplex encephalitis (HSE), the most common form of sporadic viral encephalitis seen in Europe, can affect any age group. The onset may be abrupt but is often insidious and can be quite difficult to diagnose in the early stages because hallucinations, personality change, and psychiatric disturbance resulting from frontal and temporal lobe damage may mimic psychosis or drug abuse. When seizures, further focal signs of hemiparesis or dysphasia and then coma ensue, it may be too late for treatment to be effective. Finding focal signs in a patient with encephalitis makes it likely that HSV is the cause, but it is well to remember that other conditions such as cerebral abscess or granuloma, brain tumour and stroke with infection can have a similar presentation (Whitley *et al.* 1989). The encephalitis of chicken pox differs from the others in attacking the cerebellum and has a good prognosis.

Rabies is hardly a common disease in Britain and is mentioned briefly as a reminder that the exotic can appear on the doorstep—I have seen two cases in Birmingham. The infection is contracted abroad from an animal bite three weeks to three months before, on average, but it may have been so long before that it has been forgotten. The initial symptoms are non-specific as for other forms of encephalitis, soon to be followed by symptoms and signs of cerebral irritation and excitement, then 'hydrophobia' with laryngeal and pharyngeal spasm succeeded by convulsions, coma and death.

Management

Once a diagnosis of encephalitis has been considered, investigation must be carried out rapidly to exclude other conditions and to confirm the diagnosis. Blood tests are not of initial diagnostic use but may be helpful in retrospect to demonstrate a rise in viral titres. Biochemical upset should be corrected. It is prudent to set up blood cultures, and if there is a history of travel abroad, it is imperative to have blood smears examined for malarial parasites. Brain imaging should be carried out to determine if there is space occupation or areas of focal necrosis or infarction in the temporal lobes to suggest herpes simplex encephalitis (HSE). MRI is much more sensitive than CT in demonstrating abnormalities of encephalitis but there are restrictions which limit its usefulness, as described above. This is one of the few circumstances in which the EEG may be diagnostically useful. In encephalitis, the EEG is abnormal with diffuse slow wave activity and sometimes seizure activity which is quite non-specific. In HSE, however, there may be focal abnormality arising from the temporal lobe with high voltage spike and slow wave complexes which, although not pathognomonic is highly suggestive of the diagnosis. It is usually necessary to examine the

CSF to exclude bacterial meningitis after appropriate precautions have been taken. In most viral encephalitides the cell count is raised with mononuclear cells predominating. Red cells may be found if there is necrosis, as with HSE. Protein is raised and glucose is normal. In the past, brain biopsy was used to confirm the diagnosis of HSE. I believe this is no longer justifiable, unless to exclude other pathology such as abscess or granuloma, because treatment of HSE now is relatively effective and does not carry the severe toxic side-effects of previous regimens. As with other varieties of CNS infection, the application of PCR and other techniques to detect viral antigen in CSF is promising.

The treatment of viral encephalitis is symptomatic, with analgesia for headache, anticonvulsants for seizures, and the maintenance of adequate hydration and electrolyte replacement and nutrition. In practice, most neurologists give dexamethasone to reduce brain swelling if it is suspected. Acyclovir is given relatively freely to most patients in whom no aetiology has been established or in whom HSE is suspected. It should be given as early as possible in a dose of 10 mg/kg body weight intravenously by infusion, 8-hourly for 10 days.

AIDS

Infection of the CNS is a very frequent accompaniment of AIDS. Indeed, entry of the HIV virus to the CNS appears to be an essential part of its ecology. In many AIDS patients this invasion remains asymptomatic, sometimes for years; in others, clinical manifestations occur at, or soon, after seroconversion. When immune defences have been destroyed in the later stages of AIDS the neuraxis is vulnerable to infection by a wide range of organisms. In practice in Britain, when such infection occurs in a patient already known to have AIDS, the patient will usually be referred directly to an AIDS or infectious diseases doctor and the neurologist's involvement will be minimal. However, the initial presentation of AIDS may be with just such an infection which may present to the neurologist, and the message is that AIDS must be considered in the differential diagnosis of a large number of infectious syndromes, particularly if there is anything atypical. Then, testing for HIV must be carried out as a matter of urgency, after appropriate counselling, which may not be possible if the patient is confused or unconscious. In such circumstances I have found it useful to invoke the services of the local AIDS team whose members can cope sympathetically with such eventualities.

A list of the infections which may occur in AIDS patients is listed in Table 15.4. A complete description of all these syndromes is beyond the scope of this review. For further details the reader is referred to Sande and Voberding (1995). The aseptic meningitis of AIDS occurs at about the time of seroconversion or later and there are no specific features. Because HIV invades the neuraxis early and persists there, CSF studies cannot confirm that HIV causes a particular syndrome. Cryptococcal meningitis can vary in severity from a very mild syndrome to severe meningoencephalitis. CSF in the former may be almost normal. Search should be made for the organism with Indian ink preparations and here correlation with the bacteriology laboratory is essential. Cryptococcal antigen should be sought in CSF and in serum. It is almost always present in the blood of patients who have cryptococcal meningitis and this may be useful in screening out suspects. Treatment is with amphotercin which is highly toxic and it is prudent to ask advice about dosage schedules from AIDS doctors. Meningitis which is caused by TB or syphilis may behave in an aggressive fashion in AIDS patients, and there is some evidence that the disease processes are modified in this direction by the HIV virus. Treatment must be correspondingly aggressive. Diagnosis of other forms of fungal meningitis will depend upon geographical location.

Toxoplasmosis in AIDS patients usually takes the form of focal brain disturbance. In some there may be a fulminating diffuse encephalopathy with poorly defined microabscesses on brain imaging. In areas of high HIV prevelance this is often the presenting manifestation of AIDS. The clinical findings are varied. There may be mental disturbance and psychiatric disorder, seizures, focal weakness, sensory deficit, or cerebellar disturbance. Brain imaging with MR is the modality of choice and characteristically shows multiple, bilateral, hypodense, enhancing lesions with predilection for the basal ganglia and white/grey matter confluence (Ciricillo and Rosenblaum 1990). If only one lesion is seen there is a fair chance that it may not be due to toxoplasma but to lymphoma and biopsy should be undertaken. If multiple lesions are evident treatment should be given with pyrimethamine and sulfadiazine. These drugs are toxic and may cause marrow supression, therefore close monitoring is necessary. Improvement should be expected after two weeks. If there has been none, biopsy

Table 15.4 Infections in AIDS

Meningitis: common
Aseptic

Meningitis: uncommon
TB
Syphilis
Histoplasmosis
Coccidiodomycosis

Encephalitis
Toxoplasmosis
Cytomegalovirus
Herpes simplex
AIDS dementia complex
PMLE (Progressive multifocal leuko encephalopathy)

Focal brain disease
Toxoplasmosis
TB abscess
PMLE
Cryptococcoma
Herpes simplex encephalitis
Varicella-zoster encephalitis

should be done. Encephalitides associated with cytomegalovirus (CMV) and herpes simplex virus (HSV) have no specific features.

MALARIA

This is not a common disease in Britain but it is the most common parasitic disease world-wide and is imported to Britain with increasing frequency—between 12 and 20 people die from it here each year, usually because it has not been diagnosed in time. Cerebral malaria is due to infection by *Plasmodium falciparum*. Female *Anopheles* mosquitoes inject sporozoites into the blood when they bite humans. These are hoovered up by the liver where asexual reproduction takes place following which motile merozoites are released into the blood where they invade red cells and undergo further asexual reproduction. The progeny from this rupture from the red cells and invade other red cells at 48-hour intervals and this dispersal is accompanied by fever. The parasites within red cells induce changes within the cells which make them adhere to vascular endothelium where they congregate in small cerebral venules to produce congestion and hypoxia. Simulaneously, immune-mediated inflammation is taking place with the release of vasoactive substances which cause further endothelial damage. These changes result in the clinical manifestations of cerebral malaria.

Those who are most at risk of developing severe malaria are pregnant women, the immunosuppressed, and the emigrant returning home after a long time away from his native country, whose immunity has lapsed. Asia, Africa, Central and South America, the Middle East, and Eastern Mediterranean should be regarded as potentially infective zones and anyone returning to Britain from these areas who falls ill with an influenza-like syndrome or encephalopathy should be suspected of suffering from malaria and treated accordingly. Death can occur within 72 hours if it not recognized and even if treatment is given the mortality rate may approach 50%. The presentation may be with non-specific influenza-like symptoms. The conscious level becomes depressed, convulsions commonly occur, particularly in children, and there is evidence of an acute organic brain syndrome. Anaemia, jaundice, and hepatosplenomegaly may be found.

Diagnosis is by demonstration of the parasite on blood smears. Thick and thin smears should be taken, the laboratory alerted and the films looked at by an experienced microscopist. If no parasites are seen treatment should be given and the blood examined every 4–6 hours for the next two days. Discussion with an expert in tropical diseases is appropriate. Electrolytes, blood gases, and sugar levels must be closely monitored. There is seldom need to examine the CSF if the diagnosis is confirmed, but this may be necessary if meningitis is suspected in which case the usual precautions are observed. Pyogenic meningitis and Gram-negative septicaemia are recognized accompaniments of cerebral malaria. CT imaging shows no specific pattern and is commonly normal without evidence of cerebral oedema. Nevertheless, CSF pressure is high. Unfortunately, routine administration of dexamethasone has not improved the prognosis. Patients with suspected malaria should be nursed in an intensive care unit.

Resistance to chloroquine of *P. falciparum* is widespread. Quinine is therefore the drug of choice. Check if any has been given in the preceding two days. If not, it is given by *slow* intravenous infusion after an initial loading dose has been administered. It *must not be injected as a bolus*. It may be necessary to double the loading dose for patients who have come from Southeast Asia. The dose commonly used is 5 mg/kg body weight infused over 2 hours every 8–12 hours. An antifolate metabolite, doxycycline or pyrimethemine-sulfadoxine, should also be given. In severe cases exchange transfusion may be necessary, and dialysis may be needed for renal failure. Gram-negative septicaemia and hypoglycaemia should be looked for.

INTRACRANIAL SUPPURATION

By convention, included under this heading are brain abscess, subdural empyema, and extradural abscess. Some features are common to all three yet their clinical profiles are sufficiently distinct to merit separate description.

BRAIN ABSCESS

This is an uncommon condition in general neurological practice—the incidence is estimated to be 1 per 10 000 admissions to a general hospital, or about 5 cases in 1 million population each year (McClelland *et al.* 1978). This is certainly an underestimate. Some go undiagnosed and are found at necropsy and personal experience suggests that AIDS and other diseases causing immunosuppression provide a fertile mileu for the development of suppuration. The organisms which cause brain abscess, and their variety increases year by year, reach the brain by travelling in the bloodstream, by direct extension from an adjacent focus of infection, or by direct implantation following a compound skull fracture or penetrating injury. In a fifth of all cases the source of the infection cannot be identified. Abscesses caused by middle ear disease occur in the temporal lobe or cerebellum, paranasal sinusitus spreads to affect the deeper regions of the temporal lobes and the frontal lobes, and blood-borne abscesses are often multiple and have a tendency to occur at the grey/white matter border where blood supply is relatively poor. Chronic pulmonary sepsis, cyanotic congenital cardiac disease, pulmonary ateriovenous fistulae, and dental caries are common sources of haematogenous abscesses. In any case of suspected abscess diligent search must be made for potential foci of infection, and when found they must be eradicated forthwith or reinfection may occur.

Brain abscess may affect any age group. Commonly, the presentation is as an emergency with features suggestive of a space-occupying lesion which mimics a brain tumour. The combination of rapid onset of raised intracranial pressure (ICP), focal neurology, and signs of infection is characteristic but unfortunately occurs in only about half of all patients. Headache is a common symptom and epileptic convulsions which are commonly generalized but may be focal, complicate up to one-third of cases. Focal signs point to the area of the brain which is affected. Neck stiffness is present in 25% of cases as a consequence of incipient coning, coexistent meningitis, or an inflammatory reaction in the CSF. In young children, vomiting, fits, and an enlarging head may suggest brain tumour. Sometimes the signs of the predisposing infection mask progression of the abscess. In others the onset is insidious, over weeks or months, with no evidence of infection. I have seen one case whose presentation was of headache and personality deterioration for some months, and who had a chronic frontal lobe abscess with a very thick capsule. He had suffered a fracture of his skull and nasal bones 16 years before in a road traffic accident and this was the likely source of infection. The differential diagnosis of brain abscess is therefore very wide and includes tumour, stroke, encephalitis, and meningitis. It might be expected that fever would be a feature of brain abscess. It does occur in about two-thirds of cases but is commonly intermittent. The absence of fever and signs of infection does not exclude brain abscess as a diagnosis (Chun *et al.* 1986; Mampalan and Rosenblum 1988).

As soon as an abscess is suspected the diagnosis must be confirmed immediately and treatment commenced as soon as possible because, as in other forms of neurological infection, delay worsens the prognosis. Help will be required from other disciplines and it is essential that the radiologist, neurosurgeon, and bacteriologist are alerted to the problem and briefed as soon as possible. Precise localization of the lesion or lesions, because they are often multiple, particularly those which are spread haematogenously, is best achieved by CT scanning. MRI may provide more detailed information of white matter abnormality but has constraints when used on a confused and restless patient and is not often available for emergency use. Interpretation of the CT appearances must be correlated with the stage of evolution of the abscess. At first there may be a low density area of cerebritis with surrounding oedema which can be readily misinterpreted as an intrinsic neoplasm or infarct. As the abscess matures the abnormal area will absorb contrast in a patchy fashion and later as encapsulation takes place, ring enhancement becomes evident. Interpretation of these changes which are often subtle and subject to timescale variation dependent on the virulence of the causal organism requires a degree of experience and it is always informative to discuss them with a neuroradiologist. Do not forget to look for evidence of infection in the sinuses and middle ear and for fractures. If a brain abscess is suspected, lumbar puncture should never be undertaken. Blood cultures and cultures from any obvious source of infection should be made.

When the diagnosis has been made, discussion with a neurosurgeon is appropriate. Not all agree when and if surgery should be carried out and which techniques should be used. If head trauma has taken place then toilet and debridement of the wound is necessary. Multiple lesions and deeply situated ones may be best left alone and treated on a 'best guess' basis of likely aetiology. Stereotactic biopsy may be appropriate if precise identification of the organism is needed and is said to be successful in 95% of cases. Space occupation requires surgical drainage. No matter which mode of treatment is used, the intracranial contents should be closely monitored by serial imaging and if the abscesses do not diminish in size, aspiration should be carried out. If the patient is immunosuppressed, stereotactic aspiration should be used to allow organism identification.

Results from treatment with antibiotics alone without aspiration are encouraging (Boom and Tuazon 1985).

Successful identification of the organism after aspiration has a better chance of success if the bacteriologist is involved from the beginning because he can arrange to receive the specimen straight from theatre and set up special cultures which are necessary for anaerobic, fastidious, and exotic organisms, including fungi. Abscesses from the ear often have a mixed flora of streptococci, enterobacteriaceae, and *Bacillis fragilis*. Sinus infection commonly spawns *Strep. milleri* and *Bacteroides*. Congenital heart disease is likely to be associated with *Strep. viridans* and microaerophilic and anaerobic streptococci, pulmonary disease with anaerobes, streptococci, actinomycetes, and fusobacteria, and dental sepsis with these organisms and *Bacteroides*. Those who are immunocompromised may have a wide range of fungi—*Toxoplasma* and *Nocardia*. Penetrating head wounds grow staphylococci, streptococci, and *Claustridium*.

Antibiotic treatment is started as soon as specimens have been obtained or the decision has been made not to aspirate. The favoured empirical regime at present is penicillin, 24 mega units iv (intravenous) daily, with chloramphenicol 1g iv every 6 hours, and metronidazole. For staphylococci, a choice of one of flucloxacillin, fusidic acid, nafcillin, or vancomycin should be used. In cases with AIDS, treatment for toxoplasmosis should be given and if the toxoplasma serology test is negative biopsy of the lesion should be carried out. The length of time for which treatment is given depends on the clinical and radiological response. Dexamethasone and mannitol are used for acute reduction of raised ICP. Anticonvulsants are given for epilepsy and may need to be continued for some years later because the risk of seizures following successful treatment of brain abscess is not insubstantial.

SUBDURAL EMPYEMA

This is a much rarer entity than brain abscess. Infection spreads between the arachnoid and dura from infection in the paranasal sinuses or middle ear, or from osteomyelitis of the skull. Meningitis may be complicated by subdural effusions which become infected. Sometimes, infection is blood-borne. It is a disease of the young; 50% of cases are aged less than 20

years, 75% are less than 30. Males are affected more than twice as frequently as females. Presentation is as an emergency and by contrast with brain abscess, pyrexia and clinical evidence of infection is usually present. There may be signs of raised ICP, meningitis, and focal neurology. Epileptic seizures are more common than with brain abscess, are more likely to be focal and occur in as many as two-thirds of patients in the acute phase (Cowie and Williams 1983). Signs of local infection in sinuses, mastoid, or skull are common. The diagnosis is confirmed by brain imaging with CT or MR as available. Classically, there is a low density, peripheral, extracerebral collection over the surface of the hemispheres or in the parafacine area, with a peripheral rim of enhancement following injection of contrast. Bilateral lesions may show no shift of midline structures. Osteomyelitis of the skull, sinus infection and fluid levels, and otitis media may be visualized. Cultures should be taken from sites of obvious infection and from blood. Lumbar puncture must not be carried out. Treatment is surgical to remove pus, preferably by craniotomy, eradication of foci of infection, and antibiotic treatment appropriate to the organism or organisms isolated. Aerobic and anaerobic streptococci, staphylococci, *Proteus*, and *Pseudomonas* cause adult infection; *H. influenzae*, pneumococci and Gram-negative bacteria infect infants and children. Epileptic sizures are so common that regular, prophylactic anticonvulsant medication should be given to all cases.

EXTRADURAL ABSCESS

Extradural collections of pus occur as complications of adjacent infection which may be bacterial or fungal in the paranasal sinuses, skull bone, or mastoid. Signs of local infection are prominent and signs of neurological dysfunction are uncommon. Local headache and tenderness with pyrexia and malaise are common. Diagnosis is confirmed by CT or MR imaging and treatment is by surgical removal of infected material and administration of antibiotics which have the capability to penetrate bone.

Spinal infection results from hamatogenous spread of a pathogenic organism from the primary source, which may not be clinically evident, to the vertebrae to cause osteomyelitis which then affects the spinal cord, or to the epidural and neural structures directly. The original source may have been cellulitis, wound infection endocarditis, pelvic sepsis, pneumonia, or intravenous drug addiction. With the spread of immune suppression such cases are being seen more commonly. Exradural abscess is the commonest form, subdural is rare, and intraparenchymal cord abscess is exceptionally rare. Mid and lower thoracic and upper lumbar region are the favoured sites and any age group may be affected with most cases presenting between the ages of 20 and 50 years. Staphylococci are the commonest infecting bacteria followed by Gram-negative organisms from the pelvis and urinary tract. Tuberculosis, brucellosis, and various fungi may be pathogens. The first symptoms are of localized back pain followed by radicular discomfort and accompanied by signs of infection. If not recognized and treated at this stage, signs of cord or cauda equina dysfunction ensue. Spinal imaging with MR is the investigation of choice and CT is effective. Isotope bone imaging may highlight areas of increased signal before bony changes are established by other imaging modalities. Advice from a neuroradiologist is recommended. Treatment is with a combination of surgery; to obtain material for culture, to remove cord compression, and to stabilize the spine; with administration of antibiotics with the property of penetrating bone if there is osteomyelitis. Rehabilitation should start during the acute phase with appropriate input from experts.

REFERENCES

Boom, W. H. and Tuazon, C. V. (1985). Succesful treatment of multiple brain abscesses with antibiotics alone. *Rev Infect Dis*, **7**, 189–99.

Cabral, D. A., Flodmark, O., Farell, K., and Speert, D. P. (1987). Prospective study of computed tomography in acute bacterial meningitis. *J Pediatr*, **111**, 201–5.

Chun, C. H., Johnson, J. D., Hofstetter, M., and Raff, M. J. (1986). Brain abscess. A study of 45 consecutive cases. *Medicine*, **65**, 415–31.

Ciricillo, S. and Rosenblaum, M. L. (1990). Use of CT and MR imaging to distinguish intracranial lesions and to define the need for biopsy in AIDS patients. *J Neurosurg*, **73**, 720–4.

Cowie, R. and Williams, B. (1983). Late seizures and morbidity after subdural empyema. *J Neurosurg*, **58**, 569–73.

Cuevas, L. E. and Hart, C. A. (1993). Chemoprophylaxis of bacterial meningitis. *J Antimicrob Chem*, **31**, S79–91.

Desforges, J. F. (1992). The use of molecular methods in infectious diseases. *New Engl J Med*, **327**, 1290–7.

Feigin, R. D. and Shackelford, P. G. (1973). Value of repeat lumbar puncture in the differential diagnosis of meningitis. *N Engl J Med*, **289**, 571–4.

Hambleton, G. and Davies, P. A. (1975). Bacterial meningitis. Some aspects of diagnosis and treatment. *Arch Dis Child*, **50**, 674–8.

Horwitz, S. J., Boxerbaum, B., and O'Bell J. (1980). Cerebral herniation in bacterial meningitis in childhood. *Ann Neurol*, **7**, 524–8.

Kaplan, S. L. and Fishman, M. A. (1987). Supportive therapy for bacterial meningitis. *Pediatr Inf Dis J*, **6**, 670–7.

Kaplan, S. L. and Fishman, M. A. (1988). Update on bacterial meningitis. *Child Neurol*, **3**, 82–93.

Katz, D. A., Berger, J. R., and Duncan, R. C. (1993). Neurosyphilis. A comparative study of the effects of infection with human immunodeficiency virus. *Arch Neurol*, **50**, 243–9.

Klein, N. J., Heyderman, R. S., and Levin, M. (1992). Antibiotic choices for meningitis beyond the neonatal period. *Arch Dis Child*, **67**, 157–61.

Lebel, M. H., Freij, B. J., Syrogiannopoulos, G. A., Chrane, D. F., Hoyt, M. J., Stewart, S. M. *et al.* (1988). Dexamethasone therapy for bacterial meningitis. *New Engl J Med*, **319**, 964–71.

Lorber, J. and Sunderland, R. (1980). Lumbar puncture in children with convulsions associated with fever. *Lancet*, **1**, 785–6.

Mampalam, T. J. and Rosenblum, M. L. (1988). Trends in the management of bacterial brain abscess; a review of 102 cases over 17 years. *Neurosurgery*, **23**, 451–8.

McClelland, C. J., Craig, B. F., and Crockard, H. A. (1978). Brain abscesses in Northern Ireland: a 30-year community review. *J Neurol Neurosurg Psychiat*, **41**, 1043–7.

Minns, R. A., Engleman, H. M., and Stirling, H. (1989). Cerebrospinal fluid pressure in pyogenic meningitis. *Arch Dis Child*, **64**, 814–20.

Odio, C. M., Faingezicht, I., Paris, M., Nassar, M., Baltodano, A., Rogers, J. *et al.* (1991). The beneficial effects of early dexamethasone administration in infants and children with bacterial meningitis. *New Engl J Med*, **324**, 1525–31.

Pickard, J. D. and Czosnyka, M. (1993). Management of raised intracranial pressure. *J Neurol Neurosurg Psychia*, **56**, 845–55.

Quagliarello, V. and Scheld, W. M. (1992). Bacterial meningitis: pathogenesis, pathophysiology and progress. *New Engl J Med*, **327**, 864–72.

Rennick, G., Shann, F., and de Campo, J. (1993). Cerebral herniation during bacterial meningitis in children. *Brit Med J*, **306**, 953–5.

Rutter, N. and Smales, O. R. (1977). Role of routine investigations in children presenting with their first febrile convulsion. *Arch Dis Child*, **52**, 188–91.

Sande, M. A. and Volberding, P. A. (1995). *The medical management of AIDS*, (4th edn). W. B. Saunders, Philadelphia.

Shaked, Y. (1991). Rickettsial infection of the central nervous system: the role of prompt antimicrobial therapy. *Q J Med*, **79**, 301–6.

Sze, G. and Zimmerman, R. D. (1988). The magnetic resonance imaging of infections and inflammatory diseases. *Radiol Clin North Amer*, **26**, 839–59.

Townsend, G. C. and Scheld, W. M. (1993). Adjunctive therapy for bacterial meningitis: rationale for use, current status and prospects for the future. *Clin Inf Dis*, **17**, S537–49.

Tunkel, A. R. and Scheld, W. M. (1993). Pathogenesis and pathophysiology of bacterial meningitis. *Clin Microbiol Rev*, **6**, 118–36.

Wallgren, A. (1925). Une nouvelle maladie infectieuse du systeme nerveux central? (Meningite aigue). *Acta Paediatr Scand*, **4**, 158–82.

Whitley, R. J. *et al.* and the NIAID Collaborative Antiviral Study Group (1989). Diseases which mimic herpes simplex encephalitis: diagnosis, presentation and outcome. *JAMA*, **262**, 234–9.

16 *The value of a clinical genetics unit*

Sarah Bundey and Ian Sutton

Although neurological disorders that are caused by single genes are individually rare, collectively they form an appreciable part of neurological practice, so that about 1 per 1000 of the population suffers from a genetic neurological disorder and about 5 per 1000 are at high risk of developing or transmitting a serious neurological disease (Table 16.1). Such diseases usually cause chronic disability and so contribute unduly to neurological practice.

The rate of progress in the field of neurogenetics is remarkable. Several times a week, a new advance is reported concerning the molecular analysis of neurological disorders. How do these advances affect our understanding of genetic diseases and their clinical management? Clinical genetics units provide a co-ordinated service employing doctors, nurses, cytogeneticists, and molecular scientists. The clinicians are responsible for organizing genetic clinics, for ensuring that families understand the courses of action available, for keeping in contact with families through genetic registers, and for recalling patients should new advances occur which would be of relevance to their lives. Clinicians work closely with scientists to ensure that the most reliable and up-to-date advice is given to patients. Of course, doctors from other specialities also have access to the laboratory services provided and the scientific staff make it clear what tests are available, and what their limitations and reliability are.

THE GENETICS CLINIC

The aims of genetic counselling are to identify individuals at high risk of transmitting a serious disorder, and to offer information and advice on reproductive options. In these ways couples are helped to achieve their desired number of healthy children. The most important aspect is to ensure a correct diagnosis of the index patient and this is often aided by cytogenetic and/or molecular investigations; such tests can also be used to recognize asymptomatic gene-carrying relatives who carry the same mutation. Indeed, the burgeoning number of molecular tests that are now available for diagnosis and carrier detection have transformed the work pattern of clinical geneticists. This now has a greater emphasis on counselling for the psychological effects of familial diseases.

In X-linked disorders (e.g. Duchenne muscular dystrophy) and autosomal dominant disorders (e.g. Huntington's disease, HD), relatives outside the nuclear family will often be at high risk, and so genetic counsellors have to ensure that they are contacted and counselling offered (see Box 1). On average, for each living index patient with an X-linked or autosomal dominant disorder, there will be about six relatives to whom genetic information should be offered (Table 16.2).

The question of whether to test healthy relatives for a disease mutation must be carefully considered for each individual, since it may not always be wise to know a future that cannot be altered. Experience with HD shows that about 20% of those at high risk choose to have presymptomatic

Table 16.1 Approximate incidences and prevalences of some neurological disorders and estimates of numbers of 'at-risk' relatives per 100 000 of the population

Disease	Birth frequency[a]	Prevalence[a]	Relatives at risk*
X-linked muscular dystrophy	17	6	54
Myotonic dystrophy	14	7	37
Facioscapulohumeral muscular dystrophy	3	2	18
Spinal muscular atrophy	10	1	18
Hereditary neuropathies	25	20	180
Huntington's disease	33	7	65
Tuberous sclerosis	8	7	28
Neurofibromatosis type 1	40	20	80
Numerous rarer genetic diseases	50	20	72
Approximate totals	200	90	552

* Of 1 in 10 or greater, for being affected or for being carriers (estimated from figures in Table 16.2).
[a] Data from many sources, particularly Emery (1991), Royal College of Physicians (1991).

When you refer a patient for genetic counselling, please give full name, date of birth, together with maiden name if the patient is female. This is particularly important when referring for an X-linked disease. For example, most Duchenne brothers of women of childbearing age will now be known to one of the 23 regional genetic centres in the United Kingdom, and most recently diagnosed Huntington's disease patients will have been registered with a clinical genetics unit.

Table 16.2 Numbers of relatives at high genetic risk for different types of genetic diseases

Type of disease	Average number of relatives per family*
Inherited autosomal dominant condition	6–9
New dominant mutation	2
X-linked disorder in which new mutations are rare	6
X-linked disorder in which new mutations occur	3
Autosomal recessive condition	3

* Who have a greater than 1 in 10 risk for developing, or being a carrier for, the named disease.

testing, partly to plan their own futures, partly to know what to tell their children, and, increasingly, to discover their genetic status before having children.

Usually, the asymptomatic relatives who are tested will be adults, but from time to time there will be an indication to test asymptomatic children for genetic disorders. Such indications include the availability of strategies which affect the course of the disease (such as Wilson's disease or Von Hippel–Lindau disease), early diagnosis leading to useful information for the rest of the family, and assistance with the choice of a career.

THE CYTOGENETICS LABORATORY

Chromosome analysis is worth doing on neurological patients in the following situations:

(1) a female has an X-linked disorder;
(2) a patient has unexplained mental retardation;
(3) a major central nervous system malformation is present;
(4) two genetic conditions coexist in the same individual.

Some chromosomal aberrations are submicroscopic and if one is suspected on clinical grounds then the technique of fluorescent-*in-situ* hybridization (FISH) may be available. In FISH, a cosmid or a plasmid containing a probe for a specific chromosomal segment hybridizes to the patient's chromosomes, and fluorescent colouring shows whether the correct number of copies is present and whether there has been any rearrangement. For example, a deletion of chromosome 17 in the region p13.3, which has given rise to lissencephaly, may be too small to be seen on routine karyotyping, but can be recognized using a cosmid containing part of the lissencephaly gene, when only one copy, instead of two (one on each of the chromosomes 17), will fluoresce (Reiner *et al.* 1993 and Fig. 16.1). Another deletion syndrome associated with neurological problems is that of microcephaly, blepharimosis, and spastic diplegia with a deletion at 3q22 (Jewett *et al.* 1993).

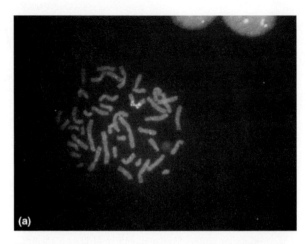

Fig. 16.1(a) FISH analysis of a patient with lissencephaly due to a deletion of 17p13: (a) shows a normal control with two fluorescent spots on each chromosome 17.

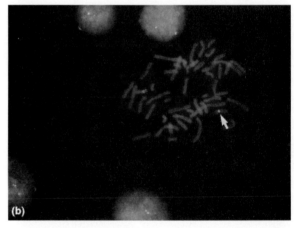

Fig. 16.1(b) Shows the patient's chromosomes with one chromosome 17 (marked with an arrow) lacking a second fluorescent spot.

THE MOLECULAR DIAGNOSTIC LABORATORY

Molecular techniques can help the neurologist by confirming the clinical diagnosis, or by testing healthy relatives to discover if any carry the same mutation that is present in the index patient. However, there are limitations to these services, as some genes and their mutations have not yet been identified, and even when a gene has been cloned, mutation analysis may be difficult, tedious, or just not helpful as some disease-causing mutations may reside outside the gene (e.g. in a promoter region). In addition, although some diseases may generally be associated with the same pathological mutation, such as HMSN (hereditary motor and sensory neuropathy) type Ia in other diseases there is a different mutation for each family. The current state of play for mutations for some neurological disorders is summarized in Table 16.3.

Table 16.3 Analysing mutations in some neurological disorders

Disease	Chromosomal location of gene	Nature and frequency of common mutation	Technique used to detect it	Ease of test	Nature of other mutations	Comments
Duchenne muscular dystrophy	Xp21	Deletion in 60–70%	Multiplex PCR	SF	Point mutations duplications	
Becker muscular dystrophy	Xp21	Deletion in 80%	Multiplex PCR	SF	Point mutations	
Huntington's disease	4p16.3	Increases in CAG repeats in ?100%	PCR	SF	Not yet found	Small overlap between affected and normal
Myotonic dystrophy	19q13	Increases in CTG repeats in ?100%	PCR and Southern	SF	Not yet known	
Facioscapulo-humeral muscular dystrophy	4q35	Deletion in 86–95%	Double Digestion with EcoRI and BlnI	Moderately difficult	Not known	Need to use linkage analysis in families lacking the rearrangement
HMSN 1a	17p11–12	1.5Mb duplication in majority	Dosage analysis of markers in region	SF	Point mutations	Several phenocopies
HNPP	17p11–12	1.5Mb deletion in majority	Dosage analysis of markers and Southern	SF	Deletion, Insertion	Deletion of PMP-22 gene which is duplicated in HMSNla
HMSN1b	1q22–23	Point mutations in majority	SSCP	Moderately difficult	Deletions	
CMTX	Xq31.1	Point mutations in majority	SSCP	Moderately difficult	Deletions	Consider testing in patients negative for PMP-22 duplication No male-to-male transmission
Familial amyloid polyneuropathy	18q11.2–12.1	Point mutations	Digestion with Nsil, Sspl, and PvuII/Direct sequencing	SF		Often no family history in affected individuals
VHL disease	3p25	Deletions in 20%	Southern blotting	SF	Point mutations	80% of mutations detected using blotting and hetero-duplex analysis
NF type 1	17q11	Various	PTT+ Many	Difficult		
NF type 2	22q12	Various	SSCP	Difficult		
AR spinal muscular atrophy	5q13	Deletion of exons 7 & 8 in SMN gene	PCR & Southern blotting	SF	Various	Dominant SMA is not linked to this locus
Familial Alzheimer's	14q14	Various	rtPCR/direct sequencing	Difficult	?	
Familial motor neurone disease	21q22	Point mutations	SSCP	Difficult	Deletion	
Mitochondrial myopathy	Mt DNA	Deletions in majority	Southern blotting	SF	See Table 16.5	Need to examine MtDNA from muscle

Table 16.3 (*cont.*)

Disease	Chromosomal location of gene	Nature and frequency of common mutation	Technique used to detect it	Ease of test	Nature of other mutations	Comments
Leber's hereditary optic neuropathy	Mt DNA	11778bp point mutation	Digestion with Sfa N1	SF		>90% of cases due to 11778 and 3460 mutations
		3460bp point mutation	Digestion with BsaHI	SF		
MELAS	Mt DNA	3243bp point mutation in 80%	Digestion with Apa 1	SF	Various	Poor phenotype/ genotype correlation
		3271bp point mutation in 10–15%	Digestion with Afl1	SF		
MERRF	MtDNA	8344bp point mutation	Digestion with BgLI or CVjJI	SF		
NARP/ Leigh's	MtDNA	8993 bp point mutation	Digestion with HpaLI or AvaI			
Paramyotonia Congenita/ HyperPP	17q23–25	Point mutations	Digestion with NsiI and TaiI	SF		Clinical service detects codon 704 (NsiI) and codon 1592 (TaiI) mutations accounting for 80% of cases
HypoPP	Iq32	Point mutations	Digestion with TspRI and NcoI	SF		Clinical service detects codon 528 (TspRI) and codon 1239 (NcoI) mutations accounting for 80% of cases
Myotonia congenita	7q35	Point mutations	Direct diprimer sequencing	SF	Deletions in AR form	AD form (Thomsen's) and AR form (Becker's)
Episodic ataxia Type I	12p13	Point mutations	Direct diprimer sequnecing	SF		

Note: PCR testing available for all diseases in Table 16.4 (Myotonic Dystrophy and FRAXA may require additional Southern blotting).

Abbreviations: SF, straightforward; HMSN, hereditary motor and sensory neuropathy; MELAS, mitochondrial myopathy, encephalopathy, lactic acidosis, and stroke-like episodes; NF, neurofibromatosis; PCR, polymerase chain reaction; SSCP, single-strand conformation polymorphism; VHL, Von Hippel–Lindaun; HNPP, Hereditary neuropathy with liability to pressure palsies; CMTX, X-linked Charcot-Marie-Tooth; PTT, protein truncation test; MERRF, myoclonic epilepsy with ragged red fibres; NARP, neurogenic muscle weakness, ataxia and retinitis pigmentosa; HypoPP, hypokalaemic periodic paralysis; HyperPP, hyperkalaemic periodic paralysis; rtPCR, reverse transcription polymerase chain reaction.

Molecular investigations can be divided into 'easy' and 'difficult', with the caveat that techniques are changing rapidly, and what is difficult one month may become easy the next.

The simplest types of mutation to recognize are partial gene deletions, other rearrangements such as duplications, and expansions of trinucleotide repeats. Other types of mutations require extensive and careful analyses.

MUTATIONS THAT ARE 'EASY' TO RECOGNIZE

DELETIONS

These can be exemplified by mitochondrial DNA and by the dystrophin gene. Mitochondrial DNA is a circular molecule of about 16 kilobases (kb). If it is cut with a restriction enzyme that recognizes only one site within it, the circular molecule will be linearized and will produce one band, 16 kb in length, which can be detected using Southern blotting. However, if a proportion of the MtDNA molecules contain a deletion, then there will be the 16 kb band, together with one or two smaller bands (which move faster on the gel) representing the deleted molecules.

Deletions of the dystrophin gene occur in two-thirds of boys with Duchenne muscular dystrophy and in about 80% of males with Becker muscular dystrophy. As the gene is about 2400 kb in length, it is difficult to study in a single manoeuvre. However, the deletions usually affect certain exons (or coding regions) and sets of oligonucleotide primers have been designed to pick out these exons. Then, the DNA between the primers is increased several thousand fold using the polymerase chain reaction (PCR), and this increased amount can be directly visualized on a gel to see if the normal array of bands is present, or if one or more bands is missing, indicating deletions of exons. In about one-seventh of instances, a deletion within the dystrophin gene will produce a novel junctional fragment, also easy to recognize on a gel.

OTHER DNA REARRANGEMENTS

Other rearrangements that can be detected using relatively simple DNA analysis techniques are the gene duplication of HMSN1 (Lupski *et al.* 1991; Raeymaekers *et al.* 1991), and the 4q35 deletion of facioscapulohumeral muscular dystrophy which results in altered restriction enzyme fragments following EcoRI/BlnI digestion (Tamil *et al.* 1998).

TRINUCLEOTIDE REPEATS

These form a type of pathological mutation that was never envisaged before being found near the fragile-X gene in 1991 (Oberle *et al* 1991; Yu *et al* 1991; Verkerk *et al* 1991). Since then trinucleotide repeats have been observed in a total of 11 neurological diseases (Table 16.4). One feature that distinguishes these diseases is a change in manifestation between generations, usually with increasing severity and with earlier age of onset in the most recent generations. This is clinically most evident in myotonic dystrophy, but there are also small anticipatory effects in Huntington's disease (Ridley *et al.* 1988), in the spinocerebellar ataxias (Zoghbi *et al.* 1988) and in dentatorubro-pallidoluysian atrophy (DRPLA) (Naito and Oyanagi 1982).

Trinucleotide repeats are present in controls, but are much longer in patients, particularly those with early onset (Table

16.4). In two of these diseases (bulbospinal neuronopathy and Huntington's disease) the repeats lie within the gene, but in myotonic dystrophy and the fragile-X syndrome, the repeats lie outside the gene. The mechanism for the pathological action of the expanded series of trinucleotide repeats is not certain, but in myotonic dystrophy the amount of transcript produced by the protein kinase gene is reduced, and in the case of bulbospinal neuronopathy and Huntington's disease the long string of glutamine coded for by the series of CAG repeats could produce a rigid arm that alters binding to other intracellular proteins (Li *et al.* 1995).

The length of a series of trinucleotide repeats can be simply recognized in the laboratory using appropriate primers and the PCR method, and comparing the amplified DNA with control amplified DNA of known length.

The implication of the above three types of mutation (partial deletions, other rearrangements, and trinucleotide repeats) is that having been recognized in the laboratory, the techniques can be simply applied to asymptomatic relatives. When applying such tests to relatives, attention should be paid to the social and ethical implications.

MORE DIFFICULT WAYS OF RECOGNIZING MUTATIONS

Diagnoses of other types of mutation can be carried out in various ways, using certain basic principles. First, is the problem of size. Genes can vary in length from a few thousand base pairs to tens or even hundreds of thousands of base pairs. As mutations may consist of only a single base change, mutation analysis can only be carried out using small fragments of DNA. Therefore, the first stage is to cut the appropriate segment of DNA into small manageable fragments.

Table 16.4 Trinucleotide repeats in neurological disease

Disease	Type of repeat	Range in controls	Range in affecteds	Change in		Correlation with clinical severity	Reference
				Female meiosis	Male meiosis		
Fragile-X syndrome: FRAXA	CGG	0–50	200–4000	+++	+/-	No	Yu *et al.* (1991)
Bulbospinal neuronopathy	CAG	12–30	40–62	+	+	No	La Spada *et al.* (1992)
Myotonic dystrophy	CTG	5–27	50–2000	++	+/-	Yes	Harley *et al.* (1992)
Huntington's disease	CAG	11–34	33–100	+	++	Yes	MacDonald *et al.* (1993)
Dentatorubro-pallidoluysian atrophy (DRPLA)	CAG	7–23	49–75	?	+	Yes	Nagafuchi *et al.* (1994); Koide *et al.* (1994)
Spinocerebellar ataxia 1	CAG	25–36	43–81	?	+	Yes	Orr *et al.* (1993)
Spinocerebellar ataxia 2	CAG	15–29	35–59	+	+	Yes	Pulst *et al.* (1996); Sanpei *et al.* (1996); Imbert *et al.* (1996);
Spinocerebellar ataxia 3	CAG	13–36	68–79	No	No	Yes	Kawaguchi *et al.* (1994)
Spinocerebellar ataxia 6	CAG	4–16	21–27	No	No	Yes	Zhuchenko *et al.* (1997)
Spinocerebellar ataxia 7	CAG	7–19	37–130	+	++	Yes	David *et al.* (1998)
Friedreich's ataxia	GAA	7–30	200–1000	+	+	Yes	Campuzano *et al.* (1996)

Secondly, the appropriate fragment of DNA that contains the gene, or part of it, has to be amplified so that techniques can be applied in the laboratory. Amplification may be carried out using the polymerase chain reaction (PCR), or by inserting the DNA segment into a bacterial or plasmid host, which replicates itself, and in so doing, replicates the human DNA.

After this, techniques can be applied to the selected and replicated segment of DNA. These techniques depend on the observation that even a single base change will affect pairing and other behaviour of a strand of DNA, under defined experimental conditions. Thus, SSCP (single strand conformation polymophism) makes use of the fact that a single base alteration in a single strand of DNA will affect its conformation and hence its mobility on an electrophoretic gel. Another technique (heteroduplex analysis) arises from the observation that a single base change in one strand of double stranded DNA will result in the formation of a heteroduplex, which will have a different conformation, and therefore different mobility, than a homoduplex composed of matching stands of DNA. Another technique uses denaturing gels, and the fact that the rate of denaturation of DNA duplexes will be affected by single base changes as well as by other factors such as temperature; this is called DGGE (denaturing gradient gel electrophoresis). Yet another technique uses the observation that certain chemicals are specific about the points at which they cut DNA, and so the cleavage products vary according to the specific bases that are present; this is the technique of CCM (chemical cleavage mismatch). Another method utilizes the synthesis of oligonucleotides that perfectly match a particular stretch of DNA (ASO, allele specific oligonucleotides). Such use of oligonucleotides can produce PCR products only if matching is totally accurate. Moreover, these primers can be constructed so that they only recognize mutations; this is called ASA (allele specific amplication). An extension of this method uses the observation that if a mismatch is present, it will affect the alignment of DNA and oligonucleotide on a nylon membrane. These 'screening' techniques will detect the presence of a mutation with varying degrees of success. For example, SSCP will detect 80–90% of point mutations.

Some point mutations in genes alter an enzyme restriction site, either by removing a site, so that an unusually long fragment of DNA is produced, or by conferring an extra restriction site, so that an extra and shorter band is produced. As there is a large number of these restriction enzymes which recognize and cut a specific DNA sequence, it is often possible to find one that will identify a point mutation that has been discovered through DNA sequencing. In this way, the MERRF (myoclonic epilepsy and ragged red fibres) is diagnosed by using the enzyme CviJI which recognizes the mutant DNA sequence AGCC but not the normal wild-type sequence: AACC. As the A to G mutation occurs at bp 8344, the mutation has taken that name (Shoffner *et al.* 1990). Similarly, the MELAS (mitochondrial myopathy, encephalopathy, lactic acidosis, and stroke-like episodes) mutation may be dia-

gnosed by using the restriction enzyme ApaI which cleaves the mutant sequence GGGCCC but not the wild-type sequence GAGCC, where adenine is present at position 3243 (Goto *et al.* 1990). In like fashion, the NARP (neurogenic atrophy and retinitis pigmentosa) mutation may be diagnosed using the restriction enzyme AvaI, since the mutation creates a new cleavage sequence: CCCGGG in which thymine has been changed to guanine at bp position 8993 (Holt *et al.* 1990).

The amyloid neuropathies that are caused by point mutations in the transthyretin gene can also be recognized using their altered restriction sites for specific enzymes (Benson 1991, Riley *et al.* 1995).

Further ways of initiating the search for point mutations are the protein truncation test (Roest *et al.* 1993) in which shortened gene products are identified, or by looking for abnormal transcripts of messenger RNA in blood samples (Roberts *et al.* 1992).

If a mutation is novel, then it must be shown to be pathological, either because it impairs the protein product or because it is present in all affected members of a family and absent in unaffected members. If, in these ways, the mutation can be shown to be pathological rather than having a neutral effect, then strategies can be developed (as they were with the mitochondrial point mutations described earlier) to find a simple method of recognizing the same mutation in relatives.

Many of these more sophisticated techniques are only applicable to research. For service use, it is only practical to screen for the most common mutations. While these will reveal mutations in most patients, there will always be some patients with novel mutations not detected by screening. Moreover in some conditions, like Lesch–Nyhan disease and adrenoleucodystrophy, every family seems to have a different mutation and so analysis is impossible in a service laboratory.

When requesting tests, it is important to understand what is easy and what is difficult, what tests have to be sent elsewhere, and what tests require immediate action rather than being left over a weekend. Clinical, molecular, and cytogeneticists are only too pleased to give advice, particularly as everyone realizes that techniques change rapidly and what is impossible one year becomes routine the next. Table 16.3 is only a guide to what is available; it cannot replace discussion with colleagues.

Blood samples should be sent to the laboratories in the correct tubes. For chromosome studies, fresh blood in heparin is required. For certain diagnoses, it is wise to collect blood into EDTA at the same time for DNA studies. DNA studies require 10 ml of blood in EDTA. The DNA can then be extracted and stored for many years. DNA can also be extracted from post-mortem tissues that have been preserved in formalin, although only PCR analysis is possible. However, fresh blood is required if the DNA is to be used for pulsed field gel electrophoresis, or if RNA is to be extracted. Please discuss with the laboratory staff if there is any doubt.

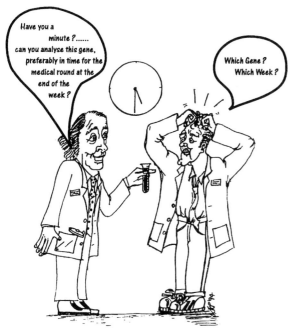

Mutation Analysis can take
a long time
SOME PRACTICAL EXAMPLES

The patterns of changing management of disease, and patterns of parental behaviour can be seen by the following examples.

VON HIPPEL–LINDAU DISEASE (VHL)

Offspring of patients with VHL disease have a 1 in 2 risk of carrying the gene, with an expected natural history that half such gene carriers will be dead by the age of 50, usually of metastases following renal carcinoma, or of complications following cerebellar or spinal haemangioblastomas, and a risk that one-third of gene carriers will be visually impaired through haemorrhage of a retinal angioma or associated retinal detachment (Harding and Robertson 1984; Maher *et al.* 1990). The aim of screening pre-symptomatic relatives is to improve the mortality and morbidity of silent VHL lesions.

Without genetic tests, screening is offered to all offspring of patients. Protocols vary in detail but usually consist of six-monthly ophthalmological assessments, yearly clinical assessments, and two-yearly examination of the abdomen by ultrasound or magnetic resonance imaging (MRI), to detect tumours of the kidney, adrenal, or pancreas. The ophthalmological examination is the most important, as retinal angiomata are usually asymptomatic initially, and appropriately timed laser or cryotherapy will prevent the complications of haemorrhage and detachment, which otherwise lead to some loss of vision. If an abnormality is found to be present, the patient is a gene carrier. If not, he or she would in the past have

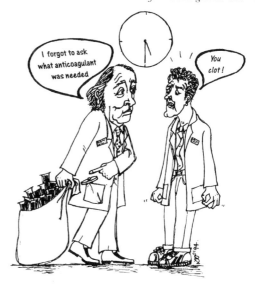

Please discuss first

had to have had continued surveillance. However, now that the VHL gene has been cloned, molecular diagnosis can be offered to asymptomatic relatives, if the mutation in the index patient is known.

The gene for VHL disease was discovered in 1993 through a combination of mapping strategies, and a search for altered fragments of the candidate region in 221 VHL patients (Latif *et al.* 1993). The gene conforms to the older hypothesis of a tumour suppressor gene (based on age of onset distribution) since its mutations result in loss of a transcript that is normally present in the brain and kidney. Mutations can be identified in about 80% of patients by a strategy of Southern blotting to detect deletions followed by heteroduplex and SSCP scanning of the remaining patients to detect the majority of point mutations (Maher *et al.* 1996). Subsequently, relatives at risk can be tested for the mutation present in an affected member of the family. Without a living affected individual, or available pathological tissues from a deceased relative, pre-symptomatic testing is not available. In the 20% of families whose mutation is not identified, prediction with linked markers may be possible.

As a result of molecular pre-symptomatic testing, resources for screening may be directed at mutation carriers, while those without a mutation in the VHL gene can be reassured. Thus, recognition of mutation carriers will not only improve the accuracy and efficiency of management, but allows prospective parents to plan their families in a more informed manner, and to have pre-natal diagnosis if they wish it.

DUCHENNE MUSCULAR DYSTROPHY (DMD)

Genetic counselling for DMD has passed through several stages, starting with genetic risks being calculated on the basis of the pedigree and the mean of three creatine kinase estimations (1965–73), followed by the offer of fetal sexing in an at-risk pregnancy (1973–85), followed later by the offer of accurate or nearly accurate pre-natal diagnosis using DNA techniques, (1985–present). The last stage and the most important one is the development of accurate tests to recognize carrier females using a variety of DNA techniques. The effects of these measures can be followed through the West Midlands DMD register, 1976–90 (Bundey and Boughton 1989 and unpublished observations). Initially, there was a fall in the number of pregnancies to women at high (1 in 10 or greater) risk of being carriers. Then there was a small increase in the number of pregnancies (and of terminations) as fetal sexing became available and gradually, socially acceptable. Later, there was a marked increase in the numbers of pregnancies as those women who had refrained from pregnancy now chose to undertake pregnancy once pre-natal diagnosis was available; this increase was accompanied by a concomitant rise in terminations of affected males. Finally, the situation has levelled off, with most women at risk choosing to have approximately two healthy children. During this time, the number of familial cases of DMD has fallen, to about one-third of its original level. A similar pattern of behaviour has been described for autosomal recessive disease (Modell and Kuliev 1993).

The DNA procedures undertaken with a new DMD family are as follows.

DNA from the affected body is searched for deletions using a multiplex PCR method. If a deletion is found, female relatives are studied to see if they are carriers. This is easy if a novel junctional fragment is produced by the deletion, as occurs in about one-seventh of instances. Otherwise, suitable polymorphic repeats from the deleted segment are studied to see if the female has one band or two. If she has two bands, then she must be heterozygous, showing that she cannot have a gene deletion at that point. If she has one band only, she could be either homozygous or hemizygous, and study of her parents should be able to differentiate these two possibilities. Otherwise, pulsed field gel electrophoresis may recognize DNA fragments of different lengths from her two X chromosomes, which could only occur if a deletion was present.

No deletion will be found in the dystrophin gene of about one-third of DMD boys, and in this situation a muscle biopsy should be carried out to confirm the diagnosis by demonstrating abnormalities in the expression of dystrophin.

Strategies then have to be used to search for a point mutation in the dystrophin gene, which is 150 times longer than a molecule of mitochondrial DNA. A useful technique here is to look for a truncated protein product which would have been produced by a point mutation resulting in a STOP codon). The protein product may be investigated using the protein truncation test (PTT) (Roest *et al.* 1993). In this test, RNA is isolated from lymphocytes, reverse transcribed, amplified by PCR and then incubated with a promotor/translation kit which allows the polypeptides to be assembled. Any alteration in the length of the polypeptide series indicates

a pathological, truncating mutation. An extra advantage of this test is that in a woman, with two X chromosomes, or in any patient with an autosomal mutation, two lengths of polypeptides will appear, one long, normal and slow moving and the other short, abnormal and fast moving; these can be easily visualized on a gel.

Finally, if all these methods fail, linked and intragenic DNA markers can be used to follow the 'at-risk' X chromosome through families; this technique carries a small risk of error because of recombination.

If the mother of a DMD boy is found to be a carrier through molecular studies she can be offered pre-natal diagnosis in a subsequent pregnancy using one of the techniques described above. If she is considered not to be a carrier, there is still a 10% chance that she might be a mosaic for the mutation in her ovaries and so there is a 5% risk of a second affected boy. Such risks change with the structure of the pedigree. Sisters of DMD boys cannot be mosaics: they are either carriers or are not carriers.

HUNTINGTON'S DISEASE (HD)

Before 1983, when Gusella and his team found an approximate location of the HD gene on the distal part of the short arm of chromosome 4, genetic advice to healthy relatives was based on the ages at which they remained healthy and on their genetic relationship to affected relatives. Such information was followed by a decrease in the number of children born to at-risk relatives (Carter *et al.* 1983; Quarrell *et al.* 1988). However, accurate genetic information can now be given as a result of the discovery that a series of CAG repeats within the HD gene is expanded in patients and in pre-symptomatic gene carriers, with very little overlap with the numbers found on normal chromosomes (MacDonald *et al.* 1993). All HD patients have an expanded series of repeats. Exceptionally, a patient clinically diagnosed as HD is shown to have another dominant disorder such as DRPLA (dentatorubro-pallidoluysian atrophy) (Warner *et al.* 1994).

While the length of CTG repeats in myotonic dystrophy gives some idea of the phenotype, there is little correlation in Huntington's disease. A length of 100 CAG repeats in a fetus at risk for HD indicates onset during childhood. However, repeat lengths of 40–70 give very little idea of prognosis or age of onset (Duyao *et al.* 1993). Thus, when carrying out pre-symptomatic testing on individuals at risk for HD, it is important to emphasize that it is not possible to predict when the disease will develop. As most individuals requesting the test are healthy adults, any who carry the HD mutation are likely to have repeat lengths in the lower end of the affected range, and occasionally in the overlap range with normals.

The proportion of at-risk individuals who request to be tested is about 20%, twice as high as the number previously requesting predictive testing using linked markers. It is important that a protocol recommended by the World Federation of Neurology is followed. This consists of two to three counselling sessions before the final decision is made and blood taken, and it ensures that counselling and support is available after the result has been given.

There could be a dramatic fall in the incidence of HD if the majority of gene carriers request testing, and then either plan to have no children or to have only healthy children. The incidence of new cases could be restricted to those whose mutation has been inherited from a parent not affected before death.

FACIOSCAPULOHUMERAL (FSH) MUSCULAR DYSTROPHY

The majority of patients with FSH muscular dystrophy can be shown to have a deletion at 4q35 using the probe p13E-11. Following simultaneous digestion with EcoRI and Bini affected individuals are shown to have smaller restriction fragments. This deletion does not appear to disrupt a transcribed gene, but possibly influences function of proximally located genes (Tawil *et al.* 1998). It can be tested for without the necessity of blood from other relatives, which is helpful as about 10% of cases represent new mutations (Bakker *et al.* 1996). Molecular testing may also be useful for pre-natal diagnosis. However, translocations between 4q35 and homologous regions on 10q can complicate interpretation of the Southern blot.

HEREDITARY MOTOR AND SENSORY NEUROPATHY (HMSN)

HMSN (or Charcot–Marie–Tooth disease, CMT is a hereditary motor and sensory neuropathy which is heterogeneous. Subdivisions may be made according to the speed of motor nerve conduction velocities. Patients with velocities less than 38 metres per second are said to have a demyelinating type of neuropathy and linkage studies have defined two loci on chromosome 17 (HMSN1a, or CMT1a) and chromosome 1 (HMSN1b, or CMT1b). Patients with normal or only mildly reduced motor nerve conduction velocities have an axonal type of neuropathy for which several loci are thought to be involved but none has yet been defined. Patients with intermediate nerve conduction velocities may have the X-linked dominant form of HMSN in which males are more severely affected than females. This type is due to mutations in the X-linked connexin-32 gene (Bergoffen *et al.* 1993).

Ninety per cent of cases of HMSN1 are caused by a mutation in the PMP22 gene on chromosome 17, and the most common mutation, and one that is readily identified in a DNA laboratory, is a duplication of the gene (Patel and Lupski 1994). If a duplication is absent then there may be a point mutation in PMP22 or alternatively the causative gene may be P_O on chromosome 1 (PMP22 and P_O are myelin protein genes that are only expressed in the peripheral nervous system). If the family is large enough, linkage studies may determine which locus is responsible for its HMSN. In practice, however, there is rarely an urgent clinical need to find a muta-

tion should the 17p duplication be absent; although the test is useful in an isolated case if clinical signs raise the possibility of an inflammatory neuropathy. About 10% of patients with the 17p duplication have no affected parent and are affected by new mutations (Blair *et al.* 1996). Only a very few laboratories would currently be prepared to look for point mutations in the genes for peripheral myelin proteins, should the 17p duplication be absent. No molecular tests are currently available for HMSN2.

NEUROFIBROMATOSIS (NF)

The genes which cause NF types 1 and 2 are large, and difficult to study by molecular techniques. Only one or two laboratories in the United Kingdom are undertaking mutation analysis and then only on selected cases, and with the anticipation of very long delays before results are available. Therefore, at present, the management of NF1 and NF2 is essentially a clinical one, and these are conditions for which joint clinics, or at least consultation between neurologists, neurosurgeons, and clinical geneticists are useful (see Huson and Hughes (1994) for helpful advice). There are two clinical situations where mutation analysis is particularly valuable. One of these is when assessing the offspring of a patient with NF2, because often there are no cutaneous manifestations. Knowledge of whether a relative has an NF2 mutation is important for deciding how often to perform scans to look for a vestibular schwannoma. The second situation is when somatic mosaicism is a possibility. For example, neurofibromas or schwannomas which affect only spinal roots and which are without manifestation elsewhere in the body, may represent the mosaic manifestation of the NF1, or more likely, the NF2 gene. From the point of view of genetic counselling it is important to know whether or not an NF mutation is in the lymphocytes of these patients (and therefore, by implication, in the germ line) and so a request for mutation analysis is justified.

AUTOSOMAL RECESSIVE DISEASES

In autosomal recessive conditions, genetic counselling is straightforward: all parents are heterozygous carriers and other couples in the family will be at neglible risk of having similarly affected children unless they are consanguineous or the condition is exceedingly common. The parents, however, may be interested in pre-natal diagnosis, and here clinical geneticists will be able to provide the most up-to-date information. For example, the recessive forms of spinal muscular atrophy have at last become amenable to molecular analysis and parents who have had one affected child may now be offered pre-natal diagnosis in subsequent pregnancies by searching for deletions of exon 7 +/– exon 8 of the survival motor neurone (SMN) gene on 5q13 (Rodrigues *et al.* 1995*a,b*).

MITOCHONDRIAL DISEASES

Indications for requesting analysis of mitochondrial DNA are listed in Table 16.5. Older children and adults with mitochondrial disease almost always have ragged red fibres on a muscle biopsy and it is unusual to find an abnormality of mitochondrial DNA in their absence. However, in some patients with mitochondrial myopathy a mitochondrial DNA abnormality can only be demonstrated in mitochondria extracted from muscle, and so it is worthwhile to send both blood and muscle for analysis. The tests carried out on mitochondrial DNA would always include a search for deleted molecules, as well as tests specific for particular mitochondrial point mutations, as indicated by the clinical picture. Not all pathological mutations of mitochondrial DNA have been identified, so about 20% of patients may have to be labelled as 'mitochondrial disease' without a specific diagnosis.

MULTIFACTORIAL CONDITIONS

Already there are clues to understanding some of the multifactorially caused neurological disorders. For example, individuals who are poor at oxidizing debrisoquine have an increased risk of developing parkinsonism (Armstrong *et al.* 1992; Smith *et al.* 1992). Familial motor neurone disease is associated in about one-fifth of patients with one of a variety of mutations in the Cu/Zn superoxide dismutase gene; these mutations alter its structure and probably its protective effect against free radicals (Deng *et al.* 1993). Some patients with motor neurone disease, but no affected relative, also have a mutation in their superoxide dismutase gene. Alzheimer's disease is caused in 5–10% of instances by a major predisposing dominant gene; the amyloid precursor protein gene and the pre-senilin genes 1 and 2 have so far been identified but there are others (Goate *et al.* 1991; Levy-Lahad *et al.* 1995; Sherrington *et al.* 1995). In the majority of patients with Alzheimer's disease the role of genetic factors is unknown. However, in both late-onset familial and sporadic cases of Alzheimer's disease the onset of symptoms occurs earlier in individuals possessing the ε4 allele of the APOE gene. This effect is dose-related with individuals homozygous for the ε4 allele developing disease at an earlier age than heterozygotes (Blacker *et al.* 1997). Currently, mutation analysis of the pre-senilin-1 gene is available and use of modified Huntington's disease counselling protocols is recommended in individuals seeking predictive testing. Genetic testing should be restricted to individuals in autosomal dominant early-onset families and the role of APOE testing remains under investigation (Post *et al.* 1997). No laboratory is undertaking service analysis for mutations of the amyloid precursor protein or presenilin-2 genes, even when there is a dominant family history. However, this is one field where future technological advances are likely to become available and be of great help in delineating subtypes of Alzheimer's disease in individual patients.

The observations described above will ultimately lead to a fuller understanding of multifactorial conditions and to

Table 16.5 Indication for requesting analysis of mitochondrial DNA

Indication	Possible abnormalities found
Leigh's encephalopathy	8993, 8344
Neurological symptoms with lactic acidosis	MtDNA depletion; 8993
Myopathy with external ophthalmoplegia and/or ragged red fibres on biopsy	Multiple deletions or a single one duplication of MtDNA. 3243, 3250, 3251, 3302, 15990
Sideroblastic anaemia	MtDNA deletion
Sudden onset of optic neuropathy ± vascular congestion around disc	11778, 3460, 14484
Myoclonic epilepsy	8344, 8356
Unexplained stroke-like episodes	3243, 3271
Unexplained encephalopathy ± dementia	3243, 3271
Diabetes and deafness	3243
Ataxia with other features	8344, 8993
Retinitis pigmentosa with deafness or with neurological features	8993; MtDNA deletion
Cardiomyopathy with metabolic abnormality	3260, 3303, 9997

strategies of prevention. If, for example, the mechanism whereby parkinsonism is partially caused by variation in xenobiotic metabolism, perhaps exposure of causative environmental agents could be minimized. With sporadic motor neurone disease and a mutation in the Cu/Zn superoxide dismutase gene, we should learn what is the mechanism by which such patients are affected but their relatives are not. Are there therapeutic strategies? What about the other enzymes that protect against free radicals? Can we help or learn from patients with sporadic forms of Alzheimer's disease? Female monozygotic twins of patients with multiple sclerosis have a 40% risk of being similarly affected. Can their autoimmune system be modified sufficiently to prevent disease, or is it too late once their twin has been diagnosed? These are some of the exciting questions for the future.

CONCLUSIONS

The main ways in which clinical geneticists can help patients with neurological diseases is by giving them an accurate diagnosis, explanation, and options for planning their families. This alone will lead to a reduction in the birth incidence of dominant and X-linked disorders, for it has been observed since genetic counselling first started (in 1946 in the United Kingdom) that most couples given high risks for transmitting serious and chronic disease to their offspring, choose to limit their families, or to have pre-natal diagnosis followed by selective termination of affected pregnancies. This has been demonstrated, for example, with Duchenne muscular dystrophy, in which the birth incidence of familial cases has dropped to about 30% of its original level. The current commonest cause of familial cases is delayed diagnosis of the index patient, so that a younger affected brother has already been born (Bundey and Boughton 1989; Norman *et al.* 1989).

Secondly, clinical geneticists can help advise and give information to members of the extended family who are at risk of developing or transmitting a serious genetic disorder. It is difficult for a hospital consultant to arrange such help for a family. Thirdly, the identification of novel genes by genetic research is leading to a remarkable increase in knowledge about the genetic control of early development and cellular processes. Such studies should lead to an understanding of how the genotype influences a clinical picture, to an understanding of why some individuals who carry dominant genes do not get ill, and conversely, why other individuals who carry mutations are the only ones in their family to become ill. An understanding of the complicated relationships between gene and disease will certainly lead to prophylactic and therapeutic strategies.

A neurologist may therefore wish to use the services of a clinical genetics unit for:

(1) genetic counselling of an index patient and his/her immediate and extended family;

(2) molecular or chromosomal diagnosis of a specific disease or of a predisposing factor; and carrier testing of relatives;

(3) maintaining contact with families so that they can be told of new advances and so that young members can be counselled when they become adults;

(4) holding joint clinics with neurologists so that patients and their families can receive co-ordinated management. Examples are clinics for Huntington's disease and neurofibromatosis.

ACKNOWLEDGEMENTS

I am grateful to the following: Dr Martin Giles for his advice on this manuscript; Dr D. Pilz, A. Long, and Dr. Maltby for Figure 16.1; Ms L. Philbin for her excellent cartoons.

REFERENCES

Armstrong M, Daly AK, Cholerton S, Batemass DH, Idle JR (1992). Mutant debrisoquine hydroxylation genes in Parkinson's disease. *Lancet* **339**, 1017–18.

Bakker E, Van der Wielen MJR, Voorhoeve E *et al.* (1996). Diagnostic, predictive and prenatal testing for facioscapulo humeral muscular dystrophy. *J Med Genet* **33**, 29–35.

Benson MD (1991) Inherited amyloidosis. *J Med Genet* **28**, 73–8.

Bergoffen J, Scherer SS, Wang S *et al.* (1993). Connexin mutations in X-linked Charcot–Marie–Tooth Disease. *Science* **262**, 2039–42.

Blacker D, Haines JL, Rodes L *et al.* (1997). Apo-E and age at onset of Alzheimer's disease: The NIMH Genetics Initiative. *Neurology* **48**, 139–47.

Blair IP, Nash J, Gordon MJ, Nicholson GA (1996). Prevalence and origin of *de novo* duplications in Charcot–Marie–Tooth Disease Type 1A. *Am J Hum Genet* **58**, 472–6.

Browne DL. Gancher ST, Nutt JG *et al.* (1994). Episodic ataxia/ myokymia syndrome is associated with point mutations in the human potassium channel gene, KCNA-1 *Nature Genetics* **8**, 136–40.

Bundey S, Boughton E (1989). Are abortions more or less frequent once prenatal diagnosis is available. *J Med Genet* **26**, 794–5.

Campuzano V, Montermini L, Molto MD *et al.* (1996). Friedreich's ataxia: autosomal recessive disease caused by an intronic GAA triplet repeat expansion. *Science* **271**, 1423–7.

Carter CO, Evans KA, Baraitser M (1983). Effect of genetic counselling on the prevalence of Huntington's chorea. *BMJ* **286**, 281–3.

David G, Durr A, Stevanin G *et al.* (1998). Molecular and clinical correlations in autosomal dominant cerebeller ataxia with progressive macular dystrophy (SCA7). *Hum Mol Genet* **7**(2), 165–70.

Deng H-X, Hentati A, Tainer JA *et al.* (1993). Amyotrophic lateral sclerosis and structural defects in Cu, Zn superoxide dismutase. *Science* **261**, 1047–51.

Duyao M, Ambrose C, Myers R *et al.* (1993). Trinucleotide repeat length instability and age of onset in Huntington's disease. *Nature Genet* **4**, 387–92.

Emery AEH (1991). Population frequencies of inherited neuromuscular diseases—a world survey. *Neuromusc Disorders* **1**, 19–29.

Goate A, Chartier-Harlin M, Mullan M *et al.* (1991). Segregation of a missense mutation in the amyloid precursor protein gene with familial Alzheimer's disease. *Nature* **349**, 704–6.

Goto Y, Nowaka I, Horai S (1990). A mutation in the tRNA[leu(UUR)] gene associated with MELAS subgroup of mitochondrial encephalomyopathies. *Nature* **348**, 651–3.

Gusella JF, Wexler NS, Conneally PM *et al.* (1983). A polymorphic DNA marker genetically linked to Huntington's disease. *Nature* **306**, 234–8.

Harding P, Robertson DM (1984). Von Hippel–Lindau disease; a familial, often lethal, multi-system phakomatosis. *Ophthalmology* **91**, 263–70.

Harley HG, Rundel SA, Reardon W *et al.* (1992). Unstable DNA sequence in myotonic dystrophy. *Lancet* **339**, 1125–8.

Hayasaka K, Himoro M, Sato W *et al.* (1993). Charcot–Marie–Tooth neuropathy type 1B is associated with mutations of the myelin Pô gene. *Nature Genetics* **5**, 314–4.

Holt IJ, Harding AE, Petty RKH, Morgan-Hughes JA (1990). A new mitochondrial disease associated with mitochondrial DNA heteroplasmy. *Am J Hum Genet* **46**, 428–33.

Hudson AJ, Ebers GC, Bulman DE (1995). The skelctal muscle sodium and chloride channel diseases. *Brain* **118**, 547–63.

Huson SM, Hughes RAC (1994). *The neurofibromatoses: Pathogenetic and clinical overview.* Chapman and Hall, London.

Imbert G, Sandou F, Yvert G *et al.* (1996). Cloning of the gene for spinocerebellar ataxia 2 reveals a locus with high sensitivity to expanded CAG/glutamine repeats. *Nature Genetics* **14**, 285–91.

Jewett T, Rao PN, Weaver RG, Stewart W, Thomas IT, Pettenati MJ (1993). Blepharimosis, ptosis, and epicanthus inversus syndrome (BPES) associated with interstitial deletion of band 3q22. *Am J Med Genet* **47**, 1147–50.

Kawaguchi Y, Okamoto T, Taniwaki M *et al.* (1994). CAG expansions in a novel gene for Machado–Joseph disease at chromosome 14q32.1. *Nature Genetics* **8**, 221–7.

Koide R, Ikeuchi T, Onodera O *et al.* (1994). Unstable expansion of CAG repeat in hereditary dentatorubral-pallidoluysian atrophy (DRPLA). *Nature Genetics*, **6**, 9–13.

La Spada AR, Roling DB, Harding AE *et al.* (1992). Meiotic stability and genotype-phenotype correlation of the trinucleotide repeat in X-linked spinal and bulbar muscular atrophy. *Nature Genetics* **2**, 301–4.

Latif F, Tory K, Gnarra J *et al.* [total of 33 authors] (1993). Identification of the Von Hippel–Lindau disease tumor suppressor gene. *Science* **260**, 1317–20.

Levy-Lahad E, Wasco W, Poorkaj P *et al.* (1995). Candidate gene for the chromosome 1 familial Alzheimer's disease locus. *Science* **269**, 973–7

Li X-J, Li S-H, Sharp A H *et al.* (1995). A huntingtin-associated protein enriched in brain with implications for pathology. *Nature* **378**, 398–402.

Lupski J R, Montes de Oca-Luna R, Slaugenhaupt S *et al.* (1991). DNA duplication associated with Charcot–Marie–Tooth disease Type I A. *Cell* **66**, 219–32.

MacDonald ME, Andrews CM, Duyao MP *et al.* (for the Huntington's Disease Collaborative Research Group) (1993). A novel gene containing a trinucleotide repeat that is expanded and unstable on Huntington's disease chromosomes. *Cell* **72**, 971–83.

Maher ER, Yates JRW, Harries R *et al.* (1990). Clinical features and natural history of Von Hippel–Lindau disease. *Quart J Med* **77**, 1151–63.

Maher ER, Webster AR, Richards FM *et al.* (1996). Phenotypic expression in Von Hippel–Lindau disease: correlations with germline VHL gene mutations. *J Med Genet* **33**, 328–32.

Modell B, Kuliev AM (1993). A scientific basis for cost–benefit analysis of genetics services. *Trends Genetics* **9**, 46–51.

Nafaguchi S, Yanagisawa H, Sato K *et al.* (1994). Dentatorubral and pallidoluysian atrophy expansion of an unstable CAG trinucleotide on chromosome 12p. *Nature Genetics* **6**, 14–18.

Naito H, Oyanagi S (1982). Familial myoclonus epilepsy and choreathetosis: hereditary dentatorubral-pallidoluysian atrophy. *Neurology* **32**, 798–807.

Norman AM, Rogers C, Sibert JR, Harper PS (1989). Duchenne muscular dystrophy in Wales: a 15 year study, 1971 to 1986. *J Med Genet* **26**, 560–4.

Oberle I, Rousseau F, Heitz D *et al.* (1991). Instability of a 550-base pair DNA segment and abnormal methylation in fragile X-syndrome. *Science* **252**, 1097–102.

Orr HT, Chung M-Y, Banfi S *et al.* (1993). Expansion of an unstable trinucleotide CAG repeat in spinocerebellar ataxia type 1. *Nature Genetics* **4**, 221–6.

Quarrell OWJ, Tyler A, Jones MP, Nordin M, Harper PS (1988). Population studies of Huntington's disease in Wales. *Clin Genet* **33**, 189–95.

Patel PI, Lupski JR (1994). Charcot–Marie–Tooth disease: a new paradigm for the mechanism of inherited disease. *Trends in Genetics* **10**, 128–33.

Post SG, Whitehouse PJ, Binstock RH *et al.* (1997). The clinical introduction of genetic testing for Alzheimer's disease: An ethical perspective *JAMA* **227**, 832–6.

Pulst S-M, Nechiporuk A, Nechiporuk T *et al.* (1996). Moderate expansion of a normally biallelic trinucleotide repeat in spinocerebellar ataxia type 2. *Nature Genetics* **14**, 269–76.

Raeymaekers P, Timmerman V, Nelis E *et al.* (1991). Duplication in chromosome 17p11.2 in Charcot–Marie–Tooth neuropathy type 1a (CMT1a). *Neuromuscular Disorders* **1**, 93–7.

Reiner O, Carrozzo R, Shen Y *et al.* (1993). Isolation of a Miller–Dieker lissencephaly gene containing G protein B-subunit-like repeats. *Nature* **364**, 717–21.

Reilly MM, Adams D, Booth Dr *et al.* (1995). Transthyretin gene analysis in Europe patients with suspected familial amyloid polyneuropathy. *Brain* **118**, 849–56.

Reiter LT. Murakami T, Kocuth T *et al.* (1996). A recombinational hotspot responsible for two inherited peripheral neuropathies is located near a marineer trasposon-like element. *Nature Genetics* **12**, 288–97.

Ridley RM, Frith CD, Crow TJ, Conneally PM (1988). Anticipation in Huntington's disease is inherited through the male line but may originate in the female. *J Med Genet* **25**, 589–95.

Roberts RG, Bobrow M, Bentley DR (1992). Point mutations in the dystrophin gene. *Proc Natl Acad Sci USA* **89**, 2331–5.

Rodrigues NR, Owen N, Talbot K, Ignatius J, Dubowitz V, Davies KE (1995a). Deletions in the survival motor neuron gene on 5q13 in autosomal recessive spinal muscular atrophy. *Hum Mol Genet* **4**, 631–4.

Rodrigues NR, Campbell L, Owen N, Rodeck CH, Davies KE (1995b). Prenatal diagnosis of spinal muscular atrophy by gene deletion analysis. *Lancet* **345**, 1049.

Roest PAM, Roberts RG, Sugino S, Van Ommen G-JB, den Dunnen JT (1993). Protein truncation test (PTT) for rapid detection of translation-terminating mutations. *Hum Mol Genet* **2**, 1719–21.

Rogaev E, Sherrington R, Rogaeva E *et al.* (1995). Familial Alzheimer's disease in kindreds with missense mutations in a novel gene on chromosome 1 related to the Alzheimer's disease type 3 gene. *Nature* **376**, 775–8.

Royal College of Physicians of London (1991). *Purchasers' guidelines to genetic services in the NHS*. London, RCP.

Sanpei K, Takano H, Igavashi S (1996). Identification of the spinocerebellar ataxia type 2 gene using a direct identification of repeat expansion and cloning technique, DIRECT. *Nature Genetics* **14**, 277–84.

Sherrington R, Rogaev E, Liang Y *et al.* (1995). Cloning of a gene bearing missense mutations in early-onset familial Alzheimer's disease. *Nature* **375**, 754–60.

Shoffner JM, Loth MT, Lezza AMS, Seibel P, Ballinger SW, Wallace DC (1990). Myoclonic epilepsy and ragged-red fibre disease (MERRF) is associated with a mitochondrial DNA tRNA^{lys} mutation. *Cell* **61**, 931–7.

Smith CAD, Gough AC, Leigh PN *et al.* (1992). Debrisoquine hydroxylase gene polymorphism and susceptibility to Parkinson's disease. *Lancet* **339**, 1375–7.

Strittmatter WJ, Saunders AM, Schmechel D *et al.* (1993). Apolipoprotein E: high avidity binding to beta-amyloid and increased frequency of type 4 allele in late onset familial Alzheimer disease. *Proc Natl Acad Sci USA* **90**, 1977–81.

Tawil R, Figelwicz Griggs RC *et al.* (1998). Facioscapulohumeral dystrophy: Adistinct regional myopathy with a novel molecular pathogenesis. *Ann Neurol* **43**, 279–82.

Verkerk AJMH, Plovottl M, Sutcliffe JS *et al.* (1991). Identification of a gene (FMR-1) containing a CGG repeat coincident with a breakpoint cluster region exhibiting length variation in fragile X syndrome. *Cell* **65**, 905–14.

Warner TT, Williams L, Harding AE (1994). DRPLA in Europe. *Nature Genetics* **6**, 225.

Wijmenga C, Hewitt JE, Sandkuijl LA *et al.* (1992). Chromosome 4q DNA rearrangements associated with facioscapulohumeral muscular dystrophy. *Nature Genetics* **2**, 26–30.

Yu S, Pritchard M, Kremer E *et al.* (1991). Fragile X genotype characterised by an unstable region of DNA. *Science* **252**, 1179–81.

Zoghbi HY, Pollack MS, Lyons LA, Ferrell RE, Daiger SP, Beaudet AL (1988). Spinocerebellar ataxia: variable age of onset and linkage to human leukocyte antigen in a large kindred. *Ann Neurol* **23**, 580–4.

Zhuchenko O, Bailey J, Bonnen P *et al.* (1997). Autosomal dominant cerebellar ataxia (SCA6) associated with small polyglutamine expansions in the α_{1A}-voltage-dependent calcium channel. *Nature Genetics* **15**, 62–9.

17 | *Neurological problems in the elderly*

Douglas G. MacMahon

The increasing profile of elderly people in society and the burgeoning interest in the study of diseases of old age amongst the medical profession has increased the attention not only to the general needs of elderly people, but also to the specialized clinical needs for diagnosis, treatment, and rehabilitation of the individual elderly patient. Specifically, in this chapter, I will present an introduction to the impact of neurological diseases upon this growing sector of the population.

The whole area provides a minefield for the unwary. In no area of clinical practice are the clinical skills of a practitioner challenged so comprehensively as in the diagnosis and management of disorders of the nervous system in the aged. Difficulties abound; history may not be easily forthcoming, examination may be fraught with the 'red herrings' of normal ageing, the presentation may differ from the classical, and co-existent disease may confound. In terms of management, prospects may either be underestimated, or conversely fail to be achieved, and some investigations or treatment may be too hazardous to be justified. Finally, ageist prejudices need to be overcome in both the lay public and in fellow professionals. Yet, in spite of, or perhaps because of, these innate difficulties, the challenge is one worthy of a respectful, informed, and sensitive response rather than a prejudiced one based on the single biological variable of age alone. Thankfully, in many significant domains, technological, or therapeutic advances have come to the clinician's rescue, and we can confidently anticipate other areas in which assistance will shortly be at hand. However, throughout this chapter there is a recurring theme that a sound clinical approach is the prerequisite of effective diagnosis and management.

The chapter concludes with an examination of falls, a common presentation for many neurological conditions, and perspectives on several of the neurological conditions that are found frequently in the elderly population.

THE CHANGING DEMOGRAPHY AND ATTITUDES OF THE AGEING POPULATION

Any attempt to describe the features specific to the ageing patient is frustrated with the problem of defining the meaning of the term 'the elderly'. Chronological age alone is a poor marker for the physiological or pathological changes seen in the older population. The innate heterogeneity of *homo sapiens* applies to this, as any other sector of the population. Many octogenarians can, through a propitious set of genetic codes, attention to diet and exercise, and a fortuitous measure of good luck, continue to outdo some of their younger counterparts in many tests of mental or physical function.

The increasing life expectancy which has occurred through medical, social, and economic progress in the past millennia has changed the shape of the survival curves with a progressive rectangularization. The question of survival needs to be balanced by an examination of quality, that is, whether survival into late life is as a healthy, active, independent member of society, or as a handicapped, confused, and dependent soul. There appears to be a marked gender difference in this aspect of gerontology, with females more likely to survive longer, but also more likely to do so in a more disabled state than are males. Recent calculations suggest that in the United Kingdom although life expectancy for men at age 65 is 13.4 years and for women 17.5 years, the difference in 'Disability-free life expectancy' (the average number of years that a person of a given age may expect to live free of disability) is much less, at 7.7 and 8.9 years, respectively, hence the mean expectancy of disabled life is 5.7 and 8.6 years respectively (1).

The late 20th century has also seen a marked change in the socioeconomic profile of the population, with a conspicuous rise in not only the numbers of very elderly people (i.e. those over 80 years) living in the community, but also in elderly persons (particularly women) living alone, or in some form of institutional care. This phenomenon is seen in most Western countries, and also increasingly now in other societies. It represents the combined effects of a number of factors: the loss of the extended family, the rise in marital breakdown and divorce, and the gender differences in survival which result in increased widowhood.

In the United Kingdom, despite the increase in the availability of residential and nursing homes at the expense of long-term hospitals, the percentage in any form of institutional care remains low by international comparison at 5–6%, even in advanced old age. The impact of the community care assessment and management control arrangements arising as a result of the National Health Service (NHS) and Community Care Act of 1990 has slowed the expansion of the residential sector, with increased interest in the facilitation of non-residential options for care and treatment in the community.

The other domain in which considerable change is being felt is in the increased awareness and rising expectations of patients themselves, and of their family, and informal carers. Nurtured by the media and political initiatives such as 'patients' charters', the concept of choice is now encouraged in the health environment. Better information through television, press, and other media, has consequential effects on perceived needs and expectations. In the United Kingdom, the introduction of the NHS reforms and the Community Care Act, and their progressive implementation has produced the beginnings of a fresh culture in which old assumptions are increasingly being challenged. For how much longer will former 19th-century workhouses, without privacy or dignity be acceptable venues for the delivery of modern health care? Unless health professionals themselves, in tandem with managers, react to changing circumstances, the public may themselves exercise democratic power to produce change. The rising profile of the 'Gray Panthers' in the United States suggests that a realization of the voting power of the oldest generations may have been underestimated. One questions how long it will be before similar movements develop greater prominence in Europe?

There tends to be a nihilistic approach to older patients in many circles. However, ageism has no place in the modern practice of medicine. Access to diagnostic tests or treatment must be based on a philosophy which recognizes the integrity of the individual, their rights, and their needs. Attempts to ration care using parameters such as 'qualys' (quality of life adjusted years) have been shown to disadvantage the elderly (2). Therefore, in the absence of an agreed tool, a clinical assessment of need, and a realistic appraisal of potential for gain must underpin resource allocation. The professions are increasingly encouraged to contribute to this debate by turning their attention to outcome measurement and clinical audit.

In Western societies, the diseases affecting the neurological system of older people are together responsible for more suffering, anguish and disability than those affecting any other system. Akhtar *et al.* (3) showed that the neurological diseases were the single largest cause of disability and dependence, counting for 48% of the disability (defined as requiring assistance to live in their own homes) and 93% of dependence (disability for self-care) in their community study of 808 people over 65 years of age. In addition to the human suffering, it would follow that they are the greatest cause of resource consumption for health and social service agencies, for individuals, and also for their families. All physicians, not only geriatricians, but also neurologists, general physicians, and general practitioners, therefore need to be aware of the significance and conversant with the management of these disorders.

THE SPECTRUM OF NEUROLOGICAL DISEASES IN THE ELDERLY

The aetiology of these causes of disability is wide and largely unknown. We have some understanding of the risk factors for the vascular insults which cause cerebrovascular disease, demonstration of the association between apo-lipoprotein E4 and Alzheimer's disease suggest a genetic component, and possible chromosomal and environmental clues suggest the causation of Parkinson's disease, at least in some cases. Specific sensory damage to sight or hearing and the age-associated, but less progressive and usually less handicapping conditions of cervical spondylosis, essential tremor, epilepsy, and autonomic dysfunction are also frequently encountered. Additional legacies of handicap from diseases striking in middle or earlier life such as disseminated sclerosis, neuropathies, and head injuries, each contribute to the picture of geriatric neurological practice. They each may present in a multitude of ways, some classical, but often in a non-specific manner, such as with falls or failure to cope. Taken together they frequently culminate in admission to hospital or entry to residential or nursing care.

Their presentation is also widely disparate. The drama of an acute insult, such as a stroke, rightly attracts a huge medical response. However, the more subtle onset of the chronic neurodegenerative diseases is much less likely to receive similar attention, and not only the magnitude but also the quality of response may be inadequate. A common complaint of elderly people is that they are dismissed from their doctor with a cursory platitude such as 'it's your age, what can you expect?' A diagnosis based on traditional history and examination, backed up where necessary by investigations and a timely explanation in appropriate terms, must surely be the appropriate response from a modern professional rather than such a nihilistic cliché.

PREVALENCE

There are considerable difficulties in quantifying the exact prevalence of each of these disorders, since definitions and methods differ. There have been numerous surveys, quoting from one by Broe (4) shows the ranges of the common giants (Table 17.1) which gives an idea of their relative prevalence. Although each disease is often seen in its 'pure' form, one feature of geriatric medical practice is the frequency with which multiple pathology is found, both within the nervous system, and also in other systems.

Parkinsonism is a particular case which exemplifies the overlap between normality and pathology in advanced age.

Table 17.1 Prevalence of neurological diseases in the elderly: literature reviews

Disease	Prevalence per 100 000	Ref.
Dementia (mild–moderate)	5400–52 700	(5)
Epilepsy	200–500	(6)
Motor neurone disease	9–19	(7)
Parkinsonism	80–1400	(8)
Primary central nervous system tumour	20–90	(9)
Stroke	2930–7000	(10)

The overall prevalence of signs of parkinsonism in an elderly population rises from 14.9% in the population aged 65–74, 29.5% for the 75- to 84-year-olds, and 52.4% for those 85 and over. This is not just a casual observation, but one with sinister implications—those with signs of parkinsonism had an age-adjusted mortality twice that of those without signs, and this excess risk is strongly related to gait disturbance (11, 12).

PATHOLOGY OF NORMAL AND ABNORMAL AGEING PROCESSES

A degree of cerebral atrophy, as measured by brain volume and weight at necropsy, is seen with advancing age, the rate of loss of brain mass accelerating beyond the sixth decade. Several studies have suggested a gender differentiation with a greater loss in women than men. Computerized tomography (CT) has confirmed these data *in vivo* and show an exponential increase in ventricular size in addition to reduced cortical volume.

Neuronal cell loss also accompanies ageing, most marked in the neocortex and hippocampus, sparing other discrete areas such as the mammillary bodies, and certain cranial nerve nuclei. Locus coeruleus loses up to 50% of its dopaminergic neurones by the age of 85, and the cerebellar Purkinje cells depreciate at approximately 2.5% per decade, mainly after 60 years of age.

Senile plaques and neurofibrillary tangles are seen with increasing frequency as age advances, but are not universal. Whether they are a marker of a disease process rather than a normal feature of old age is a matter of conjecture. They have different distributions—tangles being found more commonly in the hippocampus, and plaques in the cortex, although both have wide and overlapping distribution. They are a consistent feature of senile dementia of Alzheimer's type (SDAT) and several other neurodegenerative diseases, in which plaques and tangles are accompanied by reactive gliosis and cell loss. Amyloid protein and its precursors are also identified in SDAT, and may be implicated in its pathogenesis, indicating the probability of a genetic cause in many cases.

The ageing brain is also characterized by changes in neurotransmitter concentrations. Broadly, the cholinergic and monoamine neurotransmitters (dopamine, noradrenaline, and 5-HT or serotonin) are present in lower concentrations than in younger adults. In contrast, increased monoamine oxidase B levels have been frequently observed and there are also variable changes in the glutamate and gamma aminobutyric acid (GABA) systems. Neuropeptide levels are not appreciably different in older individuals. The implications of all these variations in healthy ageing, in benign ageing processes, and in pathological states remain controversial.

NEUROLOGICAL SIGNS IN NORMAL AGEING

Certain characteristics of ageing make archetypes inevitable. The image of the stooped elderly woman, with wasted muscles

and dementia is a powerful one. The tendency to pigeon-hole patients on superficial impressions must be recognized and resisted, as it would be when treating any other population group to avoid making judgements based on prejudice rather than rational thought. Indeed, the very signs which modern Western society interprets as a sign of weakness, fallibility, and impending senility, in many Eastern cultures are recognized paradoxically as signifying wisdom and therefore command respect, much as they did in earlier times in Western society when the elderly population was so very much smaller.

Physical signs may be found from perfectly natural ageing, from new morbid incidents, and also the legacy of disabling illnesses and trauma of the past. Neurological signs that may frequently be found in the absence of disease, and thereby could be interpreted as signs of normal ageing include an abnormally flexed posture, loss of ankle jerks, reduced vibration sense, an action tremor, benign memory loss, and a deficiency of upward gaze. Table 17.2 shows many of the other common features include wasting of the intrinsic hand muscles, especially the dorsal interossei, with relative preservation of power. Tone is commonly increased, particularly in the legs. The gait characterized by more sway, a shorter pace, and is associated with an increased tendency to fall.

Complex signs may therefore be found even in patients without neurological diseases. When a disease process is also present, diagnosis may be made more difficult by the nonspecific presentation of disease in older people. In addition, sensory impairment affecting vision or hearing through cataract, glaucoma, macular degeneration, or presbyacusis, etc., are all common concomitants of ageing. Despite these practical problems, accurate diagnosis, even if of multiple pathology, is still a prerequisite of good management.

SENSATION

Although the examination techniques are the same, interminable patience may seem to be required in checking modalities of sensation unless a more simple pragmatic methodology is used. It is often best to relate a sensory examination to its medical context: after a stroke, relevant findings would be hemianaesthesia or sensory inattention, whereas in

Table 17.2 Neurological signs in the elderly: literature reviews

Feature	Maximum quoted prevalence	Ref.
Hand muscle wasting	77%	13
Limited upward gaze	20%	14
Loss of tendon jerks	70% ankle, 26% knee	15
Loss of vibration sense	100% (legs >arms)	14
Loss of pain, touch, or temperature sense	24%	16
Rest tremor	43% arms, 7% head	13
Short stepping gait	56%	13
Sluggish pupillary responses	34%	13

a patient complaining of numbness, examination of the specific modalities of sensation in the affected area, combined with a discrimination between dermatome or peripheral nerve distribution is required. Searching for a sensory level may often be more productive than endlessly checking each dermatome, and the thumb-finding test may be a better way of determining position sense than repetitive checking of the position of metacarpal or metatarsal in thumb or toe, respectively. Normal ageing is often accompanied by loss or reduced perception of vibration sense, joint position sense, and two point discrimination.

MOTOR POWER

Tests of power for individual muscles or groups need to be related to the strength of the individual, but are otherwise similar to those in younger adults. The distribution of the weakness, coupled with the associated signs (plantar responses, fasciculation, sensory loss) help to distinguish between pyramidal tract and lower motor neurone or peripheral nerve lesions.

CO-ORDINATION

Testing co-ordination is an important part of the clinical examination. At its crudest, it can be checked, as can motor power, by asking the patient to walk, and perform other complex tasks. Finer testing may well need to follow, to distinguish between the various causes of ataxia, with formal testing of cerebellar and extrapyramidal tract function. The 'Get-up and go' test correlates well with formal tests of gait and balance and is useful for ambulant patients.

REFLEXES AND PRIMITIVE SIGNS

Ankle reflexes become increasingly difficult to elicit in older patients, but their loss is not universal and may indicate the presence of a neuropathy. Loss of other tendon reflexes because of age alone is even less common, and a cause should normally be sought. An extensor plantar reflex (Babinski test) is most unusually due to age alone. Jaw jerks, glabellar tap response, snout reflex, and grasp reflex are found increasingly commonly in the very elderly, whereas their presence in younger patients would indicate a specific disease, their finding in old (particularly very elderly) people is sometimes otherwise inexplicable. It remains contentious whether they are found in neuropsychiatrically normal old people, since positive findings correlate with formal tests of cognitive impairment, and with the presence of clinical features of dementia and other neurodegenerative diseases.

FUNCTIONAL ASSESSMENT OF MENTAL AND PHYSICAL STATUS

Assessment of the abilities of the individual should ideally be tailor-made for that patient in their own environment. In the clinical context, standard scales of impairments or disabilities are normally used, and their use is now widely accepted. None gives absolute results, all are subjective, and coloured by value judgements, and all should therefore be cautiously interpreted. Subject to these caveats, they allow a necessarily crude assessment of individual skills, and a broad measure of comparability of dependency. The introduction of the standardized assessment protocols has lead to a widespread utilization of these scales in geriatric medicine. The commonest scales in regular use are the Barthel Activities of Daily Life Index (BAI) (18, 19; Appendix 1), which measures performance in 10 areas necessary for normal personal care, and the Abbreviated Mental Test Score (AMTS) (20; Appendix 2), with 10 questions covering the domains of orientation, short- and long-term memory, and recall; or the more comprehensive 30-point Mini-mental Test Score (MMTS) (21). In addition, other specific scales may be needed to complement the Barthel and MTS scales in certain disease areas. Examples include the Glasgow Coma Scale (22); the Universal Parkinson's Disease Rating Scale (UPDRS) (23) and Webster Scale in Parkinson's disease (24); the MRC 0–5 point grading of motor power (25); and the Geriatric Depression Scale (26). More sophisticated instruments are also commonly used in specialist departments, for expert administration by therapists or psychologists.

DIAGNOSIS

The establishment of a formal diagnosis may be more difficult, but remains as essential in older individuals as it would rightly be considered in younger ones. Most conditions can be treated, many retarded, and some cured once they have been correctly diagnosed. Even if the prognosis is bad, this at least can be confronted by patient or carer to allow them the chance to address unfinished business, and if necessary, attend to matters such as the preparation of a will. Failure or erroneous diagnosis prevents appropriate treatment, can cause iatrogenic disease through injudicious prescribing, and prevents forward planning, causing much avoidable resentment.

A full treatment history, including non-prescribed medications, is required to investigate the possibility of iatrogenic disease. Commonly prescribed drugs with neurological side-effects include the phenothiazines (particularly those used as vestibular sedatives such as prochlorperazine) causing extrapyramidal signs and symptoms, phenytoin (ataxia, nystagmus), benzodiazepines (drowsiness), oral hypoglycaemics (neuroglycopaenia, blackouts, confusion), antihypertensives (lethargy, hypotension, depression, etc.).

ASSESSMENT IN DOMESTIC CIRCUMSTANCES

The clinical examination may have to be performed in a variety of environments; hospital, day hospital, and in a variety of venues within the loosely used term 'community', including the patient's own home. Examination in a formal environment may well make the clinician's task easier, but the pragmatist will also wish to see how the patient manages in their own home, be that a house, apartment, or residential establishment. In addition to the clinical, relevant functional information can be gleaned, one can also assess the domestic circumstances, obtain the story of family or carer to complete the clinical picture (important for fits, faints, collapses), and pick up other clues of incontinence, nutrition, alcohol, medication, and assess other risk factors for falls. An inspection of the contents of the refrigerator and even the dustbin can be revealing in cases of suspected malnutrition or alcohol abuse. Finally, the services of an occupational therapist can render further assistance in a formal home visit or assessment, particularly if adaptations are required, or to reduce risks of falls by removal of hazards.

INVESTIGATION

Most patients will merit simple haematological (full blood count with MCV and viscosity or erythrocyle sedimentation rate, ESR) and biochemical screening (glucose, electrolytes, renal, and liver profiles) to exclude metabolic, nutritional, or secondary causes of non-specific symptoms. The value of routine tests of syphilis serology is doubtful, although best not omitted in old sailors, or those with oddly reacting pupils. Vitamin B_{12} levels are not routinely justified, but should be obtained in patients with neuropathy and macrocytosis or other suspicion of subacute combined degeneration.

Modern imaging techniques have revolutionized the investigation of neurological illness, and the elderly have benefited as much as any other group. Computerized tomography (CT), nuclear magnetic resonance imaging (MRI), Doppler ultrasonography, and more recently functional imaging techniques using single photon emission computerized tomography (SPECT), and positron emission tomography (PET) have allowed non-invasive investigation for a range of suspected pathologies, and spared the more invasive tests such as lumbar puncture and arteriography.

Lumbar puncture is now rarely indicated, other than in the investigation of suspected Guillain–Barré syndrome, neurosyphilis, and infections such as meningitis. In most cases, a CT scan is the investigation of choice in cerebrovascular disease, tumours, and other suspected mass lesions presenting with upper motor neurone signs. In dementia, a CT scan can give useful anatomical evidence, but the correlation between intellectual impairment and cortical width is not close, and scans showing mild degrees of atrophy should be interpreted cautiously.

An electroencephalogram (EEG) may be helpful in the investigation of epilepsy, and electromyogram (EMG) in neuropathies and wasting conditions such as motor neurone disease.

TREATMENT

Once the diagnosis has been established, treatment needs to be planned. Depending on circumstances, it will often need to be a joint process employing the skills of not only the medical profession, but also the nurses, therapists, social workers, and especially, the patient and carers, in varied proportions at each stage. I shall, somewhat arbitrarily, divide this into three phases; acute, rehabilitation, and longer-term care. The diagnostic mode should not automatically lead to a therapeutic one. For example, the discovery of a trivial tremor necessitates a diagnosis, but will not necessarily merit treatment, unless there is evidence of functional impairment, and only then once an accurate diagnosis has been made.

ACUTE CARE

Clearly, the first priority after establishing a diagnosis is to arrange for any appropriate specific therapy. In the elderly patient, the background morbidity will also need to be recognized—the known decrease in renal function should be considered in the selection of an appropriate antibiotic, diabetes mellitus has a prevalence of 10% in elderly inpatients and should be tested for, and treated when appropriate. In addition, ethical, social, and moral factors, and a realistic assessment of the prospects of cure are all important considerations at this early stage. In addition, there is an important need to avoid complications such as contractures or decubitus ulceration as well as avoiding unnecessary instrumentation such as catheterization.

A functional approach should be adopted from the outset—either in the outpatient setting or at the point of admission. The two vital components are what effects this new problem has upon the ability to manage at home and what was the previous (premorbid) ability.

When the patient is able to stand, blood pressure should be recorded in both lying and standing positions, and examination is incomplete without a check on balance and gait.

REHABILITATION

The overall aims of the rehabilitation phase is to reduce disability, and alleviate handicap. A subsidiary aim from the patient's perspective, but of increasing importance to hospital management is to reduce reliance on intensive, and hence expensive, hospital resources. The two skills necessary to achieve effective rehabilitation are multidisciplinary management, and discharge planning. Treatment goals need to be planned individually, reviewed regularly, and revised accordingly. One person (normally described as a key worker) takes overall responsibility for this process at any particular point in time. This person will often change during the process as will the priorities. The culmination of the hospital stay is necessarily the discharge, but especially with complex cases, this will need extensive planning, which starts at, or even before, admission.

A full assessment is mandatory before attempting rehabilitation. To be comprehensive, aspects of impairment, disability, and handicap all need consideration. *Impairment* is defined as the damage incurred, in this case, to the nervous system. *Disability* is the effect of that impairment on the functional abilities of the person (i.e. ability to arise from bed, walk, dress, wash, make a meal and control hygiene and elimination). In many ways, it is more relevant than the impairment from the patient's perspective, and also for their caregivers, but harder to be objective about and quantify. *Handicap* is the summative effect of the impairment and its handicap produces on the patient's life. It includes the social perspectives which impact on the quality of life.

The impairment can be assessed by examination and investigation, and the disability assessed by enquiry of the patient and carers, coupled with observation by medical, nursing staff, with skilled assessment by the occupational therapist. Handicap is much more subjective, and influenced by the interaction between the environment and the patient.

LONGER-TERM CARE

For any physician, addressing the urgent needs of an acute illness takes priority over planning for the longer term. Decisions on placement should never be rushed, and must involve a full assessment of medical, social, and personal factors. The needs of carers, as well as the wishes of the patient must also be addressed. Not infrequently, it is an acute event which prompts a review of circumstances which have been inadequate for some time, ultimately culminating in a change of domicile, or entry to care.

In general terms, one should start with the assumption that old patients are as keen and able to return to their own homes as are younger ones. If new disability has been caused, then a formal appraisal is required. A case conference may be necessary to ensure that all alternatives have been explored, and that all parties are agreed with the plan. Only if there is no alternative should a change of residence be initiated.

If longer-term residential or nursing home care is required, this should be carefully planned, with the patient fully involved in the planning process. This normally entails a full discussion with the matron or manager, and a visit to the home to mutually assess suitability. Exceptionally, a long-term hospital continuing-care bed may be available if the medical or nursing needs dictate. Otherwise, consideration to the benefits of longer-term involvement of the hospital (specialist) team needs to be balanced against the transport, and resource considerations.

THE COST–BENEFIT CONCEPT

In the modern health care environment, consideration of the costs of treatment raises two concepts: first, the efficacy of treatment to cure or combat disability; and second, the measurement of benefit against cost. Cost in this context, relates to the total cost to not only to the individual, but also to the caregivers, be they informal (family, spouse, neighbours, and friends) but also to the statutory services; health, social services, and other agencies, such as social security (benefits) and insurance agencies.

Considering the costs separately, any treatment has an overt cost, for medication this would be the costs of the drugs and any pharmacy dispensing charge against which prescription charges may be offset. However, the total cost includes the cost of treating or compensating for side-effects, which may arise from interactions or poor compliance, both of which are more common in older people, and the costs of monitoring, such as anticonvulsant levels.

Any change in physical or mental status may alter the capacity of caregivers to cope, (e.g. alleviation of physical handicap may prevent the need for institutionalization, or reduce caring costs in the community), while the onset of dementia, hallucinations, and other psychiatric disorders may provoke admission to care, and a rapid escalation of cost.

Any putative benefits therefore need to be carefully assessed against this background. Many studies have shown an increased prevalence of adverse drug reactions in the elderly. Concomitant medication becomes more likely as the prevalence of coexistent disease rises, and drug interactions therefore become more frequent. Additionally, compliance may be poor. These interrelated and interdependent factors tip the balance against unwarranted use of medication, and also favour non-pharmacological treatments where possible. Physiotherapy, dietary modification, and behavioural methods may therefore need to be employed more liberally than in younger patients. The special skills required in these professions in handling older patients has also become increasingly recognized.

TERMINAL CARE

Whether in hospital or in the wider community, special care needs to be taken to recognize when curative treatment is no longer feasible, and when attention must turn to palliation. The elderly are more likely to uphold ethnic or spiritual traditions, and these demand full respect. Families may find especial difficulty in accepting the imminent demise of an elderly relation when the normal reactions of sadness and upset may be complicated with guilt or repressed fear. Living wills are becoming more popular, and demand respect, if not slavish adherence, and the ethical issues raised by them, as with demands for euthanasia can stress even the most experienced practitioner. In older patients one anticipates higher prevalence of malignancies, particularly secondary tumours, from all the common sites. These include bronchus, breast, stomach, as well as primary astrocytomas and gliomas.

Attention to hydration and nutrition are essential, and may entail the use of subcutaneous fluids, or percutaneous endoscopic gastrostomy (PEG) when the oral route becomes impossible as in advanced motor neurone disease, pseudobulbar palsies, etc. Careful explanation of the distress caused by dehydration is required to avoid the charge of inappropriate treatment.

The avoidance of malnourishment will avoid unnecessary suffering by reducing the chance of pressure areas breaking down. Opiate analgesia may need to be employed, either by oral route, or by subcutaneous infusion by syringe driver with antiemetics, benzodiazepines, and TENS (transcutaneons electrical nerve stimulation) in some circumstances. Other forms of drug treatment should be rationalised. Best practice requires the careful consideration of the multidisciplinary input into a full care plan to which the patient and carers contribute, and with specialist support from Macmillan (palliative care) nurses.

SPECIFIC NEUROLOGICAL DISEASE AREAS

FALLS

These are a major cause of home accidents in elderly people and a common presentation of many disease processes. They are not only a serious problem to the individual who falls, to their formal and informal carers, but also to the health and social services because of the resources consumed as a consequence of investigation and treatment of their consequences. Distinguishing those due to neurological rather than cardiovascular or other systems can take much time and effort.

Only a small proportion of falls come to medical attention. A tiny minority will need hospital treatment, but the risk of hospitalization doubles from the eighth to ninth decades: 19/1000 per year of those age of 70–74 increasing to 42/1000 per year of those aged 80–84. However, even a relatively trivial fall may trigger a vicious spiral of failing homeostatic mechanisms, consequential social withdrawal, and further disease and disabilities, such as decubitus ulceration, or incontinence.

It must be stressed that although falls are associated with ageing they are not just an inevitable consequence of old age. Epidemiological data have been gathered in three distinct populations of old people—those in the general community, residents of institutions, and those presenting to medical attention. Community surveys suggest fairly consistent fall rates for the over 65 year age group of around 30% per year (Table 17.3). Within this heterogeneous group of elderly people fall rates double from age 60 to 85 years. Recall bias may explain some of these differences. A cohort of community subjects in San Francisco were followed carefully over one year and although 59% were identified by the monitors as falling, only 45% of the patients could recall the fall, with men significantly less likely to recall falls than women.

The importance of advanced age, female gender, cognitive impairment, and functional disability was recognized from

Table 17.3 annual rate of falls in the community (Population aged over 65 years)

Community	Year	Fall rate (per annum)	Ref.
Newcastle England	1981	28%	(27)
Gisborne, New Zealand	1981	34%	(28)
Chepstow, Wales	1984	28%	(29)

the earliest epidemiological studies. A further important factor is drug therapy, with longer-acting sedatives and tricyclic antidepressants being particularly associated with falls. Almost any acute illness in the frail elderly may precipitate a fall. High risk is also associated with patients who have neurological impairment (particularly where balance is impaired as in Parkinson's disease), those with cognitive impairment (dementia, toxic confusion), and those with wasting disorders (e.g. neoplasia, malnourishment). Fractures are thought only to occur in some 5% of all falls in the community.

The more vigorous elderly show a different pattern of falls, with a lower overall rate of falls but a greater danger of serious injury when falling. About 25–50% of falls occur outside the home, and are associated with greater damage. They are more common in men, and occur in more robust persons than those who fall in the home. Those occurring indoors have a higher mortality.

A history of falls should prompt a careful history and examination with a view to identification of reversible risk factors. In many of those at risk a multitude of factors will be found. The relative contributions of ageing, disease, and lifestyle may be impossible to disentangle. The 'over 75 assessment' might be a suitable vehicle for case finding in those at home, but a history of falls would need to be specifically sought because of the tendency to under-report. In long-term hospital and nursing home practice, the management of falls and accidents has been highlighted as a key area of quality assessment.

Features of the fall (or falls) such as their frequency, situation, circumstances, and associated symptoms are important. Initially, emphasis should be targeted at detecting treatable conditions; arrhythmia, postural hypotension, Parkinson's disease, vitamin B_{12} deficiency, osteomalacia, normal pressure hydrocephalus, joint disease, etc. The rationalization of drug therapy is the most easily achieved and of immediate relevance to the physician.

In simple terms, trips and slips are the commonest causes of single falls. However, whether these environmental factors are a preventable cause of falls remains controversial. Campbell, in New Zealand (1990) (28) found that despite vast numbers of potential hazards on home assessment they could rarely be implicated in the fall, and that when falls did have an environmental cause this was often everyday objects such as a bed leg, or a chair in its usual position. In the home, few falls occur on the stairs, but are more likely to result in a serious injury.

Specialist clinics targeting those with symptoms associated with unsteadiness or falls have been proved successful in both evaluating and treating patients who fall. Kenny (30) in Newcastle has raised awareness of the importance of assessing both the cardioinhibitory and vasodepressor components of the carotid sinus syndrome. The finding of this syndrome in a quarter of referrals for dizziness, syncope, and falls is impressive since pacing may be curative. Tilt tables and formalized gait assessment can be used to further elucidate mechanisms in recurrent fallers.

Physical training programmes have many advocates, particularly in retirement communities in the United States. There is evidence that muscle strength can be improved even at advanced old age, with proportional changes similar to those in younger individuals undergoing training. Recent studies have shown that attention to the multiple causes of falls can reduce their prevalence. The multiple risk factor intervention approach in the FICSIT trials (31) showed considerable reduction by focusing attention on medication education, and nutrition, and especially when combined with a modest exercise programme including Tai Chi.

Environmental adaptation has a logical appeal, but household clutter may provide familiarity and therefore have an important place in navigation. The provision of stair rails, bath and toilet aids, and alarm systems to the frail elderly or those with disabilities remains an important part of maintaining safety and restoring confidence. Similarly, attention to lighting, vision, chiropody and footwear, and avoidance of trailing wires and loose rugs has common sense appeal.

In addition, fractures are more likely to occur in the presence of weakened bone such as in osteoporosis. Evidence is accruing that fractures can be prevented by calcium and vitamin D supplementation (1.2 grams and 800 Units daily, respectively) (32) in nursing home residents, and by treatment with bisphosphonates in established cases. In high-risk groups, or frequent fallers, the innovative 'hip protector' has shown promising results in those able to wear it (33).

ORTHOSTATIC (POSTURAL) HYPOTENSION

Although not perhaps strictly a disease of the nervous system, the examination of an elderly person complaining of neurological symptoms is incomplete until the blood pressure has been recorded in both sitting and standing positions. The presence of a fall of 20 mm of systolic blood pressure is suggestive of significant postural (or orthostatic) hypotension, which merits further investigation. The causes are legion (see Table 17.4) and in many cases will be found to be due to the complications of immobility or of an alternative medical diagnosis, such as electrolyte imbalance or myocardial ischaemia. The elderly are much more sensitive to modest falls of blood pressure, it is presumed because of decreased cerebral autoregulation. Precipitating factors that need to be considered include cardiovascular causes—such as following a

Table 17.4 Causes of postural (orthostatic) hypotension

Neurodegenerative
Multisystem atrophy (MSA) (includes Shy–Drager syndrome)
Parkinson's disease
Autonomic neuropathy (including diabetes)
Paraparesis

Cardiological
Heart failure
Myocardial infarction
Pulmonary embolism

Metabolic
Hypovolaemia (acute > chronic), anaemia, Addison's disease
Electrolyte abnomalities (hyponatraemia, hypokalaemia, etc.)

Iatrogenic
Hypotensives, vasodilators
Antiparkinsonians, dopaminergics, antidepressants, phenothiazines

Miscellaneous
Prolonged recumbency
Following intercurrent illness (e.g. influenza)

myocardial infarct or ischaemia, arrhythmia, or outflow obstruction such as that due to aortic stenosis.

Environmental causes are common, due to excessive heat, and consequent vasodilatation. Especially notable in this regard is the use of hair dryers, hot baths, and prolonged standing such as at church services. Hypovolaemia from blood or fluid loss is a potent acute or chronic cause for its development. Among the various metabolic causes, hypokalaemia, and hyponatraemia are the most common. Finally, the neurological causes include extrapyramidal disorders (Parkinson's disease, multisystem atrophy (MSA)—including Shy–Drager syndrome), peripheral and autonomic neuropathies (e.g. diabetes), and a variety of iatrogenic causes including antiparkinsonian drugs, antihypertensives, and tricyclic antidepressants.

Treatment should initially be directed at the underlying cause and only if this has proved unrewarding should specific hypertensive agents be given. Physical treatment methods should normally be tried before pharmacological ones. Supportive elastic stockings (correctly fitted) to reduce venous pooling in the legs is a reasonable first measure. Elevation of head end of bed is also effective, and is thought to work by re-education of the baroreceptor reflexes. When these measures are insufficient, normal practice is to start with fludrocortisone (usually with potassium supplements) unless this is contraindicated because of pre-existent oedema or cardiac failure. Often drugs will be required—if fludrocortisone is ineffective or provokes cardiac embarrassment, pindolol, an adrenergic beta-blocker with high intrinsic sympathomimetic action (ISA), may be of use (in the absence of airways obstruction), sympathomimetics such as caffeine and ephedrine have been advocated. Non-steroidal anti-inflammatory drugs (flurbiprofen, indomethacin) may occasionally be useful by virtue of prostaglandin inhibition.

PARKINSON'S DISEASE AND OTHER MOVEMENT DISORDERS

Parkinson's disease (PD) is a progressive neurological syndrome which is characterized by the cardinal clinical signs of tremor, rigidity, akinesia, and disturbance of posture, balance, and gait. Surveys have shown the prevalence to be age-related, rising from 0.06% at the age of 65 to 2% of the population aged over 80 years. It is therefore a common disease amongst the elderly (see Table 17.1). Many of the features of extrapyramidal disease may be seen in the normal population—isolated features of the signs of Parkinson's disease may be found in up to 90% of a normal elderly population.

In addition to classical idiopathic Parkinson's disease, there are also a number of syndromes in which parkinsonism is accompanied by additional signs—often called '***Parkinson's plus syndromes***'—Multisystem atrophy, Steele–Richardson–Olszewski syndrome, Shy–Drager syndrome, striatonigral degeneration, etc. (Table 17.5).

Microscopic examination of the basal ganglia shows depigmentation and degeneration of neurones with Lewy bodies—intracytoplasmic inclusions of 3–20 μm size composed of proteins, free fatty acids, sphingomyelin, and polysaccharides. Immunocytochemical studies have shown monoclonal antibody responses to tubulin, neurofibrillary tangles, and ubiquitin, but not tau protein, in contrast to Alzheimer plaques. Lewy bodies were originally thought to be

Table 17.5 A clinical classification of parkinsonian syndromes

Idiopathic Parkinson's disease
Brainstem Lewy body parkinsonism
Familial (juvenile) Parkinson's disease

Symptomatic (secondary) parkinsonism
Post-encephalitic
Toxic
– Exogenous (e.g. manganese, carbon monoxide, MTPT, drug-induced)
– Endogenous (Wilson's disease)
Traumatic
Neoplastic
Pseudoparkinsonism
– Arteriopathic parkinsonism
– Normal pressure hydrocephalus

Parkinsonism in neuronal system degenerations
Multiple system atrophy
Striatonigral degeneration
Shy–Drager syndrome
Olivopontocerebellar atrophy
Progressive supranuclear palsy
   (Steele–Richardson–Olszewski syndrome)
Pallidonigral degenerations (e.g. Hallenvorden–Spatz disease)
Corticobasal degeneration
Diffuse Lewy body disease
Alzheimer's disease

pathognomonic of PD, but are now recognized to occur with normal ageing, and also in greater numbers in a range of diseases, including diffuse Lewy body disease and dementia of the Lewy body type (34).

There are differences between younger and older patients with this disease. Whether these differences are qualitative or quantitative remains contentious. However, a higher incidence of dementia in older cases than in younger ones is clearly apparent. Prognostic features for the development of dementia are age (both at onset and at time of entry), duration of PD, and disability. Motor fluctuations are said to occur less often, but with careful observation, can be seen in up to 50% of elderly patients. The response to treatment is probably as good in the elderly as in the younger patient with idiopathic PD. A lesser response should raise the question of Parkinson's plus syndromes (e.g. Steele–Richardson–Olszewski), Alzheimer's, or Lewy body dementia or cerebrovascular disease.

Treatment follows similar lines to that of the younger patient (35,36). In the United Kingdom, a multidisciplinary approach to treatment is preferred, and geriatricians are developing improved models of care—specialist clinics and specialist nursing in particular (37). Treatment is covered in detail elsewhere. The principles are no different in the elderly—levodopa (L-dopa) combined with a peripheral dopa decarboxylase inhibitor (Madopar, Sinemet) remains the treatment of choice. It is normally started when deteriorating function becomes apparent. In older patients, this may be earlier from diagnosis than in younger ones, in view of the relatively lower risk of them developing severe motor fluctuations, and from the higher relative risk that they carry of mortality from other diseases or the development of dementia. Normal starting doses are 62.5 mg tablet or capsule 3 times a day, increasing gradually up to a total dose of 400–600 mg levodopa daily in divided doses. Recent trial data have shown a much lower incidence of motor fluctuations in patients treated with doses of levodopa less than 500 mg daily, either of conventional or controlled release (CR) preparations than was expected from earlier trials in which 10% per annum cumulatively developed them. The CR preparations can be used to control fluctuations, and may also provide a smoother rise in levodopa blood levels which can be an advantage in very sensitive patients. If this proves insufficient, adjunctive treatment with the selective monoamine oxidase inhibitor, selegiline, can be considered. The safety of this drug has been questioned since the publication of the UK PDRG trial in 1995 (38). For older patients, or the very frail, the dose of selegiline may need to be reduced to 5 mg or less. The direct agonists (pergolide, bromocriptine, ropinirole, cabergoline, pramipexole) are effective in add-in therapy, but their use may be more difficult because of the higher risk of provoking postural hypotension and confusion. Consideration of their use in earlier stages may be worthwhile in biologically, rather than chronologically young patients. Dosage changes should be very gradual and the smallest effective dose should be used. Apomorphine by subcutaneous injection (and covered with domperidone to prevent nausea) is used in patients who have become refractory to oral medication.

Anticholinergic (antimuscarinic) drugs are best avoided, especially in older patients because of their poor tolerance. Amantidine has a limited place, again because of side-effects (ankle oedema and confusion are frequently encountered), its limited duration of action, and its renal excretion which is reduced in older patients.

MOTOR NEURONE DISEASE

Although numerically rare, with a prevalence of between 9 and 19 per 100 000 in the general community and an annual adjusted mortality rate of approximately 1 in 100 000, this condition has a peak incidence in the sixth decade. It is important to recognize the features of this disease of unknown aetiology in order to best plan for the care needs of the individual and also because it features amongst the differential diagnosis of a number of conditions in which weakness or dysphagia present in the older patient. Pathologically, it is characterized by progressive degeneration of anterior horn cells and of the pyramidal tracts. The pathological features are most marked in the cervical and lumbar cord and in the cranial nerve nuclei in the brainstem. Peripheral nerves show atrophic changes and distal muscles show pathological features of atrophy.

The clinical presentation of motor neurone disease (MND) is extraordinarily variable with three characteristic classical syndromes, between which there is enormous overlap. Two-thirds of patients will present with features of progressive muscular atrophy (PMA), in which the most characteristic feature is lower motor neurone loss most marked in the distal limbs. A rarer presentation is with progressive bulbar palsy (PBP) in which the onslaught of symptoms primarily affects the cranial nerve nuclei and patients classically present with features of a bulbar palsy (i.e. slurring of speech, difficulty chewing and swallowing, dribbling, or recurrent chest infections). The third classical presentation is termed amyotrophic lateral sclerosis (ALS) in which upper motor neurone signs predominate, at least initially. These three presentations are not exclusive and most patients will have features of more than one.

The patients complaints will often relate to the type of presentation. PMA will usually present with weakness but that might present with difficulty in mobility, in altered gait, falls or difficulty with feeding or dressing. In contrast, the patient with classical PBP may have difficulty with phonation, with slurring of speech, particular difficulty in pronouncing consonants, and difficulty with chewing and swallowing food. Often solid food is more easily swallowed at first, whereas liquids may provoke unpleasant choking attacks, but latterly solid food becomes difficult to swallow as well. Food may be regurgitated or inhaled and breathlessness may supervene because of weakness of the intercostal and diaphragmatic musculature.

Although the disease primarily affects the motor neurones, patients will not infrequently complain of sensory symptoms, either as a consequence of the atrophic muscles or fasciculation, and others will complain of paraesthesiae, formication, or other sensory symptoms. If, however, these are accompanied by sensory signs alternative diagnoses should normally be sought since the signs are almost exclusively related to motor neurone damage, from upper and lower motor neurone dysfunction in varied proportions. Commonly, one sees wasting of the intrinsic hand muscles extending more proximally to affect the lower arm, which initially may be asymmetrical. Fasciculation is often a predominant feature, particularly in the affected muscles, but often also elicited in apparently normal ones. Reflexes are usually accentuated when upper neurone involvement is predominant but conversely may be diminished in lower motor neurone predominant cases. While lower motor neurone signs may be seen in the legs it is more common to see upper motor neurone signs predominating here with spasticity even amounting to a spastic paraparesis with extensor plantar responses. Bulbar palsy similarly may be either predominantly lower motor neurone with predominant wasting of the tongue and muscles of the face and jaw, and a fasciculation of the tongue being predominant features. The upper motor neurone variety of pseudobulbar palsy may present similarly but without the wasting of the tongue, which may be stiff and pointed and clumsy. Dysarthria predominates and takes a distinct course from bulbar palsy but often expert assessment is needed to differentiate between the two. As with limb involvement often there is a mixture of upper and lower motor neurone disease.

Differential diagnosis

Although a typical advanced case with a full house of symptoms and signs can be straightforward to diagnose, earlier in the course of the disease and in those patients with non-specific symptoms and signs, differential diagnoses may be extensive. It is important to exclude syringomyelia and cord compression due to cervical spondylosis, tumours, or root compression, especially if sensory loss is minimal. This is especially so in patients presenting with a spastic paraparesis in which investigations should normally exclude cord compression before alighting on the diagnosis of MND. Other conditions which may present in a similar fashion include demyelination, peripheral neuropathy, subacute combined degeneration, neurosyphilis, and a variety of metabolic and endocrine disturbances including osteomalacia, diabetes, hyperthyroidism, and carcinomatous myopathy. Within the nervous system, in addition to syringomyelia and syringobulbia, myasthenia gravis and thyrotoxicosis are worthy of exclusion.

Investigations

In classical cases, few investigations may be called for, other than those to exclude the conditions referred to above. It is normally wise to check on a blood glucose, urea, full blood count, and ESR (or viscosity), thyroid function tests and syphilis serology, and a chest X-ray together with X-rays if cord compression or root entrapment is suggested. Nuclear magnetic resonance (NMR) has reduced the need for myelography and can be invaluable in the diagnosis of syringomyelia as well as cord compression. An EMG showing fasciculation and fibrillation potentials is confirmatory. Muscle biopsy is rarely helpful. Creatinephosphokinase (CPK) is usually mildly elevated in contrast to polymyositis and other myopathic conditions in which higher levels are seen.

Management

The place of specific drug treatment for MND is gradually emerging. Currently, the antiglutamate drug, Riluzole, is restricted to specialist units for use in early ALS. Improved survival times and slower deterioration have been demonstrated in trials. In addition to any current or future drug treatment, the patient and their carers will need extensive support throughout the duration of the disease which, although typically two to three years, may be as long as ten. Various symptomatic treatments may be required such as benzodiazepines for spasticity and cramps, tricyclic antidepressants for depression and drooling, and analgesics may be helpful for discomfort. Maintenance of adequate caloric intake and hydration becomes an increasingly major problem as the disease progresses. Initially, the assistance of a dietitian and speech therapist should be sought, and modification of the consistency of the food with thickening of fluids and avoidance of food liable to aggravate dysphagia, such as mixed texture or dry foods. A liquidizer can be helpful and good positioning can assist swallowing. Later, a fine bore nasogastric tube, or a PEG may allow adequate nutrition and hydration to be maintained towards the terminal stages.

The intellect is normally preserved throughout, which often leads to a very distressing state, not only for the patient but also their near family. Time taken to explain the diagnosis and its implications and also offering sympathetic help can often allay some of the worst fears of the patient and his/her family. Exercise should be encouraged and the advice and guidance of a physiotherapist skilled in such matters can often be of great value, to maintain functional independence as long as is possible. Skilled nursing care is vitally important to avoid the secondary effects of pressure and contractures and also to supervise feeding procedures. In the later stages of the disease the experience of trained palliative care nurses can often be very beneficial to the maintenance of the patient at home, hospital ward, or nursing home.

EPILEPSY

In contrast to many conditions which are exclusively or predominantly found in the elderly, epilepsy can occur at any age, and the differences between presentation and management depend more on the circumstances than any more fundamental age-related difference. Estimates of prevalence are difficult with a wide variance between different surveys, typically about 3–4% will have a fit at some time in their life but the prevalence of active epilepsy is much lower at around 0.5%. The incidence follows a U-shaped curve with a second peak of incidence from the sixth decade, rising from 11.9 per 100 000 between 40 and 59 to 82 per 100 000 in those over 60.

Differentiation of epilepsy from other causes of faints and blackouts in older patients may make the diagnosis long delayed. An adequate history may not be forthcoming but should be sought, not only from the patient, but also from family, friends, or even such sources as the home help, warden, or other frequent visitor. The only type of fit which is not seen in the elderly is 'petit mal' but surveys of epilepsy in elderly people have suffered much from selection bias and it is difficult to be categorical about the classification of fits arising from these surveys. The majority are undoubtedly grand mal seizures, with a mixture of partial or secondary focal seizures and occasional somatosensory or temporal lobe epilepsy and very rarely epilepsy partialis continua, which may masquerade as a movement disorder which will respond to anticonvulsant medication.

Aetiology

In contrast to younger patients with epilepsy, the commonest cause of epilepsy in the elderly is cerebrovascular disease, accounting for more than half the cases. The incidence of epilepsy following stroke may be as high as 10%. The remainder are due to cerebral tumours, senile dementia, and toxic or metabolic causes, such as drugs, alcohol, uraemia, myxoedema, hypoxia, hypoglycaemia, hyponatraemia, hepatic failure, and hypocalcaemia. Before ascribing epilepsy to idiopathic, one should consider whether there may have been an early history of fits in childhood, or in younger life which has been forgotten, and attention should also be placed on the drug sheet, since drug-induced epilepsy can be provoked by a wide array of drugs, particularly aminophylline, analgesics, tranquillizers, and antidepressant and anaesthetic agents.

Investigations

As with the investigation of other causes of faints and blackouts, a general review is required to see if the aetiology can be easily explicable. Monitoring of blood sugar, ECG, and simple screening of metabolic data to exclude the common secondary causes of epilepsy should always be undertaken. A 24-hour ambulatory ECG may be helpful to exclude arrhythmias. An EEG may confirm the diagnosis of epilepsy, particularly if characteristic spike and wave discharges are seen. A negative EEG does not exclude the diagnosis and other information that may be obtained from the EEG may include the finding of a focal abnormality, which suggests the need for further investigation. Controversy surrounds the need for a CT scan. There is little doubt that scanning increases the frequency by which a definitive diagnosis can be made, however, the frequency by which the scan would actually change management is likely to be much lower. Depending on clinical circumstances a CT scan is desirable unless there is a clear-cut diagnosis possible by alternative means and certainly in recurrent fits one would be ill advised to omit this valuable investigation.

Management

Another controversial area is whether a patient who presents in later life with their first fit should be started immediately on an anticonvulsant. There is no doubt that anticonvulsants are as effective in older patients as in younger patients but their tolerance is probably lower. In the absence of definitive results of trials, the pragmatic clinician would often wait until a second or subsequent fit occurs, rather than initiating treatment after a single fit, unless there is a clear-cut aetiological reason, such as trauma or neurosurgical procedures, or to avoid the onset of epilepsy in a patient with an inoperable brain tumour. The choice of anticonvulsants is similar to that in younger patients. For patients with grand mal epilepsy three drugs are commonly used: phenytoin, carbamazepine, and sodium valproate. Phenytoin has the advantages of familiarity and cost, but has a wide array of neuropsychiatric side-effects which may be rather commoner in older patients than younger ones. Its use needs to be monitored and a high threshold of suspicion, particularly if the patient complains of loss of balance or starts to fall. Clinical response should be monitored and anticonvulsant levels may be helpful to check that therapeutic levels have been achieved without toxicity. An initial dose of 200 mg of phenytoin is often sufficient, with small increments thereafter, often 25 mg at a time, to avoid swinging from an inadequate to a toxic dose. For these reasons, other drugs and some of the newer agents are often preferred. Anticonvulsants are usually continued lifelong once started, therefore the choice of anticonvulsant needs to be carefully considered in the light of the individual circumstances, including compliance, other medication, and tolerability. Consideration also needs to be given to the effect of the prescription of an anticonvulsant on the metabolism of other drugs, since these drugs are potent enzyme inducers and may destabilize patients on a number of drugs including anticoagulants, antibiotics, and oral hypoglycaemics.

CEREBROVASCULAR DISEASE

This is the commonest cause of new onset neurological disease in the elderly population and covers a multitude of syndromes and presentations. A hemiplegia is often the most dramatic and devastating form of stroke disease. Transient ischaemic attacks, as their name implies, are short-lived events with full recovery occurring in less than 24 hours. Reversible ischaemic neurological deficit (RIND) is used to describe the intermediate conditions which resolve between 24 hours and 3 weeks after onset, usually with full functional recovery. Finally, cerebrovascular disease may present with dementia which is considered below.

As in younger patients, cerebrovascular disease may take the form of thrombosis, embolus, or haemorrhage. Cerebral thrombosis usually occurs on the background of atheromatous arterial disease. Internal carotid arteries are the most common but atheroma may also attack the circle of Willis and the basilar circulation. Cerebral emboli are increasingly recognized as causes of stroke, arising either in the heart from a mural thrombosis or in the fibrillating atrium, from the aorta or carotid vessels. Cerebral haemorrhage is the last of the three main causes of cerebrovascular disease and most commonly takes the form of a spontaneous intracerebral haemorrhage but bleeding can also occur from arteriovenous malformation or from rupture of a Berry aneurysm causing subarachnoid haemorrhage, with its characteristic abrupt onset with headache, photophobia, and rapid loss of consciousness. A chronic subdural haematoma (unilateral or bilateral) characteristically presents in an insidious manner, often following a relatively minor head injury, which frequently has been long forgotten. Suspicions should be aroused if there is evidence of fluctuating levels of consciousness, with variable mental state, and transient long tract signs. A CT or NMR scan is necessary to prove the diagnosis, and neurosurgical referral is required unless it is felt that either the patient would not withstand the trauma of surgery or if the premorbid state did not justify the intervention.

Prevention

No consideration of cerebrovascular disease would be complete without consideration of the role of the physician in prevention of stroke, the prevalence of which rises from an annual incidence of less than 10 in 100 000 per year below the age of 40, to more than 2000 per 100 000 at the age of 85. While ageing itself is inevitable, there is strong epidemiological data to link stroke with the presence of hypertension and aggressive treatment of hypertension in middle and later life is justified to reduce the prevalence of the disabling effects of stroke. Aspirin has been shown to have a positive secondary preventative role in cardiovascular and cerebrovascular disease. More recently, the relevance of atrial fibrillation has been recognized and, in the absence of any contraindicating factors, prophylactic controlled anticoagulation with coumarin anticoagulants, such as warfarin, is indicated to reduce the prevalence of stroke in patients with atrial fibrillation. Other risk factors include diabetes, polycythaemia rubra vera, and coronary artery disease but there is only limited data to suggest that interventions in these conditions will reduce risk of further stroke.

Clinical syndromes vary with the distribution of the interruption to the arterial circuit and is traditionally divided into carotid territory and vertebrobasilar territory infarction. The carotid territory syndrome can be further divided into those of the anterior cerebral circulation, middle cerebral, and internal carotid artery. Anterior cerebral artery interruption is characterized by profound loss of motor and sensory function in the leg, often associated with urgency of micturition, or urinary incontinence, intellectual impairment, and often emotional upset which can be vividly described as emotional incontinence. Middle cerebral artery syndromes are characterized by a hemiparesis with hemisensory loss affecting mainly the face and arm with relative sparing of the leg. A homonymous hemianopia may be present and in dominant lesions a dysphasia which is usually of mixed receptive and expressive type and in non-dominant lesions sensory inattention and neglect of the affected side, often associated with apraxias. Internal carotid artery syndrome usual produce a combination of anterior and middle cerebral arteries, therefore with a profound loss of both arm and leg, usually associated with homonymous hemianopia. An ipsilateral Horner's syndrome may also be associated.

Vertebrobasilar syndromes are usually divided into those affecting the brainstem and those affecting the posterior cerebral artery distribution. The former are characterized by pupillary changes if the midbrain is affected, horizontal gaze palsy if the pons is affected, often with facial weakness or sensory loss, accompanied by a quadriparesis or hemiparesis. A variety of this syndrome traditionally known as a posterior inferior cerebellar artery syndrome, produces ischaemia of cranial nerve nuclei of V, VI, VII, IX, and X with cerebellar ataxia and an ipsilateral Horner's sign and a contralateral spinothalamic loss in the arm and leg but usually without hemiplegia. A complete basilar artery occlusion produces a fatal flaccid tetraplegia with loss of brainstem reflexes. A posterior cerebral artery lesion may be confined to the visual field defect, since this is the artery which supplies the occipital lobes as well as the upper part of the brainstem and medial surface of the temporal lobe. Cortical blindness can be diagnosed with the demonstration of blindness in the presence of normal pupillary responses. A rare variant is Anton's syndrome in which the patient presents with cortical blindness, confabulation, visual hallucinations—often with denial of the blindness. Infarction of the thalamus may also be produced by posterior cerebral artery occlusion, in which pain is predominant and often gentle sensory stimulation will be interpreted as painful.

Management of stroke will be described elsewhere. In general terms, in the acute phase it is important to establish an accurate diagnosis and exclude other causes such as hypoglycaemia which may mimic cerebrovascular disease very closely. Nursing care must be of the highest quality to avoid secondary problems and should be guided by a multidisciplinary team management, involving the physiotherapist to avoid further damage to shoulder or hemiplegic limbs. Gradually, as the case progresses the rehabilitation team will take an increasingly active part working towards the eventual discharge of the patient.

Prognosis

Adverse prognostic signs are the occurrence of loss of consciousness, the presence of urinary incontinence, a complete hemiplegia associated with loss of positional sense or sensory neglect, and inability to sit unaided. Prognostication is not an exact science, however, and the wise clinician will usually not issue a clear prognosis until several weeks have elapsed to allow a full assessment of not only the extent of damage but also the psychological profile of the individual to see how he/she will counter his/her new disability. In most patients, recovery will be at its most rapid during the first 3 months following the ictus, but in some, it may be delayed and may not be complete by 12 months. The organization of rehabilitation services to allow achievement of maximal recovery is a challenge to most geriatric departments.

Specific treatment

At present, no drug interventions have been proven to be efficacious in acute stroke, other than nimodipine in subarachnoid haemorrhage, and therefore, none is indicated. Anticoagulants are indicated if the stroke is embolic (in the absence of contraindications), and also in the prophylaxis and treatment of concomitant venous thromboembolism (DVT and pulmonary embolus). Aspirin is indicated in patients without evidence of intracerebral haemorrhage on CT, NMR scan, or lumbar puncture (rarely performed since the advent of scanning). Anticonvulsants may be required if epilepsy is present. The thalamic syndrome occasionally responds to carbamazepine or other anticonvulsant or antidepressant therapy.

Attention to fluid balance is important and intravenous or subcutaneous fluids may be required if swallowing is impaired. Clearly, ethical issues arise if recovery is unlikely but in patients in whom a pseudobulbar palsy is the only neurological deficit following multiple strokes, a nasogastric tube or PEG may be required to maintain hydration safely.

DEMENTIA AND COGNITIVE IMPAIRMENT

Dementia is defined as a global impairment of intellect, memory, and personality in the absence of alteration of consciousness. It becomes increasingly common rising from a prevalence of 2% at age 65 years to 20% over the age of 80. It is important to distinguish dementia, which is a chronic form of brain failure, from delirium which is the acute analogy. Confusion may be caused by almost any organic illness, and is especially likely to be provoked in the elderly. Its onset is typically abrupt, and its course much more variable than in dementia, which is much more likely to be insidious and chronically progressive. Other features suggestive of an acute confusional state are clouding of consciousness, lucid intervals, disorientation of time or place associated with impairment of recent memory, fear, bewilderment, agitation, and hallucinations or delusions. These may all occur in dementia, but are more intense, and positive dominant features of the acute rather than the chronic syndrome.

Minor degrees of memory loss become increasingly common in the ageing population, and is characterized as benign memory loss of ageing. As implied by its name, this does not usually progress to florid dementia, but because of it can be found in up to 50% of the population over 50 years of age, some cases of senile dementia of the Alzheimer's type (SDAT) will occur by coincidence.

The history is central, but may be somewhat elusive. Attempts to obtain the history directly from the patient are unlikely to be either accurate or reliable. Other sources of information include friends, family, neighbours, agencies such as social services (the home help can often be invaluable), general practitioner, or even tradesmen such as the milkman! Corroborative information may come from the physical state of the patient, the state of their dwelling, or from other sources.

Reliance on one feature alone is insufficient to establish a diagnosis, especially when the medical and social consequences can be so devastating. Cognitive decline must be distinguished from sensory deprivation due to deafness and/or visual handicap, depression, other chronic diseases, and the Diogenes syndrome. Exhaustive patience, coupled with a high index of suspicion, with judicious referral to audiologists, speech and language therapists, and ophthalmologist may be required. Rarely, severe depression may present as pseudodementia, and referral to a skilled psychiatrist and, even in suspected cases, a trial of antidepressant therapy is worthwhile.

Acute confusional states may be provoked by a wide array of aetiological factors, alone or in combination. These include infections, especially pneumonias, urinary tract infections, and rarely meningoencephalitis; injuries, particularly a head injury or hypothermia; infarction, cerebral or myocardial; alcohol or drugs; and metabolic causes, such as hypoglycaemia or hyponatraemia; and nutritional causes such as thiamine deficiency, Wernicke's encephalopathy.

The aetiology of dementia is becoming better understood with improving imaging and neuropathological attention. There is some debate about the relative frequency of the three main causes of dementia. Senile dementia of the Alzheimer's type (SDAT) is accepted as the most common, accounting for approximately half of all cases. It used to be accepted that cerebrovascular disease was the next most common, with multiple cerebral infarction alone (15%) or mixed with SDAT (a further 20%) as the next major group. It is possible to distinguish between vascular and non-vascular causes by use of the Hatchinski score. Diffuse Lewy body disease is increasingly recognized with diagnostic features including extrapyrammidal features, postural instability, visual hallucinations, and an innate variability of clinical state. The extreme sensitivity to neuroleptics is often the point at which it is clinically recognized, and has importance in terms of management. The other cases are caused by subcortical dementias (e.g. complicating Parkinson's disease), and an array of other conditions including chronic alcohol abuse, CNS infections (AIDS, Creutzfelt–Jacob disease, syphilis), normal pressure hydrocephalus, cerebral tumours, neuroglycopaenia, myxoedema, and vitamin B_{12} deficiency.

Normal pressure hydrocephalus deserves special mention, if only because of its insidious onset with a classic triad of dementia, ataxic gait, and urinary incontinence. Mild bilateral pyramidal signs may be found, often with extensor plantar responses. CT or NMR findings are diagnostic, with bilateral ventricular enlargement, but with normal cortical sulci. Lumbar puncture reveals normal pressure recordings, although with repeated monitoring may show abnormally high pressure spikes. Protein may be normal or mildly raised. Ventriculoatrial or ventriculoperitoneal shunting improves a proportion of patients, but for not those who are markedly demented for whom it may be too late.

The course of a typical case of SDAT may cover 10 years, with the first 5 to 7 being of gradually increasing loss of short-term memory, some mood disturbance—typically depression, but sometimes apathy, agitation, or indifference, and visuospatial disorientation, and progressively increasing difficulties with the activities of daily life. Ultimately, the rate of decline accelerates, with increasing disruption to normal family life, loss of language skills, dysphasia, agnosia, apraxia, incontinence, and motor impairment occurring later.

Recent research has suggested that apo-lipoprotein E4 and amyloid β-peptide are intimately linked with the pathogenesis of SDAT. These data suggest the tantalizing prospect of an understanding of the genetics of this disease, and also the possibility of presymptomatic identification and treatment. This would have clear ethical, financial, and logistic implications for the future. Meanwhile, treatment has been directed at cognitive enhancement, most effectively with anticholinesterase drugs, physostigmine, THA (Tacrine or tetrahydroaminoacridine), donepezil, and galanthamine. Side-effects have been a limiting problem for these agents but the medicine control agencies in several countries are beginning to license these drugs which appear to offer a modest improvement to some sufferers, if only by delaying deterioration for some months.

PERIPHERAL NEUROPATHY

Assessment of the patient presenting with paraesthesiae or numbness in the periphery can often produce a difficult plethora of symptoms and signs which often do not completely add up. However, broadly the investigation of a patient with these symptoms is similar to their younger counterparts. It must be remembered that there is a higher prevalence of diabetes mellitus in the elderly and quite frequently no underlying diagnosis is found. In such cases, the term 'idiopathic neuropathy' is ascribed but clearly this does not do other than satisfy the wishes of the physician to pigeon hole a condition. Occasionally, an occult carcinoma is disclosed by intensive investigation but whether this is warranted will depend upon the clinical circumstances. Drugs should always be considered as a potential cause and close attention paid to all prescribed and over the counter medications. Alcohol should be considered and the use of the CAGE questionnaire has been validated in elderly persons and should certainly be used in cases of doubt.

It should be noted that the Guillain–Barré syndrome has a second peak of incidence in older patients (45–75 years) and may be underrecognised in older groups. It follows a similar course in older patients as in younger ones. Prompt recognition of the ascending neuropathy is essential, lumbar puncture findings of raised proteins with typical dissociation from low lymphocyte count.

Management is essentially supportive. Correction of any identified deficiency is essential, but recovery may not be swift. In rapidly progressive Guillain–Barré syndromes, the peak flow rate should be monitored since ventilatory failure may develop with extraordinary speed. Mechanical ventilation may then be required until recovery follows. Prophylactic use of heparin or warfarin is sensible, and physiotherapy is important from the outset to avoid contractures, and maintain muscle bulk. The prognosis is worse in older patients, but close attention to respiratory function, and effective multidisciplinary rehabilitation will minimize the risks of mortality or of chronic sequelae.

INCONTINENCE

One of the commonest problems encountered in the management of old people is the control of micturition. Urinary incontinence is widespread, occurring in 7% of men, and 12% of women over the age of 65 years. It is a common cause of stress in both the sufferer and in their carers, and perhaps for this reason, as well as the loss of dignity and distress it causes, it is often concealed. It may be caused by a variety of provoking factors, physical, psychological, and environmental.

Transient incontinence is a common finding in any acute illness, and can be expected to settle with the provoking cause. Examples include the effects of a stroke, myocardial infarct (especially with the use of loop diuretics), respiratory or urinary tract infection, or metabolic upsets. It is of utmost importance not to compound this transient state by unnecessary catheterization, or by the imposition of immobility or restraint. Regular toileting, avoidance of constipation, and treatment of the underlying condition should produce rapid resolution. Established incontinence merits further investigation. In the neurological context, it is most likely due to lesions in the bladder or its autonomic control, the spinal cord, or a cerebral cortex. The commonest cause is an uninhibited neurogenic bladder due to cerebral degeneration or diseases, multi-infarct dementia, stroke, Alzheimer's disease (in which it is usually a late manifestation), parkinsonism, and normal pressure hydrocephalus. These can usually be distinguished on clinical grounds.

A history should first be obtained, concentrating on the awareness of the problem, its duration, the presence of bladder sensation (dysuria, urgency), and the type of leakage (steady dribble suggesting retention with overflow, leakage with coughing, laughing, or movement suggesting stress incontinence), or sudden flooding suggesting urge incontinence.

Examination should focus on the lower abdomen (a palpable bladder after voiding signifies retention), a rectal examination (for faecal impaction, anal tone, prostate size), vaginal examination for vaginitis or prolapse, and examination of the central and peripheral nervous systems for features of pyramidal, extrapyramidal, spinal cord lesions, peripheral, or autonomic neuropathy. Finally, a mental test score as an indicator of higher cortical function, together with an appraisal of affect.

Investigations should always include a urinalysis, and an MSU if obtainable. Depending on circumstances, a pelvic ultrasound, IVU, cystoscopy, and urodynamic studies may be required. Cystomanometry is a valuable procedure which can be performed as an outpatient procedure, although it rarely adds much to the diagnostic process in the presence of significant dementia.

Treatment is dictated by the findings. Urinary tract infections should be eradicated by appropriate antibiotics and copious fluids. The Royal College of Physicians (1996) (39) suggests that two-thirds of patients are likely to have incontinence cured, or alleviated by appropriate intervention. Patients with incontinence will benefit from referral to a continence nurse adviser, working closely with specialist gynaecology, urology, ward, and community nursing services.

Indwelling catheters should be avoided whenever possible, since they act as a focus for reinfection, and cause local trauma. A sheath urinal may be helpful during the early assessment period in the male, with close attention to personal hygiene. A variety of absorbent pads are available for both sexes. If a catheter is required, attention should be paid to the selection of the type of catheter system, and some patients will be able to intermittently self-catheterize, with better results than those obtained from chronic indwelling drainage.

Urinary retention should be relieved by either slow decompression of the bladder by urethral or suprapubic drainage, followed by definitive surgical treatment. Close attention to fluid and electrolyte balance is required during this phase since a degree of pre-renal uraemia can be anticipated, and relief of pressure may lead to acute tubular failure.

Bladder retraining as part of a behavioural modification programme may be helpful in cases of detrusor instability. It is helped by a diary or chart showing the progress made, and various drugs. These include anticholinergics, imipramine being commonly employed, calcium antagonists such as terodiline, alpha-blockers such as prazosin, and flavoxate. Oestrogens can be used in cases of atrophic vaginitis. Desmopressin has been helpful in patients prone to a nocturnal diuresis, but needs careful attention to electrolyte and fluid balance.

Finally, it should not be forgotten that incontinence may be provoked by an unsatisfactory environment, such as unattainably long distances between sitting areas and toilets. Attention to these apparently trivial domestic circumstances, particularly in residential homes, may avoid the development of this unpleasant and demeaning consequence.

CONCLUSIONS

The practice of geriatric medicine is not, and is unlikely ever to become a sinecure. The diagnosis and management of some of the neurological syndromes encountered among the elderly provide a challenge for even the most steadfast. However, the opportunities for the practice of good clinical medicine, together with the potential for research are vast. We can anticipate rapid advances in the science, the pathological and in the investigative techniques available to assist the clinician. We have seen a rapid expansion of the range of effective drugs in these disease areas, and can reasonably predict more treatment options becoming available as a result of progress in the understanding not only of cerebral and neurotransmitter function in normal ageing and in illness states, but also of the molecular basis of medicine and its application to neurodegenerative and cerebrovascular diseases. The major remaining challenges may well be in the application of science, be that the ability of society to afford the expensive techniques that its scientists have produced, or in the application of effective preventative strategies. One certainty remains—the practice of geriatric neurology will not be starved of patients for the foreseeable future, and wherever these patients present, doctors must be prepared with the tools for diagnosis and appropriate treatment.

REFERENCES

1. Robine JM, Blanchet M, Dowd JE. *Health expectancy.* HMSO, London. 1992.
2. Grimley-Evans J. Evidence-based and biased medicine (Editorial) *Age and Ageing* 1995; **24**: 461–3.
3. Akhtar AJ, Broe GA, Crombie A, McLean WMR, Andrews GR, Caird FI. Disability and dependence in the elderly at home. *Age and Ageing* 1973; **2**: 102–10.
4. Broe GA, Creasey H, The Neuroepidemiology of Old Age. In Tallis R (ed.) *The clinical neurology of old age.* Wiley, Chichester. 1989, pp. 51–65.
5. Henderson AF. The epidemiology of Alzheimer's disease. *Br Med Bull* 1986; **42**: 3–10.
6. Grimley-Evans J, Caird FI. Epidemiology of neurological diseases in old age. In Caird FI (ed.) *Neurological diseases in the elderly.* Wright, Bristol. 1982, pp. 1–16.
7. Li, T-M, Swach M, Alberman, E. Morbidity and mortality in motor neurone disease: comparison with multiple sclerosis and Parkinson's disease: age and sex specific rates and cohort analyses. *J Neurol Neurosurg Psychiatry* 1985; **48**: 320–7.
8. Kessler II. Parkinson's disease in epidemiologic perspective. In Schoenberg BS. (ed.). *Epidemiology of neurologic diseases. Advances in Neurology*, Vol. 19 Raven, New York. 1978, pp. 335–84.
9. Schoenberg BS. Epidemiology of primary nervous system neoplasms. In Schoenberg BS. (ed.) *Epidemiology of Neurologic Diseases.*
10. Kannel WB, Wolf PA. Epidemiology of cerebrovascular disease. In Ross Russell RW (ed.) *Vascular disease of the central nervous system,* (2nd edn). Churchill Livingstone, Edinburgh, 1983, pp. 2–3.
11. Bennett DA, Beckett LA, Murray AM, Shannon KM, Goetz CG, Pilgrim DM. *et al.* Prevalence of parkinsonian signs and associated mortality in a community population of older people. *N Engl J Med* 1996; **334**: 1611.
12. Louis ED, Marder K, Cote L, Wilder D, Tang MX, Lantigua R. *et al.* Prevalence of a history of shaking in persons 65 years of age and older: diagnostic and functional correlates. *Movement Disorders* 1996; **11**: 63–9.
13. Prakash C, Stern G. Neurological signs in the elderly. *Age and Ageing* 1973; **2**: 24–7.
14. Kokmen E, Bossemeyer RW, Barney J, Williams WJ Neurological manifestations of ageing. *J Gerontol* 1977; **32**: 411–19.
15. Klawans HL, Tufo HM, Ostfield AM, Shekelle RB, Killbridge JA. Neurologic examination in an elderly population. *Dis Nerv Syst* 1971; **32**: 274–9.
16. Howell TH. Senile deterioration of the nervous system. A clinical study. *BMJ* 1949; **i**: 56–8.
17. Mathias S, Isaacs B. Balance in elderly patients: The "Get-up and Go" test. *Arch Phys Med Rehabil* 1986; **67**: 387–9.
18. Mahoney FI, Barthel DW. Functional evaluation: The Barthel Index. *Maryland State Medical Journal* 1965; **14**: 61–5.
19. Collin C, Wade DT, Davies S, Horne V. The Barthel Index: a reliability study. *Int Disabil Stud* 1988; **10**: 61–3.
20. Hodkinson HM. Evaluation of a mental test score for assessment of mental impairment in the elderly. *Age and Ageing* 1972; **1**: 233–8.
21. Folstein MF, Folstein SE, McHugh PR. Mini-mental state: a practical method for grading the cognitive state of patients for the clinician. *J Psychiatr Res* 1975; **12**: 189–98.
22. Teasdale G, Jennett B. Assessment of coma and impaired consciousness. An practical scale. *Lancet* 1974; **2**: 81–3.
23. Fahn S, Elton RL. and members of the UPDRS Development Committee. In Fahn S, Marsden D, Calne DB, Goldstein M (ed.) *Recent developments in Parkinson's disease*, Vol 2. Macmillan Healthcare, Florham Park, NJ. 1987, pp. 153–63.
24. Webster, DD. Critical analysis of the disability in Parkinson's disease. *Modern Treatment* 1968; **5**: 257–82.
25. Wade DT. Medical Research Council grading of muscle strength. *Measurement in neurological rehabilitation.* Oxford University Press. 1992, pp. 53–4.
26. Yesavage JA, Brink TL, Rose TL. *et al.* Development and validation of a geriatric depression screening scale—a preliminary report. *J Psychiatr Res* 1983; **17**: 37–49.
27. Prudham D, Grimley Evans J. Factors associated with falls in the elderly: A Community Study. *Age and Ageing* 1981; **10**: 141–6.
28. Campbell AJ. *et al.* Circumstances and consequences of falls experienced by a community Population 70 years and over during a prospective study. *Age and Ageing* 1990; **19**: 136–41.
29. Vetter N, Lewis P, Ford D. Can health visitors prevent fractures in elderly People. *BMJ* 1992; **304**: 888–90.
30. Davies AJ, Kenny RA. Falls presenting to the accident and emergency department: types of presentation and risk factor profile. *Age and Ageing* 1996; **25**: 362–6.
31. Tinetti ME, Baker DI, McAvay G, Claus EB, Garrett P, Gottschalk M. *et al.* A multifactorial intervention to reduce the risk of falling among elderly people living in the community. *N Engl J Med* 1994; **331**: 821–7.
32. Chapuy MC, Arlot ME, Delmas PD, Meunier PJ. Effect of calcium and cholecalciferol treatment for three years on hip fractures in elderly women. *BMJ* 1994; **308**: 1081–2.

33. Lauritzen JB, Pethersen MM, Lund B. Effect of external hip protectors on hip fractures. *Lancet* 1993; **34**: 11–3.

34. McKeith IG. *et al.* for the consortium on dementia with Lewy bodies. *Neurology* 1996; **47**: 1113–24.

35. Koller WC, Silver DE, Lieberman A. An algorithm for the management of Parkinson's disease. *Neurology* 1994; **44(suppl. 10)**: S1–44.

36. Marsden CD. Parkinson's disease. *J Neurol Neurosurg Psychiatry* 1994; **57**: 672–81.

37. MacMahon DG Maguire R, Fletcher PJ. The Parkinson's disease clinic: A focal point for multidisciplinary care. *Care of the Elderly* 1990; **2**: 406–11.

38. Lees AJ. on behalf of Parkinson's Disease Research Group. Comparison of the therapeutic effects and mortality data of levodopa, levodopa in combination with selegiline, and bromocriptine in patients with early, mild Parkinson's disease. *BMJ* 1995; **311**: 1602–7.

39. *Incontinence. Causes, management, and provision of services.* The Royal College of Physicians, London. 1995.

FURTHER READING

Practical neurology. José Biller (ed.). Lippincott Raven, Philadelphia. 1997.

Epilepsy (2nd edn). A. Hopkins, S. Shorvin, G. Cascino. Chapman & Hall Medical, London. 1995.

Falls in the elderly. Joanna H. Downton. Edward Arnold, London. 1993.

Handbook of neurology. Charles Warlow. Blackwell, Oxford. 1991.

Measurement in neurological rehabilitation. Derick T. Wade. Oxford University Press. 1992.

The clinical neurology of old age. R. Tallis (ed.). Wiley, Chichester. 1989.

Stroke. A practical guide to management C. P. Warlow, M. S. Dennis, J. van Gign. G. J. Hankey, P. A. G. Sandercock, J. M. Bamford, J. Wardlaw. Blackwell, Oxford. 1996.

Standardised assessment scales for elderly people. The Royal College of Physicians of London and The British Geriatrics Society, London. June 1992.

Appendix 1

Functional assessment: Barthel Activities of Daily Life Index (BAI)

Function	Score	Description
Bowels[1]	0	Incontinent (or needs to be given enema)
	1	Occasional accident (once a week)
	2	Continent
Bladder[2]	0	Incontinent, or catheterized and unable to manage
	1	Occasional accident (maximum once a day)
	2	Continent (for more than seven days)
Grooming[3]	0	Needs help with personal care: face, hair, teeth (shaving)
	1	Independent (implements provided)
Toilet use[4]	0	Dependent
	1	Needs some help (but can do something alone)
	2	Independent (on and off, wiping, dressing)
Feeding[5]	0	Unable
	1	Needs help in cutting, spreading butter, etc.
	2	Independent (food provided within reach)
Transfer[6]	0	Unable—no sitting balance
	1	Major help (physical, one or two people), can sit
	2	Minor help (verbal or physical)
	3	Independent
Mobility[7]	0	Immobile
	1	Wheelchair independent, including corners, etc.
	2	Walks with help of one person (verbal or physical)
	3	Independent
Dressing[8]	0	Dependent
	1	Needs help (but can do about half unaided)
	2	Independent (including buttons, zips, laces, etc.)
Stairs[9]	0	Unable
	1	Needs help (verbal, physical, carrying aid)
	2	Independent (up and down)
Bathing[10]	0	Dependent
	1	Independent Bath: must get in and out unsupervised and wash self Shower: unsupervised/unaided

Notes

[1] *Assess preceding week. If needs enema from nurse, then = 'Incontinent'.*

[2] *Assess preceding week. Occasional = less than once a day. A catheterized patient who can completely manage the catheter alone = 'Continent'.*

[3] *Asses preceding 24–48 hours. Refers to personal hygeine: doing teeth, fitting false teeth, doing hair, shaving, washing face. Implements can be provided by helper.*

[4] *Should be able to reach toilet/commode, undress sufficiently, clean self, dress and leave. 'With help' = can wipe self, and could do some other of above.*

[5] *Able to eat any normal food (not only soft food). Food cooked and served by others, but not cut up. 'Help' = food cut up, patient feeds self.*

[6] *From bed to chair and back. 'Dependent' = no sitting balance (unable to sit), two people to lift. 'Major help' = one strong/skilled, or two normal people. Can sit up. 'Minor help' = one person easily, or needs any supervision for safety.*

[7] *Refers to mobility about house or ward, indoors. May use aid. If in wheelchair, must negotiate corners/doors unaided. 'Help' = by one, untrained person, including supervision or moral support.*

[8] *Should be able to select and put on all clothes, which may be adapted. 'Half' = helps with buttons, zips, etc., but can put on some garments alone.*

⁹ *Must carry any walking aid used to be classed as 'Independent'.*

¹⁰ *Usually the most difficult activity. Must get in and out unsupervised, and wash self. 'Independent' in shower = unsupervised and unaided.*

General notes

The index should be used as a record of what a patient does. NOT what they could do.

The main aim is to establish the degree of independence from any help, physical or verbal, however minor, and for whatever reason.

The need for supervision renders the patient 'NOT independent'.

A patient's performance should be established using the best available evidence. Asking the patient, friends/relatives and nurses will be the usual source, but direct observation and common sense are also important. However, direct testing is not needed.

Usually the performance over the preceding 24–48 hours is important, but occasionally longer periods are more appropriate.

Unconscious patients score 'O' throughout, regardless of continence.

The middle categories imply that the patient supplies more than 50% of the effort.

Use of aids to be independent is allowed.

Adapted from Mahoney FI, Barthel DW. Functional evaluation: The Barthel Index. *Maryland State Medical Journal* 1965; **14**: 61–5; Collin C, Wade DT, Davies S, Horne V. The Barthel Index: a reliability study. *International Disability Studies* 1988; **10**: 61–3.

Appendix 2

Mental assessment: Abbreviated mental test score

1. Age
2. Time (to nearest hour)
3. Address for recall at end of test: *42 West Street* (should be repeated by patient to ensure that it has been heard correctly)
4. Year
5. Name of place (or institution)
6. Recognition of two persons (e.g. doctor, nurse)
7. Date of birth (day and month is sufficient)
8. Year of First World War
9. Name present monarch
10. Count backwards from 20 to 1

The observer must not omit to test his/her recall by asking the patient to recall the address (3).
Scoring: Each correct response scores one mark.

Guide to rating cognitive function:

Score	Cognitive status
0–3	Severe impairment
4–7	Moderate impairment
8–10	Normal

Adapted from Hodkinson HM. Evaluation of a mental test score for assessment of mental impairment in the elderly. *Age and Ageing* 1972; **1**: 233–8.

Medical Research Council grades of muscle power

0 = no movement
1 = palpable contraction, but no visible movement
2 = movement but only with gravity eliminated
3 = movement against gravity
4 = movement against resistance, but weaker than other side
5 = normal power

Adapted from *Measurement in neurological rehabilitation*. Derick T Wade. Oxford University Press 1992.

18 | Particular neurological problems of ethnic minority groups

Bashir Qureshi

Knowledge is luggage and it is best to travel light. The aim of this chapter is to make a clinical neurologist aware of some of the different needs of various ethnic groups which may require different solutions. The patient is the most important person in medicine. Biologically there are natural differences between people, and these differences are a respectable entity in science and should not be seen as a sort of inequality. The original maxim of Hippocrates was: 'Good medicine treats an individual, not merely a disease'. It still holds true today. Every doctor should serve his/her patients according to their appropriate needs and show respect for his/her culture, religion, and ethnicity, as well as giving regard to their privacy and dignity. In this chapter I shall raise some issues in order to help a neurologist deal with patients from different cultures without giving up scientific skills, and suggest the modification of clinical methods in order to meet the patient's choice accordingly.

Management is the main emphasis of this chapter, rather than the minutiae of aetiology, pathology, disease classification, or differential diagnosis, except when it is important to management. Interdisciplinary contacts and communication with the patient will also be duly emphasized.

TRANSCULTURAL ASPECTS OF NEUROLOGY

TRANSCULTURAL MEDICINE

Transcultural medicine is the knowledge of medical and communication encounters between a doctor or health worker of one ethnic group and a patient of another. It embraces the physical, psychological, and social aspects of care as well as the scientific aspects of culture, religion, and ethnicity without getting involved in the politics of segregation or integration. (Qureshi 1994)

Scientific variables that influence a person's genetic inheritance and environment include: age, sex, social class, race, religion, and culture. Doctors have already been taking into account the first three in medical practice, and for political reasons they were taught in medical schools to disregard the latter three variables. This attitude may suit a single-ethnic clinic or practice but it is not appropriate for a multicultural delivery of care. In a multi-ethnic setting, a clinical neurolo-gist should take into account all six variables. There is a world of difference between distinction and discrimination. Positive thinking is essential.

THE BRITISH NATION TODAY

There are Britons in almost every country and people from many countries live in Britain today. This is largely for commercial, travel, and political reasons. Moreover, many patients from all over the world visit the United Kingdom for medical treatment. A large number of tourists also come to Britain every year. A neurology consultant, registrar, or senior house officer is likely to see patients from different backgrounds depending on the attendance mix of that hospital or clinic. Many rehabilitation centres will have a variable ethnic mix among their staff and patients. It is useful to know objectively what is the current position.

Broadly speaking, the British population comprises three main cultures, six major religions, four non-religious persuasions, and four ethnicities (Table 18.1). Within each of these categories there are many subsections (e.g. subcultures or cults). Classification is the only tool in epidemiology to measure populations, groups, and facts. It should not be mistaken for stereotyping. When a neurologist diagnoses epilepsy the intention is to help the patient and in no way to stigmatize him/her.

Western culture includes ethnic English, Scottish, Welsh, Irish, French, German, Dutch, White Americans, Australians,

Table 18.1 The composition of the population in the United Kingdom

Cultures
Western, Eastern, Westernized Eastern

Religions
Hinduism, Buddhism, Sikhism, Judaism, Christianity, Islam

Non-religious persuasions
Liberalism, secularism, agnosticism, atheism

Ethnic groups
Caucasian (European, Middle Eastern), Asiatic (Asian),
Negroid (African, Caribbean), Mongoloid (Chinese)

From Qureshi, B. (1994). *Transcultural medicine: dealing with patients from different cultures*, (2nd edn). Kluwer, London.

etc. It is useful to construct a general profile of a group in order to understand individual patients from that group, and also allow for exceptions because there are exceptions to almost every rule. The personality profile of this culture is vision—and hearing—then touch. These people have a firm conviction about strict personal privacy, personal choice, free speech, rigid time-keeping, appointments, meetings, fixed prices, holidays, and standing in a queue no matter how long it is. It is easier to steal a lion cub than to come between a Western person and his/her cultural traditions.

The Eastern culture includes ethnic Asians, Africans, Chinese, Middle Easterners, East Europeans, South-East Asians, etc. Their personality profile is touch—and hearing—then vision. These people are likely to believe in shared privacy, shared choice, calculated speech, flexible time-keeping, freedom from appointments, agreed rules, haggling for prices or asking for a discount, visiting relatives abroad, and not observing a queue so as to let someone go first if they are in a greater hurry.

The Westernized Easterners are a sizeable minority and make fairly vocal groups. These groups include Asian doctors, African-Asians, Caribbean-Africans, children of mixed marriages, and so on. Obviously, their personality profiles, beliefs, and behaviour will vary enormously between the two cultures with a significant slant towards the Western culture. These people are very sensitive and shrewd, and are survivors. They are business-orientated people. It is not uncommon for an Asian doctor to do locum work during his/her annual leave. Kenyan-Asians have been particularly successful in running corner shops which are open all hours. Caribbeans also tend to work overtime wherever possible. These cultural trends may help all these groups to meet the extra expenses, which they have in caring for their extended families, but 'all work and no play' must have some detrimental effect on their health, for example, in increasing incidence of tension headaches and migraine.

A neurologist's patients are likely to include followers of all the religions listed in Table 18.1. Devout followers live by their own religion, which will influence their diet, habits, conception of disease, expectation from the doctor, dress, and beliefs. It is obvious that these are significant environmental factors in the aetiology, course, and management of any disease including a neurological condition. It is, therefore, important that the neurologist has some understanding of each of these religions. A brief mention of these religions will be included in later pages.

Non-religious persuasions have no specific founders. The problem with religions was that each religion advocated to its followers that their own religion is the only right faith and all the rest are not. As a result there have been wars in the name of religion for centuries. Therefore, by evolution as a matter of political and commercial necessity, many followers from each religion turned, in varying degree, to non-religious persuasions. Four large persuasions are: liberalism, secularism, agnosticism, and atheism. These are economically and polit-

ically powerful groups. Many parliaments, governments, and organizations world-wide are led by these groups even in those countries which by name are religious societies. Such is the power of financial necessities that all countries are dependent on each other for trade. However, in Britain the Government appears to follow the philosophy of 'rational morality' when dealing with moral dilemmas including those related to medicine.

Finally, it should be remembered that anthropologists classify the human race according to the criteria of a person's colour of skin and hair, type of hair, and the facial bone structure including the shape of the eyes. They divide mankind into four races: Caucasians (Europeans and Middle Easterners), Asiatics (Asians from India, Pakistan, Bangladesh, and Sri Lanka), Negroid (Africans, Caribbeans of African origin and Black Americans), and Mongoloid (Chinese and South-East Asians). The word 'race' has been adopted by politicians and has become smeared by the inequality debate. Therefore, it is prudent to use the word 'ethnic' which is a respectable identity of a person and this has now been accepted widely. A question about ethnicity was asked in the UK 1991 Census. It cannot be overemphasized that ethnicity consists of the genetic make-up of a person and is a useful indicator in patient care because some illnesses, including neurological conditions are ethno-specific.

ETHNIC TERMINOLOGY

It is not only what one says but also how one says it, that ensures one does not injure the feelings of a fellow British citizen from another ethnic group; this forms the basis of the Race Relations Act 1976 which is monitored by the Commission for Racial Equality in Britain. Derogatory terms, such as 'coloured', 'immigrant', 'imported diseases', 'nigger', and 'half caste', should not be used. The word 'British' does not mean only Whites because ethnic minority people are also British citizens. It is best to say British White, British Asian, British African, British Chinese, etc. 'Ethnic' does not mean ethnic minority only, although some people use it implying inferior status, but this term is a respectable entity. It is better to get used to saying ethnic English, ethnic Irish, ethnic Scottish, ethnic Asian, ethnic Caribbean, etc. The term 'ethnic' was used in this manner in the UK 1991 Census.

'Afro-Caribbean' is a term now disliked by West Indians, particularly by the younger age group. They like to be called 'Africans' or 'Caribbeans' and one should recognize these identities. However, British Whites have used the term 'Afro-Caribbean' for those Caribbeans who are of African origin. This was to distinguish them from those Caribbeans who originated from the Asian subcontinent. Where appropriate this explanation should be given to a West Indian patient and he/she will happily accept it because his/her worry was that of racial discrimination by using inappropriate identity.

'Black' and 'White' are considered respectable terms. It is not the word, it is the attitude towards that word which matters. A neurologist who shows respect to his/her patient will be rewarded by good doctor–patient rapport as courtesy surely breeds courtesy.

The Commission for Racial Equality, the Registrar General, and other government organizations accept the following ethnic classifications: The ethnic majority in Britain comprises only three groups: ethnic English, Scottish, and Welsh. All other ethnic groups, including the ethnic Irish and ethnic Jews, are ethnic minorities (Table 18.2).

A child of a mixed marriage may be called by dual ethnicity (e.g. ethnic Anglo-Pakistani, Franco-Indian, Indo-Chinese, etc.). Some people adopt the ethnicity of the father but others prefer to be affiliated with the indigenous ethnicity, for example, an Anglo-African may prefer to be called ethnic English, particularly if he/she was born in England.

Any neurologist who may have queries on terminology or other related topics can contact the Commission for Racial Equality (Elliot House, 10–12 Allington Street, London SW1D 5EH; Tel. 0171 828 7022) for clarification. A research worker should do so in writing. Other sources of advice are listed in (Table 18.3).

CULTURAL ATTITUDES TO NEUROLOGICAL DISEASES

'Culture' means the customs and civilization of a particular people or group. It also includes the appreciation and understanding of the literature, art, music, and language of the

Table 18.2 Ethnic minorities in the United Kingdom

Irish	Italians
Polish	Hungarians
Jews	Australians
Afro-Caribbeans	
Asians: Indians, Pakistanis, Bangladeshies, Sri-lankans	
Chinese, Vietnamese, South-East Asians	
Cypriots, Greeks, Turks	
Other small groups	

From Qureshi, B. (1994). Transcultural medicine: dealing with patients from different cultures, (2nd edn). Kluwer, London.

Table 18.3 Sources of information on terminology and related topics

Local
Priest/rabbi/imam/pundit/giani
Racial Equality Council
Interpreter/link-worker/relative
MP/councillor/leader/friend

National
Commission for Racial Equality
Appropriate embassy
Department of Health
Voluntary organizations

From Qureshi, B. (1994). Transcultural medicine: dealing with patients from different cultures, (2nd edn). Kluwer, London.

group or society. Cultural roots run deep. No one should expect a person to totally abandon his/her cultural customs even after migration. It is in a neurologist's interests to understand other cultures, without changing his/her own customs. In this way a successful working relationship is possible in a transcultural consultation. The following 10 points can be used as basic information.

I. LANGUAGE

History taking is essential for diagnosis and a correct history is vital in neurology. A good history can only be taken if the doctor and patient are speaking the same language. However, the ***vocabulary*** of one group of people can be different from another group speaking the same language. Oscar Wilde was justified in observing that the English have everything in common with the Americans except, of course, language. The gap will be even wider if the doctor speaks one language (e.g. English) and the patient another (e.g. Polish or Urdu/Hindi).

In London, a Christian doctor asked a Muslim Arab patient 'Do you drink?'. The patient replied, 'Yes, doctor, I drink a lot, particularly with a meal'. Later on, it transpired that the doctor meant drinking alcohol and the patient meant drinking water, because alcohol is taboo in Islam. A Jewish doctor enquired of a Sikh Indian patient, 'Do you smoke?'. The answer was given: 'Please don't be rude, doctor!'. This was for two reasons: first, smoking is taboo in the Sikh religion; second, in the Punjabi language a cigarette or tobacco is drunk and not smoked. Even a westernized Easterner can misunderstand an English person. For example, a burglar alarm engineer told me after finishing his job in my house: 'Doctor, it is all set, if a burglar were to get in, the alarm will go off'. I told him point blank: 'No, that's not right, I want the alarm to go on!'. After a short reassuring look the English engineer told me that when he said 'off' in English it meant 'on', and I need not worry. I have lived in London since 1964 and wear many English hats, such as a nationally elected member of the Council of the Royal College of General Practitioners (1990–93), yet I still need help in the correct usage of the word 'the' and my pronunciation of the letter V. Many others have such problems. A neurologist should make every effort to overcome the language barrier so as to obtain a correct and complete history.

Ideally, a trained interpreter or link worker (an interpreter and also cultural translator) should be invited to interpret. The services of an appropriate interpreter, can be obtained officially through the managers who run hospitals and other neurology centres. In addition, any doctor could seek advice from a local 'racial equality officer', who is usually based in the civic centre or town hall. He or she may have some volunteers or a list of interpreters. The managers of local District Health Authorities provide paid interpreters in many parts of Britain. Another resource is the Directory of Translators and Interpretors (The Institute of Translation and Interpreting, 377 City Road, London EC1V 1NA; Tel. 0171 713 7600).

I believe that it is absolutely wrong to use a school child as an interpreter because such a child will miss school lessons, may become a truant, and may not translate or interpret skilfully enough. However, a relative or friend of the patient can be a reasonable substitute, but there is a problem in that he/she may edit, while interpreting, in the interests of family image. It is best to use a trained interpreter not involved with the family.

2. CONCEPT OF DISEASE

There are three disease concepts which are likely to be common, with a varying degree of overlap, among patients from various ethnic groups: (i) anatomical and biomedical; (ii) the Devil's curse and God's punishment; and (iii) an enemy's bewitching and casting spells. These concepts are based on modern science, religious beliefs, and old cultural traditions respectively. However, a neurologist from any ethnic group is likely to be trained with only the anatomical and biomedical model. It is a mistake to disregard or denigrate a patient's concept of disease. Even Westernized Easterners may hold any one or more of the above three concepts when consulting a Western doctor, let alone the Eastern patients who are brought up to believe in a different model of disease. There is no place for fixed ideas or overassertiveness in neurology, and a flexible and compromising sympathetic approach will be more rewarding in reaching a correct diagnosis and proposing the appropriate management.

The anatomical and biomedical model of disease is more common among Europeans, white Americans, Canadians, Australians, and Westernized Easterners. This concept of disease is based on anatomy, physiology, biochemistry, immunology, genetics, and pathological considerations. It is customary to consider symptoms as the pointers to a disease, and symptomatic treatment is considered less scientific except where a disease remains undiagnosed and its aetiology is considered idiopathic. The cure or management of the disease remains a clinician's primary aim and the patients agree to investigations before therapeutic measures. They will (usually) be content with the doctor's advice and follow it up.

The concept that disease is the Devil's curse and God's punishment is more prevalent among religious societies, such as Jews, Christians, Muslims, Hindus, and Sikhs. It is accepted that the disease is caused by the body or the mind or both going wrong, but the disorder is considered to be either brought on or influenced by the Devil's mischief or, for believers in God, by God's punishment of their sins or their ancestors' sins. Buddhists, who do not believe in a supreme being or God, and people from non-religious persuasions may attribute a disease to bad luck caused by 'nature'. The nature believers consider that the disorder is the result of the 'unkindness' of Mother Nature. These people will believe in symptomatic treatment and then investigation of the disease. These patients are likely to conform to the doctor's plan and, in addition, turn to their appropriate religious guides for healing rituals, charity, and animal sacrifices (except Hindus who believe in non-animal sacrifices such as fasting rituals).

Finally, bewitching or spell-casting by an enemy is widely believed to be the cause of a disease, misfortune, or accident by many Asians, Africans, Caribbeans, South Americans, Chinese, and South-East Asians. The more primitive the sub-culture, the more widespread is the practice of black magic, voodoo, and spell-casting by professionals, faith healers, witches, and witch doctors. The fear generated by these rituals, and the victim's superstitions, are the cause of their effects. Black magic is based on rituals involving the invocation of devils. Voodoo is a form of religion based on a belief in witchcraft and magical rites, practised by certain Blacks in America and the West Indies. These patients expect a Western doctor to provide drug treatment for symptomatic relief only. Then they are likely to consult a religious person or witchcraft professional to neutralize the spell by practices such as exorcism. They soon learn that a Western doctor will not hear of such a thing, therefore they do not tell him/her about this alternative approach to treatment. Such a patient may blame an estranged spouse, a neighbour or a relative, particularly the mother-in-law, for hiring a spell-casting specialist. It is not uncommon for an Asian young woman with a stroke or trigeminal neuralgia to tell her neurologist that her mother-in-law has possessed her husband and has also arranged to bewitch her by *tona* (an Urdu word for black magic). On the other hand, the mother-in-law may blame her newly wedded daughter-in-law for all the misfortunes. It is naïve for a neurologist to think that these emotions have nothing to do with the cause, course, and management of the disease. A listening ear and tactful intervention are required. It is best to supervise their compliance and keep an open mind in their surveillance.

3. ATTITUDES TO ACUTE CONDITIONS

Patients may vary in their attitudes, due to cultural backgrounds, to some acute neurological conditions such as pain, paralysis, head injury, or trigeminal neuralgia.

Pain is the commonest symptom in medicine and it has the mysterious power to overrule everything else in life. It can be an enemy when it is unbearable, but it becomes a friend when it is a symptom of disease and prompts a patient to see a doctor. I knew an eminent surgeon who developed renal pain which he tried to control by analgesics because his list of operations was too important to be cancelled. When the pain did not subside he was taken to a renal unit in London where a nephrectomy was performed for renal cell carcinoma and he lived a long life to tell the tale. Insensitivity to pain can be a curse, and such patients may destroy themselves for the simple reason that they lack a system to warn them of danger. Pain insensitivity can occur in lepromatous neuropathy, diabetic neuropathy, alcoholism, multiple sclerosis, nerve disorders, spinal cord injury, and congenital indifference to pain (Brand and Yancey 1993).

There are cultural variations in attitude to pain. Europeans, especially the English and Jews, will consider pain to be a symptom of a disease. They will go to see a doctor for the underlying disease to be treated and will not rush for symptomatic treatment. Stoicism is ingrained in the English character. Some Catholics, particularly the Irish, may regard pain as a process of penitence and penance. They may not take any analgesics or may not see a doctor. On the other hand, Italians, Americans, Asians, and Africans may dramatize their response to pain by free emotional expression, crying or shouting, and will ask for symptomatic relief at all cost and at once. A neurologist must keep a cool head and reassure such a patient that pain does not mean that he/she is going to die, as this is how they really feel—that the pain may lead to death eventually. Stoical patients should not be mistaken for having no pain, and dramatizing patients should not be mistaken for being in agony. An appropriate diagnosis must be made objectively while controlling the intensity of pain.

Strokes and trigeminal neuralgia carry a stigma in Eastern cultures. Asian women often wish these diseases as a curse on their enemies, including the tax man. In addition, a patient who has a severe head injury, or becomes paralysed, loses his/her social status in the extended family system. Such a patient may be stigmatized for having a curse from heaven for some misdeed, and may be considered less reliable to decide financial matters. Another problem that may arise for a young unmarried person is that an arranged marriage, the only marriage acceptable in that culture, may be jeopardized. In the case of a young woman, her parents may have to give a much larger dowry (or *jahaiz*) to the bridegroom's family, who are then responsible for the future expenses for the treatment.

Nowadays, fortunately, British neurologists are being trained not just to think of the body as a mere machine, but to appreciate the physical, psychological, and social aspects of treating a patient and his/her disease. Where a patient comes from another culture, then that variable should also be considered sympathetically. The patient should not be made to feel guilty or that he/she is at fault because of cultural differences or disadvantages.

4. RESPONSES TO CHRONIC DISORDERS

The ethnic majority is used to the benefits of social services and enjoys the nuclear family way of life. Non-Westernized ethnic minorities support their extended family systems so that the illness of one family member becomes a crisis for the whole extended family and friends. When a person from the Asian, African, Cypriot, or Chinese culture is diagnosed as having a chronic condition such as motor neurone disease, or a terminal illness such as cancer of the spinal cord, it is customary for the patient to return to his/her homeland. Female relatives, particularly sisters and daughters, traditionally take pride in nursing the terminally ill in their family, while men provide financial support. Traditional sex roles are considered part of the family honour in Eastern culture.

An English neurosurgeon told me that he had to resign from his post in Malaysia because of a cultural phenomenon. If a patient died of a brain tumour without treatment it was accepted as a stroke of bad luck and the will of God or Allah. But if the patient died after having neurosurgery then the surgeon was blamed as it was considered to be a failed operation. Such an attitude among ethnic minority groups from all religions may be encountered in the United Kingdom.

5. WHAT IS EXPECTED FROM THE DOCTOR

An English, Scottish, or Welsh patient likes to discuss a neurological problem with his/her doctor and prefers to decide on a course of action after taking some time to think about it.

This is not the case with many ethnic minority patients. An Asian, African, Caribbean, or Chinese patient expects the doctor to explain why the disease has occurred and to advise him/her what can be done to cure it. Sometimes, if a Western doctor were to ask such a patient what he/she wanted to be done, this could be taken as a lack of self-confidence on the part of the doctor, and an ethnic minority patient would ask for a second opinion, even from an alternative medicine practitioner who is considered a wise man because he can make a diagnosis without a detailed history.

A patient from an Eastern culture may have heard that English doctors can cure many 'incurable' illnesses, so it is not uncommon for ethnic minority patients to expect instant cures from a Western doctor. They may consider that the more investigations, the better the diagnosis, and the more expensive the treatment, particularly injections, the more likely it is to be effective. Tactful counselling should clarify that a Western neurologist has no magic wand.

6. CLINIC OR SURGERY VISITS

Strict time-keeping, appointment systems, sitting quietly, queueing, and meetings are English customs. In Sweden, it is said that three Englishmen landed on a desert island after their ship was wrecked. Within an hour of landing they had formed three committees. After a day they had formed another *ad-hoc* committee to oversee the work of the three committees. Unless Anglicized, this is not the lifestyle of Asians, Africans, Caribbeans, Chinese, and patients from other ethnic groups. It is not uncommon for a Somali or Bangladeshi patient to arrive one hour late for an appointment and not say sorry (another cultural difference). He or she may turn up without an appointment and request to be seen by the doctor. They do not receive English social education but can learn to observe Western customs, if someone is there to teach them.

If a child is accompanied by both parents there will be a cultural variation in history taking. In societies in which parents share the care of children equally (e.g. English or Scottish), the history will be given by both parents. In father-led societies, (e.g. Asian or Arab), the history will be given by the father. In mother-led societies (e.g. Caribbean or Orthodox Jewish), the history will be given by the mother.

7. HOSPITAL VISITING

People from a nuclear family background will abide by British hospital routines, and two visitors at a time will visit a patient by arranging it with the ward sister over the telephone. However, people from an extended family circle may not be aware of this custom. They will visit in unlimited numbers to give the patient moral support and assure loyalty. The higher the number of visitors, the higher is considered the social status of the patient. They may not telephone the ward sister beforehand and may engage the patient in tiresome non-stop conversation. The patient will not ask them to leave him/her alone out of politeness and tradition. Nevertheless, the ward sister should pleasantly advise the visitors to visit only two at a time and not to stay more than ten minutes. They will happily do so because they do intend to help the staff to help the patient.

While, say, English or Scottish visitors often bring flowers, Asians, Africans, and the Chinese are more likely to bring their own ethnic foods for the patient. These foods may interfere with the absorption of drugs or interact with drugs, and so should be checked by nursing staff.

8. ETHNIC DIETS

This is a vast subject and limited space permits me to make only three clinical points. First, in Eastern societies a food is considered 'hot' or 'cold' according to its metabolic effects. Proteins, fats, and spices are considered to be 'hot' foods. They increase the splanchnic blood flow and enhance the absorption of food, bacteria, and drugs from the intestine into the bloodstream. On the other hand, orange juice, milk, and yoghurt are considered to be 'cold' foods, and these slow down the splanchnic blood flow and reduce the rate of absorption. This widespread concept has been explained in many ways. However, a neurological disease (as with pregnancy) is considered a 'hot' condition and Asians, Africans, and the Chinese will be reluctant to give protein or a spice-rich diet. This in turn may lead to nutritional iron-deficiency anaemia. Almost every food has an effect or side-effect on the body.

Second, it is common on the Asian subcontinent for doctors, who are trained in British-style medical schools, to prescribe glucose orally or intravenously in a neurological illness. Calcium preparations and vitamin B complex, particularly B_1 and B_{12}, are also given concurrently.

Third, a hospital dietician who has some knowledge of ethnic diets should be consulted when appropriate.

9. POLITICS

This is the science dealing with realities as they present themselves. It is not uncommon for a politician to declare that

he/she will never talk to terrorists, particularly if they do not give up violence. However, when the circumstances dictate, the same politician may have to recognize the alleged terrorists as the leaders of a new nation. They solve many difficult problems by continuing dialogue, and prevent many wars. Diplomacy is still better than confrontation.

World-wide, forced integration or segregation have been found to be impractical concepts, whereas voluntary integration or segregation coupled with a working relationship has been found to be a reasonable formula, particularly in multi-ethnic communities. Birds of a feather flock together, and it is natural that people live in their own ethnic areas in Britain but travel everywhere for work. Fortunately, there are no no-go areas, but for a good working relationship different ethnic groups need to know something about each other.

For learning and practising transcultural medicine, a doctor should not get involved in the politics of integration or segregation because when something seems unacceptable one becomes angry. Learning and anger negate each other. Therefore one should keep an open mind.

10. COMPLAINTS/LITIGATION

In recent years, the doctor–patient relationship is changing into a doctor–plaintiff relationship. Britain is catching up with the United States in this area. Three transcultural points are worth a mention as certain national patterns are emerging.

First, the more articulate a person, and the better their command of the English language, the more likely they are to complain against a doctor if they are unhappy. Asians, Africans, Cypriots, and Chinese patients are less likely to complain. Westernized Easterners are more likely to complain or go for litigation if not given a reconciliatory apology at an early stage. Sometimes they may feel so angry that an apology is not enough.

Second, an African or Caribbean is more likely to complain against a doctor if the doctor did not examine the patient, because they believe in touch and an examination, no matter how brief.

Third, there is the issue of informed consent. Explaining things to a patient and getting his/her signature for a procedure is acceptable for a patient from Western culture. However, with a patient from an extended family background, it is best to explain to the patient as well as one or more members of the family, because they believe in shared consent and responsibility.

RELIGIOUS BELIEFS ABOUT NEUROLOGICAL DISEASES

Science deals with objectivity and reason whereas religion is based on subjectivity and intuition. A person needs both: scientific technology for physical well-being; and religious enlightenment for spiritual strength. It is useful for a neurologist to understand his/her patients' religious convictions or non-religious beliefs. The doctor should be free to learn from the patient directly, but the following descriptions can be used as a starting point.

THE SIX MAJOR RELIGIONS

1. Judaism is the religion of the Jewish race. Jews are a race as well as a religious group, and they are the descendants of the ancient Israelites and Hebrews. Conversion to Judaism is rare and very difficult because to be a Jew one has to be the child of a Jewish mother. The Jews believe that they are a chosen people, to spread the message, by one true God called Yahweh. They originated at the time of the prophet Abraham and they also revere the prophet Moses. Their holy book is the Torah which is made up of the first five books of the old Testament of the Bible, which are attributed to Moses. The prophet Abraham had two sons—Isaac and Ishmael. The Jews are the descendants of Isaac, and the Muslims are the descendants of Ishmael. It is relevant to note here that Jesus Christ was a Jew and there is a strong historical link between the three Abrahamic religions, i.e. Judaism, Islam and Christianity. The Jewish laws include a particular method of killing animals for meat, advocate male circumcision, and forbid eating pork and shellfish. The Jews' place of worship is called the synagogue, and there on Saturdays the men pray in special prayer shawls. The annual Jewish festivals include: Passover, Pentecost, Tabernacles, Chanukah, Rosh Hashanah, and Yom Kippur. Jews are meant to pray three times a day, preferably in the synagogue, and Saturday, the Sabbath, is their holy day. Jews have been divided into various groups: the Orthodox majority, Conservatives, Liberals, and Reform Jews (Kennedy 1984).

2. Christianity has about 900 million members world-wide and it takes its name from its founder, Jesus Christ, who was a Jewish rabbi, but his liberal attitude towards some of the Jewish laws, such as the Sabbath law, brought him into conflict with the Pharisees and Sadducees. Jesus Christ was crucified as a common criminal by the Roman governor, Pontius Pilate, on a charge of blasphemy and treason. After three days, he is said to have been resurrected and appeared alive to his disciples and met with them over 40 days before his final ascension into heaven. The majority of Christians believe in the Holy Trinity of Father, Son, and Holy Spirit (or Holy Ghost). The idea is that one God resides in three persons: the Father; the Son who became man in Jesus Christ; and the Holy Spirit who came down upon the apostles and is the energy of God which enters humans' hearts, giving them spiritual wisdom. The Bible, both the Old and New Testaments, is the sacred book of Christianity. The place of worship is called the church (or chapel), and Sunday is the holy day. Christians celebrate Christ's saving life, death, and resurrection in church services such as baptism, the Eucharist, and other sacraments. Many Christians also go to 'confession' to repent their sins.

Their main festivals are Christmas, Easter, Pentecost, and Saints' days. The main denominations are Roman Catholicism (majority), Eastern Orthodoxy, and Protestantism (the Church of England, Presbyterian, Methodist, Baptist, Calvinist, Lutheran, and the United Reformed Church).

3. Islam has about 600 million followers world-wide and it was founded by the prophet Mohammed, who was a descendant of Ishmael, in the 7th century at Mecca in Saudi Arabia. Islam means 'peace' and its followers are called Muslims. The name of the only God is Allah. The holy book is the Quran. The place of worship is called the mosque, and Friday is the holy day. Muslims believe in the five pillars of Islam:

1. *Shahada* or *Kalma*, which means the statement of faith in one God and his prophet Mohammed.
2. *Salat* (or prayer) five times a day, preferably at a mosque, and the communal prayer on Fridays. The prayer is said facing Mecca.
3. *Saum* (or fasting) in the month of Ramadan from sunrise to sunset.
4. *Zakat* (or almsgiving) by donating one-fortieth of one's income and assets to help the poor.
5. *Hajj* (or pilgrimage) to the Kaaba in Mecca once in a lifetime.

Islamic laws allow only halal (a particular way of killing an animal) meat and forbid pork, alcohol, jazz, human pictures, and idols. Muslim festivals include Eid-ul-Fitr, Eid-ul-Azha, and the birthdays of the prophet Mohammed and other holy men. The main divisions are the Sunni majority and Shia (strongest in Iran and Yemen). Wahhabis are a Sunni sect in Saudi Arabia and they control Mecca and Medina, the holiest cities in Islam. Ayatollah is a title given to Shia interpreters of the Muslim law, the Sharia.

4. Hinduism is the religion of the majority of Indians (in pre-colonial times India was called 'Hindustan' but after independence the title 'India' was retained so as to create a secular democracy). Western historians claim that Hinduism began when Aryan warriors invaded the Indus valley in northern India in 1500 BC. The Aryan religion is expressed in the oldest Hindu scriptures such as the Vedas. Hinduism has no founder and different Hindus worship various gods and goddesses representing one supreme being or God. For example, Brahma the creator, Vishnu the preserver, Shiva the destroyer, Indira the goddess of war, Agni the goddess of fire, Lakhshami the goddess of wealth. Kali is the goddess associated with death and also with creation, including fertility. Hindus believe in reincarnation and that the soul is immortal. The soul always transmigrates into successive bodies and lives in a body of a higher (human) or lower (animal) creature depending on how the person has behaved in this life. They strongly believe in the caste system. Beef in any form, including beef fat in artificial baby milk, is taboo to non-vegetarian Hindus. The majority are vegetarians. Their holy books are the Bhagavad Gita and Ramayana. The place of worship is

called the temple; there is no specific holy day during the week for some, but Tuesday is considered the holy day for other Hindus. Hindu festivals include Holi, Divali, Durga Puja, and other special days to remember various gods and goddesses. There are no main divisions but there are a few sects, for example, Shaivite (Shiva-centred) and Vaishnavite (Vishnu- or Krishna-centred).

5. Buddhism is the major religion in the populations of Sri Lanka, Tibet, Thailand, Burma, China, Korea, Japan, and South-East Asia. It was founded by Siddhartha Gautama Buddha (563–480 BC) who was a Hindu prince in Nepal. Buddha is regarded as one of a series of such beings, the next incarnation being due in AD 3000. Meditation and service form salient features of Buddhism. It is important to note that Buddhists do not believe in any gods or supreme beings, and the religion is based on Gautama Buddha's teachings. The code of morals is as follows:

1. *The five precepts*: not to kill, not to steal, not to commit adultery, not to lie, and not to take intoxicating liquor.
2. *The four sublime states*: loving kindness, compassion, appreciative joy, and equanimity.
3. *The ten transcendental virtues*: generosity, morality, renunciation, wisdom, energy, patience, truthfulness, resolutions, loving kindness, and equanimity.
4. *The noble eight-fold path*: right understanding, right thought, right speech, right actions, right livelihood, right effort, right mindfulness, and right concentration.

There is no one specific holy book, but a book of the five precepts in the Pali language can be used for oath purposes in court proceedings. The place of worship is the temple and there is no specific holy day in the week. Buddhist monks beg their food and have no personal possessions.

Buddhists believe in reincarnation and that the eight-fold path will lead them to Nirvana, a state in which man is freed from a continuous round of rebirths and the suffering involved in life. Buddhist festivals include Wasak, which is held at the first full moon of May, and other special days. The main divisions are: Theraveda, Mahayana, and Lamaism.

6. Sikhism is a monotheistic religion founded in the Indian Punjab by Guru Nanak (AD 1469–1539) who was a Hindu influenced by Islamic Sufi mysticism, particularly the mystical poet Kabir. India has 10 million Sikhs; the majority reside in the Indian Punjab. The Sikh community originated in AD 1521 when Guru Nanak settled in Kartarpur City. This community became a movement with military-style discipline. Guru Nanak believed that both Hinduism and Islam contained the truth about God, but that the message had got lost in the rituals and traditional customs of both religions. Therefore he combined the principles of both religions. Like the Muslims, he believed in one God, whom he called *Sat Nam* (True Name). From Hinduism he retained a belief in reincarnation, karma, and moksa, but he rejected all notions of the caste system and suggested that all male Sikhs should be called *Singh* and all female Sikhs should be called *Kaur*, removing their Hindu caste surnames. He frowned on idols, pilgrimages, fixed ritual prayers, and ceremonial washing. Later, Guru Govind Singh instituted the brotherhood movement of Khalsa and bound its members to wear distinctive marks of a full Sikh, the five Ks. These are: the *kesh* (uncut hair under a turban), the *kangha* (comb), *kacha* (short underwear), the *kara* (a steel bracelet), and the *kirpan* (sword). The holy book is called the Guru Granth Sahib, which has taken the place of a leader. The place of worship is called the Gurudawara. Guru Arjan Dev built the Harimandir or Golden Temple at Amritsar in the Indian Punjab. There is no one specific holy day in the week because every day is considered holy as it is created by God. Smoking is a strong taboo and other forbidden items are pork, beef, and alcohol. Many Sikhs are vegetarians. Sikh festivals include Waisakhi, Divali, and the birthdays of all ten Gurus. There are no main sections of the Sikh religion, but different Sikhs (as with Hindus) practise their religion in various ways.

RELIGIOUS HEALING ROLES

Ancient medicine has three common strands: (i) folk medicine, derived from local and family traditions associated with the use of herbs, sometimes accompanied by charms, amulets, and spells; (ii) sacerdotal medicine, mediated by priests or priest–physicians who aimed at psychological and spiritual needs; and (iii) rational medicine, stemming from observation, philosophy, and experiment (Watt 1993). A neurologist cannot practise in isolation without realizing that his art is a part of the rational medicine pioneered by Hippocrates and Galen, and that there are other alternative therapies in current use by patients, and sometimes concurrently used.

The founders of all six major religions, and their successors, played important healing roles to the extent of being called miracle workers. They treated their followers' physical, psychological, social, and spiritual ills and the discipline of neurology was no exception. In Christianity the some neurological conditions were known by their association with saints' names; for example, chorea was called St Vitus' dance or St Guy's dance, while leprosy (including neuropathy) was called St Giles' disease.

There are similar examples in other religions to demonstrate the closeness of priest–physicians and their followers who perceive they have an illness. It is unwise to think that a patient who has come to see a neurologist with scientific training has abandoned his/her religious connections. In fact, it is to a neurologist's advantage if the patient does not do so because the religious network can be used to assist the doctor in diagnosis and treatment. As a general practitioner has a list of his/her patients, the local religious guide almost invariably has a list of the households attending his place of worship. If approached, a leader of every religion can be expected to help the doctor in dealing with the patient, particularly on problems arising from some religious and medical conflict from treatment. For example, let us take the use of medicine in gelatine capsules. Gelatine capsules are made from bones and hides of animals including pigs, cows, etc. Devout Muslims, Jews, Hindus, and Sikhs may have varying degrees of reservation about using these medications and may not discuss this with a British white neurologist, out of politeness. Where it is not possible to prescribe tablets and one has to prescribe capsules, a neurologist should contact the appropriate local religious guide for help. The religious leader can persuade the patient to take capsules as is required by the doctor. The 'sanctity of life' doctrine is used in such a case.

RELIGIOUS CONFLICTS

I hope enough information has been given objectively about all major religions for a neurologist to become aware of and identify, quantify, and rectify any religious misunderstandings that may arise in a trans-religious contact. However, the following five areas, in particular, should also be considered:

1. Sex segregation has been preached by five major religions: Judaism, Islam, Hinduism, Buddhism, and Sikhism. They believe in sex roles traditionally based on the sheer physical strength of the man to be a breadwinner and the woman to be the carer of that breadwinner. Although sex segregation was a norm in Christianity, particularly in the churches, the scene is now changing. Sex segregation should not necessarily mean sex discrimination, but the debate in all religious circles is to what should be done in the future. Until this matter is resolved, it is advisable to provide a patient with a neurologist of the same sex if the patient wishes. Some patients have not been seen by a doctor of the opposite sex before and will become very tense. If a doctor of the opposite sex has to examine the patient, he/she should be counselled beforehand and time should be allowed for this to be accepted.

2. Faith in the doctor varies with the religion and how devoutly religious a patient is. A patient from a non-religious persuasion may confide in the doctor totally, but a devoutly religious person will believe that it is the God's will that brings a cure and the doctor is simply being used by God (Allah, Bhagwan, Yahweh, Sat Nam) as a tool in the process of management of the disease. A British neurologist told me that he believes in his art and that it is hard to be humble when one is so perfect in every way. I would argue that perhaps some humility on the part of a doctor would not go amiss, and each patient has a different point of view depending on his/her religious or secular convictions. It pays to respect the patient's point of view in these days of increasing consumer choice.

3. Religious health rituals vary enormously from one religion to another. Common rituals are: wearing charms, amulets, and threads blessed by a religious guide (a rabbi, priest, imam, pundit, giani, or monk); drinking holy water brought from holy lands by the pilgrims, e.g. the river Ganges (India), Spring Zam Zam (Saudi Arabia); eating blessed food from the local place of worship (a synagogue, church, mosque, temple, or gurudawara); sacrificing a lamb, sheep, or chicken to the

poor. All these rituals are aimed to protect the patient from the deterioration of his/her condition and also to persuade heavenly forces to grant recovery from the illness. A neurologist of a non-religious persuasion or another religion should avoid denigrating such rituals and encourage the patient to use them if it gives further comfort, provided that there is no health hazard; even then, a negotiated settlement should be reached. It is kind to treat a patient as humanely as the physician or neurologist would like to be treated himself. Caring attitudes are an important part of patient care.

4. Three religious customs may be encountered by a neurologist in a clinic: psychiatric illness is considered a curse by some people, and seeing a psychiatrist is taboo. Such patients may not at times differentiate between a mental and a neurological illness, or worse still, between a psychiatrist and a neurologist; many religious books are read by devotees while they are shaking their heads and even hands—such individuals may mistake parkinsonian tremors as religious shakes and may not report the condition. Finally, a religious person never visits a shrine or place of worship empty-handed—some money or food has to be taken along as a tradition. Such a person will innocently take a present to an English consultant neurologist or ward sister who may feel embarrassed, considering that it may be a bribe. Nothing could be further from the truth. Such misunderstandings should be cleared by an open and courteous dialogue.

5. A paediatric neurologist should be aware of different cultural attitudes to certain situations. Let us look at three clinical situations:

(a) A developmental neurologist may use a toolbox such as a Stycar tests box which contains a picture card with a pig on it, a doll almost appearing to be a real baby, and some 'idols' or statues of humans or animals. These things are taboo in Islam. A child may not have seen these before and the parents may even walk out of the clinic, making some excuse for the sake of politeness. Is such a test reliable or applicable for Muslim children?

(b) Toys for Christian or Hindu children are usually cuddly toys, dolls, or animals. These may not be acceptable to Muslims as they consider them a mockery of God's creative powers.

(c) Sweets are almost always expected to be given to children by a religious guide in a mosque, temple, or gurudawara. Such a child may be disappointed to see a neurologist who has no sweets to offer.

However, with tact and courtesy, all these problems can be solved.

ETHNIC PATTERNS OF NEUROLOGICAL DISEASES

Rare neurological conditions are common in a neurological clinic because the more common conditions are usually managed by a general practitioner who plays the role of gate-keeper to the hospital system. However, there are certain diseases which are rare in one ethnic group but common in another. Although these are mentioned in the textbooks, their diagnosis may be overlooked by the specialist because, unintentionally, he/she possesses insufficient information about their ethnic nature. In this section, I have selected fifteen such conditions which should be particularly borne in mind by a specialist in a neurology clinic when examining patients from various ethnic groups, overseas visitors, and those who come to Britain for treatment.

SUBACUTE COMBINED DEGENERATION OF THE NERVOUS SYSTEM

Pernicious anaemia is the most common cause of vitamin B_{12} deficiency in the United Kingdom. It is rare in Africa and Asia, except among vegetarians. The features of subacute combined degeneration of the nervous system (SCDNS) may precede or succeed the symptoms of anaemia (Swash 1992). The majority of patients with vitamin B_{12} deficiency have pernicious anaemia, which is uncommon in tropical countries and very rare in some other areas. It can cause neuropathy, optic atrophy, cognitive impairment, and SCDNS. The following five points should be remembered:

1. Ethno-specific illnesses occur in every ethnic group and, as doctors, we should help patients from all ethnic groups. An ethnic majority or minority is a politically determined entity which may influence the redistribution of NHS scarce financial resources and a fair deal is possible in serving them.

2. A European doctor, who has seen many cases of pernicious anaemia and SCDNS, may correctly diagnose European patients, but he/she may overdiagnose these conditions among Asian, African, or Chinese patients because the symptoms of many diseases overlap, especially in the early stages.

3. An Asian, African, or Chinese doctor, even in British hospitals or general practice, who is trained abroad, may have never seen either of these conditions. It is likely that such a doctor may underdiagnose these illnesses among European patients and sometimes may miss such a diagnosis altogether.

4. A doctor trained overseas may fail to recognize SCDNS in medical examinations such as for the Member of the Royal College of Physicians (MRCP). A similar situation may arise in the diagnosis of other ethno-specific illnesses.

5. When taking a history it is useful to ask a non-European patient whether he/she has ever been given Cytamen injections if at any time they have attended an Asian doctor's surgery. For cultural reasons, an Asian doctor, particularly in ethnic minority areas in Britain, may give a course of cyanocobalamin by injection for the treatment of any anaemia in order to avoid the expense of investigations and because Asian patients prefer and even insist on injection treatment.

MULTIPLE SCLEROSIS

Prevalence of this disease varies according to latitude, with high prevalence in temperate zones, but low occurrence in the tropics. The prevalence varies within Britain depending on the distance from the equator (e.g. around 30 per 10 000 in the Shetland and Orkney Islands compared with 6 per 10 000 in England). Near the equator incidence of multiple sclerosis (MS) is very low, and it increases as one moves further from the equator in both northern and southern hemispheres. The incidence and prevalence are higher in the United States and Canada than in South America. MS occurs more among Europeans than among African, Asian or Chinese people.

There are two transcultural factors involved the distribution of MS: migration and ethno-genetic factors. Migration before the age of 15 between areas of contrasting prevalence affects the risk. For example, children born in the United Kingdom of immigrants from areas of low incidence have the same risk of developing MS as the indigenous population. However, this latitude effect can be modified by ethno-genetic factors of the inhabitants. For example, in Wellington, New Zealand, there is a relatively high number of MS cases seen in those of European origin, but it is a rare disease in the Maori population. Similarly, although Japan resembles New Zealand in latitude, MS is uncommon in the Japanese. (Forsythe 1988).

JAPANESE ENCEPHALITIS

This disease is caused by an arbovirus which can be transmitted to man by mosquitoes which feed on infected birds or animals. Pigs and other domestic animals are also important sources of this infection. Inflammatory and degenerative changes are found in the brain. This condition may be encountered in Britain among visitors from Japan, the Phillipines, Taiwan, Borneo, Maylaysia, and Singapore.

Two transcultural points should be noted: this disease is spreading slowly west ward across the Asian subcontinent where there is a high incidence of subclinical infection. A neurologist should be vigilant when seeing Bangladeshis and patients from the Indian province of Bengal; some Britons go to the Pacific islands for holidays and may also be vulnerable to this disease.

KURU

This slow virus infection occurs only in the members of a cannibalistic New Guinea tribe. Kuru is thought to be transmitted as a result of eating the brains of dead tribal members. In this condition there is degeneration of the grey matter, most marked in the cerebellum, causing a progressive ataxia (Edwards and Bouchier 1991). A visitor from such a tribe might, rarely, attend a British neurology clinic.

A point to note is that many Asians eat a delicacy in Indian cuisine which is a well-cooked brain of a sheep, lamb, or cow.

Asians are the largest ethnic minority in the United Kingdom. Are they at a similar risk? If so, is the diagnosis missed? Perhaps neurology research workers should provide the answers.

OCULOPHARYNGEAL MUSCULAR DYSTROPHY

This is an autosomal dominant syndrome consisting of bilateral symmetrical ptosis and progressive dysphagia of late onset, occurring usually in patients of French-Canadian descent, and it is regarded as an infrequent cause of dysphagia in the elderly (Sinclair *et al*. 1989). Occasionally, this condition has been described in patients from other groups (e.g. English, Japanese, Spanish, Italian, and Russian) (Duranceau 1983). An overseas trained doctor in Britain might not have seen such a case in his/her training and one should be vigilant when seeing patients from these groups.

MARCHIAFAVA–BIGNAMI DISEASE

This fatal disease was originally described in heavy Chianti drinkers in Italy, but is now known to occur with other types of alcohol abuse as well. There is a massive central demyelination affecting the corpus callosum, with neuronal necrosis, and extensive degeneration in the cerebral cortex. Death occurs within weeks or months (Scadding 1990).

ALCOHOLISM

Alcohol causes a wide range of neurological effects which are well described in textbooks. The neurotoxic effects include cerebellar degeneration, dementia, peripheral neuropathy, and myopathy. The widespread destruction of myelin in the pons results in tetraparesis, dysphagia, anarthria, and death.

A few transcultural points should be borne in mind:

1. Alcohol, as a social drinking habit, is ingrained in the fabric of European culture, and pubs or wine bars are social meeting places. A neurologist from a 'dry' country should show respect about such social drinking by Europeans.
2. Alcoholism is denounced by almost all cultures and religions. It is especially taboo in Islam, Buddhism, Hinduism, and Sikhism.
3. Chronic alcoholism is the commonest cause of vitamin deficiency in Britain; the deficiency results from malabsorption or malnutrition and can cause lesions in various sites of the nervous system.
4. If a doctor diagnoses a disease caused by alcoholism, the aim is to help the patient; it should not be regarded it as a stigma. In fact, stigma should be removed from a clinical condition altogether.

CEREBROVASCULAR ACCIDENT

Cerebral infarction (80–85% of strokes), or cerebral haemorrhage (15–20% of strokes) cause damage to brain tissue.

Stroke is the third commonest cause of death in Western countries. The most common cause of stroke is atherosclerosis, and other causes include: hypertension, diabetes mellitus, hyperlipidaemia, polycythaemia, thrombocythaemia, positive family history, high alcohol intake, cigarette smoking, oral contraceptives, and trauma. In the United Kingdom, the annual incidence of new strokes is 2 per 1000, and it is a prominent cause of disability (Cull and Will 1991).

There is some evidence to suggest an ethnic predisposition. The incidence of stroke is especially high in Japan and China where cerebral haemorrhage is more common than subarachnoid haemorrhage. The highest incidence of strokes in Whites in the United Kingdom and the United States are among those of Scandinavian descent. In the United States there is a clearly higher incidence of strokes among Blacks (Nicholl and Bulpitt 1990). Neurologists at the University of Cincinnati (*New England Journal of Medicine*, 12 March, 1992) studied 266 stroke patients and found that young and middle-aged Blacks are more at risk of subarachnoid or intracerebral haemorrhage than Whites of a similar age. Blacks had twice the risk of subarachnoid haemorrhage and 1.4 times the risk of intracerebral haemorrhage, but these ethnic differences were far less marked in those over the age of 75 years.

Among the hypertensives, White patients are more likely to develop coronary heart disease and Black patients are more likely to have a stroke. Evidence is accumulating that stroke has a multifactorial aetiology and genetic, ethnic, cultural, and environmental factors, as well as differences in standards of reporting, and these factors should be taken into consideration in the diagnosis and management.

TROPICAL MYELONEUROPATHIES IN JAMAICA AND BRITAIN

Cruickshank and Beevers (1989) have described a study of 100 cases of a neuropathic syndrome of uncertain origin, and called the disease 'Jamaican neuropathy'. This syndrome is prevalent in the Caribbean, Martinique, Africa, southern India, Seychelle Islands, and Columbia. It consists of tropical myeloneuropathies of which two distinct clinical groups were identified:

1. *Tropical ataxic neuropathy*: a syndrome of posterior column and peripheral nerve signs presenting as proprioceptive disorder, sometimes with pyramidal tract signs, occurring in endemic form.
2. *Tropical spastic paraparesis*: an upper motor neurone disorder with some sensory signs in the lower limbs, occurring in either endemic or epidemic forms.

Clinically, there is often an overlap of clinical features of both conditions and the features include back pain, burning sensation in the legs, impaired vibration perception, optic atrophy, male sexual impotence, and sensorineural hearing loss. The onset of the disease is gradual in the majority of patients.

All patients have difficulty in walking due to spasticity and a few patients become paraplegic. Spasticity, leg cramps, and spasms are distressing. Pyramidal tract signs in both the upper and lower limbs can be readily demonstrated on examination. Tropical spastic paraparesis is a retroviral-induced disease and it is widely distributed in Jamaica.

Cruickshank described a study of viral transmission among relatives in Britain. It was found that 60 out of 64 first degree relatives of the Jamaican-born patients in the series were traced in the United Kingdom and Jamaica: 20–30% of those born in the Caribbean had antibodies to retrovirus HTLV-I, irrespective of their present place of residence, while none of those born in the United Kingdom, who were the children of the patients, had antibodies. He concluded that in later adulthood perhaps sexual transmission is much more important than that from breast-feeding. A British neurologist should keep track of such current knowledge, particularly when dealing with Black patients.

AFRICAN TRYPANOSOMIASIS (SLEEPING SICKNESS)

This is caused by trypanosomes conveyed to man by infected tsetse flies of either sex. These flies are only found in Africa. However, air travel has made the world a global village and not only the patient but also a fly may board a plane bound for Europe. Sometimes patients in the early stages die of intercurrent infection, but usually death occurs in the late stage when the central nervous system is involved. Trypanosomes in the brain give rise to chronic meningoencephalitis.

In the late stages of the disease caused by *Trypanosoma gambiense*, the essential feature is a change in behaviour. The psychiatric presentation may be so serious that the patient may be sent to a psychiatric hospital. Such a patient may become violent, the excitable state may resemble mania, delusions may occur, and sometimes schizophrenia is simulated (Bell 1990).

South American trypanosomiasis (Chaga's disease) is caused by *Trypanosoma cruzi*. Death sometimes occurs due to cardiac damage or meningoencephalitis.

BACTERIAL AND PARASITIC MYOSITIS

Britons travel abroad on commercial or leisure trips and many visitors from tropical countries visit Britain all year round. It is relevant to mention some communicable neurological illnesses for easy reference.

Bacterial myositis, particularly acute suppurative tropical myositis, is relatively common in tropical countries. Staphylococcus is the usual infecting organism. Proximal lower limb muscles are usually most affected (Scadding 1990).

Parasitic myositis may occur as part of a number of parasitic infections in tropical countries and none of them are common in the United Kingdom. The parasites include: cysticercosis, *Trichinella spiralis* (trichinosis), *Toxoplasma gondii*, trypanosomiasis (already mentioned). An acute myositis in a travelling business person should be fully investigated and not dismissed as a virus infection, which is an excessively used blanket diagnosis in the United Kingdom.

VIRAL ENCEPHALITIS

The following virus infections are endemic in various countries and these should be considered in a neurological differential diagnosis.

1. Omsk haemorrhagic fever is transmitted by ticks and it is endemic in Russia.
2. Looping illness is also spread by ticks and is encountered in northern Britain.
3. Yellow fever is spread by mosquitoes and it is endemic in Africa and South America. (A weekly newspaper, *Doctor*, publishes a pull-out about the endemic areas of infectious diseases and this can be consulted.)
4. Calipernia encephalitis is transmitted by mosquitoes and it is encountered in the United States.
5. Ross River fever is also spread by mosquitoes and occurs in Australia.

Patients from these ethnic groups should be investigated for the above conditions because they may visit their homelands on holiday. Environmental factors are as important as genetic inheritance in ethnic disease patterns.

TUBERCULOUS MENINGITIS

Although this is now a generally uncommon disorder in the United Kingdom, it is still a major problem in developing countries. In the past, the condition usually occurred shortly after primary infection in childhood, but nowadays it is common among adults, especially as part of miliary tuberculosis. The condition is well described in textbooks.

UK cases of tuberculosis continued to rise in 1993, up nearly 5% compared with 1992, according to the latest figures. The possible causes include the increasing elderly population, a rise in poverty and unemployment, an epidemic of cases among HIV patients, and the particular susceptibility of recent immigrants (Watson 1994).

In the United Kingdom, tuberculosis is more common among ethnic Asians, ethnic Irish, and people from the Highlands of Scotland. Ethnic Africans and Caribbeans have had rates similar to those of the White British population. A neurologist should be vigilant when examining patients from at-risk ethnic groups.

NEUROLOGICAL SARCOIDOSIS

This is a multisystem granulomatous disease. The lesions are histologically similar to tuberculosis, but it is not caused by any mycobacteria, and does not have any caseation. The extrapulmonary manifestations include the involvement of the nervous system, particularly cerebral, meningeal, cranial, and peripheral nerve involvement.

The incidence is high in some ethnic groups and rare in others. In the United Kingdom and the United States the prevalence is 15–30 per 100 000. There is a high incidence in Black Americans, West Indians living in Britain and France, and Blacks in South Africa when compared with indigenous White populations. There is a low incidence in Africans, Asians, Chinese, South-East Asians, and North American Indians. The estimate of incidence in the West Indian population living in London is over 60 per 100 000 (McNicol 1989).

Recent evidence (Winter *et al.* 1994) suggests that sarcoidosis, in Britain, is significantly more common in West Indians, Asians, and the Irish, particularly among females. In the United States, Blacks have a worse prognosis than Whites. It should be remembered that up to 7% of patients may develop neurological dysfunction and in some cases it can be the only presenting clinical feature. Neurological manifestations may include cranial and peripheral neuropathies, and granulomatous meningitis. Occasionally, space-occupying lesions can mimic symptoms suggesting a brain tumour.

LEPROMATOUS NEUROPATHY

Leprosy is a chronic granulomatous disease caused by *Mycobacterium leprae* and it is the commonest cause of peripheral neuritis in the world. The disease is found world-wide and is related to poverty and overcrowding. It is estimated that 20 million people are affected. The disease is common in tropical Asia, tropical Africa, the Far East, Central and South America, and in some Pacific Islands. It is still endemic in Southern Europe, North Africa, and the Middle East (Geddes *et al.* 1991). Visitors or migrants from these regions may attend neurology clinics in the United Kingdom. Some White British travellers visiting these areas may contract the disease.

Lepromatous peripheral neuritis leads to loss of memory, motor, and autonomic functions. The nerves most affected are: ulnar, median, lateral popliteal, sural, and facial. Although sensation is often the first to go, the nerve damage affects both sensory and motor functions in mixed nerves. Nerve involvement is typically symmetrical (Bell 1990).

Another transcultural point relates to its prevention. Although no specific vaccine is available, Bacille–Calmette–Guérin (BCG) is of some value, particularly in Africa. Mass prophylaxis is impossible but it is hoped that with improvement of socioeconomic conditions the disease may disappear. Treatment of leprosy is lengthy and often difficult, therefore an early diagnosis is essential.

An understanding of ethnic patterns of neurological conditions can give a practitioner tremendous job satisfaction and, indeed, help the patients enormously. Caring attitudes can allay fears and misunderstandings in a cross-cultural medical consultation. Good doctor–patient rapport is essential in the practice of medicine.

TRANSCULTURAL COMMENTS ON COMMON NEUROLOGICAL PROBLEMS

Of course, many diseases occur in almost all ethnic groups, but their aetiology, course, and management may show some cultural, religious, or ethnic variations. These differences cannot be ignored because neurologists are dealing with people and not just classical textbook cases. Let us take seven examples:

EPILEPSY

Epilepsy is defined as an altered state of consciousness that occurs when the brain cells electrochemically fire and discharge in an abnormal manner. This activity presents in erratic movements of the muscles of the body and also affects respiration, heart beat, blood pressure, and mental state. It is estimated that some 35 million people world-wide suffer from epilepsy (Sugarman 1984). This condition has no significant ethnic preference. The following transcultural points should be considered:

1. There is still considerable social stigma attached to epilepsy, in all cultures. This may cause difficulty in personal relationships, self-image, and employment.

2. Some patients may not seek medical care or comply with the medical treatment because of religious beliefs, prejudice, stigma, discrimination, shame, guilt feelings, poverty, or because they live in remote areas where medical help is not available.

3. Patients from all cultures may turn to alternative medicine. Those from a Western culture are more likely to use psychotherapeutic interventions such as biofeedback, hypnosis, desensitization exercises, and transactional analysis. Patients from Eastern cultures tend to contact gurus who teach yoga, transcendental meditation, and other 'belief systems' which consist of hypnotic phenomena.

4. One of the desensitization exercises which is said to be used by traditional healers in Africa and the Caribbean, consists of hanging an epileptic child upside down in a ditch. It is akin to 'flooding'. Other extraordinary methods or exorcism may be used by faith healers in China, Asia, and South-East Asian countries.

5. In the United Kingdom, the law concerning epilepsy and driving is understandably strict. A patient who has had only nocturnal fits for at least three years' duration may hold a licence. Someone who has had one daytime fit may not drive for one year. If someone has had two or more fits, the licence will be withdrawn and will not be reinstated until a fit-free period of at least two years has passed. Holders of heavy goods vehicle licences who have any fits will have their licence permanently removed (Scadding 1990). A British citizen will be advised by his doctor that he/she should not drive after a fit and that he/she should seek the advice of the licensing authority. However, a visitor

from abroad may hold an international driving licence and may not be registered with a general practitioner, and may only see a neurologist after a fit. Since the channel tunnel was opened, more people may visit Britain by car. Perhaps a vigilant neurologist will offer the same advice to overseas visitors.

MIGRAINE

This is characterized by episodic headache, which is typically unilateral. It may be accompanied by vomiting and visual disturbance. In the United Kingdom, it affects about 10% of the population and is more common in women. However, the patient may suffer from more than one kind of headache and any underlying pathology must be excluded. Studies in a rural Nigerian community and in China suggest prevalence rates similar to those in Western countries. Daily headaches may also be due to an overuse of ergotamine or analgesics on a regular basis. Three transcultural aspects should be considered:

1. Many English patients believe in self-help and they may buy analgesics over the counter for regular use, whereas ethnic minority patients are more likely to consult a doctor for a headache. Their concept of 'tension headache' is very poor because they give more emphasis to physical causes and seek a cure by drug therapy prescribed by a doctor. For them, a doctor's paracetamol is better than a chemist's paracetamol.
2. People from Africa, Asia, or South-East Asia expect, from a Western doctor, an instant cure. They have heard of their success stories in treating infectious diseases, especially in colonial times. Moreover, they may consider a headache as more serious a symptom than their Western counterparts and, naturally, they are afraid of its possible fatal consequences if the medical treatment does not cure it immediately. The British doctor should explain to them that he/she has no magic wand and that with accurate diagnosis and treatment the patient will usually get better, but it will take some time. It is reassuring to tell such a patient: 'Don't worry, you will live!' A few such patients may consider an unexplained headache an indication of imminent death.
3. Dietary factors, including chocolate, cheese, and alcohol may precipitate attacks of migraine, and may become more frequent in patients taking oral contraceptives. Dietary or medical advice based on this information is suitable for European and Westernized Eastern patients. However, a neurologist should be sensitive to the following cultural or religious aspects when dealing with patients from an Eastern culture:
   (a) Chocolates are Western sweets, whereas Asians or Africans may use their own ethnic sweets. For example, some Indian sweets are similar to chocolate in their composition. A doctor may not be aware of this.
   (b) Cheese is not a part of Indian omnivorous cuisine. Cheese (*Paneer*) is used in place of meat in a curry by vegetarians—who are mostly Hindus or Sikhs.
   (c) Alcohol is taboo for Muslims, Hindus, Sikhs, and Buddhists.
   (d) Contraception is forbidden or frowned upon by most religions. Devout followers would not hear of it but liberals from all religions may welcome it openly or secretly.

A doctor should be sensitive in asking relevant questions and when giving medical advice.

BRAIN TUMOUR

Cerebral tumours account for 2% of deaths at all ages in the United Kingdom. The following points should be remembered when dealing with ethnic minorities from an Eastern culture:

1. There is a stigma attached to the diagnosis of brain tumour in Eastern culture. The social status of the patient is diminished in the extended family circle, especially in financial matters.
2. In some societies a brain tumour is considered a curse from the Devil or a punishment from God for a wrongdoing of the patient or of his/her ancestors.
3. Dying from a brain tumour is considered a terrible death by some Eastern subcultures. A patient or relative might request the doctor not to disclose the diagnosis to other relatives or friends. He may be requested to write another diagnosis on the death certificate.

MENTAL HANDICAP

Ironically, a mentally handicapped person, in the extended family, is considered a holy man in Asian countries. It is not uncommon for a breadwinner to have the blessings of such a person before going for a day's work. On the other hand, a mentally ill person, or someone with a nervous disease is considered fit only to be cared for in a hospital or institution. Similar customs, to a varying degree, may prevail among the followers of other religions. It should be made clear that all religions teach respect for a mentally or neurologically ill person, and yet followers demonstrate the feelings described above, which are widespread. This is a sensitive issue and a neurologist should assess the situation according to the individual patient and his or her family.

NEUROFIBROMATOSIS

This is a genetic disorder of nerve tissue affecting one in 2500 people in its most common form, NF1, and 1 in 35 000 in type NF2. In the British Isles, it is estimated to affect some 20 000 people. It affects both sexes and all ethnic groups (Neurofibromatosis Association 1993).

In all cultures, the main problem is cosmetic due to the disfigurement caused by a number of lumps and bumps on the body and the face. The adverse effects on personal esteem and human relationships are noted in all ethnic groups. However, there is an additional cultural disadvantage. In societies where an arranged marriage is customary, such a disfigurement, particularly in a woman, can lead to enormous strain on the parents. They may have to give more dowry (or *Jahaiz*) to the bridegroom's family because they will have to bear all the expenses for medical and cosmetic treatment in the future. A sympathetic approach and counselling by health professionals can help such patients and their families.

HUNTINGTON'S CHOREA

This is an autosomal dominant disorder consisting of chorea and progressive dementia. The disease occurs in all ethnic groups and about 7 people in 100 000 are affected in the United Kingdom. There are about 5000 sufferers in the United Kingdom. It is a rare disorder and only a few patients will be inpatients in British mental hospitals. In Eastern societies, it is considered a frightening mental illness, particularly for children, and for sociocultural reasons such patients are sent to mental hospitals and, even in the early stages, not cared for in the community. Dementia develops in virtually all cases of the disease. The ultimate mainstay of management will be long-term hospital care. This condition is both neurological and psychological, therefore it may be considered a curse on that patient and the family. An arranged marriage in that family becomes difficult because potential in-laws stay away in order to avoid acquiring the 'curse'.

BELL'S PALSY

Idiopathic (Bell's) palsy is a common condition affecting patients of all ages, sexes, and ethnic groups. The damage to the facial nerve is responsible for the initial loss of nerve impulse conduction leading to facial paralysis.

If an Englishman or a Scot is angry, he/she may swear to release the emotional tension caused by intense anger. But other ethnic groups have different customs. For example, in an Asian culture, if someone becomes very angry with a person for some reason, the aggrieved party may wish three curses on the persecutor: 'I wish that you would get struck by lightening', 'I wish that you would break your neck', and, worst of all, 'I wish that you would have a facial paralysis'. A neurologist should be careful when disclosing the diagnosis of Bell's palsy to an Asian patient. It could be mistaken for an abuse or insult! Of course, by understanding such delicate points many misunderstandings can be avoided in a transcultural consultation.

PRACTICAL CONSIDERATIONS

History taking

Ask the patient his/her age, sex, marital status, culture, religion, and ethnicity. This information will be useful in a medical consultation. Try to pronounce a patient's name correctly. Try to assess whether a patient from another culture is trying to be economical with the truth out of politeness or in the defence of 'family honour'. Help from an interpreter or link person should be obtained if there is a language barrier.

Examination

Use a chaperone when examining a patient of the opposite sex, even if you are a woman, in a transcultural contact. Show that you are sympathetic and allow more time for undressing if relevant. Explain beforehand about the instruments you plan to use. Non-Europeans have an inaccurate concept of 'I don't know' and may guess that the answer is 'yes' or 'no'. Ensure clarity.

Investigations

Use the information in this chapter along with the knowledge in other chapters so as to plan appropriate investigations for an individual patient. Some people from non-scientific backgrounds are afraid of the sight of their blood. Ethnic minority patients may lack British social education and it is wise to explain the machines or instruments used for investigations.

Diagnosis

Scientific variables, which affect genetic inheritance and environmental factors, include: age, sex, social class, ethnicity, religion, and culture. These variables should be considered along with medical knowledge about the physical, psychological, and social aspects of a patient's problem. Scientific knowledge should not be abandoned, it only needs to be modified according to each patient's profile. It is the only way to reach an accurate diagnosis.

Management

In a transcultural medical consultation it is prudent to inform the patient fully about the planned treatment. In the case of an extended family background, it is wise to involve one or more relatives in decision-making and obtaining 'informed' consent. This will avoid a complaint or litigation which often results from hurried communication. Where a patient has a defensive or inflexible attitude every effort should be made to reach a compromise. There is no place for overassertiveness in a transcultural consultation, from either party. In fact, in this area of medicine, which presents an intellectual challenge, an accurate diagnosis and appropriate treatment can give tremendous job satisfaction to every neurologist, whatever the level.

CONCLUSION

Medicine is practised beyond textbooks and the patient is the most important person to a medical practitioner. In this chapter an effort has been made to identify and evaluate some cultural, religious, and ethnic factors that may be encountered between a doctor of one ethnic group and a patient of another in a multi-ethnic neurology clinic. This information is based on my 35 years' experience of medical practice in London, a city which has become multicultural, and also my extensive reading of the research evidence as it became available. I have followed Hippocrates' method of observation while practising medicine, so as to construct each patient's ethnic, religious, and cultural profile. As I do not belong to any pressure group intentionally, I am more willing to learn and would appreciate readers' comments on the practical value of this chapter in their practice of clinical neurology.

Research evidence is now accumulating rapidly in the management of neurological illness in ethnic minorities. For example, while writing this chapter I have received three abstracts of recent papers from the Motor Neurone Disease Association (Tel. 01604 250505). The hard evidence is as follows:

1. Motor neurone disease (MND) mortality among ethnic Asian males was only half, and for females only one-fifth, of that expected among English patients. Mortality among ethnic Caribbeans was somewhat lower than among the ethnic English. White immigrants from the Indian subcontinent had the expected MND mortality rate. This study is evidence that MND mortality is not the same in all ethnic groups (Elian and Dean 1993).

2. Multiple sclerosis (MS) mortality was low among ethnic Asians, West Indians, and Africans. MS is very uncommon in these groups even after migration to the United Kingdom. In contrast, among the UK-born children of Asians, West Indians, and Africans in the age group available for study, a high prevalence of MS was of a similar order to that occurring in the indigenous British population (Elian *et al.* 1990).

3. There has been a marked increase in reported mortality from motor neurone disease (MND), but not from multiple sclerosis (MS) in England and Wales and some other countries. An increase in MND mortality occurred in Australia and New Zealand between 1968 and 1997 and 1978 and 1987, greater than that which occurred in England and Wales, but there was no increase in MS mortality. Among the Whites in South Africa, the MND mortality was half of that in England, Australia, and New Zealand in both time periods. Moreover, both MND and MS mortality is higher in the English-speaking than in the Afrikaans-speaking Whites born in South Africa (Dean and Elian 1993).

Although the British have a reputation for resisting change, it is hoped that readers have found this chapter food for thought and will look after their patients from all cultures, with a better understanding.

REFERENCES

Bell, D. R. (1990). *Lecture notes on tropical medicine*, pp. 38–53; 233–46. Blackwell, Oxford.

Brand, P. and Yancy, P. (1993). *Pain: The gift nobody wants*, pp. 5–6. Zondervan, USA: Harper Collins.

Cruickshank, J. K. and Beevers, D. G. (ed.) (1989). *Ethnic factors, in health and disease*, pp. 170–7. Wright, London.

Cull, R. E. and Will, R. G. (1991). Diseases of nervous system. In *Davidson's principles and practice of medicine*, (ed. R. W. Edwards and I. A. D. Bouchier), pp. 859–60. Churchill Livingstone, Edinburgh.

Dean, G. and Elian, M. (1993). Motor neurone disease and multiple sclerosis mortality in Australia, New Zealand and South Africa compared with England and Wales, *Journal of Neurology, Neurosurgery and Psychiatry*, **56**, 633–7.

Duranceau, A. C. Forand, M., Fanteux, J. P. *et al.* (1980). Surgery in oculopharyngeal muscular dystrophy, *American Journal of Surgery*, **139**, 32–9.

Edwards, C. R. W. and Bouchier, I. A. D. (ed.) (1991). *Davidson's principles and practice of medicine*, pp. 881–2. Churchill Livingstone, Edinburgh.

Elian, M. and Dean, G. (1993). Motor neurone disease and multiple sclerosis among immigrants to England from the Indian subcontinent, the Caribbean, and Africa. *Journal of Neurology, Neurosurgery and Psychiatry*, **56**, 454–7.

Elian, M., Nightingale, S., and Dean, G. (1990). Multiple sclerosis among UK born children of immigrants from the Indian subcontinent, Africa and West Indies. *Journal of Neurology, Neurosurgery and Psychiatry*, **53**, 3022–50.

Forsythe, E. (1988). *Multiple sclerosis*, pp. 27–8. Faber and Faber, London.

Geddes, A. M., Bryceson, A. D. M., and Thin, R. N. (1991). Diseases due to infection. In *Davidson's principles and practice of medicine*, (ed. R. W. Edwards and I. A. D. Bouchier), pp. 134–40. Churchill Livingstone, Edinburgh.

Kennedy, R. (1984). *The dictionary of beliefs*, pp. 104–5; 36–7; 46–7; 86–7; 96–7; 174–6. Ward Lock Educational, East Grinstead, UK.

McNicol, M. W. (1989). Sarcoidosis. In *Ethnic factors in health and disease*, pp. 209–13. Wright, London.

Neurofibromatosis Association (1993). *What is neurofibromatosis?* [Leaflet: can be obtained from 120 London Road, Kingston upon Thames, Surrey, KT2 6QJ.]

Nicholl, C. G. and Bulpitt, C. J. (1990). Identifying the causes and risk factors for stroke. *Geriatric Medicine*, **20**, 57–68.

Qureshi, B (1994). *Transcultural Medicine: dealing with patients from different cultures*, (2nd edn), Preface. Kluwer, London.

Scadding, J. W. (1990). Neurological disease. In *Medicine* (ed. R. L. Souhami and J. Moxham), pp. 948, 949, 974, 891. Churchill Livingstone, Edinburgh.

Sinclair, A. J., Thomas, H., and Nicholl, C. G. (1989). A case of oculopharyngeal muscular dystrophy. *British Journal of Hospital Medicine*, **42**, 77–8.

Spokes, E. *Understanding Huntingdon's chorea*, pp. 4–5. A booklet by S K F Publications.

Sugarman, G. I. (1984). *Epilepsy handbook*, pp. 4–159. Mosby, St. Louis.

Swash, M. (1992). *Hutchinson's clinical methods*, p. 476. Baillière Tindall, London.

Watson, J. (1994). Experts' concern over TB figures, *Pulse*, **54**, 24.

Watt, J. (ed.) (1993). *What is wrong with Christian healing*, pp. 1–2. The Churches' Council for Health and Healing, London.

Winter, J., Dhillon, D., and Williams, L. (1994). Unravel the mystery of sarcoid disease. *MIMS Magazine*, 15 February, 24–9.

19 | *The relationship between neurology and psychiatry*

Tim Betts

The relationship between the disciplines of neurology and psychiatry should be strong, but is often, sadly, rather teasing. As neurology and psychiatry developed from Victorian times onward in the United Kingdom they separated. Psychiatry in particular tended to develop in isolation, not only from neurology itself, but also from general medicine. In some countries this separation did not occur or was not extreme: indeed in some parts of the world the two disciplines may be practised concurrently by the same individual.

In recent years, attempts have been made to bridge the gap between the two disciplines in the United Kingdom. Psychiatrists are moving out of their isolation into the general hospital (although some are bypassing this and going straight into the community).

The discipline of 'neuropsychiatry' has been firmly established, although some psychiatrists have always called themselves neuropsychiatrists (as, for instance, in the armed forces). Both a British Neuropsychiatry Association and an American Neuropsychiatry Association flourish (the latter with an excellent journal). Appointments in neuropsychiatry at consultant level in the United Kingdom are being made.

There has been much recent discussion about exactly what neuropsychiatry embraces. There is a division between those who feel that it brings neurological knowledge into the management of psychiatric disorder (particularly recent advances in receptor chemistry and molecular genetics) and those, probably in the minority, who feel it should bring psychological knowledge and treatment techniques into the management and understanding of neurological disease. Indeed, it has been suggested, since it is clear that the major psychotic illnesses (schizophrenia and manic depressive disorder) are chemically caused, that neurologists should take over the care of these conditions (although I fancy that few of my neurology colleagues would care to be called out to a police station at 3.00 am to examine the mental state of some recalcitrant member of the public).

Any psychiatrist reading this who feels that his/her job is threatened by a new army of psychiatrically aware neurologists should reflect that in this country there are not even enough neurologists to deal with those conditions that are properly their responsibility. Also, in the major psychoses, biologically based as they may be, it is extremely important to look at the psychological and social factors which cause the conditions to present in the way that they do in a particular individual: these social and psychological factors also help to perpetuate, exacerbate, and worsen the condition unless dealt with. Psychiatrists should also look at the large number of neuroleptically damaged shambling wrecks of people who haunt our psychiatric hospitals in order to remember that overenthusiastic medicalization of psychiatric 'illness' can be a mistake. At least one person a week dies in the United Kingdom from untoward side-effects of psychotropic (usually neuroleptic) medication.

Is it too fanciful to say that both neurologists and psychiatrists have in common the desire to assault the dopaminergic system in the brain with powerful drugs the actions of which are ill understood? The neurologist treats movement disorders with drugs that may well drive his patient insane: the psychiatrist treats insanity with drugs that may well leave behind them a movement disorder.

This chapter is about bringing psychiatric skills and knowledge to the aid of the neurologist: the *second* but, I think, more important function of neuropsychiatry.

There are four main ways in which psychiatric and neurological symptoms and signs become linked and interwoven and where, if mistakes are to be avoided, neurologists and psychiatrists must work closely together (or have good knowledge of each others disciplines—and of their limitations).

1. Psychiatric illness may present in a neurological guise (as in the somatoform disorders including conversion disorder—'hysteria').
2. Neurological disorder may present as a psychiatric state (e.g. epileptic twilight states).
3. Psychiatric symptoms may occur as the result of neurological disease (i.e. grief reactions during the onset of dementia, the behavioural changes that accompany cerebral tumours).
4. Psychological disorder may worsen or exacerbate neurological disorder: so-called psychosomatic disease (e.g. stress increasing the frequency of epileptic seizures). In this chapter I will concentrate on the first and the last of these mechanisms, mainly using epilepsy as my example because this is the neurological condition (if, indeed, it is a neurological condition) with which I am most familiar and where psychiatry has most to offer.

Psychiatric illness of all kinds can exist side by side with neurological illness, sometimes coincidentally, sometimes as the consequence of a common cerebral disorder, or the one as a consequence of the other. Psychiatrists are much more used than neurologists to consider multi-axial classification of mental and physical disorders, so that in addition to the primary disorder being classified the patient's personality, social circumstances and physical state can be taken into account within a consistent diagnostic framework. Such a multi-axial formulation is particularly important when considering the psychiatric disorders that may exist with, or be mistaken for, neurological disease. Psychiatry has complicated itself by having two disparate but widely used classifications of psychological disorder (ICD10 and DSM IV). This chapter will be based on DSM IV (APA 1994) as this classification has particularly helped our understanding of the somatoform disorders in which psychiatry and neurology are often linked.

PSYCHIATRIC DISORDERS THAT CAN PRESENT AS A NEUROLOGICAL DISORDER

Emotional distress can often present with physical symptoms. Severe depression often presents with complaints of profound feelings of ill health, pain, or even pseudodementia. Many of the symptoms of anxiety are physical (such as diarrhoea, tremor, dizziness, collapse, headache, etc.). It is not surprising, considering how poor most doctors' training is in psychiatry, that we often fail to see the emotional distress lying behind physical symptoms, or that having been assessed physically and nothing having been found the patient is dismissed as 'functional' with no further help offered. It is a fault of medical education, particularly in the United Kingdom, that mind, brain, and body are treated as though they were totally separate, when in fact their relationship is intimate and inextricable. If a patient presents with physical symptoms which after investigation seem to have no physical basis for them, the patient still has needs: a psychological cause for physical symptoms is as valid a condition, and is just as much in need of treatment as a physical disorder is. In many patients in neurological practice psychological needs and physical needs exist side by side and the patient will not be helped unless both needs are met.

The neurologist is likely to encounter patients presenting with physical symptoms that have a psychological basis for them in several distinct disorders including anxiety, depression, psychotic illness, and particularly somatoform disorders (a term which some readers may be unfamiliar since it is taken from the DSM IV classification). This classification, however, does make an otherwise confused area easier to understand and more logical.

SOMATOFORM DISORDERS

The classic somatoform disorder which, although not as common as it used to be, still excites fascination and argument is *conversion disorder.* (Betts 1997a) The old term for this is 'hysteria' but conversion disorder is much better being less pejorative and more accurately defined. 'Hysteria' is used so loosely and inaccurately as to almost to have no meaning. (Table 19.1.)

Conversion disorder involves an often sudden change in neurological function (usually loss or impairment). Except in cases where this loss of function has been long sustained and reinforced (with both primary and secondary gain), there should usually be a discernable relationship between a psychological event and the onset of the symptom. Often, but not invariably, the symptom will have some kind of symbolic relationship with the stress that caused it and can often be seen as an escape from that stress. It is important to realize that the symptom is not under voluntary control: the patient is not consciously pretending and has belief in the validity of the symptoms. Most conversion symptoms are of a neurological nature, (such as paralysis, loss of sensation, disorder of gait, loss of vision or speech). Women are much more commonly affected than men.

Conversion disorder is a symptom and not a disease: like all symptoms there are various causes. Conversion symptoms tend to occur in the predisposed. They are common, for instance, even in normal children (indeed in some ways it is useful to conceptualize conversion symptoms as the persistence into adult life of a childhood mechanism of coping with

Table 19.1 DSM IV criteria for conversion disorder

A. One or more symptoms or deficits affecting voluntary motor or sensory function that suggest a neurological or other general medical condition.

B. Psychological factors are judged to be associated with the symptom or deficit because the initiation or exacerbation of the symptom or deficit is preceded by conflicts or other stressors.

C. The symptom or deficit is not intentionally produced or feigned (as in Factitious Disorder or Malingering).

D. The symptom or deficit cannot, after appropriate investigation, be fully explained by a general medical condition, or by the direct effects of a substance, or as a culturally sanctioned behaviour or experience.

E. The symptom or deficit causes clinically significant distress or impairment in social, occupational, or other important areas of functioning or warrants medical evaluation.

F. The symptom or deficit is not limited to pain or sexual dysfunction, does not occur exclusively during the course of Somatization Disorder, and is not better accounted for by another mental disorder.

Specify type of symptom or deficit.
With Motor Symptom or Deficit (e.g. impaired co-ordination or balance, paralysis or localized weakness, difficulty swallowing or 'lump in throat', aphonia, and urinary retention).
With Sensory Symptom or Deficit (e.g. loss of touch or pain sensation, double vision, blindness, deafness, and hallucinations).
With Seizures or Convulsions: includes seizures or convulsions with voluntary motor or sensory components.
With Mixed Presentations: if symptoms of more than one category are evident.

stress). They tend to occur in people with histrionic personalities or who have been predisposed to develop the symptom because they have had a similar physical symptom in the past and have developed the potential for secondary gain from it.

Case report 1
A middle-aged man developed undoubted acute viral labyrinthitis with severe ataxia and dizziness. He recovered after a month but had to take several weeks off work as a result and lost confidence in going out for a two to three months afterwards but was supported through this difficult time by his wife. Audiological tests indicated that although he had made a full clinical recovery he had suffered high tone hearing loss in one ear and his caloric tests were still slightly abnormal.

Three years later his marriage came under strain and his wife indicated her desire to leave the marital home. He immediately became afflicted by severe dizziness accompanied by a bizarre truncal ataxia and his wife had to accompany him everywhere if he went out: he could not work and had to stay at home, although when at home his symptoms were not prominent—but he spent most of the time in bed. He refused to acknowledge the psychological nature of his symptoms but did agree to some behavioural treatment aimed at gradual exposure to venturing out of the house again. Slow progress was being made when his wife announced her intention to stay (her lover had moved away). Almost overnight his symptoms resolved.

Conversion symptoms often take the form they do because of previous illness predisposing the person to them, and often arise in an area of 'weakness' within the brain or body. This is why it is important even in patients who have an unequivocal physical disorder not to reinforce it or allow secondary gain to develop. Depression may also release conversion symptoms which will disappear when the depression is better: conversion symptoms may also be the initial presentation of psychotic illness. Organic brain disease may also present initially as an apparent conversion disorder. It is particularly important therefore when faced with somebody who appears to have an obvious conversion symptom still to do a full neurological assessment. This is particularly true because many people who are beginning to develop a neurological disorder which is *subjectively* apparent to them but not *objectively* apparent to an examining doctor may exaggerate their subjective disability; this exaggeration is picked up by the examining doctor who therefore draws the erroneous conclusion that the patient's complaint is completely functional.

The fact that both organic disease and serious psychiatric disorder can mimic, often for some time, conversion disorder explains why long-term follow-up of cases of 'hysteria' reveals that many seem eventually to develop a physical or psychiatric disorder—particularly, in the neurological field, multiple sclerosis and a cerebral or spinal tumour. In my experience, the symptoms of spinal tumours are particularly likely to be originally labelled as functional.

Case report 2
A women of 55 who was in good health and asymptomatic was told by her son that he was leaving his wife and children for someone else. She collapsed on being told and remained apparently unconscious for some minutes. She then recovered but was totally mute. On admis-

sion to a psychiatric hospital she resisted neurological examination but apart from being totally mute appeared to understand what was being said to her and would obey simple commands. Shortly after admission to hospital her muteness became selective (she would not talk to doctors but would converse in simple terms with the nursing staff). It had initially been assumed that her selective muteness was a conversion symptom symbolically related to her inability to talk about what her son had done. However, as she settled on the ward she allowed proper physical examination which revealed a right facial palsy and mild right hemiplegia. Computerized tomography (CT) examination revealed a large infiltrating tumour of the left temporal lobe which was rapidly fatal.

Recognition of conversion disorder

When called to see a patient with suspected conversion disorder (since like all somatoform disorders it rarely presents *directly* to the psychiatrist) the psychiatrist will want to obtain the answer to several questions before deciding on the best course of action for the patient. Psychiatrists have an understandable dislike of being treated merely as removal men who only come to see the 'mad, bad, and dangerous to know' to dispose of them as rapidly as possible. The psychiatrist also knows that a primary diagnosis of 'hysteria' is likely to be wrong 90% of the time if made by a general physician or surgeon and even some of the time if made by a neurologist—this is not said lightly but is based on bitter experience. An assessment of possible conversion disorder involves reviewing the answers to the following questions.

1. Is the diagnosis of a conversion symptom correct? How has it been made?
2. Is there discordance between the presenting symptoms or signs and those of known presentations of neurological disorder? Psychiatrists will accept this discordance if it is clear that a careful neurological assessment has been made and positive reasons given for this discordance. Psychiatrists also know, from their own experience, however, that neither the brain nor the mind always behave in the way neurologists expect them to or think they should.
3. Do the symptoms or signs fluctuate in intensity and duration? This is often a helpful sign of conversion disorder but can be misleading.
4. Can the patient be distracted from the symptoms or signs? This is helpful but may mislead.
5. Does there seem to have been a clear emotional precipitant? Again this may be helpful, but in itself is not necessarily diagnostic of conversion disorder; emotional stress can precipitate a transient ischaemic attack or an epileptic seizure for instance. Case report 2 illustrates this very well.
6. Is the symptom symbolic of the precipitating stress or does it resolve it in some way: is there a clear primary gain? Again apparent resolution of an emotional crisis by the symptom may be misleading: assessment of primary gain may be no more than a value judgement.
7. Does the patient show a relative indifference to the gravity of the symptom or the situation in which he/she finds him/

herself (the classical 'belle indifférence'). This must not be mistaken for denial (which can look like indifference) or for 'gallows humour'. Many people initially respond to acute disability by stoical indifference or a joking response ('By God Sir, you have lost your leg!' 'By God sir, so I have!').

Case report 3

A 19-year-old student developed complex partial seizures which involved intense anxiety feelings followed by complicated automatisms which involved undressing. She was a reserved shy girl who privately found this behaviour most distressing but maintained a public air of flippancy and denial referring to the attacks as her 'little faints'. Her flippant 'I don't care' attitude was so strong that her seizures were initially diagnosed as 'hysteria' and her denial as 'belle indifférence'. In a prolonged interview which penetrated these defences her underlying distress and shame was readily apparent and a correct diagnosis was made: her seizures came under rapid control with medication.

9. Does the symptom rapidly respond to psychological treatment (e.g. suggestion, hypnosis)? This certainly favours the diagnosis but some physical disorders have a natural waxing and waning course that may be misleading: removing stress may also remove some physical symptoms (e.g. epileptic seizures are often responsive to psychological treatment).

10. What is the cultural, educational, family, and personality background of this patient? Is there good evidence of an histrionic personality? Has he/she responded to stress with physical symptoms before? Does he/she come from a culture which sanctions such a response?

11. Is there evidence of other psychiatric disorder (e.g. depression, incipient psychosis)?

12. Is there evidence of organic brain disease?

13. In apparent *chronic* conversion disorder what is the secondary gain? Who, or what, is reinforcing the condition?

The diagnosis of conversion disorder should never be made without full assessment of the patient and should not be made purely on the possession of *one* of the above features but made on a combination of them and after due thought. Even if there is an obvious psychological component the clinician should ask 'why has this symptom or sign arisen at this particular time in this particular patient? Is there an occult organic lesion?' A conversion symptom occurring *for the first time* in middle age or older is rare in either sex and unusual at any age in men. Once a satisfactory diagnosis has been made then management can begin. Such management assumes that a full neurological and psychiatric assessment has been made and that one is dealing with a conversion symptom which is uncontaminated by other psychiatric illness: if it is occurring in the setting, say, of a depressive illness then the depression would be the primary target for treatment.

Management of conversion disorder

Gentle confrontation is needed without being either accusatory or dismissive. The negative nature of physical investigation should be revealed and then using some phrase such as 'the brain sometimes has a way of telling us when we should slow down or when we can't deal with a situation' the psychological nature of the physical symptoms should be discussed. The probable nature of the underlying emotional problem should already be known following psychiatric assessment and this can then be brought into the conversation. It should be firmly stated that no neurological or physical disability has been found and that the symptoms relate to the patient's emotions. The underlying problem causing the symptoms should be ventilated and discussed and the confident suggestion made that the physical symptom will gradually disappear. It is usually advisable not to produce an abrupt loss of the symptoms because the patient has to save face with family and friends. If the patient is aphonic, for instance, put a little pressure on the return of speech by limiting opportunities for non-vocal communication (overuse of the writing pad will slow things down too much) and start by saying something like 'most people with your condition can whisper the letter A—I think you can'. When this has been done one goes through the alphabet initially whispering, then in normal speech, then words, then sentences until the patient speaks normally. Progress is positively rewarded.

Suggestion is a very powerful therapeutic weapon: often firm, friendly reassurance is all that is needed to allow the symptoms to resolve of their own accord although support can be given by physiotherapy and occasionally hypnotic suggestion (to which most people with conversion disorder are very susceptible). If hypnotic relief for symptoms is going to be used then some knowledge of the underlying problem should already have been gained except on rare occasions when hypnosis has to be used as a form of abreaction to get at the underlying problem. Although hypnosis is a simple but valuable skill (which most doctors should know how to use) and will relieve conversion symptoms rapidly it should not be used for abreaction except by a clinician who has the clinical experience to cope with the deluge that may follow the sudden opening of emotional floodgates.

Although the emotional problem that lies behind conversion symptoms is usually easy to recognize if it is particularly disturbing or has been suppressed for a long time it may need help in order to enter the patient's conscious awareness. Hypnosis is helpful for this but needs careful use as the inexperienced can readily implant false memories as current concerns about the 'false memory syndrome' (which does exist) testify. The older literature warns that removing symptoms without removing the underlying cause can lead to symptom substitution but in my experience this is very uncommon. It is also said that if a conversion symptom is removed without the underlying problem being ventilated then serious disturbance, even suicide, may follow. Again in my experience this is unlikely.

If the underlying emotional problem which is causing an apparent conversion symptom is not fairly obvious it may well, of course, not exist. One has to guard against the danger of the 'amateur psychologist' who faced with a patient with puzzling organic symptoms can always find a psychological cause for them. Most people with genuine physical symptoms will have psychological problems which may sometimes exacerbate their symptoms. I would also warn against pressing psychological reasons for a person's symptoms (gleaned from memories of reading a paperback about Freud a few years ago) on to a reluctant patient. It is much better to allow the patient to see the connection between symptom and problem for him/herself. In conversion states any psychological reason for the functional symptom is usually very obvious: if it isn't, think again.

As symptoms resolve patients will need support as they deal with their underlying problem but the prognosis of acute conversion symptoms (provided they are confronted properly and dealt with sympathetically) is excellent. Faced with similar stress in the future the patient may develop similar symptoms, but most patients I have known who do relapse under renewed stress can usually eventually gain some insight and may actually eventually turn up in the clinic saying 'my arm is paralysed again: I must be stressed about something'. The danger for this kind of patient, of course, is that eventually he/she will develop a real physical illness. It is only too easy because they have cried 'wolf' too often in the past for the new symptom to be ignored and to be written off as another conversion symptom. Patients with histrionic personality disorders need careful assessment each time they present with a new (or even the same) symptom. Conversion symptoms sometimes become chronic. This is usually either because the underlying problem has not resolved or because the conversion symptom has been reinforced and has developed secondary as well as primary gain and the patient has entered into playing the role of a sick person. The paralysed teenager who has begun to quite enjoy being pushed around in a wheelchair by her dutiful companions is not always easy to help, especially if her family also reinforce her paraplegia as a means of keeping her at home under their control.

Managing these chronic, well-entrenched, and reinforced conversion symptoms is much more difficult. The same kind of gentle confrontation and suggestions about improvement will need to be made and exploration of the underlying problem is important (although the underlying problem may long since have resolved itself and secondary gain will be keeping the condition going). Ancillary support such as a programme of physiotherapy may well be necessary particularly for some neurological conversion symptoms (six months inactivity in a wheelchair, for instance, is going to produce its own problems of weakness and lack of co-ordination in the legs even if there was nothing originally wrong with them). Ancillary support also helps to 'save face'. Often, a much more vigorous behavioural approach may be needed in chronic conversion disorder particularly using operant conditioning (rewarding non-sickness behaviour and ignoring or 'punishing' sickness behaviour). It is important in these situations that the victim is able to save face (and may therefore need to recover slowly) and

may need to have a powerful medical reason for getting better so that medical treatment needs to be given with a lot of suggestion. Some of these patients actually do well if they can save face by going to a faith healer or even to Lourdes (but without subsequent emotional support, the effect of either 'miracle' will be unlikely to last long particularly if powerful parents are conniving in maintaining the symptoms). In chronic conversion symptoms the support and help of a psychiatric team is clearly going to be necessary and it is best if future management is discussed and the reasons for the diagnosis made clear with the team before confrontation takes place.

The prognosis of conversion symptoms although excellent for the individual acute episode is one of a tendency towards recurrence and the prognosis of entrenched chronic conversion symptoms is poor. Long-term studies have suggested that a high proportion of people who carry the diagnosis of conversion disorder eventually turn out to have a physical or psychiatric illness: the reason for this has already been discussed.

OTHER SOMATAFORM DISORDERS

As with conversion disorder the other somatoform disorders which neurologists need to know about rarely present directly to psychiatrists. The psychiatrist often arrives like the Seventh Cavalry to rescue the neurologist (or other physician) from the patient who possesses it. Unfortunately, the cavalry often circles impotently outwith the battleground because patients with somatoform disorders often refuse psychiatric assessment or treatment and so the physician or the general practitioner has to rely on his/her own resources. Since somatoform disorders often create problems which no doctor knows how to solve (or likes trying to solve) the psychiatrist is often only too pleased that the patient has refused psychiatric care and will sometimes stand on the sidelines wringing his/her hands and saying 'if only the patient would speak to me I might be able to help'.

Since the term 'psychiatrist' is often equated (both by referring doctor and by patient) with the concept of 'quack', 'mad doctor', or 'he who treats imaginary illnesses' it would be better if the psychiatrist was usually introduced with a different title or as a recognized member of the neurological team. I sharply disagree with those of my psychiatric colleagues who 'hungry for an imagined martyrdom' insist on always being referred to as a psychiatrist. Sometimes the title 'nerve specialist' or some such term (said without archly raising the eyebrows) is better.

SOMATIZATION DISORDER (FORMERLY BRIQUET'S SYNDROME)

Confusingly, this condition was also at one time called hysteria but it is not a conversion disorder, and although an odd condition, is one whose separate existence we now recognize. It is often difficult to recognize even though the patient has the characteristic multiplicity of different physical symptoms because they are presented severally and in isolation to different specialists. The syndrome is one of multiple somatic complaints without a pathological foundation. In the DSM IV criteria it is defined as a patient who has a history of many physical complaints beginning before the age of 30 and persisting for several years. A qualifying symptom must not be related to organic pathology or to a pathophysiological mechanism. If there is an underlying organic pathology, it only qualifies if it results in social or occupational impairment that is grossly in excess of what would be expected from the physical findings. The symptoms must cause the patient to seek frequent medical advice or significant or take more than just 'over-the-counter' medication. It will be seen from Table 19.2 that neurological symptoms figure strongly in this syndrome although other symptoms from other bodily systems are necessary as well. Often, the diagnosis is reasonably clear because

Table 19.2 DSM IV criteria for Somatization disorder

A. A history of many physical complaints beginning before age 30 years that occur over a period of several years and result in treatment being sought or significant impairment in social, occupational, or other important areas of functioning.

B. Each of the following criteria must have been met, with individual symptoms occurring at any time during the course of the disturbance:

  (1) *four pain symptoms*: a history of pain related to at least four different sites or functions (e.g. head, abdomen, back joints, extremities, chest, rectum, during menstruation, during sexual intercourse, or during urination);

  (2) *two gastrointestinal symptoms*: a history of at least two gastrointestinal symptoms other than pain (e.g. nausea, bloating, vomiting other than during pregnancy, diarrhoea, or intolerance of several different foods);

  (3) *one sexual symptom*: a history of at least one sexual or reproductive symptom other than pain (e.g. sexual indifference, erectile or ejaculatory dysfunction, irregular menses, excessive menstrual bleeding, vomiting throughout pregnancy);

  (4) *one pseudoneurological symptom*: a history of at least one symptom or deficit suggesting a neurological condition not limited to pain (conversion symptoms such as impaired co-ordination or balance, paralysis or localized weakness, difficulty swallowing or lump in throat, aphonia, urinary retention, hallucinations, loss of touch or pain sensation, double vision, blindness, deafness, seizures; dissociative symptoms such as amnesia; or loss of consciousness other than fainting).

C. Either (1) or (2):

  (1) after appropriate investigation, each of the symptoms in Criterion B cannot be fully explained by a known general medical condition or the direct effects of a substance (e.g. a drug of abuse, a medication);

  (2) when there is a related general medical condition, the physical complaints or resulting social or occupational impairment are in excess of what would be expected from the history, physical examination, or laboratory findings.

D. The symptoms are not intentionally produced or feigned (as in Factitious Disorder or Malingering).

of the patient's previous experience of investigations from other specialists but if the patient is presenting primarily to the neurologist there may also be evidence of an histrionic or dependent personality, a preoccupation with symptoms, and the development of a childlike, manipulative (sometimes seductive, sometimes hostile) relationship with the doctor. The other characteristic of these patients is a vague, allusive, and inconsistent history with 'unrelenting negativism'. The condition is often associated with other psychiatric conditions particularly depression, anxiety, and drug or alcohol abuse: there may be a family history of the condition.

Treatment is difficult and requires a psychiatrist who is prepared to take on such patients, develop a good relationship with them, and gradually teach them to become more psychologically aware of the meaning of their symptoms and their demands for recurrent investigations. It may not be easy to find such a psychiatrist: almost certainly some kind of bargain will need to be struck about the extent of physical investigation before the patient will accept that the symptoms are psychologically based. Even if you can find a co-operative psychiatrist the patient may not be willing to see such a paragon in which case a therapeutic alliance with a consenting general practitioner will be needed. Form frustes of somatization disorder are now considered to exist in which the very strict criteria described above do not occur but there is evidence that the condition is nevertheless present—DSM IV refers to *undifferentiated somatization disorder* for patients who do not meet the full diagnostic criteria. Care should be taken in making such a diagnosis—some physical and psychiatric disorders cause widespread somatic complaints (e.g. collagen disorders, metastatic malignancy, depression, and anxiety).

HYPOCHONDRIASIS

DSM IV defines this as a disorder where the patient is preoccupied with a fear of having a serious disease based on the patients misinterpretation of bodily sensations as evidence of physical disease. Appropriate physical evaluation must have failed to reveal any physical disorder and the belief should persist, despite reassurance, for at least six months although the belief is not delusional. Unlike somatization disorder the symptoms relate usually to only one bodily system. There are often compulsive or obsessional symptoms accompanying these beliefs as in the other somatoform disorders.

Some people with this syndrome will come the way of neurologists with some hypochondriacal belief related to neurological illness. It is important to avoid unnecessary diagnostic testing and to avoid over-aggressive medical or surgical treatment. The therapeutic aim is to help the patient tolerate and live with his/her symptoms rather than relieve them. Iatrogenic disease in this group of patients is common (and may actually reinforce the original symptoms). It is also important to remember that patients may eventually develop an organic disease and so they should not be denied access to medical care, but rather have access to a physician or a psychiatrist who is prepared to support them. Most of these patients will not see themselves as having a psychiatric problem and may refuse the services of a psychiatrist in which case a neurologist will have to hand them back with an explanation to their general practitioner. It is particularly important in this group of patients to exclude treatable psychiatric illness (such as an associated depression or even an incipient psychosis) and to be sure that one is not dealing with a hypochondriacal *delusion*. Such deluded patients *must* be seen by a psychiatrist and since they are suffering from a potentially life-threatening and potentially treatable psychiatric illness they can be persuaded to receive psychiatric care.

There are other rarer somatoform disorders such as 'body dysmorphic disorder' (with which the neurologist is unlikely to be concerned) and 'pain disorder'. This is defined as a patient who is preoccupied with a pain in one or more anatomical sites which has no organic background. Complaining must be grossly in excess of what would be expected (this is to some extent a value judgement but is usually obvious). Patients with pain disorder are particularly likely to become addicted or habituated to analgesics: pain can be a withdrawal symptom from physiological dependence on analgesics. Pain disorder is particularly common in compensation cases and therefore will often present in neurological practice or in headache clinics. Severe depressive illness is clearly part of the differential diagnosis. Treatment of pain disorder is often unsatisfactory although a combination of antidepressants and cognitive and behavioural therapy can be successful.

MALINGERING AND FACTITIOUS DISORDERS

Neither of these are common: they are separate disorders although often confused with each other. In malingering there is a voluntary and conscious production of symptoms (and sometimes signs) for gain (in order to avoid an unpleasant event like a court case or to obtain disability payments, drugs, etc.). Malingering, unless practised or polished, is usually easily detectable and is particularly likely to occur in a medicolegal context when there is a marked discrepancy between apparent distress and objective findings, and when there is poor co-operation with evaluation or treatment.

Factitious disorder is a simulated disease which does not appear to convey any advantage except assuming the sick role: the patient's motivation is often not understandable: external incentives, unlike in malingering, are absent (Kaplan *et al.* 1994). Most patients with this disorder appear driven to sustain their factitious illness by deception and lying often with considerable ingenuity. They will often inflict injury on themselves or take drugs to simulate the condition that they are pretending to have. Unless neurological symptoms present as a consequence of the self-harm that the patient has indulged in (like laxative abuse or self-induced vomiting) the commonest neurological factitious disorders are probably convulsions, pseudodementia, and recurrent self-induced hypoglycaemia causing neurological symptoms.

Treatment of factitious disorder is difficult and requires a team approach and clear knowledge in the physician's mind that there is a genuine factitious disorder present: prematurely accusing patients with puzzling symptoms that their disorder is factitious can backfire: physicians really must have positive evidence before confronting the patient (who will often just leave). Psychiatric treatment of factitious disorder is probably of no avail. Malingering will usually respond to removing the reinforcement which is keeping the condition going.

In all the somatoform disorders, a united approach with the psychiatrist being part of the team (rather than somebody called in from outside to remove the nuisance) will make management easier. Psychological disorder, those who have it *and* those who treat it, is often (wrongly) stigmatized in our society: do not reinforce stigma. Every patient with neurological disorder should have a psychological as well as a physical assessment (just as patients presenting with psychological disorder need a physical assessment). If a psychiatrist 'misses' a physical disorder presenting as a psychological one there is much criticism: the reverse does not seem to attract the same disgrace!

OTHER PSYCHIATRIC DISORDERS THAT CAN BE MISTAKEN FOR NEUROLOGICAL DISEASE

AFFECTIVE DISORDER

Affective disorder particularly depression (occasionally hypomania) complicates and exists side by side with many neurological disorders or their treatment (e.g. steroid psychoses). Because depression so often presents with somatic symptoms it is often mistaken for neurological disorder. A significant proportion of patients with apparent dementia, if followed over time, turn out to be have been suffering from a pseudodementia related to depression. Headache is also a very common symptom in depressive illness. Hypochondriacal delusions occur in depression and may be misinterpreted as a physical illness: many people who are depressed misinterpret ordinary aches, pains and twinges (that all of us have, but most of us pay no attention to) and therefore may report them to doctors: some of these will have a neurological flavour to them. It is important in assessing patients with neurological symptoms that depression is actively looked for as well. It has been suggested that the use of a depression rating scale or screening instrument would be useful in a neurological outpatients.

Since many neurological illnesses are life-threatening or cause actual or threatened loss of function, depression is often a *result* of neurological illness and it is sometimes difficult to tell which came first. Depression needs careful assessment (including suicidal intention) and a careful treatment plan. Do not just throw antidepressants at it and do not be seduced into unnecessarily prescribing the new serotonin re-uptake inhibitors: their side-effects of agitation, sleeplessness, and nausea are particularly common in neurological patients. Cognitive therapy and psychological support are as necessary as medication. Rehabilitation of patients with neurological illness is almost impossible if they remain depressed. Do seek the experience of your psychiatric colleagues.

ANXIETY

Anxiety pervades neurological practice (partly because so many neurological conditions are in themselves anxiety-provoking) and enters widely into the differential diagnosis of many neurological symptoms, particularly attack disorder, tremor, headache, dizziness, and unsteadiness. Chronic hyperventilation and acute on chronic hyperventilation produces many quasi-neurological symptoms and signs including muscle spasms and parathesiae (which, confusingly, maybe unilateral), and eventual collapse. Because anxiety so often mimics neurological disorder and is so often an understandable reaction to it, it is well worthwhile seeking the opinion of a psychiatric colleague as to whether or not the patient's anxiety is pathological and whether it needs treatment. Treatment should be by counselling, behavioural, and cognitive therapy: the use of tranquillizers or hypnotics should be studiously avoided.

A variant of anxiety is post-traumatic stress disorder: a characteristic emotional reaction following a threatening episode in the patient's life which consists of chronic hyper-vigilance, rumination about the event, sleeplessness, nightmares, and vivid flashbacks of the event. The importance to neurologists of this syndrome is that if there has been a head injury as well, the symptoms of a treatable psychiatric disorder may be mistaken for the long-term effects of concussion. Some non-epileptic attacks are also related to post-traumatic stress disorder.

ALCOHOL ABUSE

Since 3–5% of the population have problem-drinking, alcohol-related problems are going to present to the neurologist as well as to the psychiatrist and must enter into the differential diagnosis of many conditions. Many people with drinking problems have somatic complaints, particularly headache: alcohol has its own well-known effects on the central nervous system including peripheral neuropathy, cerebellar damage, and specific memory problems. Psychiatric experience would suggest that a careful drinking history should be taken from every patient undergoing neurological investigation. Consumption of over 40 units a week of alcohol will almost always be associated with a drink-related problem either physical or psychological. It is important to recognize the patient who is **binge drinking**, which can be equally damaging, although calculation of his/her weekly alcohol intake may be spuriously low.

PSYCHOTIC ILLNESS

It is unlikely that a fully fledged psychotic illness will be mistaken for anything else but psychotic people who retain insight are often well aware that their psychotic ideas or experiences are not normal and will conceal them. Particularly in the early stages of a psychotic illness somatic symptoms of all kinds are common, including neurological ones, and their delusional nature may not be initially recognized. The 'made movements' of schizophrenia have, on occasions, been mistaken for dystonias or other movement disorders.

MYALGIC ENCEPHALOPATHY AND FATIQUE SYNDROMES

This is an area of controversy in which neurologists and psychiatrists should seek to co-operate rather than disagree. There are, of course, several types of fatique syndrome and there are probably a small number of patients in whom different physical aetiologies can be discovered and effectively treated. But even if there is a physical cause for a fatique syndrome, psychological factors are bound to be operating as well to perpetuate and reinforce it: in most of the fatique syndromes psychological factors are predominant even though their presence is often hotly contested by the patient. This denial occurs because patients, like neurologists, tend to feel that psychological or emotional disorder is somehow shameful (whereas a psychiatrist tends to see it as part and parcel of human experience). This is particularly found in the myalgic encephalopathy (ME) syndrome. It may well be that we will eventually discover that the ME syndrome is triggered off by some immune response to a virus illness; many patients with ME do have a characteristic start to their illness of fever, malaise, and swollen glands.

Thereafter, however, it is likely that the chronic symptoms of this illness are an abnormal emotional reaction to the illness rather than being related to an ongoing and undetectable virus infection. Most of the chronic symptoms of ME are those of anxiety and depression: the majority of ME symptoms will respond to psychological therapy (a graded exercise programme, cognitive and behavioural therapy and, in some patients, antidepressant therapy). The alternative to not trying psychological treatment for the ME syndrome is for the patient to lie in bed for many years waiting for a recovery. I indicate to patients that almost anything is better than that and suggest that the fatique that comes with ME leads to demoralization and that is something the patient can do something about. In many patients with ME the problem is that, in addition to the depression that so commonly follows a virus infection, the patient (or his/her parents) has become phobic of physical effort and this phobia needs treatment. Some sufferers from ME and other fatique syndromes resemble patients with the somatoform disorders very closely.

NON-EPILEPTIC ATTACK DISORDER (PSEUDOSEIZURES)

I want to bring this section of the chapter to a close by considering the common and often difficult problem of non-epileptic seizures because the topic illustrates the complexities of diagnosis and management of psychological disorders which are mistaken for neurological conditions. I am going to use the term 'non-epileptic seizure' as the more commonly used term pseudoseizure is pejorative and inaccurate and merely portrays common medical attitudes to people with psychological disorders. Non-epileptic seizures are still seizures even if they are not epileptic ones. The fact that physicians label them as pseudoseizures suggests that we have placed epilepsy on a kind of exalted pedestal so that anything which is not epilepsy is automatically condemned. The term also carries connotations of deceit, although the vast majority of people with non-epileptic seizures have acquired the erroneous label of epilepsy not through pretence but through the inaccurate diagnosis of a physician. Labelling any paroxysmal disturbance in behaviour, emotion, or thinking as 'epileptic' gives it a kind of quasi-dignity (in terms of implying that it has a respectable physical cause). Medicalizing behaviour means we can treat it with medication and, if it fails to respond to medication, the physician is not to be blamed. (Betts 1997b)

It is usually said that perhaps 20% of people who carry the equally pejorative label of being 'a known epileptic' do not actually have the condition but have some other kind of attack disorder which has been misdiagnosed as epilepsy. Although this is the usually quoted figure I suspect that the percentage of people who are labelled as having epilepsy but who do not actually have it nowadays is much less, as physicians become more aware of the need to make a correct diagnosis. A recent survey in general practice of patients with new onset seizures made it clear that diagnostic mistakes can still easily be made: when proper criteria were employed for diagnosing epilepsy in the surveyed patients in about 30% of patients even a year after the onset of seizures, the actual diagnosis was still unclear. I suspect that in real life (as opposed to the artificial life of a special survey) many of those patients would probably have been given the label of 'epilepsy' and treated as such. The diagnosis of epilepsy is not easy and is often made too hurriedly and on inadequate evidence (and sometimes in the face of common sense).

Case report 4

A young man of 20, an apprentice in motor manufacturing, had been fit and well all of his life. While having a bath with his girlfriend (with all that that implies) he got out of the bath to retrieve some object from a high shelf in the bathroom and felt hot, dizzy, and sick. His girlfriend went to his aid and inadvertently did the wrong thing by holding him upright. He became intensely pale and fell, striking his head on the bath as he went down and was, for a little while, unconscious with some mild generalized twitching and was probably incontinent. A couple of days later, still feeling rather shaken, he had another episode of feeling hot and dizzy, went pale and fell to the floor but recovered after about 30 seconds. These two attacks (obviously vasovagal) were labelled as 'epilepsy' and treated with phenytoin. As a result, this young man lost his driving licence, thereby broke his apprenticeship agreement and lost his job.

The problem with the diagnosis of epilepsy is that it relies on the account of the person who has had the attack (who may remember nothing or has only a distorted memory of what happened) and the account of a witness (who is often frightened and whose account of the attack is therefore distorted by fear) which is then given to a doctor who has to make a momentous decision on the basis of what he/she has heard and against a background of whatever he/she knows about epilepsy (which sadly is often not very much). Paroxysmal changes in behaviour, cognition, or emotion, so often mislabelled as 'epilepsy', actually have a very wide differential diagnosis. It is important, having made the correct decision that the patient's attack is a non-epileptic one, to then spend time and trouble assessing what kind of non-epileptic attack it is: just to label non-epileptic attacks as 'pseudoseizures' without making further differentiation is to fail the patient. Table 19.3 illustrates some of the possible causes of non-epileptic attacks.

In my experience about 5% of non-epileptic attacks are due to some other kind of organic disorder which has been mislabelled as epilepsy, of which syncope must be by far the commonest. The majority of non-epileptic attacks are emotionally or psychologically based.

Emotional syncope (although not well described in the literature) is common as are panic attacks with hyperventilation. These attacks can resemble epilepsy quite closely if one just listens to the description and has not actually seen the attack, as the patient will describe an often sudden rising feeling of fear accompanied by tingling of the hands followed by stiffening of the fingers (sometimes just on the one side) with an eventual loss of consciousness, cessation of breathing, and sometimes a slight cyanotic tinge. Cutting-off behaviour, *the swoon* (closing the eyes and sinking to the floor) is a not uncommon response to stress and may be a specific part of a post-traumatic stress disorder (PTSD), particularly in women who have previously been sexually abused. Some women with chronic PTSD relating to abuse have flashbacks of the experience to which they show a convulsive response the so-called *abreactive attack*. I have known men have similar attacks related to previous combat experience (Betts & Duffy 1993).

Conversion disorder occasionally presents as an attack disorder although in our culture this is not very common. Usually, what is being unconsciously imitated is the patient's ideas of what an epileptic attack is like rather than what it actually is. Occasionally, patients unconsciously imitate the witnessed attack of a friend or relative and therefore may be more accurate.

Deliberate conscious simulation of epilepsy in my experience is rare as is factitious epilepsy. There are some patients with the Munchhausen syndrome who do travel the country claiming to have epilepsy. I have experience of one patient with non-epileptic attacks who I have on separate videotapes from three different hospitals, using a different name. Another variety of factitious epilepsy is the Munchhausen-by-proxy syndrome in which one or both parents deliberately induce usually anoxic seizures in their children which are very

Table 19.3 Classification of non-epileptic seizure disorders

1. Convulsive
(a) *Physical*
   (i) convulsive syncope
   (ii) cardiac dysrhythmias (e.g. Stokes–Adams attacks)
   (iii) sudden cerebral ischaemia
   (iv) hypoglycaemia
   (v) paroxysmal dyskinesias
(b) *Psychogenic*
   (i) deliberate simulation (malingering)
   (ii) unconscious simulation
   (iii) Convulsive 'tantrum'
   (iv) convulsive 'abreaction'

2. Syncopal (collapse but no convulsion)
(a) *Physical*
   (i) syncope (including postual, cough, micturition, and stretching)
   (ii) drop attacks of the elderly (aetiology unknown)
   (iii) cardiac dysrhythmias
   (iv) aortic stenosis
   (v) atrial myxoma
   (vi) 'grey out'
   (vii) mitral valve prolapse
   (viii) basilar migraine
   (ix) cataplexy
   (x) narcolepsy
   (xi) transient ischaemic episodes
   (xii) colloid cyst of third ventricle
   (xiii) decerebrate attacks
   (xiv) akinetic mutism/coma vigile
(b) *Psychogenic*
   (i) emotional syncope
   (ii) hyperventilation (panic attack)
   (iii) breath holding (in children)
   (iv) 'swooning'

3. Partial and prolonged
(a) *Physical*
   (i) cataplexy
   (ii) transient ischaemic episode
   (iii) cortical Stroke
   (iv) transient global amnesia
(b) *Psychogenic*
   (i) catalepsy
   (ii) anxiety phenomena (e.g. depersonalization, derealization)
   (iii) fugue
   (iv) unusual tics
   (v) Gilles de la Tourette syndrome
   (vi) rare movement syndromes (e.g. jumping Frenchmen of Maine)
   (vii) episodic dyscontrol syndrome

4. Sleep attacks
(a) Hypnopompic/hypnogogic hallucinations
(b) Sleep paralysis
(c) Night terrors
(d) Nocturnal anxiety
(e) Sleep walking (and variants, including violence)
(f) REM sleep disorder
(g) Hypnogenic paroxysmal dystonia
(h) Multiple sleep myoclonus

difficult to detect. There is no treatment for the Munchhausen syndrome that can be offered by psychiatrists and certainly no treatment for the Munchhausen-by-proxy syndrome: if this turns out to be the cause of a child's seizures, the child must be removed from the offending parent permanently.

Some, but not all, patients with non-epileptic attacks, in addition to the attacks themselves, will have a psychiatric disorder (including personality disorder, depression, anxiety, post-traumatic stress disorder, conversion disorder, and somatization disorder). These will obviously need treatment in addition to any specific measures applied to the seizures themselves.

In general terms, the treatment of non-epileptic attacks is to recognize them, classify them, and to then try the appropriate treatment. Recognition is often difficult. It is possible to be 100% certain that one is dealing with epilepsy, but it is rarely possible to be 100% certain that an attack is non-epileptic. If one takes investigations to the extremes of corticoelectroencephalography or even depth electrode recording one can be more certain (but not completely, as various studies have shown that the distinguishing characteristics of epilepsy and non-epilepsy blur into each other). Partial seizures do not always show up on surface electroencephalogram (EEG) electrodes even if it is possible to record a patient's seizures electrographically (and attacks are often too infrequent to justify video-EEG monitoring or ambulatory recording). Even subdural or depth electrodes may miss some partial seizures. Intrusive and invasive EEG investigations cannot be justified unless at the end of the day (having shown that the seizure *is* epileptic), one is likely to offer the patient surgery. Somewhere in the investigatory chain one has to stop and use one's clinical judgement.

Another problem is that some episodic behaviour which looks 'psychiatric' and bizarre can actually be caused by a discharging epileptic focus particularly in the frontal lobes and sensorimotor cortex. The importance of frontal seizures has only recently been recognized. Frontal epileptic discharge, even when unilateral, can cause bilateral motor behaviour. Ictal EEG recording misses many frontal seizures and an erroneous diagnosis of non-epilepsy therefore is made.

A few years ago we were almost certainly over-diagnosing epilepsy but probably are now in a situation where we are over-diagnosing non-epileptic attacks. Certainly, a lot of the referrals I get from colleagues with a confident diagnosis of non-epilepsy eventually turn out to have frontal-based epilepsy. Attacks which are brief and stereotyped are more likely to be epileptic than not: most non-epileptic attacks, apart from syncope, are prolonged and also have their own behavioural characteristics which can be recognized.

In some patients it is impossible to be certain whether one is dealing with epilepsy or not: in these patients keeping an open mind is very important. I often say 'I am not sure whether this is epilepsy or not but we have gone just about as far as we can with drug treatment: why don't we try some psychological treatment and see if it helps?' The psychological treatment of non-epileptic attacks consists of trying to define accurately the type of non-epileptic attack the person has, managing any concurrent psychiatric illness such as depression, anxiety, or conversion disorder, and applying specific behavioural and cognitive remedies to the actual attacks themselves. This often will mean the patient keeping a diary for a while so that one can identify any precipitating thoughts, flashbacks or anxiety symptoms which precede an attack and then teaching the patient a behavioural or cognitive technique which can interrupt negative thinking or crescendo anxiety. It is necessary to prevent primary and secondary gain from occurring which means it is often very important to manage the attacks within the context of the family or the environment in which they are occurring. Family anxiety often reinforces the patient's anxiety about attacks and will have to be treated. Such a psychological approach cannot be hurried—there is no instant cure and neurologists and other physicians should not expect one nor imply to the patient that one will occur.

Non-epileptic attacks often respond well to operant conditioning which means positively reinforcing non-seizure behaviour and negatively reinforcing seizure behaviour. The longer the patient goes without a seizure by and large the more he/she is rewarded: seizure behaviour itself is ignored and studiously not reinforced. In the setting both of the family or a hospital ward this may be difficult but it is essential that this is done. When operant conditioning is successful seizure behaviour will often rise to a crescendo for a few days and then drop dramatically. With a combination of behavioural and cognitive therapy and exploration of underlying issues (such as previous sexual abuse) most non-epileptic seizures have a good prognosis although they may get better in hospital only to reappear when the patient returns home (often to the very family that caused them in the first place). Although community treatment of non-epileptic seizures is slower it is often more effective (Betts 1994).

There are two particular problems non-epileptic attacks present to neurologists. The first is that the necessary confrontation with the patient that the attacks are non-epileptic should be handled in a tactful, sensitive way and not seen as an exercise in rejection. The idea that the attacks are non-epileptic should be put across in a positive way without immediate dismissal from the ward or the outpatients with the threat of being sent to a psychiatrist. Most psychiatrists are not skilled in managing non-epileptic attacks and will probably send the patient back after a month or two with a note saying 'Are you sure this is not epilepsy?' A smooth transition to a service that can cope with non-epileptic attacks is therefore needed. Since the diagnosis may still be open to question a way back into medical assessment should also be guaranteed. Some people have both epileptic and non-epileptic attacks. I personally manage non-epileptic seizures in the same clinic that I manage epilepsy and do not make any kind of pejorative distinction between them. This is probably easier for me because I treat a lot of patients with actual epilepsy behaviourally so the kind of treatment we offer patients with

non-epileptic seizures does not seem all that different from patients who actually do have epilepsy.

The second problem is that, being medically trained, neurologists sometimes want instant results in terms of managing non-epileptic attacks and this is often not possible. A proportion of people confronted properly about the non-epileptic nature of their attacks do actually just seem to stop having them. Most people with non-epileptic attacks will go on having them for a while as psychological and behavioural treatment takes some time, and these patients do need careful assessment: a lot of teamwork and patience may be needed before these attacks actually do come under control. The problem both for the neurologist and for the psychiatrist who is treating these attacks is that non-epilepsy seizure patients do tend to turn up elsewhere (in casualty or some other hospital). At which point a lot of patient work in terms of gradual reduction of anticonvulsant medication and behavioural treatment can be totally destroyed by some new and often inexperienced doctor placing the patient back on to anticonvulsant medication or interrupting treatment plans. We need to train junior medical staff and nurses to evaluate critically every patient who comes into hospital with a diagnosis of epilepsy.

PRIMARY NEUROLOGICAL DISORDER PRESENTING AS A PSYCHIATRIC DISORDER

Psychiatrists often feel out on a limb in dealing with patients whose psychiatric presentation is a little odd or whose condition is not responding to the usual treatment and often wonder whether perhaps there is some organic disease of the brain that is accounting for their patients' symptoms. 'Am I missing something physical?'—this is a real worry for the psychiatrist. There is no doubt that some neurological disorders can present psychiatrically. Huntington's disease may initially present as a psychiatric problem (personality disorder or depression) as can Pick's disease or Creutzfeld–Jakob disease. Some cerebral tumours, which disorganize a particular part of the brain, may present psychiatrically (sometimes with conversion symptoms, sometimes with an apparent depression or anxiety state—indeed tumours of the corpus callosum are well recognized for producing an anxiety state as their initial symptom). Under certain circumstances epileptic seizures may be misdiagnosed as related to psychiatric disorder or patients with frontal meningiomas may languish in mental hospitals for many years before the diagnosis is finally made. Just as every patient who has a neurological disorder needs a psychiatric assessment, so any patient with an apparent psychiatric illness needs a good physical assessment.

It is hoped that neurologists will be sympathetic to the requests of their psychiatric colleagues for neurological assessment in their patients when they have some diagnostic doubt about the cause of the patient's psychiatric syndrome. In my experience, however puzzling the patient's psychiatric symptoms are, there is unlikely to be a neurological disorder present unless there is some positive sign that it is (i.e. the pathological behaviour is really paroxysmal, episodic, and stereotyped; there are symptoms to suggest raised intracranial pressure is present; there is some degree of cognitive impairment alongside the patient's psychological symptoms.) Just asking for a computerized tomography (CT) or magnetic resonance imaging (MRI) scan on a patient whose psychosis is not behaving in the normal way is unlikely to be helpful: unless the psychosis is accompanied by organic mental symptoms or signs there is little likelihood that a lesion will be present. In Case Report 2 (p. 299), for instance, although the psychiatric picture was very typical of a conversion disorder with selective mutism, there was a physical sign present which indicated that there was probably something amiss in the brain.

PSYCHIATRIC SYMPTOMS OCCURRING AS A RESULT OF NEUROLOGICAL DISEASE

Since so much neurological illness is unpleasant, potentially lethal, and often treated by mind-altering drugs it is obvious that many patients with neurological disease will also have significant psychiatric disability as well. Unfortunately, this can go unnoticed or be disregarded but is something that does need treating or supporting for the purely practical reasons that sometimes the symptoms of grief or anxiety can be mistaken for the neurological condition that is being treated; or significant psychiatric disability will make rehabilitation difficult and impose further disability on the patient and on the patient's family. In Huntington's chorea, for instance, after it has been diagnosed, little can be done neurologically but good psychological support, judicious use of antidepressants, and behaviour modification and anxiety reduction may do a lot to keep the patient at home for longer and reduce the degree of suffering and disability and the burden on the family.

I have been recently very much impressed with the need for patients with cerebral tumours to have some kind of psychological support available. Patients who have had a cerebral tumour operated on and treated with radio- or chemotherapy may well be seeing the original neurologist, the original neurosurgeon, and a neuro-oncologist—sometimes in different hospitals, all with different teams—as well as receiving support from the general practitioner. Unfortunately, cerebral tumours often produce quite marked behavioural changes, so not only is the patient slowly dying at home but he/she may well have become difficult to live with, perhaps very obsessional, or overtly aggressive, and perhaps have a severe dysmnesic syndrome as well. The normal support services for those who are dying or who are undergoing chemotherapy (such as hospices and MacMillan Nurses) are often unable to cope with or advise about behavioural changes: psychiatric support and advice in these circumstances may be very useful, particularly liaising with and supporting the other agencies that are treating the patient.

PSYCHOLOGICAL DISORDER WORSENING OR EXACERBATING NEUROLOGICAL DISORDER (PSYCHOSOMATIC DISORDER)

Although the term 'psychosomatic' is perhaps going out of psychiatric parlance I think it still has a function to describe those conditions where emotional factors (such as stress or anxiety) precipitate or exacerbate neurological or physical disorder. This has already been touched on in a previous section but there are some neurological conditions where this particularly applies.

There is one neurological disorder, in particular, where the concept of a psychosomatic causation is particularly applicable and this is epilepsy. Although everybody would agree that epilepsy is basically a physical disorder relating to disturbances and alterations in transmitter and receptor functioning this dysfunction can be very much affected by other influences in the brain some of which are psychological. Lockard's model of the epileptic process consists of type 1 neurones de-afferentiated, chronically irritable, and continually firing, surrounded by type 2 neurones which are normal but which can be influenced by the type 1 neurones. This model is appealing and based on some scientific evidence. She further showed that type 2 neurones' propensity to respond to the chronic stimulation of the type 1 neurone (and therefore propagate seizure discharge) was very much dependent on the state of arousal in the type 2 neurones (Lockard 1980). Different levels of arousal in these neurones could inhibit recruitment into the epileptic process or aid recruitment: changing levels of arousal in these neurones altered seizure propagation. Even in those animal species where epilepsy appears to carry some biological advantage, strong inhibitory mechanisms also exist: both excitatory and inhibitory mechanisms may be to some extent under conscious control—or at least will be arousal-mediated and arousal can be brought under conscious control.

A psychological approach to reflex epilepsies makes obvious sense. Although the commonest type of reflex epilepsy (photosensitive epilepsy) is probably physiologically mediated most of the other reflex epilepsies (which include reading epilepsy, startle-induced epilepsy, voice-induced epilepsy, language-induced epilepsy, music-induced epilepsy, touch-induced epilepsy, hot or cold water immersion epilepsy, taste-induced epilepsy, sexual stimulation-induced epilepsy, and calculation-and thinking-induced epilepsy) often respond better to behavioural management (which includes mass practice, distraction techniques, and desensitization) than to anticonvulsants. Many reflex epilepsies are remarkably specific (e.g. the sight of a closed safety pin will not induce a seizure while the sight of an open safety pin will). Often, if one digs deep enough—and this often happens during a behavioural treatment regime—it becomes apparent that the triggering reflex has a psychological meaning for the patient.

It has been estimated that about 30% of people with epilepsy develop for themselves some kind of countermeasure that they employ to try to abort or modify a seizure. Often, they do not tell their medical adviser about this in case they are thought to be stupid or that they do not have genuine seizures. Sometimes, the mechanisms they use (countermeasures) can, with help and further exploration, be refined and improved. Most involve either a counterstimulus (such as clenching the hand when a Jacksonian seizure starts in that hand) or shifting concentration or attention, or by trying to relax very quickly. Most of these techniques therefore probably work by altering arousal and it may be helpful to explore, with a patient, whether increasing or decreasing arousal is better as a countermeasure.

In any patient with chronic epilepsy it is worth enquiring if they have developed any control mechanisms and if so what they are (or if there is any situation that they have learned to avoid because they know it will bring on a seizure). It is also useful to enquire tactfully whether under certain circumstances the patient can actually induce a seizure and if so how he/she does it. Not all seizures are unpleasant and some children seem to actively enjoy having them. Learning how a seizure can be provoked may be the key to learning how to control it.

One of the problems in using a countermeasure is that often if the seizure is starting and the patient is responding to an aura and they are already a little confused they may find concentration on the countermeasure difficult. I have found it useful to teach patients a method of using an olfactory stimulus (using a pleasant aromatherapy oil) to trigger off a conditioned arousal response (usually one of relaxation, occasionally one of increased arousal). This is done using a simple auto-hypnotic technique. Any patient who uses a countermeasure needs to practise it assiduously and needs support and encouragement until they have perfected the technique. One of the problems of using behavioural methods for treating seizures is that if they are successful and the seizures go away the patient often then forgets to practise. My experience is that they may need to go on practising the technique, even if they are not having seizures, for some years after seizures have been controlled. The techniques can also be used if the patient can recognize some environmental or internal cue which is likely to trigger off the seizure. There is no doubt that some patients can learn to recognize particular states of mind (e.g. sadness, anger) that make them particularly vulnerable to having a seizure. Many people with epilepsy recognize that stress may profoundly influence the frequency of their seizures (and indeed may have been the original precipitant). If a patient tells me that her first seizure occurred during her A-level exams, or following a termination of pregnancy, or on the first day of a new job I regard that as significant in suggesting that there is a stress factor in the patient's seizures which will often have to be treated if full seizure control is to be achieved. There is good scientific evidence (both in the field and in the laboratory) that there is a definite relationship between stress, emotional arousal, and frequency of seizures in some patients. Usually, stress increases seizure frequency although occasionally low arousal and relaxation may actually induce seizures. It would seem that there is an optimal level of arousal at which an individual is the least likely to have a seizure: helping the patient to find that level of arousal is useful. Patients who are stressed or anxious are likely to be hyperventilating (although they usually cannot recognize this) may indulge in alcohol, have poor sleep, and become poorly compliant with their medication. All these factors may also increase seizure frequency.

Thus, for many people with epilepsy stress management should be an important part of their treatment package. In patients who have difficult to control epilepsy I think it is often the more acceptable alternative than piling on yet more anticonvulsant medication. Stress management involves teaching breathing control, intense relaxation exercises, and cognitive therapy and is actually very similar to the techniques used in treating non-epileptic seizures and can be as effective. The following three case reports illustrate how behavioural methods are used in treating epilepsy.

Case report 5

An 18-year-old girl had had several complex partial seizures a month since the age of 12 despite taking all the usual anticonvulsants. EEG confirmed a right temporal focus for the seizures, though MRI was normal. Almost all her seizures seemed to occur when she heard music for more than a few minutes. They started with a simple partial seizure (a rising feeling of anxiety and an uncomfortable epigastric feeling), followed by unconsciousness. It is difficult to protect people from hearing music in our society: she was anyway a classical pianist and enjoyed listening to music. She was treated with a cue-controlled arousal manipulation technique using a relaxing aromatherapy oil and auto-hypnosis coupled with massed practise of specific pieces of music which were particularly likely to induce seizures. Persistent practise of these two techniques led to the complete cessation of her seizures: she is now seizure-free and can listen to music without having a seizure.

Music had been playing at the time of her first seizure and it was assumed that there was an association between this fact and her reflex epileptic response to music. However, as the treatment process continued it was discovered that at the time of her first seizure, in addition to music playing, she had overheard her parents quarrelling and it was felt likely that she had learned to associate the music with this unhappy event (since her parents subsequently separated with much unhappiness). The heightened arousal that the reawakening of the memory of this traumatic incident caused when music played was sufficient to induce her seizures.

Case report 6

This patient had right-sided motor epilepsy due a small atrophic lesion in her left hemisphere. She would have warning of the seizure by a hot tingling feeling of her right hand followed by the usual spasms of a Jacksonian seizure which would occasionally secondarily generalize. She could control progression of the seizure by clenching her right hand very hard but as soon as she relaxed her hand the seizure would continue (so, although she could delay the onset of a seizure, until she was in a position where she was unobserved, she had not got full control). Conventional anticonvulsant medication had not helped and she was being assessed for a subpial resection. During the assessment she was taught an auto-hypnotic technique to lighten and relax her right arm (rather than clench it) as soon as a seizure warning appeared. She was able to master this technique easily and found that if she was able to lighten her right arm the seizure would stop and not return and she has been seizure-free for over two years: she did not have a resection.

Case report 7

A 27-year-old nurse had juvenile myoclonic epilepsy. This came under good control with sodium valproate (although she had excess weight gain) but she would still continue to have three of four tonic clonic seizures a year. Most of her seizures occurred in the early morning although occasionally they would occur at other times of the day. On analysing her seizure diary over a period of time it became clear that the tonic clonic seizures in the daytime were always preceded by increasing levels of anxiety usually related to a rather stormy relationship with a young man. Her early morning seizures were always preceded by a poor night's sleep.

A cognitive and behavioural programme was therefore instituted to teach her to use both behavioural and cognitive cues in order to recognize when she was becoming anxious (which she was able to do), and she then had combined cognitive and behavioural therapy aimed at anxiety reduction and stopping of negative thinking leading to a further increase in anxiety. She used an auto-hypnotic cue-controlled arousal manipulation technique using a pleasant aroma whenever she felt particularly anxious or on going to bed if she had had a stressful day and was therefore likely to sleep poorly.

She has been seizure-free since using this technique. It was recognized, as the treatment went on, that a lot of her problem was related to anxiety cues increasing her fear of having another seizure: once she had developed a technique that she felt would control the seizures she lost her fear of them.

For many patients, the biggest handicap of epilepsy is loss of control and therefore any technique that leads patients to believe that they are getting some personal control over their epilepsy is likely to reduce anxiety. These techniques obviously are time-consuming and labour-intensive and cannot be used in a routine way, but are sufficiently impressive in their results to suggest that many patients with chronic epilepsy should be assessed for using some kind of technique like this. Similar techniques will work even in patients with brain damage or impaired intellect.

The success of behavioural techniques in epilepsy reinforces the view that to some extent epilepsy is a psychosomatic condition and, although a brain disorder, is powerfully influenced by the mind that is contained within that brain. One of the slogans used in my clinic is: 'Epilepsy affects the way we think, feel, and behave, but the way we think, feel, and behave can also affect the epilepsy'. Other neurological conditions, particularly movement disorders (but even such conditions as multiple sclerosis) are profoundly influenced by the patients' state of mind. Understanding that state of mind and learning how to help an individual manipulate it may have far-reaching effects on the neurological condition itself.

CONCLUSION

I have tried to show that psychiatry and neurology are inextricably interlinked. Just as a good knowledge of neurology is essential for anybody who practises psychiatry, so anybody who practises neurology must have some knowledge of the concepts and treatment skills of the psychiatrist. Being able to practise psychological skills in a medical or neurological setting actually increases job satisfaction, and difficult, emotional, or despair-inducing patients become a challenge to these therapeutic skills rather than a burden to the clinician.

REFERENCES

(APA) American Psychiatric Association (1994). *Diagnostic and statistical of mental disorders* (4th Edition). APA. Washington D.C.

Betts, T. (1994). Management of psychogenic seizures. In Wolf, P. (ed) *Epileptic seizures and syndromes.* Wiley, Chichester, U.K. pp. 649–56

Betts, T (1997a). Conversion disorders. In Engel, J. & Pedley, T. (eds.) *Epilepsy: a comprehensive textbook.* Lippincott Raven, New York pp. 2757–66

Betts, T. (1997b). Psychiatric aspects of non-epileptic seizures. In Engel, J & Pedley, T. (eds.), *Epilepsy: a comprehensive textbook.* Lippincott Raven, New York. pp. 2101–16

Betts, T. & Duffy, N. (1983). Non epileptic attack disorder (pseudoseizures) and sexual abuse: a review. In Gram, L. Johannessen, S., Osterman, P. and Silampaa, M. (eds.) *Pseudoepileptic seizures.* Wrightson Biomedical, Petersfield, U.K. pp. 55–65

Kaplan, H. Sadock, B. and Grebb, J. (1994). Factitious disorders. In Kaplan, H. & Sadock, B. (Eds.) *Synopsis of psychiatry.* (7th Edition). Williams & Wilkins, Baltimore, MD. pp. 632–7

Lockard, J. (1980). A primate model of clinical epilepsy: mechanisms of action through quantification of therapeutic effects. In Lockard, J. and Ward, A. (eds.) *Epilepsy: a window to brain mechanisms.* Raven Press, New York. pp. 11–49

FURTHER READING

The following books elaborate on the themes developed in this chapter and are worth consulting.

Betts, T. (1998). *Epilepsy, psychiatry and learning difficulty.* Martin Dunitz, London.

Betts, T. & Kenwood, C. (1992). *Practical Psychiatry.* Oxford University Press, Oxford.

Cassam, M. (1991). *Massachusetts General Hospital Handbook of General Hospital Psychiatry.* (3rd Edition). Mosby Year Book, St. Louis.

Feldman, M. & Ford, C. (1994). *Patient or Pretender.* Wiley, New York.

Mersky, H. (1995). *The analysis of hysteria: understanding conversion and dissociation.* (2nd Edition). Gaskell Academic, London.

Micale, M. (1995). *Approaching hysteria: disease and its interpretation.* Princeton University Press, Princeton, N.J.

DEFINITIONS

The World Health Organization system of classification of the consequences disease, *The international classification of impairments, disabilities and handicaps* (ICIDH) provides a model for thinking about the outcome of disease (1,2). The definitions found in this model are sometimes lengthy and over-inclusive but are valuable in conceptualizing what rehabilitation involves. They also help focus the mind on what one is trying to achieve in a rehabilitation setting. There are four components to the classification: pathology, impairment, disability, and handicap.

The first stage of classification is to identify the *pathology*, that, is the damage or abnormal processes occurring within an organ or organ system inside the body.

Clearly, in order to rehabilitate effectively an individual one has to be sure that all possible measures have been taken to stop or reverse the disease process and that one has an idea of the likely natural history of the condition. Accurate knowledge of the pathology will answer these questions. For example, there is a clear distinction in the way patients are handled in a rehabilitation service if their disease is progressive (e.g. multiple sclerosis), rather than monophasic (e.g. traumatic brain injury). Although this seems blatantly obvious it is not uncommon to find immense effort being expended on trying to achieve the impossible. It is also one of the reasons why rehabilitation cannot be totally demedicalized. The physician in the rehabilitation team has a vital role in ensuring that colleagues are properly briefed about the nature of the pathology.

The ICIDH definition of *impairment* is:

. . . Any loss or abnormality of psychological, physiological or anatomical structure or function.

In other words it is the immediate consequence of pathology as perceived by the individual. Neurological practice is geared to spotting impairments in order to make deductions about underlying pathology from them. In the same way neurologists often think about treatment at no more than the impairment level.

Disability in ICIDH is defined as:

. . . any restriction or lack (resulting from an impairment) of ability to perform an activity within the range considered normal for a human being.

Put more simply, disability is the personal nuisance caused by pathology. Examples of common disabilities include: slow walking, inability to climb stairs, needing help to eat.

Handicap is difficult to define and measure in absolute terms. It refers to the social consequences of pathology and so is determined by the patient's own roles and interactions. It is the freedom the patient has lost due to the pathology. ICIDH defines it as:

. . . a disadvantage for a given individual, resulting from an impairment or a disability that limits or prevents the fulfilment of a role that is normal for that individual.

For example, a mild hemiparesis in a professional musician will produce vastly more handicap than in a retired person with limited leisure pursuits.

Out of these concepts a definition of *rehabilitation* emerges. In the ICIDH scheme it is described as follows:

Rehabilitation is a problem-solving and educational process aimed at reducing the disability and handicap experienced by someone as a result of a disease, always within the limitations imposed both by the available resources and by the underlying disease.

Wade (3) has simplified the definition with respect to neuro-rehabilitation to the phrase 'management of neurological disability'. It is this focus on disability (as defined above) that distinguishes neuro-rehabilitation techniques from other neurological treatment modalities.

MECHANISMS OF RECOVERY FROM NEUROLOGICAL INJURY

Although our knowledge of the process of recovery from neurological injury is limited there is enough evidence to suggest that active mechanisms to correct impairment exist. It is important to be aware of these since rehabilitation strategies need to aim to work with these processes at the appropriate time. There is also a need to reverse the traditional dogma that neurological injury is irreversible and irredeemable. Although Cajal's thesis (4) that axonal growth and neuronal differentiation do not occur in the adult central nervous system still stands, mercifully, there are other means of recovery. Awareness of these recovery processes should help staff avoid from the trap of therapeutic nihilism which leads to the sorry spectacle of a disabled person managed suboptimally in an institutional setting.

Recovery processes have been usefully classified by the time from the insult that they are thought to be most active (5). These are summarized in Table 20.1

Considerable energy has been spent on optimizing the control of reversible factors in the first few hours and days post-insult (e.g. in head injury and stroke) However, all too often the importance of these in determining long-term recovery is overlooked (e.g. in head injury) (6,7). The effect of steroids in acute spinal injury is a good example of how acute 'damage limitation' can lead to significant functional gains subsequently (8).

In the days and weeks following neurological injury resetting of receptor sensitivities and neurotransmitter production rates could lead to functional improvements. Animal experiments seem to show that initial falls in neurotransmitter levels following lesion of a specific pathway can be made good within a few weeks (9,10). Likewise, the up-sensitization in basal ganglia dopamine receptors that occur in Parkinson's disease shows that alterations in receptor numbers and behaviours can have important functional results. Although there is no evidence that neuritic sprouting is functionally useful in humans its occurrence in animal models is well documented and seems to develop in phase with functional recovery (11).

In the weeks and months following injury, dramatic recovery is often seen despite the presence of extensive lesions (12). One explanation for this phenomenon is that control of one side of the body can be exerted bilaterally in the brain. Recovery of function in young patients following surgical hemispherectomy certainly suggested this might be the case. More recently, positron emission tomography (PET) studies in stroke patients who have made a good recovery clearly show recruitment of ipsilateral neurones with movements of the recovered limb (13). This is limited evidence that vicarious functioning occurs in humans (i.e. that previously uninvolved pathways can change their functional specificity to do the work of damaged neurones.

Table 20.1 Recovery mechanisms in neurological injury

Time post-insult	Recovery mechanism
Early (hours/days)	*Reversal of:*
	Hypoxia
	Oedema
	Hypotension
	Raised intracranial pressure
Medium term (days/weeks)	Receptor up-sensitization and down-regulation
	Adjustment of levels of neurotransmitters
	Neuritic sprouting
Long term (months/years)	Vicarious functioning
	Functional substitution

Functional substitution refers to the circumventing of an impairment by use of an alternative strategy. This may or may not involve the use of orthoses or prostheses. For example, the patient with an hemianopia learns to look excessively to the effected side with head-turning to overcome the limitation of visual field.

TIME COURSE OF RECOVERY AND PROGNOSTICATION

In the planning and execution of a rehabilitation programme it is important to take into account what is known of the natural history of recovery for particular conditions. Clearly, there is a huge variation in outcomes for any one neurological insult. The result will depend not only on the nature of the impairment but on the nature of the underlying pathology; the presence of other antecedent medical problems; the degree of carer support; the reaction of the individual to the problem; availability of suitable housing; funding issues as well as the treatment given. Prognostication is therefore a difficult business and there are no 'golden rules'. For certain conditions, useful studies have been completed to assess the time course of recovery and the period when the rate of recovery slows or a "plateau of disability" is reached. In stroke, for example, about half of all recovery from disability occurs in the first month and continues until about six months post-stroke. Thereafter, significant improvement is unlikely (14). This is most well established for activities of daily living but also applies to aphasia (15), arm function (16), and gait (17). An important exception is subarachnoid haemorrhage, where recovery may be more protracted and delayed, especially in young people. After spinal injury it is generally agreed that the level of injury and its grade cannot be precisely defined until six weeks after the insult (assuming there is no instability). Functional recovery may continue for as long as five months, however, particularly in cervical cord lesions (18,19).

Recovery from traumatic brain injury has been the subject of intense study. If patients are assessed on the Glasgow Outcome Scale as severely or moderately disabled at six months, less than 10% will be in a better category at one year post-injury (20). This is, of course, extremely valuable in providing a rule of thumb for planning rehabilitation and counselling patients and relatives. It has to be remembered that later recovery does occur, however, particularly in very severe brain injury. This may continue for three to four years or longer, although it is debatable whether major changes in functional outcome result (21).

DOES REHABILITATION WORK?

When one compares the dismal outcome of spinal injury earlier this century (22) and the complication rate seen in traumatic brain injury only thirty years ago (23), with the outcomes seen at present there can be little doubt that systematized, supportive care in a rehabilitation setting is beneficial. There is less compelling evidence that goal-directed, co-ordinated, team-based, client-centred programmes result in better functional outcomes, but this is probably the case for spinal cord injury (24), head injury (25), and stroke (26). There is an urgent need for objective assessment of the efficacy of a host of rehabilitation procedures; without this, there is a very real risk that resources will be reallocated when it is realized that many of the 'rehabilitation emperors have no clothes' (27).

THERAPIES AND THERAPEUTIC PROBLEMS IN NEURO-REHABILITATION

SPEECH THERAPY AND COMMUNICATION AIDS

Regrettably, many physicians complete their medical training without any formal instruction on the role and skills of speech therapists. Although a full discussion of the theory and practice of speech therapy is beyond the scope of this chapter, the practising neurologist should be aware of the contribution that speech therapists can make in the management of dysarthria and aphasia and the use of communication aids.

Dysarthria

Most patients with dysarthria would benefit from speech therapy (28). The speech therapist is able, first, to make a full assessment either descriptively or using a formal scale, for example, the Frenchay Dysarthria Assessment (29) or the Test of Intelligibility for Dysarthria (30) (these are both standardized). Following the assessment, the therapist may opt to work on intact aspects of speech to facilitate intelligibility or work on impaired functions to promote restoration. Therapy for dysarthria usually addresses, first, respiration then phonation, resonance, and then the development of facial movements and articulation. The therapist also tries to ensure that these skills are generalized to social settings other than the treatment room. The therapist guides the patient into new strategies that may alter quality but improve intelligibility (e.g. using a slower speaking rate or abnormal phrasing) (28). Changes in posture, training in non-verbal behaviour, and use of prostheses may also be recommended. For example, the patient with a palatal palsy may be unable to phonate bilabial consonants adequately but the situation may be much improved by a palatal lift prosthesis which can be produced with the help of an orthodontist.

Aphasia

There is extensive debate as to whether speech therapy for aphasia is efficacious. A recent meta-analysis of forty five studies between 1946 and 1988 concluded that the verdict on efficacy of treatment must remain open (31). But there is certainly enough evidence to suggest that attention to aphasia

seems to be more beneficial than none and that intensive treatment is associated with greater effect (32). In the last decade, application of a cognitive neuropsychological approach has been advocated to permit more accurate delineation of the impairment (33). Whether this will be of value in a non-research setting is unknown. More usually, functional communication therapy capitalizes on patients' ability to use gesture, intonation, and facial expression as well as residual language. There is some evidence that gestural communication is impaired less severely than verbal in some aphasic patients and in these circumstances the use of a sign system may be advocated. Amer-Ind (a system originally used by American Indians) is the most studied of these (34). The use of visual symbols to aid communication may also be advocated on the basis that aphasic clients can process artificial languages in advance of their natural language-processing skills (35). The Blissymbols system is one such aid—although there are many others. Studies with Blissymbols suggests that use of symbols is impaired in a similar way to primary language and so the usefulness of the system may vary from one patient to another (35).

Communication aids

These aids have developed dramatically over the last ten years in line with progress in electronic and computer technology. Several factors determine the timing of introducing an aid and the selection of the type of aid. It is desirable to use the simplest solution possible and introduce it only when it will increase independence. The temptation is often to go for technologically impressive equipment whose use is not sustainable because of complexity, user fatigue, or slow speed of processing. Communication aids are usually of three types:

(1) -direct select aids
(2) -scanning aids; and
(3) -encoding aids.

Direct select aids These are aids by which the patient selects letters or symbols directly. The simplest aid of this type is an alphabet chart and a pointer attached to a sufficiently mobile part of the body to indicate choices. Symbols may also be used to convey needs and preferences. The Stroke Association produces a helpful and widely applicable chart for this purpose. More elaborate keyboard aids with liquid crystal or paper display are available (e.g. the Litewriter SL1, Toby Churchill Ltd; the Canon Communicator, Canon plc.). A speech synthesizer may also be driven from the keyboard (e.g. Litewriter SL4, Toby Churchill Ltd.).

Scanning aids These aids offer the patient a selection of choices dynamically and the patient chooses the required letter or phrase as it is presented. This method would normally only be appropriate for severely speech impaired individuals with coexistent gross physical disability. The listener may run through a list of options and the patient signal the letter/word/phrase by an agreed yes/no signal. Certain aids may run through the list automatically and the patient can stop the cursor at the required letter or phrase (e.g. the Scanmaster). The speed of movement of the cursor may be adjusted to suit the patient's mental and physical speed of response.

Encoding aids These work by encoding words or phrases with numerical values or symbols that increase the speed of access to more complex language tasks. A basic aid of this sort would be a series of cards mounted in a pocket wallet which the patient can use to quickly communicate by. A similar aid that uses recorded speech phrases is the Parrot Communication aid. The patient can choose their most frequently used phrases which are entered into the aid and then numbered and accessed by pressing a single numerical key. More sophisticated computerized aids that encode words and phrases by topic or concept and then offer subdivisions are being developed (e.g. SAMM Communicator, Brunel University, Uxbridge, Middlesex, UK). This particular aid has the added benefit of digitally recorded speech so that the patient can use a real human voice of their choice.

Commissioning and accessing aids Whatever aid is used it is important that those with whom the patient intends to communicate with most are briefed as well. It has recently been shown that instructing carers to decrease their conversational control and provide more opportunities for the individual to use their communication aid leads to more reciprocal interaction and greater initiation by the patients (36). The patient equipment interface should be considered as part of the assessment before an aid is chosen. The help of a bioengineer should be sought early on if a special switchgear is likely to be needed. A full description of the range of available equipment is beyond the scope of this chapter but it is worth bearing in mind that novel solutions exist in this field. These include sound-activated switches, blow switches, switches activated by piezo-electric effect induced by skin creasing and wrinkling, blink switches, as well as a whole range of pressure switches which can be modified to suit whatever limited movement a patient may have in whatever body part (37).

NUTRITION AND DYSPHAGIA

The severely disabled person is at risk from malnutrition for a number of reasons. First, in the phase of acute injury or illness catabolism is increased. Coma and inanition may deprive the individual of the drive to seek nutrition. Incoordination, limb paresis, and bulbar palsy may all lead to slow and inadequate feeding. Patients and carers may loose patience and meals are therefore unfinished. Dysphagia with choking episodes may lead to a negative view of eating. Depression and drug therapy may also lead to impaired appetite. For all these reasons the clinician caring for a disabled person needs to be vigilant regarding their nutritional status. Patients with the above features should at least be weighed on a regular basis, and any deviation from ideal body mass index (BMI) should lead to referral to a dietician. Wheelchair-bound patients can be weighed on scales that take patient and chair to-

gether and these should be available in rehabilitation units or wheelchair clinics. The dietician should particularly advise regarding vitamin, trace element, and protein supplementation.

Assessment

Dysphagia may be easily overlooked in patients with extensive neurological disability (38), and may only come to the clinician's attention when there is an episode of life-threatening aspiration pneumonia, or weight loss has become marked. Where bulbar symptoms (e.g. diplopia, dysarthria, and ataxia) are present then some sort of assessment of swallowing should be made whether the patient complains of choking or not, bearing in mind that disturbance of sensation may lead to silent aspiration. Although formal clinical measures of dysphagia exist (39) their usefulness is limited and more usually a descriptive assessment by the speech therapist is more helpful. Using foods and fluids of different consistencies each phase of deglutition can be assessed. If the patient has a coexistent tracheostomy the use of weak methylene blue or blackcurrant juice in test fluids will help clarify if aspiration is occurring since this will appear in the tracheostomy secretions. Clinically impaired pharyngeal gag reflex and wet hoarseness after swallowing suggest laryngeal penetration has occurred (40). An effective cough capable of clearing the airway requires a forced vital capacity (FVC) of at least 1.5 litres (41). If FVC is found to be less than 2 litres with an impaired swallow then risk of aspiration should be considered sufficiently high for oral intake to be curtailed.

Depending on the initial findings more formal assessment of swallowing may be needed for example with milk nasendoscopy or formal videofluoroscopy and referral should be made for this purpose.

Conservative management

Where the risk of aspiration is deemed low conservative measures may be recommended to improve dysphagia. It may help to alter the consistency of food by either blending or liquidizing or adding thickeners to fluids and runny foods (e.g. Nestagel or Vitaquick). Crumbly, dry foods, and foods requiring chewing may also need to be avoided. Ensuring good upright posture with slight neck flexion to protect the airway may be helpful. Attention should be given to providing a calm environment free of distractions and feeding at a steady, unhurried pace. If fatigue when eating is marked, small frequent meals earlier in the day should be considered. Carers should be taught how to handle choking episodes with the Heimlich manoeuvre and by using nasopharyngeal suction if necessary.

Enteral nutrition

Where the risk of aspiration is deemed high and conservative measures have failed, enteral feeding should be initiated. Enteral feeding should also be initiated when coma or behavioural disturbance leads to impaired nutritional and fluid intake likely to last for more than five days. Initially, fine bore nasogastric feeding is the method of choice. Fine bore percutaneous endoscopic gastrostomy (PEG) has become increasingly available over the last few years and offers several advantages over nasogastric feeding, including improved patient comfort, lower incidence of accidental or deliberate displacement, improved cough and speech function, and improved cosmetic appearance.

Timing of placement of a PEG varies with the indication but clearly with progressive neuromuscular disease or severe brain injury the sooner the better. In stroke it is advisable to wait at least four weeks to assess spontaneous improvement but thereafter if dysphagia remains despite conservative measures PEG is recommended (42).

The procedure is relatively safe with a reported complication rate of 3% and mortality of 1% (43). Contraindications include previous abdominal surgery causing adhesions, bleeding diathesis, and severe respiratory failure. Complications include peritonitis, abdominal wall sepsis, bleeding, and transfixation of other viscera.

Late complications of PEG include gastric ulceration at the stoma site, gastric outlet obstruction if the tube migrates distally into the duodenum, leakage of gastric contents on to the abdominal wall, and fracture of the tube. In a patient with a PEG with recurrent vomiting a contrast X-ray study through the tube can be helpful in identifying outlet obstruction, gastric dilation, or oesophageal reflux. These last two problems may be helped by treatment with metoclopramide or cisapride. It is important to bear in mind that absorption of several drugs may be significantly impaired when given with enteral foods. These include phenytoin, carbamazepine, thioridazine, theophylline, iron and potassium chloride (44,45).

Airway protection

Where dysphagia is severe and aspiration risk is considered very high, steps should be taken to protect the airway; tracheostomy is indicated with placement of a cuffed tube in severe cases. In some instances, enteral feeding, curtailment of oral intake and reduction of oropharyngeal secretions using hyoscine patches (Scopoderm TTS) may suffice to prevent recurrent aspiration pneumonia. In cases of irreversible severe dysphagia, laryngeal diversion has been recommended although is rarely used (46). Cricopharyngomyotomy is only of limited use in a small number of patients found to have marked spasm of the cricopharyngeus muscle on videofluoroscopy. It is occasionally beneficial in motor neurone disease and chronic pseudobulbar palsy.

Sialorrhoea

Often, this is one of the most troublesome symptoms suffered by people with dysphagia. Treatment is far from perfect. Treatment with anticholinergic agents, particularly hyoscine as tablet or dermal patch preparation may offer some limited help. Amitriptyline may also usefully combine anticholinergic effects with sedative and antidepressant properties. Glycopyrrolate is used in the United States and has the advantages that it does not cross the blood–brain barrier and its cardiac effects are less than marked (47). Like all anticholinergics, however, it cannot be recommended where there is a history of glaucoma or urinary outflow obstruction.

More invasive methods, such as salivary duct ligation or diversion and salivary gland irradiation, may be of value when the prognosis is poor but cannot be recommended routinely.

ASSISTED VENTILATION

There has been increasing recognition of the virtue of ventilatory support for people with neurogenic respiratory failure over the last few years but Britain still lags behind Europe and the United States in provision of long-term care of this type (48). Agreed indications for long-term domiciliary ventilation include central sleep apnoea; respiratory or cardiorespiratory failure secondary to skeletal deformity; static or only slowly progressive neuromuscular disease; healed pulmonary tuberculosis treated surgically with resultant pulmonary restriction (48).

Ventilatory support for progressive neuromuscular disease is more controversial but non-invasive methods may be helpful in relieving symptoms without prolonging survival inappropriately. Patrick *et al.* (49) have developed a scale of respiratory dependence with treatment correlates. This is summarized in Table 20.2.

Table 20.2 Scale of respiratory dependence

Grade	Range of FVC (ml)	Spontaneous ventilation	Mechanical aid
0	>1500	Always	None
I	1000–1500	Always except during chest infections and minor illnesses	Non-invasive (e.g. iron lung)
II	700–1000*	Only while awake when using accessory muscles. Nocturnal mechanical assistance	Rocking bed, Cuirass shell, Tunnicliffe jacket, iron lung
III	300–700*	Part of day only. Nocturnal ventilation with some daytime support	Positive pressure mouthpiece, Nasal or mouthpiece IPPV, IPPV via tracheostomy
IV	<300	Nil. Continuous support IPPV via tracheostomy	Iron lung

* Augmented by glossopharyngeal breathing. FVC, forced vital capacity; IPPV, intermittent positive pressure ventilation. (From Patrick *et al.* 1990, See Ref. 49.)

Patients with neuromuscular weakness are particularly vulnerable to nocturnal hypoventilation since during rapid eye movement (REM) sleep respiration is dependent on the diaphragm alone. Recognition of this has led to the use of nocturnal ventilatory support as the initial level of intervention.

It is beyond the scope of this chapter to describe individual techniques in detail, however, the clinician should be aware that in addition to the traditional iron lung there are a number of other non-invasive means of support. The Cuirasse shell and Tunnicliffe jacket are smaller lightweight versions of the negative pressure 'iron lung-type' ventilators. The former is unsuitable for patients with marked deformity and those with impaired sensation (because of the risks of pressure sores). The 'rocking bed' is useful for those with primary diaphragmatic weakness. The development of safe intermittent positive pressure ventilation (IPPV) systems delivered via a mouthpiece or nasal mask has been a major advance (50), avoiding the need for tracheostomy. However, its usefulness is limited by the inability of patients to tolerate the mask in some cases.

Formal ventilation via cuffed tracheostomy tube is now used in only a very small number of patients. Providing such treatment in the community is extremely demanding, but compact, mobile systems are available (e.g. the Cavendish Wheelchair Ventilator). In high spinal injury (above C3) diaphragmatic pacing may be used to support ventilation (51). The complication rate is not inconsiderable, however, and early hopes for the technique have not been fulfilled.

ASSISTED VENTILATION: INDICATIONS FOR TRACHEOSTOMY

Indications for tracheostomy are as follows:

1. Inability to protect airway and prevent aspiration.
2. Need for continued artificial ventilatory support by positive pressure.
3. Inadequate clearance of respiratory secretions due to impaired cough.
4. Upper airway obstruction above the level of the trachea.

The first two require the use of a cuffed tube and appropriate measures must be taken to prevent tracheal necrosis secondary to cuff pressure.

PERSISTENT VEGETATIVE STATE

The term 'persistent vegetative state' (PVS) describes the outcome of severe brain damage in which a person shows no meaningful response to changes in his/her environment except at a reflex level, although they may have an established sleep/wake cycle (52). The term differentiates those in a coma who show no eye opening and no reflex response to stimulation. Criteria for the definition of the state are different in the United Kingdom compared to the United States. In Britain,

the British Medical Association recommends that the patient should be insentient for 12 months before the diagnosis is confirmed (53). Whilst the American Neurological Association suggest that the label be applied after one month, but not considered irreversible until after six months (54). The outcome of PVS has been studied by several groups. Where PVS lasts more than six months all those regaining consciousness are left severely disabled. Where PVS lasts less than six months one-third of those recovering will be left moderately disabled (55). The rate of recovery is also not predictable. In a study of 84 patients in PVS, 34 became aware by six months, a further 10 by one year, and a further 5 by three years (56). A further study of 43 patients in PVS admitted for rehabilitation found 11 of these regained awareness four months or more after suffering brain injury. Time to first response to command was four to twelve months and time to eye tracking was between four months and three years (57). Of these 11 recovering patients only 1 was unable to communicate when outcome was assessed at between 18 and 60 months. Assessment of the patient may include CT scanning, SPECT or PET, EEG recordings, and evoked potential studies. However, no single test provides conclusive prognostic information. Management of patients in PVS centres on good supportive care including enteral feeding, skin care, and provision of proper seating systems to permit upright posture which may increase arousal. (58). Coma stimulation programmes may be used consisting of visual, tactile, auditory, olfactory, and gustatory stimuli applied in a structured way. At least one randomized controlled trial has shown that such programmes may reduce the length of coma and increases the rate of emergence from it (59). Withdrawal of treatment is a controversial issue that requires consideration of any previously, expressed views of the patient, the views of significant others in the patient's life, and the body of current medical opinion. Careful re-investigation may be helpful before such decisions are made, particularly for the sake of significant others. At the present time in the United Kingdom decisions to withdraw treatment from a patient in PVS should be made in consultation with the Courts until such time as a body of experience and practice has built up which will obviate the need for a Court application in each case (53).

COGNITIVE REHABILITATION

This refers to training procedures aimed at improving cognitive impairments. The most common impairments treated are attention and concentration deficits, memory failure, neglect and perceptual problems, and problem solving and executive function deficits. As mentioned already, cognitive rehabilitation techniques are also used in the treatment of aphasia, although their role is still unclear.

The scientific basis for this type of therapy is only just starting to be established. The field has been beset by methodological problems in the published research and this leads to continued uncertainty about the validity of certain practices (60). There are few randomized controlled trials and even fewer replication studies. Single case experimental designs are frequently used with poor control and replication studies. Instrumentation for measuring outcomes and, in particular, generalization to everyday life functions is also poor. Understandably, there is considerable difficulty in performing blind assessment of treatment outcomes when involved training techniques have been used. There is some evidence that where unblinded assessments are made then observer bias favouring the treatment group occurs (61). In view of the labour-intensive and lengthy duration of interventions in cognitive rehabilitation there is an urgent need for further methodologically sound research.

Despite this there is a growing body of evidence that certain interventions are successful in reducing impairments. A full account is beyond the scope of this chapter but important examples are as follows:

1. ***Attention***: computer-administered training of selective and divided attention, attentional switching, and psychomotor speed has been shown to improve central information-processing speed and arithmetic performance in a blind, controlled trial (62). Behavioural training by goal setting has also been shown to increase attention span for reading in a single case design study (63).

2. ***Memory***: It is generally accepted that impairments of memory cannot be corrected by treatment, although use of memory aids and compensatory strategies may produce functional benefits (64). Membership of a 'memory group' may also be beneficial by reducing anxiety levels and increasing the use of memory aids (65). Limited evidence suggesting that specific tasks can be learned by severely amnesic persons has recently been published and although this is extremely encouraging it is still unclear how much functional benefit will accrue from this in everyday life (66).

3. ***Neglect and perceptual problems***: visual scanning training methods to overcome unilateral neglect may be effective in the experimental situation but generalization to other situations has not been unequivocally reported (67,68). Other techniques include limb activation on the effected side and feedback awareness training but again evidence of generalization out of the laboratory is lacking. An important advance in this field is the appreciation that inhibition of the intact hemisphere may augment function contralterally. Thus, patching of the right eye in a patient with a right hemisphere lesion has been shown to reduce the amount of left-sided neglect shown during testing (69).

Hemianopic alexia, due to post-geniculate field disorders, is amenable to treatment involving training in new eye movement strategies using computer screen text and feedback by trainers (70).

4. ***Problem solving and executive functions***: problem-solving training in a small study has shown positive effects in brain-injured persons. Replication of the work is, however, required (71).

In summary, certain impairments are amenable to cognitive rehabilitation but the scientific basis for the use of many techniques is lacking. Investment in this type of therapy should probably be concentrated in high quality controlled research studies with blinded assessments, before it is generally prescribed.

BEHAVIOURAL PROBLEMS IN NEUROLOGICAL DISEASE

Commonly, brain-injured individuals exhibit challenging or dysfunctional behaviour. Pharmacological control of difficult behaviour and prevention of self-harm and risk to others has to be tempered with the risk of inducing motor and sedative side-effects which impede recovery. Certain symptoms, however, are worth treating when it is clear that the patient's rehabilitation is being impeded by them. These include:

Agitation and aggression may usually be controlled by low doses of haloperidol or sulpiride. The latter is favoured in some units because of its supposed lower incidence of motor side-effects. Haloperidol is thought to be less sedating than other neuroleptics. Useful adjunctive drugs include clobazam as a night time dose or low dose clonazepam.

Temper and disinhibition are often improved with carbamazepine starting in low dose of 100 mg twice-daily but aiming to rise to a dose of 400 mg twice-daily or more if side-effects permit. Higher doses are usually required for optimal therapeutic effect.

Depression: difficult to diagnose in the cognitively impaired, but should be considered when performance and rapport regress. Fluoxetine and paroxetine are currently preferred because of their mildly stimulant effects and the relatively low risk of inducing epilepsy. It should be remembered, however, that none of these drugs is entirely safe in this respect. Mianserin and viloxasine may be useful alternatives.

Abulia and inanition can be serious obstacles to any form of rehabilitation. May respond to bromocriptine in relatively low dose. Side-effects of agitation and psychosis tend to be dose-related and may limit the usefulness of the drug. Fluoxetine may be a useful alternative in this case.

Schizophrenia: frank psychosis may evolve following brain injury, and require neuroleptic treatment. Sulpiride or haloperidol are the preferred agents in this case for reasons as outlined above.

Emotional lability: inappropriate laughter and crying are said to respond to serotonin re-uptake blocking drugs such as fluoxetine and paroxetine. Citalopram, which has a similar mode of action, has been shown to be effective in North America and is now licensed in the United Kingdom (72).

As a general rule, behavioural modification techniques are to be preferred to drugs when behaviour is generally dysfunctional in the absence of specific symptoms. Analysis of a patient's actions is often rewarding using, for example, an 'ABC Chart'. This simply requires all staff who witness challenging behaviour to note down the Antecedent events leading to the problem; the nature of the Behaviour and then the Consequences of the behaviour. A programme of modification therapy can then be agreed by the rehabilitation team, usually guided by a clinical psychologist. Reward for and reinforcement of dysfunctional behaviour can usually be prevented. More complex behavioural programmes may be required and these can usually only be conducted in specialized neuro-behavioural units.

URINARY CONTINENCE

Management of urinary incontinence has changed considerably in the last twenty years. Neuro-urology is now a recognized subspecialty and a number of new drugs and techniques are available. Although a full account is beyond the scope of this chapter and is more properly the domain of a specialist urologist, certain basic principles need to be considered in a neuro-rehabilitation setting (73).

The permanent indwelling urinary catheter should only be considered as a solution for incontinence as a last resort, particularly in the young. Sepsis, urolithiasis, urethral stricture, catheter hypospadias, bladder neck irritation, obstruction, and bypassing are all recognized complications. Patients find catheters aesthetically displeasing particularly with respect to sexual function. Many complications only become apparent over a lengthy period of time and the clinician may overlook the cumulative morbidity that occurs. The decision to place an indwelling catheter is often made too lightly and too quickly.

Alternative solutions depend on the nature of the underlying bladder dysfunction. The nature of this is not always predictable from the primary diagnosis. This is particularly true for multifocal neurological diseases such as multiple sclerosis and neurofibromatosis. Urodynamic studies have an important role in determining diagnosis and treatment. They can usually help distinguish between a number of possibilities including: primary detrusor instability, detrusor/sphincter dyssynergia, neuropathic bladder with overflow, non-compliant small volume bladder, bladder neck obstruction, and mechanical outflow obstruction.

Such studies initially involve measurement of urine flow rate with spontaneous voiding and measurement of residual volume. A filling catheter and pressure transducer are then passed per urethra and a pressure transducer per rectum to measure intra-abdominal pressure. The bladder is then filled to capacity and note is made of baseline bladder stability and the volumes at which reflex bladder contractions occur. Pressures generated during voiding both within the bladder and at the external urinary sphincter are also recorded. Following this, the nature of the bladder dysfunction should become clear.

The aim of management is to obtain continence with bladder emptying leaving no appreciable residual volume. This should be achieved without the generation of sustained high back-pressures on the kidneys. How this is achieved in a particular case will be determined by the clinical history and examination and the urodynamic studies. Possible strategies include:

1. Reduction of bladder instability by anticholinergic drugs (e.g. oxybutinin, flavoxate).
2. Reduction of external sphincter spasm using alpha adrenergic blockade (e.g. indoramin).
3. Augmentation of bladder emptying using cholinergic agents (e.g. carbachol).
4. Establishment of reflex bladder emptying in response to percussion of the bladder or lower abdominal pressure (usually only appropriate in neurogenic bladder of spinally injured persons).
5. Use of intermittent self-catheterization (ISC) to ensure complete voiding in neuropathic bladder or neurogenic bladder with external sphincter spasm.
6. Use of nocturnal desmopressin (DDAVP) (either nasal spray or tablets) to prevent nocturnal enuresis. DDAVP is licensed for this purpose in patients with multiple sclerosis but may well be useful in patients with other forms of neurological dysfunction.
7. Establishment of external urinary drainage by condom sheath in men. It is vital to select the correct size appliance and observe carefully to prevent local skin complications.
8. Bladder neck resection to relieve external sphincter and outflow tract obstruction.

Other techniques under development include mechanical sphincters, electrical control of bladder function via sacral root stimulators (74), and use of intravesical capsaicin (75).

Whatever techniques are employed it is extremely important that patients are carefully followed up. Chronic retention with obstructive uropathy may be precipitated by antispasmodics. Long-term monitoring of bladder function with measurement of residual volumes and screening for hydronephrosis should be considered in patients who are using methods other than permanent catheterization. The importance of this is illustrated by the many patients with spina bifida who have required renal transplantation or chronic dialysis because of undiagnosed and untreated chronic obstructive uropathy.

The other major advance in the management of urinary continence over the last few years has been the emergence of specialist nurse practitioners acting as continence advisers. In addition to providing appropriate community follow-up for all the techniques described they can support patients and their families with advice on simple physical aids when other techniques have failed or are inappropriate.

PHYSIOTHERAPY

Although doctors widely recommend physiotherapy, detailed knowledge of the techniques used and the theoretical basis of these is rare. Physiotherapy has undergone a number of major changes over the last thirty years and methods of treatment are vastly different to those used previously. Prior to this, physiotherapy was dominated by an approach which focused on maximizing function in unaffected body parts with little regard for the dysfunctional muscles. There was widespread use of orthoses, walking aids, and rails to compensate for the impairments. This has been replaced by techniques which work towards more natural patterns of movement and posture. These newer techniques aim to minimize unwanted reflex hypertonicity and maximize motor relearning in the effected limbs, and increase the patients awareness of the limb's function.

There are several systems of physiotherapy which seek to use this concept. The most well-known methods are those described by Bobath. These were developed empirically largely from observations on children with cerebral palsy (76). Other methods are also used including the motor relearning programme (77), proprioceptive neuromuscular facilitation (78), and the approaches of Brunnstrom (79) and Rood (80).

There is a lack of adequate published data to determine the superiority of any one of these methods. There are very few clinical trials comparing these approaches to simple functional recovery programmes. The present evidence has to be regarded as inconclusive (81). More worryingly there is some evidence that the Bobath approach may actually result in longer inpatient stays without any measurable difference in outcome (82). Undoubtedly, the newer approaches are more sophisticated and time-consuming but what is not yet clear is whether they result in genuine long-term functional gains.

OTHER PHYSICAL THERAPIES

Heat may be applied to tissues superficially by packs or immersion in water or wax. Deeper structures may be warmed by use of therapeutic ultrasound or microwave or short wave diathermy. There is some animal evidence that connective tissues become more elastic with heat. In humans heat may result in a reduction in joint stiffness, pain, and swelling and the resulting hyperaemia may also be associated with accelerated wound healing. There may be concomitant reduction in associated muscle spasm. Recommendations for the use of these methods have been described (83,84) but treatment remains largely empirically based. There are sufficient published results however to support the continued use of these modalities (85,86) although much more research is required to clarify the most effective methods and their indications.

SPASTICITY AND CONTRACTURES

Hypertonicity in neurological injury is both a help and a hindrance in rehabilitation. The increase in tone is frequently essential in permitting weight bearing through an otherwise paretic leg. Excess tone, however, is associated with flexor or extensor spasms which may obstruct the re-establishment of gait, cause intense pain, and ultimately result in contracture formation.

In the assessment of tone it is important to bear in mind that it may fluctuate widely depending on a number of factors including fatigue, temperature, disease state, and the motor task being performed by the patient. Decisions about treatment should therefore always be made in conjunction with the physiotherapist and carers.

Initially, excess tone should be managed by physical measures such as correct positioning and physiotherapy techniques aimed at minimizing reflex hypertonicity. Careful search should be made for primary causes of hypertonicity, particularly in patients with impaired sensation. Ingrowing toe nails, anal fissure and abscess, decubitus ulcers, and bladder calculi are all recognized causes of worsening hypertonicity, particularly in spinal injury (87).

Once drug therapy for spasticity is deemed necessary then baclofen is usually the drug of first choice. Sedative side-effects may limit its usefulness but these are usually dose-related and patients usually develop tolerance if the dose is increased gradually. Paradoxical increase in tone and rarely epileptic seizures have been reported with the drug and vigilance for these problems is required. Dantrolene is an effective drug which has a synergistic effect with baclofen by virtue of its differing site of action. Hepatotoxic side-effects have been reported particularly in women on oestrogen therapy. Careful monitoring of the liver function tests when the drug is being started is therefore mandatory. Diazepam and is a useful adjunctive treatment particularly at night but concern over dependency and excess sedation limits its usefulness. Tizanidine is used in Europe but presently is only available on a named patient basis in the United Kingdom. The side-effect profile is similar to baclofen but because the mode of action is different patients unresponsive to baclofen may benefit from a trial of the drug.

For patients with specific focal problems with spasticity, local treatment may be worthwhile. This area has recently been helpfully reviewed (88). Peripheral nerve conduction blocks with phenol or ethanol may help correct plantar flexion deformity (medial popliteal nerve) or adductor spasm (obturator nerve). The effects may last for as long as 12 months and repeat injections may be given. These will ultimately lead to a permanent nerve lesion. Motor point blocks may also serve to control hypertonicity in specific muscle groups. Botulinum toxin may also be helpful in the treatment of deforming hypertonicity particularly in the upper limb. Also control of unwanted extensor plantar response by blockade of extensor hallucis longus has also been reported with botulinum (89). Whilst the toxin is convenient and does not require such precise localization the doses needed to obtain a satisfactory effect result in it being an extremely expensive option.

For severe, drug-resistant, generalized spasticity more invasive methods may be used. Intrathecal baclofen delivered by an implanted infusion pump is now standard treatment (90,91), although the complication rate, cost, and the need for continued high level community support render it a challenging therapeutic option. Very rarely in a patient with irreversible paraplegia intrathecal phenol may be considered to produce complete lower limb flaccidity (92,93). Potential hazards of this approach include neurogenic pain and worsening of skin condition due to more profound anaesthesia.

Contractures are best managed by prevention. Early treatment of spasticity should be accompanied by a regular programme of passive stretching and where necessary regular splintage. Care should be taken at all times to monitor pressure areas when using splints and normally they are applied intermittently during any 24-hour period. The splints should be refashioned serially at regular intervals every few weeks as correction progresses. When local tone seems to be leading to potential contracture formation then consideration should be given to measures such as botulinum toxin injection or local nerve blocks. In established contractures, surgical release may be indicated in order to achieve better posture for seating and handling. Adductor and hamstring tenotomies can often give useful benefit but it is important that post-operatively control of spasticity is optimized and attention paid to passive movements and splintage.

HETEROTOPIC OSSIFICATION

This phenomenon is a rare but important complication of brain and spinal injury and rarely stroke. The cause of the condition is not known but immobility, spasticity, and decubitus ulceration are the main risk factors. These seem to lead to the necessary conditions for the calcification of the proximal periarticular muscles. Minor trauma when mobilizing the spastic limb may be the initiating factor that then leads to the process of myositis ossificans. Recurrent trauma from mobilization then perpetuates the problem.

Clinically, the patient complains of pain around the affected joint particularly on attempted mobilization. The problem usually declares itself between one and four months post-trauma. A high index of suspicion is needed to make the diagnosis early. Frequently, the calcification is not apparent on plain X-rays and CT scanning of the painful area is required.

The mainstay of treatment is to restrict mobilization of the joint concerned so that it is not moved beyond the limits of pain. Treatment with a non-steroidal anti-inflammatory drug, such as indomethacin, is also to be recommended. Avoidance of mobilization flies in the face of the usual philosophy of the rehabilitation setting but insistence on this is essential. Mobilization may proceed when there is a remission of clinical symptoms and there is no CT evidence of progression. Rarely, treatment by surgical excision followed by local radiotherapy is required for cases that do not settle on conservative

treatment. Bony ankylosis is not uncommon and in these cases surgical excision is essential to restore functional posture and movement. There was a vogue for the use of diphosphonates for the treatment of this condition but wider experience with these agents has failed to confirm any benefit (94) and they do carry a considerable risk of pathological skeletal demineralization.

SKIN CARE: DECUBITUS ULCERS

One of the major advances in the treatment of spinal injuries was Guttman's description of methods to prevent decubitus ulceration (95). Since then there have been major developments in the field such that the evolution of pressure sores in disabled patients is now regarded as a preventable adverse event.

Risk factors for decubitus ulceration include: immobility, obesity, poor nutritional state, anaemia, incontinence, impaired skin sensation, and skeletal deformity (e.g. due to contractures). The Waterlow and Norton scores (96) are useful means of checking these and quantifying risk so as to guide management.

The foundations of prevention are, first, vigilance on the part of all staff managing the patient and, second, limitation of the time spent on any one weight-bearing area. Third, regular inspection of pressure areas by both patient and staff is essential particularly when new activities are being introduced into the patient's programme. The 'safe time' on any one pressure area will vary from patient to patient dependent on their own constellation of risk factors. Initially, very short periods should be permitted of 30 minutes or less and then these should be extended depending on the outcome of regular inspection.

When a patient has been identified as being at high risk then the use of specialized mattresses and beds can be extremely helpful (97) but is no substitute for good nursing care. Static phase mattresses of the modular foam type (e.g. Propad) or of the hollow fibre-filled quilted underlay type (e.g. Spenco) form the first level of specialized bedding. Low air loss mattresses, regarded as the next level of care, function by inflation of a compartmentalized hollow nylon sac perforated with small pores from which there is a continuous air leak. These are considerably more expensive and require constant power supply and regular maintenance. The constant flow of air helps dry the skin and reduce maceration. Patients at very high risk of ulceration may require an air wave mattress or an air fluidized bed. The former consists of a series of chambers that inflate and deflate serially so as to continuously redistribute weight bearing. The latter consists of a crystalline matrix through which air is pumped at pressure to transform it into a quasi fluid phase material which uniformly distributes weight over the entire body area in contact with the mattress.

For treatment of established pressure sores regular turning and use of a high performance mattress are essential.

Nutritional status should be reviewed and high protein intake ensured by use of supplements if necessary. Low haemoglobin should be corrected. If the wound is malodorous and sloughy antibiotics should be considered, particularly metronidazole to cover anaerobes. Consideration should be given to vitamin C and zinc supplements if dietary intake is poor (98). Necrotic tissue should be removed surgically and then the wound should be dressed with dextranomer (e.g. Debrisan) or hyaluronidase (e.g. Varidase) to chemically remove remaining debris. For clean, moist wounds alginate paste and pads (e.g. Kaltostat and Intrasite gel) are useful. For more infected-looking wounds, iodinated alginate paste may be helpful (e.g. Iodosorb).

Once the wound is superficial, clean, and granulating then occlusive dressings (e.g. Granuflex) are preferable to permeable absorbent dressings to encourage rapid epithelialization.

OTHER SKIN CONDITIONS

Facial seborrhoeic dermatitis is commonly seen in patients with stroke and severe head injury. It is unclear whether this is due to excess production of sebum, alteration in its quality, or inadequate skin cleansing. The organism *Pityrosporum ovale* is believed to be responsible (99). The condition responds well to ketoconazole and hydrocortisone cream (e.g. Daktacort) plus ketoconazole shampoo.

Tinea cruris and intertrigo are also commonly encountered in patients with chronic spasticity. Treatment with a compound antibacterial, antifungal, and weak steroid is usually helpful.

CONCLUSION

Space does not permit detailed coverage of other areas of importance in neuro-rehabilitation such as environmental control systems and special seating. As with all neuro-rehabilitation interventions, multi-disciplinary team work will ensure the best possible outcome in these areas. In the last two decades there has been massire expansion in our knowledge about and techniques of neuro-rehabilitation. The prospects for further progress in the next millenium are excellent.

REFERENCES

1. World Health Organization. *The international classification of impairments, disabilities and handicaps—a manual of classification relating to the consequences of disease.* Geneva, WHO, 1980.
2. Duckworth D. The need for a standaed terminology and classification of disablement. In Granger CV and Gresham GE (ed.). *Functional assessment in rehabilitation medicine.* Baltimore, William & Wilkins, 1984: 1–13.
3. Wade DT. *Measurement in neurological rehabilitation.* Oxford University Press, 1992: 11.
4. Cajal RYS. *Degeneration and regeneration of the nervous system.* London, Oxford University Press, 1928.
5. Whyte J. Mechanisms of recovery of function folowing CNS damage. In: Rosenthal M, Griffith ER, Bond MR, Miller JD (ed.). *Rehabilitation of the adult and child with traumatic brain injury.* Philadelphia, FA Davis, 1990: 79–88.
6. Waxman SG. Functional recovery in diseases of the nervous system. In Waxman SG (ed.). *Functional recovery in neurological disease. Advances in neurology,* Vol. 47. New York, Raven, 1988: 1–7.
7. Gentleman D, Jennett B. Audit of transfer of unconscious head injured patients to a neurosurgical unit. *Lancet* 1990; **335**: 330–4.
8. Bracken MB, Shepard MJ, Collins WF et al. A randomised controlled trial of methylprednisolone or naloxone in the treatment of acute spinal cord injury. *N Engl J Med* 1990; **322**: 1405–11.
9. Reis DJ, Gilad G, Pickel VM, Joh TH. Reversible changes in the activities and amounts of tyrosine hydroxylase in dopamine neurons of the substantia nigra in response to axonal injury as studied by immunochemical and immunocytochemical methods. *Brain Research* 1978; **144**: 325–42.
10. Reis DJ, Ross RA, Gilad G, Joh TH. Reaction of central catecholaminergic neurons to injury: model systems for studying the neurobiology of central regeneration and sprouting. In Cotman CW (ed.). *Neuronal plasticity.* New York Raven, 1978: 197–226.
11. Little JW, Halar E. Temporal course of motor recovery after Brown-Sequard spinal cord injuries. *Paraplegia* 1985; **23**: 39.
12. Smith DL, Akhtar AJ, Garroway WM. Motor function after stroke. *Age and Ageing* 1985; **14**: 46–8.
13. Chollet F, Dipiero V, Wise RJ et al. The functional anatomy of motor recovery after stroke in humans—a study with positron emission tomography. *Ann Neurol* 1991; **29**: 63–72.
14. Wade DT, Wood VA, Langton-Hewer R. Recovery after stroke—the first three months. *J Neurol Neurosurg Psych* 1985; **48**: 7–13.
15. Enderby PM, Wood VA, Wade DT, Langton-Hewer R. Aphasia after stroke: a detailed study of recovery in the first three months. *Int Rehab Med* 1986; **8**: 162–5.
16. Parker VM, Wade DT, Langton-Hewer R. Loss of arm function after stroke: measurement, frequency and recovery. *Int Rehab Med* 1986; **8**: 69–73.
17. Wade DT, Langton-Hewer R. Functional abilities after stroke: measurement, natural history and prognosis. *J Neurol Neurosurg Psych* 1987; **50**: 177–82.
18. Ditunno JF, Storer SL, Freed MM, Ahn JH. Motor recovery of the upper extremities in traumatic quadriplegia: a multicenter study. *Arch Phys Med Rehab* 1992; **73**: 431–6.
19. Mange KC, Marino RJ, Gregory PC, Herbison GJ, Ditunno JF. Course of motor recovery in the zone of partial preservation in spinal cord injury. *Arch Phys Med Rehab* 1992; **73**: 437–41.
20. Bond MR, Brooks DN. Understanding the process of recovery as a basis for the investigation of the rehabilitation of the brain injured. *Scand J Rehab Med* 1976; **8**: 127.
21. Powell GE, Wilson SL. Recovery curves for patients who have suffered very severe brain injury. *Clin Rehab* 1994; **8**: 54–69.
22. Thompson-Walker J. The treatment of the bladder in spinal injuries of war. *Proc Roy Soc Med* 1937; **30**: 1233–40.
23. Rusk HA, Block JM, Loman EW. Rehabilitation following traumatic brain damage. *Med Clin N America* 1969; **53**: 677–84.
24. Oakes DD, Wilmot CB, Hall KM, Scherk JP. Benefit of early admission to a comprehensive trauma centre for patients with a spinal cord injury. *Arch Phys Med Rehab* 1990; **71**: 637–43.
25. Cope DN, Hall KM. Head injury rehabilitation: benefits of early intervention. *Arch Phys Med Rehab* 1982; **63**: 433–7.
26. Lehmann JF, DeLateur BJ, Fowler RS et al. Stroke: does rehabilitation affect the outcome? *Arch Phys Med Rehab* 1975; **56**: 375–82.

27. Wade DT. Neurologic Rehabilitation. *Curr Opin Neurol Neurosurg* 1993; **6**: 753–5.

28. Enderby P. Dysarthria. In Greenwood R, Barnes MP, McMillan TM, Ward CD (ed.). *Neurological rehabilitation*. Edinburgh, Churchill Livingstone, 1993: 335–40.

29. Enderby P. *Frenchay dysarthria assessment*. San Diego, College Hill Press, 1983.

30. Yorkston KM, Beukelman DR. A clinician judged technique for quantifying dysarthric speech based in single word intelligibility. *J Commun Dis* 1980; **13**: 15–31.

31. Whurr R, Lorch MP, Nye C. A meta-analysis of studies carried out between 1946 and 1988 concerned with the efficacy of speech and language therapy treatment for aphasic patients. *Eur J Disorders Commun* 1992; **27**: 1–17.

32. Enderby P. Speech and language therapy for aphasia. *Curr Opin Neurol* 1993; **6**: 761–4.

33. Byng S, Jones E Cognitive neuropsychological approach to acquired language disorders. In Greenwood R, Barnes MP, McMillan TM, Ward CD (ed.). *Neurological rehabilitation*. Edinburgh, Churchill Livingstone, 1993: 343–53.

34. Skelly M. *Amerind gestural code based on universal American Indian hand talk*. New York, Elsevier North Holland, 1979.

35. Funnel E, Allport A. Symbolically speaking: communicating with Blissymbols in aphasia. *Aphasiology* 1989; **3**: 279–300.

36. Light J, Dattilo J, English J, Giltierrez L, Hartz J. Instructing facilitators to support the communication of people who use augmentative communication systems. *J Speech Hearing Res* 1992; **35**: 865–75.

37. Platts RGS, Fraser MH. Assistive technology in the rehabilitation of patients with high spinal cord lesions. *Paraplegia* 1993; **31**: 280–7.

38. Hughes C, Enderby PM, Langton-Hewer R. Dysphagia in multiple sclerosis: a study and discussion of its nature and impact. *Clin Rehab* 1994; **8**: 18–26.

39. Wiles CM. Neurogenic dysphagia. *J Neurol Neurosurg Psych* 1991; **54**: 1037–9.

40. Linden P, Siebens AA. Predicting pharyngeal penetration. *Arch Phys Med Rehab* 1983; **64**: 281–3.

41. Cumming G, Semple SJG. Management of ventilatory failure. In *Disorders of the respiratory system*. Oxford, Blackwell Scientific, 1973: 203.

42. Powell-Tuck J, van Someren N. Enterostomy feeding for patients with stroke and bulbar palsy. *J Roy Soc Med* 1992; **85**: 717–19.

43. Larson DE, Burton DD, Schroeder KW, DiMagno EP. Percutaneous endoscopic gastrostomy: indications, success, complications and mortality in 314 consecutive patients. *Gastroenterology* 1987; **93**: 48–52.

44. Holtz L, Milton J, Struek JK. Compatibility of medications with enteral feedings. *J Parenteral Enteral Nutrit* 1987; **11**: 183–6.

45. Altman E, Cutie AJ. Compatibility of enteral products with commonly employed drug additives. *Nutrit Supp Serv* 1984; **12**: 8–17.

46. Carter GT, Johnson ER, Borekat HW, Lieberman JS. Laryngeal diversion in the treatment of intractable aspiration in motor neuron disease. *Arch Phys Med Rehab* 1992; **73**: 680–2.

47. Kuncl RW, Clawson LL. Amyotrophic lateral sclerosis. In Johnson RT (ed.). *Current therapy in neurologic diseases*, Vol. 3. Philadelphia, BC Decker Inc, 1990: 294–5.

48. Branthwaite MA. Mechanical ventilation at home. *BMJ* 1989; **298**: 1409.

49. Patrick JA, Meyer-Whiting M, Reynolds F, Spencer GT. Perioperative care in restrictive respiratory disease. *Anaesthesia* 1990; **45**: 390–4.

50. Carroll N, Branthwaite MA. Intermittent positive pressure vent-

51. Moxham J, Potter D. Diaphragm pacing. *Thorax* 1988; **43**: 161.

52. Jennet B, Plum F. Persistent vegetative state after brain damage: a syndrome in search of a name. *Lancet* 1972; **i**: 734–7.

53. British Medical Association. *BMA guidelines on treatment decisions for patients in persistent vegetative state*. Supplementary Annual Report of the Council. London, BMJ Publishing Group, 1993: 3–4.

54. ANA Committee on Ethical Affairs. Persistent vegetative state: Report of the American Neurological Association on Ethical Affairs. *Ann Neurol* 1993; **33**: 386–90.

55. Berrol S. Evolution of the persistent vegetative state. *Head Trauma Rehabilitation* 1986; **1**: 7–13.

56. Levin HS, Saydjari C, Eisenberg HM, Foulkes M, Marshall LF, Ruff RM *et al.* Vegetative state after closed head injury: a traumatic coma data bank report. *Arch Neurol* 1991; **48**: 580–5.

57. Andrews K. Recovery of patients after four months or more in the persistent vegetative state. *BMJ* 1993; **306**: 1597–60.

58. Andrews K. Managing the persistent vegetative state. *BMJ* 1992; **305**: 486–7.

59. Mitchell S, Bradley VA, Welch JC, Britton PG. Coma arousal procedure: a therapeutic intervention in the treatment of head injury. *Brain Injury* 1990; **4**: 273–9.

60. Robertson IH. Cognitive rehabilitation in neurologic disease. *Curr Opin Neurol* 1993; **6**: 756–60.

61. Ottenbacher KJ, Jannell MS. The results of clinical trials in stroke rehabilitation research. *Arch Neurol* 1993; **50**: 37–44.

62. Gray JM Robertson IH, Pentland B, Anderson SI. Microcomputer based cognitive rehabilitation for brain damage: a randomised group controlled trial. *Neuropsychol Rehabil* 1992; **2**: 97–116.

63. Wilson C, Robertson IH. A home based intervention for attentional slips during reading following head injury: a single case study. *Neuropsychol Rehabil* 1992; **2**: 193–205.

64. Berg IJ, Koning-Haanstra M, Deelman BG. Long-term effects of memory rehabilitation: a controlled study. *Neuropsychol Rehabil* 1991; **1**: 97–112.

65. Evans JJ, Wilson BA. A memory group for individuals with brain injury. *Clin Rehabil* 1992; **6**: 75–81.

66. Glisky EL. Acquisition and transfer of declarative and procedural knowledge by memory-impaired patients: a computer data-entry task. *Neuropsychologica* 1992; **30**: 899–910.

67. Wagenaar RC, Van Wieringen PCW, Netelenbos JB, Meijer OG, Kuik DJ. The transfer of scanning training effects in visual inattention after stroke: five single case studies. *Disabil Rehabil* 1992; **14**: 51–60.

68. Pizzamiglio L, Antonucci G, Judica A, Montenero P, Razzano C, Zoccolotti P. Cognitive rehabilitation of the hemineglect disorder in chronic patients with unilateral right brain damage. *J Clin Exp Neuropsychol* 1992; **14**: 901–23.

69. Butter CM, Kirsch N. Combined and separate effects of eye patching and visual stimulation on unilateral neglect following stroke. *Arch Phys Med Rehabil* 1992; **73**: 1133–9.

70. Kerkhoff G, Münßinger U, Eberle-Strauss G, Stogerer E. Rehabilitation of hemianopic alexia in patients with post-geniculate visual field disorders. *Neuropsychol Rehabil* 1992; **2**: 21–42.

71. Von Cramon DY, Matthes-von Craymon G. Problem solving deficits in brain injured patients: a therapeutic approach. *Neuropsychol Rehabil* 1991; **1**: 45–64.

72. van Gijn J. Treating uncontrolled crying after stroke. *Lancet* 1993; **342**: 816–7.

73. Fowler CJ, Fowler CG. Neurogenic bladder dysfunction and its management. In Greenwood R, Barnes M, McMillan TM,

ilation by nasal mask: technique and applications. *Intensive Care Med* 1988; **14**: 115–17.

Ward CD (ed.). *Neurological rehabilitation*. Edinburgh, Churchill Livingstone, 1993: 269–78.

74. Madersbascher H, Fischer J. Sacral Anterior root stimulation: prerequisites and indications. *Neurourol Urodyn* 1993; **12**: 489–94.

75. Fowler CJ, Beck RO, Gerrard S, Betts CD, Fowler CG. Intravesical capsaicin for treatment of detrusor hyperreflexia. *J Neurol Neurosurg Psych* 1994; **57**: 169–73.

76. Bobath B. *Adult hemiplegia: evaluation and treatment* (3rd edn). London, Heinemann, 1990.

77. Carr JH, Shepherd RB. *A motor re-learning programme for stroke* (2nd edn). London, Heinemann, 1987.

78. Kabat H, Knott M. Proprioceptive facilitation therapy for paralysis. *Physiotherapy* 1954; **40**: 171–6.

79. Brunnstrom S. Walking preparation for adult patients with hemiplegia. *Physical Therapy* 1965; **45**: 17–32.

80. Goff B. Appropriate afferent stimulation. *Physiotherapy* 1969; **51**: 9–17.

81. Partridge C, Cornall C, Lynch M, Greenwood R. Physical therapies. In Greenwood R, Barnes MP, McMillan TM, Ward CD (ed.). *Neurological rehabilitation*. Edinburgh, Churchill Livingstone, 1993: 189–98.

82. Lord JP, Hall K. Neuromuscular re-education versus traditional programs for stroke rehabilitation. *Arch Phys Med Rehab* 1986; **67**: 88–91.

83. Kitchen SS, Partridge CJ. A review of therapeutic ultrasound. *Physiotherapy* 1990; **76**: 593–600.

84. Kitchen SS, Partridge CJ. Review of short wave diathermy. Continuous and pulsed patterns. *Physiotherapy* 1992; **78**: 243–52.

85. Nwuga VCB. Ultrasound in the treatment of low back pain resulting from prolapsed intervertebral disc. *Arch Phys Med Rehabil* 1983; **64**: 88–91.

86. Dyson M, Franks C, Suckling J. Stimulation of healing of varicose ulcers by ultrasound. *Ultrasonics* 1976; **14**: 232–6.

87. Illis LS. Spasticity I: Clinical aspects. In: Illi LS (ed.). *Spinal cord dysfunction*, (Vol. 2). Oxford University Press, 1992: 81–93.

88. Skeil DA, Barnes MP. The local treatment of spasticity. *Clin Rehab 1994*; **8**: 240–6.

89. Giladi N, Meer J, Honigman S. The use of botulinum toxin to treat "striatal" toes. *J Neurol Neurosurg Psych* 1994; **57**: 659.

90. Penn RD, Savoy SM, Corcos D, Latash M, Gottlieb G, Parke B *et al.* Intrathecal baclofen for severe spinal spasticity. *N Engl J Med* 1989; **320**: 1517–21.

91. Patterson V, Watt M, Byrnes D, Lee A. Management of severe spasticity with intrathecal baclofen delivered by a manually operated pump. *J Neurol Neurosurg Psych* 1994; **57**: 582–5.

92. Nathan PW. Intrathecal phenol to relieve spasticity in paraplegia. *Lancet* 1959; **ii**: 1099–102

93. Kelly RE, Gautier-Smith PC. Intrathecal phenol in the treatment of reflex spasms and spasticity. *Lancet* 1959; **ii**: 1102–5.

94. Thomas BJ, Amstutz HC. Prevention of heterotopic bone formation: experience with diphosphonates. *Hip* 1987 59–69.

95. Guttman L. *Spinal cord injuries. Comprehensive management and research*. Oxford, Blackwell Scientific, 1976.

96. Barratt E. A review of risk assessment methods. *Care, Science and Practice* 1988; **6**: 49–52.

97. Young JB. Aids to prevent pressure sores. *BMJ* 1990; **300**: 1002–4.

98. Dickerson JWT. Ascorbic acid, zinc and wound healing. *J Wound Care* 1993; **2**: 350–3.

99. Cowley NC, Farr PM, Shuster S. The permissive effect of sebum in seborrhoeic dermatitis: an explanation of the rash in neurological disorders. *Br J Dermatol* 1990; **122**: 71–6.

21 | *Respiratory and swallowing disorders*
C. M. Wiles

The function of respiration is the effective utilization of oxygen in energy production and excretion of resulting carbon dioxide by the tissues of the body. Neurological disorders impinge on this process primarily by interfering with the effectiveness of *breathing*, that is, the transfer of gases between the environment and the pulmonary circulation through the mechanical actions of the respiratory muscles on the thoracic cage. The major features of neurological disease as they pertain to breathing disorder are weakness of the muscle pump and of the muscles maintaining patency of the airway both of which, alone or in combination, may result in hypoxaemia and hypercarbia. Other contributory factors in neurological disease are disturbed control of breathing, abnormal cough, dysphagia, spinal and chest deformity, and abdominal problems. Apart from respiration, breathing has an essential role in phonation and articulation.

Swallowing may be defined as the act of transferring liquid and solid material from the mouth into the oesophagus. Component muscles of the mouth, pharynx, larynx, and thorax and their peripheral innervation must participate in three functionally discrete activities—swallowing, breathing, and speech. Clearly, the differential activation and patterning of the fifty or so paired muscle groups of mouth, pharynx, and larynx (excluding respiratory muscles) during willed or subconscious behaviours related to these three activities, while at the same time preserving airway protection, requires a complex hierarchical system of neural integration (see Figs 21.1 and 21.2). Ultimately, disordered swallowing (dysphagia) results in failure of adequate nutrition and hydration, recurrent penetration of the tracheobronchial tree (aspiration) by oropharyngeal contents, or escape of oral contents from the mouth externally (drooling) or into the nasopharynx.

Both swallowing and breathing disorder may be perceived as resulting in a graded series of functional problems. Impairment of function may occur without any overt clinical complaint (subclinical) although unnoticed compensatory behaviour (e.g. minor alteration of diet, alteration of head posture) may occur. As function worsens symptoms may develop (with more or less disability) but the patient is still able (subconsciously or consciously) to compensate to an extent and breathing or nutrition are maintained with adequate airway protection. Ultimately, compensatory mechanisms fail and, without intervention, respiratory failure, aspiration, or inadequate nutrition and fluid intake supervene. The degree of compensation that can be achieved in swallowing and breathing disorder is highly dependent on whether one or both are impaired. Dysphagia is less likely to cause major clinical problems in the presence of a normal larynx, respiratory muscle pump, and lungs (and hence normal cough). A very low vital capacity due to muscle disease is more likely to be tolerated if the swallowing mechanism and larynx are normal. For convenience, disorders of breathing and swallowing will be considered separately, but the functional interrelationship which springs from shared neuroanatomical pathways, muscles, and physical structures should always be considered in the individual patient.

CLINICAL ANATOMY AND PHYSIOLOGY

RESPIRATION

Inspiration and expiration (Roussos 1982)

Inspiration depends primarily on diaphragm (innervation C3-C5) contraction and descent: as the diaphragm contracts and flattens it displaces the abdominal contents downwards thus increasing the anteroposterior and lateral diameters of the abdomen. It tends also to elevate the lower ribs (thus expanding the lower rib cage) to an extent which depends on the compliance of the abdominal cavity. At the same time the external intercostal muscles (innervation T1-T12) contract and result in stiffening of the muscles of the chest wall and outward movement with an increase in the antero-posterior and lateral diameters of the upper chest. The sternomastoids (C2/3) and scalene muscles (C3-8) contribute to upper chest expansion in exercise or if other muscles are weak.

These muscular actions increase pleural negative pressure which draws air through the nose or mouth, oro- or nasopharynx, and into the larynx and bronchial tree. Air inflow through the nose is limited by the variable resistance of the anterior nares and a pressure gradient exists between the atmosphere and the nasopharynx and oropharynx which tends to collapse the upper airway on inspiration. This tendency is opposed by active contraction of muscles of the tongue (XII nerve) and oropharynx and larynx (X nerve) some of which thus have a patterned respiratory cycle to maintain airway patency. The volume of gas inspired for a given inspiratory pressure depends on the lung structure and its elastic recoil, and the size, shape, stability, and mechanical properties of the thoracic cage including the diaphragm. The spinal column, shoulder girdle, and ribs may be physically distorted (e.g. kyphoscoliosis) as a result of muscle weakness or imbalance particularly during the growth period causing restriction of lung volume: in addition, chronic muscle weakness with reduced rib movement is associated with reduced chest wall compliance and increased work of breathing. Finally, abdominal muscle stiffness or raised intra-abdominal pressure, by increasing load on a weakened diaphragm, may have a critical effect on inspiratory capacity particularly in the supine position (Goldman 1982).

Expiration is largely a function of passive elastic recoil of the lungs and chest wall during quiet breathing. More energetic or controlled expiration is achieved by the use of internal intercostal muscles (T1-T12), and abdominal muscles (T7-T12) which by reducing the lateral and anteroposterior diameter of the abdomen constrain the abdominal contents and push the diaphragm upwards. Other accessory expiratory muscles include those inserted into the shoulder girdle notably the clavicular head of pectoralis major (C5- 7), latissimus dorsi, and teres major (C5-C7) which can effectively compress the upper and lateral chest. Activation of these 'accessory' groups is normally most prominent during coughing when forcible expiration (initiated reflexely or volitionally) builds up pressure behind a closed glottis prior to explosive release. Deglutition is associated with a brief central apnoea which, in the majority of swallows, is preceded and followed by expiration (Selley *et al.* 1989a, b), thus refilling the pharynx with air from below and preventing aspiration of residues in the pyriform fossa or laryngeal aditus. Finally, controlled expiration also plays an essential role in the phonatory and articulatory aspects of speech.

Neural control (Berger et al. 1977; Loh 1986)

Alpha (α)-motor neurones for the respiratory muscles are in the cervical and thoracic anterior horns and for associated muscles related to airway patency in the pons and medulla (cranial nerves V, VII, IX–XII). Spinal integration of chest wall, muscle, and lung afferents plays an important role in the patterning of the breathing. The drive to α-motor neurones is *at least* dual in origin. First, rhythmic breathing activity and non-rhythmic breathing reflexes (e.g. cough, deglutition apnoea) are driven from centres in the medulla and pons. Second, non-rhythmic voluntary or behavioural breathing activity is activated via corticobulbar and corticospinal pathways while emotionally related breathing (e.g. in laughing or crying) may utilize other corticomedullary pathways (see fig. 21.1).

Neurones of the 'dorsal respiratory group' (DRG) in the nucleus of the tractus solitarius and the 'ventral respiratory group' (VRG) in, or closely adjacent to, the nucleus retroam-

bigualis, nucleus ambiguus, and nucleus retrofacialis establish respiratory rhythm modified by afferent impulses from the chest wall, respiratory muscles, chemoreceptors (e.g. carotid body), tracheobronchial, laryngeal, pharyngeal, and nasal receptors. These 'respiratory centres', and thus respiratory rate, depth and frequency, are modulated by hypoxia, mainly via afferents in the IX and X cranial nerve from the carotid bodies, and by changes in $P_{a}CO_2$ and pH via local medullary chemoreceptors. Efferent activity mainly passes in crossed pathways in the ventrolateral cervical spinal cord adjacent to the spinothalamic tracts (Nathan 1963). This pathway is predominantly active in response to metabolic stimuli and is dominant during quiet breathing and sleep. Reflex respiratory activity related to deglutition, vomiting, sighing, reflex coughing, hiccoughing, yawning, and some aspects of speech is integrated via these brainstem centres: the efferent pathways for such non-rhythmic respiratory activities may be selectively interrupted in the spinal cord.

By contrast, manoeuvres such as voluntary inspiratory or expiratory breath-holding, hyperventilation, or voluntary (as opposed to reflex) coughing, which are behaviourally rather than metabolically determined, activate the respiratory α-motor neurones via crossed corticobulbar and corticospinal pathways and thus pass in the ventral pons and pyramids of the medulla to the dorsolateral spinal cord. Individual case studies suggest that emotional activation of respiratory muscles, as in laughing or crying, may occur via cortical pathways distinct from the corticospinal tracts. Descending pathways from centres in the pons and the cerebral hemispheres can influence and override both the rhythmic and non-rhythmic generation of inspiratory and expiratory neuronal activity in the medulla.

Bilateral hemisphere disease may prolong apnoea after hyperventilation and is one factor in periodic (Cheyne–Stokes) ventilation. The latter condition is caused by instability of medullary control mechanisms caused by impaired descending neurogenic drives, drugs or sleep, and prolongation of 'lung-to-chemoreceptor' circulation time: the hyperpnoeic/ apnoeic cycle length is usually shorter (e.g. >40–50s) when the cause is primarily neurological. Central pontine injury rarely results in uninhibited hyperventilation and apneustic or gasping (prolonged inspiratory or expiratory pauses) breathing is associated with disconnection of the 'pneumotaxic' centre in the pons. Rapid respiratory myoclonus or 'diaphragmatic flutter' may occur sometimes with similar movements of eyes, tongue, pharynx, larynx, and palate in various disorders involving the olivary and dentate nuclei and connections. Medullary disease may result in breathing which is irregular in depth and/or rhythm (ataxia), hiccups, hypoventilation, or apnoea.

Respiratory failure

Conscious patients with neurological disease usually develop respiratory failure because of impaired ventilation due prim-

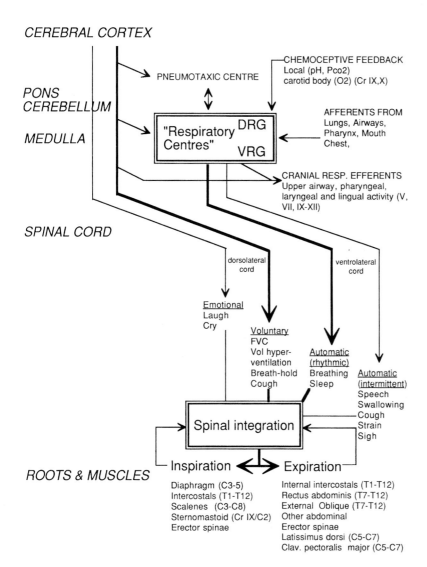

Fig. 21.1 Mechanisms in the *control of breathing.*

arily to weak muscles. Weak respiratory muscles cause a fall in total lung capacity with a rise in residual volume at the expense of either inspiratory or expiratory reserve capacity, or both. Peripheral airway collapse and atelectasis together with reduced chest wall and pulmonary compliance increase the work of breathing. Even with initially normal lungs peripheral collapse gives rise to ventilation–perfusion mismatch and increased physiological dead space which rises in relation to tidal volume. Pao_2 starts to decline largely because of shunting of unoxygenated blood through poorly ventilated lung bases and areas of peripheral collapse. Breathing frequency increases and so does the work of breathing. When respiratory muscle strength further declines to less than a third of normal, ventilation can become insufficient to prevent $Paco_2$ from rising.

Other factors contribute to hypoxia and hypoventilation even without primary lung disease. These include retained secretions due to poor cough, infection, or pulmonary oedema

all of which promote ventilation–perfusion mismatch. Associated kyphoscoliosis (low VC) or pharyngeal airway obstruction, laryngeal dysfunction (stridor or cord paresis) or recurrent aspiration may contribute. Sleep also plays an important role in potentially exacerbating the effects of respiratory muscle weakness and in emphasizing disorders of respiratory muscle control mechanisms.

Sleep

Because Pao_2 normally tends to fall and $Paco_2$ to rise slightly in sleep, particularly in rapid eye movement (REM) phases, any tendency to oxygen desaturation or hypoventilation may be exacerbated at night (Stradling and Phillipson 1986). Factors directly or indirectly associated with neurological disease contribute to disturbed gas exchange in sleep (see Table 21.1b) most notably the interaction of supine posture with diaphragm weakness (Newsom Davis *et al.* 1976), apnoeic episodes related to upper airway obstruction or vocal cord dysfunction (causing stridor) and, less often, disorders of central drive. Lack of or disturbed deep (phase III/IV) and REM sleep results in daytime symptoms which may thus be the presentation of nocturnal respiratory insufficiency. These include awaking unrefreshed perhaps with headache, poor concentration, daytime drowsiness, and 'nodding off', intellectual impairment, and affective disorder. In addition, nocturnal hypoxia may result in pulmonary and systemic hypertension, secondary polycythaemia, cardiac dysrhythmias (rarely sudden death), and less effective respiratory function in the day thought in part to be caused by 'fatigue' of residual respiratory muscles. Airway protection or assisted breathing during sleep alone can have dramatic day and night time benefits for such patients. How much of this benefit is due to improved sleep quality, to improved chest/lung compliance or to the resting of putatively fatigued respiratory muscles remains enigmatic.

Respiratory muscle strength

Information about respiratory muscle strength can be gained from measuring lung volumes, flow rates, or making pressure measurements. The forced vital capacity (FVC) gives information about both inspiratory and expiratory muscles but is also influenced by postural, pulmonary, and chest wall factors: however, these composite determinants make it a valuable measurement clinically. Weakness of the diaphragm cause an excessive fall in FVC on lying supine (>20%). FVC (a volitional corticospinal mediated event) may, however, be entirely normal in patients with disordered metabolic control of breathing. In contrast, FVC may be low in corticospinal tract disease while reflexely induced lung volumes (e.g. following airway irritation may be much higher). Thus interpretation of this measurement at the bedside must be tempered by knowledge of the neurological signs. Forced expiration is effort-dependent only in the upper quarter or so of the total lung capacity: at lower lung volumes dynamic airway compression during expiration limits flow which is determined more by the elastic recoil properties of the lungs and chest wall. Standard peak flow rates in expiration thus give little information about inspiratory capacity or inspiratory (or expiratory) muscle strength. Measurement of the peak pressure which can be obtained at the mouth with an open glottis on inspiration and expiration (maximum inspiratory and expiratory mouth occlusion pressures) and assessment of transdiaphragmatic pressure during a sniff or maximum inspiration with pressure balloons in the stomach and oesophagus give the most direct information about respiratory muscle strength (Green and Moxham 1985). The phrenic nerve and diaphragm can, to some extent, be objectively assessed using electric or magnetic stimulation and some attempts at cortical stimulation to assess central conduction time have been successful in man (Murphy *et al.* 1990; Hamnegard *et al.* 1996).

SWALLOWING (LOGEMANN 1988 B; DONNER *ET AL.* 1985)

Swallowing is needed not only for the effective transfer of food and fluid from the mouth into the oesophagus, but also for the clearance of saliva, expectorated material from the airways, secretions from the naso- or oropharynx, and vomit or regurgitated matter from lower down the digestive tract. In the absence of swallowing, material in the mouth can only escape by falling out of the mouth (drooling) or by gravity into the airway or oesophagus.

Preparation to swallow

The preparation of a bolus in the mouth (oral preparatory and oral phases) is an important preliminary to triggering of the swallowing reflex (deglutition). Thus the type of food, its consistency, temperature, taste, and the circumstances and posture in which it is eaten may help or hinder deglutition. Eating and drinking are social events as well as being essential for nutrition. The physical arrangements for eating, the company, and social interactions at meals are potentially problem areas for the individual with dysphagia: modification or restriction of the social role of eating due to slowness, clumsiness, or embarrassment may be an early compensatory mechanism in dysphagia but it is also a handicap and source of distress. Containment of food and liquid in the oral cavity and mastication of solid material to a suitable consistency will depend on the state of the dentition (if any), the ability to secrete adequate quantities of saliva, the organization and strength of chewing movements (temporomandibular joints and muscles of mastication), and of muscular control of the lips and cheeks (facial muscles). The muscles of the tongue play a crucial role in manipulating and positioning the bolus for deglutition and impaired speed and co-ordination of tongue movement is a major factor in neurogenic dysphagia. Cognitive, visual, somatic, gustatory, and olfactory sensory cues as well as emotional factors presumably play a role in patterning the appropriate deglutitive response to a particular bolus.

Deglutition

The oral phase of swallowing leads into triggering of deglutition. That deglutition may be triggered reflexly is clear since it occurs in decerebrate man. It is unclear whether patterned sensory stimuli around the pillars of the fauces or leakage of small amounts of material into the oropharynx are the primary stimulus. Receptors sensitive to taste, to water, to the speed of movement of material at the junction of oral cavity and pharynx, and the summation of such afferent input over a more or less wide area of the oropharynx appear to trigger, via sensory fibres in the V, VII, IX, and X cranial nerves, a series of events co-ordinated by neurones in the medulla. However, deglutition is under powerful voluntary/behavioural modulation and to what extent such descending influences trigger it under normal eating conditions is unclear: certainly, anxiety for example may effectively inhibit it.

The pharynx and larynx can be regarded as muscular tubes suspended from the base of the skull and the mandible through structures such as the hyoid bone, thyroid and cricoid cartilages and their suspensory muscles and ligaments which provide support, mobility, and assist patency. At the start of deglutition the hyoid is both elevated (by stylohyoid and digastric) and pulled anteriorly (mylohyoid and geniohyoid). The thyroid cartilage and laryngeal structures are lifted by muscle contraction from the hyoid (thyrohyoid), skull base and mandible: the laryngeal opening is tucked under the tongue base and tilted posteriorly while the epiglottis inverts by a combination of hyoid movement and contraction of the thyroepiglottic muscle to approximate the arytenoid cartilages. The soft palate abuts the posterior wall of the pharynx (Passavant's ridge) sealing off the nasopharynx. The tongue strips the bolus backwards along the hard palate and, acting as a piston, drives it into the oropharynx which may or may not still contain air. Breathing is inhibited in expiration and the aditus to the larynx is sealed by closure of the vocal cords, apposition of the false cords with ejection of air from the vestibule and epiglottic descent. The epiglottis helps to deflect food and liquid away from the laryngeal aditus through the lateral recesses of the pharynx (valleculae and pyriform fossae) which become opened up. The onward movement of the bolus is assisted by negative pressure in the closed hypopharynx (generated by upward, anterior laryngeal movement) and gravity. Laryngeal movement, bolus presentation, and neural inhibition trigger cricopharyngeal relaxation. The pharyngeal peristaltic wave (not the principal driving force for the bolus) sweeps the pharynx and its recesses clean after the bolus has passed. Cricopharyngeus and the upper third of the oesophagus are composed of striated muscle merging into smooth muscle lower down. The whole oesophagus receives autonomic innervation and the level of sympathetic tone may be an important factor in determining the capacity of the cricopharyngeal sphincter to relax. Once the bolus has passed into the oesophagus, the upper sphincter closes, the larynx actively descends (sternothyroid, sternohyoid), and the airway opens with the resumption of breathing in the expiratory phase thus filling the pharynx with air from below (Ardran and Kemp 1967).

Neural control (Miller 1982)

The sequence of events triggered in deglutition is far from fixed in all individuals and there are numerous variations in, for instance, initial oral positioning of the bolus and related tongue movement, the timing of soft palate movement, the initial direction of hyoid movement, the completeness of closure of the laryngeal aditus, and the patterning of the respiratory cycle before and after deglutition. However, there appears to be evidence for a central control mechanism for swallowing in the medulla related to the nucleus of the tractus solitarius. Like breathing, swallowing may occur volitionally, in response to behavioural or emotional stimuli, or subconsciously in a rhythmic or non-rhythmic manner. The final common efferent pathway involves motor impulses in cranial nerves V, VII, IX–XII, and upper cervical segments together with co-ordination of head movements and breathing activity. Predominantly crossed supranuclear control is exerted from the posteroinferior region of both frontal lobes via corticobulbar fibres and the basal ganglia but integrated reflex swallowing can occur in the absence of such pathways. As with breathing the swallowing centre in the medulla appears to be closely linked to centres of control in the pons and to be influenced by peripheral feedback from relevant receptive fields on the face, in the mouth, pharynx, palate, tongue, larynx, and airway (see Fig. 21.2).

Posture and movement of the head and neck are of importance in achieving a satisfactory swallow: some patients with major oral phase problems use neck extension to 'throw' the bolus backwards while others with lack of neck mobility (e.g. ankylosing spondylitis, dystonic retrocollis) or neck muscle weakness (e.g. myasthenia, motor neurone disease, myotonic dystrophy) must move the trunk or manually support or lift the head/neck to effect a swallow. In unilateral tongue or pharyngeal weakness rotational movements of the neck to the ipsilateral side may be employed subconsciously or therapeutically to compress the paretic side and direct swallowed material to the functional side of the pharynx. Obstructions in the oro- and hypopharynx or the upper oesophagus (stricture, web, pouch or external compression due to retropharyngeal or vertebral disease) may impede smooth peristaltic propulsion of food as well as misdirecting it. Failure of upward movement of the pharynx and larynx early in deglutition due to local non-neurological disease, tethering due to previous surgery or instrumentation may impair protection of the laryngeal opening and impede cricopharyngeal relaxation. Finally, inability to hold the breath during a swallow due to a low inspiratory reserve volume, to generate a cough of adequate strength (due to low vital capacity or laryngeal incompetence), or impaired integration of the respiratory pattern with deglutition may all increase the likelihood of laryngeal penetration and aspiration.

CLINICAL ASSESSMENT OF RESPIRATION AND SWALLOWING

The clinician should ask three questions:

1. Is there a relevant problem with swallowing or breathing?
2. How severe is it?
3. What are the component factors contributing to it?

The terms 'respiratory failure', 'dysphagia', and 'aspiration' are merely descriptive labels: full diagnosis requires clarification of the underlying causes and is a necessary step in planning the best management of the patient.

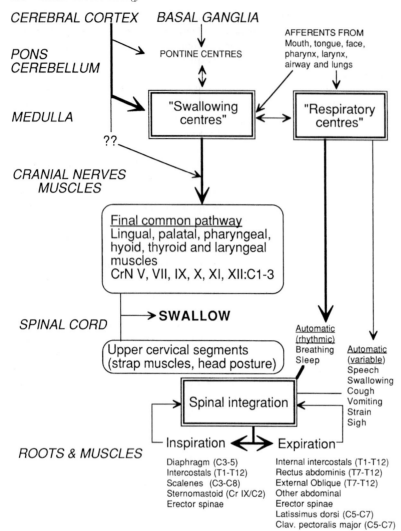

CEREBRAL CORTEX   BASAL GANGLIA

PONS
CEREBELLUM

MEDULLA

??

CRANIAL NERVES
MUSCLES

SPINAL CORD

ROOTS & MUSCLES

Fig. 21.2 Mechanisms in the *control of swallowing*.

RESPIRATION

Acute situation

Patients with incipient or actual acute hypoxic respiratory failure (Pao_2<60 mmHg) may be distraught and agitated and can manifest bizarre behaviour. Their distress is frequently compounded by choking on oropharyngeal secretions due to poor swallowing, aspiration, and a weak cough. The patient may be disturbed, restless and may refuse to sit or lie down. They prefer to sit rather than lie down and may sit gripping the chair or bed with both arms to fixate the shoulder girdle. Their attempts to breath in the face of acute neuromuscular weakness may be misinterpreted as hyperventilation due to 'hysteria', a situation well recognized in the polio era but today also seen with Guillain–Barré syndrome and myasthenia gravis.

Tachypnoea with activation of accessory muscles of respiration, including the alae nasi (a useful cranial nerve sign), is obvious; the patient is frequently sweating and the pulse rapid. Speech may be soft and only a few words managed with each breath: rarely, the patient may be speechless due to breathlessness: the quality of speech or the typical noise of stridulous breathing may suggest laryngeal dysfunction (structural or due to vocal cord paresis). Observation of the anterior abdominal wall (ideally in the supine patient) shows paradoxical inward motion on inspiration in selective or dominant diaphragm weakness (Goldman 1982): however, this sign depends on sufficient pleural negative pressure being generated to cause upward movement of the diaphragm into the chest and thus may be absent in extremis. In high thoracic or low cervical spinal cord lesions recession of the intercostal muscles is prominent reflecting significant intrapleural negative pressure generated by diaphragmatic activity: expiration is predominantly due to elastic recoil and cannot be actively assisted because of weakness of the abdominal and chest expiratory muscles which have a predominant thoracic innervation:

the cough in this situation is therefore poor. Such patients may prefer to lie down as expiration is then assisted by pressure on the diaphragm from the abdominal contents. In high or mid cervical lesions the diaphragm may be more or less compromised depending on the level and inspiration thus impaired with the sign of intercostal recession being lost due to low pleural negative pressures. The pectoral muscles may in this situation act as important muscles of expiration (De Troyer *et al.* 1986).

Recognition of acute respiratory failure depends on considering the possibility in *all* patients with new acute paralysis or an exacerbation of weakness in a patient with chronic paralysis. Appropriate investigations include measurement of vital capacity, blood gases, and oxygen saturation. A chest X-ray helps to exclude pneumothorax and parenchymal disease (in this context most often due to aspiration), pulmonary oedema, pulmonary emboli or infection, or unrelated abnormality: rarely, an unexpected retrosternal thyroid or bronchial carcinoma will be demonstrated. If the patient has severe parenchymal disease the assessment of the degree of muscular weakness by measuring vital capacity will be thwarted: in this situation measurement of maximum inspiratory or expiratory mouth occlusion pressures or transdiaphragmatic pressure give the only clear guide to muscle weakness but necessitate patient co-operation. In the presence of an upper motor neurone lesion forced vital capacity (a voluntary manoeuvre) may underestimate the functional capacity of the lungs and chest in response to reflex or metabolic stimulation. Endoscopy may be required to exclude obstruction and it is particularly important to consider this in the non-ventilated patient with a tracheostomy or endotracheal tube *in situ*.

Subacute/chronic situation

Many patients present with symptoms directly or indirectly related to respiratory insufficiency in a less acute manner. Typically, they may complain of restlessness at night with poor broken sleep, bad dreams, a preference for sleeping propped up, and a tendency to wake in the morning feeling unrefreshed with headache that may resolve after being up and about for an hour or two. Such patients may feel somnolent during the day, less intellectually competent than usual, and may be moody and depressed. Information should be obtained from any sleeping partner about restlessness, snoring, and other noises during sleep and wakefulness. A history of neuromuscular disease in the individual and their family is sought. It should be appreciated that nocturnal respiratory insufficiency or resulting daytime somnolence may be the *presenting feature* of a number of disorders most notably myotonic dystrophy, acid maltase deficiency, and motor neurone disease (Howard *et al.* 1988, 1993).

A final group of patients who present with respiratory insufficiency are those who have been ventilated either following an 'acute' pulmonary or cardiac condition or in relation to a general anaesthetic for surgery but cannot subsequently be weaned. Although the context is different the assessment is similar with a clear history from a relative or partner concerning events prior to ventilation being imperative.

Examination of such patients should include detailed assessment of the respiratory muscles as above. Kyphoscoliosis or spinal rigidity may be an important contributory factor and clue to an underlying neurological diagnosis. The patient may be obese, have a large thick neck, and/or have a large tongue and small oropharynx all of which may contribute to collapse and loss of patency of the upper airway in sleep with resulting obstructive apnoea. A careful search for focal muscle weakness, myotonia, fasciculations, and minor neurological signs such as a jaw jerk, impaired tongue movement, or brisk reflexes in wasted muscles will pay dividends in a few cases. In patients already known to have a neurological disorder the examination is focused on features known to contribute to respiratory insufficiency.

Investigations will include those noted above as a baseline but evaluation is likely also to require nocturnal sleep monitoring which can range from simple pulse oximetry to full multimodal polysomnography with videotelemetry. In addition, the role of incidental or related pulmonary or cardiac disease requires evaluation. Tables 1a and b shows a list of sites of neural injury and mechanisms to be considered as potentially contributing to acute or chronic respiratory insufficiency in a patient who has possible neurological or neuromuscular disease.

SWALLOWING

Disordered swallowing is recognized to be common in many neurological diseases. While it may not be the most prominent feature, its consequences of unsightly drooling, impaired nutrition and hydration, aspiration, and pneumonia can be major. The patient may emphasize problems with swallowing fluids rather than of solids 'sticking', which is more a feature of structural disease, although striated muscle disease affecting the pharynx and oesophagus tends to lead to the complaint of solids sticking first. The site of the difficulty is often poorly localized. The patient may just be aware of having to take extra care when eating or drinking, of taking longer than everyone else to complete a meal or of the dangers of trying to talk with the mouth full. The complaint can be of difficulty chewing, of saliva, or food falling out of the mouth (drooling) or prematurely slipping into the pharynx, or of a food material collecting in between the teeth/gums and cheeks or sticking to the roof of the mouth. Residues may be left in the mouth following a swallow. During or after swallowing the patient may notice nasal regurgitation, alteration of the voice quality, or episodes of coughing or choking. By contrast, the patient may not recognize that there is a specific swallowing problem but complain of choking episodes unrelated to meals or occurring from sleep. On other occasions the sole manifestation may be repeated 'chest infections' or episodes of foreign body aspiration presenting as cough or fever suggesting

Table 21.1a Contributory factors to be evaluated in neurogenic respiratory failure

Conscious level	Reduced consciousness and related cerebral hemisphere, or brainstem signs
Respiratory muscles	Weakness: diaphragm, intercostals, abdominal muscles, latissimus dorsi, other accessory muscles
Spine	Kyphoscoliosis, rigid spine (ankylosing spondylitis, as part of myopathy), spinal fracture
Lung parenchyma and adnexae	Aspiration (associated laryngeal disease or dysphagia)
	Pneumothorax (especially ventilated patient)
	Infection due to primary agent of paralysis or an acute incidental upper/lower tract infection
	Pulmonary embolism (paralysed patient) Pulmonary oedema (cardiogenic, aspiration)
	Relevant mass lesion (e.g. thymoma, carcinoma)
	Unrelated lung disease
Heart	Related cardiac disease or incidental disorder
	myocarditis, cardiomyopathy conduction defect
Abdomen	Distension
	constipation
	intra-abdominal mass
	Abdominal surgery
Aspiration	Dysphagia
	Salivary control/drooling
	Vomiting/regurgitation of gastric contents
	Impaired laryngeal function
	Weak cough
Upper airway obstruction (increased work of breathing, increase negative pressure, and airway collapse)	Nasal
	maxillary/mandibular instability
	Oral
	tongue
	Pharyngeal
	cervical spinal column
	Laryngeal (vocal cords)
	thyroid gland/mass
	Tracheal (tracheostomy)
	foreign body obstruction
Medication	Depressants of central respiratory drive
	Recent general anaesthetic Muscle relaxant sensitivity/overdose Extrapyramidal side-effects of medication
	Increased susceptibility to medications (e.g. myasthenia gravis, myotonic dystrophy)
Disordered control of breathing	Impaired automatic (metabolic) control
	Impaired voluntary breathing manoeuvres (voluntary cough, voluntary breath-hold)
	Abnormal respiratory rhythm (e.g. apneustic breathing, paroxysmal hyperventilation)
Metabolic disorder	Hypokalemia
	Hypophosphateamia
Second supervening neurological disorder	Guillain–Barré syndrome
	Neuropathy of the critically ill (ITU patients) Stroke

Table 21.1b Respiratory and related factors contributing to daytime somnolence

Reduced awake and/or sleep ventilation due to:
1. Respiratory muscle weakness
2. Restrictive defect (e.g. kyposcoliosis)
3. Posture: orthopnoea especially with diaphragm weakness in REM sleep
4. Upper airway obstruction (obstructive sleep apnoea, laryngeal stridor)
5. Disordered central respiratory drive
6. Peripheral atelectasis and retained secretions: V/Q mismatch
7. Associated cardiac disorder with raised left atrial pressure

Related factors
1. Disrupted sleep architecture and lack of REM and phase 3/4 non-REM sleep
2. Inappropriate night sedation or other medication
3. Lack of rest for 'fatigued' residual respiratory muscles

that aspiration has occurred 'silently': this occurs even when sensory pathways from the larynx and upper airway are not primarily involved by the disease process. The nutritional intake may start to fail and fluid intake be inadequate. In the intubated patient appearance of food or liquids in the tracheal or bronchial aspirate may be the only evidence of aspiration. The gradual onset and effective compensation for some impairments means that patients may not volunteer 'abnormal' symptoms: cognitive impairment heightens this possibility.

Assessment of swallowing disorder includes an examination of the relevant cranial nerves. The muscles of mastication and facial muscles are assessed: jaw jerk and facial jerks may be indicative of an upper motor neurone lesion to the Vth and VIIth nerve nuclei. Palatal function in response to vocalization (voluntary activation) or reflex stimulation and posterior pharyngeal wall sensation (IX) to touch are tested bilaterally. The 'gag' reflex consists of a range of responses from minimal upper pharyngeal contraction and palatal elevation in response to vigorous stimulation of the posterior pharyngeal wall to an immediate major contraction of these muscles with head withdrawl, lacrimation, coughing, retching, or vomiting on simple depression of the tongue or even on anticipation of contact. Sensory loss, depression of consciousness, or loss of lower motor neurone units or muscle fibres may reduce the response. With adequate stimulation it is rare for the gag reflex to be repeatedly absent in the alert healthy adult (Hughes and Wiles 1996*b*). Palatal and oropharyngeal muscle contraction is often reduced on voluntary activation in an upper motor neurone lesion while there may be a brisker than normal reflex contraction. However, the presence or absence of a 'gag', while giving information of value about IX and X nerve function does not reliably predict the adequacy of the swallowing reflex nor liability to aspiration.

The tongue is assessed for bulk, the presence of fasciculations, chorea or tremor and the range, direction and rapidity of lateral, up and down, and protrusive movements. The quality of speech may predict laryngeal competence and pooling of secretions in the upper larynx or at the vocal cords. Paresis of the vocal cords causes a harsh dysphonia or whispered speech while pooling in the laryngeal vestibule gives rise to a 'wet-hoarse' quality of voice. A 'bovine' cough quality indicates inadequate glottic closure and the patient may have difficulty 'clearing the throat'. Full examination of the pharynx and larynx requires the help of the ENT surgeon with direct or indirect endoscopy. This is important for full evaluation of vocal cord movement and for the exclusion of structural disease. Examination of the head and neck posture, and the range and strength of neck movement is also undertaken.

Although the above features may give important clues to swallowing disorder their absence does not exclude a swallowing problem. Direct observation of the patient swallowing is of primary importance. This test must be tailored to the individual situation. Necessary prerequisites are an alert cooperative patient and a suitable posture. It is clearly inappropriate to ask a severely breathless dysphagic patient to drink a glass of water, whereas such a test may well be appropriate in a patient who is usually eating full meals but who is under suspicion of having problems related to dysphagia. If in doubt, the patient should be asked to make a 'dry' swallow first followed by small volumes of water (e.g. 2–3 ml) given on a spoon. Timing the ability to clear larger measured volumes of water while counting the swallows provides a simple quantitative test of swallowing capacity which can be expressed in terms of predicted norms as well as a valid qualitative test of function (Hughes and Wiles 1996a). The rise and fall of the hyoid and larynx during the swallow are observed, any coughing or spluttering during or after is noted. The patient is requested to speak after swallowing to assess any pooling at the vocal cords. While the above tests may reasonably be carried out by medical staff, more detailed assessments are in the domain of the speech and language therapist whose assistance should be sought in problematic cases.

A dietary assessment of intake is necessary in many patients with dysphagia but simple measurements of fluid balance, nutritional status including skin condition, weight, body mass index, plasma proteins, and the exclusion of common deficiency states are of importance.

Although clinical examination may lead to a strong suspicion of disordered swallowing or aspiration radiological investigation can be a useful complementary tool. Plain chest radiography may confirm aspiration but the videofluoroscopic examination (see below) is especially helpful although

Table 21.2 Contributory factors to be evaluated in neurogenic dysphagia

Central control disorder	Behavioural disorder psychiatric disease Orolingual apraxia Coma Pontomedullary disease Cerebellar ataxia Akinesia Movement disorder chorea, tardive dyskinesia dystonia
Weakness of face, mastication, oral, palatal, and pharyngeal muscles	Upper or lower motor neurone lesion
Laryngeal competence	Vocal cord paresis Akinesia/dystonia surgery, infiltration, extrapyramidal disorder/drugs, multisystem atrophy
Sensory loss in oral cavity, pharynx, larynx, and airway	Neurogenic 'Desensitization' associated with tracheostomy, oro- or nasotracheal intubation, Repeated oropharyngeal suction ?Nasogastric intubation
Posture of trunk, head, neck	Freedom of neck movement collar, traction, dystonia ankylosing spondyltis Neck extensor or flexor weakness rigid spine anterior osteophytosis
Restricted movement of hyoid and larynx	Muscle weakness Previous anterior neck or pharyngeal/laryngeal surgery Endotracheal intubation
External compression of pharynx, oesophagus	Cervical spine osteophytosis (Forestier's disease) Thyroid or parathyroid or lymph node mass Retropharyngeal mass
Intrinsic oral, pharyngeal, oesophageal, or laryngeal disease	Candidiasis or other infection (related pain), mass, pharyngeal pouch, stricture Cricopharyngeal spasm Gastro-oesophageal reflux, hiatus hernia
Associated or incidental cardiopulmonary disease	Breathlessness Cough
Associated or incidental breathing disorder	Respiratory reserve (VC) Expiratory muscle strength Effectiveness of cough Artificial breathing support
Associated speech disorder	Dysphonia Dysarthria

Table 21.2 (*cont.*)

	Dysphasia
	vocal aid
Medication	Anticholinergics
	Dopamine-blocking agents
	Botulinus toxin

only providing a brief, albeit detailed, snapshot of the swallowing mechanism (Kidd *et al.* 1993). Table 21.2 shows a list of factors and diagnoses to be considered as potentially contributing to acute or chronic dysphagia in a patient who has, or possibly has, a neurological or neuromuscular disease.

CAUSES OF DISORDER

RESPIRATION

The causes of neurogenic or neuromuscular respiratory disorder may be conveniently subdivided by the causative anatomical site of injury or disease, bearing in mind that occasionally mild neurological disorder will be associated with intrinsic cardiopulmonary or chest wall disease and precipitate the need for intervention (Hughes and Bihari 1993). Important causes of neurogenic breathing disorder are shown in Table 21.3 according to site of causation. Most such disorders may be analysed in terms of combinations of factors outlined in Table 21.1a.

SWALLOWING

Conventionally, neurogenic swallowing disorders have been considered as being caused by disease either of the brainstem, the lower cranial nerves or, neuromuscular mechanisms. Although not exhaustive Table 21.4, indicates a wider differential diagnosis including the important categories of cerebral hemisphere lesions and diseases of the extrapyramidal system including parkinsonism and dystonia. Table 21.2 indicates the contributory factors to causation—often multiple in any given disorder.

INVESTIGATION OF CAUSE

Diagnosis of the cause of respiratory insufficiency proceeds along standard paths once it is appreciated that the patient has a breathing problem possibly of neurogenic origin. Although this may be obvious, the patient who presents having had a respiratory arrest or who fails to wean following an anaesthetic can present a difficult diagnostic challenge. Often, a detailed history from a relative is helpful in clarifying the duration of the underlying problem and whether the present situation is entirely new or an exacerbation of a longstanding disorder—a distinction critical to correct diagnosis. Motor neurone disease, botulism, myasthenia gravis, myotonic dystrophy, and a Chiari malformation are conditions particularly notable for presenting with respiratory insufficiency with,

Table 21.3 Causes and features of neurogenic breathing disorder

Disorder	Cause	Features
Cerebral hemispheres	Cheyne–Stokes ventilation	Bihemispheric disease Diencephalic compression Prolonged circulation time Hypoxia
	Post-hyperventilation apnoea ?Hyperventilation syndrome	
Basal ganglia disease	Irregular breathing Abnormal timing of inspiration, tremor, aspiration Paresis of vocal cord abduction (laryngeal stridor)	Chorea Dystonic movement disorder Parkinsonism Multisystem atrophy
Pons	Apneustic breathing Paroxysmal breathing disorder Neurogenic hyperventilation Impaired or lost voluntary/ behavioural respiratory control	Infarction or haemorrhage Trauma/distortion Multiple sclerosis Encephalitis (polio, rabies, etc.) Tumour/surgery
Medulla/foramen magnum	Hiccoughs Failure of all drive to breathing or erratic irregular breathing Failure of metabolic drive to breathing (Ondine's syndrome) associated aspiration	As for pons Also: syrinx Chiari malformation Drug overdose Brainstem degenerations Rheumatoid disease
High cervical cord (C1–3)	Failure of inspiration and expiration, absent cough Anterior cord lesions:- loss of metabolic control alone	Spinal trauma Ant. spinal artery syndrome Multiple sclerosis Transverse myelitis Tumour Bilateral cordotomy
Mid/low cervical lesions	Inspiration: diaphragm-dependent Expiration weak (pectoral-dependent) or absent Cough weak	Spinal trauma (Ankylosing spondylitis) Extradural cord compression Transverse myelitis Tumour Ant. spinal artery syndrome Syrinx, Multiple sclerosis Motor neurone disease

Thoracic lesions	Variable impairment of inspiratory and expiratory function Loss of abdominal muscle expiratory function	As for cervical cord
Anterior horn cell	Dysfunction depending on distribution	Genetic disorder (spinal muscular atrophy) Motor neurone disease and variants Poliomyelitis Tetanus
Motor nerve	Dysfunction depending on distribution but diaphragm commonly affected	Genetic neuropathy (e.g. HMSN) Guillain–Barré syndrome Porphyria Toxic neuropathy (arsenic, hexacarbon) Brachial plexus neuropathy Paraneoplastic neuropathy or neoplastic infiltration Neuropathy of the critically ill Surgical injury to phrenic nerve
Neuromuscular junction (NMJ)	Usually bulbar and respiratory impairment plus ocular involvement	Botulism, botulinus toxin Other toxic agents Lambert–Eaton syndrome Drug-induced blockade or poisoning at NMJ Myasthenia gravis
Muscle disease	Variable distribution of respiratory and bulbar weakness depending on specific disease	Duchenne Emery–Dreifuss Myotonic dystrophy Facioscapulohumeral Periodic paralysis Mitochondrial Nemaline rod Rigid spine Toxic (drugs, poisons) Metabolic (potassium, phosphate) Inflammatory myopathy

sometimes, only minor associated neurological signs: multisystem atrophy and laryngeal dystonia can present with stridor: Guillain–Barré syndrome may be triggered following surgery or an illness necessitating admission to the ITU and can thus present quite unexpectedly. Critical illness neuropathy may be an important cause of failure to wean from ventilation in the context of multisystem illness and sepsis (Wiles 1996).

Table 21.4 Causes of neurogenic dysphagia

Coma/impaired conscious level	Drugs/overdose Trauma Stroke Other
Cerebral hemisphere	Stroke (especially frontal) Bilateral pyramidal tract lesions (e.g. multiple infarcts), demyelination, motor neurone disease Space-occupying lesion 'Cerebral palsy'
Basal ganglia/extrapyramidal	Parkinsonism Multisystem atrophy Movement disorder chorea dystonia
Cerebellar pathway disease	Spinocerebellar degeneration Multiple sclerosis
Brainstem	Infarct or haemorrhage Encephalitis Multiple sclerosis Space-occupying lesion Degeneration Chiari malformation/syrinx
Brainstem nuclei	Motor neurone disease Other degeneration Fazio–Londe Vialetto–van Laere Poliomyelitis
Cranial nerves (V, VII, IX–XII)	Guillain–Barré syndrome Other inflammatory Neoplastic infiltration (including recurrent laryngeal) Surgical division of recurrent laryngeal or vagus Sarcoidosis Diphtheria Degeneration
Neuromuscular junction	Botulism, botulinus toxin Lambert–Eaton syndrome (dry mouth) Myasthenia gravis
Muscle disorder	Genetic myotonic facioscapulohumeral oculopharyngeal Mitochondrial Congenital Acquired inflammatory myopathy (notably inclusion body)

The type and severity of breathing disorder can usually be readily established clinically by examination and a few simple investigations including forced vital capacity, peak inspiratory and expiratory occlusion pressures, blood gas measurement, and oxygen saturation monitoring during sleep. These tests allow voluntary/behavioural and metabolic disorder to be distinguished, clear weakness of the breathing muscles, and severe obstructive or central sleep apnoea to be identified. More detailed function tests including full sleep polysomnography may be required and the assistance of a respiratory physician with more sophisticated pulmonary function testing and transdiaphragmatic pressure testing may be required to clarify the contribution to symptoms of intrinsic lung disease and muscle weakness if both are present. Laboratory investigation may include imaging of the brain especially the posterior fossa and foramen magnum, nerve conduction studies and electromyogram (EMG), edrophonium test, examination of the cerebrospinal fluid (CSF), and biopsy of muscle or nerve, together with blood investigation as the clinical circumstances dictate.

Although reflex swallowing may persist in coma or the persistent vegetative state, aspiration is a common event in the patient with a depressed level of consciousness whose airway is unprotected: a tendency to vomit and the disorganization of the respiratory cycle in relation to deglutition probably accounts for this. Decompensated swallowing disorder may only present gradually with recurrent pulmonary episodes, failure of nutrition, and weight loss. If the patient complains of a swallowing problem or of the consequences of dysphagia and is known to have a disorder (see Tables 21.2 and 21.4) of potential relevance then a degree of dysphagia compensated or otherwise should be assumed, even if the standard neurological examination appears unremarkable. If the patient does not complain of dysphagia but has potentially related symptoms *and* a condition recognized to cause dysphagia then direct observation of the swallowing process supplemented by videofluoroscopy is of particular importance. With most cases of dysphagia not clearly linked initially to neurological disease, a preliminary assessment by an ENT surgeon with barium or endoscopic studies to exclude gastroesophageal disease is an essential prerequisite to detailed neurological assessment. In the ITU patient who is intubated the extent of secretions and saliva visualized or aspirated from above the endotracheal cuff and from the oropharynx gives some index of swallowing capacity. Introduction of small amounts of a dye such as methylene blue into the mouth and later inspection of bronchial or tracheal aspirate may give an obvious indication of aspiration.

Videofluoroscopy can be useful in defining the detailed impairments in dysphagia, notably the detection of silent aspiration, and the timing relationships of various aspects of swallowing: the technique only samples a few swallows under controlled circumstances and findings must be interpreted in this light. The standard barium swallow is *not* the appropriate investigation. Small amounts of liquid barium or non-ionic contrast media and a series of semi-solid and solid foodstuffs made radiopaque with contrast are best administered by a speech therapist and radiologist working together: the passage of material is monitored by cine- or videofluoroscopy and

recorded for later frame-by-frame analysis. In an undiagnosed case contrast should be followed down the length of the oesophagus into the stomach to exclude intrathoracic or lower sphincter pathology. Videofluoroscopy can have an additional role in teaching swallowing techniques with varying food consistences.

For oesphageal disorders manometry (sometimes combined with contrast radiology) of the oesophagus and its sphincters is of diagnostic value but the place of this for routinely investigating pharyngeal dysfunction is unclear. Twenty-four hour pH monitoring in the oesophagus is of assistance in diagnosing acid reflux. Other techniques are being used to study swallowing for research purposes including ultrasonography, radionuclide scanning, and electrical impedance tomography: the simultaneous monitoring of phase of breathing and of deglutition marked either acoustically by the swallowing sounds or by electromyography (EMG) may prove of considerable interest in neurogenic dysphagia (Tarrant *et al.* 1996). Cortical magnetic stimulation of the brain has recently been used to study neural mechanisms of dysphagia, and in conjunction with modern scanning techniques may shed light on mechanisms of impairment and recovery (Hamdy *et al.* 1996).

MANAGEMENT

SEVERITY, MONITORING, AND INITIAL MANAGEMENT

The urgency of breathing and swallowing problems is usually inversely related to its duration. Acute problems often need urgent action and intervention. Depending on the certainty of the diagnosis the help of a respiratory physician, anaesthetist, or ENT surgeon may be required initially particularly if endoscopy of the pharynx, larynx, and trachea are required to exclude obstruction. If the patient is acutely breathless and distressed a rapid decision is required about symptomatic relief alone or in combination with life-supporting intervention. The course of action will depend on many factors, not least whether the diagnosis and overall prognosis, and wishes of the patient and family are known. By contrast, a long history of neurological disease followed by breathing-or swallowing-related symptoms may allow more time for assessment before intervention.

The initial steps are outlined in Tables 21.5a and b. Many alert, conscious patients prefer to sit or even stand rather than lie flat. With diffusely weak respiratory muscles or dominant diaphragm weakness vital capacity is improved in the erect posture. By contrast, a patient with a high thoracic or low cervical spinal cord injury with thoracic and expiratory muscle paralysis, but preservation of diaphragm function may prefer the supine position. If intubation either for airway protection or assisted ventilation are considered likely to be necessary pre-emptive transfer to the ITU should be organized so that an 'arrest' situation on the ward can be avoided and any intervention carried out electively and calmly.

Table 21.5a Immediate management of acute neurogenic respiratory distress

1. (a) Sit patient up if alert, speak to him/her, and explain what is happening
   (b) If patient already intubated and ventilated check all machine functions, connections and patency of tubes and oxygen/air supply
2. Consider upper airway obstruction: emergency endoscopy if necessary
   Examine chest and exclude pneumothorax
   Assess ability to cough
   Check circulation and BP
   Check if patient swallowing own saliva
3. Arrange portable chest X-ray, and electrocardiogram plus monitor
4. Check vital capacity (lying and sitting if possible)
5. Check blood gases and establish pulse oximetry
6. Request ITU support and intubate if necessary
7. Do not give anything by mouth
8. Do not sedate the patient until control of airway and breathing is secured

Table 21.5b Immediate management of acute neurogenic dysphagia

1. Sit patient up if alert, explain, and reassure
2. (a) check mouth and pharynx clear of obstruction, false teeth, etc.
   (b) check movements of chest and air entry
   (c) check circulation and BP
   (d) assess if patient controlling own saliva
3. If patient cannot speak or swallow acutely consider foreign body obstruction and request urgent laryngoscopy/intubation
4. Assess ability to cough and vital capacity
5. Do not give anything by mouth
6. If patient has major respiratory symptoms proceed as from (3) in Table 21.5a
7. Do not attempt to place a nasogastric tube as an emergency in the distressed patient
8. If patient unconscious, position correctly, protect airway by intubation

Traditional intubation and ventilation via a cuffed oro- or nasotracheal tube remains the safest practice in the neurological patient with respiratory failure. The use of positive pressure ventilation by nasal mask, although a useful technique for assisted noctural ventilation, may be fraught with difficulties in the emergency situation. The patient may well tolerate the face mask poorly and any tendency to aspirate due to bulbar insufficiency may be exacerbated. Negative pressure devices are better tolerated for purely respiratory failure but may also promote aspiration (see below). The management of acute respiratory distress in the conscious patient already ventilated for neurological disease is largely the province of the specialist respiratory physician or anaesthetist but disconnection (accidental or deliberate), pneumothorax, obstruction of tubing, and machine failure all need urgent consideration.

LONG-TERM MANAGEMENT

RESPIRATION (SCHNEERSON 1988)

There are a range of options available for aiding breathing in the long term: evaluation needs to include review of the opportunities for treating the underlying disease, treatment of relevant associated conditions (e.g. kyphoscoliosis), prevention of other factors relevant to breathing (e.g. abdominal distension), and constipation, weight gain, recurrent aspiration, the level of distress caused by the respiratory symptoms, and the provision of breathing aids (Smith *et al.* 1991).

Preventive measures

Kyphoscoliosis

Boys with Duchenne muscular dystrophy can be helped and respiratory failure delayed by careful attention to weight gain at an early stage and the correction of kyphoscoliosis by the Luqué procedure or Harrington rods with partial reversal of the concomitant restrictive pulmonary defect. Kyphoscoliosis is common in those chronic neurological disorders starting at or before the growth spurt at puberty and, when severe, may well be a factor in late respiratory deterioration in other conditions. Correction with modern surgical and anaesthetic techniques, although still a major undertaking, is entirely feasible but the relative importance of the spinal curve in relation to respiratory dysfunction can be hard to assess and the risks of surgery not inconsiderable. Close collaboration between orthopaedic surgeon, intensivist/ anaesthetist, and neurologist is desirable.

Weight gain and abdominal distension

Obesity not only increases the work of breathing and moving but also places extra strain on other muscle groups. Intrabdominal and abdominal wall fat masses may materially impede diaphragm function and neck deposits may promote any tendency to upper airway collapse and obstructive apnoea. Long-term dietary and nutritional advice given early is relevant. Abdominal distension due to constipation and 'wind', a distended bladder, or paralytic or obstructive ileus may all have an important deleterious effect in patients whose breathing is marginal due to muscle weakness. Abdominal surgery may be particularly problematic from this point of view.

Medication and anaesthesia

Sedative medication and alcohol excess have a potentially serious depressant effect on breathing during sleep in patients with muscle weakness. The drive to breathing may be suppressed but also airway control may be impaired and obstructive episodes promoted. If breathing is impaired further in sleep the negative effects in the day can more than outweigh any benefit of night sedation and may be hazardous. Certain groups of patients notably those with myotonic dystrophy, myasthenia gravis, and central disorders of respiratory control have special potential problems with general anaesthetics and it is of importance that an anaesthetist experienced in managing such patients is involved.

Obstructive sleep apnoea

In some patients with nocturnal hypoventilation due to neuromuscular disease obstructive apnoea plays a role in worsening symptoms. Medical measures to prevent this component include weight loss, treatment of upper respiratory tract and nasal obstruction, sleeping on the side rather than the back, and the use of drugs such as protryptiline which suppress rapid eye movement (REM) sleep. Nasal continuous positive airway pressure (nasal CPAP) is useful if recurrent obstruction is a major problem including those patients where obstruction is precipitated by negative pressure ventilation. Tracheostomy remains a useful option in severe upper airway obstruction whether associated with typical sleep apnoea or laryngeal cord paresis, stridor, or dystonia, in which case it may be the only feasible way to prevent life-threatening hypoxaemia.

Aspiration

Recurrent aspiration may be a preventable cause of pulmonary deterioration. Diagnosis depends on a high level of clinical suspicion supported by videofluoroscopy. In the ITU patient who is intubated with a cuffed endotracheal tube aspiration is still quite possible (Cameron *et al.* 1973): frequent movements of the tube and connections occur due to patient movements, nursing, and physiotherapy procedures: swallowing is inhibited by the splinting effect of the endotracheal tube and cuff restricting upward movement of the larynx during deglutition, the balloon itself may cause partial backward obstruction and loss of normal glottic airflow may cause sensory impairment. Naso- or orotracheal tubes have an effect over and above a tracheostomy tube because of their presence in the mouth and pharynx. If a patient is felt to require a cuffed tube for airway protection (because of dysphagia and aspiration) rather than for ventilation (for which it is not always necessary) then oral feeding and fluids should be generally discontinued.

Recurrent chest infection and pulmonary embolism

It goes without saying that smoking is a preventable cause of lung deterioration. Prompt treatment of chest infections with antibiotics, physiotherapy, and temporary or increased mechanical breathing support if necessary all play a role in minimising the deleterious effect of these episodes. Patients with critical respiratory function are helped by regular review from an expert physiotherapist along with the monitoring of pulmonary function and muscle strength.

Patients with ventilatory failure due to acute spinal cord injury or neuromuscular disease have an appreciable risk of deep venous thrombosis related to lower limb paralysis. Most notable are those with cord transections and Guillain–Barré syndrome. Anticoagulation in the early stages may prevent later impairment of lung function due to embolism. How

long such anticoagulation should continue in the presence of prolonged paralysis is uncertain but three to six months is commonly suggested.

Breathing aids (Branthwaite 1991; Schneerson 1991)

Breathing aids may be required in the short term to get over an acute chest infection or other crisis in the weak or paralysed patient but we are concerned here with the longer-term management of the patient at home. The primary purpose of a breathing aid is to reduce symptoms and disability and to aid rehabilitation into the community. Whether such aids should be introduced to treat abnormalities of blood gases (e.g. nocturnal desaturations) in the absence of related symptomatology is a matter for research and discussion. The provision of a tracheostomy tube alone, by reducing anatomical dead space and resistance to breathing, obviating upper airway obstruction and improving access to the bronchial tree for suction of secretions may be all that is necessary to maintain adequate ventilation. A speaking valve on the inner tracheostomy tube in this situation allows speech in the usual way. Further aids to support ventilation may be divided into oxygen supplementation to raise the inspired oxygen concentration, and ventilatory support: the latter is subdivided into positive pressure ventilation (via a face mask or tracheostomy tube) or negative pressure ventilation.

Establishing a patient on a domiciliary breathing aid is a truly multidisciplinary task—much more than simply the provision of kit for the patient to take home. Detailed discussion about the implications of such devices with the patient and carers is essential. Matters which may be perceived as trivial by health professionals, by comparison with the disease process, include the loss of independence, the appearance of a mask and (sometimes noisy) ventilator in the bedroom, the possible need for separate beds or rooms, and the effect on sex life. The balance of advantage and disadvantage needs to be weighed up on an individual basis.

The degree of ventilator dependence is important: completely dependent patients require a reserve machine immediately available in case of failure, together with an emergency power supply and an experienced carer to provide immediate help if the patient cannot react themselves. Patients with complete ventilator dependence may include those with high tetraplegia (C1–3) or medullary disorders. Those who are not ventilator-dependent can be expected to spend much of the day off a ventilator due to the improved quality of night-time sleep which they experience when on the machine. In this group machine or power failure gives a longer period to rectify matters. Proper arrangements for machine servicing, for replacement of tubes and connections, and an emergency contact number at the centre responsible for the patient are essential. The co-operation of the general practitioner and local nursing services also needs to be enlisted. Psychological needs of patients and their carers, largely related to increased feelings of dependency, need to be appreciated and many will benefit from regular hospital admission to their base unit for review of ventilation arrangements, physiotherapy review, and respite. The provision of a second portable ventilator may greatly enhance quality of life by facilitating holidays or stays with family and friends. Ventilator-dependent patients require a breathing device incorporated into their wheelchair for daytime use.

Clearly, there is a strong case to be made for domiciliary ventilation services to be centralized on a regional basis with each unit having sufficient experience, patients, and resources to justify a comprehensive 24-hour service.

1. *Positive pressure*. Glossopharyngeal or 'frog' breathing is a technique which those with weak respiratory muscles but competent bulbar function can learn (Schneerson 1988). It consists of using the muscles of the pharynx and mouth to pump air into the lungs and was found to be of value in the polio era. It may allow the patient with weak respiratory muscles to periodically improve their vital capacity by about a litre and is thus a valuable aid to opening up peripheral areas of collapse, and assists coughing. The increased chest expansion achieved probably helps to increase chest wall compliance and reduce the work of breathing.

Intermittent positive pressure ventilation by nasal mask (and thus without airway protection) has been used increasingly frequently in recent years. The technique may not be appropriate for those with severe swallowing disorder and poor airway control nor for those who are ventilator-dependent but appears to be most useful in patients with nocturnal hypoventilation with secondary daytime symptoms who have relatively preserved bulbar function including speech and swallowing. The great advantage is its non-invasive nature. Complete lack of use of the arms due to weakness is a disadvantage because the patient is reliant on a carer to adjust the face mask if it is uncomfortable. Failure to adjust the mask or a poorly designed mask can cause troublesome pressure sores on the bridge of the nose. Some individuals dislike wearing a face mask and cannot tolerate it, but time spent 'fiddling' with the mask in the early stages is usually worthwhile. A few patients with structural disease of the nasal cavities will not be suitable and some require a chin strap to prevent the mouth from falling open when asleep, with loss of inspiratory pressure.

Classical intermittent positive pressure ventilation via a tracheostomy with a cuffed or uncuffed tube is still used. This procedure tends to be used for patients who are ventilator-dependent or who require airway protection or frequent bronchial toilet due to secretions. If the patient has preserved bulbar function, for example, high (C1–3) tetraplegia, ventilation should ideally be carried out through an uncuffed tracheostomy tube. This allows voice preservation in the expiratory phase of the cycle. Some cuffed tracheostomy have 'vocal aids' which allow a stream of air to be directed inwards above the cuff and thus up through the larynx but voice quality is poor. Even if bulbar function is imperfect it is uncertain whether a cuffed tube is the best option for the long-term since, as noted above, the cuff does not provide complete airway protection and perhaps impairs residual swallowing capacity further. From the patient's point of view the preservation of speech is a major concern and should not be relinquished easily! A variety of machines are available, some portable and some of which can be incorporated into a wheelchair. Proper management, cleaning, and changing of the tracheostomy tube is essential.

2. *Negative pressure*. One of the most physiological methods of long-term negative pressure ventilation is via the technique of diaphragm pacing with implanted electrodes (Glenn and Phelps 1985). Many neurological patients are not suitable for this technique because the pathogenesis of their disease or injury has destroyed the lower motor neurones or neuromuscular mechanism. Patients with injury to metabolic control pathways (Ondine's syndrome) or isolated high cervical tetraplegia with preservation of phrenic motoneurones may be suitable.

A rocking bed tilts the supine patient up and down +/– 30 degrees from horizontal about 13–22 cycles per minute. The abdominal contents push the diaphragm up on head-down tilt thus facilitating expiration and fall away again on head-up tilt, thus allowing diaphragm descent and inspiration. Patients with nocturnal hypoventilation due to dominant diaphragm weakness can be suitable for using this at night (or for a rest in the day) instead of a normal bed. The technique is probably not suitable for those with very weak limbs, those who are ventilator-dependent, or who suffer from motion sickness! The bed itself is somewhat cumbersome and noisy and requires reasonable space around it to manoeuvre. It is, however, simple and reliable and leaves the patient easily accessible.

Other negative pressure techniques all depend on artificially developing a negative pressure around the patient's chest and upper abdomen using a moulded shell (cuirasse), a jacket over a frame (Tunnicliffe jacket), or the traditional iron lung. The iron lung, developed in the days of the poliomyelitis epidemics, is a highly efficient form of negative pressure ventilation which also allows access to the patient through side ports and may allow turning for chest physiotherapy, pressure relief, etc. Its use is highly specialized and available through a few experienced units in the United Kingdom. The cuirasse and Tunnicliffe jacket are effective nocturnal breathing aids but can be difficult to fit properly and the weak patient may need considerable assistance getting into the device satisfactorily. All negative pressure devices suffer from two potential disadvantages which should be assessed before prescription. The first is that aspiration may be promoted and thus reasonable bulbar function is important. The second is that any tendency to upper airway obstruction may be increased although this is not a problem if the patient has a tracheostomy. The techniques have the advantage of being non-invasive (although inconvenient) and of allowing normal speech. Only the iron lung is really suitable for the ventilator-dependent patient.

SWALLOWING

As with breathing disorder the management of neurogenic dysphagia is a multidisciplinary effort involving the patient, the family or carers, speech/language therapist (Logemann 1988*a*), and dietician, in particular. The natural history of dysphagia in the particular disorder needs to be considered: thus aspiration and dysphagia commonly resolve after stroke (Wade and Hewer 1987; Kidd *et al.* 1995). Many factors other than the purely medical influence the options which a patient will consider for eating and drinking. Enjoyment of food and drink is an important experience *per se* for many and, unlike breathing, has not only a life-sustaining role but also an important social role which many are not happy to relinquish because of what may be perceived as theoretical risks. Dietary and swallowing advice are not once-and-for-all interventions and need repeated reassessment in the light of changing circumstances. In addition, the need to preserve speech communication becomes a relevant issue in most patients.

Symptomatic

Having determined the specific cause of dysphagia and the level of speech and respiratory impairment, if any, nutritional status is assessed. Although some patients may be able to maintain adequate intake under normal metabolic conditions, they may not be able to manage the increased intake necessary in the presence of sepsis, pressure sores, or injury, and a temporary period of gastric intubation or parenteral feeding may be appropriate. Evaluation of breathing and swallowing disorder can take several days or even weeks and nutritional status must not be allowed to deteriorate while a long-term solution is under consideration.

The chances of improving oral intake in any patient are improved by certain simple but essential preliminary points often neglected in hospital. Most healthy people have difficulty eating and drinking when lying semi-supine or with their neck extended. The patient needs to be sat up, preferably out of bed at a table, in a comfortable chair. Dentures, if needed, should be properly fitting and oral hygiene optimal. Drugs which impair the production of saliva (e.g. anticholinergics), cause sedation or have a dopamine-blocking action (especially neuroleptic medication) should be stopped unless absolutely essential: by contrast, dopaminergic medication in Parkinson's disease should not be withdraw suddenly because of the risk of exacerbating dysphagia. Consideration needs to be given to the ability of the patient to self-feed and to the implements required—commonly relevant in the multiply-disabled neurological patient. If the patient needs feeding a sympathetic approach free from distraction is essential. Talking while eating increases the likelihood of aspiration. Patients may be embarrassed at their disability and need reassurance and the opportunity to eat out of the sight of passers by. Swallowing is a process notoriously sensitive to emotional status and tension, anxiety, or agitiation may significantly impair swallowing ability. Finally, food consistency and type needs careful evaluation.

In patients at risk of aspiration (whether improving or deteriorating) the speech therapist and dietician assess the types of consistency and taste which can be coped with and need to be personally involved in the initial stages of feeding *and* in close collaboration with nursing staff. A variety of manoeuvres are available to reduce the chances of aspiration. These include facilitating the swallowing reflex by the use of cold stimulation of the faucial arch and palate: an extension of this technique is the use of a palatal loop prosthesis which requires an orthodontic assessment. This device which is fitted to the teeth supports the paretic soft palate thus reducing the chance of nasal regurgitation but also may facilitate the swallowing reflex. Turning of the head and neck to one side may facilitate the safe passage of material through the non-paralysed side of the pharynx. The technique of a supraglottic swallow whereby the patient makes a deliberate inspiration, closes the glottis, then swallows, then breathes out may help prevent aspiration: teaching patients to voluntarily maintain laryngeal lift and backward tongue pressure after swallowing perhaps also helps. When the neck muscles are severely weak so that head posture cannot be maintained a neck support can assist swallowing. If, despite these efforts, there is evidence of clinically detrimental aspiration or inadequate hydration or nutrition other measures may be called for.

Salivary drooling can be a troublesome symptom particularly in cerebral palsy, extrapyramidal disease, and motor neurone disease. Loss of spontaneous swallowing related to bradykinesia particularly is associated with facial and lip diplegia or akinesia often underlie the problem. Salivary production may be temporarily reduced with anticholinergic drugs such as atropine or hyoscine: we have found the cautious use of glycopyrrolate subcutaneously (administered by nurse, carer, or patient) very useful although it is a non-licensed indication: more permanent ablation of saliva by radiotherapy or surgery is occasionally used. However, the consequences of a dry sore mouth, prone to infection, with thick tacky saliva may be less preferable than the social embarassment of drooling. Alternatively, the advice of an orthodontist may be sought, the possibility of a palatal training loop considered, and some have had success with diversion of the submandibular ducts.

Intubation (Wollman et al. 1995; Finucane and Bynum 1996; Norton et al. 1996)

In an acute new case at risk of serious aspiration, oral feeding and fluids should cease immediately: the usual immediate alternative is gastric intubation unless there is a major reason why enteral feeding should not be undertaken, in which case parenteral fluid and feeding is necessary. In chronically deteriorating dysphagia gastric intubation is less of an immediate necessity unless the patient has an acute pulmonary complication or is otherwise ill. The options need more careful consideration.

It is not always appreciated that establishing gastric feeding does not of itself fully protect against the possibility of aspiration (Logen and Weinryb 1989). Aspiration of saliva and nasal secretions, and aspiration of regurgitated or vomited stomach contents remains possible. Factors, apart from laryngeal dysfunction, which potentially make aspiration more likely are impaired consciousness (including sleep), hiatus hernia, incompetent gastro-oesophageal junction, previous cricopharyngeal myotomy, supine position, and lying on the left side so that the stomach contents lie in the fundus. Gastric feeding should normally be undertaken in the awake sitting patient or, if lying, turned on the right side to promote passage into the duodenum. Duodenal or jejunal intubation may be necessary in recurrent gastric regurgitation (Lazarus *et al.* 1990).

There are a wide range of artificial feeds of differing consistency, osmolality, and nutritional value and cost. The advice of the dietician is invaluable in determining which is the most suitable on an individual basis for the long term.

1. Nasogastric tube. Some patients find even fine-bore modern nasogastric tubes unpleasant and, if confused, often pull them out. The facial appearance, soreness of the anterior nares, the need to tape the tube to face, and the pharyngeal irritation, all make for an unsatisfactory long-term choice of feeding route. The tube itself probably has some inhibitory effect on the swallowing mechanism and the presence of a foreign body in the pharynx makes aspiration more likely. In patients with hiatus hernia, the tube may show a particular propensity to be regurgitated. However, the nasogastric tube is usually easy to replace, is easily removable, and cheap.

2. Percutaneous endoscopic gastrostomy (PEG). Delivery of adequate nutrition has been greatly improved by the advent of percutaneous endoscopic gastrostomy. Gastric endoscopy is necessary to place a fine bore tube through a small abdominal puncture and can be undertaken without general anaesthetic. Currently further endoscopy may be necessary to remove the gastrostomy tube but systems are now available to avoid this. The technique has the advantage of avoiding a tube on the face and in the pharynx. The whole system once placed is less conspicuous to the patient and the observer. There is often a need for sedation at the endoscopy and for some patients with combined respiratory and bulbar disorder this constitutes an additional hazard which in the context of a disabled neurological patient can be life-threatening. The patient and carer need to be warned about this and the implications of, for instance, needing to intubate the airway seriously considered. Placement in this context thus requires endoscopy, anaesthetic back-up, and hence hospitalization.

Serious complications of the procedure seem generally uncommon, however. In a number of centres the PEG has become the method of choice for gastric feeding and is undertaken in preference to nasogastric feeding at the earliest opportunity despite greater overall cost. Uncommonly, a formal laparotomy may need to be undertaken for gastrostomy usually because a history of previous surgery, abnormal anatomy (e.g. hiatus hernia or gastic resection), or technical difficulty with endoscopy.

Surgery

ENT surgeons obviously have considerable experience in dealing with aspiration and airway protection and their advice may be invaluable. A number of surgical procedures are available which may reduce the likelihood of aspiration and promote passage of food and liquid into the oesophagus. Cricopharyngeal myotomy has been widely used in neurogenic dysphagia but the criteria for effective use remain debated. If the predominant problem is at the oral stage of swallowing, as is often the case with, for instance, motor neurone disease, the procedure seems unlikely to help. If only small boluses can be presented to the pharynx or there is marked impairment of hyoid/laryngeal lift, the cricopharynx will not open in the normal manner but this does not give rise to the typical radiographic appearances of cricopharyngeal spasm on videofluoroscopy and myotomy is less clearly beneficial. Cricopharyngeal myotomy is most useful in patients who have a well-preserved oral phase and effectively triggered swallowing reflex, but radiological evidence of spasm when presented with an adequate bolus.

As has been emphasized earlier tracheostomy *per se* can do little to improve swallowing and may worsen it. Its principal merit in the current context is to improve access to the bronchial tree and trachea for suction purposes and to act as a port for ventilation if required. The cuffed tracheostomy tube does not reliably prevent aspiration. Further, a cuffed tube reduces the opportunity for and potential quality of speech. These considerations also apply to the placement of a so-called minitracheostomy which can have a major inhibitory effect on residual swallowing.

If the vocal cords are unilaterally or bilaterally paralysed, injection of teflon may help approximation and improve airway protection during a swallow (Woo *et al.* 1992). Various operations are sometimes undertaken on the epiglottis or false vocal cords to make laryngeal closure and protection more effective. Finally, formal operations may be undertaken to close the larynx *in situ* or to perform a laryngectomy with fashioning of an end-tracheostome for breathing. The latter procedure, in the context of progressive neurological disease, is only likely to be considered for intractable symptomatic aspiration or laryngeal spasm causing choking when there is irrecoverable loss of speech but reasonable respiratory function and relatively minor general disability. In the face of severe recurrent aspiration which has not responded to conventional therapy and, in a patient who may otherwise have reasonable quality of life (despite loss of speech), active consideration should possibly be given to these heroic measures more often than is currently the case in the United Kingdom (Baredes 1988; Blitzer *et al.* 1988).

COMBINED SWALLOWING AND BREATHING DIFFICULTY

Many neurological patients have combined disorders of breathing, speech, and swallowing. No simple rules can be applied to the wide range of clinical circumstances which this group encompass but the contributory factors for each patient need to be worked out and listed, bearing in mind each of the three major functional components (breathing, swallowing, and speech) and the options for management determined (see Table 21.6). It is essential to assess the *cumulative* burden of handicap which may accrue with these disorders. Taken alone, coping with anarthria requiring a communicator, dysphagia requiring a gastrostomy, or nocturnal respiratory insufficiency requiring a breathing aid may be quite tolerable for an otherwise able-bodied individual. In combination, however, or if individually added to *other* physical, mental, or social adversity, the burden of handicap may be altogether too much for some personalities to support even with good home care and effective hospital support (Glenn *et al.* 1980).

Table 21.6 Factors to be considered in long-term breathing or swallowing intervention

---

1. Does the patient have relevant symptoms and signs which may be effectively and most appropriately alleviated by mechanical intervention?
2. The underlying diagnosis and prognosis
3. Swallowing function
4. Respiratory function
5. Speech function
6. Other illnesses or injuries
7. The level of general physical disability especially mobility and use og arms
8. Cognitive and sensory disability
9. Are there preventable, reversible, or remediable factors which may alleviate the need for major intervention?
10. The domestic circumstances of the patient:
    (a) physical
    (b) relatives and carers
    (c) domiciliary availability of professional support (e.g. speech therapist physiotherapy, occupational therapy, general practitioner)
11. The level of hospital support and backup available
    (a) Medical (e.g. anaesthetic, ENT, neurological)
    (b) ITU facility for rapid admission and contact
    (c) Machine maintenance and servicing
    (d) Access to tubes, connections, suckers, etc.
    (e) Expert dietary, speech therapy, physiotherapy, and occupational therapy advice
12. Cost (funding) and availability of suitable equipment (e.g. ventilators)
13. Will the intervention change the end-point of the disease process?
14. Has the situation been fully explained to the relevant individuals more than once?
15. What are the considered and informed wishes of the patient and relatives?

Without either or both of the latter such disabilities become insupportable. In determining whether to intervene with mechanical swallowing or breathing aids on a long-term basis the factors summarized in Table 21.6 can usefully be enumerated and weighed up. The great variation between individuals and their level of support at home needs to be appreciated: the less robust the personality of the individual patient the greater the level of support both from hospital, community, and home is required.

REFERENCES

Ardran, G. and Kemp, F. (1967). The mechanism of the larynx. II. The epiglottis and closure of the larynx. *British Journal of Radiology*, **40**, 372–89.

Baredes, S. (1988). Surgical management of swallowing disorders. *Otolaryngologic Clinics of North America*, **21**, 711–20.

Berger, A. J., Mitchell, R. A., and Severinghaus, J. W. (1977). Regulation of respiration: III. *New England Journal of Medicine*, **297**, 194–201.

Blitzer, A., Krespi, K. P., Oppenheimer, R. W., and Levine, T. M. (1988). Surgical management of aspiration. *Otolaryngologic Clinics of North America*, **21**, 743–50.

Branthwaite, M. A. (1991). Non invasive and domiciliary ventilation: positive pressure techniques. *Thorax*, **46**, 208–12.

Cameron, J. L., Reynolds, J., and Zuidema, G. D. (1973). Aspiration in patients with tracheostomies. *Surgical Gynaecology and Obstetrics*, **136**, 68–70.

De Troyer, A., Estenne, M., and Heilporn, A. (1986). Mechanism of active expiration in tetraplegic subjects. *New England Journal of Medicine*, **314**, 740–4.

Donner, M. W., Bosma, J. F., and Robertson, D. L. (1985). Anatomy and physiology of the pharynx. *Gastrointestinal Radiology*, **10**, 196–212.

Finucane, T. E. and Bynum, J. P. (1996). Use of tube feeding to prevent aspiration pneumonia. *Lancet*, **348**, 1421–4.

Glenn W. W. L, Haak B., Sasaki C., and Kirchner J. (1980). Characteristics and surgical management of respiratory complications accompanying pathologic lesions of the brainstem. *Annals of Surgery* **191**: 655–63.

Glenn, W. W. L. and Phelps, M. L. (1985). Diaphragm pacing by electrical stimulation of the phrenic nerve. *Neurosurgery*, **17**, 974–84.

Goldman, M. D. (1982). Interpretation of thoraco-abdominal movements during breathing. *Clinical Science*, **62**, 7–11.

Green, M. and Moxham, J. (1985). The respiratory muscles. *Clinical Science*, **68**, 1–10.

Hamdy, S. Aziz, Q. Rothwell, J. C. Singh, K. D. Barlow, J. Hughes, D. G. *et al.* (1996). The cortical topography of human swallowing musculature in health and disease. *Nature Medicine*, **2**, 1217–24.

Hamnegard, C.-H. Wragg, S. Kyroussis, D. Mills, G. H. Polkey, M. I. Moran, J. *et al.* (1996). Diaphragm fatigue following maximum ventilation in man. *European Respiratory Journal*, **9**, 241–7.

Howard, R. S., Loh, L., and Wiles, C. M. (1988). Respiratory complications and their management in motor neurone disease. *Brain*, **112**, 1155–70.

Howard, R. S., Wiles, C. M., Hirsch, N. P., and Spencer, G. T. (1993). Respiratory involvement and its management in primary disorders of muscle. *Quarterly Journal of Medicine*, **86**, 175–9.

Hughes, R. A. C. and Bihari, D. (1993). Acute neuromuscular respiratory paralysis. *Journal of Neurology, Neurosurgery and Psychiatry*, **56**, 334–43.

Hughes, T. A. T. and Wiles, C. M. (1996*a*). Clinical measurement of swallowing in health and in neurogenic dysphagia. *Quarterly Journal of Medicine*, **89**, 109–16.

Hughes, T. A. T. and Wiles, C. M. (1996*b*). Palatal and pharyngeal reflexes in health and in motor neuron disease. *Journal of Neurology, Neurosurgery and Psychiatry*, **61**, 96–8.

Kidd, D., Lawson, J., Nesbitt, R., and MacMahon, J. (1993). Aspiration in acute stroke: a clinical study with videofluoroscopy. *Quarterly Journal of Medicine*, **86**, 825–9.

Kidd, D., Lawson, J., Nesbitt, R., and MacMahon, J. (1995). The natural history and clinical consequences of aspiration in acute stroke. *Quarterly Journal of Medicine*, **88**, 409–13.

Lazarus, B. A., Murphy, J. B., and Culpepper, L. (1990). Aspiration associated with long-term gastric versus jejunal feeding: a critical analysis of the literature. *Archives of Physical Medicine and Rehabilitation*, **71**, 46–53.

Logemann, J. A. (1988*a*). The role of the Speech Language Pathologist in the management of dysphagia. *Otolaryngologic Clinics of North America*, **21**, 783–8.

Logemann, J. A. (1988*b*). Swallowing physiology and pathophysiology. *Otolaryngologic Clinics of North America*, **21**, 613–23.

Logen, R. and Weinryb, J. (1989). Aspiration pneumonia in nursing home patients fed via gastrostomy tubes. *American Journal of Gastroenterology*, **84**, 1509–12.

Loh, L. (1986). Neurological and Neuromuscular Disease. *British Journal of Anaesthesia*, **58**, 190–200.

Miller, A. J. (1982). Deglutition. *Physiological Reviews*, **62**, 129–84.

Murphy, K., Mier, A., Adams, L., and Guz, A. (1990). Putative cerebral cortical involvement in the ventilatory response to inhaled CO_2 in conscious man. *Journal of Physiology*, **420**, 4–18.

Nathan, P. W. (1963). The descending respiratory pathway in man. *Journal of Neurology, Neurosurgery and Psychiatry*, **26**, 487–99.

Newsom Davis, J., Goldman, M., Loh, L., and Casson, M. (1976). Diaphragm function and alveolar hypoventilation. *Quarterly Journal of Medicine*, **45**, 87–100.

Norton, B., Homer-Ward, M., Donnelly, M. T., Long, R. G., and Holmes, G. K. T. (1996). A randomised prospective comparison of percutaneous endoscopic gastrostomy and nasogastric tube feeding after acute dysphagic stroke. *British Medical Journal*, **312**, 13–16.

Roussos, C. (1982). The respiratory muscles. *New England Journal of Medicine*, **307**, 786–97.

Schneerson, J. (1988). *Disorders of ventilation*. Oxford: Blackwell Scientific.

Schneerson, J. M. (1991). Non invasive and domiciliary ventilation: negative pressure techniques. *Thorax*, **46**, 131–5.

Selley, W. G., Flack, F. C., Ellis, R. E., and Brooks, W. A. (1989*a*). Respiratory patterns associated with swallowing: Part 1. The normal adult pattern and changes with age. *Age and Aging*, **18**, 168–72.

Selley, W. G., Flack, F. C., Ellis, R. E., and Brooks, W. A. (1989*b*). Respiratory patterns associated with swallowing: part 2. Neurologically impaired patients. *Age and Aging*, **18**, 173–6.

Smith, P. E. M., Edwards, R. H. T., and Calverly, P. M. (1991). Mechanisms of sleep disordered breathing in chronic neuromuscular disease: implications for management. *Quarterly Journal of Medicine*, **81**, 961–74.

Stradling, J. R. and Phillipson, E. A. (1986). Breathing disorders during sleep. *Quarterly Journal of Medicine*, **58**, 3–18.

Tarrant, S. C., Ellis, R. E., Flack, F. C., and Selley, W. G. (1997). Comparative review of techniques for recording respiratory events at rest and during deglutition. *Dysphagia*, **12**, 24–38.

Wade, D. T. and Hewer, R. L. (1987). Motor loss and swallowing difficulty after stroke: frequency, recovery and prognosis. *Acta Neurologica Scandinavica*, **76**, 50–4.

Wiles, C. M. (1996). Neurological complication of severe illness and prolonged mechanical ventilation. *Thorax*, **51**(**suppl. 2**). S40–4.

Wollman, B., D'Agostino, H. B., Walus-Wigle, J. R., Easter, D. W., and Beale, A. (1995). Radiologic, endoscopic and surgical gastrostomy: an institutional evaluation and meta-analysis of the literature. *Radiology*, **197**, 699–704.

Woo, J. S., Van Hasselt, C. A., and Chan, H. S. (1992). Teflon injection for unilateral vocal cord paralysis and its effect on lung function. *Clinical Otolaryngology*, **17**, 497–500.

22 | *Muscle spasticity*

Richard J. Hardie

It is conventional in clinical neurology to distinguish between upper and lower motor neurone features in patients with significant motor weakness in order to establish an accurate differential diagnosis. Muscle spasticity is the commonest and perhaps most reliable clinical sign of the upper motor neurone (UMN) syndrome, signifying pathological involvement of the central nervous system (CNS), along with a characteristic pyramidal pattern of weakness affecting certain muscle groups more than others, tendon hyperreflexia, clonus, and also extensor plantar or Babinski responses (Table 22.1).

Other associated positive features may include exaggerated autonomic and cutaneous reflexes with pain and the release of so-called flexor spasms, and also other forms of increased muscle tone ranging from mobile dystonia through rigidity to fixed deformity, and even contracture. Possibly more disabling is the tendency for abnormal patterns of muscle contraction to occur during voluntary movement, including simultaneous co-contraction of agonist and antagonist muscles at the same joint or of multiple muscle groups in the same (overflow) or contralateral limb (synkinesia) and certain reflex patterns of gross movement known as associated reactions.

As well as weakness, the UMN syndrome comprises negative features that are harder to define. Thus, following a cerebral stroke, patients may exhibit fatiguability and impaired

Table 22.1 Features of the upper motor neurone syndrome

Positive	Negative
Muscle spasticity	Muscle weakness in pyramidal pattern
Tendon hyperreflexia	Fatiguability
Clonus	Impaired timing and sequence of movements
Babinski responses	Impaired dexterity
Pain	Loss of learned motor programmes
Exaggerated autonomic and cutaneous reflexes	
Spontaneous flexor spasms	
Dystonia and abnormal postures	
Co-contraction– agonist/antagonist overflow synkinesia	
Associated reactions	

dexterity with defects in timing and sequencing of movements, presumably due to loss of specialized learned motor programmes with retention of less complicated semi-volitional movements.

Spasticity is distinguished from rigidity by the clasp-knife phenomenon and the increased dynamic sensitivity of stretch reflexes, apparent clinically by the excessive amplitude of the tendon reflexes (hyperreflexia) with clonus and the irradiation or spread of reflexes. Although there is no electromyographic (EMG) activity in spastic human muscles at rest, a rapid (dynamic) stretch elicits a reflex contraction whose force is proportional to the velocity of stretch but suddenly diminishes or gives way beyond a certain point, hence the term 'clasp-knife phenomenon'. This is best appreciated clinically in certain lower limb muscles such as the gastrocnemius and quadriceps.

The confusing term 'upper motor neurone' is unfortunately a firm part of the clinical vocabulary. Strictly, it may refer to any neurones descending from above to influence the spinal lower, alpha motor neurones, but conventionally it is used synonymously with corticospinal or pyramidal tract neurone. Similarly, although 'extrapyramidal tracts' technically describes any descending pathway outside the medullary pyramids, it has come to imply only those originating from the basal ganglia. The anatomical arrangements in humans are such that pathological processes seldom if ever damage the pyramidal system anywhere along its course without also damaging adjacent parapyramidal tracts. Hence it is unwise ever to equate the clinical UMN syndrome with selective damage to the corticospinal tract which alone, it has been concluded, is unlikely to play a major role in the production of spasticity (Brown 1994).

Although often easy to detect and recognize, spasticity is still poorly understood and difficult to manage clinically. One reason may be that pure spasticity seldom occurs in isolation; for example, many children with developmental disabilities have a combination of other motor impairments including dystonia and choreo-athetoid involuntary movements. The underlying mechanism may well be important, for spasticity following an acute event such as stroke or CNS trauma may require different management from that in progressive degenerative disorders. Some authors believe that spasticity after spinal cord damage differs clinically from that of cerebral origin. Furthermore, clinical assessment may not correlate well with neurophysiological or biomechanical evaluation in the laboratory, and the functional relevance of spasticity must always be considered. Thus, measures to reduce spasticity will not correct other aspects of the UMN syndrome, may not necessarily improve activities such as walking, and may even make things worse.

PHYSIOLOGY

PERIPHERAL MECHANICAL FACTORS IN SPASTICITY

Direct measurement of the resistance to slow passive stretch at the elbow or ankle of hemiparetic stroke patients has recently confirmed the importance of mechanical changes in the musculo-tendinous unit itself. Although secondary to the neurological impairment, there is good evidence of alterations in muscle protein synthesis and fibre morphology as well as in tendon compliance and peri-articular connective tissue (Thilmann *et al.* 1991; O'Dwyer *et al.* 1996). Contractures are commonly associated with long-standing and severe spasticity, when even soft tissue calcification can occur, but the extent to which less severe mechanical changes might be prevented by early intervention in hypertonia is unknown.

THE ALPHA-SKELETOMOTOR NEURONE

There are numerous inputs, perhaps about a dozen, on to the lower motor neurones which are in the anterior horn of the spinal cord and comprise what Sherrington termed the 'final common pathway' for all nervous influences on skeletal muscle. These inputs determine both the number of motor neurones recruited at a given spinal segmental level and their rate of discharge, the output which in turn affects the force of muscle contraction. These neurones have extensive dendritic trees and enormous numbers of synaptic connections which provide infinite variation of resting membrane potential.

There is some evidence to suggest excessive alpha-motor neurone excitability in spasticity, perhaps by failure of normal GABA-mediated presynaptic inhibition. However, there is no EMG activity at rest and the abnormalities seem to be rather of sensitivity of segmental stretch reflex activity. The following discussion is a very simplified account of the complex anatomy and physiology of a typical spinal segment.

THE MONOSYNAPTIC SEGMENTAL STRETCH REFLEX

The fundamental unit mediating the tendon jerks examined by clinicians is the monosynaptic segmental stretch reflex arc whereby muscles are held at constant length and movement is restrained. If the muscle is stretched quickly, the primary annulospiral ending (ASE) situated in the muscle spindle is lengthened and the type Ia afferent neurone is stimulated. Via a monosynaptic connection, excitatory amino acid receptors on the alpha-efferent lower motor neurone activate the main

or extrafusal muscle fibres which develop the tension necessary to resist attempted movement (i.e. a negative feedback loop).

Within the muscle spindle (intrafusal) there are also a few weak muscle fibres unable to develop significant tension. Between the two contractile ends of the spindle is a capsule filled with nuclei (the nuclear bag) that contains not only the ASE but also the secondary endings of smaller type II afferents, descriptively termed 'flowerspray endings'. The spindles have an efferent nerve supply of their own, fusimotor fibres belonging to the type A-gamma. Since the spindles are attached at either end to the sides of the extrafusal fibres or to the tendon, the intrafusal fibres lie in parallel to the rest and undergo identical alterations in length.

Normally, tonic activity in the gamma-efferent system maintains tension in intrafusal fibres and hence on the ASE. Afferent impulses from the stretched ASE stimulate the alpha-efferent in turn, contributing to the normal muscle tone which resists passive lengthening. Whereas stimulation of the gamma-efferents cannot lead to detectable muscle contraction, it does increase the tension on the ASE. If the whole muscle is now lengthened the degree of afferent activity is significantly enhanced, so the resulting muscle contractions will be more marked and occur at a lower threshold.

Conversely, if gamma-efferent activity is abolished, as for example in the acute spinal animal, the intrafusal fibres are slack and considerable stretch of the whole muscle will be required to stimulate any afferent discharge from the ASE. Tonic discharge in the alpha efferents is considerably reduced (i.e. hypotonia and the threshold of the stretch reflex correspondingly increased, as in hyporeflexia). The normal gamma activity or 'fusimotor bias' in effect presets the sensitivity of the negative feedback loop reflex arc and constitutes a servo-mechanism whereby the afferent signal may be amplified or attenuated.

Although regulation of muscle length by the monosynaptic segmental stretch reflex used to be considered the principal mechanism of load compensation during motor actions, whereby muscle force was adjusted according to externally applied loads, the gamma-operated reflex is probably more important in the stabilisation of posture (Davidoff 1992). Similarly, although increased fusimotor bias is often assumed to be an important factor determining spasticity, there is little data to support this (Burke 1983).

OTHER SEGMENTAL REFLEXES

Golgi tendon organs (GTO) are proprioceptors lying at the origin or insertion of small groups of extrafusal fibres into a tendon or aponeurosis. In contrast to spindles, they respond not to passive stretch but to active muscle contraction. Whereas type Ia afferents discharge mainly in response to rapid phasic muscle stretch detected by the primary ASE, secondary flowerspray endings within muscle spindles have little dynamic sensitivity but their response slowly adapts to steady stretch and is carried via type II afferents. These, and type Ib afferents from GTOs, make mainly disynaptic connections onto motor neurones whereby flexion and extension in reciprocal muscle groups are co-ordinated, but do not seem themselves to contribute to spasticity. The reflexes of spastic muscles in response to stretch are facilitated at rest, a phenomenon which progressively diminishes and is believed to be mediated by type II and III non-spindle afferents.

SPINAL INTERNEURONES

These provide a further intricate network in addition to the alpha-motor neuronal dendritic arborization whereby different peripheral afferent systems and descending supraspinal pathways converge to influence segmental efferent activity. Many neurotransmitters are believed to be involved including glutamate, aspartate, and a wide range of neuropeptides. There are three groups of interneurones that are particularly important.

Before they exit the spinal cord, alpha-motor neurone axons give rise to recurrent cholinergic collateral branches that stimulate nicotinic receptors on the inhibitory interneurones known as Renshaw cells. These synapse in turn with the original as well as other synergistic alpha-motor neurones to provide negative feedback known as recurrent inhibition, probably mediated by glycine receptors, although they have other more diverse connections as well.

Not only do afferent type Ia neurones from ASEs directly stimulate alpha-motor neurones innervating the stretched muscles, but they also give rise to collateral branches that excite inhibitory interneurones acting, probably also via glycine receptors, on alpha-motor neurones to antagonist muscles. This is termed 'reciprocal inhibition'. Other collaterals from both type Ia and GTO (type Ib) afferents ('autogenic inhibition') stimulate non-reciprocal group I inhibitory interneurones acting on agonist alpha-motor neurones, probably via GABA receptors. There is good clinical evidence for increased recurrent inhibition via Renshaw cell activity in human spinal cord injury (Shefner *et al.* 1992) and reduced reciprocal inhibition may also contribute to spasticity.

Electrical stimulation of a large range of afferent neurones is known to mediate a pattern of excitation and inhibition that results in ipsilateral flexion of a limb and crossed extension. In the intact animal, these exteroceptive reflexes would withdraw the limb from the stimulus and increase support provided by the opposite limb to maintain stance. Afferents belonging to both types II and III, and coming from cutaneous and joint receptors as well as muscle spindle secondary endings, presumably share common interneuronal projections with polysynaptic connections at segmental level and are often termed 'flexor reflex afferents'. However, their precise action depends upon descending suprasegmental influences.

Enhanced transmission in flexor reflex pathways in the recovery phase from cord injury after spinal shock is thought to account for the often distressing problem of flexor spasms. Cutaneous reflexes appear in which noxious stimuli or even light touch results in withdrawal of the limb and may be accompanied by emptying of the bladder or rectum (the mass reflex).

The overall effect then in spasticity is a pathological increase in the response of alpha-motor neurones to proprioceptive input mediated by the so-called propriospinal interneurone system, which acts as an excitatory system and recruits widely from other surrounding motor neurones. There is evidence for abnormal excessive gain of the stretch reflex rather than a reduction in the response threshold during passive stretch (Thilmann *et al.* 1991), although this is disputed and there are undoubtedly even more complex changes in reflex activity in spastic limbs during active movement (Ibrahim *et al.* 1993; Ada *et al.* 1998).

DESCENDING SUPRASPINAL INFLUENCES

Focal lesions of the cerebral motor cortex alone do not seem to lead to spasticity. Ablation of Brodmann area 4 in monkeys results in a contralateral flaccid hemiplegia with hyporeflexia, and isolated lesions of the premotor cortex are associated with subtle impairments of learned and other movements. Furthermore, sudden interruption of UMN pathways in the brain or spinal cord immediately results in flaccid paralysis and absent tendon reflexes. This state of cerebral or spinal shock is thought to be due to the abrupt cessation of tonic bombardment of spinal neurones by descending impulses both excitatory and inhibitory, and may last several weeks. The later development of spasticity presumably reflects release of pathological mechanisms by damage not just to the corticospinal tracts but also more widely to other subcortical or more caudal structures.

Various brainstem structures give rise to several different pathways that descend into the spinal cord and exert facilitatory or inhibitory influences upon segmental reflexes. These include the reticular formation and the vestibular and red nuclei, although the clinical relevance of the numerous descending tracts distinguished on anatomical and pharmacological grounds remains uncertain (Brown 1994). Normal muscle tone is determined by a balance of their activity, and thus different clinical pictures may result from certain patterns of pathological involvement (Fig. 22.1). The ventromedial reticular formation exerts a powerful inhibitory effect, for which input from the cerebral cortex seems to be essential and without which therefore spasticity results after vascular or traumatic lesions of the frontal cortex or internal capsule. This inhibitory pathway descends principally in the dorsal reticulospinal tract (DRST) which, judging from the results of cordotomies in neurosurgical patients, runs in the dorsal half of the lateral columns of the human spinal cord (Brown 1994). Facilitatory effects on muscle tone arise from other parts of the reticular formation independent of any cortical input and descend in the ventral reticulospinal tracts (VRST). Thus, damage to the ventral parts of the spinal cord alone is not normally associated with spasticity.

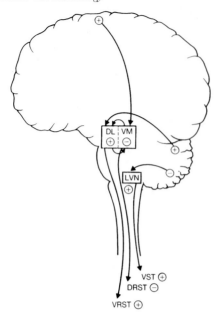

Fig. 22.1 Central influences on the segmental stretch reflex. DL, dorsolateral reticular formation; VM, ventromedial; LVN, lateral vestibular nucleus; VRST, ventral reticulospinal tract; DRST, dorsal reticulospinal tract; VST, vestibulospinal tract. (Reproduced with permission from: Hardie, R. J. and Lees, A. J. (1992). Control of movement and its clinical disorders. In *Neurosurgery–the scientific basis of clinical practice*, (2nd edn), (ed. H. A. Crockard, R. D. Hayward, and J. T. Hoff). Blackwell Science, London.

Flexor reflexes, which produce limb withdrawal in response to noxious stimuli, are normally suppressed by the activity of the DRST and are typically released by spinal cord damage affecting the lateral columns. The Babinski response is actually part of a generalized withdrawal response disinhibited by interruption of UMN pathways. Decerebrate rigidity seems to arise because of loss of inhibition of facilitatory descending projections and a generalized increase in gamma-efferent activity particularly in the extensor muscles. The flexor reflex afferents are effectively switched off and the clinically characteristic posture of opisthotonus and rigid extension of all four limbs may result.

Although spindle sensitivity is normal, established spasticity can be reduced by interruption of dorsal root inputs to the propriospinal interneurone system, which facilitates alpha-efferent activity when deprived of supraspinal influences. Plasticity within the spinal cord including terminal sprouting of axons and the development of receptor hypersensitivity is believed to mediate the delayed appearance of spasticity and hyperreflexia after complete transection of the cord. The prominence of often severe flexor spasms in this clinical setting suggests that they are normally inhibited by the VRST as well as the DRST.

It is also perhaps worth mentioning here the possible contribution of cortical plasticity to the UMN syndrome. Following various types of insult to the brain or spinal cord,

functional imaging and magnetic stimulation studies have shown alterations in regional blood flow, metabolic rate, and somatotopic organization of the sensorimotor cortex with reductions in the size of the cortical representation areas of weak and/or spastic body parts. To what extent this may be reversed by, for example, sensory stimulation, active physiotherapy, or other interventions is not known, but worthy of study.

MANAGEMENT OF MUSCLE SPASTICITY

Spasticity never occurs in isolation, and it affects all aspects of human movement. It has great pathological heterogeneity and is difficult to define and measure. Therefore, a functional problem-orientated approach to its management is recommended. Because of the complexities of assessment and treatment, collaboration in difficult cases is important within a multidisciplinary team combining the skills of clinical neurology and paediatrics, nursing, physiotherapy, occupational therapy, orthotist, and rehabilitation engineer. Orthopaedic or neurosurgical expertise may also occasionally be necessary.

ASSESSMENT

Physicians are trained to differentiate motor impairments caused by weakness, spasticity, ataxia, bradykinesia, and various types of involuntary movement. However, it may be impossible to evaluate clinically the relative severity of two types of motor impairment in combination. Objective methods of assessment, where these exist, have usually been developed and standardized in those with one relatively isolated impairment, and cannot be used to diagnose or differentiate other types of motor disorder.

As discussed in the introduction to this chapter, spasticity is just one component of the UMN syndrome with a wide range of other complex motor deficits already listed in Table 22.1. Many diverse factors including fatigue, pain, and anxiety influence the level of spasticity, extrapyramidal rigidity may coexist and thus objective measurement is extremely difficult (DeSouza and Musa 1987). Most therapists and physicians attempt to grade spasticity clinically on a simple semi-quantitative (but non-linear) scale from absent through mild and moderate to severe. The Ashworth scale, with several arbitrary intermediate points defined (Table 22.2), has been developed for research purposes and has good inter-rater reliability (Bohannon and Smith 1987). Some variability can be eliminated by testing under uniform conditions at consistent times of the day.

There is only limited correlation between spasticity and various electrophysiological measures, such as amplitude and latency of the H and tonic stretch reflexes, F waves, and central motor conduction time. Such quantitative methods are also time-consuming and hence of little practical value. Biomechanical measurements of resistance of a body part to passive movement generally require complex apparatus, with

Table 22.2 Ashworth scale of muscle spasticity

0. Normal muscle tone
1. Slight increase in muscle tone (e.g. catch and release or minimal resistance during part of the range of motion)
2. Moderate increase in muscle tone through most of the range of motion, but affected part(s) easily moved
3. Severe increase in muscle tone making passive movement difficult
4. Affected part(s) rigid in flexion or extension

There is also a 6-point modified Ashworth scale used by some authors (See Wade, 1992).

the notable exception of the Wartenburg knee pendulum test, which describes passive movement restraint as the angular displacement of a limb when it is left to oscillate freely. However, most fail to take account of other variables such as joint contractures and muscle viscoelasticity although, theoretically at least, EMG silence in an antagonist muscle during passive movement excludes spasticity as the cause of increased resistance. Electromechanical measurement of torque during controlled displacement at a particular joint and of voluntary force production is measurable experimentally but so far has no practical clinical application.

Furthermore, the functional relevance of spasticity measurement remains doubtful, not least because it may differ between passive and active movement. In patients with UMN lesions therefore, spasticity should be viewed as one of many possible factors limiting the development of normal voluntary movement. It can sometimes actually be beneficial, and its clinical assessment must be conducted with all this in mind.

The consequences of spasticity can best be considered to form a hierarchy of motor impairments and disabilities (Table 22.3). In addition to the standard evaluation of posture

Table 22.3 Hierarchy of motor impairments and disabilities

Spontaneous motor phenomena:
  clonus
  flexor/extensor spasms
Passive movements:
  resistance to passive stretch
  range of motion
Posture:
  postural tone and deformity
  maintenance of stability
  postural reflexes
Active movements:
  force
  range of motion
  speed of initiation and action
  synergistic agonist and/or antagonist movements
  synkinetic (contralateral) movements
  accuracy and adaptability
Manual dexterity
Maintenance of static and dynamic balance
Personal care skills
Transfers and mobility
Ambulation

and range of movement in all joints, physiotherapists have introduced a number of reliable and validated methods of bedside spasticity assessment, mainly examining effects on normal voluntary movements (de Neve *et al.* 1992). The Bobath method incorporates a qualitative judgement of ability to perform particular movements, either in isolation or in opposition to defined patterns of spasticity. The more quantitative Motor Club assessment was developed to follow the pattern of recovery after stroke, and evaluates the ability to perform a series of normal movement patterns and also certain functional activities mainly relevant to physiotherapeutic goals. Various other validated generic measures of disability in performance of activities of daily living such as the Barthel scale are available to complete the hierarchy of assessments (see Wade 1992).

Finally, the temporal aspects of spasticity must be considered. This is particularly important in children still undergoing motor development, but short-term improvements may occur at any age after some interventions without being sustained. Hence, long-term prospective studies are essential and should assess the incidence of late complications in what is after all usually a chronic condition.

GOAL-SETTING

Having assessed the individual patient's problems, the problem-orientated approach requires careful selection and prioritizing of treatment goals before planning appropriate intervention. The usual complaints of patients with spasticity are the so-called negative symptoms of weakness, fatiguability, and lack of dexterity and it is debatable whether they will improve with specific treatment to reduce spasticity, although positive symptoms such as fixed deformity and painful flexor spasms may be relieved. Moreover, spasticity may sometimes be beneficial, for example, in the leg extensors enabling a person to stand or even walk, and the value of any treatment questioned. Landau (1977) warns about spasticity 'the fable of a neurological demon and the emperor's new therapy'. Possible treatment goals are listed in Table 22.4.

INTERVENTIONS

A wide range of interventions for the relief of spasticity is available and often used, perhaps reflecting the failure of any one of them to be outstandingly successful. They constitute a hierarchy of measures including basic physical therapy

Table 22.4 Possible goals in the treatment of spasticity

General aim	Specific areas
Improve function	ambulation, manual dexterity, speech, sphincters
Improve cosmesis	Posture, deformity, clonus
Reduce pain	Flexor spasms, mass action
Reduce complications	Contractures, tissue damage, chest and bladder infections

techniques, pharmacological intervention, and a variety of more invasive nerve blocks and surgical procedures. These will be considered individually but are invariably used in combination and aggressive preventive measures before spasticity becomes fully established and disabling are still the most likely to improve outcome.

Prevention

The importance of minimizing secondary mechanical changes to muscles and tendons has already been mentioned, although the time course of their natural development has not been well studied. Many factors known to make established spasticity worse may also initiate it by increasing afferent input. The avoidance of nociceptive stimuli during the acute phase of cerebral or spinal cord injury, with scrupulous attention to care of the skin, bladder, and bowels, may minimize the eventual level of spasticity. In addition, proprioceptive facilitation in the early stages may be valuable by maintaining joint mobility and promoting the development of helpful extensor synergies. Until more effective neuroprotective treatment is developed to ameliorate the underlying pathology however, prevention often remains more a desirable rather than achievable goal.

Physical measures

As has already been shown, the intensity of spasticity varies greatly according to a wide range of factors including diverse afferent inputs and fluctuations in endogenous influences such as arousal and activity levels. Even modest exercise increases spasticity and is best avoided if practicable before bathing, transferring, or retiring to bed, for example, where spasticity interferes with these activities.

Not only does spasticity vary spontaneously but it may also be altered considerably by changes in position of adjacent or affected body parts. Attention to principles of positioning patients can reduce muscle tone and associated complications such as the development of painful contractures or skin breakdown. If walking is difficult, subjects spend excessive periods supine or sitting, and daily programmes should promote periods of standing and of lying on either side and prone. Positioning aids can be made or are available commercially, such as pads, wedges, low-pressure seating cushions, and standing frames. The selection of an appropriately designed wheelchair or other seating system is very important, and lumbar extensor muscle activity can be altered greatly by adjusting head position and seat angles.

Nociceptive stimuli can make established spasticity markedly worse. These include bladder infections, faecal impaction, pressure sores, paronychia, or even tight clothing, and should be avoided or removed. Patients must be educated accordingly. Various physical therapies such as massage, vibration, cold and heat have been advocated, but the most effective seems to be prolonged passive stretching of spastic muscles (Tardieu *et al.* 1988). Apart from preventing contractures, an essential management aim, this diminishes spasticity for hours afterwards and can be taught and done twice daily at home, whereas the application of ice gives only temporary benefit. Time spent daily in a standing frame is of course a form of passive stretching, which is complementary to positioning techniques. Different methods of electrical stimulation and/or EMG biofeedback have been claimed to reduce spasticity but objective evidence is lacking.

There is little or no objective evidence about the value of or indications for splints or plaster casting, another form of passive stretching, in spastic limbs. They should certainly be as precise and close-fitting as possible and ideally the patient's skin should be free from breakdown in those areas to be covered. Some stretching of soft tissues must be possible to achieve anything useful and therefore a minimum adequate range of motion is necessary, unless prevention of an existing deformity worsening is the only goal.

Casting is traditionally recommended for those with generalized or more severe spasticity and functional abilities already limited. Serial casting with solid plaster cylinders can be extremely effective at reducing contractures provided that circulation and sensation is checked regularly. Each cast is changed after 4–10 days until no new gain in range of motion is achieved. Removable bivalve casts can then be made of a more durable material such as fibreglass or polypropylene to maintain those gains.

Many different upper limb splints have been devised, some based on theoretical principles of reflex-inhibiting postures advocated by various schools of physiotherapy. The cubital fossa or palm are the commonest sites of skin breakdown because of a combination of sustained pressure, poor ventilation, and inadequate hygiene which can be prevented by appropriate orthoses.

DRUGS

Oral drugs

Three drugs, each with a different mechanism of action, are widely used orally. They are likely to vary in their efficacy against spasticity of different neurophysiological origins (Young 1989).

Benzodiazepines, such as diazepam, are believed to facilitate GABA neurotransmission and thus presynaptic inhibition of stretch reflexes. They act centrally at various supraspinal levels and at both pre- and postsynaptic sites mainly in the spinal cord. Diazepam is of greatest clinical value in those with spinal spasticity due to partial spinal cord lesions, provided drowsiness is tolerated. The anti-spasticity effect lasts longer than the immediate sedative action so it is best taken as a single daily dose at bedtime. The average dose is about 15 mg daily. However, well-known complications of chronic therapy exist, and many patients feel too drowsy. Few other benzodiazepines have been studied in any detail.

Baclofen is an analogue of GABA with both pre- and postsynaptic actions that inhibit alpha- and gamma-motor neurones. It was an early and successful 'designer drug'. GABA itself does not cross the blood–brain barrier so pharmacologists tried introducing lipophilic substituents such as a phenyl nucleus to the basic amino acid molecule. Beta-phenyl-GABA was found to be orally active but, when other structurally related compounds were synthesized, the addition of a halogen substituent conferred greater efficacy. Thus, beta-4-chloro-phenyl-GABA emerged as a potential GABA-mimetic, for which the partial acronym baclofen was coined.

It was introduced into clinical practice in the 1970s, and since then considerable doubts have emerged as to its true mechanism of action. Bicuculline is classically an antagonist at GABA receptors but at similar concentrations does not antagonize the actions of baclofen. It is now generally agreed that baclofen probably acts mainly on presynaptic terminals in the spinal cord to depress the release of some as yet unidentified excitatory transmitter. However, a population of GABA receptors in the mammalian nervous system has been identified that is pharmacologically distinct and insensitive to bicuculline, so it is possible that baclofen exerts some of its action through these GABA-B receptors.

It has proved particularly effective against flexor spasms in spastic legs and also relieves pain, while causing less sedation than other centrally acting drugs (Young 1989). Although generally well tolerated with few adverse effects, large doses are often required and dose-limiting sedation is often encountered. Other adverse effects include muscle weakness and fatigue. Thus, low daily doses (e.g. 10–15 mg) should be used initially and gradually increased according to response. Optimum benefit usually occurs from 30 mg to 80 mg daily.

The infusion of baclofen directly into the lumbar subarachnoid space produces cerebrospinal fluid (CSF) levels of the drug that are 10 times higher than those achieved by oral administration, even though the amounts infused are 100 times less than those taken by mouth. Thus, it has also been administered intrathecally with some success for periods of a year or more via an implantable pump which can be programmed to produce steady-state CSF concentrations (Ordia *et al.* 1996).

The drug remains stable and soluble in the pump reservoir at body temperature and does not produce cognitive side-effects in therapeutic doses, although inadvertent overdose may result in reversible respiratory depression or coma and careful dose titration is required (Teddy *et al.* 1992). Most studies have concentrated on lower limb spasticity in spinal cord injury, although limited experience suggests comparable benefit in cerebral lesions (Becker *et al.* 1997).

Dantrolene acts directly on muscle, inhibiting excitation/contraction coupling by depressing calcium release from the sarcoplasmic reticulum. Its peripheral site of action means that it should be effective in unselected cases of spasticity of any aetiology, although it also means that weakness is the commonest unwanted result. It is therefore probably of most use in those patients with good strength who are limited by their spasticity, or those with complete paralysis. Treatment is usually started at 75 mg daily with average optimal daily doses of 100–200 mg up to a maximum of 5–10 mg/kg body weight. Because of a relatively high (1–2%) incidence of hepatic toxicity, liver function should be monitored regularly.

Other oral drugs. Many other drugs have been tested for antispasticity efficacy. Those that have some limited actions include morphine, phenothiazines, tetrahydrocannabinol, and clonidine. The most promising newer agent is tizanidine which, like clonidine, is a centrally acting alpha-2 agonist (Young 1994). It is believed to inhibit preferentially polysynaptic spinal transmission by reducing release of excitatory amino acids, and has been claimed to cause little muscle weakness. Although it has been available in North America and certain European countries for many years, experience in the UK is limited.

Nerve blocks

While more conservative measures are naturally preferable, the judicious use of proximal motor nerve or more distal branch ('motor point') blocks can be simple and effective provided the critical muscle can be identified by EMG. Injection of local anaesthetic can be tried initially to produce transient weakness although temporary sensory loss will also occur. If beneficial, ethanol or 5% phenol will produce chemical neurolysis with a similar motor effect lasting for several months. Motor point blocks reduce dynamic stretch reflexes and clonus with relative sparing of voluntary movements, and selective blockade of gamma-efferents has been suggested as the possible mechanism. Repeated or more concentrated injections may be used to produce irreversible nerve damage in selected cases.

Motor point blocks are particularly useful in preventing deformity, since the muscle is effectively paralysed, but function may also be improved. They may permit proper fitting of an orthosis, relieve painful muscle spasms, or even improve walking. The most commonly performed blocks are to triceps surae, the hip adductors and the finger and wrist flexors. Non-selective infiltration of muscle, and direct injection of one or more spinal roots or peripheral nerve trunks, can also be done using the same techniques. Serious complications are uncommon in experienced hands but unwanted weakness and peripheral oedema do occur. If major nerve trunks are injected that contain significant numbers of cutaneous sensory fibres, there is also a significant chance of painful dysaesthesia, although these may be temporary.

Because of the risks of non-specific damage, particularly to sphincter function, intrathecal neurolysis by injection of phenol around the cauda equina was usually restricted to relief of spasticity in those already incontinent or catheterized but baclofen is now usually preferable.

Botulinum toxin

Botulinum toxin type A (BTX-A) is a potent neurotoxin which binds irreversibly to presynaptic cholinergic neurones and prevents calcium-mediated transmitter release, thereby producing non-depolarizing blockade at motor endplates. When injected into muscles, it produces temporary weakness usually for up to three months. Although it has been more widely used in focal dystonias, it is also of benefit in the relief of spasticity (Dunne *et al.* 1995). BTX-A dosage is usually expressed in biological units known as mouse units based on the mean lethal dose (LD50) for laboratory mice. Confusingly, there are two different pharmaceutical preparations currently available whose potencies are not directly equivalent, both freeze-dried and requiring dilution in saline. There is uncertainty about the best method of delivering BTX-A regarding optimum dilution and the number of injection sites per muscle, but the toxin seems to diffuse adequately within the tissue to produce dose-dependent weakness. Dosage is usually estimated according to the relative mass of the target muscle.

Its current high cost would prove prohibitively expensive if large doses were used to weaken several large powerful proximal muscles. However, smaller doses injected into upper limb muscles are very effective at relieving pain as well as spasticity and can, paradoxically, actually increase grip strength by unmasking underlying voluntary movement (Simpson *et al.* 1996).

Evidence is rapidly accumulating that BTX-A is excellent at relieving pain in one of the most distressing complications following stroke, the hemiplegic shoulder. As well as analgesia and improving cosmesis and hygiene, for example, by releasing chronic finger flexion and preventing fingernail trauma to the palm, BTX-A injection may bring about more sustained functional improvements. It is claimed that the treatment may break the vicious cycle whereby chronic spasticity shortens muscles and increases spasticity further, permitting residual volitional movement to bring about active stretching. If supplemented by regular passive stretching by orthoses and intensive physiotherapy, benefit may last much longer than the duration of any paralysis induced by BTX-A and perhaps even be permanent. Its role in the management of children with spastic gait disorders is discussed further below.

Although EMG guidance may be helpful in localizing specific hypertonic muscles, and even more precisely the motor points and end plates within them, it is not absolutely necessary. BTX-A injection technique, in contrast to the more traditional nerve blocks, requires little special equipment and can be learnt relatively easily. Although the two have not been formally compared in a clinical trial, it seems likely that BTX-A is destined to become much more widely used.

Surgery

Surgical lengthening or division of soft tissues may offer a more radical treatment when contractures are present. The indications include cosmesis, correction of deformity and to improve function. However, much weakness may be revealed if a muscle is lengthened that has undergone major histological transformation. For best results, patients should have relatively static deficits and be sufficiently co-operative with active therapy and exercises before and after surgery.

Many different procedures have been described for the correction of various deformities, especially of the foot and ankle. These include subtalar fusion or triple arthrodesis, section or lengthening of the Achilles tendon, and section or transfer of the tibialis posterior tendon. Section of the tendons of the hamstrings, obturator, or iliopsoas muscles may be contemplated in severe deformities due to spasticity (Fig. 22.2). Peripheral neurectomy can also be undertaken and, although associated with marked muscle atrophy and sensory loss, is sometimes technically easier, for example in the relief of hip adductor spasms by obturator neurectomy.

More invasive surgical procedures such as selective dorsal rhizotomy or myelotomy of the adjacent dorsal root entry zone preferentially interrupt afferent input from nociceptors and muscle spindles, thereby eliminating flexor and tendon reflexes without causing complete deafferentation of the limb. Such ablative procedures and older operations such as cordectomy are irreversible and are now rarely, if ever, justified. Electrical stimulation of dorsal columns or cerebellum via implanted electrodes has been tried in very small uncontrolled studies over many years with rather disappointing long-term results but is still undergoing evaluation.

SPASTIC GAIT PATTERNS AND THEIR MANAGEMENT

THE ADULT HEMIPLEGIC GAIT

One of the most important functional goals in the rehabilitation of an adult patient following a hemiplegia is the restoration of independent walking. This requires intact body balance, adequate proprioception, and selective control of

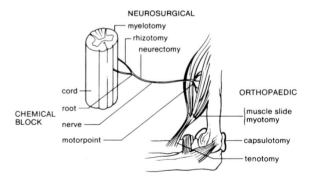

Fig. 22.2 Surgical methods of relieving spasticity. Reproduced with permission from: Hardie, R. J. (1995). Principles of neurological rehabilitation. In *Neurology in clinical practice*, (2nd edn), (ed. W. G. Bradley, R. B. Daroff, G. M. Fenichel, and C. D. Marsden). Butterworth-Heinemann, Boston.

lower limb movement to provide the normal sequential, asynchronous but posturally related changes at the hip, knee, and ankle during both stance and swing phases of gait with a smooth continuous flow from one step to the next.

The natural hemiplegic gait is characterized by abrupt simultaneous extension of hip, knee, and ankle in a single primitive mass movement. Although spasticity may not be evident with the patient supine or sitting, the act of standing erect and attempting to walk brings out the positive support reaction which physiotherapists refer to as the extensor pattern. Fortunately, this does at least provide lower limb stability during stance, but it provides characteristic obstacles too.

Some of the most obvious features of the hemiplegic gait result from overactivity in plantarflexors of the ankle. Apparent foot drop or equinus deformity interferes with toe clearance during the swing phase which, combined with failure to flex the knee, leads to compensatory circumduction of the hip and upward tilting of the pelvis. Initial contact with the floor is with the toes or a flat foot rather than the normal heel strike which is important for shock absorption of the impact forces. Supination of the foot caused by asymmetric actions around the subtalar joint, notably excessive contraction of soleus, provides an additional varus component to the foot deformity.

During midstance in the normal gait cycle, gradual ankle dorsiflexion allows the centre of gravity to move smoothly ahead of the stationary foot but spasticity prevents this and also the natural roll on to the forefoot ('heel off') and flexion of the knee prior to the toe-off phase. The overall effect is to restrict trunk progression and contralateral step length, with the tendency to retropulsion diminished by compensatory forward flexion of the trunk.

THE SPASTIC DIPLEGIC GAIT

As with the hemiplegic gait, the most obvious features result from overactivity in plantarflexors of the ankle with striking equinovarus deformities. Children with cerebral palsy commonly have Achilles tendon contractures and a toe stance, taking weight only on the forefeet with the hips and knees flexed in a crouching posture reinforced by pain and spasticity in the hamstrings. Exaggerated hip adduction ('scissoring') is common, causing a narrow support base, difficulty with swing phase, and skin shear over the medial aspects of the knees.

As described earlier, although BTX-A causes local paralysis of injected muscles, it can actually bring about improvements in function if the correct hypertonic muscles are selected. Promising results have been reported in young children with cerebral palsy and diplegic gait patterns after BTX-A injections into the calf muscles (Graham in press). Equinus deformity can be corrected, allowing improved active dorsiflexion during the swing phase and a normal heel strike rather than toe walking. These improvements cannot be achieved after the age of 5-6 years, and the value of prophylactic injections to prevent the development of contractures is currently under investigation. BTX-A injections into the hamstrings have

been reported to be of benefit in reducing crouching, particularly post-operatively after adductor release, and it may have a diagnostic role in pre-operative assessment to select those cases most likely to improve after surgery.

GAIT ANALYSIS

Technological advances have allowed the development of highly sophisticated gait analysis laboratories in which computerized kinematic motion analysis of anatomical landmarks is combined with surface EMG recordings. Such observations are already being applied for pre- and post-operative orthopaedic surgical assessment. The sheer volume of data acquired during a few short timed walks across a standard force platform is beguiling, but the technique has major limitations currently in terms of validity, reproducibility, etc. Nevertheless, it has great potential for the future.

ORTHOTIC INTERVENTIONS

There is an extensive literature, but a paucity of compelling objective evidence, about orthotic interventions to improve gait pattern in spastic lower limbs. The field is complicated because of the heterogeneous nature of clinical material incorporating varied combinations of weakness as well as spasticity and other problems. The biomechanics of the lower limb is extremely complex and changes in the tone or alignment at one joint causes secondary changes at all the others. As well as correcting foot drop, there may be permanent equinus deformity due to spasticity and/or contracture in the calf muscles, subtalar instability, and greater problems more proximally to be taken into account. The aim should be to restore the normal loading pattern and alter the ground reaction force closer to the plane of the hip, knee, and ankle joints.

The simplest remedy is a lightweight polypropylene ankle–foot orthosis (AFO) to correct marked foot drop. Important considerations when casting the AFO are incorporating a full sole plate to resist spasticity in the ankle plantar flexors, with sufficient lateral calcaneal control to prevent additional varus deformity. If necessary, the sole plate can be trimmed back behind the metatarsal heads to avoid exacerbating spasticity by excessive plantar skin stimulation. It may not be possible to get the foot plantigrade if the Achilles tendon is shortened, and a heel raise may also be required. A plastic AFO will only be successful if it is worn in conjunction with a shoe that has good contact in the instep region.

In general, adults after stroke or head injury do not tolerate lower limb orthoses well, although some well-motivated patients do persevere and benefit. However, it is also surprising what can be achieved by simpler and more cosmetic measures such as wearing modern footwear designed for athletic sports. Greater success is claimed in children suffering from cerebral palsy. Paediatric orthotics is a highly specialized art as well as science but in experienced hands great functional gains can be achieved by correct prescription. One reason is that orthotic stabilization of more proximal joints can be achieved. However, as the child grows and muscles become stronger, the mechanical advantages are lost because of the increasing strength and weight of an orthosis required to resist powerful spastic flexion at the hips and knees.

CONCLUSION

Spasticity is a well-recognized clinical entity which is nevertheless still poorly understood and hard to define. Indeed there is probably no such thing as pure spasticity given the heterogeneity of neurological disorders with which it may be associated. While clearly pathological, its presence is not necessarily disabling. In some cases, spasticity may actually be essential to permit standing or walking, activities which may be impaired by well-intentioned antispasticity medication. Coexistent negative features of damage to the corticospinal and parapyramidal tracts are common and include weakness, fatiguability, and impaired accuracy of fine movements. These are usually responsible for the majority of the resulting disability, and do not respond to treatment.

If specific interventions are required to reduce spasticity, then a problem-orientated approach is recommended. A comprehensive assessment of the full hierarchy of motor impairments and disabilities is an essential preliminary, and objective evaluation of each intervention is desirable where possible. Management should also be planned according to a hierarchy, selecting from a range of simple preventive and physical therapeutic measures before pharmacological agents and more invasive surgical procedures are contemplated. Particular attention should be paid to the analysis of the gait pattern and the use of orthoses. Because of the complexities of assessment and treatment, an interdisciplinary team approach is desirable. Although often time-consuming, the rewards of successful spasticity management can be considerable.

REFERENCES

Ada, L., Vattansilp, W., O'Dwyer, N. J. and Crosbie, J. (1998). Does spasticity contribute to walking dysfunction after stroke? *Journal of Neurology, Neurosurgery and Psychiatry*, **64**, 628–35.

Becker, R., Alberti, O., and Bauer, B. L. (1997). Continuous intrathecal baclofen infusion in severe spasticity after traumatic or hypoxic brain injury. *Journal of Neurology*, **244**, 160–6.

Bohannon, R. W. and Smith, M. B. (1987). Interrater reliability of a modified Ashworth scale of muscle spasticity. *Physical Therapy* **67**, 206–7.

Brown, P. (1994). Pathophysiology of spasticity. *Journal of Neurology, Neurosurgery and Psychiatry*, **57**, 773–7.

Burke, D. (1983). Critical examination of the case for or against fusimotor involvement in disorders of muscle tone. *Advances in Neurology*, **39**, 133–50.

Davidoff, R. A. (1992). Skeletal muscle tone and the misunderstood stretch reflex. *Neurology*, **42**, 951–63.

De Neve, P., De Vleeschhouwer, J., and van Lacre, M. (1992). Evaluation of motor function in hemiplegia. *European Journal of Physical Medicine and Rehabilitation*, **6**, 137–41.

DeSouza, L. H. and Musa, I. M. (1987). The measurement and assessment of spasticity. *Clinical Rehabilitation*, **1**, 89–96.

Dunne, J. W., Heye, N., and Dunne, S. L. (1995). Treatment of chronic limb spasticity with botulinum toxin A. *Journal of Neurology, Neurosurgery and Psychiatry*, **58**, 232–5.

Graham, H. K. (1997). Botulinum toxin A in cerebral palsy: indications and outcomes. *European Journal of Neurology*, **4** (suppl. 2), S15–22.

Hardie, R. J. and Lees, A. J. (1993). The control of movement and its clinical disorders. In *Neurosurgery—the scientific basis of clinical practice* (2nd edn), (ed. H. A. Crockard, R. Hayward, and J. T. Hoff), pp. 290–310. Blackwell, Oxford.

Ibrahim, I. K., Berger, W., Trippel, M., and Dietz V. (1993). Stretch-induced electromyographic activity and torque in spastic elbow muscles. *Brain*, **116**, 971–89.

Landau, W. M. (1977). Spasticity: the fable of a neurological demon and the emperor's new therapy. *Archives of Neurology*, **31**, 217–9.

O'Dwyer, N. J., Ada, L., and Neilson, P. D. (1996). Spasticity and muscle contracture following stroke. *Brain*, **119**, 1737–49.

Ordia, J. I., Fischer, E., Adamski, E., and Spatz, E. L. (1996). Chronic intrathecal delivery of baclofen by a programmable pump for the treatment of severe spasticity. *Journal of Neurosurgery*, **85**, 452–7.

Shefner, J. M., Berman, S. A., Sarkati, M., and Young, R. R. (1992). Recurrent inhibition is increased in patients with spinal cord injury. *Neurology*, **42**, 2162–8.

Simpson, D. M., Alexander, D. N., O'Brien, C. F., Tagliati, M., Aswad, A. S., Leon, J. M. *et al.* (1996). Botulinum toxin type A in the treatment of upper extremity spasticity: a randomized, double-blind, placebo-controlled trial. *Neurology*, **46**, 1306–10.

Tardieu, C., Lespargot, A., Tabary, C., and Bret, M. D. (1988). For how long must the soleus muscle be stretched each day to prevent contracture? *Developmental Medicine and Child Neurology*, **30**, 3–10.

Teddy, P., Jamous, A., Gardner, B., Wang, D., and Silver, J. (1992). Complications of intrathecal baclofen delivery. *British Journal of Neurosurgery*, **6**, 115–8.

Thilmann, A. F., Fellows, S. J., and Garms, E. (1991). The mechanism of spastic muscle hypertonus: variation in reflex gain over the time course of spasticity. *Brain*, **114**, 233–44.

Wade, D. T. (1992). *Measurement in neurological rehabilitation*. Oxford University Press.

Young, R. R. (1989). Treatment of spastic paresis. *New England Journal of Medicine*, **320**, 1553–5.

Young, R. R. (ed.) (1994). Role of tizanidine in the treatment of spasticity. *Neurology*, **44**(suppl. 9), S1–80.

FURTHER READING

Barnes, M. P., McLellan, D. L., and Sutton, R. A. (1993). Spasticity. In *Neurological rehabilitation*, (ed. R. Greenwood, M. P. Barnes, T. M. McMillan, and C. D. Ward), pp 161–72. Churchill Livingstone, Edinburgh.

Brown, J. K. (1993). Science and spasticity. *Developmental Medicine and Child Neurology*, **35**, 471–2.

Glenn, M. B. and Whyte, J. (ed.) (1992). *The practical management of spasticity in children and adults*. Lea and Febiger, Philadelphia.

Little, J. W. and Massagli, T. L. (1993). Spasticity and associated abnormalities of muscle tone. In *Rehabilitation medicine: principles and practice* (3rd edn), (ed. J. A. DeLisa and B. M. Gans), pp. 666–80. Lippincott, Philadelphia.

Spasticity Study Group (1997). Spasticity: etiology, evaluation, management and the role of botulinum Toxin type A. *Muscle and Nerve* Suppl. 6, pp. S1–232.

23 | *Bladder, bowel, and sexual problems*

Michael Swash

The bladder, bowel, and sexual organs are involved in many neurological diseases (Henry and Swash 1992). They are also affected in local disease processes, and it is not always easy to separate these processes; indeed they may coexist. Therapy is concerned with the restoration of function. It is not always necessary to restore normal function, and it is often not possible to do this. In the management of bladder, bowel, and sexual disorders it is often sufficient to restore function sufficiently to allow the patient to achieve social confidence. It is often neither necessary nor possible to address the precise physiological deficit in order to achieve this. Since the bladder, bowel, and pelvic floor sphincters share related innervations, they are involved together in many neurological disorders. Management of one aspect is therefore often relevant to management of another.

BLADDER AND BOWEL DISORDERS

Generally, consideration of bladder and bowel disorders involves the two related functions of retention and voiding urine and faeces, respectively.

CENTRAL NERVOUS SYSTEM LESIONS

Incontinence and retention may be caused by disrupting descending and ascending pathways concerned with the modulation of sphincter control, or by interfering with central control processes in the brain that integrate the functional systems necessary for defecation and micturition (Table 23.1). Upper motor neurone lesions with respect to the urethral and anal sphincters are located in the brain, brainstem or spinal cord rostral to the Onuf nucleus in the sacral cord, which innervates the smooth and striated peri-urethral and anal sphincter muscles (see De Groat 1990).

Voluntary control of the bladder and rectum consists of the two processes of *storage* and *voiding*. Both are represented in the cortex, and subserved by separate but related descending pathways, subject to feedback modulation by sensory input, and by conscious decision-making regarding the appropriateness of time and opportunity for socially acceptable micturi-

Table 23.1 Neurological causes of incontinence and retention of urine and faeces

Upper motor neurone lesions	Lower motor neurone lesions
Cerebral disorders	*Conus medullaris lesions*
Dementia	Ischaemia
Cerebrovascular disease	Spinal dysraphism
Hydrocephalus	Degenerative disease (e.g. primary autonomic failure)
Multiple sclerosis	Multiple sclerosis
Tumours (especially frontal)	
Traumatic encephalopathy	
Cerebral infections	
Brainstem lesions	*Cauda equina lesions*
Infarction	Lumbosacral trauma
Tumours	Lumbosacral disc prolapse
Infections	Lumbar canal spondylosis
	Lumbosacral canal stenosis
	Ankylosing spondylosis
	Chronic arachnoiditis
Spinal cord lesions	*Peripheral nerve lesions*
Trauma	Proximal diabetic neuropathy
Cord compression	Lumbosacral plexitis
Multiple sclerosis	Intrapelvic trauma/haemorrhage
Infarction and ischaemia	Childbirth-associated injury
Viral myelitis	Metastases and infections

tion or defecation. Sexual function is modulated by similar processes (Lundberg 1992). Kleist (1922) reported that the bladder and rectum are represented on the medial surfaces of the cerebral hemispheres, with motor and sensory representation adjacent to each other across the Rolandic fissure. This observation was confirmed by Penfield and Rasmussen (1950). However, discrete lesions at this site have not been reported to cause sphincter dysfunction.

Frontal lesions, particularly when located on the inferior or medial surfaces of the frontal lobes are well-known causes of incontinence, or of loss of socially appropriate micturition and defecation behaviour. Thus, meningiomas arising from the falx, or from the olfactory groove, particularly if there is bilateral frontal lobe compression, may present with incontinence. A similar disturbance of sphincter control, consisting of incontinence without embarrassment, occurs in people with *dementia, cerebral vascular disease involving frontal lobes, or after head injury.* In addition, many people with chronic diffuse brain degenerations develop faecal impaction, perhaps because they are relatively inactive physically, or their diet is bland, and there is overflow incontinence through a patulous anal sphincter; the sphincter relaxes because the anal canal is loaded with faeces—the recto–anal reflex. This reflex is a normal component of the initial phase of defecation induced by rectal filling. Faecal impaction may itself lead to retention of urine with subsequent leakage during coughing.

Urinary incontinence and faecal incontinence are frequent problems in people with *multiple sclerosis* (Goldstein *et al.* 1982; Betts *et al.* 1993). In this disease there are lesions in the brain and spinal cord that may interrupt the ascending sensory and descending motor pathways that modulate the storage and voiding of urine and faeces, leading to incontinence, or to retention of urine or faeces (often termed constipation, although this term really has a different clinical meaning). *Hydrocephalus* may cause incontinence from damage to sphincter pathways, assumed to be due to the increased ventricular size impinging on these pathways as they pass round the lateral surface of the dilated ventricular system. In *spinal cord injury* there is direct damage to the spinal afferent and efferent pathways for sphincter control, and a combination of retention, with overflow incontinence, develops. Multiple sclerosis, hydrocephalus, and spinal cord injury are associated with corticospinal tract degeneration and signs of spasticity and weakness in the lower limbs, with extensor plantar responses. It is important to recognize that the pathways subserving sphincter control are located more medially in the cord (Nathan and Smith 1951, 1958), and that corticospinal tract damage is not itself correlated with sphincter dysfunction. This is best exemplified by familial spastic paraplegia, a disorder in which there may be profound corticospinal tract dysfunction without sphincter abnormality.

In any chronic neurological disease the development of sphincter dysfunction is followed by secondary dysfunction of the bladder and bowel, respectively. For example, when there is retention of urine the bladder wall becomes stretched, losing its compliance and sensitivity to filling, and promoting a tendency for the bladder to become larger and less able to generate adequate detrusor activity, and less able to empty the bladder properly (see Mundy *et al.* 1994). Similarly, rectal distention associated with faecal retention leads to a desensitized rectum and so to less sensitivity to the usual stimuli to promote a call to stool, and persistence of abnormal bowel habit, and impaction. These secondary functional effects can be prevented, and improved when they have developed, by appropriate attention to achieving full bladder and bowel emptying. Intermittent self-catheterization has been particularly successful in achieving full bladder emptying in neurogenic bladder disorders, and so in restoring continence, and especially in restoring the sensation of bladder-filling, for example, in patients with incomplete spinal cord syndromes due to trauma, multiple sclerosis, and other causes.

PERIPHERAL NERVOUS SYSTEM LESIONS

Sphincter control systems may be disrupted by lesions in the afferent and efferent pathways in the peripheral nervous system in the *lumbosacral nerve roots* in the spinal canal, due to spondylosis, sacral meningomyelocele, or trauma. This may also follow pelvic disease involving the *pelvic plexus*, such as diabetic proximal neuropathy, metastases, haemorrhage or trauma. Stretch-induced damage to the *pudendal innervation* of the pelvic voluntary sphincters can also lead to sphincter denervation and incontinence. Direct *damage to the sphincters* from instrumentation, or trauma during childbirth may also lead to incontinence; this is usually associated with partial denervation of the sphincters from accompanying pudendal and intrapelvic nerve damage (Snooks *et al.* 1984*a*, *b*, 1985).

Sphincter dysfunction from peripheral nerve damage, as in central nervous system (CNS) lesions, is associated with secondary damage to the bladder and rectum due to overfilling. There is therefore the same need to protect these organs by intermittent catheterization and by regular manual evacuation of faeces. These measures result in a greatly improved functional capacity in these organs, and thus in quality of life for the patient.

BLADDER DISORDERS: THERAPEUTIC INTERVENTIONS

The management of bladder dysfunction in neurological disease is essentially empirical (Table 23.2). A classification of voiding disorder based on lesion location, or pathway dysfunction is not of practical significance, since dysfunctional syndromes cannot reliably be related to lesion location. This reflects the long CNS pathways from the cortex to the bladder detrusor and urinary sphincters, and the importance of semi-automatic mechanisms in the brainstem (pontine) voiding and storage centres. In addition, the dual functions of storage and micturition are accomplished by the coordination of autonomic and somatic nervous system activity, interacting at multiple segmental levels in the CNS.

This empirical approach has become generally accepted since its development by Lapides and colleagues (see Kendall and Karafin 1974). Although most neurologists would prefer to attempt a lesion-based, or physiologically-based classification of bladder disorders, and to plan therapy according to principles derived from such an approach, this has proven impractical. The term 'neuropathic bladder' itself illustrates this difficulty. To a neurologist the term 'neuropathic' implies an abnormality of innervation, especially of the lower motor neurone component, but to the urologist the word 'neuro-

Table 23.2 Empirical classification of bladder dysfunction

Sensory paralytic bladder
Motor paralytic bladder
Autonomous neuropathic bladder
Uninhibited neuropathic bladder
Reflex neuropathic bladder

pathic' is used more widely to describe any bladder abnormality due to neurological disease, at any level in the nervous system, and including both sensory and motor syndromes. The description of abnormalities in micturating cystograms by urologists into obstructive and neuropathic bladder syndromes illustrates this usage, with the addition of 'unstable bladder syndromes', and recognizable patterns of abnormality such as detrusor failure, sensory defects, and detrusor–sphincter dyssynergia. These functional descriptions do not correlate with specific neuropathological abnormalities, or neurological disorders, and some (e.g. unstable bladder and minor degrees of detrusor–sphincter dyssynergia), appear to occur in normal individuals. The classification based on cystometric criteria given in Table 23.2 is described and correlated with the neurological lesions. It will be seen that there is scope for considerable overlap in the data. The International Continence Society (1988) recommended a slightly different description, which omits sensory bladder disorder, and delineates weakness of the bladder sphincter mechanism as an important subgroup. Although the latter is common and important in urogynaecological practice, due to childbirth-induced trauma and denervation of the voluntary sphincter, it is not a primary feature of neurological disease.

Sensory paralytic bladder

In this syndrome the bladder is insensitive to filling pressure (stretching), so that it becomes overfilled. Enlargement of the bladder results in overstretching of the detrusor muscles of the bladder wall, causing a hypotonic bladder. This can occur from sensory neuropathy as in diabetic neuropathy, and other proximal neuropathies. The classical, now rare cause, is tabes dorsalis. The bladder has a large capacity, and there is poor vesical contraction. The commonest cause is overfilling of the bladder, for example, in patients with acute retention (e.g. in acute myelitis, multiple sclerosis, or acute neuropathy). When the acute overfilling is relieved, and the bladder allowed to resume a normal pattern of filling and voiding, with avoidance of a residual urine by intermittent catheterization, bladder function is restored. If bladder overfilling is allowed to persist the functional loss of normal sensation may not recover, leading to permanent functional deficits in micturition with a persistent residual urine, and a propensity to develop recurrent urinary tract infections.

Motor paralytic bladder (detrusor hypokinesia)

Loss of the parasympathetic outflow to the bladder detrusor causes failure of bladder contraction and painful retention of urine. Bladder sensation is present, but vesical contraction is absent. There is a secondary increase in bladder volume and impairment in bladder sensation from overstretching. This is a rare functional syndrome.

Autonomous neuropathic bladder

The bladder has no motor or sensory innervation. The urethral sphincter is also denervated. All components of the peripheral innervation of the bladder have been destroyed. This is a complication of central disc protrusion with compression of the cauda equina or conus medullaris, of tumours of the conus or cauda equina, and of intrapelvic malignancy. It may occur in multiple sclerosis when there is demyelination of the conus region of the cord. The bladder is large and hypotonic, and sensation and vesical contraction are both absent.

Uninhibited neuropathic bladder

The lesion is in the descending pathways from the pontine centre that integrates detrusor and sphincter contraction and relaxation; these consist of autonomic (parasympathetic) output to the detrusor muscle, and corticospinal inhibitory and excitatory output to the external bladder sphincter muscle. There is inability to suppress the voiding reflex more than briefly, resulting in urgency and perhaps urge incontinence. This is a common problem in multiple sclerosis, and in other spinal cord disorders, including cord injury and cord compression syndromes. The syndrome is sometimes termed *detrusor instability*. It may also occur with lesions in the corticospinal pathway in the deep cerebral white matter, and brainstem. The bladder has a low capacity, sensation is present, and there is uninhibited detrusor contraction from low volumes and low filling rates, usually with complete bladder emptying.

In *sphincter–detrusor dyssynergia* there is detrusor instability, with premature induction of voiding detrusor contractions, but these are accompanied to a varying degree by contraction of the external urinary sphincter. Micturition therefore occurs in short uncontrolled spurts, and the bladder pressure rises and falls in response to detrusor contractions against urethral resistance. Minor degrees of this phenomenon often occur in normal subjects.

Reflex neuropathic bladder

This is the pattern of abnormality found in complete cord lesions, above the T10 level, that leave the sacral parasympathetic and somatic innervation of the bladder detrusor and urethral sphincter intact. The sensation of bladder filling, a small fibre input to the sacral cord, is absent and the bladder is of large capacity, with a resultant hypotonic contraction. Bladder contractions are uninhibited, however, because the small fibre sensory input to the sacral segments results in unmodulated reflex detrusor contraction in the absence of descending inhibition. The bladder empties frequently but incompletely.

A SIMPLE FUNCTIONAL APPROACH TO BLADDER DYSFUNCTION

It is helpful to consider bladder dysfunction in terms only of its two functions of *storage* and *voiding* (Table 23.3), without detailed consideration of lesion location, or of neurophysiological aspects. Although the urodynamic classification described above is useful in understanding bladder dysfunction, there is overlap between the phenomena described.

Table 23.3 Functional classification of bladder dysfunction

Failure to store
Failure to void
Failure to store and void

Failure to store urine

The bladder is uninhibited with detrusor–sphincter dyssynergia. The patient benefits from measures to increase the capacity to store urine, and to inhibit the micturition reflex. Without appropriate management there is a risk that increased intravesical pressure may be transmitted to the upper urinary tract, leading to hydronephrosis, and renal failure. The presentation is usually with urgency and frequency, rather than incontinence. Failure to store urine almost never occurs as an isolated dysfunction without associated impairment of voiding.

Clean self-catheterization (CISC)

This is a major management strategy in this group of patients (Lapides *et al.* 1974; Blaivas *et al.* 1984). The first step is to discover whether or not there is a residual urine. The residual urine can be measured directly by catheterization, or by transabdominal ultrasound. If there is a residual urine of greater than about 100 ml, daily intermittent self-catheterization should be considered. This will empty the bladder fully, restoring the normal emptying behaviour of the bladder, and increasing the interval between calls to void. Full emptying of the bladder by intermittent catheterization improves its sensation and, most importantly, its contractility, resulting in more effective emptying during voiding (Betts *et al.* 1993).

Sometimes, bladder emptying can be enhanced by the use of transabdominal vibration (Das Gupta *et al.* 1997). Anticholinergic drugs (e.g. propantheline) are then more likely to be effective in reducing detrusor hyperreflexia, and urgency.

Pharmacological intervention

Drug Therapy is often useful, but only when the question of a residual urine and its management has been resolved, as above:

(1) a smooth muscle relaxants: oxybutyin (Ditropan), imipramine, flavoxate (Urispas);

(2) anticholinergic drugs: propantheline, atropine (?), tricyclic antidepressants.

Oxybutynin, 2.5–5 mg twice daily is used to reduce detrusor contractility (see below). Oxybutynin should not be used prior to elimination of the residual urine volume by self-catheterization, since this medication will cause an increase in the volume of the residual urine, leading to further deterioration in voiding, with urge or overflow incontinence.

Other conservative measures

Other measures have been recommended but are generally not effective. These take the form of general advice, as follows:

1. Bladder training programme, with encouragement to try to delay micturition.
2. Fluid restriction during critical times of public activity, to reduce urine production. Generally, this proves relatively ineffective and impractical for most people.
3. Avoid sudden exposure to cold, or changes in posture, especially to the erect posture, which increases sensory input from the activation of sensory receptors in the trigone of the bladder.
4. Void regularly.

Reduction in urine volume

This can be achieved by the use of the antidiuretic hormone, DDAVP, 2.5–5 µg, administered as a spray or intranasal solution, at night. This is a simple method of preventing interruption of sleep by urinary urgency, simply by preventing urine production. Clearly, this should not be used continuously, and should be reserved for nocturnal use. It is a useful adjunctive therapy to other measures.

Reduction in bladder sensitivity

Bladder sensitivity can be reduced temporarily by the instillation of a dilute solution of capsaicin, a pepper derivative that stimulates and then reduces the activity of unmyelinated C-fibre afferent endings in the bladder by competitive blockade, so reducing the sensitivity of the bladder (Chandirami *et al.* 1996). This method of treatment is not established in routine use, but does appear to benefit a minority of patients with detrusor hyperreflexia. The improvement lasts from six weeks to six months (Fowler *et al.* 1994).

Increasing urethral resistance

Increasing urethral resistance is not appropriate for the management of storage disorders due to neurological disease, since there is risk to the renal tracts from increasing bladder and ureteric pressure.

Surgical augmentation of the bladder

This has been used as a last resort to increase bladder impedance, and to reduce its sensitivity to filling, and its contractility. After such a procedure it is sometimes necessary to resort to manual expression of urine (Credé manoeuvre), or intermittent self-catheterization, in order to achieve complete bladder emptying. The bladder is augmented by the addition of an ileal loop cystoplasty.

FAILURE TO EMPTY THE BLADDER

This is potentially the most serious bladder dysfunction because of the risk of reflux, renal tract destruction, and chronic urinary tract infection. As discussed above, failure to empty usually occurs in association with dysfunctional storage of urine. From the viewpoint of the urologist, failure to empty can be due to outlet obstruction, with a high pressure system, or to detrusor failure, with weak bladder contraction. Incoordination of bladder contraction and sphincter relaxation, detrusor–sphincter dyssynergia, may also be a cause in neurological disease. The distinction between these dysfunctional bladder syndromes is made by micturating cystography.

The compliance of the bladder varies during the process of filling. At first, the compliance is very high, so that filling is accompanied by an imperceptible increase in pressure but, as filling proceeds, the pressure gradually increases. As the elastic properties of the bladder wall are exceeded by increasing volumes the compliance decreases. The rate of change of compliance is dependent not only on the physical properties of the bladder wall, but on the rate of filling; with faster rates of filling the compliance rapidly decreases. At a certain point, sensory input from bladder stretch receptors triggers the generation of detrusor contraction, leading to a rapid rise in bladder pressure. The latter induces rhythmic detrusor contractions, leading to the initiation of the micturition reflex. In the presence of sensory disturbance, or failure of detrusor contraction because of local pathology, especially overstretching of the bladder wall, this process is impaired and bladder compliance remains high even with large bladder volumes, leading to failure to empty.

Cholinegic drugs

Cholinegic medications have been used to encourage bladder emptying, but these may induce painful bladder contractions, and they may raise intravesical pressure, leading to pressure back-up in the renal tract. This treatment is not recommended.

Reduction of outlet resistance

This is a feasible management strategy when there is an increased outlet resistance, as in men with neurological disease in whom there is also prostatic obstruction. This may be accomplished with sympathetic alpha-blocking drugs such as phenoxybenzamine 10 mg twice-daily. Phenoxybenzamine interferes with tonic closure of the bladder neck. Prazosin may also be used, although there is a potential side-effect from hypotension. Striated muscle relaxants, such as dantrolene, or baclofen, have little practical effect. Surgical treatment (e.g. by prostatectomy in the male) has the risk of causing incontinence. If this is acceptable, it may be controlled (e.g. in the paraplegic), by an external collecting device.

Passive emptying of the bladder

Emptying the bladder by intermittent self-catheterization is the more logical approach. This results in alleviation of the problem of a residual urine, and allows the bladder to recover tone, as a prelude to the resumption of normal detrusor tone and contractility. Intermittent self-catheterization has a small risk of infection. Rhame and Perkash (1979) noted about 20–30 infections per 100 days in patients with spinal cord injury managed by intermittent catheterization, but the risk is probably less now than it was twenty years ago, particularly in the contemporary context of self-catheterization.

Permanent indwelling catheterization

Permanent catheterization is necessary in a number of patients in whom detrusor contractions never recover. This outcome depends on the underlying pathology, and is more likely in chronic multiple sclerosis than in acquired autonomic neuropathies. In patients with functionally complete spinal cord injury permanent catheterization is frequently needed.

Urinary diversion

Diversion of the urine by ileal bladder collection, or ureterostomy, may be acceptable as a last resort.

URINARY RETENTION IN YOUNG WOMEN

In this rare disorder there is inability to void, without local or neurological cause. Although this disorder has often been ascribed to psychogenic causes, usually in the absence of any overt evidence to support this hypothesis, electromyographic (EMG) evidence suggests that it may arise from abnormal contraction of the external urinary sphincter, with bizarre high frequency EMG activity recorded from this muscle, even during the resting state (Fowler *et al.* 1985). The aetiology of this disorder is unknown and treatment is unsatisfactory. Recently, S2 nerve root stimulation has been suggested as a means of overcoming this abnormal striated sphincter muscle activity (Fowler 1997).

STRESS URINARY INCONTINENCE

It is important to remember that women with voiding abnormalities may have an associated idiopathic disorder of micturition, with stress incontinence, superimposed on their neurological disorder. The development of unexpected stress urinary incontinence after treatment of the neurological voiding disorder must then be managed according to established surgical principles, which involve restoration of the normal anatomy of the pelvic floor sphincters and bladder neck.

BOWEL DYSFUNCTION: THERAPEUTIC INTERVENTIONS

The basic classification of defecatory disorders in neurological disorders follows that of urinary voiding disorders. There is a similarly organized central control system, involving the Onuf nucleus in the sacral cord, and pathways in the spinal cord and in the brainstem and brain, with similar localization as for the urinary system.

FAECAL INCONTINENCE (see TABLE 23.4)

This is a difficult problem to manage (see Henry and Swash 1992). When it occurs in neurological disease it is a feature of lesions of descending pathways modulating parasympathetic

Table 23.4 Multifactorial causes of incontinence

Incontinence in the elderly
Incontinence in confusional states
Faecal impaction
Immobility
Rectal prolapse
Anorectal, vaginal and perineal discomfort and pain
Constipation

activity, or innervating the pelvic striated sphincter muscles, especially the puborectalis and external anal sphincter muscles that close the anal canal and maintain continence. As in the urinary system there is co-ordination between contraction of the rectum and left colon, which are innervated by parasympathetic nerves from the sacral outflow, and the pelvic floor striated sphincters that are innervated by somatic efferents from the Onuf nucleus at the S2 level in the spinal cord.

Faecal incontinence is a feature of failure of the striated sphincters, which is due to denervation of these muscles in *neuropathies*, or in lesions of the *conus medullaris* or *cauda equina*. It may also occur with intrapelvic lesions that damage the *lumbosacral plexus*, including immune plexopathies, diabetic neuropathy, CIDP, metastatic infiltration, or trauma. Overaction of the peristaltic contraction of the gut may also lead to incontinence by overwhelming the striated pelvic floor sphincters, as in severe diarrhoea. This is particularly likely to occur when the sphincters are weakened, as in *women after childbirth* in whom there is often neurogenic weakness of these muscles, or there may be traumatic tears in the external sphincter itself. Thus, the pre-existent state of the pelvic floor is important in considering the outcome of neurological disease affecting the pelvic floor musculature.

Faecal incontinence may also occur in *myotonic dystrophy*, in which there is degeneration not only of the striated sphincter muscles but also of the unstriated smooth involuntary musculature of the gut, including the internal anal sphincter muscle. Faecal incontinence is not a feature of other myopathies.

In *Parkinson's disease*, constipation is a major problem, and later in the disease incontinence of urine and of faeces may develop, in association with involvement of the autonomic nervous system, with postural hypotension, and sexual dysfunction. Constipation in Parkinson's disease is partly the result of involvement of gut neurones in the degenerative process, with Lewy body inclusions in the enteric neurones, and partly the result of obstruction of defecation by failure of relaxation of the external anal sphincter and of the pelvic floor muscles, a dysfunctional problem that can be relieved by L-dopa or dopaminergic agonists. The importance of this obstruction of the pelvic outlet in the disease, causing failure of defecation rather than constipation is uncertain.

In paralytic disorders, including *motor neurone disease, peripheral neuropathies*, and *myopathies*, as well as *multiple sclerosis* and *cerebrovascular disease*, constipation is a common and uncomfortable problem. When there is disease of the spinal cord, involving descending and ascending pathways that are concerned with parasympathetic pathways to the gut, constipation may be the result of loss of the parasympathetic innervation of the gut. The upper gut, including the stomach, jejunum, and ileum are innervated by the vagus nerve, and the left colon by the parasympathetic outflow from the sacral cord. Thus, impaired descending colon motility may result from low cord lesions, and upper gastrointestinal dysfunction from high cord lesions. Since the gut has a rich non-cholinergic and non-adrenergic innervation, and its own nervous system in the enteric neurons, these parasympathetic effects have proven difficult to detect in spinal cord-injured people. Constipation may be an early feature of multiple sclerosis, however, perhaps because of cervical cord involvement. In gastrointestinal practice constipation has been defined as straining at stool more than 25% of the time, or two or fewer bowel motions per week. In neurological patients the alternative definition, that constipation is a subjective feeling of a full bowel, is probably more appropriate.

Management

The management of bowel disorders is essentially symptomatic. Attention to diet is important in preventing constipation but mobility and exercise, when possible, are even more effective measures. A high roughage diet, with at least one helping of fresh fruit, and of vegetables, daily is useful.

Laxatives are used when essential:

(1) bulk-forming drugs (e.g. bran, ispaghula husk, methylcellulose);
(2) stimulant laxatives (e.g. bisacodyl, danthron, docusate sodium, glycerol, and senna);
(3) faecal softeners (e.g. liquid paraffin);
(4) osmotic laxatives (e.g. lactulose, magnesium salts, rectal phosphates).

Manual evacuation

The rectum should be evacuated manually when there is impaction of faeces, and a patulous anus. The latter results from reflex dilation of the internal anal sphincter because the rectum is full and, if not relieved, leads to overflow incontinence of faeces.

In patients with spinal cord injury it is important to protect the bowel, as well as the bladder, from the effect of impaction and dilatation with faecal content in the acute stages, in order to encourage the development of intrinsic rhythmic defecatory activity. The latter often reappears, with a frequency of one or two motions a week, which is usually entirely acceptable.

SEXUAL DYSFUNCTION

Sexual problems (see Lundborg 1992) are a feature of a number of different disorders, including endocrine disease, hypothalamic dysfunction, limbic and temporal cortical lesions, including limbic epilepsy, and peripheral nerve lesions, especially involving the autonomic nervous system. In addition, psychological disorders, especially depression and anxiety, may lead to sexual dysfunction. These are summarized in Table 23.5. A simple way to distinguish psychogenic from organic male impotence is to ascertain whether nocturnal penile tumescence occurs, as shown by the presence of erections on wakening in the morning; if morning erections occur, the impotence is likely to be psychogenic. Although psychogenic impotence used to be thought common, it is now recognized as relatively rare, accounting for only about 15% of cases. (See also Table 23.6.)

Table 23.5 Sexual dysfunction in neurological disorders

Endocrine disorders
Hypothalamic–pituitary tumours
  suprasellar tumours
  pituitary tumours with hyperprolactinaemia
  rhinencephalic malformations
  Kallman's syndrome

Stroke
Hemiplegia, associated with loss of self-esteem, depression, and
  side-effects of antihypertensive drugs
Sexual dysfunction more marked after right than left hemisphere
  stroke

Head injury
Diencephalic, mesial basal-frontal and temporal-limbic damage
Frontal lobotomy leads to sexual disinhibition

Epilepsy
Seizures may occur during sexual intercourse
Sexual phenomena may be a component of an epileptic seizure
Epilepsy may be associated with decreased sexual activity interictally

Parkinson's disease
Decreased sexual desire is common, and may respond to L-dopa
Failure of erection and orgasm is characteristic of multiple system
  atrophy

Multiple sclerosis
Erectile failure and loss of orgasm occur commonly
Associated bladder and bowel problems are frequent

Spinal cord injury and malformations
Conus lesions cause loss of reflex erection, lubrication, ejaculation,
  and orgasm
Sacral cord lesions may cause sacral sensory loss without sexual
  dysfunction

Pelvic pain
Perineal pain in women is associated with loss of sexual function

Polyneuropathy
Erectile dysfunction is common in diabetic polyneuropathy
Loss of erection and ejaculation is a presenting feature of familial
  amyloid polyneuropathy
Acquired demyelinating polyneuropathies are large fibre disorders,
  and do not involve sexual function

Table 23.6 Clinical evaluation of impotence

Do nocturnal and morning erections occur?
Does orgasm occur?
Is sperm ejaculated?
Can erection be induced by masturbatory activity?
Is there a neurological disease present?
Is there pelvic, spinal, or femoral vascular disease?
Is there any intrapelvic cause for sexual dysfunction?
Is penile and perineal sensation intact or disturbed?
Is there any other feature of sympathetic or parasympathetic dysfunction?
Consider imaging pelvis and lumbosacral spine
Consider neurophysiological evaluation, e.g.
  pudendoanal reflex latency
  bulbocavernosus reflex latency
  pudendal sensory evoked responses
  anal sphincter EMG
Advise on physical measures (e.g. vibration)
Reduce stress levels
Avoid drugs likely to inhibit erection (e.g. beta-blockers)
Try pharmacological therapy (see text)

Sexual disorders may be devastating for both the patient and their partner, and this aspect of clinical practice should not be ignored. In some neurological disorders the neurological disability itself leads to sexual difficulties. For example, if there are contractures of limbs, or spasms, it may be difficult to assume the appropriate posture for successful and pleasurable sexual intercourse. In others, for example, multiple system atrophy (MSA), primary autonomic failure (PAF), and familial amyloidotic polyneuropathy, sexual dysfunction including loss of erection and orgasm are primary features of the disease. In stroke there is uncertainty as to whether the cerebral lesion itself leads to sexual dysfunction, or whether this follows secondary loss of self-esteem, depression, and anxiety consequent on the stroke itself, and its effect on the patient's lifestyle. In epilepsy and hypertension, drug therapy may diminish the sensitivity of sexual responsiveness. Erectile dysfunction may occur, in addition, from local vascular disease, without the necessity for any neurological lesion.

PENILE ERECTION

Penile and clitoral erection (Andersson and Wagner 1995) occurs when the smooth muscle of the cavernosal arteries, and their helicine branches (Wagner *et al.* 1982), relaxes following reduction in tonic resting norepinephrine (α_1-receptors) released from sympathetic nerve endings (Brindley 1988). This smooth muscle relaxation is mediated by nitric oxide released through a cyclic guanosine monophosphate induction mechanism, probably mediated by non-adrenergic, non-cholinergic nerves (Burnett *et al.* 1993). During penile erection there is passive occlusion of venous drainage from the corpora cavernosa caused by occlusion of these veins against the surrounding tunica albuginea and by active neurally mediated closure of these veins. Clitoral erection follows a similar mechanism.

Seminal emission (ejaculation) occurs from rhythmic contraction of the bulbocavernosus, ischiocavernosus, and periurethral striated sphincter muscles, innervated by the pudendal nerves, following contraction of the smooth muscle of the epididymis, vas deferens, seminal vesicles, and the prostate gland, innervated by the sacral parasympathetic outflow (Brindley 1988).

MANAGEMENT OF IMPAIRED ERECTION

There are several ways of achieving some restoration of function in men with impaired penile erection. The use of a penile vacuum pump, applied to the penis, will lead to erection (Salvatore *et al.* 1991), which can be maintained to a degree dependent on the presence of some residual innervation and reflex pathway in the cavernosal nerves. In the presence of severe vascular disease in the pelvis and femoral circulations, also, this method may fail. It is relatively non-invasive and often acceptable. Surgical treatment was formerly used, by inserting pumpable or fixed intrapenile prostheses (Brindley 1994) to achieve penile erection and firmness. This is a procedure that is permanent, and which is only indicated if all other measures have failed.

Intracorporal injection

Improved understanding of the pharmacology of penile erection has led to new and far less invasive therapies. The injection of drugs that relax cavernosal smooth muscle has proved efficacious in inducing sustained penile erection (Brindley 1986). The first such substance to be used was papaverine (40–80 mg) which, injected into one corporal body will pass through vascular connections to the other side of the penis and induce erection. Patients are advised to use this therapy once or twice weekly. A combination of papaverine (40 mg) and phentolamine (1–2mg) has also been recommended. There is a risk of the induction of corporal fibrosis, perhaps related to the acid pH of the papaverine solution used, and haematoma may occur (Levine *et al.* 1988). Priapism occurs in about 1–4% of patients, especially when higher doses are used. Abnormalities in liver enzymes have been reported. The recommended dose varies from patient to patient and should be ascertained by self-injection under medical supervision during the educational phase of the use of this therapy. Alpha adrenergic agents, (e.g. phenylephrine), given by intracorporal injection, is the treatment of choice to relieve drug-induced priapism (Dittrich *et al.* 1991).

Intracorporal injections of alprostadil (Caverject) a synthetic prostaglandin E$_1$ derivative, have replaced papaverine for most patients, except perhaps those who wish to induce penile erection only rarely, because it is unlikely to induce priapism, and long-term usage has not been associated with the development of fibrosis. Linet and Ogrinc (1996) observed a linear dose response to 2.5, 5, 10, and 20 μg doses, with erections lasting 12–44 minutes. Men with neurogenic erectile failure required smaller doses than men with vascular causes.

Other therapies for induction of penile erection

Oral yohimbine, an alpha-adrenergic compound, has a weak effect in inducing erection, particularly in men in whom spontaneous or sexually induced penile erection is not entirely absent. A dose of about 20 mg (0.3mg/kg body weight) is used. Because it may induce hypertension (it raises the blood pressure by 10–30 mmHg at this dosage) it should not be used in hypertensive men, or in men with tetraplegia, or high spinal paraplegia.

Alprostadil may be administered by transurethral, rather than by intracorporal injection, using a special applicator, using a dose of 125–1000 μg. Padma-Nathan *et al.* (1997) reported 66% satisfactory erections occurred 10–7 minutes after the application, and 64% of 461 men using this medication at home reported satisfactory intercourse, compared to 19% using placebo. Adverse effects consisted of pain, minor urethral trauma, and dizziness. Priapism, fibrosis, or haematoma did not occur.

A further advance has been the introduction of sildenafil (Viagra) a novel compound that can be taken orally (Boolel *et al.* 1996), and that inhibits the hydrolysis of cyclic AMP, thus potentiating and prolonging the action of nitric oxide on the corpora cavernosa, inducing and prolonging erection. It has been shown to be effective in a dose of 50 mg in men without neurological dysfunction and is currently undergoing trials in men with spinal cord injury and with multiple sclerosis.

ORGASM

Male and female orgasm, and male ejaculation, are absent when there is severe sacral root or pudendal sensory loss, and are also impaired or lost when there is a parasympathetic lesion. Sympathetic lesions usually spare orgasm, but prevent ejaculation, since the prostatic and epididymal innervation is lost. Treatment is difficult, but a combination of psychological management, a penile vibrator, and physostigmine, with metoclopramide, to diminish the emetic effect of this drug, may be effective. Yohimbine may also be effective and does not cause nausea or vomiting. The dopamine agonists, apomorphine and bromocriptine, may also be useful, as has been reported in Parkinson's disease, and selegiline may have a mild beneficial effect on orgasm.

Brindley (1981) introduced the method of electrical stimulation of pelvic autonomic nerve fibres, using a transrectal technique, in patients with spinal cord injury, and showed that regular use of this technique induced ejaculation, and improved the sperm count in men with paraplegia. If the sympathetic innervation of the testis is destroyed sperm will not be ejaculated, although orgasmic movements will occur.

SOME PRACTICAL CLINICAL PROBLEMS

There are several common clinical disorders of bladder, bowel, and sexual function. A summary of their management will be given here.

MULTIPLE SCLEROSIS

Micturition disorders are almost always present in advanced stages of the disease (Betts *et al.* 1993), and may develop in the early phase of the disease when there is demyelination in the conus medullaris or in the spinal cord. Urgency, hesitancy, frequency, and incontinence all occur (Patti *et al.* 1997). Detrusor hyperactivity, with urge incontinence, often associated with detrusor–sphincter dyssynergia is the commonest urodynamic pattern, but a flaccid areflexic bladder is also common. In disabling urge incontinence sacral root stimulation has been used (Vodusek *et al.* 1986). Urinary dysfunction is correlated with the presence of corticospinal tract signs.

Constipation is a feature in 36%, and 30% experience faecal incontinence (Chia *et al.* 1995); some have both these symptoms. Bowel dysfunction does not correlate with urinary tract dysfunction.

Sexual disorders are common, especially when there is spinal disease, occurring in two-thirds of men with the disease. Loss of libido, physical difficulties associated with spasticity, loss of erection, and anorgasmia are all common (Betts *et al.* 1993). Management of these problems (Fowler *et al.* 1992) is summarized in Box 1.

SPINAL CORD INJURY, AND OTHER MYELOPATHIES

The problem in these patients is similar to that in multiple sclerosis, and the same principles underlie management. In partial lesions, it is essential to adequately empty the bladder in order to avoid overstretching, and to encourage the restoration of sensation and cyclic bladder emptying (Creasey 1994). Bowel function usually develops into a pattern of bowel motions about twice a week, and dietary management should be adjusted accordingly. In high spinal lesions, although there is no conscious sensation of bowel movement or anal sphincter activity, movement of the patient may induce bowel opening. Patients with low spinal lesions may have an abnormal parasympathetic outflow, leading to low rectal pressures, and poor responsiveness of the anal sphincter to changes in posture. In spinal injury, retraining methods may be helpful in improving bowel control, by teaching the patient to recognize impending bowel activity (Glickman and Kamm 1996).

Urinary symptoms are managed by clean intermittent self-catheterization, with oxybutynin, to control urgency. Sacral root stimulation has proven a great benefit to some of these patients (Brindley and Rushton 1990). Management of these problems is summarized in Box 2.

PARKINSON'S DISEASE

Urgency and frequency of micturition are features that develop during the course of the disease. Chandirami *et al.* (1997) reported these symptoms in 85% of their patients, but incontinence did not occur. Urinary retention in men is associated with coincidental prostatism; this should be treated medically whenever possible (e.g. with Proscar). Transurethral prostatectomy should be avoided because of the risk of post-

---

Box 1 Bladder, bowel, and sexual problems in multiple sclerosis

> *Bladder problems*
> measure post-void residual by ultrasound or catherization
> if greater than 100 ml, consider CISC
> then use oxybutynin or flavoxate for urgency
> DVAPP for urgency at night may help sleep
> for persistent unmanageable incontinence consider urinary diversion
>
> *Bowel problems:*
> for incontinence:
>   modify diet, or use codeine phosphate
> for constipation:
>   modify diet,
>   use bulking agents, osmotic laxatives, or stimulant laxatives
>
> *Sexual disorders*
> intracavernosal or transurethral injection of alprostadil (Caverject)
> oral Sildenafil (Viagra)
> *Always* explain the problem, in detail, to the patient and their partner

---

Box 2 Bladder, bowel, and sexual problems in spinal cord injury

> *Bladder care*
> aim is to achieve urine storage at low pressure, and to regularly empty the bladder completely
> clean intermittent (self, if possible) catheterization is useful
> reflex voiding requires a low urethral resistance (e.g. by sphincterotomy)
> sacral anterior root stimulation may achieve bladder emptying, and continence; the posterior roots are divided to deafferent the bladder and promote storage
> artificial sphincter implants have a small place in management eg, in spina bifida
> treat urinary tract infections
>
> *Bowel care*
> Diet, laxatives, suppositories, digital stimulation of the anal canal manual evacuation may be necessary when the rectum is hypotonic in low sacral lesions
> enemas should *not* be routine
>
> *sexual function*
> reflex erection may occur in up to 70% of men with spinal injuries
> vibrators and vacuum devices may assist reflex erection
> intracorporeal injection has given way to trans-urethral and oral methods (Sildenafil) for achieving erection
> seminal emission usually requires trans-rectal pudendal/autonomic nerve stimulation
> female fertility is normal once menstruation is re-established after injury
> pregnancy and childbirth are also normal, although autonomic dysreflexia may occur during delivery when the lesion is rostral to T6; epidural anaesthesia will prevent this

operative incontinence. If there are associated autonomic features (e.g. failure of penile erection or postural hypotension), this risk is greater (Chandirami *et al.* 1997). In patients with clinical features suggestive of multisystem atrophy (MSA), especially failure to respond to dopaminergic agents, loss of penile erection, a significant post-micturition residual volume, and incontinence or urinary symptoms preceding the onset of parkinsonism, operative treatment of prostatism or urinary retention is not indicated, and catheterization may be required as a last resort.

Constipation also occurs frequently and may respond to dopaminergic treatment (Mathers *et al.* 1988). Sexual dysfunction in Parkinson's disease suggests a diagnosis of MSA, but may develop in the late stages of the idiopathic disease; it may improve with dopaminergic therapy. Pathological confirmation of the diagnosis in these cases is lacking.

PERIPHERAL NEUROPATHY

The primary onset of loss of erection and orgasm, with retention or incontinence of urine is a feature of hereditary autonomic neuropathies (e.g. familial amyloidotic polyneuropathy), and of acquired neuropathies with prominent autonomic involvement, especially diabetic neuropathy. The Portuguese type has been treated by liver transplantation to reverse the metabolic error. Intermittent self-catheterization is necessary to ensure adequate bladder emptying and to reduce the frequency of urinary incontinence. Constipation is a feature of all these neuropathies. The sexual disorder can be managed by intracavernosal injection as described above.

DRUG-INDUCED DYSFUNCTION

In any patient with disturbed bladder, bowel, or sexual dysfunction consider the drug history before setting out on a series of complex neurological investigations (Wein and van Arsdalen 1988). This is important even when there is an evident neurological cause, since drugs such as beta-blockers, hypnotics, and antidepressants frequently interfere with these functions.

PSYCHOLOGICAL DISORDER

It is very uncommon for psychological disorder to cause urinary, bowel, or sexual dysfunction. In the past, desperate clinicians have ascribed undiagnosable and ill-understood disorders of these functions to 'functional' causes. This is nearly always a wrong diagnosis, and it does not lead to resolution of the patient's symptoms.

CONCLUSION

The simple, step-wise approach to bladder, bowel, and sexual disorders outlined in this chapter will greatly aid management of these disorders. It is important to ask patients about these aspects of their bodily functions since these disorders are important to their quality of life.

REFERENCES

Andersson K-E, Wagner, G. (1995). The physiology of penile erection. *Physiological Reviews*, **75**: 191–236.

Betts CD, D'Mellow MYT, Fowler CJ. (1993). Urinary symptoms and the neurological features of bladder dysfunction in multiple sclerosis. *Journal of Neurology, Neurosurgery and Psychiatry*, **56**: 245–50.

Blaivas JG, Holland NJ, Geiser B, LaRocca N et al. (1984). Multiple sclerosis bladder; studies and care. *Annals of the New York Academy of Sciences*, **436**: 328–46.

Boolel M, Gepi-Attee S, Gingell JC, Allen MJ. (1996). Sildenafil, a novel effective oral therapy for male erectile dysfunction. *British Journal of Urology*, **78**: 257–61.

Brindley GS. (1981). Electroejaculation: its technique, neurological implications and uses. *Journal of Neurology, Neurosurgery and Psychiatry*, **44**: 9–18.

Brindley GS. (1986). Pilot experiments on the actions of drugs injected into the human corpus cavernosum penis. *British Journal of Pharmacology*, **87**: 495–501.

Brindley GS. (1988). The actions of parasympathetic and sympathetic nerves in human micturition, erection and seminal emission, and their restoration in paraplegic patients by implanted electrical stimulators. *Proceedings of the Royal Society B*, **235**: 111–20.

Brindley GS. (1994). Impotence and ejaculatory failure. In *Handbook of neuro-urology*, (ed. DN Rushton), pp 329–48. Marcel Dekker, New York.

Brindley GS and Rushton DN. (1990). Long term follow up of patients with sacral anterior root stimulators. *Paraplegia*, **28**: 469–75.

Burnett AL, Tillman SL, Chang TSK. (1993). Immunohistochemical localization of nitric oxide synthase in the autonomic innervation of the human penis. *Journal of Urology*, **150**: 73–6.

Chandirami VA, Peterson T, Duthie GS, Fowler CJ. (1997). Urodynamic changes during therapeutic instillations of capsaicin. *British Journal of Urology*, **77**: 792–7.

Chia YW, Fowler CJ, Kamm MA, Henry MM, Lemieux MC, Swash M. (1995). Prevalence of bowel dysfunction in patients with multiple sclerosis and bladder dysfunction. *Journal of Neurology*, **242**: 105–8.

Creasey GH. (1994). Managing bladder, bowel and sexual function after spinal cord injury. In *Handbook of neuro-urology*, (ed. DN Rushton), pp. 233–51. Marcel Dekker, New York.

Das Gupta P, Haslam C, Goodwin R, Fowler CJ. (1997). The 'Queen Square bladder stimulator'; a device for assisting emptying of the neurogenic bladder. *British Journal of Neurology*, **80**: 234–7.

De Groat WC. (1990). Central neural control of the lower urinary tract. In *Neurobiology of incontinence*. CIBA Foundation Symposium **151**, pp. 27–56. Wiley, Chichester.

Dittrich A, Albrecht K, Bar-Moshe O. *et al.* (1991). Treatment of pharmacological priapism with phenylephrine. *Journal of Urology*, **146**: 323–4.

Fowler CJ. (1997). Communication to the British Society for Clinical Neurophysiology, London.

Fowler CJ, Kirby RS, Harrison MJG. (1985). Decelerating burst and complex repetitive discharges in the striated muscle of the urinary sphincter associated with urinary retention in women. *Journal of Neurology, Neurosurgery and Psychiatry*, **48**: 1004–9.

Fowler CJ, VanKerrebroeck PEV, Nordenbo A, Van Poppel H. (1992). Treatment of lower urinary tract dysfunction in patients with multiple sclerosis. *Journal of Neurology, Neurosurgery and Psychiatry*, **55**: 986–9.

Fowler CJ, Beck RO, Gerrard S, Betts CD, Fowler CG. (1994). Intravesical capsaicin for treatment of detrusor hyperreflexia. *Journal of Neurology, Neurosurgery and Psychiatry*, **57**: 169–73.

Glickman S, Kamm MA. (1996). Bowel dysfunction in spinal cord injury patients. *Lancet*, **347**: 1651–3.

Goldstein I, Sirohy MB, Sax DS, Krane RJ. (1982). Neurourologic - abnormalities in multiple sclerosis. *Journal of Urology*, **128**: 541–5.

Henry MM and Swash M. (1992). *Coloproctology and the pelvic floor*, (2nd edn). Butterworth-Heinemann London.

Kendall AR and Karafin L. (1974). Classification of neurogenic bladder disease. *Urologic Clinics of North America*, **1**: 37–44.

Kleist K. (1922). Kriegsverletzungen des Gehirnes. In *Handbuch der Arztlichen Erfahrungen im Weltkrieg 1914/1918*, Vol 4, *Geistes- und Nervenkrankheiten*, (ed. K Bonhoeffer), pp. 1343–69. Leipzig-Verlag, Leipzig.

Lapides J, Diokno AC, Lowe BS, Kalish MD. (1974). Follow-up of unsterile, intermittent self-catheterisation. *Journal of Urology*, **111**: 184–188.

Levine SB, Althof SE, Turner LA. *et al.* (1988). Side effects of self administration of intracavernous papaverine and phentolamine for the treatment of impotence. *Journal of Urology*, **141**: 54–7.

Linet OI and Ogrinc FG. (1996). Efficacy and safety of intracavernosal alprostadil in men with erectile dysfunction. *New England Journal of Medicine*, **334**: 873–7.

Lundborg P-O. (1992) Sexual dysfunction in patients with neurological disorders. *Annual Reviews of Sex Research*, **3**: 121–150.

Mathers SE, Kempster PA, Swash M, Lees AJ (1998) Constipation and paradoxical puborectalis contractions in animus and Parkinson's disease: a dystonic phenomenon?

Mundy AR, Stephenson TP, Wein AJ (ed.) (1994). *Urodynamics: principles, practice and application*, (2nd edn). Churchill-Livingstone, Edinburgh.

Nathan PW, and Smith MC. (1951). The centripetal pathway from the bladder and urethra within the spinal cord. *Journal of Neurology, Neurosurgery and Psychiatry*, **14**: 262–89.

Nathan PW, and Smith MC. (1958). The centrifugal pathway for micturition within the spinal cord. *Journal of Neurology, Neurosurgery and Psychiatry*, **21**: 177–89.

Padma-Nathan H, Hellstrom WJG, Kaiser FE, *et al.* (1997). Treatment of men with erectile dysfunction with trans-urethral alprostadil. *New England Journal of Medicine*, **336**: 1–7.

Patti F, Ventimiglia B, Failla G, Genazzani AA, Reggio A. (1997). Micturition disorders in multiple sclerosis patients: neurological, neurourodynamic and magnetic resonance findings. *European Journal of Neurology*, **4**: 259–65.

Penfield W and Rasmussen T. (1950). *The cerebral cortex of Man*. Macmillan. New York.

Rhame FS and Perkash I. (1979). Urinary tract infections occurring in recent spinal cord injury patients on intermittent catheterisation. *Journal of Urology*, **122**: 669–73.

Salvatore FT, Sharman GM, Hellstrom MD. (1991). Vacuum constriction devices and the clinical urologist: an informed selection. *Urology* **38**: 323–7.

Snooks SJ, Barnes PRH, Swash M. (1984*a*). Damage to the innervation of the voluntary anal and periurethral striated sphincter musculature in incontinence; an electrophysiological study. *Journal of Neurology, Neurosurgery and Psychiatry*, **47**: 1269–73.

Snooks SJ, Swash M, Setchell M, Henry MM. (1984*b*). Injury to the innervation of the pelvic floor sphincter musculature in childbirth. *Lancet* **ii**: 546–50.

Snooks SJ, Henry MM, Swash M. (1985). Faecal incontinence due to external anal sphincter division in childbirth is associated with damage to the innervation of the pelvic floor musculature. *British Journal of Obstetrics and Gynaecology*, **92**: 824–8.

Vodusek DB, Light JK, Libby JM. (1986). Detrusor inhibition induced by stimulation of pudendal nerve afferents. *Neurourology and Urodynamics*, **5**: 381–9.

Wagner G, Bro-Rasmussen F, Willis EA. *et al.* (1982). New theory on the mechanism of erection involving hitherto undescribed vessels. *Lancet*, **i**: 416–18.

Wein AJ, van Arsdalen KN. (1988). Drug-induced male sexual dysfunction. *Urologic Clinics of North America*, **15**: 23–31.

24 | *Neurological disease and driving*

C. J. Earl

In many people's lives the ability to drive a motor vehicle is as near a necessity as anything can be. Anyone who is unable to drive may be obliged to make profound changes in his or her way of life. The severity with which this disability strikes in a particular case will of course depend on circumstances. There are those who are employed as drivers, there are others whose employment makes driving a near necessity, and many whose family commitments (e.g. school journeys), make life without driving extremely difficult. The situation for professional drivers may be complicated by the fact that some of them need to be in possession of a licence, which will entitle the holder to drive large goods vehicles and passenger-carrying vehicles, when regulations are particularly strict. This chapter will consider some of the important factors which neurologists need to take into account when advising patients. Because driving is controlled by systems of licensing which vary from country to country the legal requirements referred to here are those of the United Kingdom, but principles adopted in most developed countries are similar.

Patients who suffer from neurological illness may be even more dependent for mobility on driving than a healthy person because of disability due to their disease, and it may be especially unfortunate that this very disability may make driving unsafe.

In the United Kingdom, the decision to withdraw a driving licence is made by the Secretary of State for Transport on the advice of the Medical Advisers at the Driver and Vehicle Licensing Agency (DVLA). There is also a Panel of Honorary Medical Advisers to the Department. This Panel advises the Secretary of State on matters of principle and provides guidelines for the Medical Officers at the DVLA in Swansea. Sometimes, individual cases are referred to members of the Panel and cases presenting problems of particular difficulty may be referred to a meeting of the whole Panel.

A publication by the Medical Branch of the Driver and Vehicle Licensing Agency (DVLA 1998) summarizes the advice which the Medical Branch has received from the Secretary of State's Honorary Medical Panels. This is a most useful summary and certainly one to which neurologists will find helpful to refer.

Decisions on diagnosis must, of course, be made by the clinicians concerned with the care of the patient and it would be very exceptional indeed for the Medical Officers at the DVLA or members of the Panel of Honorary Medical Advisers not to accept the diagnostic conclusions of the clinicians in charge of the patient. But it often happens that for one reason or another doctors are uncertain about the nature of episodes of altered consciousness or of the risks of driving with a particular disability due to neurological disease, and wish to share the responsibility about the decision on fitness with Medical Officers at the DVLA or members of the Panel of Advisers. It is very rare for disagreement to occur between the Panel and the clinicians involved on the facts or clinical diagnosis but sometimes the considered view of the Panel on potential risks in a particular clinical situation may differ from the views of the clinician in charge of the patient.

It is important that medical advisers, whether general practitioners or consultants, should be aware of their responsibilities in respect of the advice about driving they give to patients who consult them. They are obliged to offer advice if they believe it to be necessary and not only if they are asked. Thus, a patient who presents with 'dizzy spells' may never have thought that the episodes might in any way affect his/her ability to drive safely, but if the doctor comes to the firm conclusion that the episodes are attacks of minor epilepsy the patient must be told this, advised not to drive, and informed of his obligation to notify the DVLA. The doctor will be wise to make a note of the advice given in the patient's records. The family doctor who is uncertain about the true nature of some transient alteration of consciousness and is unable to come to a definite conclusion will usually seek a second opinion, and if it is appropriate he/she will advise the patient not to drive until this opinion has been obtained. A consultant may be able to come to a definite diagnosis, but if not, must decide in such a case whether on the balance of probabilities the patient should be regarded as unfit.

Where patients are suffering from some persistent disability there is usually little problem for the physician in deciding what to advise and the patient will usually understand the reasons for the decision. Where the illness leads to episodic disturbances of function such as loss or alteration of the state of consciousness, transient dysfunction of limbs, or temporary loss of vision or hearing it may be more difficult to decide what is appropriate.

PAROXYSMAL DISORDERS

ATTACKS OF LOSS OR ALTERATION OF CONSCIOUSNESS

The commonest type of loss of consciousness and one which many people experience in their lives is simple syncope. The attacks are often precipitated by sudden pain, the sight of blood, or even an account of some unpleasant happening. In this type of syncope loss of consciousness is preceded by a warning, which may last for some minutes, of malaise, sweating, pallor, and slowing of respiration. The pulse is slow and blood pressure falls. It is generally accepted that a liability to such attacks of simple syncope is unlikely to cause a disturbance of consciousness which will lead to loss of control of a vehicle. If the doctor is quite satisfied that an attack of loss of consciousness is due to this cause the patient may be advised to continue driving. Diagnostic problems may be encountered in some cases where a patient at the end of an attack of typical syncope has some convulsive movements. These are well known to occur and are the result of severe generalized cerebral ischaemia. It may be difficult sometimes to be absolutely sure of the nature of attacks of this pattern but careful questioning of the subject and of witnesses will usually lead to the truth being established. Patients who have attacks of this sort are not regarded as suffering from epilepsy and are therefore not subject to the regulations related to epilepsy.

A fairly common and dangerous form of syncope is cough syncope. This affects patients with chronic obstructive airways disease during a paroxysm of coughing and may cause sudden loss of consciousness while driving, since such paroxysms may occur at any time. A single episode of sudden loss of consciousness without any special distinguishing clinical features and often without witnesses may cause a driver to seek advice. Clinical examination and full investigation may fail to reveal any possible cause. It has been advised in cases of this sort that driving should cease until a year has passed without recurrence of an attack.

Paroxysmal disturbances of cardiac rhythm are a much rarer cause of syncope. Syncope from this cause often happens without warning and can readily cause loss of consciousness while the patient is driving a motor vehicle. Confirmation of the diagnosis in such cases can be obtained sometimes by a prolonged electrocardiographic (ECG) recording or by more sophisticated intracardiac rhythm recording. Once the diagnosis is established the attacks can often be prevented by appropriate cardiac pacing or drug therapy, and decisions about resumption of driving will depend on expert cardiological advice.

EPILEPSY

Drivers who develop a liability to attacks of epilepsy are not allowed to hold a driving licence and must be advised not to drive and to report the facts to the DVLA. This is because epilepsy is a disability specifically prescribed by the regulations.

For ordinary (non-vocational) licences these were amended recently and now allow resumption of driving by patients with epilepsy after a period of freedom from attacks of one year. The special regulations about sleep epilepsy remain unchanged. Thus, those who suffer from attacks *only* during sleep may drive once they have demonstrated that the pattern of attacks occurring only in sleep is a persistent one by having suffered from such attacks during at least three years before they apply for a licence. The occurrence of a seizure while awake will at once bring patients into the group bound by the ordinary regulations.

The more stringent regulations covering drivers holding vocational licences were relaxed to some extent in January 1993, and the requirements are now in line with those of many countries of the European Union and are similar to recommendations made by the Federal Transport Commission in the United States. A Group II licence may now be held by a person with a history of epilepsy provided that:

(1) the applicant has been free from epileptic attacks for at least 10 years;
(2) has not taken antiepileptic medication during this 10-year period; and
(3) does not have a persisting condition giving rise to an increased liability to seizures.

The last condition will limit the automatic application of the new less strict regulation in patients with a fixed intracranial abnormality. In this type of case the Department will require an opinion from an appropriate consultant before the application is granted.

In other situations where there is an increased risk of the development of seizures the Panel has given advice which ordinarily the licensing authority will follow. For example, patients who have undergone craniotomy involving the supratentorial compartment of the skull and who have never suffered from epilepsy will be barred from driving for a time. Patients in whom the presence of an intracerebral glioma has been demonstrated will be advised that they must not drive because whether or not they have had epilepsy in the past there is a serious risk that epilepsy will develop at some time in the future. Where a diagnosis of glioma has been made, either on radiological or histological grounds, patients will be advised that they should not drive for a period of at least four years. Patients who have suffered from severe head injuries where there have been penetrating wounds of the dura or evidence of local brain damage or intracerebral haematoma will be denied an ordinary driving licence until the passage of time has demonstrated that they can be safely assume to have no significant liability to epilepsy. Details of the regulations in particular types of cases will be found in the relevant chapters in MCAP (1995)

Benign supratentorial tumours which have been completely removed do not usually present serious problems. If epilepsy has occurred as a symptom of the tumour then the epilepsy regulations must apply and in any case craniotomy with opening of the dura will lead to temporary revocation of a licence.

Stopping anticonvulsant medication

Many patients who have suffered from epilepsy and whose attacks have ceased for the required period have their driving licences restored. Some, aware of the consequences of a further seizure, will wish to continue with medication for a much longer period, some will even choose to do so indefinitely. Others may wish to discontinue taking their drugs, and if drugs are discontinued there is an increased risk of seizure recurrence MRC (1991). Patients who discontinue antiepileptic medication should be warned of this and the advice of the Medical Officers at the DVLA at the present time is that driving should cease for a period of six months after the reduction in the dose of medication begins.

CEREBROVASCULAR DISEASE

Cerebrovascular disease with cerebral haemorrhage or cerebral infarction needs careful consideration. It has been advised that after an event of this sort at least one month should elapse before the patients should drive, and this of course is provided that clinical recovery is satisfactory and that there is no persisting neurological deficit causing loss of impairment of the patients ability to control a vehicle. Episodes of transient ischaemia which have ceased and which have been absent for a period of four weeks may also be disregarded.

GIDDINESS

The guidelines from the DVLA Medical Branch include 'disabling giddiness' as a reason for withdrawing a driving licence and this must be regarded as important. However, the significant qualification here is the word 'disabling'. In terms of driving giddiness (vertigo) is rarely disabling for the driver in the true sense of the word, but if in a particular case the doctor does feel honestly that this is so he must advise his patient accordingly. However, in most neurologists' experience this is very rarely necessary.

OTHER PAROXYSMAL DISORDERS

Migraine

The visual disturbance or the motor and sensory symptoms that may occur in association with attacks of migraine are not ordinarily symptoms which lead to increased risk in driving—provided of course that the patient, if driving at the onset of the attack, is ready to stop driving until the visual symptoms have passed.

Tonic spasms of multiple sclerosis

These phenomena are well recognized although not common manifestations of multiple sclerosis. They tend to occur in bouts lasting for a period of weeks. During this time they may be very frequent (many times a day). They tend to affect the arm and leg on one side, which usually assume a 'tetanic' posture lasting for some seconds. They are often readily controlled by carbamazepine. They have been classified as 'non-epileptic seizures' (Gilliatt and Roberts 1986). While the bout of attacks is occurring the patient should not drive, but driving may be resumed when the attacks have ceased.

EXCESSIVE SLEEPINESS

There is no doubt that many road traffic accidents occur as the result of excessive sleepiness and accidents of this sort may be much more frequent than can be proven. Excessive sleepiness may sometimes be physiological, precipitated by a period of lack of sleep caused by excessive hours of work or other simple reasons. There are other situations where the daytime sleepiness must be regarded as pathological (e.g. sleepiness resulting from obstructive sleep apnoea, narcolepsy and hypersomnia as a result of medication, either prescribed or taken on the patient's own initiative). These conditions may respond to appropriate treatment.

This type of disability is often beyond medical control unless the somnolence brings the patient to his/her doctor, and mild degrees of excessive somnolence are unlikely to lead to this. Where patients do complain of excessive sleepiness they must be questioned carefully about its occurrence during driving and if it seems to the doctor that there is a truly increased risk of the patient falling asleep while driving the patient must be advised not to drive and to report the facts to the DVLA.

Cases of this sort usually need to be dealt with on an individual basis once they are reported, and often they are referred to members of the Panel of Advisers. Once the hypersomnolence can be controlled the patient may have his/her licence restored, but again ascertainment of the facts in this sort of case may be very difficult.

PERSISTING DISABILITIES

DEMENTIA

Patients with dementia can present some of the most difficult cases in which to come to a decision about driving which is fair to the patient and not excessively risky for other users of the road. Very often the patient's family will raise this question and will often seek the doctor's help in persuading the patient that driving is unsafe. Where this has happened there is little difficulty in coming to the right decision. Where the patient has no family or close friends the doctor is reliant on the observations he/she is able to make himself. It will be clear that severe forms of dementia will render a patient unfit to drive since there may be disorientation and serious loss of judgement. Where intellectual deficit is less severe and personality changes are not so obvious the problem is much more difficult. In these cases a doctor's opinion may often have to be based on a brief and limited period of observation but sometimes it may be helpful to require such patients to undergo a driving test at an appropriate Centre.

A recent multicentre collaborative study in the United States (Drachman and Swearer 1993) considered the relative accident rate in drivers in whom a diagnosis of Alzheimer's disease had been made. The conclusions of the study can be quoted verbatim:

The present study demonstrates that patients with AD who drive under usual self and family imposed restraints represent a statistically modest crash risk, well within the level for normal young adult drivers. The risk remains low on average for two to five years at which time the majority have stopped driving.

PHYSICAL DISABILITIES

Most neurologists will find little difficulty in advising patients who suffer from persistent physical disabilities about their driving. In many cases there is no serious risk in driving where the disability is a fixed one. Where the doctor believes that there is a significant risk in allowing a disabled person to drive, the driver should be advised to report his disability to the DVLA. The Medical Officers in such cases will advise that the only practical way of dealing with such problems is to arrange for an assessment to be made at one of the many special Centres at which such assessments can be carried out. A list of Centres in the United Kingdom can be found in the guide published by the DVLA in 1998 and up-to-date information may be obtained directly from the DVLA in Swansea.

PARKINSON S DISEASE

Since it has become possible to provide very effective treatment for Parkinson's disease with preparations of L-dopa a new episodic phenomenon has been frequently observed in patients who have been taking L-dopa preparations, usually for some years. These phenomena are sometimes described as 'on–off' phenomena which may cause severe temporary incapacity in terms of movement. While the advice to patients with mild Parkinson's whose symptoms are well controlled with medication is usually that they are able to drive, the development of 'on–off' symptoms with the sudden onset of immobility which may result may need very careful assessment.

VISUAL DISTURBANCES

Impairment of vision may be a symptom of neurological disease and may have important effects on driving ability. The requirements relating to visual acuity are well known as far as they affect ordinary drivers—the ability to read a standard number plate at 25 yards (22.5 metres)—which corresponds to vision of between 6/9 and 6/12. The requirements for Group II drivers are stricter and more complicated and current regulations need to be consulted in particular cases.

Visual field defects, in particular where they are homonymous, are frequently encountered in patients with diseases of the nervous system, most frequently in patients who have suffered vascular lesions involving the central visual pathways. The minimal field for safe driving is defined as:

At least 120 degrees width on the horizontal and at least 20 degrees from the central fixation point above and below the horizontals on any meridian measured by perimetry using a 3 mm test object at 1/3 metre (or equivalent perimetry) (DVLA, 1998, p. 20).

Testing the field of vision with both eyes open is generally acceptable. It is clear therefore that the dense homonymous hemianopia or quadrantanopia detectable on confrontation using finger movements will disqualify a person from holding a licence. If the field defect is not so dense it will need full assessment by perimetry before driving can be allowed. It must also be remembered that the field within the peripheral limits of vision must also be normal so that an homonymous scotoma may be a serious disability for driving even though the peripheral limits of the field appear normal. Some patients with a left hemianopia from a lesion in the parietal lobe may be quite unaware of the field loss.

THE PATIENT WHO CONTINUES TO DRIVE

It is important that a doctor should know what would be the wise course of action when confronted with the situation where a patient who has been advised not to drive for medical reasons continues to do so. Most doctors would have little difficulty in the case of a bus driver or the driver of a large goods vehicle. After due warning to the patient, preferably in writing, it would be the duty of the doctor to inform the Licensing Authority. Few doctors would take a different view and would be prepared to justify their decision if necessary. Where an ordinary driving licence is held many doctors have in the past taken the view that confidentiality should prevail. However, there is no doubt that in some circumstances the doctor's public duty may override his responsibility to the patient, and it is possible that a doctor might be regarded as having some responsibility for any harm that might result to property or to a third party in an accident where the patient's disability had played an important part in causing an accident. It is also important to remind patients that if they have been advised not to drive for medical reasons their insurance policy may be invalidated. Knowledge of the effect on insurance cover is often more persuasive than the simple fact of disobeying regulations laid down by the Department of Transport.

REFERENCES

DVLA (Driver and Vehicle Licensing Agencies) (1998). *At a glance guide to current medical standards of fitness to drive*. Driver Medical Unit DVLA, Swansea.

Drachman, D. A. and Swearer, J. M. (1993). *Neurology*, **43**, 2448–50. 1993

Gilliat, R. W. and Roberts, R. C. (1986). Syncope and non-epileptic seizures. In *Diseases of the nervous system*, (eds. Asbury A. K., McKhann G. M. and McDonald W. I.) W. B. Saunders, Philadelphia and William Heinemann, London

MCAP (Medical Commission on Accident Prevention) (1995). *Medical aspects of fitness to drive*. HMSO, London.

MRC (Medical Research Council Anti-Epileptic Drug Withdrawal Group) (1991). Randomised study of anti-epileptic drug withdrawal in patients in remission. *Lancet*, **337**, 175–80.

25 | *Dying from a neurological disease*
David Oliver

Although all patients will die, health care professionals often have little preparation in how to care for a dying patient. The care of patients dying with a neurological disease will present many different challenges, depending on the nature of the disease process. There may be a clear terminal phase, such as with an incurable and progressive disease like motor neurone disease or cerebral tumour. There may be a slow decline when the control of the disease process fails, such as end-stage Parkinson's disease, or death may be unexpected, such as a cerebrovascular accident. A particularly challenging area of care can be when the patient has altered mental capacity due to brain damage. All these patients will require different treatment, but in all cases the aim of treatment will have changed from curative to palliative.

Palliative care has been defined as

. . . the active total care of patients whose disease is not responsive to curative treatment, where control of pain, of other symptoms and of psychological, social and spiritual problems is paramount, and where the goal is the achievement of the best quality of life for patients and their families (WHO 1990).

It is the openess with which these various aspects of the patient and their family are considered that is so important in the care of a dying patient. So often, the dying patient becomes isolated—frightened to express fears and worried by the reaction of both family and professionals.

The attitudes to care are the same whether there has been a longer terminal stage, such as in multiple sclerosis, or a sudden deterioration, as in an acute head injury with severe brain damage. The 'whole patient' in the context of the family must be considered.

It is also essential that the approach of death is recognized in the terminal phase of a progressive illness or when active curative treatment is no longer appropriate in an acute episode (Dunlop 1993). A patient may not be treated in an appropriate way if the seriousness of the condition is not recognized. However, if the preparation of patient and family is to be co-ordinated and facilitated all involved in the patient's care need to be aware and agree to the change from a more active and curative approach to a caring and palliative approach.

Deaths from neurological disease account for approximately 15% of all deaths in the United Kingdom—in 1991 there were over 87 000 deaths from neurological disease, cerebro-vascular disease, cerebral tumour, and head injuries (OPCS 1993). However, there is very little or no information on the care of the dying patient in the main neurological textbooks. This may reflect current practice of the relatively rare resource of the neurologist being used to diagnose and assess patients, but the follow-up and care in the final stages being with the primary health care team or the general medical services. The management of the late stages of neurological disease may not be undertaken by a neurologist, who may be less aware of the clinical features and dilemmas in the care of these patients as death approaches. It is hoped that this chapter will be of help in coping with the problems in the terminal stages of neurological disease, as neurological services become more involved in the continuing care of patients.

PATIENT CONCERNS

The most important task when confronted with a patient with advancing disease is the careful assessment of their particular needs and concerns. These may be physical, psychological, social, and spiritual (Saunders *et al.* 1995). Only after this assessment should treatment be given. The treatment will need to be individualized to each patient and these areas of concern need to be assessed.

PHYSICAL PROBLEMS

There are many different physical problems to be faced in the care of patient with progressive disease. Some will be specific to a particular disease process, whereas some, such as pain, will be common to many different illnesses.

The distress caused by particular symptoms can often be overlooked by professional carers, as patients may not like to 'bother the doctor' or see these symptoms as a necessary part of the condition (Dunlop 1993). Several surveys have shown unrecognized and uncontrolled symptoms. Wilkes found, in a study of a large group of terminally ill people, that general practitioners reported uncontrolled pain in 26% of the cases, whereas 52% of the patients and 54% of the family carers reported pain (Wilkes 1984).

Symptoms that may be troublesome are discussed below.

Pain

Careful assessment of the cause is essential as pain can be due to musculoskeletal causes, cramp, nerve damage (neuropathic pain), bed sores, or skin pressure from immobility. Specific regimes may be helpful—non-steroidal anti-inflammatory drugs (NSAIDs) for musculoskeletal pain; muscle relaxants for cramp; antidepressants or anticonvulsants for neuropathic pain.

The pain due to continuous skin pressure may be best helped by regular analgesics. Although simple analgesics, such as paracetamol, can be sufficient opioid medication may be necessary if there is only a limited response. If oral medication can be taken the opioid of choice is morphine. This can be given as an elixir (Oramorph) starting at a dose of 5 mg on a regular 4-hourly regime, or as a modified release tablet (MST Continus or Oramorph SR tablets every 12 hours or MXL—morphine sulphate—capsules every 24 hours) starting at 20 mg over 24 hours. Morphine is available in suppository form if oral medication is difficult due to dysphagia. Parenteral medication may become necessary and diamorphine is the opioid of choice as it has a higher solubility and thus the dose can be given in a smaller volume. Diamorphine can be given as an intramuscular injection every 4 hours or by continuous subcutaneous infusion using a portable syringe driver (Oliver 1988). The infusion allows the medication to be given with little distress to the patient and eases the pressure on nursing staff as the infusion is primed every 24 hours. The dose will depend on the previous oral opioid regime—the total oral morphine dose over 24 hours is divided by three to give the 24-hour dose of diamorphine in the infusion (Oliver 1988).

Opioid medication may cause nausea and vomiting in about 30% of patients and an antiemetic, such as metoclopramide 10 mg four times a day or haloperidol 1.5 mg once or twice a day, may be necessary. This may be prescribed routinely for a few days, after which it can be stopped as the nauseating effect of opioids appears to be transient, or a supply given to the patient for use if necessary. Antiemetic medication can be included in a subcutaneous infusion, such as haloperidol 5–10 mg over 24 hours. Constipation is the other important side-effect of opioids and can be prevented by the concurrent use of aperient medication, such as co-danthramer or lactulose with sennoside.

Opioids have been shown to be effective and safe in motor neurone disease (Oliver 1993, 1996) and if the dose is carefully titrated to the patient's pain their use can be very effective and reduce distress.

Dysphagia

Neurological illness may affect swallowing and specific treatment may not be available. Certain techniques can be helpful in aiding feeding (Summers 1981) but other feeding measures, such as nasogastric tube or gastrostomy may need to be considered. Assessment as to the appropriateness of such procedures is necessary, and in the terminal stages of a progressive illness it may be inappropriate to interfere and unnecessarily prolong the patient's dying.

However, a percutaneous endoscopic gastrostomy can be inserted with little distress to the patient and can be very helpful in maintaining a good nutritional intake and relieve the distress of problems with feeding (Iftikar and McIntyre 1990; Park *et al.* 1992). This technique causes fewer problems than nasogastric feeding, in particular less secretions and a reduced risk of aspiration (Norton *et al.* 1996; Scott and Austin 1994).

When swallowing is reduced drooling of saliva may occur. This is particularly distressing and may be helped by an anticholinergic, such as atropine or hyoscine. This can be given as a sublingual tablet, such as hyoscine hydrobromide (Kwells) 0.3 mg 8-hourly, by injection, such as hyoscine hydrobromide 0.4–0.6 mg every 4 hours or as a continuous subcutaneous injection, at a dose of 0.8–2.4 mg over 24 hours (Oliver 1988). Tricyclic antidepressants can also be helpful in reducing secretions.

Muscle spasm

With rigidity, the patient may develop muscle spasm, which may become painful. Muscle relaxant medication, such as dantrolene sodium, which acts directly on skeletal muscle, or baclofen, which inhibits spinal transmission, or diazepam, which is often sedative, can be useful. Physiotherapy can also reduce spasm and discomfort (O'Gorman and Oliver 1998).

Dyspnoea

The involvement of respiratory muscles in neurological disease, such as motor neurone disease, can lead to dyspnoea and ventilatory problems. Careful assessment is necessary before appropriate treatment is commenced. Although ventilation may be possible in some cases, there is a need for discussion and debate before this is started as many ethical and social dilemmas are raised (Oliver 1993). Opioids are effective in the control of dyspnoea and reduce the subjective distress experienced by the patient (Oliver 1993, 1996).

Seizures

As a patient deteriorates there may be an increased risk of a fit, for instance, intracranial pressure increases as a cerebral tumour enlarges. Prophylactic treatment with anticonvulsants may prevent a fit, which can be distressing not only for the patient but also the family. If there is a risk of a fit it can be helpful to provide diazepam enemas so that the family or other close carers are able to take action to stop a fit should this occur.

Incontinence

Many patients fear urinary and faecal incontinence and the ensuing loss of dignity. Sphincter function may be affected in neurological disease, especially as deterioration occurs. The use of a condom catheter or urinary catheterization can be helpful and may reduce the risk of bed sores, although there is an increased risk of infection. Antimuscarinic medication, such as flavoxate, may be helpful if there is unstable detrusor activity.

Faecal incontinence may be more difficult to control, but it is essential to exclude faecal impaction before treating with antidiarrhoeal medication. Incontinence may also be related to poor mobility when the patient may merely be unable to reach the toilet in time. This loss of dignity and control can be eased by ensuring that a patient can call for help and is able to be aided or move him/herself appropriately.

Pressure sores (decubitus)

Skin damage may occur when a patient becomes less mobile and capillary pressure is increased and ischaemia ensues, particularly over bony prominences, especially if there is friction on the skin from lifting or turning. There is an increased risk when there is reduced sensation, incontinence, poor nutritional status, steroid therapy, and reduced mobility (Kaye 1992). Many of these factors may become important in a patient with advanced neurological disease and the aim should be to attempt to reduce them. In a dying patient prevention may be limited and once established healing may be very difficult, so that comfort becomes the primary aim of care. Specific dressings and topical care are helpful and pressure relieving mattresses may aid the patient's comfort.

Constipation

Any patient taking a reduced diet, which may have a reduced fibre content, may develop constipation. Various medications, such as analgesics and anticholinergics, can increase the risk. Constipation should be prevented, if possible, by the administration of aperients. Local rectal measures, suppositories, and enemata, may be necessary for certain patients, especially when there is weakness of anal tone when aperients may cause anal leakage and incontinence.

Confusion

Acute delirium, may be seen, with clouding of consciousness in a previously lucid person associated with disorientation, sleep disturbance, reduced attention, incoherent speech, altered psychomotor activity, and memory impairment. Dementia, with loss of intellectual ability, memory loss, personality change, cortical function changes, such as aphasia, and loss of intellectual abilities in the presence of unimpaired consciousness may occur in progressive disease (Fainsinger *et al.* 1993).

Acute delirium may be caused by many different factors, such as infection, fear, medication, metabolic disturbances, hypoxia, and dehydration and a careful assessment of the patient is essential to allow the appropriate treatment of a reversible condition. General measures, such as adequate lighting, explanation, and management by only a few carers, to minimize confusion, can all be helpful to the patient. However, sedation may become necessary and haloperidol may be necessary to reduce the distress to the patient and their family. On occasions, further sedation, by a phenothiazine or benzodiazepine may be needed, although on many occasions, support and listening may be sufficient. Rarely, it may become necessary, after discussion and involvement of the wider interdisciplinary team, to sedate a distressed patient by parenteral medication. This may become the only way to reduce the distress of the patient and the distress caused to the family and other carers (Murphy 1993).

Anxiety and depression

Any patient facing a progressive illness causing disability and physical distress and maybe with the knowledge of impending death, may experience varying moods and feelings. Many patients may talk of feelings of depression, but it is often very difficult to differentiate this from the natural sadness which would be expected from a debilitating illness. Many of the symptoms of depressive illness, such as appetite loss, insomnia, weakness, reduced libido, constipation, and weariness may be found as part of the symptomatology of the illness itself (Stedeford 1994). Certain factors that may be indicative of depression include reduced mood, reduced interest, agitation or psychomotor retardation, reduced self-esteem, and feelings of worthlessness and hopelessness (Hodgson 1993; Stedeford 1994). If these features predominate, antidepressant medication should be considered, commencing at a low dose initially and slowly increasing.

Anxiety may occur as the seriousness of the illness is realized and faced. In addition to feelings of anxiety there can be profound somatic symptoms, such as sweating, palpitations, dyspnoea, or diarrhoea. Listening and explanation of these symptoms may be effective but anxiolytic medication, such as benzodiazepines or phenothiazines, may be needed (Hodgson 1993). Relaxation techniques can also be very helpful.

EMOTIONAL CONCERNS

Any person facing change in their lifestyle as a result of illness may experience varied emotional reactions. It is important to allow patients during the disease process to express these fears, and this need is even more important as deterioration occurs and death approaches.

Diagnosis

There is increasing evidence that patients with life-threatening illnesses do realize the seriousness of the illness, even if this has not been openly expressed. Hinton showed that 66% patients with advanced cancer knew of their diagnosis and realized that they were dying whereas only 54% had told their family and only 28% had talked of dying to professional carers (Hinton 1980). Openess and sharing within the family is important so that the patient is not left with the 'conspiracy of silence' when a patient is not made aware of the diagnosis or 'the conspiracy of speech' (Carey 1986) when the patient is told of the diagnosis but with an unrealistic view of the prognosis.

Openess and listening to the patient's own suspicions and fears is essential, so that information can be given sympathetically and be heard by the patient. There may be a need to repeat the message on many occasions as the shock of the news itself may block out all the information given. The patient's questions need to be answered honestly and appropriately, allowing he/she to absorb the new information both intellectually and emotionally (Ransohoff 1978).

Families may try to prevent knowledge being imparted as they may try to protect the patient from the shock that they have experienced. However, the seriousness of the news will often be imparted to the patient by other means, by nonverbal communication and from the stress and anxiety of the family. If at all possible the patient should be told with their family so that these problems are lessened.

The actual knowledge of the diagnosis brings with it fears and apprehension. There is a need for the caring professionals to listen to these fears and help to allay any that may be unrealistic. Often details of neurological disease in the press or lay medical books can be overinclusive and even inaccurate so that needless fear is engendered. Patients need opportunities to share these fears openly. The situation may be more complex with certain patients where the capacity to learn more about the diagnosis is restricted by mental impairment. The truth may need to be modified if the patient's ability to understand is altered, as if too much information is given further distress may be caused.

In all communication with patients the prime aim must be to be truthful, for if there is deceit there can be loss of confidence in the integrity of the professional if the lie is found out.

Disability

If there is increasing disability as the disease progresses the patient may have increasing fears of these changes and of resulting dependence. These fears need to be expressed and shared and all the carers, both family and professional, need to be aware so that these feelings can be minimized. Some patients may fear the thought of becoming a 'vegetable' (Ransohoff 1978). There may be opportunities to discuss the future with the patient and some reassurance may be offered that there would not be extensive and inappropriate treatment in the future. It may only be possible to listen and hope to help the patient make the most of the remaining abilities, whether physical or mental.

Fears of mental deterioration

As physical abilities fail fears may arise that mental deterioration may develop. Although these changes may occur in certain neurological disease, such as multiple sclerosis, this may be rarer and is unlikely in other disease processes such as motor neurone disease. Clear explanation and a sharing of these concerns may be needed, and for all patients, reassurance that the symptoms will be helped and reduced to the minimum can be helpful.

Sexuality

With increasing disability and maybe neurological changes sexual performance may become affected. Moreover, the fear of the loss of sexual powers can lead to their loss due to performance anxiety. Delicate discussion may be necessary to allow a patient and their partner to express these fears and problems. Altered sexual behaviour may become necessary, such as a change in position for intercourse, or the consideration of mutual masturbation as an alternative way of expressing their sexual feelings together. A couple may need counselling to cope with these changes.

Fear of death

Each individual has his/her own views of the meaning of life and of death. This may be expressed in a religious certainty of 'heaven' or thoughts of oblivion. Each person's own belief system may result in anxieties, which all need to be shared—there can never be a set answer.

Fear of dying

As many people have never been involved with a dying person or been with anyone at the time of death there may be many fears of this 'unknown'. These fears need to be shared and reassurance given that symptoms, such as pain, can be controlled.

SPIRITUAL CONCERNS

Patients facing progressive disease and death will often have many questions in their minds of a more spiritual nature. These spiritual issues are not necessarily 'religious' but relate to more basic beliefs about the meaning of life and the greater moral issues (Doyle 1992). These thoughts may be of 'Why me?' or a search for existential meaning to the suffering experienced in the illness.

Some people may be supported by their religious beliefs, although this cannot be assumed, as these beliefs are sorely tested by the disease and the resulting distress. A religious leader may be able to provide extra support to patients and become an invaluable member of the caring team. There are no easy answers, but time to share there concerns may be helpful in meeting these important spiritual needs (Doyle 1992). Some patients need to share their experiences and to know that others have been in the same position before (Doyle 1992). On occasion, a team member will be able to help the patient make their own connections within their own experiences.

When considering spiritual issues it is essential to ensure that all the cultural aspects of care are considered. These may be related to specific religious practices but may also be deeply felt within the culture of the patient and his/her family. As death approaches consideration of these issues is necessary so that the care offered is of the best to the patient. If these aspects of care are ignored and cultural customs denigrated, either intentionally or unintentionally, great distress may be caused (Neuberger 1993).

FAMILY CONCERNS

The majority of patients are part of families and these family members, whether spouse, partner, child, brother, sister, or parent, are very much involved in the patient's disease. Some of the fears experienced by a family will be similar to those of the patient but there may be certain specific concerns for family members.

Fear of the illness

A family may, in a similar way to the patient, fear and avoid the diagnosis and the illness. As has been discussed the patient and the family need the opportunity to discuss the diagnosis and the prognosis as openly as possible. Many fears about the illness may be expressed and any myths or unreasonable fears can be clarified. If at all possible, and where the patient's intellectual abilities are not greatly affected by the disease, the patient and family should be seen together so that there is less opportunity for misunderstanding and conflict within the family (Buckman 1993).

Fear of death

Many people, even in old age, may have never been with a dying person or seen a dead body, and when the death of a family member appears to be approaching many fears may develop. There may be specific fears, such as of pain or breathlessness, or a more general concern that they do not feel able to cope with death itself. Family attitudes may vary greatly and there is a need to allow these concerns to be shared and expressed.

Communication

It is important to allow communication to continue within a family. There may be a physical problem, such as dysarthria or dysphasia, causing problems in speech but there may be barriers to openess leading to increasing problems within the family relationships. If there has been an element of deceit, with the hope of protecting the patient from the pain of the diagnosis, communication can become strained when the reality is exposed. Sharing these feelings within the family can be helpful, so that all can be open with each other.

If a patient becomes more disabled the whole family may become isolated, as it becomes increasingly difficult to leave the house. This isolation can be exacerbated if, due to fears of the disease or its effects, such as the wasting and possible drooling in advanced motor neurone disease, other family members or friends avoid the situation and find it difficult to visit. Support of the carers so that they are able to care for the patient is essential and carers need time for themselves, so that they can retain their strength to cope with the full-time caring load (Kinsella and Duffy 1979).

Finance

As the disease progresses finances may become strained, as part-time working, early retirement, or long-term sickness absence reduces the family income. Moreover, a partner may also be forced to take leave of absence or retirement to care for the patient. These changes can have profound effects on a family and need to be addressed.

Children

Many families suppose that children should be protected from the feelings and fears as a parent or other close family member deteriorates. However, there is much evidence showing that children of all ages sense that all is not well, although the full extent of their knowledge will depend on their emotional development and previous experience (Stedeford 1994; Ward 1992). Thus, it is important to include children in the care of a dying patient and help them to talk about their perceptions and fears. An open approach within the family and by health care professionals may allow a child to express their feelings and the child should be included within the family (Monroe 1993).

After the death, children should be included in the rituals, such as attending the funeral, if they wish. If a child is excluded there is evidence that there can be increased problems in bereavement (Black 1987).

Decisions in treatment

In the care of a patient dying from a neurological disease there may be many occasions when very difficult management decisions need to be made, for instance, in the decision to start, stop, or alter the dose of corticosteroids in a patient with a cerebral tumour. Although it may be the ideal to include both the patient and family in this decision-making process this can be a cause of great stress and concern. On occasions, the family may be faced with a decision, such as those relating to ventilation or removing ventilatory support in a patient with severe brain injury or the giving of permission for organ donation in a patient who is brain dead, and very careful discussion is necessary. A family may feel threatened and very vulnerable at this time and undue guilt may be engendered if the family are left to make a decision alone. Involvement with close discussion can allow the family to be involved but without the need to carry the load unaided.

Most patients will be part of a wider social network, family, or friends, and there will often be many people who will be affected by the problems caused by the disease. The inclusion of these people in the care of the patient is important, as the aim in the care of any patient, and particularly a dying patient, is to treat the 'whole patient' and this should be in the context of the 'whole family'. All families will be different and there are many individual family coping mechanisms which all need to be respected. Their needs may be very profound and time with the family, to explain, involve, and support, will help to ensure that the family unit is kept together and does not become split.

INTERDISCIPLINARY TEAM CARE

The assessment and subsequent treatment of a patient with a neurological disease will be greatly improved by the co-ordinated response of a wider interdisciplinary team. All members of the team are able to offer their own expertise and experience to the benefit of the whole team and the patient. However, it is essential that this is co-ordinated, so that there is not unnecessary duplication or ommission and a 'key worker' approach, when one member of the team co-ordinates the patient's care, can ensure the best possible care (Newrick and Langton-Hewer 1984).

The various disciplines involved in the patient's care may include:

Medical care—providing the medical assessment and advice on the medical care, including symptom control, assessment of the progression of the disease.

Nursing care—assessing the patient's and families particular needs and planning the care and support needed to eliminate or reduce the effects of these needs.

Physiotherapy—assessment of the patient's physical condition and capabilities. This may include the maintenance of mobility, the reduction of stiffness or contractures by regular passive movements, maintenance of joint mobility, and minimizing the effects of the disease process (Oliver *et al.* 1986).

Occupational therapy—assessment of the patient's needs to maintain his/her lifestyle. This may include the assessment and provision of aids for daily living, such as special feeding aids, aids to help with toileting, mobility aids, and adaptions to equipment and housing to allow a patient to function as fully as possible in his/her own environment. Mobility aids may become increasingly important as deterioration occurs with a progression from simple aids, such as a walking stick, to a wheelchair.

Social worker—assessment and help with a patient and his/her family's needs and concerns can be provided by a social worker. These needs may be of a practical nature, such as advice on benefits and other social security aspects, but will also include the counselling and support, especially of children, within the family.

Speech and language therapist—many patients with a neurological disease will develop speech problems, such as dysphasia, dysarthria, or more complex problems. A therapist can assess these problems and provide not only advice but communication aids, varying from a spelling or communication board to computer communication systems. The therapist may be able to assess swallowing problems and advise on possible treatment options.

Dietician—assessment of a patient's nutritional needs and advice on the choice and preparation of food when eating is difficult due to dysphagia or disability can be provided by a dietician. If gastrostomy or nasogastric feeding are necessary the dietician has a crucial role in ensuring the successful implementation of a feeding regime.

Chaplain—a religious leader, appropriate to the patient's needs, may be able to offer support to a patient and family. They may be able to address deeper spiritual needs as well as to provide religious support.

Specific support groups—there are many specific support groups for patients with neurological disease, such as the Motor Neurone Disease Association or the Multiple Sclerosis Society, and these groups can provide support and help to patients and their families. Patients may benefit from meeting other patients and sharing their experiences, and the groups may provide useful information, such as booklets and advice sheets.

There is therefore a need for a interdisciplinary assessment of patients and a close working relationship, based on mutual respect of each professional's expertise. Team members may vary in their involvement at different stages of the disease and the co-ordinator ('key worker') may need to ensure that all the team are kept updated.

There is also a need to support each other, as certain members of the team may find the patient's deterioration more stressful. If the other team members are aware of these potential problems there can be a sharing and support of each other. When a patient dies there may be a profound sense of loss within the team and time needed to share these feelings to ensure that the team continues to function as effectively as possible.

TERMINAL CARE

As a patient deteriorates there is an even greater need to ensure that all the symptoms and other problems are controlled and addressed. Any treatment should be appropriate to the patient's needs and unnecessary investigations, which do not lead to any change in the management of the patient, and procedures should be avoided. For instance, intravenous infusions may not be appropriate in a person who is imminently dying, as the discomfort of the procedure outweighs any potential benefits when dehydration causes few symptoms apart from a dry mouth (Micetich *et al.* 1983; Stone 1993). This should be considered on an individual basis, but in the palliative care of a patient with an incurable and progressive disease the most appropriate treatment may be mouth care rather than the use of intravenous fluids (Dunlop *et al.* 1995; Dunphy *et al.* 1995; Randall and Downie 1996).

During this period both the patient and family may wish to undertake specific aims. These may include preparations for the continuing deterioration or impending death, such as the writing of a will or ensuring the family, including children, are prepared. There may also be the wish to undertake a specific visit, fulfil a particular wish, or relive previous experiences. Families may require increasing support to cope duing these preparations and they may all need help to share their feelings and concerns.

Other preparations may be needed as death approaches to ensure that all involved are aware of the situation. It is essential that all the health care professionals continue to communicate well so that they are all aware of their own roles. There is often a reluctance to admit that death is approaching and staff who have cared for a disabled patient for some time may try to ignore the real position, as they develop similar feelings as the family. Only if there is an agreement that death may be near can the most appropriate treatment plan be made, as if there is disagreement within the caring team, the patient and family may feel insecure and the quality of care in the terminal phase may be less effective.

The place of caring may need to be discussed. The majority of seriously ill patients wish to remain at home (Dunlop *et al.* 1989; Ashby and Wakefield 1993) but this may become very difficult if serious problems, such as severe pain, confusion, or incontinence, develop. Discussion about admission to hospital, nursing home, or on occasions a hospice may be necessary. There is no single answer for all patients and only by individual discussion between the patient and family will these problems be resolved. Locally available resources will also vary and need to be taken into consideration.

Many hospices are able to take patients with terminal malignant disease, motor neurone disease, and other terminal illnesses. Most hospices would be able to provide advice on symptom control and the care of terminally patients and their families even if they cannot admit the patient. Many hospices can help with advice on symptom control and support of patients and their families at home. A hospice home care team of nurses, with the support of the wider multidisciplinary team, can provide support for the primary health care team at home. Macmillan Nurses are also based in the community to help and be a resource in the care and support of patients requiring palliative care.

If the patient and his/her family wish to remain at home the primary health care team, of general practitioner and community nurse, can support the patient, but there is a need to ensure that there is good communication with the services that have also been involved with the patient so that everyone is aware of the problems and the needs of the patient and family.

There may be particular fears and concerns that need to be addressed, such as the fear of choking that often occurs when a patient becomes dyspnoeic, as in motor neurone disease. Explanation of the symptom and careful symptom control can be very helpful in allaying these fears, but it is often advantageous to provide medication for emergency use at home. The Breathing Space Pack, developed by the UK Motor Neurone Disease Association, provides advice on the medication that can be of help in an emergency and provides a box so that the medication can be safely stored in the patient's home after discussion between the patient, family, and doctor (Oliver 1993). An intramuscular injection of an opioid, such as diamorphine or morphine 5–10 mg, a tranquillizer, such as midazolam 5–10 mg or chlorpromazine 12.5–25 mg and an anticholinergic, such as hyoscine hydobromide 400–600 µg, will usually control severe symptoms in the emergency situation (Oliver 1994). Often, the patient can return to their regular medication but if parenteral medication becomes necessary intramuscular injections may be continued. A subcutaneous infusion using a portable syringe driver can allow parenteral medication to be continued with little discomfort to the patient and with less strain on home nursing resources (Oliver 1988).

In neurological disease very specialized care may be needed with certain patients. For instance, in a patient with a persistant vegetative state there may be many very difficult decisions as to how far active treatment should continue. Although it can be argued that the withdrawal of treatment, such as hydration and feeding, is 'the withdrawal of useless, non-beneficial treatment—albeit in the knowledge that this will lead to the underlying condition causing the patient's death' (Gillon 1993), others may see these actions as the 'opening of the back door to euthanasia' (Spencer 1993). There are no clear answers and careful discussion with all the family and carers can allow the elucidation of the most appropriate course of action (Andrews 1993). In the future there may be a greater opportunity to consider the patient's own views on some of these problems if the patient has completed an Advance Directive (Living Will) so that their intentions in the event of a serious illness are clearly declared (Oliver 1993). However, conflicts may occur between the patient's expressed wishes and the family's hopes. There are no easy answers and each patient will require an individual assessment.

The care of the patient and family when there is brainstem death is also complex. Before the tests to establish that the criteria for this condition are met, the clinicians should explain the procedure and the implications of the results. If the tests confirm brainstem death, discussion of the possibility of organ donation may be suggested. There is evidence that organ donation can be very helpful to families in their bereavement, although there be initial reluctance by both the professional health carers and the family to initiate this discussion (Tymstra *et al.* 1992; Peters and Sutcliffe 1992). However, the family may remain very shocked especially when there has been a sudden deterioration and all staff must be aware of the grief and disbelief that may be shown and be able to cope with the potential anger of the family (Ransohoff 1978).

BEREAVEMENT

Bereavement care starts well before the death of the patient and the involvement of the family in the patient's care and the encouragement of the expression of feelings will facilitate the later grieving process. Following the death, the family will still require support as grief is experienced and help may be needed to encourage and facilitate its expression (Worden 1991; Oliver and McMurray 1993). Extra help, from a counsellor, clinical psychologist, or psychiatrist, may be necessary for some families.

CONCLUSION

The care of a dying patient requires a careful approach which includes everyone, patient, family, and other carers. The aim is to allow patients and their families to maintain control of their lives and the carers need to listen to them before imposing ideas and plans (Hodges 1992).

There is no way to alter the inevitable, that death is approaching, but the care offered can allow a patient to live as full a life as possible, and live with dignity until they die.

REFERENCES

Andrews, K. (1993). Patients in the perspective vegetative state: problems in their long term management. *British Medical Journal*, **306**, 1600–2.

Ashby, M. and Wakefield, M. (1993). Attitudes to some aspects of death and dying, living wills and substituted health care decision-making in South Australia: public opinion survey for a parliamentary select committee. *Palliative Medicine*, **7**, 273–82.

Black, D. (1987). Family intervention with bereaved children. *Journal of Psychology and Psychiatry*, **28**, 467–76.

Buckman, R. (1993). Communication in palliative care; a practical guide. In *Oxford textbook of palliative medicine*, (ed. D. Doyle, G. W. C. Hanks, and N. Macdonald), pp. 47–61. Oxford University Press.

Carey, J. S. (1986). Motor neurone disease—a challenge to medical ethics. *Journal of the Royal Society of Medicine*, **79**, 216–20.

Doyle, D. (1992). Have we looked beyond the physical and psychosocial? *Journal of Pain and Symptom Management*, **7**, 302–11.

Dunlop, R. (1993). Wider applications of palliative care. In *The management of terminal malignant disease*, (3rd edn), (ed. C. Saunders and N. Sykes), pp. 287–96. Edward Arnold, London.

Dunlop, R. J., Davies, R. J., and Hockley, J. M. (1989). Preferred versus actual place of death: a hospital palliative care support team experience. *Palliative Medicine*, **3**, 197–201.

Dunlop, R. J., Ellershaw, J. E., Baines, M. J., Sykes, N., and Saunders, C. M. (1995). On withholding nutrition and hydration in the terminally ill: has palliative medicine gone too far? A reply. *Journal of Medical Ethics*, **21**, 141–3.

Dunphy, K., Finlay, I., Rathbone, G., Gilbert, J., and Hicks, F. (1995). Rehydration in palliative and terminal care: if not—why not? *Palliative Medicine*, **9**, 221–8.

Fainsinger, R. L., Tapper, M., and Bruera, E. (1993). A perspective on the management of delirium in terminally ill patients on a palliative care unit. *Journal of Palliative Care*, **9**, 4–8.

Gillon, R. (1993). Patients in the persistent vegetative state: a response to Dr Andrews. *British Medical Journal*, **306**, 1602–3.

Hinton, J. (1980). Whom do dying patients tell? *British Medical Journal*, **281**, 1328–30.

Hodges, J. (1992). Death, the unexpected certainty: anticipatory grief work in the hospital setting. *Palliative Medicine*, **6**, 179–81.

Hodgson, G. (1993). Depression, sadness and anxiety. In *The management of terminal malignant disease*, (3rd edn), (ed. C. Saunders and N. Sykes), pp. 102–30. Edward Arnold, London.

Iftikar, S. Y. and McIntyre, A. S. (1990). Percutaneous gastrostomy; an alternative endoscopic approach. *British Journal of Surgery*, **77**, 1062.

Kaye, P. (1992). *A to Z of hospice and palliative medicine*. EPL Publications, Northampton.

Kinsella, G. J., and Duffy, F. D. (1979). Psychosocial readjustment in the spouses of aphasic patients. *Scandinavian Journal of Rehabilitation Medicine*, **11**, 129–32.

Micetich, K. C., Steinecker, P. H., and Thomasma, D. C. (1983). Are intravenous fluids morally required for a dying patient? *Archives of Internal Medicine*, **143**, 975–8

Monroe, B. (1993). Social work in palliative care. In *Oxford textbook of palliative medicine*, (ed. D. Doyle, G. W. C. Hanks, and N. Macdonald), pp. 569–70, Oxford University Press.

Murphy, M. (1993). Confusion. In *The management of terminal malignant disease*, (3rd edn), (ed. C. Saunders and N. Sykes), pp. 131–8. Edward Arnold, London.

Neuberger, J. (1993). Cultural issues in palliative care. In *Oxford textbook of palliative medicine*, (ed. D. Doyle, G. W. C. Hanks, and N. Macdonald), pp. 507–13. Oxford University Press.

Newrick, P. G. and Langton-Hewer, R. (1984). Motor neurone disease; can we do better? A study of 42 patients. *British Medical Journal*, **289**, 539–42.

Norton, B., Homer-Ward, M., Donnelly, M. T., Long, R. G., and Holmes, G. K. T. (1996) A randomised prospective comparison of percutaneous endoscopic gastrostomy and nasogastric tube feeding after acute dysphasic stroke. *British Medical Journal*, **312**, 13–16.

O'Gorman, B. and Oliver, D. (1998). Disorders of nerve I: Motor neurone disease. In *Neurological Physiotherapy*, (ed. M. Stokes), pp. 171–9. Mosby, London.

Oliver, D. (1988). Syringe drivers in palliative care; a review. *Palliative Medicine*, **2**, 21–6.

Oliver, D. (1993). Ethical issues in palliative care—an overview. *Palliative Medicine*, **7**(suppl. 2), 15–20.

Oliver, D. (1994). *Motor neurone disease*, (2nd edn). Royal College of General Practitioners, Exeter.

Oliver D. (1996). The quality of care and symptom control—the effects on the terminal phase of ALS/MND. *Journal of the Neurological Sciences*, **139**(suppl.), 134–6.

Oliver, D. and McMurray, N. (1993). Bereavement—whose responsibility? *Palliative Medicine*, **7**(suppl. 2), 73–6.

OPCS (Office of Population Censuses and Surveys) (1993). *Mortality statistics—cause*. Series DH2 No. 18. HMSO, London.

Park, R. H. R., Allison, M. C., Lang, J., Morris, A. J., Danesh, B. J. Z. et al. (1992). Randomised comparison of percutaneous endoscopic gastrostomy and nasogastric tube feeding in patients with persisting neurological dysphagia. *British Medical Journal*, **304**, 1406–9

Peters, D. and Sutcliffe, J. (1992). Organ donation: the hospice perspective. *Palliative Medicine*, **6**, 212–16

Randall, F. and Downie, R. S. (1996). *Palliative care ethics. A good companion*, pp. 124–6. Oxford University Press.

Ransohoff, J. (1978). Death, dying and the neurosurgical patient. *Journal of Neurosurgical Nursing*, **10**, 198–201.

Saunders, C. M., Baines, M., and Dunlop, R. (1995). *Living with dying. A guide to palliative care*, (3rd edn), pp. 45–56. Oxford University Press.

Scott, A. G. and Austin, H. E. (1994) Nasogastric feeding in the management of severe dysphagia in motor neurone disease. *Palliative Medicine*, **8**, 45–9.

Spencer, S. J. G. (1993). Inconsistency and confusion cloud the debate. *British Medical Journal*, **307**, 202.

Stedeford, A. (1994). *Facing death. Patients, families and professionals*, (2nd edn). Sobell, Oxford.

Stone, C. (1993). Prescribed hydration in palliative care. *British Journal of Nursing*, **2**, 353–7

Summers, D. H. (1981). The caring team in motor neurone disease. *Hospice—the living idea*, (ed. C. Saunders, D. H. Summers, and N. Teller), pp. 148–55. Edward Arnold, London.

Tymstra, Tj., Heyink, J. W., and Prium, J. (1992). Experience of bereaved relatives who granted or refused permission for organ donation. *Family Practice*, **9**, 141–4.

Ward, B. (1992). *Good grief. Exploring feelings, loss and death with under 11's and adults*. Jessica Kingsley, London.

WHO (World Health Organization) (1990). *Cancer pain relief and palliative care, Report of the World Health Organization Expert Committee*. Technical Report Series 804. World Health Organization, Geneva.

Wilkes, E. (1984). Dying now. *Lancet*, **i**, 50–2.

Worden, J. W. (1991). *Grief counselling and grief work*, (2nd edn). Tavistock/Routledge, London.

Michael Donaghy

British neurologists are in the throes of confronting issues which could profoundly alter their role in providing health care. Their specialty is already the most diagnostically diverse in internal medicine. They must keep abreast of a rapidly expanding repertoire of treatments, be alert to the ever-widening implications of genetic diseases in neurology, and be prepared to enjoin patients with ever more detailed and precise discussion of prognostic, ethical, and legal issues. The value of such diverse activities is difficult to quantify, yet neurologists must now justify their worth to their paymasters, who increasingly are fundholding general practitioners.

The role of neurologists is not merely to see today's patients. They are also responsible for training the neurologists of tomorrow, for ensuring that all medical students understand the rudiments of neurology, and for advancing understanding of disease processes and their treatment. Methods for teaching medical students must change so as to acknowledge the move of neurological practice to an outpatient setting. Furthermore, these methods should recognize openly that few students will become specialist neurologists. The quest to unravel the biological bases for neurological diseases faces an increasingly tight and questioning grasp on the availability of biomedical research funds. Academic neurologists should recognize that society is becoming interested in reducing the burden of neurological disability by approaches which are no longer founded in the dogma of cell biology, but which involve practical measures, such as reducing road traffic injuries.

THE RANGE OF NEUROLOGISTS' FUNCTIONS

No single individual can undertake effectively the whole range of duties for which neurologists are responsible. The clinical duties include general neurology and subspecialty services. Educational roles include undergraduate teaching, postgraduate training, and continuing education. Biomedical research is becoming increasingly specialized, and moving away from the bedside. The health care funders will demand more and more outcomes research, and only by participating can neurologists ensure that this asks the right questions and employs reliable methodologies. The advent of market-

orientated health care demands increased involvement by neurologists in management and administration. Each group of neurologists must apportion these various responsibilities among themselves and be prepared continually to redefine their individual responsibilities in response to a constantly changing environment. The neurological community can only provide these disparate services if its neurologists are specialized into three broad types, and if these neurologists interact within regional neurological centres.

CLINICAL DUTIES

It is clinical practice which is the essence of a neurologist's work. The majority of neurological problems fall within a relatively small grouping of diseases, yet the overall diagnostic scope of neurology is enormous. Many of the rarer or diagnostically complex disorders cause particularly significant disability, often in youngish patients. Such patients may require advice from subspecialists concerning precise diagnosis and prognosis, possible genetic implications, and treatment prospects.

General neurological practice

Most, if not all, neurologists should have a general neurological practice with referrals direct from general practitioners—9.5% of the British population consult their general practitioners (GPs) about a neurological symptom each year, and about 7% of these are referred on to hospital consultants, mainly neurologists (Hopkins 1989). The proportion of patients referred to consultant neurologists seems likely to increase in response to various pressures. On the one hand, GPs feel increasingly uncertain in the face of the diagnostic complexity of neurology and the ever-growing threat of litigation resulting from delayed or non-referral. On the other, patients are better educated about health matters due to broadcasting and journalism, and increasingly demand that their GP obtains an expert's assessment of their symptoms. As Hopkins (1989) estimates, only a small shift in referral practice could submerge the already hard-pressed consultant neurologist services in the United Kingdom. Although we have yet to attain the goal of a full-time equivalent neurologist per 200 000 of the population (Langton-Hewer and Wood 1992), most of the 230-odd British neurologists are aware that referral rates are soaring with outpatient waiting times often exceeding six months. More neurologists will be required, in turn imposing severe demands training programmes. In reality, a goal of one neurologist per 100 000 population seems a more appropriate aim for the provision of general neurological services.

The problem is compounded by a rapidly changing notion of what a neurologist should achieve during each outpatient consultation. Gone are the days, thankfully, when the neurologist could merely look up from the referral letter and say 'Your general practitioner says you have had a fit', examine the patient's fundi and plantar responses, before saying 'I'll arrange a scan and write to your doctor' as he moves to a similar consultation in the adjacent room on his way to 'achieving fifteen new patients for the morning'. Patients and their GPs now expect and deserve a considered diagnostic assessment, followed by full discussion of the diagnosis and prognosis, or of the diagnostic possibilities, what investigations may be necessary, how work or driving may be affected, any genetic implications, recommendations for treatment with frank advice about possible side-effects, and even informal counselling about coping with the psychological consequences of an unpalatable diagnosis. On average, such consultations take at least half an hour. Yet, it is a rewarding mode of practice; and not one for the 'fifteen new patients a morning' neurologist.

In general neurological practice, approximately 75% of the new patient referrals fall within only ten clinical problem or diagnostic areas. The commonest conditions, in rough order of frequency, are:

Headache
Epilepsy and blackouts
Cerebrovascular disease
Peripheral and cranial nerve disorders
Sciatica and lumbar disc disease
Cervical spine disorders
Multiple sclerosis
Disequilibrium
Parkinson's disease
Dementia (Hopkins 1989; Stevens 1989; Perkin 1989).

Such lists are valuable in guiding training both for would-be neurologists and for medical students, many of whom will encounter neurological problems in general practice or general internal medicine.

However, there are important reasons why all neurologists must continue to be more broadly trained, rather than aiming to become 'bare-foot' practitioners skilled only in these ten conditions. First, the majority of these clinical problem areas already contain a considerable differential diagnosis, resolution of which may be important for specific treatment and prognosis. For instance, those occasional patients whose cerebrovascular disease is due to vasculitis deserve better than aspirin therapy; the various types of headache require differing treatments and have varying morbidities; and peripheral

neuropathy encompasses over a hundred possible diagnoses which include eminently treatable disorders. Second, the less frequently encountered 25% of referrals include some notably serious and disabling diseases which may strike at a young age, posing particularly expensive and demanding diagnostic exercises, and require specialized advice about treatment, prognosis, genetics, or ethical issues. Third, many patients referred to neurologists either never attain a formal diagnosis of a recognized neurological disease or they have psychologically determined somatic symptoms. Such patients pose considerable diagnostic uncertainty for the GP. Neurologists are crucial to resolving this uncertainty by recognizing that the patient has neither the symptoms nor signs of any serious neurological disease, and by eliciting the subtle inconsistencies so typical of psychologically based symptoms.

The numerical pressure of new patient referrals often prevents British neurologists from following up an appropriate proportion of their patients. Of course, most referrals only need to be seen once in the neurology clinic. The consultant's initial letter should anticipate any likely 'set plays' in the patient's future management. Most GPs are adept in manipulating the commonly used drugs in epilepsy and Parkinson's disease, and in targeting support care to patients disabled by diseases such as multiple sclerosis. Thus, in a GP-based health care system, it is appropriate for neurologists to transfer back care for most patients after only one consultation, with a recommendation for re-referral if difficulties arise. Many such difficulties can be resolved by communication between the GP and neurologist rather than by another clinic appointment. Yet, there will always be a group of patients who do require regular follow-up. These include those with difficult epilepsy or movement disorders, those on immunosuppression for neuromuscular or vasculitic disorders, and some patients with a particular need for pastoral support from a specialist in neurology; these often include patients who are health care workers.

A number of pressures are responsible for the increasing shift of neurology from the ward to the outpatient clinic. Definitive, noninvasive diagnostic investigations, such as magnetic resonance imaging (MRI), have made many admissions unnecessary. Health care purchasers are exerting pressure to promote a shift away from expensive inpatient facilities. Patients now object to inpatient stays made unnecessarily long by failure to prebook investigations or by their neurologist apparently needing time 'to think'. Neurologists should support these moves; a consultant neurologist in a consulting room is cheap, and can provide prompt and direct care, when compared to inpatient facilities. Neurologists should ensure that savings derived from the contraction of inpatient facilities are converted into an increased number of consultant neurologists, so that prompt outpatient appointments are widely available. However, there are invisible costs associated with the increasingly sophisticated nature of modern outpatient care. In particular, neurologists now spend far longer discussing the interpretation of scans with their neuroradiological colleagues. The resultant correspondence with GPs and patients has become more complex as subtle explanations must be conveyed using the written, rather than the spoken, word. All this takes time.

Subspecialty services

A glance at any neurology reference text will show the enormity and variety of neurological disease. No single neurologist can now master the entire subject. Neurologists should aim to be competent in handling the commoner general neurological problems, and couple this to a special interest in a more specialized clinical area. As diagnosis, prognostication, treatment, and genetic implications become more complex and detailed, neurologists will wish to refer a small, but significant proportion of their caseload to colleagues more expert in that particular subspecialty. Commonly encountered examples include clinics for difficult epilepsy, movement disorders, peripheral neuropathy, muscle disorders, neurogenetics, and dementia. Furthermore, if specific treatments are proven to be effective for commoner diseases, neurologists may have to evolve subspecialty services for these: possibilities include thrombolysis for cerebrovascular disease, interventional angiography for cerebral aneurysm, and beta-interferon therapy for multiple sclerosis. Inevitably, the provision of such highly specialized services will be predominantly the responsibility of neurologists based in a regional centre.

However, there is another type of subspecialty service which neurologists could usefully provide, particularly those who are based in district general hospitals. Examples include neurological rehabilitation and stroke services (Greenwood 1992; Selzer 1992), clinical neurophysiology (Gutmann *et al.* 1991), and geriatric neurology (Whitehouse 1991). As numbers of consultant neurologists expand, with an ever-increasing presence in district general hospitals, there may be a need to develop training schemes which lead to dual accreditation in neurology coupled with one of these other specialties. This would benefit the local patient population by increasing the range of clinical services available to local doctors. The added responsibilities would justify appointment of pairs of neurologists to the larger district hospitals, thereby expanding local neurological services, minimizing professional isolation, and allowing the dovetailing of leave so as to maintain constant neurological cover for that hospital.

Inpatient neurological services

Despite the shift of neurological care to outpatients, and the growth of subspecialty referral services, there will remain a continuing need for neurological inpatient services. Highly specialized inpatient care will always be required for patients with acute, potentially serious or disabling conditions such as stroke, acute spinal cord lesions, Guillain–Barré syndrome, myasthenia gravis, status epilepticus, raised intracranial pressure, and neurological infections. Britain is already losing the truly general physician from its university hospitals. This poses a pressing question about who should be primarily responsible for inpatients with acute neurological disease. Traditionally, such patients have been admitted and managed by general physicians who request for neurologists to provide inpatient consultations, or to take over inpatient care, in only a small proportion of these patients. There will be increasing pressures for expanded neurological services to assume primary responsibility for the admission of all patients with acute neurological disease to university hospitals.

Inpatient consultations form an important part of a neurologist's work, and few neurologists have been specifically trained to provide the crisp and practical advice which is required. District general hospital physicians frequently ask their neurological colleagues for advice about clinical problems which span the whole range of neurology; such consultations are also required in university hospitals. There is also a need for some university hospital-based neurologists to develop liaison with particular non-neurological specialties. Neurological complications in transplant recipients, in patients with rheumatological disease, or in patients with HIV infection represent examples.

TYPES OF NEUROLOGIST, AND REGIONAL NEUROLOGICAL CENTRES

From the foregoing, it will be evident that the needs of neurological patients will be best served by three types of neurologist, who interact with each other in a regional neurological centre incorporated into a university hospital. These different prototype neurologists should be seen as stereotypes merely for the purposes of discussion. In reality, many will have roles which overlap in varying manners and degrees. The regional neurological centre should be the clinical focus for managing the local population's general neurological disease, offer subspecialty services, and provide specialized facilities, such as neurological intensive care and investigational facilities for patients referred from a much wider area. This area should include at a minimum the district general hospitals (DGHs) of neurologists affiliated to that centre and is likely to serve a population of 2.5–7.5 million. The centre should also contain the regional neurosurgery, neuroradiology, neurophysiology, neuropathology, and neuropsychology services so as to allow appropriate multidisciplinary consultation both for the provision of patient care, and for education. Ideally, such regional centres should be located in a university hospital where academic clinicians are particularly likely to develop subspecialty clinical services. The need to provide a range of subspecialty referral services should be satisfied by recruiting or training consultant staff in specific areas. The centre should provide an educational focus for training would-be neurologists, teaching neurology to medical students, and for the continuing education needs of consultant neurologists and their colleagues in related disciplines. All neurologists should be affiliated to such a centre even if based in a DGH.

Centre-based neurologists

These would be primarily responsible for providing general and subspecialty clinical services at that regional centre. They might carry out 'satellite' clinics and inpatient consultations once or twice weekly at a nearby DGH, but should not have inpatient responsibilities at that hospital. They should have a prominent role as academic clinicians, and may be employed primarily either by the National Health Service, or by the university; split funding arrangements would be most appropriate in the future. Their academic roles will include teaching and training at undergraduate and postgraduate levels, development of subspecialty services, and clinically based research or collaborative research with basic scientists.

District general hospital-based neurologists

These would attend primarily to in and outpatients at their DGH. They may develop subspecialty roles relevant to their DGH, such as provision of neurophysiology or rehabilitation services. They should be formally attached to a regional centre for a minimum of one whole day per week so as to care for patients from their district who have more complex disorders, for their own continuing education needs, and so as to avoid long-term professional isolation. Such activities should be funded by their own DGH.

Clinical scientists in neurology

This group constitutes the final category. They are likely to be few in number and many would be funded by research organizations and charities rather than by the universities. Their primary role will be to undertake research into fundamental mechanisms of disease, or to develop novel approaches to investigation or treatment. If appropriately trained they may undertake limited clinical and educational roles in parallel with their centre-based colleagues. The clinical service should not become dependent on them, given that their research tenure may be insecure, and their research commitment may demand considerable flexibility in their commitment to clinical and educational activities.

EDUCATION

Neurologists have four potential roles in educating other doctors in addition to the education of nurses and paramedical workers. Of these, their role in clinical audit, and in attempts to change clinical practice by outcome measures, will be discussed later.

UNDERGRADUATE EDUCATION

All medical students should rotate through an attachment to the neurology department of a university hospital, a situation only provided in approximately two-thirds of British medical schools (Wilkinson 1990). Neurologists should recognize that few students will wish to become neurologists. Consequently, they should devise an approach to teaching neurology which arms students for careers in disciplines such as general practice, psychiatry, or other branches of internal medicine. Those few who are intent on a neurological career usually make their special interest and aptitude clear and are particularly diligent about self-education. Greater emphasis needs to be given to outpatient teaching, so that students can encounter the common problems, such as headaches and blackouts, which form such a large proportion of neurological referrals. In these days of burgeoning medical knowledge and expectation, guidance about the core curriculum would be valuable. Undergraduate teaching should be a specific duty of academic clinicians in university neurology centres, be they employed by the National Health Service or by universities. Such teaching should not be undertaken primarily by those who are biologically based neuroscientists rather than fully practising clinicians (Menken 1990).

Exposure to neurological inpatients will remain important. First, they provide a source for students to practise eliciting abnormal physical signs. Second, they allow students to encounter patients with serious disabling conditions, such as multiple sclerosis, stroke, and brain tumour. Third, they provide an opportunity to learn the elements of history taking from patients with established disease, unfettered by the time constraints and unpredictability of the outpatient department.

Most students are daunted by the breadth and complexity of the neurological history and examination as usually listed in textbooks or student handouts. Neurologists should indicate both explicitly and by example that neurological diagnosis is an exploratory exercise based on a small selection from the range of possible questions and physical signs. Thus, students need to be familiarized with the concept of a '5-minute neurological examination' that focuses on the clinical problem confronting them. For instance, if the urological house surgeon (or indeed consultant) merely examined the ankle jerks, plantar responses, and sacral sensation in patients with apparent prostatism, they would unmask the true problem in many of those with neurogenic bladders who are liable to be inconvenienced even further by urological surgery. The shift of emphasis in teaching to outpatients will require changes in the way in which consultants allocate their time to clinics; medical schools will have to provide the financial resources necessary to pay for the teaching component of outpatient time.

POSTGRADUATE TRAINING

There are likely to be continuing pressures for expansion of consultant neurologist numbers and these will have to be trained by the existing neurologists. Any deregulation of the current state monopoly on health care in Britain would require more formal assessment of whether and when a trainee has qualified as a specialist neurologist. In the future, this might be determined by examination, coupled with rotation through a formally accredited training structure, rather than by the current *ad-hoc* arrangements which pertain in Britain. In any event, there will be a shift away from our tradition of simply exposing trainees to a busy clinical service, and expecting knowledge to follow by osmosis. Of course, supervised clinical practice will always remain fundamental to neurological training.

In the future, there will be increased pressures to create formal training programmes. These will be designed both to cover subject matter central to neurology, and to provide an introduction to overlapping specialties such as neurophysiology, neuropathology, neuroradiology, paediatric neurology, and neurosurgery. To provide for this, training rotations may need to incorporate time for 'day release' for educational activities and block attachments to paraneurological specialties. This will create funding problems given the dependence of current service provision on the clinical activity of trainees. Regional neurological centres should aim to develop coordinated four- or five-year training programmes to replace the current appointments to separate registrar and senior registrar posts—all too often in different places. It must be acknowledged that any formalization of training would embody the notion that most trainees would reach a time when they are certified as 'trained'. Yet, in the absence of a professional outlet to 'office practice' they would have nowhere to go at the end of their training programmes, thereby clogging the training programme.

CONTINUING EDUCATION

Knowledge, technology, and therapy are changing rapidly in modern neurology, as are concepts of how to use these advances most appropriately. For trained neurologists in post, it is vital to provide a regular formal opportunity to keep up to date. Traditionally, this has been achieved by every neurologist attending the weekly case conference at his/her local regional centre, and by attending national or international conferences or symposia once or twice a year; clinical audit provides a recent addition to these educational activities. District general hospitals should recognize their responsibility for keeping their neurologists trained by funding their weekly attendance at the regional neurological centre's continuing education programme.

RESEARCH, AND THE OUTCOMES MEASURES MOVEMENT

Neurologists can contribute to the research development of their subject in three ways. Clinical scientists, and some academic clinicians, may investigate basic biological mechanisms underlying disease processes. Many neurologists will participate in clinical research, be it in reporting a series of cases illu-

minating particular diseases, by participating in multicentre clinical trials, or by providing clinical input to basic science research programmes. These important matters are considered elsewhere in this volume. A third area has assumed great prominence: *outcome measures*.

The outcome measures initiative is seen by many as the 'Holy Grail' which underlies modern cost-effective health care. Put simplistically, this initiative considers that a series of practice guidelines can be developed as a result of collecting data about the quality of treatment outcomes (i.e. mortality rates; complication rates; measurement of reversal of disability; or quality adjusted life years), or about the impact of investigations (i.e. Is MRI scanning necessary to diagnose multiple sclerosis? Does the electroencephalogram influence the diagnosis of adult epilepsy? Is CT (Computerized tomographic) brain scanning worthwhile in diagnosing chronic headache?) (Weingarten *et al.* 1992). These guidelines could be used to alter neurologists' practice so that they practise in a more cost-effective manner.

Such changes in clinical practice could be effected in one of two general ways (Greco 1993). First, managerial coercion could be imposed in the form of administrative rules, financial incentives, or financial penalties (or combinations of these). One anticipates that such bureaucratic measures would be most effective in a fee-for-service office practice setting. The second method would employ a combination of education, feedback, and participation by physicians in an effort to achieve rational change. This will be familiar as the approach embodied in the current National Health Service clinical audit initiative. At its most mundane level, this is exactly what responsible physicians have tried to achieve informally for decades by reading textbooks and academic articles, by clinical case discussions, and by academic meetings (Tanenbaum 1993).

Neurologists should be cautious about the outcomes movement. First, all neurologists are aware how it has been necessary to conduct enormous, carefully designed, and costly multicentre trials in order to answer relatively straightforward clinical questions. These have included whether the outcome of cerebrovascular disease is improved by extracranial-intracranial vascular bypass operations (EC/IC Bypass Study Group 1985) or carotid endarterectomy (North American Symptomatic Carotid Endarterectomy Trial Collaborator 1991; European Carotid Surgery Trialists' Collaborative Group 1991); whether Guillain–Barré syndrome recovers better with plasma exchange (French Cooperative Group on Plasma Exchange in Guillain–Barré Syndrome 1987; McKhann *et al.* 1988), or intravenous immunoglobulin (van der Meché *et al.* 1992); or whether acyclovir influences survival and outcome in herpes encephalitis (Whitley *et al.* 1986). All to often, one hears unrealistic and ill-considered predictions that, as a result of clinical audit, a single doctor can answer questions more complex than these by simply reviewing retrospectively some hospital case records in his/her spare time. Neurologists need to participate in outcomes research to ensure that the methodology is sound, the questions are appropriate, and the answers valid.

Second, neurologists must be aware that outcomes research often tries to impose a unidimensional solution on a multifaceted problem. For instance, health care purchasers, patients, and neurologists may all have conflicting views on the worth of intensive investigation to confirm the diagnosis of multiple sclerosis, still considered an incurable disease. The purchaser may regard money spent diagnosing incurable diseases as a waste. Yet, the patient may value an indisputable diagnosis as an explanation for symptoms, as a basis for taking important life decisions, and as a foundation on which to be eligible for future therapeutic developments. And the neurologist may wish to exclude alternative diagnoses, even if unlikely, to address the patient's inevitable questions from a position of complete diagnostic confidence, and to guard against legal retribution because of wrong diagnosis.

Third, in the current medicolegal climate, few physicians will wish to be bound by practice guidelines which embody statistical approaches that dictate strategies for investigation or treatment which, with hindsight, may be seen as inappropriate to a particular patient.

Fourth, the scope of neurological disease is huge with a disproportionate apportionment of costly clinical activity to a relatively small group of rarer but serious diseases. How can practice guidelines be developed that cover all such diseases? And even if such guidelines were developed, how could neurologists be expected to wade through the morass of regulatory bureaucracy that would follow? Outcomes research and managerial implementation of practice changes are vast and expensive bureaucratic exercises which could only be judged as effective if they accrued a clinical value which at least equals the cost of the process. And neurologists must participate in determining whether that is indeed the case. They should be prepared to wield Occam's razor in order to avoid being stifled by mountains of overlapping, and potentially contradictory, guidelines.

What should be the role of neurologists in developing practice guidelines? They should ensure that outcomes research addresses issues of real concern to patients and their doctors. They must prevent the setting of tangential agendas by those primarily concerned with controlling expenditure rather than with the quality of medical care. The discipline of outcomes research is in its infancy, and should be welcomed by neurologists as a potential methodology for answering important questions about their clinical activity; but first they must be convinced that this methodology is valid (Kassirer 1993). Participation in the development of practice guidelines will be time-consuming for neurologists. It should be co-ordinated by national professional bodies, such as the Association of British Neurologists and the Royal College of Physicians in Britain, or by the American Academy of Neurology and American Medical Association, rather than being attempted in a half-hearted manner at a local level (Rosenberg and Greenberg 1992; Menken 1992). The climate of change in health care

is such that neurologists will ignore involvement in these issues at the peril of their patients' welfare, their own vocational fulfilment, and the rational development of clinical neurology.

THE NEUROLOGIST'S LEADERSHIP ROLE

Neurologists should strive to retain an executive role in managing their clinical service. The imposition of market-orientated health care, in a climate of restricted funding, necessitates that specialties like neurology manage their activities within strictly defined budgets. It will involve decisions about the best deployment of clinical activity within the overall range of possible neurological services that could be offered. This may include judging the different values to patients of the medical, nursing, and technical staff of the specialty, or of the relative merits of out and inpatient care. Neurologists must retain a hand in these fiscal decisions so that they continue to address needs relevant to patients (Williams 1992). Thus, within each regional centre, one neurologist should devote a significant part of his/her time to the clinical direction of his/her department. Whether this role is executed as a rotating chairman elected from within his colleagues, or as a clinical director appointed by hospital managers to act in an executive role, will vary from hospital to hospital.

The academic activities of a neurology department also need leadership and must be co-ordinated with the clinical activity. Britain and the United States have taken different approaches as to whether the same person should direct both the clinical and academic activities of a neurology department. In many American university medical centres one individual performs both roles, but the combined weight of scholarly, clinical, fiscal, and managerial activities now threatens the viability of this unified task (McKhann 1989). British university hospitals still have to evolve a modern structure for managing their clinical and academic activities. In order to prevent the impossibility of a single pair of shoulders bearing an unsustainable load, we should aim to develop two parallel management structures, for academic and clinical activities, respectively. Each would be responsible for a particular number of salary sessions for academic or for clinical duties respectively, and employ medical staff for a fixed number of sessions in each mode.

Professional bodies such as the Association of British Neurologists or American Academy of Neurologists will play an increasing role in defining how neurological health care can and should be provided. They will need to act as rational advocates of the interests of patients in the face of strict fiscal control; often, they will act in concert with patient charities. They will need to participate in the regulation and provision of postgraduate training so as to ensure the succession of trained neurologists. Finally, they must advise on standards of professional activity, and resist erosion of these standards by those acting from positions of ignorance or fiscal interest.

REFERENCES

1. EC/IC Bypass Study Group (1985). Failure of extracranial-intracranial arterial bypass to reduce the risk of ischemic stroke: results of an international randomized trial. *The New England Journal of Medicine*, **313**, 1191–200.

2. European Carotid Surgery trialists' Collaborative Group (1991). MRC European carotid surgery trial: interim results for symptomatic patients with severe (70–99%) or with mild (0–29%) carotid stenosis. *Lancet*, **337**, 1235–43.

3. French Cooperative Group on Plasma Exchange in Guillain–Barré Syndrome (1987). Efficiency of plasma exchange in Guillain–Barré syndrome: role of replacement fluids. *Annals of Neurology*, **22**, 753–61.

4. Greco, P. J. (1993). Changing physicians' practices. *New England Journal of Medicine*, **329**, 1271–4.

5. Greenwood, R. (1992). Neurology and rehabilitation in the United Kingdom: a view. *Journal of Neurology, Neurosurgery and Psychiatry*, **55(suppl.)**, 51–3.

6. Gutmann, L., Bell, W. E., and Scheiber, S. C. (1991). Added qualification in clinical neurophysiology. *Neurology*, **41**, 1171–2.

7. Hopkins, A. (1989). Lessons for neurologists from the United Kingdom third national morbidity study. *Journal of Neurology, Neurosurgery and Psychiatry*, **52**, 430–3.

8. Kassirer, J. P. (1993). The quality of care and the quality of measuring it. *New England Journal of Medicine*, **329**, 1263–5.

9. Langton-Hewer, R. and Wood, V. A. (1992). Neurology in the United Kingdom: II. A study of current neurological services for adults. *Journal of Neurology, Neurosurgery and Psychiatry*, **55(suppl.)**, 8–14.

10. McKhann, G. M. (1989). Clinical departmental director: manager or scholar? *Annals of Neurology*, **26**, 779–81.

11. McKhann, G. M. Griffin, J. W., Cornblath, D. R. *et al.* (1988). Plasmapheresis and Guillain–Barré syndrome: analysis of prognostic factors and the effect of plasmapheresis. *Annals of Neurology*, **23**, 347–53.

12. Menken, M. (1990). The changing paradigm of neurologic practice and care. Implications for the undergraduate curriculum. *Archives of Neurology*, **47**, 334–6.

13. Menken, M. (1992). Practice guidelines in neurology. Will they get us where we want to go? *Archives of Neurology*, **49**, 193–5.

14. North American Symptomatic Carotid Endarterectomy Trial Collaborators (1991). Beneficial effect of carotid endarterectomy in symptomatic patients with high-grade cartoid stenosis. *New England Journal of Medicine*, **325**, 445–53.

15. Perkin, G. D. (1989). An analysis of 7836 successive new outpatient referrals. *Journal of Neurology, Neurosurgery and Psychiatry*, **52**, 447–8.

16. Rosenberg, J. and Greenberg, M. K. (1992). Practice parameters: strategies for survival into the nineties. *Neurology*, **42**, 1110–15.

17. Selzer, M. E. (1992). Neurological rehabilitation. *Annals of Neurology*, **32**, 695–9.

18. Stevens, D. L. (1989). Neurology in Gloucestershire: the clinical workload of an English neurologist. *Journal of Neurology, Neurosurgery and Psychiatry*, **52**, 439–46.

19. Tanenbaum, S. J. (1993). What physicians know. *New England Journal of Medicine*, **329**, 1268–71.

20. van der Meché, F. G. A., Schmitz, P. I. M., and the Dutch Guillain–Barré Study Group (1992). A randomized trial comparing intravenous immune globulin and plasma exchange in Guillain–Barré syndrome. *New England Journal of Medicine*, **326**, 1123–9.

21. Weingarten, S., Kleinman, M., Elperin, L., and Larson, E. B. (1992). The effectiveness of cerebral imaging in the diagnosis of chronic headache. *Archives of Internal Medicine*, **152**, 2457–62.

22. Whitehouse, P. J. (1991). Geriatric neurology. *Neurology*, **41**, 1169–70.

23. Whitley, R. J., Alford, C. A., Hirsch, M. S. *et al.* (1986) Vidarabine versus acyclovir therapy in herpes simplex encephalitis. *New England Journal of Medicine*, **314**, 144–9.

24. Wilkinson, I. M. (1990). A survey of undergraduate teaching of clinical neurology in the United Kingdom 1990. *Journal of Neurology, Neurosurgery and Psychiatry*, **54**, 266–8.

25. Williams, I. R. (1992). Neurology in the market place. *Journal of Neurology, Neurosurgery and Psychiatry*, **55(suppl.)**, 15–18.

Coping with contracting in a changing National Health Service

Ian Williams

At the Rubicon, Caesar hesitated, staggered by the enormity of his enterprise. Plutarch (*c*.100/1884) tells us that after much rumination and discussion with advisers and friends Caesar cried out, 'The die is cast!' crossed the river, and then advanced rapidly.

In years to come it may be apparent just how much rumination and discussion took place before the changes to the National Health Service (NHS) were announced in 1989. There had been increasing debate about the funding of the service; in the press and professional journals there had been many articles comparing health care provision and funding around the world. Inadequacies in the availability of care had been highlighted, much to the discomfort of the government. To health economists and thinking members of the health professions change was both inevitable and desirable. However, so far as is known, few of these experts were asked to give evidence or advice and the public debate on restructuring the NHS in the United Kingdom was minimal. Those who had looked for change were left wondering whether the new NHS would deliver the improvements they had been looking for and whether their views had been considered. Whatever the answer it was certainly true that after the announcement events moved very quickly.

THE CHANGING NHS

Caesar had the advantage of knowing where he was going. Crossing the Rubicon was a means to achieving a goal which was itself the purpose of the venture. There were many opportunities to restate or redefine the role of the NHS and to link changes in the structure of the service to changed goals, but they were not taken. Change appears to have been the goal rather than the means to the goal. It is true that politicians encouraged us to believe that the changes were made in order to make the service more responsive, more efficient, and more accountable. They also assured us that health care would remain free for all at the point of delivery. Admirable goals in themselves, of course, but none of this addressed the question of what the NHS was there for. A reorganization which does not take time to decide what the service is for, but prescribes a new structure and funding mechanism is in grave danger of losing its way: it is, however, less likely to recognize

that it is lost. Because the destination has to be deduced from the present direction of travel it is extremely difficult to know when the direction is wrong!

This was a curious situation. At the beginning of the decade Sir Douglas Black (DHSS 1980) had produced a report which could have been the basis for a fundamental review of the successes and failures of the NHS, leading to reform and restructuring to create a service which would deliver better health for all. Instead, that report was ignored. A consideration of the Black Report would have led the government of the day to look at housing, employment, education, and the health service together, and to review the contribution of each to the health of the nation. The shelving of the report was a political decision which had little to do with the importance of the health issues raised. It was the same government which, nearly 10 years later, produced the White Paper on the Health Service (HMSO 1989), and introduced changes with so little obvious debate. From the emphasis on the means of delivering care rather than on the aims of the service one can only deduce that again the motive was predominantly ideological.

The United Kingdom had not been alone in questioning its system of funding and managing health care: many other countries were, and still are, facing similar challenges. Costs were rising at a time of relative economic stagnation. Rationing, whether by default or by design, was on the agenda. In the United States at that time, roughly 35 million people had no health care coverage despite an annual expenditure of about 13% of the gross national product (GNP) on health (Enthoven and Kronick (1991). In comparison, everybody in the United Kingdom had access to health care for just over half that proportion of a much smaller GNP. In terms of access the United Kingdom was delivering a better service at lower cost. Indicators of health in the UK population seem not to have suffered. Part of the explanation for this difference in expenditure lay in administrative costs which were much higher in the United States than in the United Kingdom, largely because of the multiplicity of sources of payment and the insurers' demand for prior approval and monitoring of treatment. It should then come as no surprise that the changes in the NHS have greatly increased the administrative costs within Trusts through the introduction of contracts and the proliferation of purchasers.

CHANGING SOCIETY

Another phenomenon that was occurring in many countries was the political emphasis on consumerism, the individual, and the importance of the market. Enthoven, along with many others, believed that the market was the best way of providing a high quality health care system (Enthoven and Kronick 1989). He suggested that informed consumer choice coupled with economic incentives and managed competition would deliver high quality care at relatively low cost. However, his views should not be accepted without challenge. The free market rewards those with economic power at the expense of those who have no purchasing power. Unless the incentives and the management of the market are sensitively deployed those most in need will have least say and be most at risk. The nature of the economic incentives and the parameters governing the management of the market will, in the main, be determined by politicians and those with economic power. At best, the chronically ill or disabled members of society will depend on the benevolent paternalism of the wealthy, powerful, and politically well-connected members. At worst, their needs will be ignored. The existence of such a large body of people with no access to health care in the United States should serve as a reminder that the market is not benevolent. Thus, in the market-driven health service in the United Kingdom, the government still determines the extent and range of the service provided but uses a less direct, less accountable, and inevitably more bureaucratic and more costly mechanism.

It is, of course, right that health care should be subject to political control: in the United Kingdom, funding is almost exclusively through taxation collected by the central government. Health is only one of the claims on that income. In such a situation one would hope that there would be a clear statement of health care policy with extensive public discussion leading to agreement or at least an electoral mandate. Informed public debate has not really taken place in this country. At the time of the White Paper on the NHS in 1989 neither the government nor the opposition parties focused on the aims of the service and the need to improve care for the most vulnerable groups in society. Fears that the creation of NHS Trust hospitals would be the beginning of the end of the NHS dominated the limited public debate. The loss of clear public accountability of purchasers and the extreme sensitivity of the new market structure to direct political pressures were barely recognized. Short-term contracts and performance-related pay for senior managers together with the loss of locally accountable health authorities and their replacement by boards appointed through patronage, put enormous power into the hands of the Secretary of State.

For the health care professionals, the health economists, and the general public there is a real challenge. The new NHS presumably exists to provide the full range of health care (including prevention, education, and promotion) necessary to meet the needs of the population as efficiently and as effectively as possible. If this is so the real health needs of the population must be identified and politicians must be persuaded to ensure that these needs are met. The experience in Oregon shows that it is far from easy to have the local, public debate and even harder to get the politicians and professionals to agree the action which might follow. All those involved in health care as consumers, purchasers, or providers must constantly insist that this debate does take place, is well informed, and is followed by action.

CHANGE IN THE MEDICAL PROFESSION

In many debates that challenge the status quo, and consequently the status of professionals, the medical profession has been less than helpful. This response probably results more from a desire to protect the interests of the patient than from any inherent negativism, but it is often reactionary and is rarely based on the patients' own assessment of need. The stress in the new NHS on the short term and pressure to introduce locally determined pay, performance-related pay, and short, fixed-term contracts for senior doctors could make it more difficult to gain their co-operation. Doctors will be forced to put their own rewards even higher on the agenda and are likely to be less sensitive to the general needs of patients or the service. In order to achieve change which is beneficial to patients and to the community as a whole, doctors will have to become more flexible. The role of doctors and the way in which they contribute to health care are not immune to change: health care and medicine are not synonymous. It still remains to be seen whether the profession will meet this challenge and whether change will be facilitated or impeded by the recent changes in the NHS. Some consultants have chosen to resist changes proposed within their hospital: medical directors, chief executives, and chairmen of boards have been the casualties. The abolition of regional health authorities and the dissolution of medical advisory structures has further narrowed the view of doctors. There are now few opportunities for the development of strategy and for recognizing the interdependence of different sectors. Competition rather than co-operation is the mood.

Change was occurring before the reform of the NHS and it must continue if the important issues in health care are to be tackled. For the medical profession, the test will be whether it acts in the interest of patients and the community or whether it defends its own interest. The real test of the reforms, with the emphasis on the market, will be the extent to which necessary change has occurred which could not, or would not, have taken place had the reforms not been introduced.

THE PURCHASER

The purchaser has been given an impossible role. The tools required to undertake the task satisfactorily have not yet been developed. A group of people who used to run hospitals, and were criticized for doing that badly, have been told to assess the health needs of the population and then look for the most effective and efficient way of meeting those needs. Barely had the ink dried on the documents setting out this agenda for needs-based, local purchasing when a set of central directives giving a different agenda for purchasing against nationally determined targets arrived: the flow of paper continues. Purchasers should be forgiven for failing to get the government's act together!

Whatever the imperfections of the system, it has to be made to work. It will take many years yet to develop the necessary tools to assess need and adequate measures of outcome. Some purchasers have, in the meantime, taken the easier path of negotiating contracts based solely on financial criteria or activity volume defined in a very narrow way. The tight financial limits on purchasers were bound to encourage this. However, they must be drawn into the more useful, if more difficult, work of defining need, quality of life, and outcome as enthusiastic partners.

Some health authorities came together or employed agencies for the purpose of negotiating contracts. While the process consisted of agreeing numbers and cost, with some central quality targets, there was no reason to object to the obvious savings in time and manpower that this could achieve. However, as contracting began to develop a more detailed, local flavour it was no longer appropriate to enlist another agency to undertake the negotiation. Agreeing a contract has important practical implications apart from the agreement itself. The conversations between purchaser and provider create a relationship in which problems can be explored and solutions found. Such a relationship has, however, proved difficult to achieve in the face of continual changes in the purchasing role and structure.

Not all purchasers are health authorities. Universities, colleges, research funds, and private health insurers could all be purchasers. Fundholding general practitioners (GPs) are certainly purchasers even if they are also undoubtedly providers. This ambiguous role of the GP could threaten the new NHS: very close monitoring will continue to be necessary. There is ample evidence that the practice of doctors is changed by financial incentives or opportunities (Levinsky 1993). Already the rules concerning funding of some GP enterprises have had to be changed and there are still reports of large sums of GP fundholders' money remaining unspent.

Some of the government's keenest hopes for the reforms were for changes brought about by switches of GP contracts. To a limited extent such changes have happened. This has usually been beneficial to the patients of the practice involved but has not necessarily taken into account the needs of other practices or of the provider unit. Removal of one block of work is unlikely to allow any significant reduction in overheads: these will then have to be shared among the other purchasers. Co-operation between specialties can be damaged if support for one is reduced; hospitals can lose viability without another institution being able to take on their remaining

work. In one way or another some form of co-operation between such small volume purchasers has to take place.

For small specialties, the GP fundholder poses a different problem. How should the provider respond to so many purchasers? A tertiary provider could have well in excess of 100 GP practice purchasers and 10 or 20 health authorities. To agree contracts with each would entail the completion of at least two GP agreements every week and one or two major purchaser agreements every month. Without an army of staff this would be impossible. Again it will probably be necessary for GP purchasers to find a way of acting along with major purchasers if they are to take part in the contract negotiations with multidistrict specialties. Advice from the NHS Executive suggests that such purchasing could be arranged through a single major purchaser. This may not be acceptable to GPs who value their freedom to win the best deal for their patients. A mechanism which is practical and gives purchaser and provider a role in setting the level and quality of care still has to be found. In the meantime a great deal of patience and understanding will be needed.

Eventually, the purchaser places the contract, the provider delivers the service. It is unfortunate that the user of the service is not yet aware that the extent and quality of the service are defined by the purchaser. The public invisibility of the purchaser is a source of frustration to the provider who is in contact with the patient. Inevitably, the provider is seen to be at fault if care is rationed or refused. A public education programme could help purchaser and provider cope with complaints and could be helpful in informing the contracting negotiations more generally.

As the tools become available and purchasers gain confidence the contracting process will become more useful and could become an important instrument for changing the pattern of health care in the United Kingdom. Purchasers and providers have a responsibility to use the contracting process to improve the health of the nation.

THE PROVIDER

It will come as a surprise to many providers to learn that their own problems and inadequacies were at least as great as those of the purchasers. The questions were not all for the purchaser. How would the provider respond to a well-constructed request to tender for the provision of a service to meet a well-defined health need within set quality and time standards? The absence of such clear requests has allowed providers to ignore their own inadequacies so far. Providers will only be able to respond appropriately to need when they can define their own practice in terms of outcome, efficiency, quality, and value for money. Until then providers should be thankful that contract negotiations have been concerned largely with numbers of patients treated and total cost.

For many providers the introduction of the contracting process was a sideshow accompanying their preparations for their change to an NHS Trust hospital. Although the 'opting out' of Trust hospitals was seen to be a major threat to the survival of the NHS, it was always likely to be less significant than the separation of purchaser and provider. The negotiation of contracts is vital to the survival of hospitals whatever their size and complexity. Without a satisfactory agreement they cannot provide a service or pay their staff. Many staff at all levels in the service have not yet fully recognized this fact. Survival demands that all staff do come to recognize the importance of contracts and the factors which purchasers see as important.

Purchasers do not always speak the same language as consultants: they are less likely to be taken in by dogmatic assertions, and wish to see evidence. Within the hospital, professionals of all disciplines will have to recognize the change in perspective. Quality, to the consultant, may mean using the latest and most expensive equipment; the purchaser is almost always more interested in whether patients are seen on time in the outpatient clinic and whether the GP receives a letter within a few days.

These different approaches are not mutually exclusive. Purchasers expect to be able to buy the best treatment available: but they will need to be persuaded that the more expensive treatment is better and that no matter how expensive the treatment the patient is still treated with respect and dignity.

This is a new task for providers. They still have to develop the skills and gather the information to enable them to present a good case to purchasers. This will entail a review of all professional practices within the unit, a determination to identify and perform only those procedures which have been shown to be effective, and a willingness to listen to the purchasers' agenda.

Such a review could well open up opportunities to provide care in a very different way. It could also lead to the development of guidelines for the management of some conditions. Such guidelines and protocols could govern the stage at which referrals should be made and would identify the resources required for the agreed investigation and treatment of a wide range of disorders. They could also form the basis of training and continuing medical education. Brook (1989) believes that, in the United States, the use of guidelines based on even the present state of knowledge would not only improve care but release very significant resources. Can providers, or the doctors they employ, ignore this possibility? Purchasers certainly will not.

For many years the NHS has operated on the basis of clinical freedom for doctors to practise the kind of medicine they thought necessary. This has led to significant advances in investigation and treatment but has also led to a rather unquestioning attitude to the introduction of new procedures and medications. Much that is now established practice has been adopted as standard treatment without adequate assessment. The frequency with which individual procedures are used varies widely from place to place without any obvious reason and without apparent impact on the health of the population. Even where there are good studies which define the indica-

tions for particular procedures they are not always followed. Medical staff, even senior consultants, will have to recognize that clinical freedom is not the freedom to misuse or misapply resources.

For the provider the contracting process will force a review of practice which is long overdue. Professional jealousies, restrictive practices, and privileged hierarchies cannot be protected from change. Such an agenda is threatening to many within the service despite the opportunities to provide better care at lower cost.

Changes in practice will be made more difficult by the many other changes which also have to be accommodated. The reduction in junior doctors' hours and the restriction in the number of junior doctors will inevitably alter the pattern of care. Consultants appointed after much shorter periods of training will be less able to cope with the range of activities required. Older, more experienced consultants are unlikely to relish the thought of continuing to work longer hours than their junior staff. So far, it is not possible to see a solution to this dilemma. If a solution leads to a diminution in the standard of care neither providers nor purchasers will be happy and some consultants will be tempted to increase their commitment to private practice or take early retirement from the service. This would leave even fewer experienced consultants available to NHS provider units.

It will, in any event, be necessary for providers to address the issue of consultant contracts and the more difficult problem of private practice. Most consultants undertake some private practice: some of this is within the Trust hospital and some in private rooms and hospitals. In accepting private patients for investigation and treatment consultants are effectively competing with the Trust for business. There can be few businesses that will allow employees to use the facilities of the company to take their business away from them! Although this is a parody of the present situation in most Trusts, it would become a major problem if the volume of private medical care were to increase. Some consultants are already taking significant business away from their Trust and some form of action might not be far away.

Salaries and rewards will also become an increasing issue for providers. Some specialists are more restrictive than others, some used to longer hours than others, but all receive the same salary. It may be possible to argue, in defence, that different salaries for different specialties would adversely affect recruitment and the ability to provide a service. A single national pay scale for consultants certainly prevents leap-frog pay awards to retain essential staff. If providers begin to bid against each other for staff in shortage specialties, the cost will increase without an increase in the overall level of service.

It is much more difficult to defend the poor use of time and resources. Purchasers will not continue to pay over the odds for contracts: providers will find it hard to justify consultant contracts with few committed sessions in the outpatient clinic or the operating theatre. The consultants and other professional staff will have to recognize that they are employed by the Trust to fulfil a contract with a purchaser. Setting this alongside their obligation to provide the best health care available to each individual patient will be a continuing source of tension.

Contract negotiation will force providers to change. Much of the change will be welcomed by those who wish to improve care but will threaten those who look for an easy life or who ignore the claims of patients to have the best and most appropriate treatment. Change will take place: it will either be managed through informed debate or enforced through budgets. Providers in all specialties should commit themselves to the former so that finance serves the service and not vice versa.

CONTRACTING

Having split the NHS into two parts, neither of which had any responsibility for the other, it was necessary to find a way in which the parts could do business with each another. Individual relationships were to be defined in quasi-legal contracts which would embody agreements between a purchaser and a provider to deliver an agreed type of care to an agreed number of people, within defined standards, for an agreed cost. This arrangement, in theory at least, gave purchasers great responsibilities but equally great freedom while applying considerable control over the providers. Properly employed this mechanism could be a useful tool for achieving fundamental changes in patterns of care.

In the market model, the government had found a way of widening the opportunities for change. Nothing and nobody would be protected from the influence of the market. There could, for example, be no guarantee that hospitals with a long tradition of excellent service, but no longer serving a local or national population, would attract purchasers in the future. In large cities with falling populations expenditure on health, based on capitation, would fall and some hospitals, even London teaching hospitals, might well have to close. Need rather than availability would drive purchasing. For some groups of patients, however, the market could not guarantee that any kind of service would be available. People with chronic progressive disease or very uncommon diseases could be vulnerable to purchasing decisions based on outcome or volume. Neurologists might then consider that the whole specialty of neurology would be particularly at risk!

Although the idea of contracting or commissioning is sound it has to be recognized that techniques for measuring health need and health gain are relatively poor, particularly in the area of chronic progressive disease. This undermines the most important currency for the evaluation of contracts leaving cost and volume as the most commonly used determinants. Over the last forty years knowledge of health need in an area has come largely from providers as they have identified and sought to remedy problems.

The public health function has, since its heyday a century ago, largely failed to take on this task at the local level. Prim-

ary, secondary, and tertiary care have developed through the efforts of those involved but, outside a few academic centres, the analysis of health need has not paralleled this. Growth and development have been provider-driven not because of any deviousness on the part of those providing the service but because they have been active in finding solutions to the problems they encountered. They will wish to remain active in finding solutions to such problems as they encounter.

There are now signs that the new public health function is becoming significantly more extensive and better supported. Unless this development continues purchasers and providers will be left in the dark. Until the purchasers can ask the right question the providers can only guess at the right answer. Finding the right questions will depend on co-operation between purchasers and providers and may require considerable investment in research.

Health gain has proved equally difficult to define and measure, especially in the context of chronic progressive disease. How do you recognize the success of an intervention in the face of relentless deterioration of function and progressive loss of independence? In the absence of clear measures of health gain, contracts have been judged centrally against efficiency ratios, volume per unit cost, etc., without any real reference to the quality or nature of the service provided. This situation is understandable but it has led to frustration among people who find their energies diverted from the search for techniques and language which could define need and measure gain, to sterile mechanical measurement against crude, centrally determined performance targets. In the end, such figures show what we already know and add nothing to health care. They may indeed divert not just the energy of the health professionals but also the attention of the general public and politicians. The definition and attainment of health gain are too important to be lost in party political jousting.

In concentrating on health gain it is, however, possible to focus on some individual and local problems to the detriment of other issues. Somehow the notion of national health must be established within the context of local contracting. The health of individuals does depend on the health of the nation: the health service must recognize and respond to the needs of society and not be diverted into responding only to the needs of the more vocal middle class.

Champions of the contracting process will counter that there have been great changes in practice and that these have been to the benefit of patients. It is true that there have been improvements for patients: it is not clear that most of these have anything to do with the contracting process. For the very considerable investment devoted to agreeing and managing contracts there is, as yet, very little to show which could not have been obtained without the additional expenditure. On the contrary, arbitrary definitions, the expectation of increasing efficiency year after year, and unrealistic targets demean the relationship between provider and purchaser. Both parties see the problem but neither is free to change the nature of the relationship. The contracting process can only get better.

The contract finally agreed defines the health care to be provided for the local population. It is an agreement to use public funds to improve the health of the nation. Whatever its faults it is now the only way of distributing funding for health care in the United Kingdom. Public understanding of the issues and the respective roles of purchaser and provider would probably be improved if the contract were to be a public document. The actual text may well intimidate the man or woman in the street but a summary in plain English giving information about the range of facilities available, the quality standards agreed, and the limitation on access or volume should be provided. Such information could help considerably in future discussions about priorities, increase accountability and might just bring public expectations of providers closer to the level of service which has been purchased.

CONTRACTING FOR NEUROLOGY

The government White Paper and the subsequent reforms arrived at an inconvenient time for neurology! Few specialties can have changed so much in so short a time. New investigations, new treatments, and new diseases have arrived. More importantly the diagnostic process and the necessary skill base have changed with a consequent change in the role of the neurologist. Instead of being wholly preoccupied by the obscure and incurable the neurologist now devotes much of his time to the continuing care of people with common and treatable disorders. The diagnosis is now the beginning not the end of the process: it is the context in which care is provided.

Sadly for the neurological showman, the new imaging techniques have dispelled some of his mystique: he is no longer held in such awe. His brilliant diagnosis may be subjected to a more objective analysis than he might wish, and that analysis may well be in the hands of those whom he has mocked in the past. The image and standing of the neurologist is no longer safe. Descent from the pedestal does, however, create an opportunity for neurologists to practise in a different and better way but poses a threat to those who do not wish to change.

Neurologists have come to recognize that people with incurable illnesses do not disappear after the diagnosis has been made. The quality of life can be changed by the attention or lack of attention from specialists. Many neurologists have also come to recognize that health care is not only provided by doctors. Team work, multidisciplinary practice, nurse specialists, and case management are developing. Most neurologists have heard the language, some have begun to explore new patterns of practice. The new pattern involves co-operation with the voluntary sector and crosses the boundaries between primary, secondary, and tertiary care. This progress must not be discarded no matter how difficult it is to sustain: it must be incorporated into the contract negotiations.

The timing of the changes was also inconvenient for neurology because of the relative immaturity of its internal political structures. The Association of British Neurologists had only recently begun to express views on the practice of neurology and had not yet grown bold enough to challenge political decisions. At this stage in its development it was more likely to behave in a protective manner than to look for innovative alternatives to traditional patterns of care. Colleges and government departments have tended to seek opinions from respected senior members of the specialty, colleagues with vast experience. The proximity of retirement, however, sometimes alters perspective. There is a real need for a broader, more open discussion both within the specialty and more widely, to explore new opportunities. In an increasingly diverse health service with increasing financial constraints we must be free to think the unthinkable.

Not everybody agrees that neurology is valuable. In some areas general physicians are still protective and neurosurgeons are not always to be relied upon for unqualified support! Neither in the centre nor in the district general hospital (DGH) can the neurologist be assured of an uncritical welcome. The mixture of common and uncommon diagnoses which makes up neurological practice poses an organizational dilemma. Should the neurologist be in the DGH with the general physician or in the centre with the neurosurgeon? It does not make good sense to have large numbers of patients travelling to the centre, but neither does it make good sense to isolate the neurologist in a DGH without adequate support or investigational facilities.

Almost all neurologists spend some time in a centre and some in the DGH but there are many different patterns. These will ultimately be reflected in the contract but that contract is only the seal on an agreed pattern of care. The contract will only be signed if neurologists can win support for their model of care. Institutions will only survive if they can persuade purchasers that they provide a valuable service in a manner acceptable to patients and at a cost that can be afforded. Inevitably, this requires information and marketing but it also requires the provider to provide a service which is genuinely useful and acceptable.

The utility of neurological care has been questioned in the past and this doubt persists in some quarters despite the change in the specialty. Unless neurologists are out and about listening, giving advice, education, and support to GPs, purchasers, patients, and carers they will not change opinions. The ivory tower is not the place to win contracts. Purchasers, hard pressed for cash, will not continue to spend money where they can see no gain. There are already examples of purchasers changing providers or insisting on a different pattern of care.

It is not easy to convince everybody of the value of neurologists. Neurologists have come into the field of some of the common disorders rather late. General physicians and geriatricians have had to look after patients with stroke and Parkinson's disease for a very long time. They are not amused to be told that these are now neurological disorders, unless the patient requires long-term care! If contracts to provide a service for patients with these disorders are to be won neurologists will have to spell out very clearly the contribution that they can make and the reasons why purchasers should pay them, rather than anybody else, to provide the service.

For some patients, co-operation with colleagues in other specialties is required. Discussion and agreement with each of these colleagues and their Trust are needed before purchasers will agree a contract. When facilities belong to another Trust separate payments and agreements are usually needed adding further to the administrative burden of the contracting process.

Patients and carers have a view on the quality of the neurological service as have the charities and self-help groups. Listening to their point of view may be uncomfortable but the purchasers hear it; it is as well to be prepared. We have to acknowledge that we have not been perfect.

Only after careful and detailed analysis of the potential benefits of neurological care can the provider design a service and enter into productive contract negotiations. After five years of the new NHS the contracts agreed look very different in different parts of the country and even in different parts of the same region. A study of the reasons for this could shed some light on the way in which purchasers define health need and providers deliver health gain.

COPING

The continuing changes in neurology, the relative weakness of its specialty structures, the tendency for financial targets to take precedence over patient care, the obscuring language of the reforms and the contracts, and the none-too-subtle pressures on the negotiators are all part of the scenery. Debates about the best way of providing a neurological service will continue. Contracting has to take account of all this but it can still provide a stimulus to continue to improve and develop a service that is of value to the patient, the carer, the GP, and other professionals, and is seen to be good value for money. Notwithstanding these opportunities it has to be recognized that the contracting process, and especially the GP fundhold-

ing scheme, has increased the administrative burden enormously. Every Trust employs accountants and clerical staff to operate the contract merry-go-round. Clinicians have become impatient with the mechanistic process that sometimes defies logic.

It would be easy, and to some extent understandable, to let the imperfections of the contracting process thwart development. During the last six years there have been opportunities to use the contracting process to improve care and there can be little doubt that they will continue. In order to recognize and take advantage of these opportunities neurologists must be prepared to devote time and energy to the organization of the service. They must ensure that they, and the managers and negotiators, are well informed, understand the issues, and have sensible proposals which put patients first. This will continue to be a demanding and sometimes unrewarding task: not every attempt will succeed, compromise is never popular and few wish to lose sight of their own dreams. But the prize of better care, provided in a new way, and secured through contracts is too important to lose. Even the most difficult battles must be fought, and if possible, won to give patients, carers, and the population as a whole, a better deal.

REFERENCES

Brook, R. H. (1989). Practice guidelines and practising medicine. *Journal of the American Medical Association*, **262**, 3027–30.

DHSS Department of Health and Social Security (1980). *Inequalities in health. Report of a research working group*, (D. Black, Chairman). DHSS, London.

Enthoven, A. and Kronick, R. (1989). A consumer choice health plan for the 1990s: universal health insurance in a system designed to promote quality and economy: I. *New England Journal of Medicine*, **320**, 29–37.

Enthoven, A. C. and Kronick, R. (1991). Universal health insurance through incentives reform. *Journal of the American Medical Association*, **265**, 2532–6.

HMSO (1989). *Working for patients*. HMSO, London.

Levinsky, L. G. (1993). The organization of medical care. *New England Journal of Medicine*, **329**, 1395–9.

Plutarch (1884). Life of Julius Caesar in *Plutarch's lives*, (Langhorne translation). Frederick Warne, London. (Original work *c*.100).

28 | Commissioning

Jonathan R. Cook and Daphne I. Austin

OVERVIEW

The 1990 National Health Service (NHS) and Community Care Act (1) introduced distinctive new roles for health authorities and providers of health care. Health authorities were given the responsibility of securing health care for the population they served by purchasing services from hospitals and community health services both within and outside their geographical boundaries. Providers of health care, on the other hand, no longer directly managed by their host health authority, could be paid directly for treating patients who resided in other health authority areas. In addition, general practitioners (GPs) were allowed and encouraged to hold their own budgets and act as purchasers for their own patient population.

This fundamental change in the organisation of the health service was characterized and discussed in terms of the 'internal market'. A market in health care exists when there are both purchasers and providers of health care who act relatively independently of each other and have the freedom to negotiate which services are purchased and provided. The term 'internal' was applied to this market because the purchasers and most of the providers lay within the public sector.

The White Paper *The New NHS: Modern and Dependable*, published in 1997, ended the internal market by stating that competitive relationships would be replaced by co-operation and partnership and that service reconfiguration would not be achieved by success or failure (i.e. hospitals closing down because of reduced contract income), but through planning with an inclusive process of dialogue and decision making (2).

However, although 1998/99 was to become the last year of operation of general practitioner fundholding, the 1997 White Paper did confirm the roles of commissioners and providers within the NHS. Now, general practitioners acting together in a primary care group (PCG), based on natural communities of between 75 000 and 150 000, are taking the lead commissioning role. Health authorities will continue to have a commissioning role mainly in relation to specifying the strategy for health gain in the Health Improvement Programme (HImP). Health improvement programmes are a combination of health and health care strategies and will, to a large extent, set the framework for the more detailed commissioning decisions of the PCGs. Furthermore, HImPs will be signed up to by both PCGs and providers.

The role of health authorities in commissioning will vary and be dependant on the PCGs in their district. Currently four PCG levels have been proposed. Level 1 is advisory leaving the health authority to undertake commissioning on the PCG's behalf. Level 2 requires the PCG to undertake most of the commissioning work, with health authority support only. The exception to this is specialized services which will continue, in most districts, to be commissioned by the health authority. At the time of writing this chapter it is uncertain what the nature of levels 3 and 4 PCGs will be as the legislation for these bodies is not yet in place. It is proposed that they will be completely independent of the health authority while level 1s and 2 remain as sub-committees of the health authority.

The organizational structures and working relationships of the NHS are becoming increasingly complex. Consequently, never has it been more important for different parts of the service to work cooperatively and constructively with each other. This chapter aims to introduce to health care professionals some of the concepts, principles, and the language of commissioners. In doing so it is hoped that this chapter will make a contribution to breaking down some of the barriers that exist as a result of the cynicism and poor regard which permeates through many of the relationships between health care professionals and managers, and between commissioners and providers. These barriers which arise, in part, from a lack of understanding of each other's roles, hinder the ability of the NHS to provide better care.

It is impossible to cover all aspects of commissioning. Important areas such as managing change in a complex professional and political climate, the use of mechanisms to improve services (particularly in reducing clinical variation and getting evidence-based practice), and monitoring the care provided are not covered. It will also become apparent on reading this chapter that the knowledge base of commissioners is drawn from disciplines which are either not covered or only superficially in the training of health care professionals. Examples include epidemiology, management and organizational theory, political and social studies, and economics. In addition, commissioners adopt a population approach as opposed to focusing on individual patients' needs. Together these create a different ethos which belies the fact that commissioners and providers all share the fundamental aim of improving health care and patients' and carers' experience of it.

It is difficult in these rapidly changing times to maintain the relevance of some material which is so clearly influenced by policy decisions of the government of the day. While some of the contents presented may become out of date fairly quickly many of the general principles which are presented will remain applicable whatever organizational structure and health policies are in place.

THE ORGANIZATIONAL STRUCTURE OF THE NHS

Each successive shift in ideology and resultant change in health policy has been accompanied by changes in the structure of the NHS. Fig. 28.1 illustrates the three main structures which have existed over the last decade during which time two major white papers on the NHS have been published.

HEALTH CARE COMMISSIONING IN ITS WIDEST CONTEXT

Before describing the commissioning of health care it should be appreciated that the provision of health care is but one part of a wider strategy aimed at improving health. The concept of 'health' is broad (i.e. physical, psychological, and social), and because social factors and social policy have a significant influence on health it follows that much health-promoting activity falls outside the NHS.

A health (as apposed to a health care) strategy should encompass the entire range of health interventions available. These have been broadly classified into the three categories shown below. Box 1 gives an outline of the possible contents of a health strategy designed to prevent strokes.

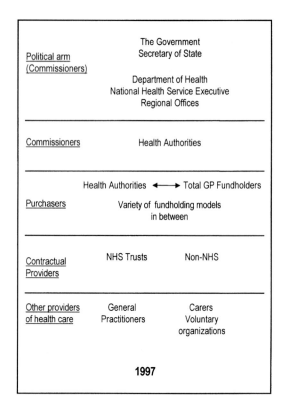

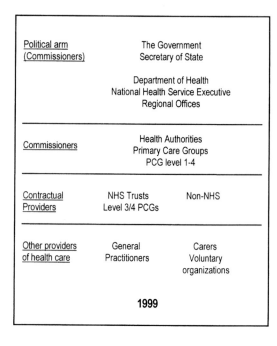

Fig. 28.1 Organizational structure of the National Health Service in 1997.

Primary prevention

Interventions which are aimed at preventing a disease or illness developing. This is done by altering either personal or environmental risk factors. Primary prevention strategies include a diverse range of interventions targeted at either entire populations, groups, or individuals. Examples are health protection and economic measures, community development, and health promotion clinics.

Secondary prevention

Interventions which are aimed at preventing the serious consequences of a disease or illness once it has developed. Included are screening and the proactive management of chronic disease.

Tertiary prevention

Interventions which are aimed at 'damage limitation' with the view to improving outcome (mortality, morbidity, and quality of life) when serious complications arise. These include the acute, curative, and rehabilitative therapies together with palliative care.

AN OVERVIEW OF THE ACTIVITIES OF COMMISSIONERS

Commissioning involves the development and implementation of a health care strategy for a given condition, groups of conditions, or client group within a defined population (Fig. 28.2). This defines the strategic framework within which purchasing should take place. The aim of this is to determine the services that are required and the minimum standards they should meet. Within this function is the important task of managing what could be considered *strategic risks* of which four are of particular importance:

1. The risk of *inadequate supply* of services (including provider instability and inequity issues).
2. The risk of *uncontrolled provider proliferation* which may lead to there being more providers than required which can result in a distortion of purchasing priorities, greater overall costs for a particular service, and poorer quality services.
3. The risk of *failure to contain interventions* which are of marginal health benefit or which distort purchasing priorities.
4. The risk of having *poor quality services*.

As well as *defining* strategic parameters, commissioners have an active role to play in *delivering* a strategy by working directly with both providers and purchasers of health care.

Purchasing can be seen as an operational function in which a strategy is translated into an actual service. Purchasing therefore involves securing services in the quantity, quality, and configuration required. The boundary between commissioning and purchasing is blurred.

Contracting is the process by which formal agreements are made between purchasers and providers. Although primarily

Box 1 Key elements of a health strategy aimed at reducing the incidence and long-term health consequences of acute cerebrovascular disease (3)

Primary prevention

Health protection measures:
Banning tobacco product advertising
Tax on tobacco products
Enforcement of law to prevent retailers selling cigarettes to people under 16 years of age
No-smoking areas
Medicolegal action against the tobacco industry

Health promoting measures
Educating children and parents on the health effects of smoking
Counter-advertising
Promoting a negative image of smoking (e.g. 'kissing an ashtray')
Promoting keeping fit and weight reduction

Secondary prevention
General practitioners advising their patients to give up smoking
Programmes to help children, teenagers, pregnant women, and other adults to give up smoking
Screening for, and good management of, hypertension
Good management of transient ischaemic attacks
Prophylaxis in high-risk patients

Tertiary prevention
Access to facilities to make accurate diagnosis in acute cases of stroke
Appropriate surgical intervention for subarachnoid haemorrhage
Well-organized acute management and rehabilitation.

---

a mechanism to achieve budgetary control, a formal agreement can also be used as a lever to implement strategic goals.

The terms 'purchasing' and 'contracting' are rapidly losing favour following the 1997 White Paper and indeed are no longer 'official'. The terms nevertheless represent functions which have changed little over time. Pre-1992, when hospitals were directly managed units, there was 'health service planning'. District health authorities in those days had an annual business cycle whereby detailed plans for service development were drawn up followed by negotiations with hospital management as to what funding was available and the nature and scale of services which were to be provided. During the years of the internal market there was a greater division of function and the more formal contractual arrangements led to the introduction of the terms commissioning, purchasing, and contracting. In an attempt to move away from the philosophy of Thatcherism the Labour government, in 1997, adopted a new set of terms—'the service and financial framework' replaced the annual purchasing plan and 'service level agreements' replaced contracts. It also became acceptable, once again, to use the term planning. The vocabulary used within the NHS sets the tone and culture of the organization and is therefore of great significance.

The shortcomings of the language, past and present, used to describe the various activities of commissioners is, however,

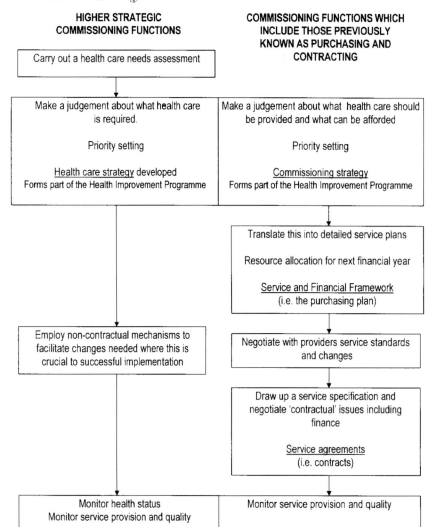

HIGHER STRATEGIC COMMISSIONING FUNCTIONS

Carry out a health care needs assessment

Make a judgement about what health care is required.

Priority setting

Health care strategy developed
Forms part of the Health Improvement Programme

Employ non-contractual mechanisms to facilitate changes needed where this is crucial to successful implementation

Monitor health status
Monitor service provision and quality

COMMISSIONING FUNCTIONS WHICH INCLUDE THOSE PREVIOUSLY KNOWN AS PURCHASING AND CONTRACTING

Make a judgement about what health care should be provided and what can be afforded

Priority setting

Commissioning strategy
Forms part of the Health Improvement Programme

Translate this into detailed service plans

Resource allocation for next financial year

Service and Financial Framework
(i.e. the purchasing plan)

Negotiate with providers service standards and changes

Draw up a service specification and negotiate 'contractual' issues including finance

Service agreements
(i.e. contracts)

Monitor service provision and quality

Fig. 28.2 Overview of commissioning

problematic which has been only too apparent while writing this chapter. Pre-1999 there was confusion over the terms commissioning, purchasing, and contracting as no nationally accepted definition existed. Although the terms purchasing and contracting have been removed no words have replaced them; rather all these activities have been subsumed into the word 'commissioning'. It is possible nevertheless for different aspects of commissioning to be functionally separate. For example GP fundholders mostly did contracting. Service reviews, HNA or the development of service standards based on the best clinical evidence was generally absent from much of the purchasing undertaken by them. With the development of PCGs the commissioning and purchasing activities are closer together. However in the area of specialised services, if PCGs are to be involved in securing services for their population it will be mainly in a contractual and not a commissioning sense, the latter being undertaken by health authorities, consortia and overseen by regional commissioning Lora.

THE COMMISSIONING PROCESS

HEALTH CARE NEEDS ASSESSMENT

Commissioning decisions should be informed decisions. The information needed to do this is generated from a process called health care needs assessment (HNA).

A working definition of the term 'health care need' in the context of a HNA is '*the ability to benefit from a health care intervention at reasonable risk and reasonable cost*' (4). In this sense a health care need is different from a health problem which exists for the individual and their carers regardless of whether or not there is an effective intervention. A health care need is also different from a demand to provide a service as the intervention requested can be ineffective, inappropriate for the condition, or have an unacceptable cost–benefit ratio. Further, the services available are not always the most appropriate to best meet need.

There are a number of models available for carrying out HNAs (5, 6). Most comprehensive models are a synthesis of three distinct but complementary approaches. These are epidemiological, comparative, and corporate in nature. The *epidemiological approach* uses epidemiological information, research-based evidence, and economic evaluations to describe the burden of disease or illness to a population and the effectiveness of interventions. The *comparative approach* directs purchasers to a common standard in terms of what is provided, how much is provided, and the quality of that provision. Comparing local services with those of other districts also encourages a cross-fertilization of ideas and the dissemination of good practice. Long term, this approach should also facilitate the move towards a more uniform quality of care within the NHS and equitable access to health care. The *corporate approach* takes into consideration the views of all the groups that have an interest in the service. This includes politicians, the public, professionals, purchasers, providers, patients, and their carers.

The epidemiological approach is considered, by some, to be an ideal rational approach to prioritizing the services to be funded with the comparative and corporate approaches only being used when epidemiological information is lacking. While it is true that epidemiology should be the foundation of any HNA, the other two methods gather different but equally valuable information and so should be considered an integral part of developing local services.

Epidemiological assessment

The stages of an epidemiological assessment are described in brief below. Technical details can be found elsewhere (see References). It is important to utilize fully the scientific literature and routine data sources and to have a detailed understanding of the limitations of the data used. Common sources of information are listed in Box 2. An increasingly important source of information is the number of national initiatives to review scientific evidence. These have experts reviewing both published and unpublished studies in a systematic way (including carrying out meta-analyses) in order to establish the effectiveness of given interventions. An example is the Cochrane Centre in Oxford which undertakes systematic reviews of randomized controlled trials.

Step 1. Define the condition of interest

At the outset, the condition of interest should be defined in clinically accurate and meaningful terms. For example, when considering what services to purchase for stroke patients two different classifications can be used. In the acute stage underlying pathology (i.e. thrombotic infarct, haemorrhage, tumour) will dictate early management and therefore the services provided. In the rehabilitative stage, however, it is the patient's functioning and prognosis that determine management rather than the underlying cause (7).

Box 2 Sources of epidemiological information

Published work (surveys, studies, economic evaluation)
Unpublished work
Database of good quality studies (e.g. Cochrane Centre Database, Oxford)
Office of National Statistics
Census data
Surveys (e.g. General Practitioner Morbidity Survey, General Household Survey)
Routine surveillance (e.g. mortality statistics)
Korner data
Central surveillance systems (e.g. PHLS infectious disease surveillance, cancer registries)
General practitioner databases
Local disease specific registers
Local surveys
Guidance documents from the Department of Health
Expert Advisory Committee reports
Reports from the Royal Colleges

Step 2. Describe the epidemiology

Next, it is important to have an overview of the extent of the problem within a given population. Purchasers need to know how many people are at risk of developing the condition, how many are suffering from it, how often complications arise, whether there are certain groups of people who are more likely to get the disease and whether there are likely to be more or less people in the future needing treatment. The minimum information needed is:

1. The incidence of the condition. This is the number of new cases that occur in a year in a given geographic area.
2. Changes in incidence in time, place, and person. This includes identifying the variables associated with differences in incidence such as sociodemographic, environmental, behavioural, or personal. The key is the identification of factors which can be manipulated to influence incidence.
3. The mortality associated with the condition and in particular an estimation of preventable premature death.
4. The prevalence of the condition. This is the number of people with the condition at any one point in time in a given geographical area.
5. The morbidity of the condition. This involves identifying the incidence and prevalence of specific complications and the associated disability.

Step 3. Establish which health care is effective and what it costs

Having identified the problems, the next step is to assess the intervention options available. Each intervention is assessed with respect to effectiveness. Questions that need answering are:

1. Is the intervention effective?
2. What are the risks?
3. Is the intervention more effective than others aimed at treating the same specific problem?

4. Do some patients benefit more than others, and can variables be identified which predict ability to benefit?
5. How does the intervention compare economically with other interventions aimed at the same specific problem?
6. How does the intervention compare economically with others which operate at a different level of prevention (i.e. prevention versus treatment)?
7. Is the intervention effective in all or only some health care settings?

It is worth saying more about economic evaluation at this point. It is important to view economic evaluation as a tool to aid purchasing decisions rather than providing the solution to difficult resource allocation issues. It is also important to appreciate that economic evaluations are not always entirely objective because value judgements are integral to the methodology in the case of cost–benefit and utility studies. There is often confusion about the different types of evaluations carried out, all of which measure very different things (8).

Cost-minimization analyses simply compare the cost of providing services which have the same aim but without reference to clinical outcome. For example, generic versus named prescribing.

Cost-effectiveness analyses identify the costs associated with achieving a specific clinical goal. This enables the identification of the intervention which is most effective at achieving that goal at least cost. An example of this would be comparing two drug treatments for epilepsy or, on a more complicated level, comparing the management of epilepsy by GPs with that of neurologists in order to achieve patient acceptable control of epilepsy. In this type of evaluation the two interventions being compared have the same clinical aim and the costs considered purely financial.

Cost–benefit analyses aim to identify how to maximize benefit for a given level of resource. These entail more detailed analysis than those used in cost-effectiveness analyses. A wider view is taken of what costs and benefits are (e.g. time off work, travel costs to the family, psychological complications of treatment, quality of life, social functioning) but both are still expressed in financial terms. These studies also allow a comparison to be made between interventions which have different clinical goals. *Cost–utility* analyses are similar to cost–benefit analyses except that benefits are expressed in some measure of health gain, such as QALYs (quality adjusted life years), rather than money.

All economic evaluations should provide a clear definition of the intervention in question, the service setting in which it is being delivered and the methodology used to calculate costs.

Step 4. Consideration of organizational and quality of care issues

The way in which a service is delivered can influence health outcome. For example, evidence to date suggests there is a net health gain if rehabilitation services for stroke patients are delivered in a stroke unit compared with providing them in a general medical setting (Cochrane Database, Oxford). It is

important, therefore, that the HNA includes a review of good practices which improve health outcome.

Comparative assessment

The next stage of the HNA moves away from the literature in order to look at the services currently being provided. This requires the service to be disaggregated into its basic elements which are then described in quantitative and qualitative terms. A useful framework is to look at the organization's structures, processes, and outcomes (9) (Table 28.1). Traditionally, most emphasis has been on the structure and process of a service. This is understandable as they are generally more easily measured. However, better direct outcome measures are needed.

Having gathered this information the local service is then compared with the services provided in other districts and with national statements on service standards produced by professional of other bodies where these are available. Consideration should also be given to whether the service is at an appropriate level for the local epidemiology of the condition and an explanation sought for significant differences in expected and actual levels of service provision.

Corporate assessment

The third and final stage of the health needs assessment involves obtaining the views of groups that have an interest in the local service (Fig. 28.3). The purpose of this is to:

1. Gain a professional view on the effectiveness of interventions when the scientific evidence is lacking.
2. Obtain a consensus view on the priority that the service should be given when considering resource allocation.
3. Identify ways in which to develop the service locally.
4. Identify possible blocks to implementing any health care strategy.

Integral to developing a corporate view is some assessment of the major forces which continually shape health care (10).

Table 28.1 Some elements of a health care service

Structures/inputs
Service configuration
Manpower including skill mix
Buildings
Equipment
Financial costs

Processes
Activity undertaken; type, volume, case mix, and by whom
Referral patterns
Relationships between different departments
Clinical practice (including variations)
Patient perceptions

Outcomes
Health outcome (including variations)

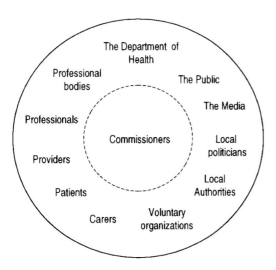

Fig. 28.3 Stakeholders in health care.

Three particularly stand out:

1. *Technological developments*. The overall cumulative effect of recent developments are leading to both decentralizing and centralizing forces. In the first instance, improved technology is making it safer to carry an increasing amount of care in a non-acute, outpatient or community setting and, in some instances, by non-specialist staff. Complex work, on the other hand, is requiring more specialist equipment and skills leading to the concentration of some services in fewer larger major acute hospitals.

2. *Manpower trends* such as:

(1) an increasing demand for a consultant provided service;
(2) increased subspecialization within the medical profession;
(3) changes to the training and terms and conditions of employment of junior medical staff;
(4) skill substitution with GPs taking on some tasks previously undertaken by the consultants and nurses and paramedics taking on some tasks previously undertaken by doctors.

Together, these reinforce the trends outlined in 1.

3. *Health policy*. Health policies such as the primary care-led NHS, the purchaser-provider split, and the private finance initiative will exert their own effect on what health care is provided and how it is delivered.

Pitfalls of health care needs assessments

It is clear to anyone who has undertaken a HNA that the above description represents the ideal. The reality is often quite different. There are three major obstacles. The first is the time taken to undertake a HNA which means that commissioners can realistically only review a few services at any one time. The consequence of this is that many services are developed in a strategic vacuum. The second problem is that

external events can often precipitate major strategic decisions without recourse to the above process and worse, frequently override potentially more rational decisions (e.g. the site of a new hospital). Such events are usually of a political or financial nature, and often both. The third major difficulty is poor information. Deficits encountered include:

1. Rudimentary knowledge of the epidemiology of many diseases.
2. Inadequate information on the effectiveness of health care interventions. Many new technologies and drugs have been introduced without having been fully evaluated. Despite widespread acceptance that this situation is undesirable neither the medical profession, commissioners, or provider management appear to be able to halt premature introduction of some medical developments at present.
3. Inadequate clinical outcome data.
4. Inadequate information on the services currently being provided.
5. Poor data quality with data being incomplete and inaccurate.

A few cautionary notes can be made regarding the use of data. Care should be taken when deciding what data to collect and how it is to be used. Collection of masses of data that tells us nothing or is not used is wasteful of resources. Data is also a powerful tool and should not be used indiscriminately. A point that has already been made is that information is an aid to improving health services but cannot be a substitute for careful decision-making. Finally, while it is understandable that there is a focus on quantitative data, good qualitative data should be neither ignored nor undervalued. The danger in doing so is that only that which can be easily measured will be given priority for funding. It may have to be accepted ultimately that some things that have value cannot be adequately measured.

The outcome of a health care needs assessment

The outcome of a HNA should be:

1. An understanding of the nature and size of the health problem including current and future service needs.
2. A hierarchy of interventions in terms of their ability to produce health gain and the costs incurred in doing do so.
3. An understanding of the current service being provided together with an assessment of its quality.
4. A view on what a model service looks like and what changes and developments are potentially achievable in the short-, medium-, and long-term locally.
5. Acceptable quality standards.
6. Preliminary costings.

This information forms the basis of the health care strategy which defines the health care needs for the population and the standards services should meet. This strategy has then to be translated into tangible services.

COMMITMENT OF RESOURCES

Before detailed planning can be undertaken it is necessary to determine what resources can be committed to implementing the health care strategy. This in turn is dependent on the resources that commissioners have available to them and the priority the service has in relation to others competing for resources. In coming to resource allocation decision commissioners must reconcile many demands and needs.

Identifying resources available

Generally, a purchaser will be allocated funds as follows: last years allocation *plus* an inflation adjustment (based on general inflation in the economy) *plus* new monies. The move towards distributing funds within the NHS on a fair shares basis (known as capitation funding) rather than on a historical basis means, however, that in recent years some districts have received less money than previously. The capitation formula (which has varied year to year) takes into account the total population, the age and sex distribution of that population, and incorporates some measure of social deprivation which is known to closely reflect poor health (11).

Having received a budget the purchaser will divide it broadly into four categories:

1. Funds to support existing services.
2. Funds to support cost pressures. These are increased costs beyond inflation such as funding the 'new deal' for junior doctors.
3. A contingency fund for unexpected costs.
4. Funds for new developments.

Traditionally, developments arose out of new monies. This need not be so. With the financial constraints being experienced resources to developed services will increasingly have to be generated in ways other than additional funding from central government by:

(1) providing existing services more efficiently;
(2) providing services in a radically new and cheaper, but clinically sound way;
(3) stopping activity which has low health gain;
(4) reducing effective interventions but which have a high cost–benefit ratio;
(5) raising money from donations (directly or indirectly) through voluntary organizations.

New developments can also be financially cost-neutral by changing the nature and emphasis of the work of health care professionals. A decision also has to be made as to whether new money generated out of one service can then be spent on another. This is understandably unpopular with providers and there is a danger of demotivating professionals. The most controversial example of this is the shift in funding from secondary to primary care.

Priority-setting

Whatever the resources available, purchasers need to set priorities. No single methodology has been established, and priority-setting, in the United Kingdom has occurred in a piecemeal manner and lacks central direction (12). Other countries have tried priority setting exercises on a large scale of which the State of Oregon's is the most comprehensive and controversial (13).

It is disappointing to both commissioners and purchasers that the government has failed to give them the tools needed to accomplish good strategic and financial control. In order to do this, one of the tools they need is to be able to ration openly and honestly. This is not to say that many purchasers are not committed to the concept of a comprehensive NHS but they see that it is not possible to provide every single intervention, regardless of cost or efficacy. For example, in the field of neurology, purchasers would wish to see a good rehabilitative and palliative care services for individuals with amyotrophic lateral sclerosis. They would not accept, however, that the drug Riluzole, whose effectiveness is at best marginal and cost-effectiveness ratio poor, should be automatically funded. For a district of half a million this drug has the potential to commit about £50 000–£70 000 (at 1997 prices) of a commissioner's budget. To date an absolute ban on the drug is not seen as being politically acceptable. Commissioners therefore find it difficult not to fund Riluzole. In funding it, however, they have to delay other developments or cut back on other services; in other words, they have to ration covertly. The issue for commissioners is not the difficulty of the fact that choices have to be made but that rationing has to be done covertly and often at the cost of those patients who have the least power in society.

It is the difficulty in recognizing and accepting rationing as an integral part of the NHS past, present, and future, which causes many of the problems in both managing and providing health care. Rationing is fortunately becoming increasingly overt and while it is recognized that this is difficult, uncomfortable, and not without its own costs in terms of the relationship between the NHS and patients, more openness is welcomed by many (14–16) (Table 28.2). Underpinning resource allocation issues is the ethical concept of justice. Justice can be considered to be the *'the fair adjudication between competing claims'* (17). There is no single interpretation of what is fair but rather interpretation reflects the value system adopted (see Box 3). It is important to appreciate that ethical standards are subject to individual interpretation and are not absolute.

Until the NHS reforms in 1991, service planning reflected the historical patterns of service provision which were heavily

Table 28.2 Levels at which rationing occurs

Governmental	Unconscious	Overt
District	Conscious	Covert
Service		
Patient (18)		

Box 3. Classification of moral philosophies which underpin different interpretations of what is just (adapted from Gillon) (17)

Libertarian theories
These protect the individual's personal liberty to life and acquisition of possessions, if by doing so they do not violate others. Adaptation of this principle underpins the free market approach to health care.

Utilitarian theories
These support the view that people deserve to have their welfare maximized. The distribution of resources should be in accordance with the greatest good for the greatest number. Maximizing health gain reflects this philosophy.

Marxist theories
These support the view that people deserve to have their needs met. The distribution of resources should be in proportion to the individual's need. Meeting medical need (often in terms of illness severity) reflects this philosophy.

Rawls' theory
Rawls combined the philosophy of individual freedom and utilitarian approach. The two underlying principles are first, that people should have maximum liberty compatible with the same degree of liberty for everyone and second, deliberate inequalities are unjust unless they work in favour of the least well-off.

Theories of merit
These support the view that people should receive what they merit either as an individual or the individual's value to society.

---

influenced by the interests of the medical profession. The prevailing value system was health care need (in terms of severity) and merit. In recent times this has been replaced by greater value being placed on maximizing health gain and countering inequalities.

The absence of an agreed ethical framework within which to allocate resources adds to the problem facing commissioners when trying to prioritize services. A public debate is required in order to establish a societal view on the role of publicly funded health care and the values that will underpin future decisions on how resources are to be shared. However, the reality is that there are no easy or rational solutions to the issue of priority-setting. Consequently, it is vital that mechanisms exists which allow a wide, continuous, and well-informed public debate to occur.

Part of the rationing debate is the issue of consulting and involving the public (and patients) in resource allocation issues; something to which the present National Health Service Executive is committed. While some purchasers may share this view, it is in fact difficult to implement public consultation in a meaningful way. This is in part because of the technical complexities of the issues under consideration. More problematic, however, is the difficulty of getting a representative view. The public is not a homogenous group and represents as complex a range of interests as those within the NHS. Factors such as age, circumstance, and experience of illness all shape individual values. Views can therefore change over time. In

addition, individuals can simultaneously hold contrary views particularly when considering the individual's position as a taxpayer compared to their position as a user of the service (19, 20).

The increasing democratization of the NHS will lead, nevertheless, to more open decision making and greater public involvement.

THE COMMISSONING STRATEGY

The outcome of the HNA indicates the needs of the population and the standards commissioning services should meet. The strategy is a more detailed plan about how this is to be achieved and in what order of priority. The latter should define:

1. Details of what services are to be provided and the order of priority in which developments are to occur.
2. Identification of key changes to the services.
3. The timescale for implementing these changes.
4. What resources will be required to achieve this.
5. Definition of the quality standards which are to be adopted

The commissioning strategy for an individual service forms an integral part of the HImP, which year on year is implemented by means of the Service and Financial Framework (SaFF).

SERVICE AND FINANCIAL FRAMEWORK

The SaFF is produced by the health authority in the autumn each year. This document contains a portfolio of service agreements which are provider based. It will contain:

(1) activity and financial information;
(2) detail changes in investments;
(3) identify cost improvements expected to release funds to be either reinvested in the provider or elsewhere.

The SaFF also takes into account the national priorities and guidance which is issued annually by the NHS Executive. National priorities include a wide range of objectives across many policy areas. The main long-term national policies are Our Healthier Nation targets, Patients' Charter standards, waiting time guarantees, financial, and activity targets. In addition, there are medium-to short-term priorities of which current examples are:

1. To give greater voice and influence to users of NHS services and their carers in their own care.
2. To work with other agencies, to ensure that integrated services are in place to meet needs for continuing health care and to allow elderly, disabled, or vulnerable people to be supported in the community.
3. To develop NHS organizations as good employers.

Health authorities, whose performance is monitored by the Regional Offices of the NHS Executive, are required to make progress on these priorities. However, health authorities also have local objectives and inevitably tension develops between national and local priorities. As the former take precedence, commissioners are sometimes left with limited financial resources to achieve local objectives.

Following the consultation exercise, commissioners have to finalize the details of the service agreements for the coming year. This is done in the fourth quarter (Fig. 28.4). The SaFF is produced in the autumn and the financial allocation to PCGs is usually notified in November. This means that in the third quarter of the financial year, when the first meetings with providers take place concerning the service agreements for the next year there is no certainty about the resources that will be available. Generally, this means that from January through to March, there are fairly intense rounds of negotiations between commissioners and providers about the key areas of change and the resources associated with these changes.

In March, the service agreements are signed off by both the purchasers and providers. In some areas of the country there is an encouragement to obtain the signatures of clinicians to contracts although this is usually only the signature of the clinical director. However, when there has been a particularly

difficult negotiation concerning any one specialty or a significant development is to take place, all consultants in that specialty may be asked to sign the service agreement or they may themselves wish to sign the agreement.

HEALTH SERVICE AGREEMENTS BETWEEN COMMISSIONERS AND PROVIDERS

Health service agreements are relatively simple documents drawn up and agreed by the providers and commissioners of health care. The agreement has four components: (1) a definition of the service provided; (2) the volume of workload to be undertaken; (3) a quality specification, and (4) a financial value.

Definition of the service to be provided

The agreement has to state what is being bought by the PCG or health authority and provided by the hospital. In terms of the definition of the service, most agreements will contain a simple 'prose' description such as 'neurology is the diagnosis and treatment of neurological disease by consultant neurologists and his/her junior medical staff in association with the

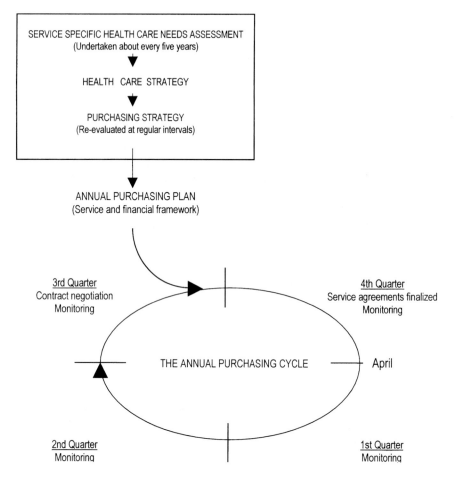

Fig. 28.4 The annual purchasing plan and cycle, and the relationship between strategy development and contracting.

related specialties of neurophysiology, neuroradiology, neuropathology, neuro-ophthalmology and neurosurgery'. The work undertaken by neurologists is often defined very simply in measurable units such as:

(1) elective inpatient finished consultant episode (FCE);
(2) emergency inpatient finished consultant episode;
(3) elective day case finished consultant episode;
(4) new outpatient consultation;
(5) repeat outpatient consultation

These measures have come under considerable criticism as it has been recognized they do not accurately reflect the work undertaken. Other tools will gradually be developed to look at different aspects of the work done but measures of activity will nonetheless remain important for both the management of a service and for the purposes of evaluating the service agreement.

Volume of work

The volume of work to be undertaken in the period of the agreement, a minimum of one year and usually three years, is specified in the categories of inpatient FCE, day case FCE, and outpatients. In the absence of a recent HNA the most important determinants of the volume of activity to be bought in a year are: the volume agreed by the commissioners and provider in the previous year; the actual volume undertaken in the previous year; and the maximum waiting times which were achieved at those volumes. Many commissioners will analyse the past trend in activity to make a projection of the level of activity for the next year. They will also take into consideration trends in the waiting list size and maximum waiting times.

The commissioner, in negotiation with the hospital, will then attempt to buy a level of outpatient and elective activity which is sufficient to meet the agreed waiting time standards. The calculation of the volumes of activity necessary to achieve these standards has to take into account the fact that a proportion of outpatient and inpatient work is deemed to be of high clinical priority (even if not classified as emergency work) and will be seen much earlier than 'routine' cases. Therefore, emergencies and clinically determined 'urgent' work will always take priority over the routine cases and, if the activity volumes which have been agreed are too low, the waiting time for routine cases may extend beyond the maximum waiting time standards set.

Quality specification

All quality specifications in contracts include National Patient Charter Standards (21) along with the local standards which may improve upon these standards (e.g. shorter waiting times). Patient Charter Standards cover a whole range of issues, for example:

1. Waiting times (for elective treatment, outpatients, when at a clinic, assessment in accident and emergency, on a trolley).
2. Cancellation of appointments, admission to hospital.
3. Patients' rights (privacy, taking part in research, single sex accommodation).
4. Information available to patients.
5. The discharge process.

In addition, specifications which reflect key issues may be included. For example, the manpower and physical capacity which should be employed in the diagnosis, treatment, and rehabilitation might be specified. This may include stating the types of staff and their qualifications involved for different conditions. For example, in stroke rehabilitation the paramedic input should include physiotherapy, occupational therapy, speech therapy, and social worker time. Equally, the process of care can be included such as a crude approximation of the 'average treatment profile' expected for a given condition which will outline what tests should be done for diagnosis, what forms of treatment, discharge planning, and continued rehabilitation post discharge in the community. Clinical guidelines which are expected to be followed may also be specified. The agreement will also require providers to submit information on their audit programme. It is the commissioner who ultimately pays for audit and as such that should have opportunity to specify audits which should be undertaken to achieve strategic goals. Finally commissioners may request information on specific outcomes for example in surgical specialties the unit's risk stratified mortality rates and survival.

The description of inputs to and the process of service provision has not been favoured by all commissioners and providers and can be completely absent from agreements. It is the provider's responsibility to have in place appropriate operational policies to provide the services set out in its prospectus. An extreme interpretation of this approach is that the inputs and process of service provision is solely a concern of the provider while the commissioner's role is to monitor outputs. The counter-perspective is that the main outputs currently monitored are crude and not clinically relevant. There is therefore an obligation on the commissioner to negotiate with the provider the most critical inputs and stages in the process of service delivery.

Finance

The agreement will include the financial sum to be paid to the provider. The total financial sum is calculated by multiplying the price of each unit of activity by the volume purchased. The annual financial sum paid by the purchaser for the volume of neurology activity agreed in the contract will not be recognized easily by the neurologist even if he/she has a good knowledge of the departmental budgets. The main reason for this is that all of the running costs of the hospital, including

Table 28.3 Maxwell's six aspects of quality (22)

Clinical effectiveness	The ability of the service to deliver health gain and avoid an unacceptable range of clinical outcomes
Efficiency	The efficient use of all the resources available (manpower, financial, equipment)
Equity	That the service is equitable (however defined)
Appropriateness	This has two elements. Appropriateness as it relates to effectiveness refers to whether patient selection ensures treatment results in benefit and excludes those that have little hope of benefiting (allocative efficiency) Appropriateness as it relates to efficiency refers to patients receiving effective health care in a setting that optimizes service efficiency
Acceptability	That the service is acceptable to the patient (thereby facilitating access)
Accessibility	Ensures that the service is accessible to the patient in terms of location, physical accessibility, opening time, availability of information, and the nature of the interaction between service providers and patients

overheads such as management costs, must be recovered through the prices charged. The price of a neurology inpatient stay, for example, is derived by adding a share of the overhead costs for running the hospital to the costs of providing the neurology service and then dividing this total cost by the number of neurology inpatient stays per year.

TYPES OF HEALTH SERVICE AGREEMENTS

There are several terms used to describe different types of health service agreements. Essentially, however, there are only two categories. The first is a 'block' agreement which does not allow any variation in the financial value of the agreement no matter how much change there is in the volume of activity undertaken. The second is a 'variable' agreement which allows the financial value to vary to reflect the level of activity undertaken.

In 1991/92, which was the first financial year in which health service agreement operated, most agreements were of a 'block' nature. By the mid 1990s most agreements included the ability to vary payment to reflect the actual volume of activity undertaken in order to give a degree of financial security to both parties. This is achieved by agreeing a financial value in relation to an 'indicative' volume of activity. The hospital and the commissioner then agree how much the activity may vary from the 'indicative' level before discussions take place on a financial adjustment to the agreement. For example, if a hospital was to be paid to undertake 1000 inpatient finished consultant episodes (FCEs) with a 5% margin or 'tolerance' level, this would mean that the unit could undertake 950 FCEs or 1050 FCEs before any financial variation

would take place. For activity levels outside the 5% margin the hospital and the commissioner would need to negotiate payment to compensate the relevant party for under-or over-performance. These financial adjustments are usually at a price significantly lower than the average FCE price. In the example given, if the average price for a neurology FCE was £1000 per case, then a 'marginal' rate for such an FCE could be as little as 15% of the average price; this price would be based on the consumable cost of treating a case. However, a marginal price in excess of 50% of the average price may be charged in instances where the provider has made clear to the commissioners that the indicative activity agreed in the contract was at the upper limits of its capacity and additional cases would require more capacity to be employed, for example additional nursing staff.

The different types of 'variable' agreements which exist reflect the degree to which the financial payments will vary with the changes in the levels of activity undertaken. Another illustration of this is when commissioners pay all of the fixed and semi-fixed costs in relation to the estimated annual workload agreed at the beginning of the year (and this payment will not change whatever the actual volume of activity) but the variable costs of providing the service are paid throughout the year in relation to the actual number of cases undertaken each month or financial quarter. In a 'cost per case' contract the purchaser pays for each case undertaken at full average price. This type of contract was commonly used by general practitioner fundholders.

It is important to recognize that in all types of service agreements emergency work has to be undertaken by providers, and commissioners must make payment for this. In fact, most agreements include separate volumes for elective and emergency care. Although the provider may need to exceed the agreed volume for emergency care, the volume of elective care cannot be exceeded by the provider unless the commissioner has agreed to pay for this additional activity (or the provider does so at its own cost).

CASE MIX

Commissioners and providers have stopped using simple block agreements and introduced variable payments for the volume of work done because commissioners wish to obtain 'value for money' and hospitals want the correct financial recompense for their work. However, these objectives cannot be achieved unless the agreement identifies the different types of cases treated which use more or less resources. Therefore a variable agreement needs to take into account the change in the case mix of the service. Certain conditions and their degree of complexity will use up different amounts of resources. For an individual case, the amount of resource employed is mainly determined by the length of stay in hospital. Agreements should therefore specify the price and volume for each category of cases. If commissioners understand the nature of the service provided and their associated costs they can, with confidence, make explicit decisions about the control and expansion of activity when setting priorities.

In contrast to neurosurgery, where case mix prices have been developed because of the relative ease of classification of surgical procedures and associated costs, neurology has been difficult to define in terms of resource usage. Consequently, agreements usually only include one average price. Within neurology, an 'average treatment profile' for an inpatient case would be fairly meaningless because there is such a range of conditions with different treatments. Under these circumstances it is difficult for either party to the agreement to know if 'value for money' has been achieved even if the total agreed level of activity has been undertaken.

Developments in case mix have occurred in some neuroscience units in those areas of work where services are more costly than average. A good example of this is the neurological assessment of intractable epilepsy for neurosurgical treatment.

There has been a national requirement to introduce casemix costing through the use of health care resource groups (HRGs) which have been developed by the Royal Colleges and professional associations with the assistance of the National Case Mix Office (23). Figure 28.5 gives an example of HRGs for the nervous system. HRGs have been designed to contain conditions, procedures, and treatments which are sufficiently similar in clinical terms and consume similar amounts of resource. The total number of FCEs (finished consultant episodes) for each HRG can be agreed in the contract at a given price. This is not meant to be prescriptive to the last detail of the work to be undertaken but will allow for better monitoring of resource use. Also, where priority has been allocated to certain types of cases, purchasers can monitor more closely whether or not their objectives are going to be achieved.

Both commissioners and providers in their respective roles have to identify and then implement the action which needs to be taken to ensure the terms of the contract are met. As a first step to doing this, the unit's performance must be monitored continually. Monitoring the contracted performance includes activity and finance, waiting times, and quality.

MONITORING THE SERVICE AGREEMENT

Activity and financial monitoring

In a specialty like neurology the hospital will send to the Commissioner information on outpatients attendances, inpatient, and day case treatments every month. For both outpatient attendances and admissions there is a contract minimum data set for each patient containing details such as name, address, date of birth, and clinical data including diagnosis, the consultant responsible, procedures undertaken, length of stay, method of admission, and discharge from hospital. There will be a count for the month of the volume of new outpatient attendances, elective inpatient and day cases, emergencies, and possibly the number of bed days.

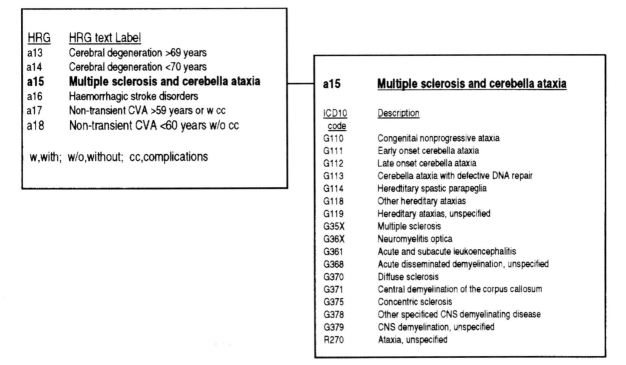

Fig. 28.5 Selected health care resource groups (HRGs) for neurology.

Alongside the activity monitoring, there will be a financial appraisal depending on the contract type. If the agreement includes variation in the payment for greater or less activity against the anticipated activity level for that period and these variations have been agreed with the commissioner, then a financial adjustment will be made. It should be noted that, if within a agreement, there are financial penalties for poor performance against waiting time standards, then these should be included in the amended payments for that period.

Waiting times

The national Patient Charter Standards will be regularly reported to the commissioner including the following:

1. Maximum waiting times for inpatient or day case treatment.
2. Maximum waiting times for a first outpatient appointment.
3. Waiting time from the appointment time to be seen in the outpatient clinic.

Monthly waiting time monitoring will usually include the actual waiting time experience during the month of people admitted to hospital or seen in outpatients, the current length of wait of people on the waiting list, and the expected waiting time of people with a booked outpatient appointment.

Quality

There are formal monitoring requirements under the Patient Charter Standards. In addition to these returns the hospital will make a whole range of returns depending on the particular method of quality specification agreed by the unit and its main commissioner. There may also be intermittent quality assurance exercises. These are more labour-intensive and still not widely used.

Service agreement review meetings

It is very important that the commissioner and provider meet regularly to discuss contract performance against the terms of the service agreement. For both the commissioner and provider, these meetings are time-consuming but for any relatively large contract it is important that the commissioner meets not only the corporate hospital management but each clinical directorate within the hospital on a quarterly basis. By meeting with the clinical directorates, any significant variation in performance can be discussed, understood, and action agreed. Ideally, it would be useful to meet quarterly with representatives from each specialty, however, for most hospitals and commissioner there are too many service agreements to make this possible.

Managing variance in service agreements

In terms of resource flexibility, there is very little on either the commissioner or provider side that can be achieved during the financial year. If, within a service agreement, there is significant under or over performance, then increases or decreases in payments will be made. Furthermore, commissioners will be reluctant to enter into any negotiations about increases in payments which will follow through to the next financial year. This means that the commissioners will not want to enhance a service in-year because they do not know whether the following year's resource allocation will include any development resource. Therefore, the commissioner's flexibility is limited to what is termed, 'non-recurrent expenditure'. This cash may be available because of underperformance at other hospitals or underperformance in other clinical directorates in the same hospital or through slippage on development schemes across the whole range of services. It is likely that the officer of the PCG or health authority who is responsible for service agreements will be able to take decisions on small levels of additional non-recurrent expenditure without seeking the formal approval of the PCG board or health authority. It should be recognized, however, that most health authorities will commit all of their recurring expenditure at the beginning of the financial year because the identified demands for recurring expenditure very often exceed the resource available; it is difficult to justify holding back recurring resource at the beginning of the year on the assumption that higher priorities for resources will emerge later in that year.

Most hospitals will have contracts with many commissioners. Although a commissioner will only be interested in the activity undertaken by the hospital for patients who are registered with the relevent PCGs, the hospital may choose to manage the performance of each specialty for all commissioners rather than by individual commissioners. This issue has been fairly contentious. For example, it is possible that a neurology department must see 100 new outpatients a month and may meet this target but, if this target is made up of several commissioners then performance may exceed target for some and be insufficient for others; during the contract period if this balance between commissioners does not even out then the unit will need to manage its workload. Some units have been reluctant to introduce this, often because clinicians believe this interferes with clinical prioritization. From the unit's financial position, if commissioners with excess activity have not agreed to pay for additional work then their elective activity should be controlled during the rest of the period of the service agreement to meet the agreed contract level, and any purchasers receiving too little activity may agree to action that increases activity in order to meet contracted levels, thus reducing waiting times.

It is not possible to state how commissioners and providers resolve variances but Table 28.4 sets out some examples of commissioner responses to variances in provider activity performance.

From the above it is clear that the options available for negotiation when contract variances occur in service agreements, must be explicit in the document and that the

Table 28.4 Contract variance: provider and purchaser

Provider's activity performance	Commissioners response
Underperformance on elective activity	Reduce payments
	Encourage more elective activity thereby reducing waiting times
	If emergency activity is above agreement then offset against elective activity
Overperformance on elective activity	Increase payments if there was prior agreement to exceed targets with the provider, no additional payments without prior agreement
	Trade-off increase in elective activity if there is under performance on emergencies
	Require provider to manage elective workload to contracted level; this must be done throughout the year to avoid significant restriction late in the year; commissioner must accept the possibility of increase in waiting time, which may breach standards

clinicians who provide the service must be party to the agreement on volumes of activity and waiting times. In general, the most likely in-year contract management issues are the following:

(1) increases in emergency activity;
(2) under/over-performance on elective treatment;
(3) breeches of local and national waiting time standards, (this can occur even when elective contract targets are being met by the provider);
(4) introduction of new techniques and drugs which, despite all efforts, still occur without warning;
(5) dramatic price changes on consumables.

Depending on the specific clauses in the service agreement the overall financial position of both parties and the maturity of the relationship between commissioner and provider, these issues may be more or less amenable to solution.

The preceding sections have described what is involved in the commissioning process from the most strategic elements of health care needs assessment for the population as a whole, through to a description of the key components of the health service contract between a commissioner and provider. It is hoped that most of the people who are currently involved in the different stages of this process will recognize these descriptions. Nevertheless, within this central framework, there will be considerable local variation, for example, in the types of professions directly involved in negotiations concerning activity and finance.

KEY STRATEGIC ISSUES IN NEUROLOGY

A systematic strategic approach to developing services has not been feature of the NHS. The 1990s have seen the beginnings of such an approach with the introduction of commissioners, a strengthened public health perspective, and increased emphasis on good management which aims to deliver better integration of the activities of the organization. The Calman–Hine Report on Cancer Services has also made a significant contribution to this process (24). This document heralds the first national framework for mainstream services developed by the Department of Health with the view to imposing more sensible planning and standardized service delivery.

The possibility of a national service framework for neurology services brings to the fore two key strategic issues in neurology. The first is the question of what the service configuration for neurology should be in future. Consideration needs to be given to the relationship between the small number of specialized neuroscience centres, perhaps serving a catchment population of several million, and local district hospitals. Since the London Service Reviews which took place in 1992 in response to a perceived need to rationalize services, the 'hub and spoke' model has gained favour for a number of services (25). This comprises a highly specialized centre (the hub) which has strong and formalized relationships with smaller centres providing services to a district level (the spoke). There are many interpretations of the hub and spoke model but the two most basic are either: having consultants based in the hubs and outreaching to districts (usually in the form of an outpatient clinic) or having consultants based in districts with 'in-reach' to hubs to enable them to maintain a specialty interest and reduce professional isolation.

There is no single solution to the 'best' service configuration but it is fair to say that many districts which are at some distance from tertiary centres wish to see a more district based neurological service for diagnosis and support for the management of common neurological conditions. As such a good proportion of the work of a neurologist will in future be considered core district services. In very densely populated areas the travel time to a specialist neuroscience centre may not differ significantly from that of the travel time to the local hospital. In this situation commissioners would need to evaluate the benefits of undertaking neurology within the local hospital. In such a situation pricing may prove the deciding factor as routine work in specialist centres is generally more expensive. Such a centre would need therefore to be able to price different categories of neurological work to ensure that the overhead costs related to expensive support facilities which accompany neuroscience centre status are apportioned accurately to the different types of care undertaken. This must be done to ensure that the cost of treating common neurological disease will be more or less the same as the local hospital. It is likely, however, that in most instances commissioners will wish to buy an appropriate-case-mix from each tier of the service.

Decisions about service configuration cannot be made without examining the future role of the neurologist. This is the second major strategic issue in neurology. A significant proportion of services for neurological patients at a district level fall into the realm of rehabilitation and palliative care. It is uncertain at present whether the specialty of neurology can meet these needs. Commissioners are therefore faced with two options. First to maintain the established pattern of working for neurologists and for rehabilitation to be undertaken by specialists in that field some of whom may come from a neurology background. The other alternative is to encourage and support neurologists to take over the total care of patients with neurological conditions. If this is to be the case then neurologists will need to address the challenging re-training issues this model requires.

Professional bodies have argued the case for more neurologists on the basis that the United Kingdom has one of the lowest numbers of neurologists per head of the population in the Western world (26, 27). However, international comparisons can be misleading as they do not always compare like with like. Neurologists in countries other than the United Kingdom may have a much broader spectrum of care. Without a clear view on the remit of the neurologist discussions on consultant numbers are somewhat meaningless.

DISCUSSION

There has been considerable and far reaching change in the NHS since the beginning of the 1990s. Change is likely to be an ongoing feature of the NHS for many years to come. Many of the innovations that have been introduced are not unique to the United Kingdom but are part of a more general phenomena as Western nations strive to control the costs of health care. The internal market however was, until recently, unique to the United Kingdom.

It is possible to identify a number of themes in today's NHS which will be of ongoing relevance for decades to come. The first and probably the most important is cost containment. Initiatives which have been introduced to achieve this include; resource management by clinicians, general practitioner fundholding, generic prescribing, and efficiency drives. Linked to this is the issue of rationing. The move to more explicit rationing is being seen as many as an end to a comprehensive NHS and as such has led to widespread resistance. The idea that rationing is a new phenomena is false and there is plenty of evidence, for those wishing to look, to give weight to the argument that rationing has always been a feature of the NHS. The most obvious is the waiting list and the historical pattern of funding and service provision which led to those areas with the greatest healthcare need getting the least funding. Less obvious are service development decisions whether it be at a commissioner level or at a provider level. It is clear that these require choices to be made with some services being relatively underdeveloped and as such rationed,

albeit by default. It is explicit rationing which is the new feature of the NHS rationing per se.

Another ongoing theme will be pressure on professionals to have a better evidence base to their practice and reduce unacceptable clinical variation. To achieve this there will be demand for improvements in NHS information systems and audit. An inevitable consequence will be increased accountability of the medical profession to both the NHS as employer and society at large. Closely related to this is clinical governance.

Finally there are a number of relationships which will continue to dominate the NHS and health policy:

The relationship between primary and secondary care. Fundholding was designed to change the balance of power within the NHS which in part it has done. It also gave rise to the notion of a primary care led NHS which aims to make the primary health care team the main locus for service provision and decision making regarding initiating clinical care and therefore resource allocation. In this context the acute sector becomes a supporting service to primary care and not the other way around. This has led to a different sort of tension between primary and secondary care and one task is to ensure that the two work more closely together with better management of the interface.

The relationship between the health authority and primary care groups. Health authorities are going to increasingly take on purely a strategic, supportive, and monitoring role. A key challenge for health authorities will be ensuring the implementation of strategies in the absence of any budgetary control.

The relationship between commissioners and providers. The internal market has led to a deterioration, in many instances, in the relationship between these two groups. There is now a desire for closer working although some tension is inherent by virtue of the different roles they play.

The relationship between different trusts. The internal market has fostered greater competition to a level which is unsustainable and undesirable in the context of a publicly funded health care system which aims to be equitable needs rather than supply driven, support provider stability (but not complacency) and which has only a fixed amount of money available to it. There will be increased emphasis on co-operation. Furthermore, changes to service standards will require smaller hospitals to either merge or collaborate more closely if they are to survive at all. This will result in hub and spoke models developing on a much more local level with larger district hospitals supporting smaller ones.

The relationship between the patient and health care services and individual doctors in particular. The public is becoming more knowledgeable and empowered to challenge medical opinion. Services will be required to be more patient focused and this will lead to a maturing of the relationship between doctors and patients.

The relationship between medicine and society. It has already been said that the complete freedom of the medical profession is being challenged and eroded. There is no doubt that the public have lost some faith with the profession and doctors, will in future, be required to be more corporate in their thinking and behaviour and be more accountable.

The relationship between health care professionals themselves. Skills mix issues and changes in areas of responsibility both within professional groups and across them will undoubtedly be on the agenda in order to make services more efficient and address manpower problems.

The relationship between the private and public sector. The use of private health care is increasing by both individuals and by commissioners. While the two systems have lived side by side since the inception of the NHS attitudes to private health care remains ambivalent and governmental policy in this area remains noticeably absent.

It is impossible to describe the NHS landscape of the next decade. It is the nature of organizational change in the NHS that changes reflect a cyclical pattern. The cynic may interpret this as events coming full circle and that change occurs for the sake of change. There is no doubt that the pace of change today is overwhelming at times. However, close examination of these cycles indicates that we never quite come back to where we started. For example the changing structure of the NHS over the last decade has seen the merger of health authorities into larger organizations, the creation of very small fundholders and now the creation of primary care groups which, in some instances, cover similar areas to the original health authorities. Only the foolish would believe that this represents a replication of the old area health authorities. Big cultural changes have occurred in the intervening time.

In any analysis it is clear that the NHS is built upon relationships and as such will more or less succeed or fail on the strength of the key relationships described above. It is these relationships which observers will watch with the greatest of interest.

REFERENCES

1. *Working for patients: The NHS and Community Care Act.* HMSO, London (1989).
2. *The New NHS: Modern and Dependable Government White Paper.* HMSO London, 1988.
3. Wade, D. T. *Stroke (acute cerebrovascular disease).* In *Health care needs assessment*, Vol. 1, (ed. Stevens, A. and Raftery, J.). Radcliffe Medical Press, Oxford (1994).
4. Stevens A. *Needs assessment. Health Trends*, 1991, **23**, 20–3.
5. *Health care needs assessment*, Vol. 1, (ed. Stevens, A. and Raftery, J.). Radcliffe Medical Press, Oxford (1994).
6. Holton, S., Stevenson, C., and Thomas, J. *Commissioning Health Care: A basic guide to health needs assessment, intervention planning and outcome monitoring (PHIS Project).* School of Postgraduate Studies in Medical and Health Care (1993).
7. As for (3).
8. Drummond, M. *Principles in economic appraisal in health care.* Oxford University Press (1980).
9. Donebedian, A. *Explorations in quality assessment and monitoring. In*
The definition of quality and approaches to its assessment, Vol. 1. Michigan Health Administration Press, Oregon (1980).
10. *Annual Health Report of the Director of Public Health.* Worcestershire Health Authority, UK (1996).
11. *Inequalities in health: The Black Report and the health divide,* (ed. Townsend, P., Davidson, N., and Whitehouse, M). Penguin, London (1990).
12. *Patterns of priorities: a study of the purchasing and rationing policies of a health authority.* NAHAT Research Paper 7 (1992).
13. Honigbaum, F. *Who shall live? Who shall die? Oregon's health financing proposals* King's Fund College Papers No. 4 (1992).
14. Menzel, P. T. Some ethical costs of rationing. *Law Medicine and Health Care*, 1992, **20**, 57–66.
15. Taylor, T. R. Pity the poor gatekeeper: a transatlantic perspective a cost containment in clinical practice. *BMJ*, 1989, **299**, 1323–5.
16. *Rationing dilemmas in healthcare.* NAHAT Research Paper 8. (1993).
17. Gillon, R. *Philosophical medical ethics.* Wiley, Chichester, UK.
18. Klein, R. Dimension of rationing: Who should do what? *BMJ*, 1993, **307**, 309 11.
19. Lomas, J. Relunctaar rationis: public aspect to health care priorities *J Health Serv Res Policy*, 1997 **2**(2): 103–111.
20. Doyle C. Rationing health care: who should come first? *Daily Telegraph*, 12 September (1994).
21. *The Patient's Charter: Raising the standard.* HMSO, London (1991).
22. Maxwell, R. Quality assessment in health. *BMJ*, 1984, **288**, 1470–2.
23. Information Management Group. *HRG: Healthcare Resource Groups*, Version 2.0. NHS Executive, London (1994).
24. *A policy framework for commissioning cancer services.* A Report by the Expert Advisory Group on Cancer Services to the Chief Medical Officers of England and Wales (1995).
25. Neurosciences Review Group. Hide, R. (Chair). *Report on an independent review of specialist services in London: Neuroscience.* HMSO, London (1993).
26. Langton-Hewer, R. and Wood V. A. Neurology in the United Kingdom: II. A study of current neurological services for adults. *Journal of Neurology, Neurosurgery and Psychiatry*, 1992, **55**(suppl.), 8–14.
27. ABN (Association of British Neurologists). *Neurology in 1988 and beyond.* ABN, London (1988).

FURTHER READING

Coast, J., Donovan, J., and Frankel, S. (ed.). *Priority setting: the health care debate.* Wiley, Chichester, UK (1996).
Department of Health documents relating to *Health of the Nation* (accidents and cerebrovascular disease). HMSO, London
Drummond, M. *Principles in economic appraisal in health care.* Oxford University Press (1980).
Effective health care bulletin series. Published by the School of Public Health of Leeds, Centre for Health Economics, University of York and the Research Unit of the Royal College of Physicians
Gale, G. and Grant J. *Managing change in a medical context.* The Joint Centre for Educational, Research and Development in Medicine, London (1990).
Gillon, R. *Philosophical medical ethics.* Wiley, Chichester, UK (1990).
Glennerster, H. Matsaganis, M., and Owens, P. *Implementing General Practitioner fundholding: Wild card or winning hand?* Open University Press, Mitton Keynes, UK (1994).
Handy, C. *Understanding organisations.* Penguin, London, UK (1985).

Inequalities in health: The Black Report and the health divide (ed. Townsend, P., Davidson, N., and Whitehouse, M.). Penguin London (1990).

Klein, R. *The politics of the NHS, (2nd edn). Longman, Harlow, UK (1990).*

The Wessex toolkit for health care needs assessment. Radcliffe Medical Press, Oxford 1993.

Klein, R., Day, P., and Redmayne, S. *Managing Scarcity: Priority setting and rationing in the national health service. Open University Press (1996).*

The Health of the Nation: Key Area Headbook Coronary Heart Disease and Stroke. Department of Health Jan 1993.

Our Healthier Nation. Department of Health 1998.

29 Translating clinical research and technological developments into changes in practice

S. B. Blunt and C. Kennard

RESEARCH AND HEALTH CARE: THE PRESENT SITUATION

It is acknowledged that 'Research is essential to any strategy to improve health' (1) and the Medical Research Council has as its ultimate objective 'the maintenance and improvement of human health' (2). And yet, there has been a feeling that clinical and managerial decisions in the National Health Service (NHS) are not always based on reliable research. Likewise, there are many areas where, despite good evidence from clinical trials, for example, concerning the benefits or otherwise of a particular treatment, clinical practice is slow to change. The problem of incorporating new research and technological developments into health care within the NHS is further complicated by the limitation of resources: Archie Cochrane identified the dilemma in 1972 (3), when he questioned how a system (the NHS) with limited resources might finance a free, comprehensive, and effective health care system accessible to all? He drew attention to our great collective ignorance about the effects of health care, and explained how evidence from randomised controlled trials could help us to use limited resources more rationally. Cochrane recognised that individuals who want to take more informed decisions about health care did not have ready access to reliable reviews of the available evidence. He suggested that the randomized controlled clinical trial was the type of research most likely to ascertain whether a treatment was effective or not. Cochrane further noted that, bearing in mind the limited resources, only treatments proven to be of benefit should be used, and those which had not should not. He proposed that treatments/care of unknown efficacy should be supplied only within the confines of a trial.

Doctors and health care providers operating within a health care system have a responsibility to provide the highest quality of medical care within the financial constraints. Ideally, health care provided within the NHS should be of proven efficacy; it should be as economical as possible; there should be clear clinical policies on as many aspects of treatment as possible; health care providers must be aware of what the public's needs and purchaser's expectations are. Purchasers, managers, and patients must be aware of the difficulties sometimes encountered in drawing up hard guidelines for management of certain conditions; they must also be aware of the constraints placed on health care providers by limited financial resources. Purchasers must also be aware that efficiency and accessability are in the long term perhaps not as important as the provision of appropriate and effective care (4). As if fulfilling the prophetic nature of Cochrane's report, today, cost-effectiveness of all aspects of patient care is at the forefront of the minds of many clinicians, purchasers, and managers. Furthermore, the public expects more from health care providers than ever before, not only in terms of access to new (and often expensive) treatments, but also the expectation that a particular treatment has been shown to work. With the availability of medical information on computer networks, the public is also becoming increasingly informed (often with misleading data) about treatment options. This makes it even more important that doctors should be able to support their clinical practice with reliable reviews of research on the subject.

These various pressures on clinical practice may have massive implications for the nature of medical research carried out. There are several different types of medical research each with their own merit, and each with varying relevance to clinical practice. The following are some examples of the type of research that might be carried out:

1. Clinical research directed with a particular problem or treatment in mind whose outcome may have a direct bearing on the management of today's patients (e.g. the randomized clinical trial).
2. Clinical research which may be relevant at some later date (or future generations) to patient management, but which is not problem-driven.
3. Technological advances whose introduction into clinical practice will affect patient care (e.g. MRI scanning, radiosurgery, functional neurosurgery, gene therapy).
4. Technological advances which increase understanding of normal functions as well as pathological states, but whose findings may not be of relevance to immediate patient management (e.g. functional imaging with positron emission tomography, PET).
5. Basic research which is relevant to clinical situations (such as molecular genetics).
6. Basic research which, whilst increasing further understanding, may not contribute readily to patient health.

Funding bodies are more likely to finance research which is clearly of direct relevance to clinical problems, current patient care, or research whose outcomes can be readily translated into clinical practice. This should not mean, however, that very basic research should be neglected. It is here that some of the fundamental breakthroughs have occurred and which have gone on to have major impacts on clinical practice. Bearing in mind these different types of research, therefore, an ideal system should operate where there is a flow of information driven by clinical problems:

Problem identification in health care
↓
Research strategy and commissioning of work in context of previous works on the subject
↓
Outcomes
↓
Evaluation of findings in context of previous works on the subject (i.e. reviews)
↓
Dissemination of information to clinicians/purchasers/managers/patients
↓
Audit of uptake and efficacy in terms of change in practice.

If such a system is to work, it is important that clinical needs should be fed into the earliest stages of research, producing 'problem-oriented' research. The fruits of the research are then more likely to be fed back in to the health care system. This should not, however, mean that research driven by curiosity alone (rather than for specific problem-solving) should not continue. Such research can yield unforeseen information which may be relevant and beneficial to health care; the discovery of penicillin is an obvious example of such work. Nevertheless, research can only be translated into clinical practice if it is clinically relevant, and therefore at least some research should be 'directed'.

The eventual outcome of individual research trials must be assessed in the context of previous trials, and the conclusions must then find their way into clinical practice, where relevant. The usefulness of systematic reviews here cannot be overemphasized (5). Thus, there are many examples where a number of small trials have been singularly unconvincing, but a systematic review of all trials has gone on to show a clear benefit of treatment: examples include effects of stroke units on mortality (6) and steroid treatment of children with meningitis reducing complications such as deafness (7). Unfortunately, there has been some resistance of some clinicians, in other medical specialities, to incorporate evidence from systematic reviews into routine clinical practice (8). This gap between research findings and changes in clinical practice emphasizes the importance of continuing medical education for clinicians. But continuing medical education alone is not sufficient. There must be some means of auditing to what degree information obtained from such education is then put into effect as changes in clinical practice.

The extent to which a particular effective treatment has been taken up is often not known. For example, to what extent have the benefits of anticoagulation in atrial fibrillation, or endarterectomy in carotid stenosis been disseminated to general practitioners, hospital doctors, and other health care workers? To what extent has clinical practice been altered by such knowledge? What proportion of patients presenting to the general practitioner with transient ischaemic attack are being referred for vascular screening? Is such information even known? This problem of clinical guidelines based on current research reaching practising clinicians is clearly evident at the hospital consultant level. A recent survey by the Stroke Association of acute stroke treatment in UK hospitals showed that there was great uncertainty amongst key clinicians about the value of all available forms of treatment for stroke (9). This sort of survey exposes the defects that exist both in educating clinicians and in translating acquired knowledge into clinical practice. This raises two most important question of how widely clinical practice (and changes in clinical practice on the basis of recent research) is audited on a national scale, and what is done about deficiencies that are so revealed.

Clinical research is usually funded by medical charities, or centrally by government funds. The above examples, in which treatments for clinical problems have been established in randomized clinical trials and yet in which the translation of the findings into clinical practice remains unknown raise important questions. First, how well and how reliably are the results from clinical trials reviewed and condensed into an accessible form for busy clinicians; second, what measures are available to ensure that key clinicians take up this information; third, what measures are in place for auditing how well such information is incorporated into clinical practice; finally, what is done about areas in which clinical research does not seem to have altered clinical practice appropriately?

Are there lessons to be learnt from the drug industry regarding the way in which treatments are advertised and presented to clinicians, and their utilization taken up? There are several poignant examples where drugs have been heavily advertised by the pharmaceutical industry with the main targets being the patient and the practising clinician, using data which may have been based on single clinical trials rather than systematic reviews. For example, the prescription of selegiline in the treatment of Parkinson's disease underwent a massive increase following the preliminary publication of the DATATOP study in 1989 (Parkinson Study Group, Ref. 10), which suggested a possible role of selegiline in slowing progression of disease. The increase in use of this drug seemed to become widespread among general practitioners and hospital physicians, and even patients were asking for the drug. The reasons for the successful (and possibly premature) incorporation of selegiline into the general regime for Parkinson's disease were: (a) the neurological world was delighted to be able to offer a possibly protective treatment to patients; and (b) the company producing selegiline was quick to market the product widely and effectively on the strength of what at first seemed to be sound and encouraging research. With the recent publication of further studies, however, suggesting that the apparently beneficial effects of selegiline might be explained on a symptomatic basis alone (Parkinson Study Group 1993, Ref. 11), and that the addition of selegiline to an L-dopa treatment regime might increase mortality (12), one wonders to what extent its use will now change in the opposite direction. Similarly, the use of sumatriptan might not have been introduced so widely into clinical practice, had it not been for the huge publicity given by the drug company, at all levels of the NHS, quite apart from patient-directed advertisement. More recently still, patients with multiple sclerosis are obtaining information about possible benefits of beta-interferon directly from the pharmaceutical industry, and via media press, rather than through more conventional medical channels, and before completion of sufficient trials of the drug. The pharmaceutical industry has an impressive ability to spread information to both health providers and patients. Until recently, however, there has been no comparably efficient and fail-safe mechanism(s) for ensuring the translation of appropriate clinical research into practice within the health service system.

To maintain high standards of medical care, doctors use a variety of methods to keep up-to-date with recent developments in treatment and technological advances. Much of this is self-driven and includes reading books and journals; attending conferences and clinical meetings; using computer systems; and satellite transmission. However, with the huge amount of medical literature published daily, it is not possible for individual clinicians to keep up with the latest developments and to decipher what of the many articles available are worthy of influencing their practice.

If we look in more detail at the methods currently used by clinicians to 'keep-up' with current developments within a speciality (such as neurology), there have been several rather haphazard methods (see below).

Medical literature

Conscientious neurologists devour the neurological press and good quality medical journals. But how reliable is the information derived from single studies which may have referred back to only a proportion of previous relevant studies? Also, not all research articles are well conducted, and the information and conclusions reached by the authors of the article may not be accurate in relation to other work in the field. Results of original papers can therefore be misleading. It may be difficult for the reader to disentangle the sometimes conflicting information, often from poorly performed research, from the plethora of published data that is available. One way of circumventing this is the publication of regular review articles provided by an expert panel, and giving an overall consensus

and recommendation for clinical practice within particular areas. However, even review articles can be selective about what is included. It is important that such reviews should take into account all published literature. Counsell *et al.* (5) suggest that up-to-date systematic reviews of all trials are the only way to keep doctors well and clearly informed of the important clinical developments that are worthy of changing clinical practice. The best use of available data can save time and resources if each new trial is reviewed in the context of previous similar studies. The Cochrane collaboration (see below) will help to ease the task of reviewers.

Regional centres

These provide an environment where related specialities (such as neurology, neurosurgery, and neuroradiology) come together to mutual advantage. Within these specialities, individuals with particular subspeciality interests can contribute to raising the level of expertise within the centre. Such an environment would encourage the existence of speciality clinics where up-to-date information can be more readily utilized in clinical practice. The dissemination of information through formal and informal discussion occurs. Regional centres are also important as they can provide a more organized postgraduate education system than might exist in a smaller unit. Thus, regular lectures by visiting and local speakers on particular areas of recent change are of great use, as are journal clubs where important articles are brought to general attention. Some neuroscience centres organize teaching courses and meetings with information about management and research developments in particular areas.

The pharmaceutical industry

The role of the pharmaceutical industry has been mentioned in the context of marketing drugs. However, it also plays an important role in problem-directed research, can assist with the funding of research fellows and research nurses, and is enormously effective at publicizing results for its own benefit, and in auditing to what extent its particular product has been introduced into clinical practice.

HOW CAN TRANSMISSION OF INFORMATION BE IMPROVED?

Acknowledging that there is a problem in the translation of research findings and technological developments into clinical practice is a major step in improving the situation. There are various areas that need to be tackled to improve the current situation. Figure 29.1 illustrates a way in which such a system might operate.

PROBLEM-DIRECTED RESEARCH

Changing the ethos surrounding research

An awareness among clinicians of the importance of research findings in affecting clinical practice must be encouraged.

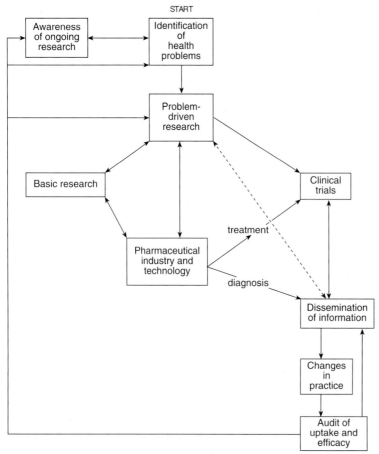

Fig. 29.1 Transmission of information. Health problems should be identified and used to drive research. Basic research should continue, and a link between this and more clinically relevant research and developments should be maintained so that information can be transferred rapidly between the two. Information derived from these research sources can be channelled into clinical trials. The information from these areas must then be collated in a usable form and distributed to those clinicians for whom the information is relevant. Systematic reviews of clinical trials and CME (continuing medical education) are of importance here. Changes in practice should occur where appropriate, and these changes should be monitored. At the same time, the efficacy of the given change or treatment should be assessed in the wider clinical setting. This can then be fed back into the system to affect the driving research forces. Throughout this whole system, however, there has to be an ethos among medical practitioners, that research is relevant to clinical care.

This may require a change in attitude towards research and researchers among many clinicians. In today's climate of NHS reforms and cost-effectiveness, the evidence for and against particular treatments and interventions becomes even more important. Research should no longer be regarded as a luxury, but as something that is important not only for scientific advancement, but also for efficient health care in both the short and long term.

Related to this ethos favouring research is the role of education: at the undergraduate level, teaching should shape attitudes to create a receptive attitude towards knowledge and developments; in addition, relevant skills for acquiring information rapidly and efficiently (such as computer skills) are important (13). Similarly, at the postgraduate level, a more formalized programme of continuing medical education should exist for hospital doctors, as was recently introduced by the Royal Colleges (see below).

What should be researched?

The subject matter of the research is of obvious importance: topics that are not relevant clinically will not be translated into changes in clinical practice. Related to this is the overall im-

pact in terms of size of a clinical problem: research outcomes that affect common conditions are more likely to be widely publicized. Advisory committees involved in sponsoring research must be aware of ongoing research, and of areas in the basic sciences that are potentially clinically relevant. Individuals directing research projects, and organizations involved in their funding (and therefore to some extent in determining its direction), must work closely with health departments and respond to perceived major areas of health problems (e.g. AIDS, stroke). Specific studies can then be undertaken with these areas in mind, so accelerating their incorporation into clinical practice.

Basic medical research should be directed with a view to its immediate or future clinical relevance. This is a key factor in speeding up the process of applying scientific and technological advances to clinical practice. Technological advances must be utilized in the appropriate clinical setting; this requires interaction between many different scientific disciplines (consider PET units). If the developments are to be of clinical benefit, it seems sensible that clinicians should be involved at the earliest stages of such development. Likewise, close collaboration between industry and research bodies, and academic units will speed up the development of technological advances which might be of practical value in health care. Technological developments, together with appropriate technical and specialist support, especially where they can profoundly influence both the quality and efficiency of medical care (such as the use of magnetic resonance imaging, MRI) must be made available on a national basis particularly to regional centres.

Which individuals and organizations should undertake research?

Who should do the research if its clinical relevance, and its incorporation into clinical practice are fundamental? The role of the research neurologist, academic units, and regional neuroscience centres are important not only in directing the nature of research, but also in participating in research and ensuring its accurate interpretation and appropriate dissemination amongst other practising neurologists and health care workers. For example, basic scientists working in isolation from clinical settings, or physicists developing instruments without directed clinical applications, will be of little use to health care. Links between clinical and research departments must be strong, and there must be key individuals whose responsibility it is to maintain a flow of information between the two.

There has been a tradition in neurology, and one that is spreading in many specialities, that doctors in training should undertake a period of research and completion of a higher degree, before becoming eligible for a consultant post. Whether this universal requirement is necessary or beneficial to either the individual or to the practice of medicine is uncertain. There can be no doubt that key individuals, who are interested in research, and are good at it, should be encouraged to pursue research projects, and academic careers. On the other hand, for individuals who have no enthusiasm for pursuing research, or who are unlikely to be good at it, perhaps their energies could be better employed in clinical service while the funding that would otherwise have been allocated to their research project could be diverted elsewhere.

With the limitations in funding for research, there is some support for the view that obligatory research degrees should be questioned. This approach might reduce the amount of poor quality research being produced. A recent survey suggested that most consultant physicians who did not pursue an academic career felt that the time spent doing research had not been of significant use (14). Furthermore, it has been suggested that 'too much time is spent on ill considered, ill conceived research' (Professor Michael Peckham, Director of Research and Development in the NHS 1993). And yet 'high quality clinical researchers are like gold dust' (15).

PRODUCTION OF ACCURATE SUMMARIES OF DATA AND APPROPRIATE CLINICAL GUIDELINES

Recently, the importance of collating data from all clinical trials, interpreting each study in the context of previous work on the subject, and producing informed recommendations about optimal clinical practice in the light of research findings has become apparent. Randomized clinical trials are among the most powerful tools available to clinicians for testing new procedures, validating old ones, and comparing alternatives. But how correctly are the results reported (16,17), then analysed, and if deemed valuable, how effectively, accurately and efficiently are the results translated into clinical practice? Ketley and Woods (18) have highlighted some of the problems which might be encountered today: despite demonstration of clear short-and long-term benefit on mortality (in this case in the use of thrombolytic therapy for acute myocardial infarction) from several good trials, there is a reluctance among clinicians to put treatment into practice; furthermore, there was a time-lag of two to three years before a significant increase in use of the method was seen. Counsell *et al.* (5) suggest that one way of providing accurate and useful advice for best clinical practice is to employ systematic reviews of all past, ongoing studies of a particular topic, and they point out the dangers of conventional incomplete reviews.

Centrally organized information systems

Systematic reviews of all available trials can dramatically shorten the time taken to show a significant effect (or lack of) for a given treatment. Centrally organized efforts are now underway to ensure that outcomes of research are available to the relevant clinicians (and managers, purchasers, and possibly patients). Ideally, these efforts should include blanket recommendations and 'best approach' strategies for particular clinical problems.

The Cochrane Centre was set up in October 1992 by the NHS Research and Development (R&D) Programme. The main task of the Centre is to facilitate and extend the creation of systematic reviews of randomized controlled trials (RCTs) evaluating health care. The aim is to make essential information available to those who make health decisions, so that the best decisions can be made. The information is made available on computer disk (regularly updated) and in published books. The Centre works together with the Clinical Trial Service Unit at Oxford University to establish an up-to-date database of reviews of RCTs, making them readily available electronically. The Centre also keeps an up-to-date record of all published clinical trials, and of those in progress. It will disseminate some of its data via an online journal *Current Clinical Trials*. Within a year of launch of the Cochrane Centre an international Cochrane collaboration evolved with centres in Scandinavia, Canada, and the United States, with further centres planned in Italy and Australia. Reviews are prepared by small groups working in an area of common interest under supervision of an editorial board. All groups will be registered with the Cochrane Centres. Individual diseases, types of treatment, or whole specialities may be covered. The Centres will also help to ensure that the results of each review are widely disseminated so that clinical practice and research can be directed appropriately. It will be interesting to observe whether there is resistance among some neurologists and neurosurgeons to alter practice according to centrally derived directives, as there was amongst obstetricians following systematic reviews prepared by the Pregnancy and Childbirth Group (8).

A new centre has also been created by the NHS R&D Programme in York to commission expert research reviews, and the existing 'Health care effectiveness bulletins' will be taken into this. The York centre will also concentrate on the regular transfer of information to users. This will include not only those involved in making clinical decisions, but also those involved in purchasing contracts. The centre will concentrate on the skills required to ensure that research information moves into practice. Awareness is simply not enough: 'Encouraging NHS staff to play a part in setting agenda, and when appropriate, participating in the conduct of research and development are potent ways of promoting the use of research data' (Professor Michael Peckham, Director of Research and Development in the NHS, 1993). The Medical Research Council also has as one of its objectives, to improve the mechanisms for the dissemination of information about the outcome of MRC-supported clinical research.

DISSEMINATING INFORMATION FROM SYSTEMATIC REVIEWS

Continuing medical education (CME)

The importance of CME was stressed in a *Lancet* editorial in 1993 (20). The Royal College of Physicians issued a booklet in June 1994 (21), which recommended the introduction and implementation of a CME system for consultants and staff or associate grade specialists. The aim of this system is that the problems facing clinicians in acquiring, updating, and disseminating their medical knowledge, and the pressures felt from patients and purchasers in this direction are addressed. The importance of maintaining the highest possible standards of practice and continuing to develop professionally is stressed. A number of activities have been recognized for CME. For *internal CME*, these include grand rounds, clinical and interdisciplinary meetings, specialist meetings and audit, and hospital postgraduate meetings. *External CME* activities include college-based educational events, specialist society or association meetings, international/overseas meetings, national audit meetings, professional development courses, teaching/presentations at approved meetings, examining of postgraduates, etc. All consultants are now issued with a CME diary which is to be completed each year. The recognition of CME will be made by the issue of a certificate at the end of each five-year period following participation in CME by individuals. The Colleges recognize that introduction of CME will require major reorganization and reallocation of resources to enable specialists to take sufficient study leave, to pay for courses, and to fund extra staff to cover their duties when away from their workplace.

Specialist associations, charities, international, national, and local hospital meetings

Specialist associations may also have a valuable role to play in targeting its members with guidelines about management of particular conditions, and 'alerts' of important developments. An example of this is the work of the Association of British Neurologists in relation to the use of beta-interferon and copolymer-1. The outcome of consensus meetings and statements could also be made available to the general neurologist via this route. Individual hospitals and departments might consider adopting 'treatment protocols' for individual clinical problems. Practice guidelines may improve clinical practice when introduced in the context of rigorous evaluations (22,23). Making research-based information available to purchasers and patients (e.g. with videos, leaflets) will be a useful method for increasing awareness and decision-making. Certain charities and associations are already extremely good at increasing patient awareness of new developments in a particular field.

AUDIT OF CHANGE IN CLINICAL PRACTICE

Centrally organized methods aimed at auditing to what extent recent research developments have been incorporated into clinical practice should be established on a national scale. Local intradepartmental audit systems could also improve efficiency. A further step is to measure outcomes routinely once the changes have been implemented, and to have a system whereby these can be fed-back into the system driving the research.

SUMMARY

The problems that face health care today need to be identified. Research must then be directed with the aims of providing solutions to particular problems so that clinical decisions can be based on the best possible information available. This requires a close collaboration between key clinicians with an interest in research, and the various research bodies as well as government health departments. The ability to base clinical practice on reliable research-based information also requires a close communication between industry, where many of the technological advances arise, and the clinical needs. The infrastructure of research training and research facilities needs to be optimized so that the most appropriate individuals for pursuing careers in research are encouraged and given appropriate incentives. The outcomes of research, new technological developments must then be accumulated and summarized in a way that makes them readily incorporated into clinical practice; this may require an active presentation of data to heads of departments and individual clinicians. Treatment protocols and clinical policy guidelines may be considered for individual diseases. Time must be made available to specialists to participate in CME. The needs of purchasers, the increasing demands and pressures of a knowledgeable public must be continuously borne in mind. Finally, the uptake of relevant information into changes in practice needs to be audited to assess how effective the whole process is.

REFERENCES

1. *The Health of the Nation: a strategy for health in England*, HMSO, London (1992). Research for health. Department of Health, 1993. Michael Peckham.
2. MRC (Medical Research Council) *Scientific strategy*. MRC, London (1993).
3. Cochrane AL. *Effectiveness and efficiency. Random reflections on health services*. Nuffield Provincial Hospitals Trust, London (1972).
4. Harris A, Shapiro J. Purchasers, professionals and public health. *BMJ* (1994), **308**, 426–7.
5. Counsell CE, Fraser H, Sandercock PAG. Archie Cochrane's challenge: can periodically updated reviews of all randomised controlled trials relevant to neurology and neurosurgery be produced? *JNNP* (1994), **57**, 529–32.
6. Langhorne P, Williams BO, Gilchrist W, Howie K. Do stroke units save lives? *Lancet* (1993), **342**, 395–8.
7. Schad UB, Lips U, Gnelm HE, Blumberg A, Heinzer I, Wedgwood J. Swiss meningitis study. Dexamethasone therapy for bacterial meningitis in children. *Lancet* (1993), **342**, 457–61.
8. Paterson-Brown S, Wyatt JC, Fisk NM. Are clinicians interested in up to date reviews of effective care. *BMJ* (1993), **307**, 1464.
9. Lindley RI, Amayo EO, Marshall J, Sandercock PA, Dennis M, Warlow CP. Acute stroke treatment in UK hospitals: the stroke association survey of consultant opinion. *J. Roy. Coll. Phys.* (1995), **29**, 479–84.
10. Parkinson Study Group (1989). Effect of deprenyl on the progression of disability in early Parkinson's disease. *N. Engl. J. Med.* (1989), **321**, 1364–71.
11. Parkinson Study Group (1993). Effects of tocopherol and deprenyl on the progression of disability in early Parkinson's disease. *N. Engl. J. Med.* (1993), **328**, 176–83.
12. Lees AJ. Comparison of therapeutic effects and mortality data of L-dopa and L-dopa combined with seregeline in patients with early, mild Parkinson's disease. *BMJ* (1995), **311**, 1583–4.
13. Williams JG. *et al.* Collecting, communicating and using information: the educational issues. *J. Roy. Coll. Physicians* (1992), **26**, 385–7.
14. Harvey RF, Burns-Cox CJ, Heaton KW. The MD thesis in the training of a consultant physician. *J. Roy. Coll. Physicians* (1992) **26**, 380–2.
15. Smith R. Academic medicine: plenty of room at the top. *BMJ* (1993), **306**, 6.
16. Munro AJ. Publishing the findings of clinical research. *BMJ* (1993), **307**, 1340–1.
17. Herxheimer A. Publishing the results of sponsored clinical research. *BMJ* (1993), **307**, 1296–7.
18. Ketley D, Woods KL. Impact of clinical trials on clinical practice: example of thromolysis for acute myocardial infarction. *Lancet* (1993), **342**, 877–8.
19. Herxheimer A. Randomised controlled trials: the Cochrane Collaboration. *J. Roy. Coll. Physicians* (1993), **27**, 180.
20. Editorial. Continuing Medical Education. *Lancet* (1993), **342**, 1497–8.
21. *Continuing medical education for the trained physician*. A report by the Royal Colleges of Physicians of Edinburgh, Glasgow and London, June 1994.
22. Grimshaw JM and Russell IT. Effect of clinical guidelines on medical practice: a systematic review of rigorous evaluations. *Lancet* (1993), **342**, 1317–22.
23. Hayward RSA *et al.* More informative abstracts of articles describing clinical practice guidelines. *Annals of Internal Medicine* (1993), **118**, 731–7.

It is easy to underestimate the value of patients in the learning of clinical neurology. The current emphasis on identification of one session per week for education activity for all medical staff brings to mind tutorials, seminars, talks, and various other forms of classroom activity. In reality, the educational resource from which we learn most is our clinical contact with patients. Patients stimulate all the activities required for accurate diagnosis, challenge our knowledge, test our management skills in sorting out their illness, and measure our powers of communication and explanation to provide satisfaction. Medical education relies heavily on patients, and this is particularly true in a very clinical speciality like neurology.

The use of a matrix (shown in Fig. 30.1), is extremely valuable when considering any aspect of medical education, whether it be the whole undergraduate medical course on the one hand, or an individual session such as an afternoon visit to a neurological rehabilitation unit, on the other. In this chapter, the matrix will be used to cover the different categories of students trying to learn and understand neurology, and in each instance the important place of patients in the learning process will be defined. Most often there will be something to mention in most of the boxes of the matrix for each category of learner. The place occupied by patients in the educational process is highlighted. Areas of weakness or difficulty in providing first class educational experience for each category, within the NHS in the late 20th century, will also be identified.

The categories of learners which will receive attention are as follows:

(1) pre-clinical medical students,
(2) clinical medical students,
(3) SHOs (senior house officers) with MRCP (Member of the Royal College of Physicians) examination in mind
(4) trainee neurologists and specialist registrars,
(5) established neurological consultants,
(6) other hospital specialists and general practitioners.

PRE-CLINICAL STUDENTS (FIG. 30.2)

Although moves are afoot to improve the integration of the pre-clinical and clinical parts of the medical student's curriculum, progress is slow. Even when achieved there will be a need to think of ways to expose, with benefit, large groups of students early in their course to patients with common neurological disorders.

Exposure of young medical students, while they are learning anatomy, physiology, biochemistry, pharmacology, pathology, to patients who have been specially selected to illustrate the clinical relevance of anatomical, physiological, biochemical, pharmacological, or pathological knowledge, is extremely encouraging and motivating. The most commonly used format for this is the clinical demonstration of a patient, his/her investigations and treatment, to a large number of students in a large lecture theatre. Very careful explanation to the patient is essential. He or she needs to be given space, status, and opportunity to speak during such a session. The teaching neurologist should be experienced, able to present the case so that it is entirely comprehensible to clinically naïve intelligent minds, and able to create an atmosphere of informality on such a large stage which enable the students to ask questions freely of the patient and teacher. It is unlikely that most young neurologists-in-training can carry this off. It is a job for the established neurological clinician.

There is no real difficulty in providing such sessions since they are infrequent and very economical in terms of the number of teachers and patients for the number of students to be educated. There may be logistical problems in taking partially disabled patients to the preclinical students' large lecture theatre, and in demonstrating physical signs which are small (e.g. nystagmus, an extensor plantar response), to a very large group of students, but usually these can be overcome using modern technology.

The demonstration of exemplary neurological patients on videotape to pre-clinical students, by staff from the pre-clinical disciplines, has its attractions. In some instances, it may spare embarrassment of the patient. The interactive vitality provided by the presence of the patient in person is lost however, the sense of complete reality is missing, as is the clinical input from a practising neurologist.

CLINICAL STUDENTS (FIG. 30.3)

The main item students want to learn from neurologists, and which neurologists want to impart to clinical students, is the ability to perform a competent neurological examination.

	Factual knowledge	Clinical and other skills	Attitudes
Aims			
Learning methods			
Assessment			

Fig. 30.1 The matrix (see text).

The skills of history taking and of formulation of a diagnosis, and familiarity with the common neurological disorders and emergencies, are also very important, but the ability to do a reliable neurological examination ranks highest. It is a tool which will last.

The learning of any practical skill (e.g. to drive a car, to examine the nervous system), requires teacher, learner, and hands-on experience with the instrument or person on which the skill is to be mastered. No substitute to this apprenticeship model (requiring neurologist, student, and patient with a neurological disorder) works better for students in their acquisition of skill in neurological examination. Videotaped demonstration of neurological examination should be used as a supplementary resource, rather than a replacement for supervised hands-on experience.

Figure 30.3 highlights the importance of patients in the learning of clinical neurology by clinical students. The student needs to learn about the common neurological disorders and emergencies, and the best stimulus to learn about these is first-hand contact with patients suffering from them. Their clinical skills are best learnt by rehearsal and practice on inpatients and outpatients, with supervision and demonstration by experienced neurologists. Correct attitudes will be acquired by exposure to able staff performing well in the clinical setting. Patients with neurological disorders are important in the assessment of students' knowledge and clinical skills after a period of neurological instruction.

Currently, in the United Kingdom, there are many problems in providing such neurological learning experience for clinical students. In some London schools there is an inadequate number of patients to exemplify the common neurological disorders and emergencies. Throughout the United Kingdom there is a reduction in the duration of neurological ward admissions (for good reasons), so there are greater problems in exposing clinical students to neurological inpatients. In the outpatient clinic, the number of patients to

	Factual knowledge	Clinical and other skills	Attitudes
Aims	To integrate the student's knowledge of the individual pre-clinical disciplines: neuroanatomy neurophysiology neuropharmacology neuropathology To emphasize the relevance of the above to the management of patients with neurological disorders	To provide early experience of 'the clinical method', used by clinicians	To motivate the student's learning of the pre-clinical disciplines
Learning methods	Demonstration of carefully selected neurological patients to groups of pre-clinical students at the relevant moment in their pre-clinical course		
Assessment	Student and clinical neurologist can assess the value of the pre-clinical courses, from the point of view of clinical relevance		

Fig. 30.2 Pre-clinical students (shaded area indicates direct involvement of patients in the learning process).

be seen by one neurologist, and the size of the room in which he/she sees them, limit student exposure to neurological outpatients. There is a greater tendency to appoint neurologists to district general hospitals with a toehold in the local regional neurological centre/teaching hospital. This means that neurological instruction of clinical students, to some extent, needs to be relocated in the district general hospitals, where patients with common disorders are seen by neurologists who are interested in patients with common neurological disorders. There are good reasons for keeping some neurologists interested in common neurological disorders at the teaching centres. Teacher time to watch students performing neurological examinations, and to hear their diagnostic formulations, is short. Students may easily find their neurological instructors under considerable strain and pressure in outpatient clinics, threatening their role-model function for engendering ideal attitudes towards patients and colleagues. Time may be inadequate for assessment of students by neurologists

at the end of a period of clinical attachment to the neurology department, and for comprehensive feedback of student comment about the neurology teaching programme.

For all these reasons, in the financial atmosphere surrounding health care provision current in the United Kingdom and likely to remain, the needs of students must be emphasized loudly and constantly by neurologists with responsibility for clinical student teaching, particularly the proper provision of neurological consultant time and accommodation in the outpatient clinic.

SENIOR HOUSE OFFICERS WORKING FOR THE MRCP EXAMINATION (FIG. 30.4)

Some SHOs will do an attachment in neurology for three to six months as part of a rotation, a few will do a six-month neurology post in its own right, and some will not hold a

	Factual knowledge	Clinical and other skills	Attitudes
Aims	To enable the student to learn about the common neurological disorders and the common neurological emergencies	To reinforce the importance of accurate history taking To learn how to perform a neurological examination To develop the student's ability to make an appropriate differential diagnosis and management plan	To demonstrate the importance of developing a good relationship with patients and colleagues To encourage self-criticism and audit To promote a lifelong self-learning habit
Learning methods	Centred on patients, not diseases Centred on individual students as much as possible Small groups, not large lectures Text-books 'On-call' experience, if possible	Practice on inpatients and outpatients Student's performance is watched and checked Students observation of experienced neurologists at work	Example of neurologists, at work Teachers actively promote self-learning
Assessment	Of students MCQ with subsequent explanation of the correct answers	'Short case' assessment by clinical neurologists	Open applause, but private confidential criticism
	Of teaching Comprehensive uninhibited commentary by the students		

Fig. 30.3 Clinical students (shaded areas indicate direct involvement of patients in the learning process).

specifically neurological post at all. For all SHOs, however, their experience of common neurological conditions and emergencies is likely to be predominantly inpatient-based rather than outpatient-based. From the point of view of passing the MRCP examination, this bias towards inpatients is acceptable, since the clinical part of the MRCP examination relies considerably on patients with neurological conditions who are often seen in the wards. SHOs do not obtain a very full look at neurology (most of which is handled in the outpatient clinic), but this is not crucial from the point of view of the specific objective of passing the MRCP examination.

Whether they are in a neurological SHO post or not, the SHOs' neurological clinical skills will be rehearsed by presentation of inpatients they have seen, either in formal clerking of inpatients, in their involvement in the management of neurological emergencies admitted under the care of their consultant, on specific MRCP small group teaching ward rounds, or occasionally in presentation of a patient at departmental or hospital meetings. All of this patient-based learning must be complemented by learning in seminars and from textbooks, and this must be actively encouraged and promoted by senior neurological staff. Development of good attitudes will depend on the example and private comments of consultant staff.

The introduction of individual training programmes for SHOs is undoubtedly helpful in giving greater prominence to the educational needs of SHOs. Concurrent with this development, however, is an underestimation of what factual knowledge and clinical skills SHOs can learn from their clinical activity with neurological patients, and an overestimation of what they might learn from classroom sessions during a formal, hospital, educational half-day. For the time being, preparation for success in the MRCP examination is still going to depend on the availability of neurological inpatients, and of senior and middle-grade neurological staff to guide and correct SHOs rehearsing their knowledge and skills in relation to these patients.

	Factual knowledge	Clinical and other skills	Attitudes
Aims	To become very familiar with the common neurological conditions and emergencies To become familiar with the rare classical neurological disorders, over-represented in the MRCP examination To pass the MRCP examination	To rehearse history taking and neurological examination to a high level of competence To make sensible, safe differential diagnoses and management plans To become able explainers and communications To pass the MRCP examination	To have good relationships with patients and colleagues, with a developing sense of responsibility towards both To be self-critical and open to audit To be an able self-learner
Learning methods	Predominantly inpatient-centred On-call experience for neurological emergencies Small groups Text books	Presentation of inpatients on consultant ward rounds on specific MRCP teaching ward rounds at department or hospital meetings Observation of experienced neurologists at work	Example of consultants and specialist registrars at work Active stimulation of self-learning
Assessment	MRCP examination Consultant commentary and reference	MRCP examination Consultant commentary and reference	Open applause and confidential criticism by consultant Consultant reference

Fig. 30.4 Senior house officers working for the MRCP examination (shaded areas indicate direct involvement of patients in the learning process).

TRAINEE NEUROLOGISTS AND SPECIALIST REGISTRARS (FIG. 30.5)

Figure 30.5 shows that the knowledge, skills, and attitudes to be learnt by neurological trainees is becoming more defined, and different from the groups considered hitherto. Factual knowledge is required about all common, rare, and emergency neurological conditions to a high level of sophistication. Familiarity with knowledge in the associated neurological disciplines is necessary, and the need to keep all this knowledge up to date becomes paramount. In addition, skills other than those directly relating to patient management need to be developed, in NHS business/management, in teaching, and research. An increasing sense of responsibility and awareness of being a member of a team become important attitudinal aspects of training.

Supervised care with progressive assumption of responsibility, for outpatients, routine and emergency inpatients, supported by active learning from textbooks, journals and meetings, is the optimal method of learning. In practice, trainees may not be given enough time to present their thoughts to senior staff on diagnosis and plans for management with regard to inpatients. Trainees might feel their efforts to be redundant, unless specifically sought by consultants. With regard to neurological outpatients, the monitoring of trainees' diagnostic and management skills is probably poorly supervised, and there may be too much responsibility given to trainees in the care of outpatients too soon. Although the exposure of trainees to patients is excellent in the United Kingdom compared with many European countries, the degree of supervision probably leaves a lot to be desired. Within the United Kingdom the Patients' Charter may enable patients to demand to be seen by consultant staff rather than trainees before long. A greater degree of supervision of trainees in the outpatient clinic seems inevitable, and more attention will have to be given to this as neurology becomes more and more an outpatient speciality.

	Factual knowledge	Clinical and other skills	Attitudes

Aims	To become extremely well-informed about all common, rare and emergency neurological conditions
	To have a good working knowledge of the associated disciplines: N-surgery, N-physiology, N-pathology, N-radiology, N-rehabilitation, N-genetics, N-psychology, paediatric Neurology etc
	To have a working knowledge of NHS business/management
		To become extremely able in diagnosis, management, explanation and communication, in relation to patients with all neurological disorders
		To be able in teaching
		        research
		        N.H.S management
			To be aware of the importance of good relationships, and of being a team member
			To be self-critical, and active in the practice of audit
			To become fully responsible for the neurological service provided
			To remain a lifelong self-learner

Learning methods	Supervised care of routine and emergency inpatients, and of out patients, with increasing delegation of responsibility by consultants. Trainee's thoughts to be actively sought by consultants.		Example of consultant neurologists at work
	Active learning from text books, journals and meetings Rotation around the associated neuro-disciplines Attendance at departmental and hospital management meetings	Attendance at medical teaching courses is rare Research training goes well N.H.S. management training is in its infancy	Encouragement of self-criticism and and it by consultant neurologists Consultant commentary, open applause, private criticism
Assessment	No exit examination of trainee neurologists in the UK (yet) Informal and formal two-way discussions between consultants and trainees Consultant references Length of time in post R.C.P. inspection of training departments and accreditation of trainees		

Fig. 30.5 Trainee neurologists and specialist registrars (shaded areas indicate direct involvement of patients in the learning process).

Within the United Kingdom, of the other non-clinical skills to be developed in trainees, there is no doubt that research skills do best. Most trainees in neurology spend a significant period of time in research and most obtain higher degrees indicating success in this. Attendance at research-orientated meetings is commonplace. The skills of teaching neurology and of managing a neurological department do not fare so well in training programmes. Most trainees teach but receive no instruction in how to teach. It is not yet customary to involve trainees in management meetings, or for them to attend management courses.

Currently, formal assessment of neurological trainees at the end of their period of training is not yet very robust. Informal and formal discussion between consultant and trainee occur.

Individual training posts are inspected by the RCP (Royal College of Physicians) at regular intervals. Perhaps the greatest indicators of the performance of an individual neurological unit in training neurologists is the quality of applicants to work in that unit, and their subsequent success in being appointed to senior posts.

ESTABLISHED NEUROLOGICAL CONSULTANTS (FIG. 30.6)

Here, the main objectives are to maintain competence and excellence in the different areas of endeavour and to remain enthusiastic and well informed. Some personal professional development, in post, is vital.

	Factual knowledge	Clinical and other skills	Attitudes
Aims	To remain up-to-date in knowledge of all neurological disorders. To have a working knowledge of developments in the associated neurological disciplines. To remain informed in changes in N.H.S. management and health care delivery	To remain able in the care of patients with neurological disorders, taking pains to prevent any decline in standards. To develop in teaching, research, management, or some other special professional interest	To retain enthusiasm. To be Hippocratic in terms of the next generation of doctors and neurologists. To remain self-critical and open to audit. To engage in lifelong self-learning
Learning methods	No neurologists in isolation. Joint ward rounds. Weekly attendance and involvement in the local neuroscience centre. Attend neurological and general medical educational meetings. Retain time in the week for reading in the library. Interact with managers	Joint meetings and ward rounds with other neurologists. Give and take second opinions in difficult cases. Audit. Seek feedback on quality of clinical performance, and of non-clinical activities (e.g. teaching and training)	
Assessment	There is a case for certification and re-certification. The rate of case referral to an individual neurologist is some measure of his clinical performance. The quality and number of recruits to junior posts is some measure of the neurologists' clinical performance and care over training. Maintenance of a strong place in the undergraduates teaching programme is some measure of the quality of neurological teaching offered. Survival of the neurological unit and service, or its development and expansion, is some index of the management ability within the unit.		

Fig. 30.6 Established neurological consultants (shaded areas indicate direct involvement of patients in the learning process).

No neurologist should work in isolation any longer, since this must make regular audit of a neurologist's knowledge and clinical performance very difficult. Each neurologist should spend a minimum of one day a week in the local neuroscience centre and become thoroughly involved in the educational activity occurring there. Regular attendance at local neurological departmental meetings, hospital general medical meetings, and national symposia, are important ways of remaining up to date in terms of knowledge, apart from ready access to neurological journals.

Keeping the clinical performance of an individual neurologist and his/her team up to the mark in terms of diagnostic accuracy, treatment efficiency, communication to patients, general practitioners, and other referring doctors, is the essence of informal or formal clinical audit. Informal audit is well achieved by joint ward rounds with other consultants and at meetings within a neuroscience centre. The giving and taking of 'second opinions' on difficult cases is another way of measuring overall clinical performance.

Since there is no certification of clinical neurologists in the United Kingdom there is no question yet of re-certification. One cannot avoid the argument that the aim of re-certification to maintain clinical competence is a good one. Maintaining competence in non-clinical areas, teaching of students and supervision of trainees, research, and management capability, is not at all formalized. Developing a system for open feedback from students and trainees, and listening to the criticisms of the teaching and training programmes offered by the medical school and the Royal College of Physicians, must help.

To a certain extent neurologists should worry about their competence if case referral to their service is low, and recruitment to their trainee posts is poor, and if they become aware of pressure from the medical school to marginalize their contribution to the clinical students' programme. The chief threat to neurologists being able to ensure their competence, and their ability to remain up to date, is time. This threat is increased rather than decreased by the new market system of UK health care. Neurologists must do all they can to ensure that their job plans contain sufficient time for education and audit activity, and for the non-clinical tasks which have to be accomplished.

OTHER HOSPITAL SPECIALISTS AND GENERAL PRACTITIONERS

The aim here is to enable general practitioners and other hospital specialists to look after patients with the common neurological disorders, either entirely, or after initial diagnosis and management suggestions by the neurologist. Furthermore, the criteria for the appropriate referral of neurological patients and emergencies to neurologists must be established and updated. The main instruments of learning are the interactions between hospital specialists and general practitioners with neurologists in letters, in phone calls, and in consultation notes with respect to ward referrals. The regular attendance at meetings where neurological patients or topics are being presented to other hospital specialists or general practitioners is important, whether they be in the local hospital, at special symposia, or in residential general practitioner refresher courses.

Two problems exist which tend to perpetuate ineffectiveness of non-neurologists in taking care of neurological problems. First, it is easy for neurologists to write congratulatory letters to colleagues but very difficult, at a personal level, and in medicolegal terms, to write critical letters or notes. Second, meetings tend to be attended by the excellent, well-motivated hospital specialists and general practitioners and not by less able, less enthusiastic colleagues in these disciplines . . . ignorance is bliss!

Many episodes of acute and long-term illness involve more than one member of the caring professions but structured, multidisciplinary approaches to the care of people with long-term neurological conditions have been the exception rather than the rule. This chapter focuses on the experience of the Neuro-care Team which has been active in Romford, Essex, England since late 1985 and thus has many years' experience of a team approach to neurological disease.

The Romford Neuro-care Team's objective is to provide a co-ordinated, flexible, high quality service to a group of people who face the prospect of increasing disability from illnesses for which there is presently no cure and which have no clear pattern of progression.

THE MEDICAL CONDITIONS INCLUDED

When the project began in 1985, it was confined to people with Parkinson's disease and entirely funded by the Parkinson's Disease Society. That was, however, a pilot project and the extension of its principles and approach to other neurological conditions was intended from the beginning. That extension (funded jointly by the health authority and the relevant voluntary organizations) was achieved in April 1990 and, from that date to the present, the service has been offered to newly diagnosed people with motor neurone disease, multiple sclerosis, dystonia, and ataxia, as well as those with Parkinson's disease. Responsibility for providing and managing the service passed to the BHB Community Health Care Trust in April 1993. Table 31.1 shows the total number of

Table 31.1 All patients ever in the Neuro-care project and status at 31 December 1996

	Current (31/12/96)	Dead	Moved away/ withdrawn	Total
PD	195	33	11	239
MS	83	0	0	83
MND	11	31	5	47
DYS	33	0	0	33
ATAX	5	0	2	7
Total	327	64	18	409

PD, Parkinson's disease; MS, multiple sclerosis; MND, motor neurone disease; DYS, dystomia; ATAX, ataxia.

patients in the project from its beginning in December 1985 to 31 December 1996.

It is clear therefore that this team approach is limited to the main progressive motor disorders. The services of the team were offered to every newly diagnosed person with one of these conditions in Dr Leslie Findley's clinics and wards in Oldchurch and Harold Wood Hospitals in Essex. The only grounds for exclusion were severe mental illness or confusion.

CHARACTERISTICS OF THE TEAM

A TEAM FOR OUTPATIENTS

Most health professionals have experienced teams within the hospital setting where both the patients and team members are on the same site and communication is relatively easy. However, people with progressive neurological conditions do not spend most of their time in hospital and, significantly, the group with which we started—those with Parkinson's disease—are usually diagnosed and treated as outpatients. Because of this and because of the high hopes for L-dopa treatment which had been current in the 1970s, very few people with Parkinson's disease had had access to anyone other than the neurologist and the general practitioner (Oxtoby 1982).

Even after six years involvement with other conditions, the Neuro-care Team was still a mainly outpatient service. Only 10% (53/513) of the co-ordinator/counsellor's 1992/3 contacts were in the ward and, although no comparable figures have been collected since, there is no reason to think that the position in 1996 was radically different.

A TEAM TO BRIDGE THE HOSPITAL/COMMUNITY DIVIDE

People with progressive neurological conditions need access to specialized diagnosis and treatment at the beginning of their illness and from time to time thereafter. They also need to be encouraged to carry on with normal life in their families and communities rather than to see themselves primarily as patients. The idea therefore was to have a team which would be able to provide the necessary bridge between the two health systems without being limited to either. Being a special project rather than part of the statutory services made this early attempt at 'seamless care' more feasible. The challenge now is to see if a service located within a community health care trust can continue to deliver this seamless care.

A TEAM FOR EVERYONE WITH A RELEVANT DIAGNOSIS

The incentive for the original project came from the survey on the needs of people with Parkinson's disease (Oxtoby 1982) and from members of the Parkinson's Disease Society who talked about the sort of service they needed and the ways in which their experience of medical care had fallen short of their hopes and needs. Most of their experiences were replicated in accounts of patients with other progressive conditions. Some of these needs were concentrated around the time of diagnosis and related to the way in which the diagnosis was given. Lack of access to information, to counselling, and to advice on other sources of help also caused concern. We did not think that access to such help should be limited to people who contacted the relevant voluntary organization or to those perceived by the doctor as being 'in need', but should be available to all patients diagnosed as having a progressive and incurable condition as a standard component of the diagnostic procedure. As a couple facing motor neurone disease recalled, 'We gave the impression we were handling it but, deep down we were devastated. We definitely needed to speak to someone professionally to reassure us or whatever'.

A CO-ORDINATED TEAM

Teams for inpatients are often heavily dependent on the willingness and ability of the consultant to co-ordinate the activities of the various personnel. We realized that our mainly outpatient team, facing much greater barriers to effective communication, would not succeed unless this task was clearly defined and allocated to one person. From 1985 to 1993 we chose to combine the role of co-ordinator with that of social worker or counsellor and this proved to be a very satisfactory solution. It worked because the co-ordinator/counsellor was present in clinic when the diagnosis was given and when patients returned for their follow-up appointments. She was therefore available when required and there were no logistical problems in sending for her or in asking patients to find her afterwards. Nor was there any suggestion that access to her services implied a failure to cope. She was able to copy the basic record sheet containing clinical and social information to other members of the team so that everyone got identical information and had no need to repeat the same questions. It worked because the counsellor was not seen as a competitor or threat by other team members and because her dual role gave patients a choice about how to use her. Especially at the post-diagnosis interview, she could be used as a counsellor by those who wished to share their feelings of sadness, relief or anger, or as a co-ordinator by those who were only able, at this stage, to cope with practical matters like how

the team operates and when visits will be made. Since 1993, the co-ordination role has been combined with one of nurse specialist and this has allowed these important advantages to be retained.

A TEAM WITH THERAPISTS AND DIETITIAN

As the honeymoon with L-dopa came to an end, both patients and doctors were coping with the realities of its reduced effectiveness and increased side-effects in the longer term. Patients and relatives were asking for access to therapists and dietitians but finding these difficult to obtain. When referrals were made, the therapists often felt that they were too late in the disease process for much to be achieved. Interest in earlier referral to therapists thus came from several quarters and its implementation was a key feature of the Parkinson's Disease Pilot Project. Patients with other conditions are not routinely referred for therapy assessments but are referred selectively as soon as a need is identified. Such constructive intervention can be a visible proof of 'something being done', despite the fact that several of these conditions have no specific treatment.

Emphasis on the need for a dietitian came from people with Parkinson's disease and also from the Parkinson's Disease Society which received many enquiries about foods, diets, and supplements. There was a growing awareness among health professionals of how widespread and distressing was the problem of constipation and so there was a greater interest in encouraging patients to increase their intake of fluids and high fibre foods. The dietitian also has an important contribution to make in multiple sclerosis and in advanced stages of motor neurone disease.

A TEAM WITH NURSING INPUT

Before 1993 we were often asked why the core team did not include a nurse. The answer was that one was not required in the early days when the team was working almost exclusively with new Parkinson's disease outpatients. The sister and staff in the outpatients' clinic were very supportive and provided any nursing expertise which was required. This pattern of building close relationships with existing nursing staff continued throughout the extended project with nursing staff in the neurology wards and in the hospice becoming important partners in the Neuro-care enterprise. At one stage, a bid was made for a specialist neurology nurse with a dual neuro-care *cum* educational role but funds were not available. It was felt that such a person would make a very valuable contribution to the team especially as the contacts with severely disabled patients increased. He or she would provide a resource for nurses caring for neurological patients in the community and in medical and surgical wards where understanding of the needs of neurological patients is often limited. As already indicated, a new way of meeting this need was found in 1993 when the post of Co-ordinator/Counsellor became vacant and was filled by a nurse specialist. The post of Nurse/Co-ordinator has proved very beneficial in improving liaison with medical and other nursing staff. The Team works closely with local social service departments when additional social work involvement is required.

A LESS HIERARCHICAL TEAM

It was agreed from the beginning that the Neuro-care Team would be more flexible than many inpatient teams in that, once a patient had been identified as falling within its remit, anyone could propose new initiatives (although new drug regimes are decided only by medical staff) or make referrals to other team members. This arrangement saves time because everything does not have to go back to the consultant and it provides added interest and responsibility for the other team members. Consultations between team members take place at the regular team meetings and through informal direct contacts.

A TEAM INVOLVING THE PATIENT AND FAMILY

Giving a voice in their own care to people with neurological conditions was an important objective from the beginning as was the involvement of close relatives. It was recognized that most motor disorders result in people feeling a loss of control over their own bodies and that the job of the helping professions should be to offset this sense of loss of control rather than, as sometimes happens, to compound it. Provision of information, courteous and caring attitudes, and involvement in decision-making are all part of the Team's approach to ensuring that the patient's voice is heard. Unless patients choose otherwise, a member of the family or a friend is invited to be present during outpatient consultations and when the diagnosis is given in hospital to those admitted for diagnostic tests. Opportunities are also available for both patients and relatives to see team members separately if they so wish.

A TEAM WHICH RECOGNIZES THE ROLE OF THE GENERAL PRACTITIONER

It was no part of the Neuro-care Team's aims to undermine or detract from the general practitioner's (GP) role in patient care and considerable attention was paid to ways of keeping the GP informed and involved. A letter explaining the Neuro-care Team approach goes to the GP with the first report from the consultant and the GP is encouraged to contact the team with queries or concerns. Patients are told during the diagnostic consultation that their GP will be kept informed and that they might want to discuss the diagnosis and its implications with him/her. Later, when one member of the team is identified as the 'key worker' for a particular patient, he/she makes a personal contact with the GP of any patient who is seriously ill or disabled.

TEAM ACTIVITY

The first objective of the team is to give the diagnosis in a patient-oriented, honest, and caring way. In order to learn how to do this, many discussions were held with the consultant neurologist, relevant voluntary organizations, and individual patients. The result was a series of scripts for giving the diagnosis and aides-mémoires for easy reference in clinic or ward. Given that these patients are likely to require medical supervision for the rest of their lives, great importance is attached to the character of this first contact. Apart from ensuring that the setting is appropriate (not a ward round) and that there are a minimum of interruptions, there are three basic rules:

1. Find out what the patient and relative are expecting.
2. Having named the condition, find out what the patient and relative(s) know about the condition before providing further information.
3. Offer time for questions immediately, but also offer a further opportunity at the next appointment when the patient has had time to think things over and to formulate ideas.

Strategies of care for each of the neurological conditions were also devised and Table 31.2 sets out the original programme for patients with Parkinson's disease.

The team has tried to meet the needs of its clients, or to refer them on to other specialist workers (e.g. phychologists, local social workers, or continence advisers, if this seemed appropriate). Thus Tables 31.3 and 31.4, which are extracted from the audit of team activity for 1992/3,[1] are an indication, not just of the level of activity, but of the scale of need. During 1992–3 the team had a full-time co-ordinator/counsellor and quarter-time posts in physiotherapy, occupational therapy, and speech and language therapy. Contacts with the dietitian have not been included because only minimal cover was available.

Tables 31.3 and 31.4 highlight the variation between conditions in the intensity of demand. The much shorter timescale in motor neurone disease means that the demands for care at all stages of the disease can be more easily charted and a more detailed account of the team's approach to this group of patients can be found in Oxtoby and Eikaas (1993). By the end of the year, team resources were stretched to their limits and discussions were underway about future arrangements.

ADVANTAGES OF THE TEAM APPROACH

ACCEPTABILITY

All the evidence suggests that this way of working is very acceptable to clients. Table 31.1 indicates that of 409 patients ever identified as within the team's remit, 327 (80%) were still

---

[1] No later figures are available because statistics have been collected in a different way by the community healthcare trust.

Table 31.2 Original programme[a] of contacts with team members: Parkinson's disease patients

	Initial assessment[b]	Feedback[c]	Continuation
Outpatient clinic[d]	Examination Diagnosis Discussion Information	Questions Discussion Info. re. medication	Medication at optimum, Discussion Info. re. future team contacts[e]
Co-ordinator/ counsellor's room	Time for reaction/ clarification Family situation charted Info. re. team and 1st therapy assessments Voluntary organization named	Listening, discussion More info. re. voluntary organization	Explanation of second assessments —role of key worker

[a] Since 1993, the programme has had to be trimmed. Home visits are now only made to people unable to attend a special therapy assessment clinic.

[b] The interval between assessment and feedback is usually 3–4 weeks, and during this time the patient is visited at home by the physiotherapist and occupational and speech therapists who offer advice on self-help and complete a professional assessment which is fed back though the co-ordinator/counsellor to the whole Team. A dietary diary is also completed and returned to the dietitian for comment.

[c] The interval between feedback and continuation is longer and more variable (between 3 and 9 months). There are further OP visits and contacts with team members as indicated by clinical developments and individual needs.

[d] The co-ordinator/counsellor is present in the consulting room when the diagnosis and ensuing explanation is given. Patients are always encouraged to bring a relative or friend along with them so that they are supported during and after the 'telling'.

[e] Once optimum is reached and a key worker has been appointed, the objective is to reduce outpatient visits to one per year so that patients are encouraged to continue with normal life and the pressure on clinics is reduced.

in contact at the end of 1996; 64 (16%) had died and of the other 18 (4%) no longer in touch, most had moved away or, exceptionally, had the diagnosis changed at a later date. Only one or two had voluntarily withdrawn from contact with the Team.

Table 31.3 Number of face-to-face contacts by medical condition and team member (1 April 1992–31 March 1993)

	PD (n = 106)	MND (n = 18)	MS (n = 25)	DYS (n = 6)	ATAX (n = 3)	Total (n = 152)
Incl. deaths	1	5	0	0	0	6
C/C	279	99	114	13	8	513
OT	53	49	20	2	4	128
SLT	50	86	13	0	0	149
PT	70	37	21	2	0	130
Totals 1992/3	452	271	168	17	12	920
Average per patient	4.3	15.1	6.7	2.8	4.0	6.1

C/C, co-ordinator/counsellor; OT, occupational therapist; SLT, speech and language therapist; PT, physiotherapist.

THE DELIVERY OF SUPPORT AND INFORMATION

People with these incurable conditions are supported through the weeks and months around diagnosis, their emotional, social, and practical problems are acknowledged and they get to know the people to whom they can turn for help. We hope that, by being informed about these sources of help, patients and families will press for and obtain the services they require and avoid the feelings of helplessness which can accompany chronic illness.

EDUCATION IN SELF-HELP

Feelings of being 'in control' are also encouraged by patients having the opportunity to learn from the therapists and the dietitian about things which they can do to help themselves. A man with Parkinson's disease who first encountered speech therapy during an intensive therapy course some years after being diagnosed wrote;

The last two weeks have proved to me that I can still speak intelligently. We have the rules, formula, and exercises. It is up to us but should it be? What a lot of heartache would be saved by referral at diagnosis being made mandatory (Parkinson's Disease Society 1991).

CONTINUITY OF CARE

The team approach and especially the role of the co-ordinator/counsellor or nurse/co-ordinator provides continuity of contact—a commodity in short supply for many people receiving health care in either hospital or community. The symptoms experienced by people with long-term neurological conditions are often difficult to describe and there are special advantages in meeting the same person in the ward, the clinic and, when necessary, at home.

IMPROVED TELLING OF THE DIAGNOSIS

It is interesting that relatively little attention has been paid until recently to how to minimize the distress caused by unwelcome news. No one questions that it is important to minimize the physical pain inseparable from treatments like injections even though such physical pain is often of shorter duration than the psychological pain caused by news of an incurable illness. Of course, there are no easy answers and this team does not claim to have the solution but only to have listened to patients and to be trying to do things better. There was some encouragement (although the finding is not statistically significant) from an independent interviewer study of the Parkinson's Disease Pilot Group and a group of newly diagnosed patients in another hospital (Oxtoby and Findley 1990)—77% of the pilot group were satisfied with the way the diagnosis was given compared with 63% of the comparison group, even though a quarter of the latter group had been given the diagnosis in the more favourable setting of a private consultation or domiciliary visit.

Table 31.4 Numbers and percentages of patients requiring high level input* by medical condition and team member (*n* = 160) (1 January 1992–31 March 1993)

	PD1		PD2		PD3		MND		MS		DYS		ATAX	
	n	%	*n*	%	*n*	%	*n*	%	*n*	%	*n*	%	*n*	%
C/C	10	32	14	29	5	18	12	63	15	60	0	0	2	66
OT	8	26	1	2	2	7	9	47	6	24	1	17	2	66
SLT	6	19	10	21	1	4	12	63	1	4	0	0	0	0
PT	7	23	9	19	3	11	11	58	10	40	1	17	0	0
n =	31		48		28		19		25		6		3	

* All patients requiring home visits apart from those which are an integral part of the early PD assessments or the key worker role. Considerable additional liaison/referral work even without home visits. Delivery of/referral for therapy services.
PD1, Parkinson's disease pilot patients diagnosed before 1988; PD2, PD patients diagnosed 1988–91; PD3, PD patients diagnosed January 1992–31 March 1993.

IMPROVED MANAGEMENT OF MOTOR NEURONE DISEASE

There is widespread recognition of the rapidly changing requirements of this group of patients and of the need to ensure speedy access to the necessary aids, adaptations, and services. There is less recognition of the very difficult and sensitive task of matching the ordering and provision of an appliance or service to the patient's or family's ability to accept and use it. Anyone with any lingering doubts on this score should read Rosalind Pegg's (1992) moving and thought-provoking account of caring for her husband. Although the team approach offers no easy solutions to this problem, it does ensure that the patient and family become well known to the team and that the chances of timing interventions appropriately are increased.

The local hospice was able to offer its highly skilled respite care to people with motor neurone disease and the team's detailed knowledge of the patients allowed very effective communication with hospice staff and facilitated both admission and discharge arrangements.

IMPROVED CONTACTS WITH THE RELEVANT VOLUNTARY SOCIETIES

A huge amount of information and long-term support is provided by the voluntary societies to those people who choose to join them. Whether and when to join is, of course, a personal decision and it was one of the Team's principles that no pressure for or against joining should be applied. People cannot, however, decide on this issue unless they know what exists and the relevant information was given to all newly diagnosed patients. The comparative study referred to above did show statistically significant differences between the two groups in knowledge of the existence of the Parkinson's Disease Society. Close co-operation between team members and the voluntary societies also facilitated additional practical and financial help for several patients.

DEVELOPMENT OF PROFESSIONAL EXPERTISE

As the medical conditions covered are relatively or absolutely rare[2], and variable in their signs and symptoms, it is difficult for GPs, nurses, and therapists to build up specialist knowledge and expertise. The team approach allows for the development of such expertise and, while concentrating on their own clientele, the team members have also become a resource for other health professionals in both hospital and community. Such a multicondition team also allows a high standard of care to people with a very variable condition like dystonia (approximately 70 per 250 000 population) and very rare conditions like the ataxias (approximately 5 per 250 000) where it is especially difficult to develop expertise.

IMPROVED JOB SATISFACTION AND MUTUAL SUPPORT FOR TEAM MEMBERS

Throughout the project, team members have expressed increased job satisfaction from working as part of a structured and co-ordinated team. This showed in the reports contributed by each Team member to the end of project report (Oxtoby *et al.* 1988) and has been a recurrent feature of internal discussions and reports. Working with people who have incurable, progressive conditions can be very stressful. The team approach means that members derive support from each other and so are more able to cope with the inevitable distress while continuing to meet the patients' and families' needs.

EFFICIENT USE OF SCARCE RESOURCES THROUGH THE KEY WORKER SYSTEM

The objective of this system is to help patients to maintain a link with the team while living as normal a life as possible in

[2] Prevalence per 250 000 of the population of: Parkinson' disease (500); multiple sclerosis (200); motor neurone disease (15) RCP 1986).

the community. Because the key worker is allocated after the early intensive work around the time of diagnosis, the team's knowledge of the patient's needs and coping strategies and of the wider family situation allows an individualized programme to be devised. The programme can range from frequent *ad-hoc* contacts with motor neurone disease patients through a contact before the annual outpatient appointments for people with well-controlled Parkinson's disease to an annual phone call (or no contact if that is the patient's clearly expressed choice), to patients with multiple sclerosis believed to be in remission. Information derived from an audit of team (co-ordinator/counsellor and therapists) activity in the 15 months up to April 1993 supported the team's claim to provide a comprehensive but time-efficient pattern of support. Only two of the 160 patients potentially in contact with the team over this period had no record of contact. One was a patient with multiple sclerosis and the other a patient with advanced Parkinson's disease who was admitted to a residential home and then died. Of the others, 64 (40%) had contact with just one team member, 43 (27%) with two, 31 (19%), with three, and only 20 (12.5%) with all four.

DISADVANTAGES OF THE TEAM APPROACH

COST

Providing this kind of co-ordinated team approach does, of course, cost money. It is easy to measure the staff and administrative costs (approximately £45 000 in 1992/3 when research expenditure was excluded), and difficult to measure the likely savings because they are spread over time and among several 'pockets'. These savings could arise from fewer outpatient consultations and ambulance journeys, from reductions in falls and accidents, and in reactive illness of both patients and carers, and from delayed requirements for long-term care. Very few of the team's clients have so far required long-term care and, even among those with motor neurone disease, there has been only limited use of inpatient or nursing home care.

THE NEED TO MAINTAIN PERMANENTLY HIGH STANDARDS OF CARE

This is only a theoretical disadvantage from the point of view of busy or overstretched staff but, once the expectations of patient-oriented care have been established, any failure to deliver can lead to acute and vocal disappointment. It is therefore especially important to put time and resources into inducting new staff (particularly junior medical staff who change regularly) and into staff training and development. Because the co-ordinator/counsellor or nurse/co-ordinator carries a particularly heavy burden of stress and sadness, it is essential that resources are put into providing this post-holder with supervision and support.

MAINTAINING THE TEAM'S REPUTATION

The reputation of the team depends on consistently high quality work from every member of the team member so careful selection and effective mutual support is essential. It is important that all team members, including medical staff, make time for team meetings and that the practical arrangements for delivery of care—in ward, community or outpatient clinics—reinforce the team's philosophy of the primacy of patient needs over those of the organization.

COPING WITH THE GROWING DEMAND

Because no one is discharged from contact with the Team, the work load grows each year. The resources allocated to the Team and the way in which its services are delivered therefore need to be regularly reviewed. The advent of Care in the Community and the major reorganization of health and social services should also make such reviews more likely. It is important in such reviews to emphasize two points: (1) people with these diagnoses are not invented by the team—they are just more visible because of the team's acknowledgement of their needs; and (2) it is extremely difficult to measure outcomes in progressive illnesses and almost impossible to find truly comparable control groups. Sadly, at the time of writing (early 1997), additional resources have not been allocated to the Neuro-care Team. Although much good work continues to be done—and Romford probably compares favourably with areas which have no initiative of this kind—the quality of the overall service has inevitably declined. There is quite a lot of talk nowadays about putting resources into rehabilitation and this is a welcome development, but for people with conditions which are progressive by their very nature, the Romford Neuro-care Team's commitment to 'prehabilitation' makes much more sense.

CONCLUSION

The nature, scope, and objectives of the Romford Neuro-care Team have been described and its advantages and disadvantages listed. I believe that the advantages greatly outweigh the disadvantages and that this way of working is helpful for patients, their families, and Team members. It is vitally important in these days of national targets and measured outcomes that patients with progressive neurological conditions are not denied appropriate care because their needs are not primarily for high-tech treatments, or because their conditions are currently neither preventable nor curable. If, because of their communication difficulties, people with these conditions are unable to make their voices heard in the battle for resources, it is vital that health and social service professionals add their voices so that the needs of this group are not forgotten.

REFERENCES

Oxtoby, M. (1982). *Parkinson's patients and their social needs*. Parkinson's Disease Society, London.

Oxtoby, M. and Eikaas, M. (1993) Multi-disciplinary management from day one: the Neuro-care approach to motor neurone disease. *Palliative Medicine*, **7**(suppl.), 31–6.

Oxtoby, M. and Findley, L. S. (1990). *Prehabilitation in Parkinson's Disease: a model for early intervention*. Society for Research in Rehabilitation—Record of Summer Meeting.

Oxtoby, M. Findley L. Kelson N. Pearce, P. Porteous, A. Thurgood, S., *et al.* (1988). *A strategy for the management of Parkinson's disease and for the long-term support of patients and their carers: End of Pilot Report*. Parkinson's Disease Society, London.

Parkinson's Disease Society (1991). *Pitstop: an intensive therapy course for people with Parkinson's Disease*. Macmillan Magazines, London.

Pegg, R. (1992). *Motor neurone disease—a carer's perspective*. Motor Neurone Disease Association, Northampton.

RCP (Royal College of Physicians) (1986). *Physical disability in 1986 and beyond*. RCP, London.

Ruth Pinder

I was absolutely stunned, so much so that driving back I had to stop because I was crying and couldn't see through the windscreen . . . My husband, who *hates* anything to do with medicine, he was reading his book when I walked in. I went over to the bar as we always had plenty of liquor, but that's not like me. I hardly ever drink without someone offering me one. And I poured myself a brandy. He said 'What's the matter?' And then, of course, it all had to come pouring out. We didn't sleep all that night.

To some extent, I suppose, the diagnosis is not a kind of crisis point usually. Patients obviously present with problems which means that now they have to do such-and-such, then they have to go home and think about it. But it's not like breaking a leg. Nothing very dramatic has to change. You don't have to think 'Well, am I going to be able to get upstairs?' because presumably that problem may have arisen, but it's not an acute problem.

This is a patient and a general practitioner (GP)[1] talking about the diagnosis of Parkinson's disease[2]. However, it hardly seems as though the two are talking about the same phenomenon. This chapter asks can we explain how, on the face of it, the two concerns seem to be so different? And, crucially, how may we bring them closer together so that GPs may respond sensitively and effectively to their patients' distress?

An obvious departure point might be to explore what was actually conveyed and understood in the doctor–patient consultation. Typically, studies on doctor–patient communication focus on this encounter, probing for instances of medical jargon, interruptions which disrupt the patient's flow of thought, the inappropriate use of body language, the effects of a doctor's 'busyness' on a patient's ability to tell a coherent story, and the influence of education and social class in determining how much information is understood and retained (Pendleton and Hasler 1983; Byrne and Long 1984; Tuckett *et al.* 1985). Such studies, provide valuable information on the success or failure of a particular communication *event*. However, we need to take a broader view. Consultations are the end, rather than the starting point of a much more complex *process* which arises

[1] General practitioners in the community probably have closer contacts with their patients than hospital physicians. Despite this advantage, GPs in this research experienced dilemmas an exploration of which I hope will yield valuable insights for their hospital colleagues.
[2] I have used the abbreviation PD for Parkinson's disease throughout the text, but retained patients' and doctors' own usage in the verbatim material.

from the many beliefs, values, and assumptions which patients and doctors bring to encounters with one another. The few studies adopting such an approach have concentrated primarily on one particular disease, cancer, (McIntosh 1977), and focused on the hospital physician (Taylor 1988). This chapter takes the unusual step of going behind the consultation to examine the ideas of *both* patients and GPs which affected their response to the diagnosis of a particular degenerative chronic illness, Parkinson's disease. Only by exploring these prior considerations, and their social and cultural underpinnings, may we hope to achieve some insight into how communication events may succeed and, sometimes, misfire.

THE MISSING DIMENSION: TOWARDS A HEALING APPROACH

I propose to explore some of the tensions and contradictions between doctor and patient perspectives by reference to a model outlined and developed by two medical anthropolgists: Kleinman (1978) and Helman (1990), which distinguishes between biomedical (or 'disease') and lay (or 'illness') explanations of ill-health. As Helman (1985) explains:

The 'disease' perspective of modern medicine is characterized by a mind–body dualism, the reduction of most ill-health to physico-chemical terms, and an over-emphasis on biological (as opposed to social or psychological) information in reaching a diagnosis . . . Biological data is /seen as/ being more 'real' and clinically significant than either social or psychological data.

My own observations also suggest that medical knowledge is primarily second, third, or 'nth-hand knowledge, which does not directly threaten doctors' bodily or emotional integrity. It forms the subject matter of a doctor's work, but does not affect his/her *raison d'être* (Pinder 1990, 1992). It may usefully be termed *experience with* knowledge.

By contrast, the lay, or 'illness' explanatory model relates to the subjective experience of ill-health. It focuses on the way patients, their families, and wider social networks perceive, live with, and respond to symptoms and disability, including judgements about how best to cope with the practical problems posed by the onset of disease. Crucially such a model has to do with '. . . categorizing and explaining, in common-sense ways accessible to all lay persons in the social group, the forms of distress caused by those pathophysiological processes' (Kleinman 1988). Being patterned in social, psychological, and cultural factors, it is both more elusive and diffuse than the biomedical approach. Furthermore, unlike the biomedical model, illness impacts directly on personal identity. It is first-hand, direct, *experience of* knowledge.

At the core of the lay model, particularly at the diagnosis of a chronic illness, are questions which not only ask 'What can be done?' on a practical level,[3] but broader questions such as 'What is going to happen to my life?', 'Why me?', 'Why now?', which highlight complex problems of meaning. In addressing these, patients attempt to restore a sense of coherence to their lives which the advent of chronic illness often so rudely disrupts (Bury and Anderson 1988; Robinson 1988; Charmaz 1991).

One of the dilemmas of modern Western scientific medicine lies in the difficulty of integrating the two approaches (Engel 1977; Capra 1985; Gordon 1988).[4] A medical culture which is geared to speedy problem-solving, impatient with 'theory', and uncomfortable with problems which cannot readily be 'cut down to size' makes attention to the complex layers of significance in which the illness experience is embedded particularly intractable. Moreover, the logic of enterprise which has seeped into all our institutions, medicine included, has scant respect for values other than a minimalist interpretation of economy, efficiency, and effectiveness. A healing approach, which is attentive to the desperation and inner moral pain of many chronically ill patients, has been lacking. As Kleinman (1988) notes:

Clinical and behavioral science research . . . possess no category to describe suffering, no routine way of recording this most thickly human dimension of patients' and families' stories of experiencing illness. Symptom scales and survey questionnaires and behavioral checklists quantify functional impairment and disability, rendering quality of life fungible. Yet about suffering they are silent . . . /yet/ it remains central to the experience of illness, a core tension in medical care.

The tensions are at their sharpest at the time of diagnosis of chronic illness such as PD, where the scope for technical intervention is comparatively limited. In trying to shed some light on the apparent disparity of the two opening quotations, an important key lies in doctors' capacity and willingness to address this missing dimension.

This chapter first explores how a group of GPs conceptualized diagnosing patients with PD, and the impact of the diagnosis on a separate group of patients with PD. I will then consider how doctors in the research study attempted to attend to the illness experience by reference to certain key

beliefs and assumptions they held about PD and PD patients, namely, questions about age, the lengthy illness careers anticipated for many patients, and the availability of a replacement therapy. The extent to which patients found these notions helpful or otherwise in their initial attempts to embark on rebuilding a sense of their own identities is discussed. I will then move on to consider how patients and doctors thought about the vital question of making sense of PD and explaining human suffering. The chapter concludes by exploring some of the ways in which biomedical and lay dialogues might better be woven together so that more effective and sensitive communication between patient and doctor may be achieved.

THE RESEARCH STUDY

As the emphasis was on eliciting complex meanings and interpretations which are largely inaccessible to measurement and statistical analysis, a qualitative approach was used, in which in-depth interviewing was the principal research instrument. This meant addressing much broader and more complex questions of 'how?' and 'why?' rather than the 'how many?' or 'how much?' issues which characterize quantitative studies. The study was interested in drawing out meanings, not mapping dimensions.

Initially, I had intended to study specific pairs of patients and their GPs. However, the first two patients I approached were reluctant to allow me to interview their own doctor. I can only speculate about their reticence: perhaps they feared that if interpretations were going to differ, their accounts might be given less credence? (Becker 1967).

This led to a major shift in the research. I turned to the much richer exercise of mapping patients' and doctors' inner dialogues across a range of responses as both parties separately confronted 'the same' disease. Thus, I was comparing and contrasting what one group of patients with PD needed from their GPs at the time of diagnosis with a different group of doctors' ideas on the subject. The context was PD.

Fifteen patients were selected from a variety of sources, including social service department day centres, local GPs, and local branches of the Parkinson's Disease Society. Four patients were 'snowballers' (friends of patients already contacted). Eighteen GPs, with declared experience in caring for patients with PD, were recruited from conferences, via personal contacts at London teaching hospitals, and, following a practice adopted by Dowie (1983), introductions from a local GP I approached.

I carried out in-depth interviews which freely encouraged patients to discuss their experiences of, and with, PD in their own homes. They were seen, on average, three times between 1985 and 1986 and contact was maintained with some patients over a much longer period. I was able to spend less time with GPs. Nevertheless, I interviewed them for a minimum of 45 minutes, mostly in their surgeries, in 1987. Some GPs

---

[3] The problem of explaining, and coming to understand, what to expect of the illness has been dealt with elsewhere (Pinder 1990).

[4] It is too simplistic to polarize sharply the two approaches. As Helman (1990) notes, doctors draw on a repertoire of interpretative models, from genetics, immunology, epidemiology, and psychology. Nevertheless, biomedicine is still the dominant paradigm (Stacey 1991).

invited me to their homes to explore the issues raised further, and this added greatly to the depth of my understanding. Prior to the interview, all GPs were asked to make a note of patients they had diagnosed and the number of patients with PD currently on their lists.

All interviews were taperecorded and transcribed unedited, yielding some 900 pages of data. Patients were invited to go through their transcripts to iron out any ambiguities and clarify interpretations. Attempts to encourage GPs to check their transcripts in the same way were successful in only three cases, and I discontinued the exercise. Those who did respond, and the four GPs who commented on earlier drafts of my work, helped modify and confirm my initial understandings.

I have dealt with the question of representativeness elsewhere (Pinder 1990). Suffice it to note there was no prima-facie reason to suggest that the impressions and perceptions illustrated here differed significantly from those of patients and GPs in the population at large. The cases studied here were representative in the more colloquial sense in that they illuminated important areas of patients' and GPs' ideas and experiences which have general applicability.

DIAGNOSIS; SOLVING THE PUZZLE

Doctors' views about the impact of diagnosis on their patients were coloured by two considerations: firstly, the well-established difficulties of diagnosing it in the first place (Duvoisin 1984; Thompson 1987); and secondly, the relationship of PD to a wider medical taxonomy of conditions which affected judgements about its seriousness.

First, because the early symptoms of PD may so readily be confused with those of other presenting complaints, doctors often stumbled on the diagnosis by chance. As one doctor described the situation:

I think the thing about Parkinson's, from the doctor's point of view, is recognizing it in the first place. It's terribly easy not to know they've got it. I happened to see a patient rather than my colleague, and the second he walked through the door I said 'That chap's got Parkinson's'. And I think it's helpful sometimes for people to see a new doctor because it often hits you, bang, just like that.

The ideal of diagnosis as a logical process, of proceeding systematically from observation to careful refinement of hypotheses (Ledley and Lusted 1959) was confounded in practice. Recognition was often quite sudden, a 'Eureka!' moment, when the pieces of a jigsaw fell into place. Although doctors in the study felt that this was not necessarily a scientific way of approaching the matter, they were nevertheless tolerant of their colleagues for 'missing' when the signs were so elusive.

Under these circumstances, it was not surprising that most doctors here experienced the diagnosis as being a relief—as much for themselves as for their patients. One doctor described a patient with giddy turns whom she had referred to an audiologist. Subsequently, the patient had returned to her care, and the mask-like face which often characterizes PD was suddenly obvious:

It was almost a relief to have something definite to tell her, and because with luck tablets might help her.
RP. And you felt . . .?
Doctor. Relief that it mightn't alter her quality of life *that* much. There *is* a positive side to it. And I think she felt that herself.

Discrete symptoms which on their own had not added up suddenly fitted a larger explanatory framework. Moreover, doctors felt that patients were as pleased as they were that the mystery had been solved: diagnosis had a legitimating function for them too. The application of biomedical skills not only confirmed doctors in their traditional role as diagnosticians. It addressed patients' concerns by giving them badly needed credibility.

Second, confirming the diagnosis gave doctors immediate access to a wider taxonomy of conditions, malignant and life-threatening on the one hand, and self-limiting and trivial on the other, which allowed them to judge the seriousness of the news they had to break. In comparing and contrasting PD with other diseases, doctors drew on shared perceptions as to its immediate danger to life, its treatability, and its implications for short- and longer-term mental and physical functioning. It was evident that for most GPs in the study, PD did not fare too badly within this hierarchy. As one doctor, with experience as a clinical assistant in neurology, explained:

I don't see it as so emotionally loaded as some things. If one puts it in the context of death in general practice, I'd prefer to be told I had Parkinson's disease than be told I was going to die. But in neurology, which of course I do a lot of, there could be a lot worse things to have, like MS, or a brain tumour, or MND. All these things are very relative.

No doctor likes giving bad news, but the news was evidently not drastically bad. Diagnosis was a relief from that point of view too.

However, some doctors were also able to relate to patients' initial feelings of shock illustrated in the introduction. One GP considered: 'Epilepsy, diabetes, PD, any of these things, are enough to scare the pants off anyone'. And another remembered as a child watching his uncle who had PD trying to drink a cup of tea and thinking '. . . This is a terrible thing he's got. That left a lasting impression really, not being able to do something as simple as having a cup of tea without spilling it'. With more direct experience of the illness, he thought that diagnosis of PD '. . . has quite horrifying ramifications in people's minds'. Although he could not directly experience the frustrations of being unable to hold a drink steady, this doctor had grasped, if only momentarily, something of the havoc PD caused to a patient's identity.

Diagnosis was thus largely a positive step for doctors. Everything flowed from that moment. They could now get down to the business of initiating treatment and monitoring progress. Without it, they were casting around in the dark, unable to draw up a coherent plan of action. How did patients respond to the news?

THE IMPACT OF DIAGNOSIS

'It was lack of hope; that was the operative word really'

For most patients in the study, diagnosis marked a significant turning point in their lives. The comparative certainties on which we predicate our lives were shattered. Nothing could ever be quite the same again, no matter how slow the progression of the disease or how mild the presenting symptoms. Diagnosis marked a transition from a past that might have been perceived as 'normal' to a future over which there now hung an ominous shadow.

No single word does justice to the complexity of patients' reactions to the news of having contracted PD or to the speed with which, in recollection, one reaction was overtaken by another. For most patients it was a time of utter turmoil.

For a few patients in the study, diagnosis was initially a relief, for the reasons that doctors had anticipated. One patient had had a trying time at work because her colleagues had thought she was malingering. Now she had a label:

I think one of the reasons I was relieved was because people were inclined to think I was saying I was ill for no reason. People can get criticized for appearing to be unwell. But if you've got a name for it, then they change their views.

A label was, to some extent, liberating: her image of herself as a hard-working, conscientious employee, but one who was legitimately ill, was restored. But her relief was short-lived. It was rapidly overtaken by feelings of shame and stigma. The word 'disease' had conjured up feelings of being unclean, and the fear of contagion lay barely concealed beneath the surface. Once again patients' identities were jeopardized.

Some patients also considered they accepted the news with fortitude and were philosophical about it at the time. One patient, hampered by the lack of speech, whispered 'I just accepted it. I'm fatalistic. I always have been'. However, the fact that some patients did not openly grieve or express much emotion about the diagnosis says little about the underlying distress the news had caused. It was evident from patients' other remarks that 'unease', and 'upset' were never far from the surface.

But shock was often paramount as the opening quotation from one patient has attested. Even though some patients knew about the disease from experiencing family or close relatives, the news that *they* had contracted it was still profoundly upsetting. One patient's mother and grandmother had had PD, yet his own identity was suddenly transformed by the news. He had, at a stroke, become 'a Shaky Bill'. Plans for the future had to be shelved.

I felt really choked when that happened to me at that period. It knocked a lot out of my life really. Just at the time when the children were grown up, the wife and myself felt we could do things together that we wanted to do without the children. We'd spent some years bringing up the children and we thought this was our time now, and then suddenly I'm a Shaky Bill.

Patients often used vivid metapahors to describe their feelings. They remembered 'feeling numb', or their minds 'being a blank' so that they 'didn't know *what* to think any more', as one patient recalled. The experience was overwhelming, almost anarchic.

In trying to understand what the words 'Parkinson's disease' might mean for their lives, patients drew on culturally available images of the disease, the initial results of which were not always comforting. One patient remembered as a child seeing '. . . a wizened old man bent over and shaking' with PD—a disease she thought '. . . had died out years ago, like quinsy'. Another thought it was '. . . a wasting disease, you just wasted away'. A flood of questions burned for an answer: was it going to affect patients' ability to work, to bring up their children? Indeed, had it been passed *on* to their children? What was going to happen to their own lives, their marriages, their futures? Any coherence to their lives was shattered.

In attempting to engage with patient's feelings, what were those redeeming features of PD which doctors felt would ease patients into their new roles? And how well did they match patients' own ideas and experiences? I will discuss first the question of the availability of a drug treatment, second the longer-term nature of PD, and third the question of age.

THE DRUG REGIME

'Having something tangible on offer'

With diagnosis, doctors could get down to the business of initiating and monitoring treatment. PD offered a model of practising medicine with which GPs in the study were entirely at home. It locked into the acute pattern of medicine in which they had primarily been trained. Having something concrete on offer took some of the sting that might otherwise have accompanied the diagnosis of such a condition from the situation. One GP spoke for several others when he said:

It makes me feel much better! It makes you feel useful in the sense of being able to give something. I think if you're comparing it to MS, it's much easier to manage than MS. It's easier to hang a discussion around a change in medication and treatment, and that forever to be talking about how someone's continuing to get worse, or to have episodes where they feel dreadful, where all you can say is 'that must be terrible', it does make you feel better to be able to give them something which might help.

The relief was palpable. Not only could doctors actively *do* something; managing treatment was also attractive because, in emphasizing the technical, less personal side of medicine, it deflected attention away from the need to confront patients' distress—and their own anxieties—more directly. However, other doctors felt less comfortable. The cost–benefit issues involved particularly troubled one GP:

Often with Parkinson's you run into a situation where there are problems with side-effects. Whether the overall benefit's good or not, the side-effects are troublesome. And then there are feelings of guilt about doing harm, dealing with patients' resentment and resistance.

They're taking treatments *you* reckon are good for them and *they* reckon aren't.

Doctors were aware that quite serious problems could be anticipated in the medium-and long-term which did not lend themselves to neat, logical solutions. Nevertheless, in the short-term, having a therapy available fitted into most doctors' immediate management plans following diagnosis. This was positive, goal-oriented medicine which doctors felt helped ease their patients' immediate distress about the diagnosis.

'I expected to be returned to normal functioning'

Having established that the disease was 'not a killer', but that its cause remained unidentified, patients wondered 'could anything be done?' Not surprisingly, the availability of a treatment helped ease patients' immediate anxieties concerning an ill-understood and potentially upsetting piece of news. It held out some promise for them to re-establish a sense of order to their lives. One patient, despite feeling intensely distressed by the diagnosis, was reassured by her doctor:

My GP said 'You've got these tablets. They're very good. They're quite new. They'll control you . . . You're lucky you've got these. Other people haven't had them'.

Patients felt that even though a cure was evidently some way off, the situation could be contained. They could be a little more optimistic. As one patient said:

It's making up for a lack of dopamine, isn't it?
RP: That's right.
Patient: I thought if I could get that back again I'd be all right. Not cured, as I say, but improved and able to lead a normal life

Armed with this expectation and reassurance from a well-respected GP, she was able to distance herself from the bleak experience of her early nursing days in the 1940s. Patients were comforted that some of the depressing images they had held of PD were not going to apply to them. Evidently the whole scene had been transformed with the advent of a replacement therapy. However, control for patients implied containment. They had little experience of medications which had troublesome side-effects and which, with time, failed to control the progression of the disease.

Moreover, the availability of a therapy did not always have a consoling effect. Far from tempering the fears aroused by diagnosis, these were compounded when patients learnt that they were to be on medication for the rest of their lives. Several patients actively disliked taking drugs and had prided themselves on 'never having taken a pill in my life, not even aspirin', as one patient explained. This new dependence had powerful symbolic meanings for patients, emphasizing the fact that they were no longer in control over their own bodies.

Such reservations apart, for most patients in the study the therapy afforded them a degree of optimism which no patient could afford to relinquish. They, too, were influenced by social and cultural expectations about progress—what Ignatieff

(1997) has referred to as 'the myth of progress'—in treating previously untreatable disorders. With medication lay the hope of re-establishing that sense of self which had been so rudely shattered. Doctors' medical knowledge was an important component in that process.

A PROLONGED CAREER

'I'd put it that the progression's rather variable'

The diagnosis of PD was also a relief to doctors because it allowed them space and time to prepare patients to make the necessary adjustments to living with a gradually disabling illness. As the opening quotation to this chapter illustrates, doctors felt that time was on their patients' sides. Moreover, seeing the diagnosis in physical rather than in symbolic terms, doctors did not feel this was an abrupt turning point in patients' lives. Time was also on their own side: they were not immediately going to be confronted with problems which might threaten their own experiential integrity. Doctors were anxious to explain to patients that:

. . . It's not an illness like cancer where you're likely to go within a year or two of diagnosis. It's a slow progressive illness which may give you many years of happy, fulfilled life . . .

as one GP put it. Several GPs made a point of trying to comfort patients with such phrases as 'you're likely to die of something else first' and 'yours is a mild case'. They were concerned at a human level to try and structure diagnosis for patients as positively as possible. Spinning out time in this way gave both patients—and, doctors hoped, themselves—a reprieve. They might be able to side-step having to face in their patients the longer-term implications of the disease which they knew from clinical experience might well happen. 'Let's hope he has his heart attack before we get to that stage', said one GP. Other events might easily supervene. It made sense to try and spare patients premature, and perhaps unnecessary exposure to the distressing later stage complications of the disease.

At the same time, doctors knew they could be faced with the task of sustaining the quality of care through a series of gradually deteriorating personal and family crises over time. Although GPs acknowledged that 'most general practice is chronic illness', most doctors in the study were ill at ease with the problems raised by longstanding medical conditions. One GP remembered the frustrations aroused by one patient she had treated:

I also remember the feeling, and I think you've got to be aware of it, where you actually say 'I've run out of sympathy'. It's only a temporary patch. It's just that you've run out of steam and haven't another suggestion to make.

Doctors were uncertain where to go next, how they could best help when it seemed they had tried everything there was to try and the end was not yet in sight. Time was Janus-faced.

How did the question of time affect patients?

'They gave me a good 25 years'

Doctors' reassurances that PD was not a killer, that theirs was 'a mild case' and that the disease was a long, slow process, were of some initial help to patients. One patient recalled with relief his consultant saying:

'No need to worry, you'll never die of Parkinson's'. So that's something good. I said 'I won't shake meself to death?' And he said 'No, not really'. He said it's most unusual for anyone to actually die of Parkinson's disease . . . You know you've got to be pleased when a doctor tells you you've got a disease that you're going to keep until you die but you know you're not going to die of it, at an earlier stage. We all want to live as long as we can, don't we.

Attending to cultural beliefs and expectations about longevity in the West played a major role in helping to restore this patient's sense of self. Patients' and doctors' ideas, in this instance, meshed. However, at the outset, patients did not know how slow was slow, how mild was mild. If it was not a killer, what was it? Only in gaining some answers to these questions were patients able to start restoring some order to their lives. At the time of diagnosis, these were generally unknowns.

Attempted reassurances could go astray. One patient, whose mother had had PD, and who knew what it meant at first hand, said of his consultant at the time of his own diagnosis:

He built me into this euphoric state by saying 'Well, it's a mild case'. And then when I got back home, I realized it's always a mild case to start with, isn't it.

Patients' direct experience of the disease sometimes flew in the face of doctors' attempts to reassure.

Patients had well developed ideas of their own about slowly deteriorating illnesses which were partly reflected in doctors' own discomfort. The idea of gradually losing control over one's mental and physical faculties, of being dependent in a culture which places a high premium on individual responsibility and self-reliance, was a source of disquiet for most patients. Despite the progress made by the Disability Movement in the 1990s towards reframing able-bodied attitudes towards dependency, the fear still bites deep.

I've always had this dread of long-term illness . . . My neighbour dropped down dead whilst he was putting a kettle on. What a way to go whilst you're making yourself a cup of tea!

mused one. And another, now seriously disabled and confined to a nursing home, watched his life closing in around him: 'I'd like to either die of it or be cured of it', he said. 'This hanging on is tedious, isn't it'. Diagnosis of PD awakened just such reflections. Underestimated in our culture, and only uncomfortably reflected in the views of some doctors in this study, may be the preference for a swift death rather than a protracted process of deterioration.

A QUESTION OF AGE

'I think they more or less regard it as part of the ageing process'

Several doctors referred to age as a factor in tempering the impact of diagnosis for patients. Some considered that pa-

tients were able to view the onset of PD with more equanimity as it was part of the normal biological process of growing older. As one GP put it:

Well, they know that things have been happening, like their joints are aching, things like that. I think that most of them actually accept it as one of the unfortunate things that can happen to you as you get older. And it seems to be that's the way they take it. They've seen it happen to other elderly people. And they just regard it as a bit of bad luck . . . I think I probably try to give that impression to them as well. They're not *unduly* distressed by the whole thing.

Age was not only seen to have a mitigating effect on the impact of diagnosis. Doctors considered that older people approached the onset of longer-term illness with resignation, if not gracefulness, as an inevitable accompaniment to the general slowing down of mental and physical functions. As a result, several doctors felt that PD was a much less distressing condition than other neurological illnesses, such as multiple sclerosis, which typically occur before a person's life has had a chance to flower. One GP spoke for many doctors in the group:

I don't get that tragic feeling with Parkinson's that you obviously get with MS. Because with *luck* they'll be older, they will have had some quality of life. I'm not saying for the individual person it's not tragic, but it's the overall concept. Younger people with Parkinson's in their forties or fifties are disastrous, but that's a whole different order because you're dealing with much younger people.

Doctors were not unsympathetic with their more elderly PD patients. Rather, their feelings were especially engaged with those patients disabled much earlier in life. As a comparatively young GP himself, one doctor said feelingly of one of his MS patients, 'There for the grace of God go I'. The experience was uncomfortably close to home. With older patients, it could more readily be distanced. Working *for* elderly patients rather than being *of* them, doctors' own identities were not directly threatened.

Ageing before time?

Evidence as to whether references to age helped reconcile patients to their lot was equivocal. Age *itself* was not always accepted with equanimity. The image of serene acceptance of one's years was often at odds with the actual experience of ageing. As one patient put it:

It gives me real sadness, yes. I can only put it that way. When Parkinson's came along it was a blow. I had the feeling, here was something *else* to make you feel old. What did someone say? Every day after retirement they regard it as a bonus. Every day after Parkinson's I don't regard as a bonus. Is this what you're given to finish your time off with?

Patients felt cheated that their 'third age', when they might have anticipated some relaxation of financial pressures or family commitments, was going to be marred by illness.

In some cases, patients felt prematurely aged by the diagnosis (Singer 1974). However, contrary to Singer's findings, it was not exclusively younger patients who felt bereft. There were several references to PD 'taking ten years off his life' (the wife of one 65-year-old patient); and 'suddenly getting old in one week' (the wife of a 76-year-old patient). Patients were sometimes catapulted into a role for which there had been little preparation or warning.

Although most patients agreed that to be struck down in one's forties would be a tragedy—and those few patients in the study who contracted the disease atypically early were outraged at being 'caught out'—it was far from clear whether patients were ready to define themselves as old *now*, or were any more accepting of the situation just because they were officially classed as retired. Patients might, in theory, accept the likelihood that with advancing years, illness could be expected. In practice it proved to be of little comfort when the likelihood became a reality, reinforcing already existing negative images of being old (Trieshmann 1987). No age was a good age to have PD.

COMMENT

I have explored the differing impact of diagnosis on patient and doctor and examined three of the ways in which doctors tried to translate their experience with PD into a framework which might address patients' distress, which are likely to have important implications for subsequent encounters between patients and doctors. In examining how patients considered each of these issues, it was evident that the technical aspects of healing—the drug regime—played an important part in helping patients to adjust. Patients needed the fruits of doctors' biomedical knowledge. However, patients were not always comforted by references to the slowly progressive nature of the disease; neither did their age necessarily assuage their anxieties. Further, treatment itself was only a partial and short-term answer. Later, GPs would have to confront both their own feelings of helplessness and inadequacy, as well as their patients' distress, when strictly clinical solutions ran out. However, for doctors, the problems posed difficulties in management which did not directly impinge on their identities: for patients, their very lives were at stake. Wider issues hung in the balance.

I will now briefly explore those more insistent 'Why me?', 'Why now?' questions discussed earlier which are so painfully raised by the diagnosis of PD, looking first at the way patients attempted to make sense of the experience of suffering, before considering the extent to which doctors felt they could respond appropriately.

THE MISSING DIMENSION: IN SEARCH OF COHERENCE

The questions which most troubled patients raised concerns which extended well beyond strictly biomedical ideas of causation and scientific rationality. In an increasingly secular culture, they were faced with the task of trying to make sense of what had happened to their lives now that PD had been diagnosed—a process which drew on wider concepts about the origin and significance of misfortune generally. The wife of one patient, newly diagnosed, illustrated the pain of such a quest:

So much in life hasn't gone right in these last few years that my faith in God has been very sorely tested . . . My husband's been such a good living, *decent* man, it doesn't seem fair. You look at some people you can only describe as worthless rotters, and nothing seems to happen to them. Life swims by for them. Why has it happened to him? The doctors can't explain.

It was evident from the interviews that this patient understood the nature of the illness clinically and its implications fairly well. However, not even recourse to the comparative certainties of religious belief could entirely calm her. In explaining what to expect of the disease, doctors had not felt able to engage her at this level.

Trying to understand why they, rather than someone else, had been afflicted with a chronic illness was part of the need to explain life's many other catastrophes. Patients and their families searched their biographies for pointers, an understanding of which would help render their lives meaningful once more. Was it the stress of overwork or money worries? Was there after all a genetic factor, a 'propensity to the illness' as one patient put it, at work which had been so long denied? How far had patients' own life habits contributed to the condition? Or was exposure to some toxic substance in the environment which had yet to be identified the culprit? Patients found the apparent arbitrariness of suffering particularly hard to bear. The idea of illness 'simply happening' drained all order and sense of purpose from the world.

Although patients in the research often wished to test the waters with their doctors, the problem arose of how to couch such questions in a language that was appropriate for a medical consultation. Some patients found the task daunting and unrewarding as the following conversation indicates:

Patient: I went to him with depression once.
RP: How did that go?
Patient's wife: Another pill.
Patient: He says 'How are you doing?' I tell him and there's little reaction.
RP: What do you think you're looking for that's missing?
Patient: Well, I'm looking for relief of my suffering but I don't get it.
RP: I wonder what would relieve it?
Patient: Probably the sort of thing we're doing now. Discussing it.

The apparent invitation to explore his feelings was not pursued. His doctor had responded to his 'depression' at a clinical rather than at a human level. Suffering was reduced to a biochemical problem requiring a technical fix.

Reaching within for those patients who felt that their inner distress was being addressed was often an intuitive process. One patient described how her doctor had

. . . pointed out to me a lot of people have it and some of them manage to lead normal lives, because John Betjeman did, didn't he. And he put the ideas into your mind, although I've never discussed it with him fully . . . I'm sure he must think the same things, because little things sometimes that I've said to him, and his answers . . .

RP: They've locked in together?

Patient: That's right.

It did not matter that fears remained unarticulated. Using a 'third ear', this patient's GP had shared her unspoken fears, drawing on culturally familiar symbols with which to attune himself to what was happening. Even if the response was implicit rather than explicit, these patients felt their doctors understood, as far as humanly possible, what it was 'really like'. Such understanding helped to make the illness experience more bearable.

A HEALING APPROACH: STANDING IN THE PATIENT'S SHOES

Doctors in the study trod warily on these concerns. Some GPs refused to be drawn at all—relying on the pressures of modern general practice to circumscribe their consultations. As one GP explained, the efficient practice of medicine required a certain detachment.

You should never get involved with your patients . . . there are so many diseases . . . you find you aren't working efficiently. You have to keep a distance.

However, the limitations of such an approach were painfully brought home to him with the failure of his colleagues to respond meaningfully to his wife's newly diagnosed breast cancer. In the unfamiliar role of patient, he found that the abstract language of probabilities in which the treatment options had been covered with him had little to say to the tragedy that was being played out before his eyes.

Other GPs in the study were alive to the importance of responding to patients at a deeper level, but were unsure how to approach questions of such magnitude. Somehow, the emotional vocabulary was missing. The following GP spoke for most other doctors in the study:

I think it's one of the most difficult things to do. In one way one rather dreads it, because you can do so little to help a lot of the time. I mean one can try but I think my reaction's one of inadequacy when faced with this sort of problem.

Doctors were at a loss to know how to respond. There were no rules to guide them, no protocols they could follow. Their training and clinical expertise had ill-prepared them for the need to reach within. While biomedicine provided one framework for responding to the experience of illness, this alone was insufficient.

A few doctors in the study, however, wished to be more receptive to what Young (1983) refers to as patients' inner 'language of distress'. One GP, who practised in a mission alongside fellow-Christians, had a readily available conceptual map with which to respond to his patients' pain and suffering

. . . which by no means has all the answers, but I see suffering as an inevitable sad thing in a fallen world which sometimes strikes people for reasons which are by no means their fault. And occasionally with patients I'm looking beyond the psychological and the social to the spiritual. I mean I don't force my views on patients, but that's the framework in which I do all my medicine.

This doctor was able to draw on the age-old function of religion to provide ultimate certainty amid the constraints and exigencies of the human experience. With it, he felt better equipped to mediate between the two worlds of biomedical and lay knowledge.

Other GPs in the study were obliged to consider the meaning, or meaninglessness, of the human condition without the support of such a framework. One doctor reflected:

. . . all you can offer really is time for people to come and talk to you about things. You can alleviate suffering very often just by being there yourself, and I think it's important to recognize that as an important thing to do. I know it sounds trite. I don't know whether it comes to you as you get older?

This entailed putting on one side the mantle of biomedicine and revealing something of herself as a human being to her patients. It was not an easy task.

COMMENT

The diffidence with which both patients and doctors approached wider questions of pain and suffering attests to the many difficulties both may have in communicating issues of such profound human importance. As the findings have indicated, it is no facile undertaking. Moreover, the new structural and organisational imperatives of the 1990s—the demands of the business culture, patient 'consumerism', and the movement towards evidence-based medicine—will make it harder. Most doctors in the study were profoundly ill at ease with the subject. Their training had provided them with little grounding and even fewer conceptual categories with which to respond.

Yet, as we have seen, patients were unable to embark on the task of rebuilding their lives if such ontological concerns remained unattended to, whether implicitly or explicitly. The search for predictability, the drive to impose order on disorder is fundamental to human existence. Even if adequate scientific explanations are now more readily available to explain the cause of PD, on its own. This cannot address the wider search for meaning which so concerned patients here. Meaning does not lie unambiguously on the tip of the tongue. In communicating with their patients, it is vital that doctors are alert and sensitive to this quest, and to the meanings behind the words.

CONCLUSION

I have shown how diagnosis may throw patients' lives into disarray, and have indicated some of the ways in which doctors' experience with the disease may help or hinder patients in their initial efforts to come to terms with this crisis in their lives. Thus, biomedical and lay models of illness are not incompatible: rather, the dialogue between the two needs to develop the moral sensitivity which is a prerequisite for the sensitive meeting of minds between patient and doctor. Encounters between the two worlds may initially be tragic for patients, and yet contain within them the seeds for personal growth and healing.

Healing, as more widely understood (Kleinman 1988), goes beyond strictly clinical concerns to embrace existential, social and cultural dimensions. It is both an art and a science, concerned as much with being as with doing. Essentially 'the problem of communication' in chronic illnesses such as PD is one of linking these dialogues together, so that doctors' experience with the disease more closely approximates patients' experience of the illness. Kleinman (1996) puts the matter pithily: how can doctors move more comfortably along that continuum of 'disease sans suffering, treatment sans healing?' In this final section, I will consider some of the wider tensions involved in seeking a *rapprochement* between the two, and conclude with some practical suggestions for enhancing the communication process between patient and doctor.

Part of the difficulty has to do with the dominance of science in contemporary Western thought at the same time as traditional moral and spiritual certainties are declining. As a result, experience with and experience of knowledge are often seen as representing opposite sides of the coin. One is considered to be superior, objective, rational, and reliable; the other inferior, subjective, woolly, and unreliable (Cobb and Hamera 1986). Ideally, I see them as complementary, with doctor and patient making a journey of discovery together as partners (Tuckett *et al*. 1985). This will involve some departures from the standard model of doctor–patient interaction. It means sharing each others' knowledge and experience, with mutual respect for what each can contribute. Doctors need patients' knowledge to gauge whether they are communicating effectively or not, as much as patients need their doctors' experience with the disease.

For a genuine partnership to take place, it is important for doctors to move beyond a strictly biomedical understanding to grasp something of what it is like to have PD first-hand. Here doctors face a further tension: the nearer they come to responding to patients' inner distress, the more they risk exposing themselves to the very anxieties they find so difficult to handle. Research has shown that the management of chronic and terminal illness is a major source of stress for doctors (Sutherland and Cooper 1993). In attempting to address this major dilemma, three steps are necessary.

First, it is vitally important for doctors to scrutinize, on an ongoing basis, the various judgements they use. This is not to say that there is no need for judgements. Rather, beliefs need to be adapted, modified, and redefined to remain in step with the way patients think and feel. However, such a process raises other tensions: it invites ambiguity and doubt when the pressures of work demand simplification and routinization. Yet, only with such scrupulous self-analysis may doctors be attentive to the complex, constantly evolving nature of patients' needs.

Second, and equally difficult, is the task of stepping into another's shoes. We cannot transcend the limitations of our own experience except perhaps fleetingly. This research has shown that GPs who could reach intuitively into their patients' worlds helped transform patients' ability to come to terms with their predicament. Such a process involves the development of a 'third ear'—an imaginative reaching within for those sudden shafts of light which momentarily illuminate our perceptions.

Third, as most patients with chronic illnesses live in the home, not in hospital, an appreciation of the broader social and cultural contexts in which patients' experience their illness is necessary. To communicate effectively, doctors need to draw freely on the repertoire of personal and cultural beliefs with which patients endeavour to make sense of their lives with the onset of PD. For doctors, this means squarely addressing wider questions of misfortune and suffering.

How may medical training respond to these demands? In the first place, the teaching of communication skills is now a modest but regular part of the medical curriculum. However, there is increasing awareness that such skills, on their own, fail to 'stick' (M. J. Johnston personal communication). Formal training in communication may well give students the necessary behavioural tools, but without an understanding of humanistic concepts, they are simply instruments (Arnold *et al*. 1987).

Secondly, the emotionally demanding nature of caring for the chronically ill strongly suggests that there is a need, as in other caring professions, to support the supporter. Recent research has shown the value of counselling in both the delivery and receipt of health care (Davis and Fallowfield 1991). The inclusion of core counselling skills both as an integral part of the medical curriculum, and an ongoing resource, rather than as a soft option to be tacked on at the end as a concession to liberalism, might be a way forward.

Third, far wider educational issues are at stake. One of the major problems of contemporary medical education, particularly at the postgraduate level, is the 'narrow "range of relevancies" ' which it still fosters (Pinder 1998), and its well-documented resistance to voices from other disciplines (Pietroni 1996). Developing a rounded practitioner means broadening the educational base to embrace contributions from the social sciences and humanities, thus attending to the debates about medicine which take place 'on the outside'. It means training doctors to move between 'that coherent body of explanatory knowledge which is used to predict, control and dominate the world' (science) and one which requires the individual 'to become more consciously aware of the social and cultural roots of their self-understanding' (Carr 1995). To address these questions is no easy undertaking. But can medicine afford not to?

At the end of the day, most doctors would hope to evoke a a response similar to that of the patient who said of her own GP:

I suppose there is a bond really. I feel he understands perfectly how I feel. I know when I go in he's going to understand.

ACKNOWLEDGEMENTS

This chapter is based on a study commissioned by the Parkinson's Disease Society, London, between 1985 and 1989, and I gratefully acknowledge their support. I should also like to thank Judith Monks for her helpful comments on an earlier version of this chapter.

REFERENCES

Arnold, R. M., Povar, G. J., and Howell, J. D. (1987). The humanities, humanistic behavior, and the humane physician: a cautionary note. *Annals of Internal Medicine*, **106**, 313–18

Becker, H. S. (1967). Whose side are we on? *Social Problems*, **14**, 239–47.

Bury, M. and Anderson, R. (ed.) (1988). *Living with chronic illness: the experience of patients and their families*. Allen and Unwin: London.

Byrne, P. S. and Long, B. E. L. (1984). *Doctors talking to patients: A study of the verbal behaviour of General Practitioners consulting in their surgeries*. Royal College of General Practitioners, London.

Capra, F. (1985). *The turning-point: Science, society and the rising culture*. Fontana, London.

Carr, Wilfred (1995). *For education: Towards critical educational inquiry*. Open University Press, Milton Keynes.

Charmaz, K. (1991). *Good days, bad days: the self in chronic illness and time*. Rutgers University Press, New Jersey.

Cobb, A. K. and Hamera, E. (1986). Illness experience in a chronic disease—ALS. *Social Science and Medicine*, **23**, 641–50.

Davis, H. and Fallowfield, L. (ed.) (1991). *Counselling and communication in health care*. Wiley: Chichester

Dowie, R. (1983). *General practitioners and consultants: A study of outpatient referrals*. King Edward's Hospital Fund, London

Duvoisin, R. (1984). *Parkinson's disease: A guide for patient and family*. Raven, New York

Engel, G. (1977). The need for a new medical model: A challenge for biomedicine. *Science*, **196**, 129–36.

Gordon, Deborah (1988). Tenacious assumptions in Western medicine. *In Biomedicine examined*, (ed. M. Lock and D. Gordon). Kluwer, Dordrecht, pp. 19–56.

Helman, C. (1985). Communication in primary care: the role of patient and practitioner explanatory-models. *Social Science and Medicine*, **20**, 923–31

Helman, C. (1990). *Culture, health and illness*, (2nd edn) Wright, London.

Ignatieff, M. (1997). *20:20 Vision. On the nature of suffering*. Radio 4, 29 January 1997.

Kleinman, A. (1978). Concepts and a model for the comparison of medical systems as cultural systems, *Social Science and Medicine*, **12**, 85–93.

Kleinman, A. (1988). *The illness narratives: suffering, healing and the human condition*, Basic Books, New York.

Kleinman, A. (1996) *Writing at the margin: discourse between anthropology and medicine*. University of California Press, Berkeley.

Ledley, R. S. and Lusted, L. B. (1959). Reasoning foundations of medical diagnosis, *Science*, **130**, 9–21.

McIntosh, J. (1977). *Communication and awareness in a cancer ward*. Croom Helm, London

Pendleton, D. and Hasler, J. (ed.) (1983). *Doctor–patient communication*. Academic Press, London

Pietroni, Patrick (1996). *A primary care-led NHS: Trick or treat?* (Professorial lecture). University of Westminster Press, London.

Pinder, R. (1990). *The management of chronic illness: Patient and doctor perspectives on Parkinson's disease*. Macmillan, Basingstoke, UK.

Pinder, R. (1992). Coherence and incoherence: doctors' and patients' perspectives on the diagnosis of Parkinson's disease. *Sociology of Health and Illness*, **14**, 1–22.

Pinder (1998) Thinking about how GPs think: the rationality behind 'resistance' to professional development.

Robinson, I. (1988). *Multiple sclerosis*. London, Tavistock.

Singer, E. (1974). Premature social aging: the social–psychological consequences of a chronic illness. *Social Science and Medicine*, **8**, 143–51.

Stacey, M. (1991). *The sociology of health and healing: A textbook*. Routledge, London.

Sutherland, V. J. and Cooper, C. L. (1993). Identifying distress among general practitioners: predictors of psychological ill-health and job dissatisfaction, *Social Science and Medicine*, **37**, 575–81.

Taylor, K. M. (1988) 'Telling bad news': physicians and the disclosure of undesirable information, *Sociology of Health and Illness*, **10**, 119–32.

Thompson, M. K. (1987). *Caring for your Parkinsonian patients*. Royal College of General Practitioners, London.

Trieschmann, R. B. (1987). *Aging with a disability*. Demos, New York.

Tuckett, D., Boulton, M., Olson, C., and Williams, A. (1985). *Meetings between experts: an approach to sharing ideas in medical consultations*, Tavistock, London.

Young, A. (1983). The relevance of traditional medical cultures to modern primary health care, *Social Science and Medicine*, **17**, 1205–11.

An outreach service for neurological disease

Melesina Goodwin and Amanda Powell

'The future of neurology is bright' Williams (1993). The development of new drugs and treatments for many currently incurable neurodegenerative diseases, will help to bring neurosciences into line with other fields. Future reorganization of formal health care will be based on the 'hub and spoke' principle (HMSO 1993), with fewer regional centres which will be responsible for delivering highly specialized medical, paramedical, and nursing care, and for carrying out expensive investigations and treatments. There will be a greater number of district units responsible to the local community for more generalized neurology and rehabilitation services, as treatments become less expensive and specialised they would be devolved to district level. The regional centres will be centres of excellence whose knowledge will be readily available and quickly transferable helping to ensure a more consistent level of service. However, it would be inadvisable to concentrate all the specialist resources in the regional centres. In the future more patients are likely to be treated as day cases, and hospital inpatients will be discharged home earlier with community care packages. This will require greater liaison between hospital and community services and make the role of an outreach or liaison nurse essential. This function will span the hospital and community, providing education, knowledge, advice and counselling to patients, carers, and other health professionals. These tasks will help to supplement existing services and not replace them. It is anticipated that there will be further development of outreach nurses for individual disease groups such as Parkinson's disease and Alzheimer's disease with funding from regional and district levels, but also supported by the voluntary organizations, thus ensuring a more responsive service to meet patient and carer demands. This chapter will discuss the role of outreach and its likely development in the future.

THE ROLE OF OUTREACH

There has been increasing awareness of a 'care gap' in recent years when patients are transferred between hospital and home, or visa versa Jowett (1988). A liaison/outreach role has developed in various ways across the United Kingdom to try to fill this gap. An increasing number of nurses are being employed in specifically designated hospital/community liaison posts in areas such as diabetes, stoma, and breast care. There are no central guidelines on the way they should function or their specific aims, but it is generally felt that it should include the roles of caregiver, co-ordinator, teacher, counsellor, and advocate. The outreach nurse works with a designated client group and there should be flexibility within the role, to meet their specific requirements. The role of outreach nurses as planners co-ordinators, and communicators between informal and formal carers should help to facilitate a smooth safe transfer of patients into the community or alternative institutional care (O'Leary 1990). Outreach nurses can provide vital links between community, hospital and social services, professionals, lay workers, and the voluntary organizations.

The future quality of care in the community will depend on good communication between hospitals, charity organizations and the primary health care team. Outreach nurse's build up extensive local, regional, and national knowledge and become invaluable assets to patients, carers, and health care professionals. They are qualified to undertake and reach informed decisions on the basis of the information available and therefore ensure continued appropriate care of their clients. 'Achieving the goal of seamless care requires an integrated approach' HMSO (1993). This aim will not be realized if regional centres or district hospitals and carers in the community work in isolation from each other.

The role developed within our unit was that of outreach nurse for neurodegenerative diseases including Parkinson's disease, Alzheimer's disease, Motor neurone disease, Huntington's chorea and multiple sclerosis.

These illnesses all become very disabling, are ultimately a direct cause of death and often affect people at a relatively young age. The effects on the patients and their carers or families can be devastating. The outreach service within this unit is aimed at providing support to the patient and relatives at the time of diagnosis and in the first few weeks after discharge from either hospital or outpatient clinics. The outreach nurse would be a source of information about the disease, have a link role between the hospital, and primary health care teams, and liaise with the voluntary organizations. When set up it was hoped that this role would have the greatest input in the first few weeks following discharge or diagnosis and following bereavement. It was hoped to avoid too much input in the middle stages of illness due to fear of an overwhelming caseload. It will be discussed later in this chapter the way in which the role has actually developed.

DIAGNOSIS

Occasionally, when a neurodegerative disease is first diagnosed and there is only minor disability, and with no need for input from the multidisciplinary team it is possible that a diagnosis may be given in the outpatient setting, even though this may not be ideal. Patients are then left to go home with the label of a disease that they know very little about. The initial shock of receiving the diagnosis, prevents many patients formulating the questions they may have wanted to ask, or in hindsight wished that they had asked. It is known that some of the information imparted will not have been understood or taken in (Crate 1965*a*).

Many patients and families express their feeling of abandonment and isolation even more profoundly when a diagnosis is given in the outpatient setting compared to a hospital setting. This can be highlighted in the case of one lady, who three years after a diagnosis of multiple sclerosis which was given in outpatients, still does not understand that the symptoms she experiences are due to her illness. Following diagnosis, she was never given any subsequent information or counselling and was unaware of who she should contact for further help, as symptoms became more troublesome. The outreach post has shown it is beneficial to be present at the imparting of diagnosis to hear exactly what the patient was told and to observe their response and reaction. It has highlighted the need to go back and speak to the patient and relatives, to reiterate or expand on the recently imparted information. The effect of what was said or understood at diagnosis will have an underlying effect on morale. Patients and their families will have varying interpretations which may be unrealistically optimistic or pessimistic. The outreach nurse has the skill to assess the interpretation made by the patient and family, and to assess its accuracy. It gives the opportunity for ongoing evaluation of what stage of acceptance the patient is at, and what further information they need.

Following diagnosis, patients move through various phases before they can begin to accept their illness. The stages of acceptance come in no particular order duration, or intensity. One of the first reactions is that of disbelief which is characterized by denial and avoidance. This is followed by the gradual development of awareness as patients realize the implications of their diagnosis. This may be expressed in anger which if directed inwards can result in depression. Reorganization follows as the patient accepts increased dependence and changes in identity. If the disease is a chronic illness, the patient is likely to undergo this process again and again.

Many factors play a part in determining an individuals response. These include the effects of the disability on the person, the prognosis, the likely effects on the person's way of life, their personality, and the amount of support received or available from family and professionals. Outreach gives the flexibility to offer counselling and advice dependent on individual needs. If the person is a hospital inpatient there is opportunity to build good rapport and trust, ensuring reduced feelings of isolation and abandonment on diagnosis. It is not always possible for a diagnosis to be given in this setting due to limited resources and this makes it imperative that further counselling and education is available in the home setting and is always offered.

COMMUNICATION

To allow smooth transition from hospital to community, or vice versa, good communication is essential. The Romford project has shown it is essential to identify a key worker for which the outreach role seems ideal (as discussed in Chapter 31).

There is a need to go beyond the traditional medical, surgical, and rehabilitation programmes currently available and develop new patient-centred counselling. Community services play a vital role in supporting and maintaining people with progressive neurological conditions in their local settings making it essential for good communications with specialist staff at the district or regional hospitals. The development of specialist outreach nursing services to provide effective liaison across primary and community services is therefore essential.

This liaison between hospital and community has been shown to be imperative in the provision of urgent specialist equipment such as suction machines and feeding equipment which may not be readily available in the community setting. A delay in the provision of this type of equipment can result in either prolonging hospitalization or unnecessary suffering and distress for patients and relatives. A particularly distressing situation that occurs frequently is that of the patient with bulbar motor neurone disease suffering from infrequent but severe choking attacks, which can be far less anxiety-provoking for the patient and relative if the necessary specialist equipment and knowledge has already been provided. The specialist knowledge and experience of the outreach nurse ensures forward planning so that knowledge and resources have been provided before a crisis occurs. This means the patient and carer will learn the necessary skills in a relatively calm environment which ensures maximum uptake of knowledge. As discussed previously, co-ordinating care in the community can be troublesome as policies vary from region to region as do resources and availability of equipment. Patients have described feelings of 'being in a maze' unsure of who to contact for various aspects of care.

SPECIALIST CLINICS

Following diagnosis of a progressive neurological condition, patients are reviewed at regular intervals in outpatient clinics. Some patients, throughout the progression of their disease, become disheartened and disillusioned with these visits. Expectations are high, only to wait a considerable amount of time for a brief consultation which is often not with the consultant. Travelling can also be problematic and very uncomfortable. Some patients felt they were beyond help and felt guilty taking up the doctor's time (Newrick 1984).

The development of a specialist clinic would help to reduce these problems as it would be aimed specifically at management and treatment of the specific neurological disorder. 'Specialist clinics can measure the effective management of patients with neurological disorder throughout the progression of their disease' (Mutch 1992). Specialist clinics give easy access to a neurologist who has the necessary expertise to recognise common problems that a general practitioner may have difficulty detecting, or who may not be aware of the most effective treatment. These clinics also provide an excellent opportunity for the outreach nurse to maintain contact with patients and carers, and allows time to assess routine problems and to deal with them effectively. If these clinics are to achieve maximum effect then access to members of the multidisciplinary team should be readily available. This was proved to be very successful in the Neuro-care Team project (as discussed by Oxtoby in Chapter 31)

The provision of good service builds up patient and carer trust. Patients rely on doctors to advise about the best or most appropriate treatment available. This includes information about forthcoming clinical drug trials and ongoing research.

CRISIS INTERVENTION

The outreach post ensures patients and relatives have easy access to the 'key worker', thus ensuring intervention occurs before a crisis point is reached. This situation often occurs because of a general lack of support and specialist advice available to patients and carers. Following contact with the key worker, patients and carers are more likely to initiate further contact as and when further problems arise, making it possible to prevent potential crisis situations occurring. Ideally, the outreach post should have the facility to offer continuous support throughout the disease progression.

The importance of contact with the key worker was demonstrated when the wife of a man with bulbar motor neurone disease rang to say her husband was suffering increasing problems swallowing fluids and diet. Further questioning revealed that dietary and fluid intake over the previous five days had been minimal, despite the input of both community dietician and speech therapist. This patient was reviewed on the ward that day and following discussion with him and his family urgent gastrostomy was performed. The patient continued to lead as normal a life as possible within the limitations of his disease. If the links to the outreach nurse were not available this patient's condition may have deteriorated to such an extent that gastrostomy insertion would not have been a viable option.

CARERS

All too often the attention is focused on the patient and overlooks and neglects the family carer, who has been described by Zaritt (1985) as the 'hidden victim'. With the increasing emphasis on cost-effective patient care following the White Paper 'Caring for people' (HMSO 1989), patients are being discharged into community care at a much earlier stage and are sometimes sent home to cope as best as possible with the assistance of family and friends. Family members who help with care, or, are in fact the main carer, face changes that might lead to problems of burden, fatigue, and deterioration in their own physical and mental health (Bull 1990). Bains (1984), and Cantor (1983) found that 'the emotional strain of caregiving was often greater than the physical effects'. Family members describe the activities of providing care as less burdensome than the restrictions on personal freedom imposed by the caregiving routine (cited Bull 1990).

This can bring about complete role reversal with a wife suddenly becoming the main breadwinner, decision-maker, and organizer which has traditionally and socially been accepted as the male role. If it is the female partner who is affected by illness, the male has to take on nursing and household tasks which have traditionally been the province of the female. Marriages that are already floundering can break up because of the added stress and burdens placed on them. It is commonly taken for granted that if there is not a partner, then the nearest female relative will take over the care burden, frequently impinging and trespassing into her marriage and family life. Gilhooly (1984) found that 'when there were both sons and daughters who could potentially give assistance, sons were rarely expected to give as much help as daughters'. Society's expectations are that females are better able to cope than males and there appears to be discrimination in the resources and services offered when the carer is female, with a tendency to offer more input to male carers, which shows that services are not necessarily available on a basis of need.

Carers will usually need much reassurance and psychological support so that the acceptance of help or intervention of any sort from health care professionals is not to be viewed as failure, but as a means of allowing them to continue to cope. There have been numerous studies attempting to determine what carers really need. The four main areas highlighted have included those of information, skills training, emotional support, and regular respite (Nolan and Grant 1989). Although these needs have been recognized, provision continues to be fragmented and unfortunately often only provided in crisis situations.

Social support has been defined as a set of exchanges which provides material and physical assistance, social contact, and emotional sharing. (Pilisuk and Parks 1983). Initially, following diagnosis there will be contact with numerous people and awareness that others care about them may lessen the carer's feeling of burden (Bull 1990). However, over a greater period of time, which could be the case with most neurodegenerative conditions, the number of people in the caring network might be of less importance than other types of support received (Bull 1990). In fact, some patients report feeling overwhelmed with the number and variety of different therapists. They report feeling that decisions are taken away from them, their home has become too clinical, and their privacy is invaded. The key worker with knowledge of specific problems associated with particular neurological diseases will be of the greatest benefit to the patient and carer, ensuring specific needs are addressed with the minimum disruption from the minimal number of therapists.

RESPITE

As neurological disorders progress, each stage of deterioration presents potential problems. Patients and carers are expected to cope, and come to terms with reduced independence, and changes in mobility and bodily functions. These have direct effects on their work, home life, and general lifestyle and bring about obvious fears and worries for the future. Regular respite should help relieve and reduce these stresses to enable the carer and family to continue.

Respite can be difficult if not impossible to organize for chronically ill neurological patients. A study by Cowley (1990) revealed that members of the health professions differentiate between dying patients and those dying of cancer. Presumably, the conclusion being that only patients with a diagnosis of cancer needed terminal care. It is well accepted that following a diagnosis of cancer many patients need a lot of support, information, and arrangement of services. This is provided from various sources such as Macmillan Nurses and hospice day care. However, although the need for respite is often greater in patients with neurological disorders, there are not the clearly defined support systems that are available for patients with cancer. The development of the neurology outreach post will help ensure this type of support becomes more widely available. Respite should be part of the care package available to neurological patients. Counselling provided by the outreach service can broach the subject of respite care at an early stage in the disease process. Respite can be traumatic for carers and they may have overwhelming feelings of guilt. This can result in the loss of any benefit that may have been gained. It is important to stress that the acceptance of respite facilities should not be viewed as a failure to cope but as a means of being able to continue to cope. 'For respite to be effective staff must appreciate the needs of the patients and also the worries and anxieties of the carer' (Webster 1988).

EDUCATION

The threat of illness and, later confirmation of it precipitate a series of redefinitions of the self. It is a process that allows a person to adapt and grieve for 'loss' whatever they may encompass and allows a person to adapt to illness. The patient's response to illness will vary according to his or her self-concept, severity of illness, possible changes in living patterns, and how altered function is perceived by the patient and family. Effective professional care supports and guides the patient and family as they move through the stages of adaptation (Crate 1965b). Teaching, properly timed, is a care skill that can facilitate adaptation.

There are variations in patient receptivity to teaching. During the initial stages following diagnosis denial may interfere with patients learning about their diagnosis. In the stage of denial patients suppress and distort information that has been imparted and tend to withdraw from role demands. The patient may deny illness and if the caregiver tries to force the patient to look at the illness, the patient may resist. In later stages of adaptation, the people involved become better able to consider their illness, to hear facts about it and to participate in their own care. During these later stages, one can expect the patient to be more receptive to teaching regarding diagnosis, treatment, and the possible course of their illness (Crate 1965b).

Learning is most effective when an individual is ready to learn and wants to learn. Sometimes patient's readiness comes with time and the caregiver's role is to encourage this progression. If desired change is urgent, for example, when a patient with motor neurone disease is dangerously unsteady when walking, and needs to be urged to use a wheelchair, the carer may need to directly 'supervise' to ensure learning occurs. Patients and families are sometimes unrealistic about what they can accomplish. They may not have the necessary skills, strength, or determination to care adequately for an invalid relative. The outreach nurse is responsible for helping to set realistic goals for both patient and carer, and must be skilled in providing the necessary information, advice and intervention to enable those goals to be met.

Tools for assessment of motivation and readiness to learn exist within the context of the patient–professional relationship. Rapport within this relationship is necessary to obtain evidence about motivation and determination to learn new skills and knowledge. Continuing changes in the way health care is financed and delivered have required, and will continue to require, changes in the availability of education to patients. Highly technical home care and enhanced self-care are two continuing trends that require strongly directed patient education. Education is therefore an essential health care service.

The limited contact with rare neurological diseases means that some health care professionals may not have the necessary skill to set realistic goals or advise about the likely progression or treatment of these diseases. Therefore, it is important that the outreach service can offer a programme of health care education for other professionals and also offer easy access to specialist knowledge for further advice and information.

CONCLUSION

Following implementation of the outreach post, although no official audit or statistical analysis has been carried out, patient and carer feedback is extremely positive. Medical and nursing staff also feel that the service to patients has greatly improved.

Limitations of this single post has meant that patients (with the exception of those with motor neurone disease) are generally only seen at diagnosis, in the few weeks that follow, and during the end-stage of the disease process and bereavement. It is hoped that as budget holders on a regional and district level see the positive improvement in service to patients and carers, the outreach post can be expanded to employ at least one specialist nurse per disease group. The post has highlighted that patients with neurological disease require a lot of support and intervention.

This area has up until now not been fully addressed by regional and district health authorities and the gap has been left to the voluntary organizations to fill. The pressures placed on such organizations due to an increasing elderly population will continue to stretch their limited resources, making it imperative that the health authorities address this problem.

Addendum

Since the writing of this chapter, the number of specialist nurses has increased across Neurology. Our unit now employs nurses dedicated to specific groups including two nurses for multiple sclerosis, Parkinson's disease, epilepsy, and migraine.

REFERENCES

Bains, E (1984). Cited in Bull (1990).
Bull, M. J. (1990). Factors influencing family caregiver burden and health. *Western Journal Of Nursing Research*, **12**, 758–76.
Cantor, M (1983). Cited in Bull (1990).
Crate, M. A. (1965a). Nursing functions in adaptation to chronic illness. *American Journal of Nursing*, **65**, 72–6.
Crate, M. A. (1965b). *The process of patient education*. (7th edn).
Cowley, S. (1990). Who qualifies for terminal care? *Nursing Times*, **86**, 26–29.
Gilhooly, M (1984). Cited in Goodman, C. (1986). Research on the informal carer: a selected literature review. *Journal of Advanced Nursing*, **11**, 705–12.
HMSO (1989). *Caring for people*. HMSO, London
HMSO (1993). Report of an independent review of specialist services in London. *Neurosciences*, June.
Jowett, S and Armitage, S (1988). Hospital and community liaison links in nursing: the role of the liaison nurse. *Journal of Advanced Nursing*, **13**, 379–87.
Klug Redman, B (1988). *Mosby Year Book*. London.
Mutch, W (1992). Specialist clinics: a better way to care? *Journal of Neurology, Neurosurgery and Psychiatry*, **55**(suppl.), 36–40.
Newrick, P. (1984). Motor neurone disease: can we do better? A study of 42 patients. *British Medical Journal*, **289**, 539–42.
Nolan, M. and Grant, G. (1989). Addressing the needs of informal carers: A neglected area of nursing practice. *Journal of Advanced Nursing*, **14**, 950–61.
O'Leary, J. (1990). Primary health care. Liaison nursing Forging vital links in care. *Nursing Standard*, **5**, 52.
Oxterby, M. *et al.* (1990). *A strategy for the management of Parkinson's disease and for the long-term support of patients and their carers. End of Pilot Report*. Parkinson's Disease Society, London.
Pilisuk, M and Parkes, S (1983). Cited in Bull (1990).
Williams, A. (1993). What will be now in neurology? *Update*, 629–35.
Webster, S (1988). Boosting the effectiveness of respite care. *Geriatric Medicine*, October, 81–3.
Zarrit, J. M., Zarrit, S. H. and Orr, N. K. (1985). *The hidden victims of Alzheimer's Disease. Families under stressimer's*. New York University Press.

34 | *Linking with lay societies*

Mary G. Baker and Bridget McCall

Lay societies are self-help groups set up to meet the needs of a certain group of people, such as the Parkinson's Disease Society, which was set up to help all those who have Parkinson's disease and their families. As with the Parkinson's Disease Society, they are usually founded by lay people with personal experience, to represent the needs of people who have a particular condition and to give them a voice. Lay people are usually at the heart of such organizations and play an active role in their work.

Their aims are generally to improve the information available about the condition; identify needs and signpost the way to support, help, and advice; promote the exchange of ideas between people in a similar situation; raise public awareness of the needs of the group; encourage research; and develop and influence existing services to ensure they meet the needs of their group, and to develop new services. They also allow the tales of their client group to be told, so that experience and understanding can be built upon and progress made.

Improved quality of life and the empowerment of the individual through the development of effective partnerships are the basis of most lay societies. These partnerships may be:

1. With their client group, listening to them and responding to their needs.
2. With the service providers (i.e. the power base of politicians, doctors, and all other professionals involved in the care of their clients), initiating, and developing services.
3. Between lay and professional people facilitating communication and developing links to ensure optimum standards of care.
4. With other voluntary organizations who share areas of common interest so they can develop a stronger voice and articulate needs to advocate change.

The development of information and education resources for both lay and professional people are fundamental to successful partnerships.

In this chapter, we propose to use the experience of the Parkinson's Disease Society to demonstrate how lay societies, working in effective partnerships, can produce enormous benefits for people with neurological conditions and provide an effective and wide-ranging support service for them and the professionals who care for them. The work of our Society reflects that of any other neurological voluntary organization.

To be diagnosed with a chronic neurological illness is the beginning of a long journey into the unknown. A journey that may begin in hope, pass through periods of elation and frustration, and finally end in acceptance and resignation. How a person copes on this journey is dependent on many factors— the medical and social care available; their own understanding and acceptance of their condition; and the support available to them on their journey.

A lay society is a major source of help and support to anyone embarking on this journey. People want to understand what is happening to them and how it will affect their future, so that they can make informed choices about their lives. They also need time and space to discuss any anxieties and fears they have and to raise questions. They want to talk to other people who are facing a similar future. They want the services available to cater to their individual needs and to take account of all they are as a person. They also want to promote research into their illness to improve understanding and treatments and to make their own contribution to this research.

All these needs can be facilitated by the lay society. Furthermore, the lay society gives their client group space and opportunities to tell their stories in order to increase understanding, exchange ideas, and allows them to be partners in care.

WELFARE, INFORMATION, AND EDUCATION

Most lay societies provide certain information and welfare services themselves. The nature and extent of these services varies, depending on a number of factors such as the nature of the condition, the services required, life-expectancy of people with the condition, and the resources available. Most offer extensive information and welfare advice services.

At the Parkinson's Disease Society, the operations department, which incorporates welfare, information, field and training services, responds to the individual needs of people with Parkinson's disease and their carers as well as providing advice and support to the professionals who look after them. The welfare counsellor is able to offer emotional support to anyone who is anxious about the future and wants help to come to terms with their diagnosis and living with Parkinson's disease. There are also some common problems which require sensitive handling, such as depression and problems with relationships, which people may find easier to talk about to a trained counsellor from a lay society, rather than a doctor or other professional. The counsellor also runs a helpline, staffed by trained volunteers, which offers a befriending 'listening' service to anyone who wants to talk to someone who knows something about Parkinson's disease. Many of the volunteers on the helpline have personal experience of Parkinson's disease, either through having it themselves or as a carer.

The staff within the welfare section also provide help and advice on the financial and practical issues which can affect people with Parkinson's disease and their families. It is important that people are aware of the benefits and services available to them from the health and social services and are given advice on how to access them if they are to obtain the support they need. People also need information and advice on suitable equipment to help with activities of daily living; driving and mobility; employment issues; leisure pursuits; respite care and long-term care.

The financial help provided by lay societies themselves varies from organization to organization but can be a large part of their work. They often provide finances to help with the cost of equipment, respite care etc., or else they may operate loan systems for equipment, as, for example, the Motor Neurone Disease Association does. This will depend on a number of factors including prognosis of the condition and financial resources available to the organization. The Society does not provide ongoing grants but does sometimes give one-off grants to help with specific needs. However, the Society also helps people to make application to relevant benevolent funds, such as those allied to certain professions, who give one-off and ongoing grants. Holidays are another important area. The Society runs special holidays, both in the United Kingdom and abroad, many in conjunction with the Winged Fellowship Trust, a voluntary organization which has several specialist holiday centres for people with disabilities in the United Kingdom. People may go on their own, or with their carer.

Information is a fundamental need and a service common to all voluntary organizations. For the client group, it needs to be written in layman's language and to be easily accessible. Professionals also need information to suit their particular concerns. The information provided by the Society covers all aspects of Parkinson's disease and disability in general. The requests for information come from many lay and professional sources and a number of standard publications are available to help them. However, the welfare and information sections in the Society also respond to specific requests for information not covered in the publications. These may need researching, liaising with appropriate professionals, and/or writing an individual reply. The development of information resources are also important. The Society is in the process of setting up a library, named after the famous footballer, Ray Kennedy, who has Parkinson's, which we hope in time will become an important information centre for anyone interested

in Parkinson's disease. Information databases are another innovation in many voluntary organizations. They allow the collation of information on specialist and more general subjects for easy access by both lay and professional people. They also have wide-ranging applications for access to other organizations in the United Kingdom and abroad. This enables the exchange of ideas and information on an international level, which has tremendous potential for all sorts of work including fundraising, research, welfare, information, and training. The advent of the Internet has increased this potential and many voluntary organizations now have their own 'pages' to take advantage of this. The Parkinson's Disease Society's education programme provides study days and conferences throughout the country to suit both specialized and multidisciplinary audiences. Branch seminars and workshops for people with Parkinson's disease and their carers are also held.

One of the major features of the education programme is the involvement of people with Parkinson's disease and their carers as speakers. This is always a very popular slot in the programme. Where possible they attend to talk about their own personal experiences of living with Parkinson's disease. Sometimes this is not possible, and the Society has produced a British Medical Association prize-winning video *Parkinson's disease: The personal view* which allows several people with Parkinson's disease and their carers to give voice to their own experience and concerns. This video has been used widely to enhance the knowledge of many different kinds of professionals. A second video for professionals, aimed mainly at residential and nursing home staff, has been completed, again with the involvement of people with Parkinson's.

Another area of important work of a lay organization is working with professionals to ensure standards of care and to provide ongoing education resources to enhance professional understanding and knowledge about the specific problems of people with neurological conditions. The Society has developed publications to meet the needs of specific professions, often through the establishment of working parties made up of professionals from a specific occupation with a special interest in Parkinson's disease. These working parties have identified and developed the most appropriate forms of education materials to help their profession. These working parties have included nursing, speech and language therapy, physiotherapy, and most recently, occupational therapy.

In the information developed for the therapeutic professions, the role of each profession has been highlighted as it relates to Parkinson's disease. The working parties have also addressed the concern, highlighted by a survey of the Society's members by Dr Marie Oxtoby in 1982, that very few people had access to the therapeutic professions, and doctors were not always aware of the benefits these professions could have for the management of Parkinson's disease. Study days for these professionals are an important further development of this work.

The Nurse Working Party was set up in response to letters the Society received from members, who had experienced problems when admitted to hospital. They felt that nurses did not always understand the specific problems of Parkinson's disease and the complex nature of the drug treatment, such as the individual timing and dosage required, and the complex nature of the side-effects that can occur. As a result, people often found that their drugs were taken away from them and only given at routine drug rounds. The Nurse Working Party aimed to improve the understanding of nurses through the publication of a poster highlighting four key areas that all nurses should have, and an information pack for nurses based on the activities of daily living to guide them in their work.

A Co-ordinated Care Working Party was also set up, involving neurologists, geriatricians, general practitioners, people with Parkinson's disease, and carers, looking at ways of providing seamless care, something which has become even more important under community care reforms. The group have produced a document called *Meeting a need*, which contains their recommendations for the care of people with Parkinson's disease and their carers, attractive enough to persuade the purchasers to buy, with the quality right for the people with Parkinson's disease, in the most cost-effective way.

All the services discussed above would not be possible without extensive involvement of various professionals and voluntary organizations. Access to these people is necessary to ensure up-to-date, comprehensive, and accurate information. Their involvement is needed for the education programme as speakers and participants in conferences and study days. The welfare programme needs access to them in order to provide the best services to the client group, and often the best way of helping someone is not to 'reinvent the wheel' but to refer people to specialist agencies, like the Disabled Living Foundation.

Our response to the needs of our client group does not, however, stop there. In listening to our client group, we have identified five principles which are essential to the good management of Parkinson's disease. These are:

1. Referral to a specialist with knowledge of their illness.
2. Early referral to multidisciplinary team.
3. A good telling of the diagnosis.
4. Continuity of care.
5. To be involved in the management of their care.

To respond to these needs, the Society works with professionals in existing establishments within the health and social services to set up welfare projects under the Society's research programme, to provide models of good practice for the management of Parkinson's disease, incorporating these five principles, which can then dovetail into the existing services. All of the welfare research is governed by a Welfare Advisory Panel, made up of professionals and lay people involved in Parkinson's disease.

One of the most successful of these projects has been the 'Neuro-care Team' at Harold Wood Hospital, Romford, which started as a project involving just Parkinson's disease but has now been extended to include several other neuro-

logical conditions. This project uses a multidisciplinary approach to management, involving a consultant neurologist. It has a specific telling of the diagnosis, scripted by people with a neurological condition. There is early access to the therapists; continuity of care provided by the identification of a key worker, and ongoing involvement of the patient and carer in the management of their care. (This project is discussed in more detail in Chapter 31.)

An alternative way of fulfilling the five principles is through the employment of nurse specialists in Parkinson's disease, either attached to clinics or working in the community. Previously, the Society has pump-primed two specialist nurse practitioners, one attached to the apomorphine clinic at the Middlesex Hospital in London and one at the National Hospital in London. More recently, the Parkinson's Disease Society has been involved in a nurse specialist project which finished in January 1997, involving a team of nurses working in hospitals and the community to support people with Parkinson's disease and their carers, linking them into the appropriate services and helping consultants to set up Parkinson's disease clinics. The interest in this project and the demand for the services of the nurses has been enormous. An evaluation of the project will be published in mid 1997. Another project based in Southampton, funded by the Society, showed the benefits of providing a local and integrated home-based service for elderly people with Parkinson's disease and other related chronic neurological conditions. This involved a nurse working in a role analogous with that of a community psychiatric nurse and a community occupational therapist. There have also been several welfare projects looking at rehabilitation issues, including the development of a care-users' assessment centre in Newcastle to help anyone with a disability with driving and mobility problems. This project was taken over by the Regional Health Authority in 1991.

Help for carers has been another focus of the Welfare research programme. Some projects have focused on gaining a greater understanding of the needs of carers, such as the project based at Addenbrookes Hospital, which has studied the impact of caring on the carer. We have also funded research at the National Children's Bureau looking at the needs of children who have a parent with Parkinson's disease. As a result of this research, the Society has produced a number of booklets for young carers.

Respite care is also very important for the well-being of carers. Some welfare projects have focused on this issue. A rehabilitation flat was set up at Chesterton Hospital in Cambridge to try and provide an alternative form of respite care. Many carers expressed reluctance to be separated from their partners, despite the need for respite care. The idea of the flat was to allow the carer and the person with Parkinson's disease to go together with individual care packages drawn up by the flat co-ordinator so that the carer can have a break. Opportunities were also available for the needs of both people to be assessed. This model of good practice is now being developed in other areas, most recently in Inverness.

Another response the Parkinson's Disease Society has made is to the needs of people with chronic neurological conditions who come from an ethnic minority background. This has been a response to both lay and professional needs, as several doctors expressed their concerns that they often saw patients who came from an ethnic minority background once for an initial diagnosis and then never again. They were concerned that these people were not receiving the care they needed to ensure quality of life. As this was a need common to several neurological conditions, four groups representing people with Parkinson's disease, Huntingdon's disease, motor neurone disease, and multiple sclerosis set up a joint project, with funding from the Department of Health, to look at the needs of people from ethnic minority groups who have a neurological condition. This initiative, which is now funded by Birmingham Social Services, involves two information workers who are themselves from ethnic minority backgrounds researching the needs of people with chronic illness from these backgrounds and offering them support. One of the main needs they have identified, is the need for information in appropriate languages, and have already developed booklets in Urdu, Punjabi, and Cantonese. Cassette tapes are also available in the first two languages and they have recently received a grant from the Department of Health to produce videos in several different languages.

MEDICAL RESEARCH

Research is at the forefront of most lay societies. The government is cutting back on the funding of medical research and researchers rely more and more on voluntary organizations for funding. The ARMC estimate that 85% of all medical research in this country is funded by charities and charitable trusts. Much of the understanding gained and progress made in research into neurological conditions and the treatments available to treat people who have them, would not have been possible without the support of lay societies. Not only in financial ways, but also through helping to find volunteers for clinical trials. The Parkinson's Disease Society is often approached by researchers requiring help from branches and members for their research projects. Lay societies can also help focus the research by co-ordinating and facilitating communication between researchers working on a specific condition, and in turn relaying this information to the lay person.

The Parkinson's Disease Society's medical research programme, is governed by a medical advisory panel, consisting of eminent doctors and researchers interested in Parkinson's disease. The aims of the programme is to gain greater understanding of the processes of the body involved in Parkinson's disease, in the hope that this may lead to the identification of the cause of this disease and subsequently the cure. Medical research also tries to identify new treatments for Parkinson's disease and also improve existing ones. The search for the cause has concentrated on possible environmental causes and

the possibility of a genetic susceptibility which may predispose certain people to the disease. Treatments have focused on new and improved drugs and surgical techniques such as the brain implants using fetal tissue and pallidotomy, a form of stereotactic surgery.

The Society has a Brain Research Centre situated at the Institute of Neurology in London. Tissue is donated for use after death in a similar way to most tissue and organ transplantation schemes. The Brain Bank is a major internationally renown research establishment for Parkinson's disease and much of our understanding of the nature of Parkinson's disease has come from the work which it does.

Lay societies can also prompt research, through listening to their client group and passing on areas of particular concern or of possible research interest to researchers. For instance, the Parkinson's Disease Society has identified the tremendous problems women with Parkinson's disease can experience with menstruation and gynaecological problems and have interested medical researchers in doing some work in this area.

WORKING WITH GOVERNMENT AND OTHER VOLUNTARY ORGANIZATIONS

Lay societies obviously have a lobbying role to play in representing the needs of their client group to government and statutory bodies. This can involve making representation to government on particular issues such as prescription charges or more generally by serving on government committees and advisory groups nationally and also locally through community health councils, etc. Working with other voluntary organizations is also an important factor in the effectiveness of a lay society, particularly in forging good partnerships with government and statutory bodies and seeking to influence government policy. When you take away the specific nature and problems of particular conditions, there are often many areas of common need and by combining forces, organizations can have a stronger voice and greater lobbying power.

The Neurological Charities Group is an umbrella group, consisting of 25 neurological organizations, launched at the House of Commons in February 1994. It has been set up to explore areas of common need and to develop combined responses to government policy. The Community Care legislations have brought great changes which are of concern to all the charities, especially those who are concerned with chronic neurological conditions. The Neurological Charities Group have drawn up a set of standards for services for quality of life when living with a neurological condition. This document seeks to address the 'insufficient recognition of the needs of 1.5 million people in the United Kingdom affected by neurological conditions' (1). The Group feel that standards are needed to ensure appropriate care services are considered and provided for people affected by neurological conditions. Many people do not receive appropriate health or social care services, but are forced to accept assumed solutions in response to their needs. This inhibits the right to maintain independence and achieve quality of life. Having the right package is the most appropriate and cost-effective way of giving care. The standards also seek to address the question of limited resources and the fact that provision varies between health districts and across local authority boundaries. This variation, against the right for all to receive a high standard of health and social care, necessitates an accepted national standard ensuring equity within Health and Social Care Service Provision. Existing resources must be utilized for their optimum effectiveness and service provision established according to need. This document and the work of the Neurological Charities Group has received considerable interest from government, the National Health Service Management Executive, and professionals involved in community care changes.

European legislation and issues is another area of concern to neurological organizations. In common with many neurological organizations, the Parkinson's Disease Society has collaborated with its sister organizations across Europe and formed European Parkinson's Disease Association. The aims of the Association are:

1. To distribute information and exchange experiences on all problems associated with Parkinson's disease and arising from it, in particular by organizing meetings and publishing advisory information and news material.

2. To co-ordinate and support all efforts to develop, establish, and provide basic standards in Parkinson's disease for the care and rehabilitation of patients and their carers involving all measures aimed at ensuring the highest possible quality of life. Every effort must be made to minimize the burden on the patient, family and carers by, for example:
(a) collecting and evaluating experience,
(b) co-operating with medical and nursing associations, health administrations, and government, including other organizations in Europe,
(c) promoting co-operation amongst scientific and other professional groups which contribute to the advancement of health in Parkinson's disease,
(d) promoting and encouraging research in the field of Parkinson's disease.

3. To motivate, support, and promote new national Parkinson's disease associations and existing national Parkinson's disease associations, whose priorities should include:
(a) arranging social and psychological help for all Parkinson's disease patients and their carers in each country by meeting with Parkinson's disease patients and carers from each country, and encouraging exchange of experiences,
(b) working towards optimal care and rehabilitation conditions on a national/regional basis.

The European Parkinson's Disease Association has been successful in obtaining funding from European sources to develop a number of initiatives to benefit all European people living with Parkinson's disease and there has been a great deal of interest in their activities from international sources.

EMPOWERMENT OF THE INDIVIDUAL

Empowerment of the individual is an important part of any self-help group. To feel involved and in control of your life with a chronic illness helps to keep self-esteem high. Local support groups play an important part in allowing people to be involved as well as providing them with opportunities to meet other people and share ideas. Knowledge of local services is very important and local self-help groups can provide this knowledge and often also provide welfare visitors to visit people in their home and supplement the work of the national welfare section. Local support groups also allow people to lobby for their own needs in their local areas and to promote the cause of Parkinson's disease locally.

The Society has also responded to the needs of younger people with Parkinson's disease and their carers, an often unrecognized and neglected group, through the development of a special interest group called the YAPP&RS (Young Alert Parkinson's Partners and Relatives). The YAPP&RS is run by people with Parkinson's disease and their carers and has an important part to play in giving them a voice. They have their own magazine, regional groups, a computer bulletin board, and a national conference every two years. They have been greatly instrumental in raising the profile and understanding of younger people with Parkinson's. Many other neurological charities have similar groups for younger people.

FUNDRAISING AND PUBLIC RELATIONS

Fundraising and public relations work are also a very important part of any lay society's work. Without the fundraising which voluntary organizations do, many services and vital research to improve care for people with Parkinson's disease and their carers would not be possible. Public awareness is important in order to help understanding of Parkinson's disease and to allow people a place in society. However, many lay organizations face a dilemma when mounting awareness campaigns, as it can be difficult to strike a happy medium between the need to raise funds, which is often more successful using shock tactics than through positive images, against the concern not to distress newly diagnosed people and others affected by the condition, in the general public.

CONCLUSION

As can be seen from the work of the Parkinson's Disease Society, lay societies have a vital role to play in the lives of people with neurological conditions and their families and an equally important one in liaising with and supporting professionals involved in their care. Unfortunately, all too often lay societies are viewed with suspicion or seen as being in competition with professionals or making the lay person too powerful, as this story from one of the magazines produced by the younger parkinsonians illustrates:

When I was in hospital recently and the neurologist did his first round after I was admitted and asked how I was, I replied that the dyskinesia was not as bad, but the festination was no different. He looked down at me and thundered: 'I do not like laymen quoting medical terms to me' (2).

Early referral to lay societies can be beneficial to all. Although some people may not want contact until they are ready, if they have the information they can choose when and if they want involvement. Unfortunately, professionals often make this choice for them, telling them they do not want to get involved with a lay society or simply by omitting to tell them that there is a society. Surely it is every professional's responsibility to ensure that their patients have information and access to relevant lay organizations as the choice of involvement should be the patient's. There are also tremendous benefits for the professional if they choose to make links with lay societies and it is only by working with one another that the greatest benefit to the person with a neurological condition can be achieved.

REFERENCES

1. *Living with a neurological condition: Standards of services for quality of life by the neurological charities*, September 1992, updated 1996.
2. *YapMag*, published by the YAPP&RS, Parkinson's Disease Society, London, December 1993.

Organizing neurology outpatient services

David L. Stevens

In the waiting room, the floor paint was peeling, the high panelled walls were a dirty olive colour and the large slatted benches did not provide enough space for all the patients who had come from far off.

Neurologists, like other hospital-based clinicians, routinely see patients in the outpatient department and, like our colleagues in other disciplines, we take it for granted that this is how we should deliver a service to the patients who need our help. It is a traditional way of providing a specialist service, so we convince ourselves that it is effective and appropriate. Only rarely do we stand back to have a long hard look at how this system works and hardly ever do we ask what it is like for the patients and what we really think of it ourselves.

Before going more deeply into such matters, I must acknowledge that this is not the first chapter on outpatient services in neurology that has begun with the quotation given above. It is not, as some of you might have suspected, a description of the waiting room in an outpatient clinic in a National Health Service (NHS) hospital, but a fictional account of outpatients in the book, *Cancer ward*, by Alexander Solzhenitsyn. Louis Caplan (1990) used the same quotation in his book *The effective clinical neurologist*, when he described the neurology outpatient services that are available in North America. He compared and contrasted the office-based system with the outpatient clinic and came down so firmly in favour of the former, that he was moved to write that 'clinics are ineffective, probably immoral and should be discontinued'. Those of us who generally use more temperate language, may feel that he is overexaggerating in saying this, but he could be right.

I am sure that traditional outpatient clinics survive in this country because they are the most economical method of juxtaposing a large number of patients with small numbers of skilled specialist doctors. I know of no evidence that suggests that outpatient clinics are still in general use because an enthusiastic public has deemed them irreplaceable and I have never heard any doctors argue that outpatient clinics are so enjoyable and effective that their replacement with some other technique would be regretted.

Before discussing this service in more detail, I feel that a few general comments are appropriate on why we work the way we do and why, in particular, we are, to a greater or lesser extent, the slaves of the outpatient system. At the very heart of the issue is the timetable, the creation of which is a vital part of the design of a new consultant post. It contains all sorts of details about where he or she[1] will be at 9 a.m. on Tuesday and 2 p.m. on Thursday and similar matters. Before an appointment is made this timetable has to be approved by a multitude of individuals, the majority of whom will not be involved in any way in the working of the post once the new consultant has started.

One of the central issues in timetable design is that scarce resources, both space and manpower, must be allocated to the new appointee. It appears to be the norm that there is never enough money and there are always too few facilities and people available to help the new consultant to do his job. Indeed, it is almost the rule that prior to the appointment of a new specialist, the moneys allocated for the purchase of supporting junior staff are withdrawn to reduce the cost of the appointment. The result of these constraints is that timetables and job descriptions are designed around the money, facilities, and manpower that are available and not according to an abstract concept of how best the task ahead could be done by the new appointee. Thus, the final design of a post is often an uneasy compromise between what would be best in an ideal world and what is actually possible. I am sure that the perpetuation of the traditional outpatient service has much to do with this central problem of inadequate resources, facilities, and staff. When resources are scarce and space in the outpatient department is limited, it is easier to carry on doing more-or-less what has always been done, than it is to try and break new ground and to encourage different methods.

Is there anybody that can remember being told that, when appointed as a consultant in the United Kingdom, as long as they met the targets of numbers of out- and inpatients, they could do their job in any way that they wished? I very much doubt it. Ask a version of that question of your friends in senior positions in industry or commerce (or even in health service management) and I suspect that many would say that that is precisely what was said to them when they were appointed. They were given a job to do, not a timetable. They were given the facilities and told to get on with it. Out there in the market place they are judged by results and they are not, in general, judged by whether they turn up here at 9 a.m. on Mondays and there at 2 p.m. on Tuesdays and so on.

[1] To avoid endlessly creating clumsy, but politically correct sentences: 'he' equals 'he/she', 'him' equals 'him/her', etc.

I believe that, without a lot of extravagance, there are ways in which the system can be changed and I will return to them at the end of this chapter.

THE OUTPATIENT DEPARTMENT

Next time you go to your own outpatient department, have a look around. Imagine that you are a patient with a neurological illness and that you are entering the building for the first time. (Even better, imagine that you are a foreign patient who, at home, is used to something a little different.) Is it a bright cheerful place? Are the decorations pleasing to the eye? Do the seats look comfortable and are there enough of them? Does the place have a pleasant welcoming aspect? Indeed, does it look like the smart waiting rooms found in the offices of accountants, solicitors, or other businesses in your town?

I suspect not. Instead, it will probably have a run-down institutional look, it will need decorating, the seats will be in rows and they will probably be hard and uncomfortable. It is also likely that the only decorations on the walls will be pieces of paper, stuck there with sellotape, giving naïve messages, in childlike writing, about AIDs and head lice and diabetic feet? Not as awful as the Solzhenitsyn example, but along those lines.

What of the consulting room? Is it a quiet peaceful place? Are the furnishings and decorations modern and pleasing to the eye? Are the chairs for the patient and his relatives comfortable? Is there privacy or do people keep walking in and out? Does the phone keep ringing and are there other interruptions? Ask yourself if this is the sort of environment in which you would feel comfortable answering questions about intensely personal aspects of your life? Does it resemble the place where you do your private practice or, if you don't do private practice, then the sort of place where you imagine that private practice goes on?

And then the consultation. Again, try and imagine that you are a patient, with symptoms that are to you mysterious and frightening. Having seen your family doctor initially, did you know that the person you were to see was a neurologist and do you know what a neurologist does? Did you have to wait for months for your appointment and have you had to wait for ages in the waiting room? When you get to see the doctor, is he the consultant or one of his assistants? Indeed, do you actually see the person whose name appears on your appointment card? When giving your story, did you have enough time to tell it in your own way, or were you under the impression that you were being rushed? Did the thought occur to you that you had better hurry up anyway, because there did seem to be an awful lot of people in the waiting room? Did the doctor appear to have time to really go into your story in as much detail as you wished and did you have time to ask him all those questions about the thing the lady down the road said about her friend who had numbness, 'just like yours. . .' and who died. Were you able to ask about the multiple sclerosis and

motor neurone disease that you have read about and all the other dreadful things that have kept you awake at night with worry?

The real question is: if you were ill with a neurological condition, would you like to receive your outpatient care in your own outpatient clinic? Would you like to wait for months for an appointment, sit for ages in that waiting room and reveal all your worries and anxieties in that consulting room? Would you want more time with the doctor—yourself? Would you be happy with the lightning fast production line medicine that you yourself probably deliver day in and day out? I suspect that most of us, if we are really honest, would have to answer in the negative to all these questions. In doing so, we are not calling our own sensitivity or expertise into question; instead, we are questioning the system that we are required to use when delivering cheap mass medical care to others.

WAITING LISTS

INTRODUCTION

Before we discuss the outpatient session and what goes on there, it is logical to look at what the patient experiences first, namely, the waiting list. An outpatient waiting list is made up of people who are waiting until it is their turn to attend an appointment in the outpatient department. By and large, neurologists in the United Kingdom have fairly long waiting lists. We tend to take waiting lists for granted and, in doing so, we fail to ask why we should have them in the first place. They do not have them everywhere, so why do we have them in Britain? The answer is obvious, but a brief review of the reasons why they come about is worthwhile.

Imagine that a new consultant is appointed to a particular area and that when he starts work there is no waiting list. This new consultant decides early on how many patients could be seen in the outpatient clinics that he is scheduled to hold in an average week. If the number of referrals exactly matches the number that he can see in a particular time period, then no waiting list accumulates. However, sometimes he goes on holiday and sometimes he has to miss a clinic for another reason. During these periods, the referrals continue to come in. So a waiting list starts. Increasing the numbers seen per clinic may control this situation, but there is a limit as to how much this technique can be used. If consistently more referrals come in each week than he is able to see in a week, then inevitably a waiting list will appear. Eventually, when the list becomes inordinately long, those who make referrals modify their thresholds of referral and the waiting time stabilizes. At a later date, should the waiting time fall for one reason or another, then more liberal referral habits resurface and the cycle repeats itself. I will give some evidence to illustrate the dynamics of this situation a little later.

I think it is fair to say that consultants do not deliberately create waiting lists for themselves. Instead, I believe that they accumulate because of a mismatch between the work that can be done and that which is demanded in a given time period. This is not a perception that is universally shared and there are some who express, somewhat provocatively, the view that waiting lists are created and deliberately exploited by some consultants (Yates 1987). I find it hard to believe that in neurology this is a significant issue. Instead, I believe that neurology waiting lists exist because more work is demanded of the neurologists than they can deliver.

Neurology waiting lists vary from place to place, even within the United Kingdom and, in general, the fewer neurologists in the area, the longer the waiting lists and vice versa. Countries that have a greater number of neurologists per unit population, than in the United Kingdom (e.g. United States, Canada, and most of the countries in Europe), do not have the neurology waiting list problems that we have here So, long neurology waiting lists mean that there are not enough neurologists. This is not exactly a revolutionary conclusion.

Despite this rather obvious conclusion, there is, nevertheless, a curious and somewhat irritating tradition in this country, which regards the waiting list as in some way the sole property and, therefore, responsibility of the relevant clinicians, even if he is the only representative of his discipline for a huge population. I believe that this is wrong and, instead believe that the waiting list, using current NHS terminology, is not the property of the provider of health care, but instead it belongs to the purchaser of health care, the local health authority. Clearly, it is reasonable, up to a point, to expect an individual clinician to do his best to keep the waiting lists short, but beyond that point it must be the responsibility of those who purchase hospital services to do one of two things in order to keep waiting lists down: either they must influence referral habits or they must buy more doctors.

In 1990, the British Department of Health published a document, known as the Patient's Charter, which requires, among other things, that nobody should have to wait more than 13 weeks for an outpatient appointment at a hospital. This instruction has led local purchasers to inspect the waiting lists in their area and to pay for new consultants in the specialities that have the longest lists. I believe that it is not a coincidence that there has been an extraordinary flood of new consultant neurologist appointments in this country since the publication of the Patient's Charter. In the south-west of England, where I work, there were, up to 1990, 10 neurologists serving a population of about 3.7 million and each of those had long waiting lists for outpatient appointments. Since 1990, there have been 8 new appointments in this relatively small geographical area and at the time of writing three more are being considered, so that by the end of 1998 there could be 21 of us. Neurologists who worked alone for up to 20 years (I am one of them) and who spent much of that time asking for a colleague, have finally been rewarded. I am sure that the waiting list argument has played an important part in the creation of these new appointments. There have been so many new consultant neurologist posts advertised, that it can truly be said that the Patient's Charter has not only caused an improvement in neurological services in the country, but it has also had an interesting impact on the career prospects for young trainee neurologists. None of this can be bad.

PAYING ATTENTION TO WAITING LISTS

Despite the fact that we now have more neurologists than ever before, the total number is still so small that the waiting list problem is not going to go away. This being so, I feel that some of the results of experiments that I have conducted over the years, might be of interest to other neurologists who are struggling to keep their waiting lists under control.

I have kept data on the waiting time for neurology outpatient appointments since I was appointed in 1973 and at intervals have introduced changes in practice to try and reduce the length of time people have to wait for appointments. No single manoeuvre, or combination of manoeuvres, has had a consistent or long-term effect on waiting times and some have actually had a deleterious effect.

WHAT IS THE STRUCTURE OF THE WAITING LIST?

Superficially, it seems asinine to ask about the structure of the waiting list, but this is not the case. Not all patients will wait for the maximum length of time. Politicians and health service administrators are obsessed with this maximum waiting time and it is this figure that looms large in the Patient's Charter. However, many people do not wait very long. I have not analysed this phenomenon very often, but I reviewed my 1986 figures, so that I could try and understand the dynamics of the situation.

Basically, the distribution of waiting times is trimodal. There are patients who are seen very quickly, mainly those where the referring doctor marks the letter 'urgent' and the contents make it clear that the problem is indeed urgent. Patients with papilloedema, those with newly acquired and progressive hemipareses, and others with obviously important and threatening disorders are seen at once or within a few days. Many patients in this category are referred by telephone or facsimile messages, rather than by letter. Others, where again the letter may be marked 'urgent', but where the contents indicate that the problem is not really that urgent, are seen within six to eight weeks. There are some family doctors who use the 'urgent' request rather liberally, my most extravagant example to date being an urgent paraesthesiae of the tip of one finger—extraordinary, but true. Urgent faint feelings and urgent tension headache are commonplace. These are the problems that get put into the 'soonish', rather than the urgent category. The important point here is that it is necessary to read the referral letters as they arrive in order to establish the true urgency of the problems. It is not enough to leave this to the departmental secretaries or to the clerks in the records department. I do this every day and make decisions concerning urgency on the basis of the contents of the letter and not simply because it has the word URGENT stamped in large red letters on each corner. The remainder of the patients are classified as non-urgent and they are allocated the next available space at the end of the waiting list.

ALLOCATING APPOINTMENTS

For this system to work requires an adequate supply of urgent and 'soon' appointments and it is virtually impossible to get this right. I used to allocate 50% of all appointments for such patients, but after a while that didn't work, because more and more letters were marked as 'urgent'. The appointments were rapidly filled and the 6–8 week appointments started to become 10–12 week appointments instead. Now we allocate about two-thirds of all appointments for such patients and even that does not work. Since 1990, we have had a registrar working in the department and a registrar urgent clinic has been introduced, so that patients who are seriously urgent can be seen within three working days. This is a good system, although it too is beginning to lose its effectiveness, for the urgent tension headaches are creeping in. Nevertheless, it does work fairly well and I understand that it is effective in the other centres where registrars or senior registrars offer a similar service.

WAYS OF INFLUENCING THE WAITING LIST

More patients per session

The simplest manoeuvre, if a waiting list starts to build up, is to include a few more new patients into existing clinics. The price that is paid for doing this, is that the time per patient is less. Up to a point, this is acceptable, but beyond that point it is not. We are now living in an era when patients increasingly expect to be given more time rather than less. Quite rightly, they want time to describe their symptoms, to hear about the management of their illness, and to ask questions. The Patient's Charter gives them these rights. They will not be satisfied if the time allocated is reduced. (The issue of how much time should be allocated to a new patient is discussed on pp. 69–71.)

Editing the follow-up list

After a while, a follow-up list starts to accumulate, this being made up of patients who are being regularly reviewed (see pp. 471–2). Slowly but surely, the amount of available clinic time becomes saturated. At this stage it is reasonable to review policies and to reduce the size of the follow-up component of the clinic, in order to make more spaces for new patients. This manoeuvre often involves discharging patients with complex and difficult disorders, in order to make spaces for more new patients with dizzy turns or tension headaches. That seems wrong, but it can happen.

Lengthening the session

Another strategy is to allow the clinics to go on for longer. There must be few neurologists in this country who do not smile wryly when reminded that an NHS session is considered to be a mere three and a half hours. Four and a half-or five hour-long outpatient sessions are commonplace, although with clinics like this, one wonders whether the real object of the exercise is for the staff to survive to the end, rather than for them to really make people better.

More pairs of hands

Eventually, the system becomes fully saturated and all the beneficial effects of the changes are cancelled out. At this stage it is reasonable to bring in additional pairs of hands to those already available from the consultant and (if he has one) his team of junior doctors. There is a custom in this country to employ general practitioners (GPs), in the capacity of clinical assistants or hospital practitioners, to function as extra pairs of hands in outpatient clinics. In a given geographical area there will be few, if any GPs, who have been sufficiently trained in neurology that they are likely to be really useful in the clinic, but there are some and they can help a lot. It has to be said, however, that it is a strange sort of specialist service where GPs refer patients to a specialist clinic, only for the specialist advice to come back to them from another GP. Persuading hospital administrators to pay for such clinical assistant sessions is difficult and often unsuccessful.

WHAT HAPPENS?

Some numerical illustrations

So far, all of these manoeuvres have been designed to be tried within the conventional outpatient sessions. I tried them all and the waiting lists carried on growing. These techniques can be regarded as sensible efforts to use the time available to best effect. Eventually, I came to recognize that none of them really work, although the numbers of patients seen per year rose steadily. What I am able to do here, is to illustrate some of this with numerical data. The figures refer exclusively to my outpatient service at Gloucester, which is one of the places where I work. They do not include specialist neurophysiology clinics, other clinics done elsewhere and, obviously, they do not refer to private practice. At Gloucester, I do two regular outpatient clinics a week, and in these two clinics in 1974 and 1975, I saw approximately 350 new patients and between 700 and 800 follow-up patients each year. By using some, but not all of the techniques described above, the numbers rose to 500 new patients and 2000 follow-up patients by 1980. In the same period the duration of the maximum waiting time increased from an average of 8–10 weeks in 1974 to about 22 weeks in 1980.

Extra clinics

The next possibility is to start seeing patients outside normal clinic hours. The problem here is in finding somewhere to hold the consultations. Seeing outpatients on the ward is something that I am sure all of us have tried, but I only used this technique for a very short period. The ward is there for other reasons and it is simply not the right environment for outpatient activities. It does not work. I gave it up.

In 1982, I was able to persuade the hospital authorities in Gloucester to convert an old wooden building on the hospital site into a small neurology department, with offices for doctors and secretaries and with two examining rooms. This enabled us to do extra clinics outside normal outpatient times. Some of these were short sessions with only one patient attending, but some were bigger, with up to eight or more new patients. By the late 1980s we were doing between 30 and 40 such sessions a year and seeing between 80 and 120 extra new patients a year as a result. During the same period, we reduced the intensity of the conventional outpatients to averages of 450–470 new patients and 1400–1500 follow-up patients a year. The effect of this change was to make the conventional clinics more civilized, at least in part because we reduced the follow-up load. At this stage we were seeing about 550 new and 1500 follow-up patients in approximately 130 sessions a year, 98 being routine clinics and 30 or so extra clinics. In 1980–1, before the new offices were opened, the average maximum waiting time was about 22 weeks. By the late 1980s it had risen to 28–30 weeks. So this did not work either.

Have a 'blitz'

There is another technique and this one is much beloved by ministers and people who like to get in the newspapers to show the world that they are grappling with the waiting list problem. The 'blitz'. In the first week of July 1985, at a time when the maximum waiting time at Gloucester was 22–24 weeks, we saw 64 new patients in one week and succeeded in reducing the waiting time to 11–12 weeks. During the 12 months prior to the blitz we had seen 487 new patients at this hospital. During the 12 months after the blitz we saw 654 new patients (including the 64 seen during the blitz) at the same hospital. From a maximum waiting time of 11–12 weeks after the blitz in mid 1985, it rose to 30 weeks by the summer of 1986. I have calculated that the publication of the shorter waiting times led GPs to increase their referral rates by 50%.

So much for waiting list initiatives. One really has to be very cynical about the money that is annually made available for waiting list initiatives in this country, for the evidence that it does anything other than to produce a short-term solution to the waiting list problem is minimal. One wonders if the only real benefit of this piecemeal activity is that it produces a brief spell of political advantage for those who instigated the initiative in the first place. It certainly does not provide any long-term good.

Get a registrar

In January 1990 a registrar was appointed to work with me. Before then we only had a senior house officer. The addition of an extra pair of skilled hands allowed us to do more extra clinics, including the 'urgent clinic' mentioned already. The 1993 figures indicate that at Gloucester we were seeing about 650 new and 2000 follow-up patients in 175 separate consultation sessions in the clinics, in addition to those seen elsewhere. At the end of 1993 the maximum waiting time was 20 weeks. So even having a registrar did not solve the problem.

Get another consultant neurologist

What else is there to try? Another consultant neurologist. I asked for one of those for more years than I care to remember. As a part of the 'Oh dear look at those waiting lists' Patient's Charter business a second neurologist was appointed and since February 1994 we have tried the two neurologists technique. Rather cynically, or so it seemed at the time, I indicated that rumour had it that there would be a brief honeymoon, during which the waiting list would fall for about a year and then would again rise. That prediction was correct. Down went the waiting lists and after a year they started to rise and they are now worse than they have ever been, except that now we have two of them not one.

THE CLINIC SESSION

The next topic to discuss is the outpatient session itself. The patient has survived the waiting list and now he attends the clinic. The dynamics of the outpatient session are complex and, when attempting to define what goes on during the session, it is necessary to take account of the type of clinic as well as the seniority and number of the doctors who will be attending.

Before going into details, I would like to mention a small survey that I conducted in the autumn of 1993 of my consultant neurologist colleagues in south-west England. This survey was performed exclusively to enable me to write this chapter and its main purpose was to prevent me from basing all my opinions on facts gleaned from an analysis of my own work. I felt that it would be more useful to look at a wider range of neurological practices, in the hope that my conclusions would be more representative. Fortunately, the figures that have emerged from the survey of my colleagues have revealed that, while we vary quite a lot in how we work, none of us, including myself, have emerged as so different from the average that we can be truly regarded as unrepresentative. Because I have been able to look at the work of a reasonable sample of consultant neurologists, I hope that what has emerged may be fairly representative of what happens elsewhere in the United Kingdom.

At the time when I surveyed them, there were 14 consultant neurologists in south-west England: 2 in Cornwall, 4 in Devon, 1 in Somerset, 4 in Avon (Bristol and surrounding area), 1 in Gloucestershire (myself), and 2 who serve the northern part of Wiltshire and who are based in Bath. These

14 Consultants serve a total population of about 3 700 000, which gives a ratio of neurologists to population of about 1:264 000. There is a wide variation within this large area, for the biggest population per neurologist (1:530 000) is in Gloucestershire, where I was working on my own at the time when the survey was done. The smallest average population per neurologist is in Avon, where the value is 1:205 000.

NUMBER OF SESSIONS PER WEEK

The survey revealed that the 14 consultant neurologists hold between them a total of 69 different types of clinic. Some of these are not performed every week, so the weekly average is 58.5 clinic sessions, which gives an overall average of 4.2 each. The actual numbers of outpatient sessions per week per consultant varies from 3 to 5. Here it is worth noting that the Association of British Neurologists (ABN), in a document, published in 1993, entitled 'Good neurological practice: with particular reference to job plans for consultant neurologists in the UK' (ABN 1993*a*), recommended that the timetable for a consultant neurologist should contain no more than three fixed outpatient sessions each week, although it was acknowledged that some neurologists could choose to do more. So, in common with most British neurologists, our south-western consultants are doing more clinics than is considered ideal by their professional body.

TYPES OF OUTPATIENT CLINIC

Of the total of 69 clinics performed by these neurologists, 49 are routine sessions and 20 are specialized clinics. Two of the neurologists have urgent appointment clinics and in both instances these are conducted by the registrar. Eight provide a neurophysiology service and they do clinics, not necessarily every week, at which they perform electromyography (EMG) and nerve conduction studies. Many of these neurologists also provide the only service in their area for the interpretation of electroencephalograms (EEGs) and evoked response studies. They do this because in the 3.7 million population in the area that we are discussing, there are only three consultant clinical neurophysiologists. Some of the neurologists have other types of specialized clinics. Two have regular epilepsy clinics, three hold botulinum toxin clinics, two have disability or rehabilitation clinics, one does a movement disorder clinic, and one takes part in a neuro-ophthalmology clinic. In general, these specialized clinics do not take place every week. One interesting observation on this topic is that most of these specialized clinics are held by neurologists in district general hospitals and they are not exclusive to those working at the teaching centre in Bristol.

Specialist clinics

At this point it is worth asking why specialised clinics are held at all and whether they really serve a useful purpose. In general, they are introduced because the neurologist has a particular interest in a certain type of neurological disease. Clearly, certain clinics, such as the EMG clinics described above, are introduced because there is a defined need for the service. That is not always the case and it is a little difficult to justify some of the other types of specialized clinic. The two neurologists who hold epilepsy clinics argue that the care given to their patients with epilepsy is better if the patients are all concentrated together and they support their case by arguing that certain features of the service, such as control of quality, educational activities, and the presence of a clinical psychologist can be more readily organized if all the patients are gathered together in a single clinic. Whether the patients truly benefit from these additional services and activities is not known, but the instinctive rather than the scientific answer is that they do. The same comments can be made about movement disorder clinics and other specialized clinics. This may be a topic where the auditing of these services could come up with some useful answers.

Of all the specialized clinics that involve neurologists, the easiest to discuss is the botulinum toxin clinic. Such clinics can be justified on simple economic grounds. The ampoules of the toxin are very expensive, so it is logical that several patients should attend a single session, to ensure that the best possible use is made of a costly substance. Because the toxin is expensive, the clinic will also be expensive and, because the treatment of an individual patient must be continued for many years, it is imperative that the economic implications of the service are worked out at the very beginning and that plans are agreed with the hospital administration to ensure that enough funds will be available on a regular basis for the service to be continued indefinitely. If such an agreement is not forthcoming, then the service should not be started. I know of colleagues who have initiated such a service, only to have to withdraw it at a later date, because the hospital management would not agree to provide a regular source of finance for the toxin. That is not the way in which a specialized service should ever be organized and it must be said that in a civilized society it really is deplorable that such a thing should happen anyway.

DURATION OF THE CLINICS

The terms and conditions of service that apply to consultants in the NHS, lay down that a session of work has a duration of three and a half hours. Thus, if a consultant neurologist were to be in outpatients three times a week, as recommended by the ABN, then he should be doing that type of work for ten and a half hours a week. The reality is different. All of our south-western neurologists exceed this value, for the overall average is about 15 hours and two of them put in over 19 hours a week. These values come about because almost all of them do more than three sessions a week and individual session frequently last for four hours or more.

There are two ways in which this phenomenon can be interpreted. One view is that the ABN miscalculated and it is reasonable for neurologists to do more than ten and a half hours a week of outpatient work. The opposite view says that health authorities, by employing too few neurologists, are cynically demanding more than is reasonable from those neurologists and, thereby, are shamelessly capitalizing on the goodwill of the clinicians, who find themselves working excessive hours because they feel obliged to respond to the pressures generated by patients and other doctors.

I acknowledge that some of this is somewhat intemperate, but there may be an element of truth in this analysis, because what happens elsewhere is revealing. Robust data on neurological practice in other countries is hard to come by, but the 1981 report on *Medical practice in the United States*, which contains the results of a survey conducted by Mendenhall (1981), is illuminating. The survey looked at every type of physician, among which were 3630 neurologists. The average neurologist spent 2.2 hours a day performing office examinations and treatments and 0.2 hours a day conducting outpatient or clinic examinations. Thus, from Monday to Friday, 12 hours a week is allocated to this type of work. It must be noted that to compare directly this workload of an American neurologist with that of his English counterpart is somewhat unrealistic. Of the 14 neurologists that I have surveyed, almost all have a private practice (the equivalent of the North American office practice), as well as a NHS practice, and this adds to the amount of time spent each week in outpatient activities. I have not surveyed the private practice habits of my colleagues, but it is probable that most spend between three and eight hours a week doing private practice sessions. We know from the survey conducted by Hopkins *et al.* (1989) that 15% of all new patients seen by British neurologists are private patients, so the assumption is reasonable. All of this indicates that in the United Kingdom we do considerably more outpatient work than our United States counterparts.

Before leaving this American survey, there is another interesting statistic. The average amount of time the American neurologists admitted to working each day, which includes travelling time, is seven and a half hours. Most of us would have to have long memories to remember the last time our lives were ordered thus.

PAIRS OF HANDS IN THE OUTPATIENT CLINICS

Between them, the 14 south-western neurologists, conduct an average of 58 clinics of all types each week. Details of the numbers of doctors in these clinics is given in Table 35.1. Overall, 71% were done by the consultant on his own or with the help of one other doctor. Thus, in this part of England, the vast majority of outpatient work is done by the consultant neurologist and not by junior doctors.

One interesting statistic that emerged from this study was that, in general, the number of doctors in the clinic is inversely related to the age and seniority of the consultant neurologist

Table 35.1 The number of doctors working in neurology outpatient clinics, south-west England 1993 (figures for one average week)

No. of doctors	No. of clinics
One doctor only	
Consultant	27
Registrar	2
Total	29 (50%)
Two doctors: Consultant plus:	
Clinical assistant	4
Registrar	7
Senior house officer (SHO)	7
Total	18 (31%)
Three doctors: consultant plus:	
Senior registrar/SHO	1
Registrar/SHO	5
Registrar/Clinical assistant	1
Clinical assistant/SHO	1
Total	8 (14%)
Four doctors: consultant plus:	
Senior/registrar/SHO	2
Registrar/SHO/SHO	1
Total	3 (5%)
Overall total	58 (100%)

running the clinic. Thus, established consultants had junior doctors to help them, whereas newly appointed neurologists were far more likely to do their clinics on their own. It is quite possible that the consultants who have been appointed to new jobs in recent times are being asked to work without any support from junior staff because of the economic constraints that were discussed earlier.

NUMBER OF PATIENTS ATTENDING A CLINIC SESSION

There is an enormous variation in the number of patients that are seen per session and this is a function of the numbers of doctors in the clinic, the nature of the clinic (routine or specialized), and the mixture of old and new patients. The smallest possible clinic, which does not occupy a full three and a half hour session, is when a single patient is seen in an *ad-hoc* clinic. The biggest recorded number for a clinic held in the south-west is 48 follow-up patients in one of the epilepsy clinics. Because of this wide variation, it is pointless to attempt an overall summary, although some useful data can be squeezed out of this mass of figures.

Looking at routine clinics is fairly straightforward. Of the 51 routine and urgent clinics conducted by the south-western neurologists, 22 are done by the consultant working on his own. The numbers of patients varies somewhat, as different consultants tend to set up their clinics with different patterns of attendance of new and follow-up patients. For example, one consultant considers that six new patients is all that he can see in a session whereas, at the opposite extreme, another considers seven new and eight follow-up patients to be acceptable.

Presenting this data in a form that is easy to understand is difficult, but one way of looking at the situation is to argue that a follow-up patient uses one unit of consultation time and a new patient uses two such units. In reality this fairly accurate. The range of allocation of these units for consultants working on their own is from 12 to 22 per clinic, with an average of 16. To translate this into something that makes a little more sense, and to illustrate how this device works, 16 units means that the consultant can see 8 new patients, or 6 new and 4 follow-up, 4 new and 8 follow-up, and so on. These figures represent what the average consultant neurologist in south-west England feels that he can manage in a session when he is working on his own. The same type of analysis can be done for the more complex clinics at which there are other doctors present, and an attempt to summarize this is given in Table 35.2.

Certain conclusions can be drawn from these data and some are rather obvious. Others are less so. The more doctors and the more senior the doctors in the clinic, the more patients can be seen. The consultant neurologist on his own averages 16 units of consultation time per session, but when he is joined by a second doctor, an average of 10 more is added, giving a total of 26 units. A third doctor makes a modest difference, for a consultant plus two others adds a further 7 units

to give an average of 33 per clinic. Adding a fourth makes no difference, for the average does not change. From these figures it can be deduced that a consultant plus one junior doctor is the equivalent of approximately 1.5 consultants and a consultant plus two or three junior doctors is the equivalent of two consultants. They also reveal that there is little point in there being more than two other doctors helping the consultant. These data allow calculation of the average duration of one of these units and, thereby, the average duration of new and follow-up appointments in routine clinics. The mathematics is beautifully simple. The consultants recorded the average duration of each of the 22 clinics that they performed on their own and the total comes to 87.85 hours, giving the average duration of each session as 4 hours exactly. Because the average number of units allocated by these consultants is 16 per clinic, the value of one unit (a follow-up visit) is 15 minutes and for two units (a new patient visit) is 30 minutes. It almost appears that these numbers are too neat and tidy to be true, but this is really how the calculations worked out.

By using the same technique and rather crudely assuming that if the consultant who is working with other doctors in the clinic is seeing the same number as he would see on his own (which is probably false, because he will inevitably spend some time reviewing patients seen by the others), then the duration of the units for the other doctors can be calculated. If there is one other doctor helping, the duration of the clinic is longer, for the average works out at 4 hours and 25 minutes. The average allocation of units for such a clinic is 26, which means that the second doctor does 10 if the consultant does 16 (as he would if he were on his own). This gives a value for a junior doctor unit of 26.5 minutes—as near as makes no difference—30 minutes. So a follow-up patient takes almost 30 minutes on average and a new patient takes almost an hour. These values also fit the situation with the three doctor clinics, so there is a reasonable coherence to these data. These values are summarized in Table 35.3.

These figures can be used to make a number of important comparisons. In the United States, according to the survey by Mendenhall (1981), the average neurologist spends almost 30 minutes (28.5 minutes) on an ambulatory consultation. In an average week he sees 23 such patients, giving a total of 11.5 hours of work, which fits well with the overall estimate of outpatient time for such neurologists of 12 hours (discussed earlier). The classification of patient encounters described by

Table 35.2 Details of the number of appointments, expressed as units of consultation time (see text for details), for 51 different routine clinics performed by the neurologists in south-west England

No. of doctors	No. of clinics	Units of consultation time	
		Range	Average
One doctor			
Consultant	22	12–22	16
Registrar	2	8–11	10
Two doctors: consultant plus:			
Registrar	5	30–40	34
Senior House Officer (SHO)	7	16–26	20
Clinical Assistant	4	23–30	25
Average	16	16–40	26
Three doctors: consultant plus:			
Senior registrar/SHO	1		32
Registrar/SHO	5	21–40	33
Clinical assistant/Registrar	1		35
Clinical assistant/SHO	1		32
Average	8	21–40	33
Four doctors: consultant plus:			
Senior registrar/Registrar SHO	2	25–44	32
Registrar/SHO	1		28
Average	3	25–44	32

Table 35.3 Data showing the length of consultation in routine clinics for new and follow-up outpatients by neurologists in south-west England

	Average time spent per patient (min)	
	New	Follow-up
Consultant	30	15
Junior doctor, average	60	30

Mendenhall is somewhat complex, but our new patients appear to come under his categories of 'first encounters' and 'consultative encounters', which together make up 50% of the patients seen in an average week. This means that the average American neurologist sees 12 new and 11 follow-up outpatients a week. (Compare these numbers with the British figures below.) Employing the device, of allocating units to new and old patients, it can be calculated that the American neurologists spend 20 minutes on a follow-up patient and 40 minutes to a new patient. Menken (1989) reviewed the 1985 National Ambulatory Medical Care Survey, conducted by the United States Division of Health Care Statistics and noted that the average duration of new patient encounter was 43 minutes and a follow-up patient visit was 20 minutes. Thus, there is coherence here, although these analyses appear to be a little at variance with the comments made by Caplan (1990), who speaks of a new visit lasting an hour and who implies that this time allocation is commonplace. However, it is clear from these data that American neurologists allocate 33–43% more time to their patient encounters than we do.

One area of neurological practice in the United Kingdom that is generally obscured from us is private practice. Very little published data exists about this type of practice. Discussion with colleagues reveals that it is commonplace in this type of practice for new patients to be allocated 40–45 minutes and follow-up patients 20 minutes. So, British patients, if they are seen privately, get exactly the same amount of time as their American counterparts, but 33–43% more time than if they see the consultant at the hospital.

Finally, what of the ABN's (Association of British Neurologists) view on all of this? At a time when published data on this subject were not available (as it now is), the ABN published the job plans for neurologists document (1993*a*) and recommended that outpatients be allocated time according to the values in Table 35.4. The time allocation for consultants exactly matches the figures derived from the NHS work patterns of the south-western neurologists. However, the ABN only gives advice on the time allocation for senior registrars and registrars and does not acknowledge that more junior doctors frequently help in clinics. Indeed, of the 51 routine south-western clinics discussed earlier, 17 are attended by senior house officers, 14 by registrars, and only 3 by the solitary senior registrar in this part of the country. The figures derived from the south-western data suggest that, in general, junior doctors require rather more time than the ABN recommends.

Table 35.4 ABN recommendations on the allocation of time for seeing new and follow-up outpatients (see text)

	Average time per patient	
	New	Follow-up
Consultant	30	15
Senior registrar/Registrar	40	20

There are some final comments to make on this topic and they relate to the general question of how typical are these south-western figures when compared to the generality of neurologists elsewhere in the country. Some comparative statistics are helpful here. The 14 south-western neurologists see an average of 26 new patients a week in outpatients (range 17–37). The Services Committee of the ABN (1991), found that the weekly average number of new patients seen by the 33 Neurologists in their survey was 20, with a range of 9–32. The 13 Neurologists studied by Hopkins *et al.* (1989) saw an average of 30 new patients a week (range 15–50), of whom 18 were NHS outpatients. Thus, if all of these data are accurate, the south-western neurologists are seeing more new patients each week than the other samples that have been studied. The differences are not great, but they are worth noting.

The reason for rather labouring the point in the previous paragraph is that there is another style of neurological practice, which has a very different tempo from that defined here. Some neurologists see huge numbers of patients each week and they apparently work at lightning speed. This means that they give each patient a very small amount of time. Understandably, they think that this is how everyone else practices and I have even heard some of them give the impression that they think that this is how we should all practice. We do not have any of these high-speed practitioners in the south-west, which suggests that this style of practice is pursued by a minority of consultant neurologists in this country. I have to admit that I am not comfortable with this approach and I suspect that the average patient would share my opinion, for one gets the impression that patients want more than just a diagnosis and some treatment; they want time to explain things, time to ask questions, and time to discuss the future. To deny them this facility, because you believe that a real man should see half the county by lunchtime, is to deny them an important part of a consultation with an expert.

THE FOLLOW-UP CLINIC

This is a very difficult topic and it is easy to have an attitude on this subject. There is a wide spectrum of views. At one end of this spectrum of opinion is the argument that neurologists are there to find out what is the matter with people, decide on a plan of management, and then pass the patient back to the referring doctor. This approach leads to very small follow-up clinics. The view from the other extreme is that neurological diseases are often unpleasant and complicated and that it is best for an expert (the neurologist) to keep an eye on certain patients. This approach leads to large follow-up clinics. There is no right answer, although all consultant neurologists will have their own opinion and consequently, their own system.

Examination of the habits of the south-western neurologists is illuminating. For the 14 Consultants, the numbers seen as follow-up patients in an average week is 31, with a range of 4 to 64. The 33 Neurologists in the ABN study, cited earlier, saw an average of 30 a week (range 3–67) and the 13 in the Hopkins et al. (1989) study, saw an average of 40 a week. If the age and, therefore, seniority of the south-western neurologists is taken into account, then the oldest 7 have an average of 52 follow-up patients (range 20–63) each week and the youngest 7 have an average of 25 such patients (range 4–44). The older neurologists have accumulated larger cohorts of people who they feel need watching in the clinic and they have done this by having been in their posts for many years, during which time they have had far more opportunity to pick out patients who require long-term supervision. The younger consultants, on the other hand have not yet seen enough patients to pick out large numbers, with the consequence that their follow-up clinics are smaller. Obvious, you would think—but it is not that simple.

The number of junior staff comes into the equation as well. It is traditional to argue that follow-up clinics often grow because junior doctors do not discharge patients, whereas senior doctors do. The 7 older consultants have an average of 2.0 other doctors helping them with their clinics, whereas the 7 younger neurologists have an average of 1.4. The consequence of this is that the 7 older neurologists see only 55% of the patients attending their follow-up clinics (the junior doctors see the rest), whereas the younger neurologists see 77% of their own follow-up patients. So, it is quite possible that the control of the follow-up list is more effective for the younger neurologists, because they do more of it themselves. Age and seniority may not come into it that much, although the length of time in post and the larger number of patients seen over the years must be relevant to some degree.

Before leaving this topic, it is worthwhile for us to address the whole issue of the purpose of the follow-up clinic. My own follow-up patients come into a number of categories. There are quite a few where I do not know what is the matter and I am still investigating or watching to try and find the answer. There are others where the management of their condition is so difficult that it is unreasonable to the patient or the family doctor to abandon them. This group include many patients with difficult epilepsy, some patients with brittle Parkinson's disease and others with unusual and potentially difficult conditions like myasthenia gravis. There are some patients who specifically ask not to be discharged and there are others who, whenever they are discharged, are promptly referred back again by the family doctor. Overall, I find that I discharge patients from the follow-up clinic at a rate of about 25%, meaning that a quarter of such patients are discharged at each clinic. (In this context it is worth noting that I discharge about 60% of all new patients after a single visit.) Despite these fairly aggressive policies, we see an average of 60 follow-up patients each week in all the NHS clinics that I do in Gloucestershire. Clearly, if patients were discharged even more aggressively, more time would be made in the clinics so that greater numbers of new patients could then be seen and, thereby, one could grapple more effectively with the waiting list problem. However, it does seem very unreasonable to

make space in the clinic for patients with tension headaches or faint feelings, by telling an unfortunate individual with brittle Parkinson's disease that he must go, particularly when one knows that two-thirds of patients with that disorder are referred in the first place because the family doctor has already got into difficulties.

There is no easy answer. Or is there? Ask yourself (or the general practitioners and administrators who complain that you follow-up too many people) a very simple question. Who would you (or they) like to see regularly if you (or they) had epilepsy or Parkinson's disease or multiple sclerosis? The answer you (and they) would surely give is: not an amateur, but a professional—an expert in the condition. After all, as many of us know from experience, that is what other doctors (and administrators) tend to organize for themselves, if they are unlucky enough to be afflicted with a neurological disorder. That really embodies the problem in a nutshell. What we should be organising for our patients is the sort of service that we (and those who administer the health service) would want for ourselves (and themselves) and nothing less. If we try to do that, then we must follow-up our patients.

CONCLUSIONS

There are many reasons for believing that in this country the NHS system for outpatient neurology is flawed. In earlier sections of this chapter, I have tried to illustrate the many areas where I perceive there to be difficulties. The theme which inevitably runs through almost all of these problem areas is that of economics. In essence, we are not spending enough on this particular service, with the consequence that it is not of the highest quality. I realize that this is not a conclusion that is unique to neurology, but our specialty does have particular problems, which are only now being addressed. These relate largely to manpower and in particular to the number of consultant clinical neurologists.

What I would like to do in this concluding section is to go through these problem areas and try and suggest ways in which things could be changed.

MANPOWER

I think it is legitimate to look first at consultant numbers and I believe that it is appropriate to address this topic in a chapter on outpatient services, for the bulk of our work is in seeing outpatients and if we get the numbers right for that, then they should be about right for everything else. In the past it has been extremely difficult to give a sensible answer to the question: how many consultant neurologists do we need in this country? It is clear that we need more than we have at the moment. The ABN has previously proposed a figure of 1:200 000 population. It was always clear that this figure, which was no more than a guess, was really an interim figure. Nobody knows what the ideal figure is, indeed the perfect value for today may well be the wrong one for tomorrow.

In this situation it is understandable that comparisons are drawn with the United States, where they appear to have vast numbers of neurologists. Kurtzke *et al.* (1986) have looked at the neurological manpower of the United States and have concluded that in certain areas, the neurologist:population ratio is as small as 1:34 800. It has been suggested that this may not be enough. To translate such a figure to the United Kingdom would be unrealistic and almost certainly inappropriate.

At the centre of any case that we are to make as a specialty for expansion of our numbers must be a statement on what we consider is our business, that is: what do we feel neurologists should deal with and what do we consider to be beyond our sphere of professional interest and competence? Curiously enough, there is no consensus view on this topic, although the ABN has produced a preliminary opinion (*Guidelines for the care of patients with common neurological disorders in the United Kingdom*, ABN 1993*b*). In this chapter I have not discussed the conditions that afflict the patients we actually see in outpatients, although this is a topic that I have looked at in the past (Stevens 1989) and others have done so too (Perkin 1989; Hopkins *et al.* 1989). From these analyses it is clear that for some neurological diseases we probably see all, or at least most, of the people afflicted in our catchment population (motor neurone disease, chronic myelopathy, multiple sclerosis), but there are others (most notably stroke and dementia) in which we are barely involved. If we are going to try and devise an accurate figure for how many neurologists we need, then we must begin by defining what we think we are here for, not just in general terms, but in quite specific terms. We must say whether we should be involved in the management of all patients with cerebrovascular disease, dementia, or epilepsy and so on. My feeling is that these conditions are our business and that now is the time to break away from the rather peculiar views expressed in the past that certain disorders of the nervous system (such as stroke) are general medicine and not neurology. It is very difficult to support this old-fashioned perception of our specialty. This is not the place to rehearse all the arguments on this topic, although I have addressed this subject elsewhere (the 1996 Sydney Watson Smith Lecture at the Royal College of Physicians in Edinburgh, Stevens 1996*a*), but it is enough for me to state that I believe that neurologists should do rather more neurology than has been the case hitherto. Clarification of our views on this topic facilitates the calculation of how much work will be generated for neurologists by a population of a particular size and, therefore, how many neurologists we will need to service that population. In conjunction with colleagues on the Services Committee of the ABN, I have done these calculations and the result is now in the public domain (*Neurology in the United Kingdom: numbers of clinical neurologists and trainees*, Stevens 1996*b*). The sequence that produced the answer is discussed below.

What do neurologists do now and what should they be doing?

The current clinical workload of British neurologists

This stage of the analysis involves evaluating the current pattern of clinical work of neurologists and in particular the frequency of different disorders in outpatient practice. Information is available on this topic and some of it has already been cited. (Perkin 1989; Hopkins *et al.* 1989; Stevens 1989; ABN 1991). The ABN study revealed that 16 conditions constitute 74% of the clinical workload of neurologists, with conditions like blackouts, headache, cerebrovascular disease, and multiple sclerosis predominating.

What should neurologists do?

This topic is rather more contentious. As I have indicated already, there is no clear consensus on the scope and limits of clinical neurology, that is to say, the range of disorders which neurologists should legitimately regard as their business, although such a consensus is emerging (Marsden 1981; Editorial 1994). The general impression is that the majority of neurologists believe that we should be dealing with more of the neurology in the population than has been the case hitherto.

How much neurology is there in the population?

Having established what neurologists do now and what we feel they should do in the future, the next step is to analyse how much neurology there is out there. Epidemiological data exists, although it is unlikely that it is absolutely accurate. Nevertheless, the general figures published by Kurtzke (1982) and Wade and Hewer (1987) and other more specific data concerning particular disorders (Hauser and Kurland 1975; Sandercock 1984; Sander and Shorvon 1987; Hopkins 1989; Marshall and Mohr 1993) have been useful in this context. Combining all the data contained in these sources gives a reasonable picture of the epidemiology of common neurological diseases.

How much outpatient work could be generated by patients with these conditions?

The next step is to calculate the annual workload for neurologists that could be generated by patients with neurological disease in a given population. The same sources, plus unpublished opinions of colleagues, have been used to analyse the numbers of new and follow-up consultations that could be generated. Implicit in this process is the belief that at the moment there are large numbers of people in the community who should be seen by a neurologist, but who are not seen, either because the neurology service is overloaded or because they are referred to generalists or other specialists who are not neurologists. Patients with cerebrovascular disease is an obvious example of a group of patients who could benefit from seeing a neurologist, but who at the moment do not do so.

How much time should be allocated to outpatient consultations?

The ABN has already analysed this topic (ABN 1993*a*) and additional data have been presented earlier in this chapter. The formula mentioned earlier of allocating one unit of consultation time to a follow-up patient and two units to a new patient has been employed and the duration of the units takes account of the data presented earlier on how long doctors of different seniority spend on dealing with patients in the two categories.

How much time is required for outpatient work for a defined population?

Having got this far, it is then a very straightforward business to calculate how much outpatient work could be generated by a particular population. In the ABN policy document (Stevens 1996*b*) cited earlier, the calculations were carried out for a population of 100 000.

How many hours a week should a neurologist spend seeing outpatients?

For the purposes of this analysis it has been assumed that the minimum amount of time spent in outpatients is 10.5 hours a week (3 sessions of 3.5 hours), but alternative patterns of work are also considered. The ABN publication on job plans (ABN 1993*a*) has been used as a basis for these analyses.

How many neurologists are required for a given population?

The answer to this question emerges very readily. It is easy to work out how many neurologists will be required to service the calculated demand within a population of known size. Details of the results of these calculations are given in Table 35.5, where it can be seen that the ideal consultant neurologist: population ratio lies between 1:67 000 and 1:130 000. These values must be compared to 1:200 000, which has been the target hitherto.

However, purchasers of health care are going to have to be persuaded that making additional appointments is both desirable and necessary. If we do what has always been done in the past and simply produce documents and hope that our powers of persuasion will be enough, then we will probably

Table 35.5 Work structure and number of UK consultant neurologists

Pattern of work of the consultant neurologist and of the available help in outpatients	Consultants required per 100 000	Consultants per head of population
3 clinics a week plus help from junior doctors	1.02	1:98 000
4 clinics a week plus help from junior doctors	0.77	1:130 000
3 clinics a week but no help from junior doctors	1.48	1:67 000
4 clinics a week but no help from junior doctors	1.11	1:90 000

fail, but if we do what other specialities have done in the past and become somewhat political, then we could succeed. In essence, we must persuade politicians that something drastic must be done about neurology manpower levels, so that they can apply pressure on our behalf. Shroud waving may be going too far, but a campaign will be needed. The intensity of that campaign will be a measure of our collective seriousness for the cause of improving the lot of our patients.

OUTPATIENT CLINICS: HOW TO BREAK AWAY FROM THE PRESENT SYSTEM

I have already outlined, either directly or indirectly, the aspects at fault regarding the manner in which we provide an outpatient service in the United Kingdom. What I would like to propose is a fairly simple way of breaking loose from the traditional system. In making these suggestions I have an advantage, because I now work in an environment that has the characteristics that I will describe next and which I would encourage others to mimic.

What I would like to suggest is that we cease to do outpatient clinics in the conventional outpatient department and, thereby, break away from the tradition of the fixed outpatient session. In Gloucester we have a department of neurology, where we have a sufficient amount of space to provide not only the necessary offices for the medical team (consultants, registrar, and senior house officer), but secretarial offices as well. Thus, we have ample space for the administrative and office-based aspects of our work. In addition, we have enough examining rooms and a large enough waiting room that we can conduct all our outpatient consultations within the department. The rooms are also used for a variety of other medical and paramedical activities. The regular neurology team meetings are held in the department, the neuropsychologist sees some patients there and the physiotherapist and psychologist use the rooms to run the newly diagnosed group for patients with multiple sclerosis. The secret is that this facility is exclusively for neurology and no other specialty uses the space. Consequently, we can see outpatients whenever we wish, which means that we have the ability to break away from the fixed clinic sessions that have traditionally been in our timetables. Outpatients are seen in the department almost every day, sometimes just a small number, but on other occasions in the old-fashioned large clinics. The choice is ours. Theoretically, there could be difficulties in getting other staff to support these multiple clinics, but that has not been a problem. The lady who works in the department as a clerk filing letters, collating reports, and so on, also functions as a receptionist when she is required to do so. We have a staff nurse who is officially the clinic nurse and she is almost always available to help with *ad-hoc* clinics and to act as chaperone when needed. Overall, this system works exceptionally well and it has allowed us to increase patient throughput and to structure clinics in a more sensitive way.

THE PHYSICAL ENVIRONMENT

One aspect of the new department, which has turned out to be far more interesting than we originally expected, is the reaction to the physical environment. When we were planning it, we paid a lot of attention to the design and the physical appearance of the waiting room and the offices where consultations are held. All floors are carpeted, the walls in the waiting room are wallpapered, and there are proper curtains at the windows. The colour scheme was deliberately designed to be warm, bright, and relaxing. The lighting is more subtle than is usually found in a hospital clinic. All the furniture and fittings are new. There are plants in all the rooms. There are framed pictures on the walls and not a piece of sellotape in sight. There are no health propaganda notices. The offices contain bookcases and they look homely, but business-like, and not at all like a traditional outpatient consulting room. The intention was to create a department that resembles the smart offices one finds in commercial concerns or in private hospitals and to deliberately break with traditional hospital design. We are pleased with it, for it works well and it is a pleasant environment to work in.

The difference between the new neurology department and the old outpatient department is so great that the two areas have been evaluated and patient reactions have been measured by a team of psychologists. The new department, when compared to the old outpatient department, has been shown to reduce self-reported stress levels, yet to heighten arousal and, overall, to create in the patients a high level of satisfaction (Leather *et al.* 1994). The intention, when designing the department was to try and escape from the traditional style of outpatients in order to make our lives more pleasant and we have certainly succeeded in that, but what we have also done is to make the experience of attending the clinic more pleasant for the patients as well. So it can be done. It uses space and it costs money, but I am in no doubt that it is money well spent, for the improvements in the quality of the environment have been demonstrated to be beneficial. Nowadays, we hear much about quality initiatives. This is one.

THE OUTPATIENT SESSION

Using the facility described in the previous paragraphs, we have broken away from the traditional prolonged outpatient session. Very rarely does a clinic go on for much longer than three and a half hours, although in a week we do put in more than the ABN recommended ten and a half hours (the equivalent of three sessions). This is acceptable if the individual sessions are designed not to be too intense. We are now able to do frequent *ad-hoc* clinics, with small numbers of patients, and to provide a fast track epilepsy service and an urgent patient service in a way that was not previously possible. As a result of splitting outpatient activities in this way, we are able to allocate more time to individual patients than was formerly possible. The time spent each week seeing outpatients is no longer as onerous, even though more hours are spent doing so. This is because the process of conducting the clinics has changed.

Addendum

The preceding paragraphs were initially written in 1993 and the conclusion now is the same as it was then. The department continues to work very well, even though we now have more staff. The secret is that the space is exclusively for neurology and it is not used by other hospital specialities. Thus, it is with sadness that as a footnote to my enthusiastic recommendation for this type of facility, I have to record that with the newly introduced private finance initiatives that are being explored within the NHS, a new hospital is being planned for Gloucester in which it will not be possible to have integrated departments, such as the one I have described here. Sadly, we are being told that in the new hospital we must revert to the old system of offices scattered about here and there and we must go back to having designated slots in the general outpatient department and thereby lose the flexibility that is the hallmark of the service that we are able to give at the moment.

WAITING LISTS

We still have waiting lists that are unacceptably long. From the various experiments that I have conducted over the years and which I have described in earlier paragraphs, I have come to the conclusion that the only technique that is likely to work (and we cannot even be sure of that) is to have more people seeing patients. I believe that there is a limit to how many patients one can see in a week and, although I acknowledge that different consultants have different thresholds of how many they can manage on a regular basis, we all have our limits. The critical point is that if one consistently exceeds that limit, then the job becomes too demanding and in the long run the quality of the service suffers. Clearly, the number seen must be reasonable and obviously it has to resemble the number seen by neurologists elsewhere, but it is unacceptable for us to be expected to keep on increasing the workload simply to satisfy the rather arbitrary whims of health ministers, who pluck numbers from the sky and then announce that from now on waiting times will be like this and throughput will be like that and everything will be done with an X% reduction in costs. In my view our job is to give as good a service as we can and we must leave it to the purchasers of health care to make value judgements on what they wish to do about the waiting lists. It is not pleasant to find oneself thinking of a waiting list as a political tool, but in the long run it works that way. All those new neurologists appointed in recent years appeared because of waiting lists. So, my final message on this topic is that we should worry about the quality of what we do in the consulting room and how we do it and the politicians and health managers should worry about waiting lists.

FUTURE DEVELOPMENTS

There are various ways in which the outpatient service could change in the future, all of which would improve the quality of care for patients with neurological disease. Some of these are already being tried in some centres, but so far these developments are far from universal.

Guidelines and Protocols

It is currently fashionable for specialists to be asked to prepare written guidelines or protocols to facilitate management of patients by non-experts and, in some instances, to help in the process of referral of patients to outpatient clinics. There is apparently a subtle distinction between a document containing guidelines and one that can be thought of as a protocol. The former is simply a guide, which does not necessarily have to be followed, although the contents are designed to help patient management; whereas the latter is sometimes considered to have a legal status, so that a failure to follow the rules contained within the document could, under certain circumstances, be regarded as negligent. Clearly, it is safer for all concerned to talk rather more of guidelines than protocols. So far, there are relatively few generally agreed documents of this type which refer to neurological disease, although the ABN published a document on this topic in 1993 (ABN 1993*b*). It is inappropriate to dwell extensively on this topic here, but I have done one small study which yielded rather curious results and which could be of interest (Stevens 1997). I presented 100 general practitioners with vignettes of three different types of headache: common migraine, migrainous neuralgia, and chronic daily headache, these being respectively, a common disorder with a classical pattern of symptoms, a rare disorder of the same type, and a common disorder with a pattern of symptoms that is far from classical. The same vignettes were given to 10 neurologists, in the hope that they would create between them a sort of gold standard for the diagnosis and management of these conditions. The results revealed that both groups of doctors were brilliantly accurate in their analyses of the migraine problem, but the general practitioners were not very good with the migrainous neuralgia, although (fortunately) the neurologists were very good with this one and, finally, neither group were consistent among themselves with the vignette of chronic daily headache. So, what has this to do with guidelines or protocols? Simply this: the neurologists would be able to produce beautiful guidelines for migraine, but the GPs do not need them; they could also make sets of guidelines for migrainous neuralgia, but the condition is rare, so guidelines are hardly needed, and, when it came to chronic daily headache, for which a guideline would be useful, the neurologists could not agree among themselves, so they would not be able to produce an agreed document. Perhaps this is why there are few such documents on common neurological diseases.

ONE-STOP CLINICS

This is descriptive term for a type of clinic where everything that needs to be done for a particular problem is done at a single session. An example is the breast tumour service organized by some surgeons. In such a clinic the patient is interviewed and examined, then a fine needle biopsy is performed, and the cytology is done at once, so that the result of the assessment is available to the patient during the first visit. There are several neurological disorders where this approach would be valuable. It would be ideal if patients with late onset epilepsy could be assessed clinically and then have an EEG and a scan all in one session. Similarly, patients with transient ischaemic attacks would benefit from being seen urgently and having a clinical assessment, blood tests and carotid Doppler, and other relevant studies all at a single visit. We have tried to set up both of these services and have failed to get all of the other hospital departments to put aside protected time to allow for the performance of the tests on the same day as the patient visits the clinic. The only service that we have been able to organize is the live performance of serum anticonvulsant levels in the epilepsy clinic. Clearly, there is much scope for enhancing the outpatient service in this way and I understand that in those departments, where such an approach can be organized, that the service is efficient and valuable. It is a difficult one though.

Specialist nurses

Rather like clinical assistants, it is difficult to persuade the hospital management to pay for specialist nurses in epilepsy or Parkinson's disease or other named conditions. We have tried to organize this, but have failed. I know of other neurology departments where such nurses are employed and I am told that they are very valuable and that their presence enhances the quality of care that can be given to patients. This is another topic that could be explored in the future.

The neurological network

The Association of British Neurologists has recently looked at the future organization of neurological services and has published a document entitled *Neurological services in the United Kingdom: Towards 2000 and beyond* (ABN 1997). The concept of a neurology network is introduced and it is anticipated that as more and more neurologists are appointed it will be possible to ensure that every district general hospital (DGH) in the country will have access to one or more neurologists. This will ensure that a neurological outpatient service will be available in every town and that all patients will have ready access to neurological expertise. These small DGH neurology units will be served by either a neurology centre or a centre for neurology and neurosurgery. The latter will be similar to the neuroscience centres that exist already, but the neurology centres will serve a smaller population (probably 500 000–1 000 000) than the relatively scarce neuroscience centres and they will be staffed by all of the neurologists in the surrounding area. These centres will provide a comprehensive in and outpatient service to the populace, with both general and specialized clinical services from the consultant neurologists. As more new consultants are appointed, so the service will improve, until eventually a network of DGH neurology units, neurology centres, and centres for neurology and neurosurgery is established across the country. This network should facilitate access to high quality services and expertise for all patients. It has to be acknowledged that this concept will not develop at all unless there is a radical change in attitudes from ministers and health authorities on the priorities that must be given to neurology in the future. If there is no real desire for an improvement in the service, then nothing will happen.

REFERENCES

ABN (Association of British Neurologists) (1991). *U.K. Neurologists work loads and work environments: a survey.* ABN, London.

ABN (Association of British Neurologists) (1993a). *Good neurological practice: with particular reference to job plans for consultant neurologists in the UK.* ABN, London.

ABN (Association of British Neurologists) (1993b). *Guidelines for the care of patients with Common neurological disorders in the United Kingdom.* ABN, London.

ABN (Association of British Neurologists) (1997). *Neurology in the United Kingdom: towards 2000 and beyond.* ABN, London.

Caplan, L. R. (1990). *The effective clinical neurologist.* Blackwell Scientific, Oxford.

Department of Health (1992). *The Patient's Charter.* HMSO, London.

Editorial (1994). Economic change and health service reform: likely impact on teaching, practice and research in neurology. *J. Neurol. Neurosurg. and Psychiat.,* **57** 667–71.

Hauser, W. A. and Kurland, L. T. (1975). The epidemiology of epilepsy in Rochester, Minnesota, 1935 through 1967. *Epilepsia,* **16**, 1–66.

Hopkins, A., Menken, M., and DeFriese, G. (1989). A record of patient encounters in neurological practice in the United Kingdom. *J. Neurol. Neurosurg. and Psychiat.,* **52**, 436–8.

Hopkins, A. (1989). Lessons for neurologists from the United Kingdom third national morbidity survey. *J. Neurol. Neurosurg. and Psychiat.,* **52**, 430–3.

Kurtzke, J. F. (1982). The current neurologic burden of illness and injury in the United States. *Neurology,* **32**, 1207–14.

Kurtzke, J. F., Bennett, D. R., Beringer, G. B., Goldsten, M., and Vates T. S. (1986). Neurologists in the United States: past, present and future. *Neurology,* **36**, 1576–82.

Leather, P. J., Stevens, D. L., Morrison, L., Earll, L., Watts, J., and Munir, F. (1994). *Environmental design and the stress of the hospital out-patients' visit. Comparative evaluation of two neurology clinic waiting areas: Interim summary of results.* Presentation at British Psychological Association, September 1994.

Marsden, C. D. (1981). *J. Neurol. Neurosurg. and Psychiat.* (Editorial), **44**, 1059–60.

Marshall, R. S. and Mohr, J. P. (1993). Current management of ischaemic stroke. *J. Neurol. Neurosurg. and Psychiat.,* **56**, 6–16.

Mendenhall, R. C. (1981). *Medical practice in the United States.* The Robert Woods Foundation.

Menken, M. (1989). The 1985 National Ambulatory Care Survey of Neurologists. *Arch. Neurol.,* **46**, 1346–8.

Perkin, G. D. (1989). An analysis of 7,836 successive new out-patient referrals. *J. Neurol. Neurosurg. and Psychiat.,* **52**, 447–8.

Sander, J. W. A. S. and Shorvon, S. D. (1987). Incidence and prevalence studies in epilepsy and their methodological problems: a review. *J. Neurol. Neurosurg. and Psychiat.,* **50**, 829–39.

Sandercock, P. A. G. (1984). The Oxfordshire community stroke project and its application to stroke prevention. DM thesis, University of Oxford.

Solzhenitsyn, A. (1971). *Cancer ward,* (trans. N. Bethell, and D. Burg). Penguin, London. (Original work published 1968).

Stevens, D. L. (1989). Neurology in Gloucestershire: the clinical workload of an English neurologist. *J. Neurol. Neurosurg. and Psychiat.,* **52**, 439–48.

Stevens, D. L. (1996a). *Who should manage patients with neurological disease?* Sydney Watson Smith Lecture, Royal College of Physicians of Edinburgh.

Stevens, D. L. (1996b) *Neurology in the United Kingdom: Numbers of clinical neurologists and trainees.* Association of British Neurologists, London.

Stevens, D. L. (1997). Headache: How good are we at early management? *Horizons in medicine,* Vol. 8. Royal College of Physicians of London. pp.369–78.

Wade, D. T. and Langton-Hewer, R. (1987). Epidemiology of some neurological diseases, with special reference to work load on the NHS *Int. Rehabil. Med.,* **8**, 129–37.

Yates, J. (1987). *Why are we waiting? An analysis of hospital waiting lists.* Oxford University Press.

Index

Abbreviated Mental Test Score 279
abdominal distension, and respiration 337
absence seizure 67
abulia 317
acoustic neurinoma 27, 220
acromegaly 219
acupuncture, for chronic pain 48
acute dystonia 135–6
   botulinum toxin 135–6
acute transverse myelopathy 206–9
adolescence, seizures in 68
adrenocorticotrophic hormone, and multiple
      sclerosis 115
affective disorder 303
age
   effect of illness 446–7
   and stroke 183
aggression 317
agitation 317
AIDS, encephalitis 241–2
alcohol abuse 304
   and ethnic groups 291
allodynia 43
   in trigeminal neuralgia 51
alpha-skeletomotor neurone, muscle
      spasticity 346
alprostadil 362
Alzheimer's disease 17, 165, 168, 272
amantadine 150
amaurosis fugax 15
amblyopia 7–8
amitriptyline
   for chronic pain 45
   diabetic neuropathy 52
   post-herpetic neuralgia 50
   trigeminal neuralgia 51
amyotrophic lateral sclerosis 268
anaesthesia, and respiration 337
analgesics, for chronic pain 44–5
aneurysm, optic nerve compression 12–13
anterior artery cerebral interruption 271
anterior frontal epilepsy 66
anterior ischaemic optic neuropathy 13–14
antiarrythmics, for chronic pain 45–6
antibiotics, for meningitis 237
anticholinergics, risk of 135
anticonvulsant drugs
   for chronic pain 45–6
   toxicity of 79
antidepressants, for chronic pain 45
antimuscarinic agents 150
antiphospholipid syndrome 189

Anton's syndrome 180, 271
anxiety 304
   palliative care 375
aphasia 313
apnoea 338
arachnoiditis 205
Arnold–Chiari malformation 94
arteriovenous malformations 95–6
aspiration 338
aspirin
   headache 101
   stroke 185, 186
assisted ventilation 315–16
   tracheostomy 316
ataxia, multiple sclerosis 121
athetosis 139
attention deficit hyperactivity 142
auditory disorders 29–37
   hearing impairment 29–36
   tinnitus 36–7
auras
   frontal lobe seizures 66
   temporal lobe epilepsy 65
autonomous neuropathic bladder 357
autosomal recessive diseases 255
azathioprine, multiple sclerosis 116

baclofen
   multiple sclerosis 120, 121
   spasticity and contractures 320, 351
Bálint's syndrome 17
ballism 139
Barthel Activities of Daily Life Index 262,
      277–8
Becker muscular dystrophy 250
behavioural problems 317–18
Bell's palsy, and ethnic groups 295
benign familial convulsions 70
benign intracranial hypertension 94–5
benzhexol, idiopathic torsion dystonia 133
benzodiazepines
   Huntington's disease 137
   multiple sclerosis 120
   muscle spasticity 350
beta-blockers, for headache 102
bladder disorders 355–9
   autonomous neuropathic bladder 357
   bladder sensitivity, reduction in 358
   drug-induced dysfunction 364
   drug therapy 358
   failure to empty bladder 358–9
   increasing urethral resistance 358

motor paralytic bladder 357
multiple sclerosis 363
neurological causes 355–6
Parkinson's disease 363–4
peripheral nervous system lesions 356
peripheral neuropathy 364
reflex neuropathic bladder 357
self-catheterization 358, 359
sensory paralytic bladder 357
spinal cord injury 363
stress urinary incontinence 359
uninhibited neuropathic bladder 357
urinary retention in young women
      359
urine storage, failure of 358
urine volume, reduction in 358
blepharospasm 136
   botulinum toxin 136
blood pressure 97–8
border zone infarcts 181
botulinum toxin
   acute dystonia 135–6
   muscle spasticity 352
   spasticity and contractures 319
   torticollis 211
bowel disorders 355–6
   diet and laxatives 360
   faecal incontinence 359–60
   multiple sclerosis 363
   neurological causes 355–6
   peripheral nervous system lesions 356
   peripheral neuropathy 364
   spinal cord injury 363
brain abscess 243–4
brainstem gliomas 221
breathing aids 338–9
Briquet's syndrome 301–2
bromocriptine 149
Brown–Sequard syndrome 200, 201
bruit 187
   asymptomatic 188
bulbospinal neuronopathy 251
butyrophenone
   acute dystonia 135
   Huntington's disease 137
   symptomatic dystonia 134
   tics 141

cabergoline 149
caeruloplasmin 131
Caisson's disease 202
callosotomy, for surgery 84

capsaicin
  chronic pain 47
  diabetic neuropathy 52
  post-herpetic neuralgia 51
carbamazepine
  chronic pain 46
  diabetic neuropathy 52
  epilepsy 80
  trigeminal neuralgia 51
cardiac disease, and stroke 183
carers, help for 453
carotid
  endarterectomy 186
  stroke 179
catechol-*O*-methyl transferase inhibitors 150
Cawthorne–Cooksey exercises 27–8
central pain 49–50
cephalosporin, meningitis 237
cerebral
  angiography, and stroke 184
  anterior artery cerebral interruption 271
  haemorrhage 190
  infarction, causes of 189
  internal carotid artery syndrome 271
  metastases 217
  middle cerebral syndromes 271
  venous thrombosis 189
cerebrospinal fluid, meningitis 234–40
cerebrovascular disease
  and driving 369
  in the elderly 270–1
  and ethnic groups 291
cervical
  compression, signs and symptoms of
    197–8
  dystonia, and botulinum toxin 136
  lesions, indicators of 197
  spondylosis 211
Charcot–Marie–Tooth disease 106–7, 130,
    255
charities *see* self-help groups
chest infection 338
childhood
  epilepsy 64
  seizures in 68
chlormethiazole, delirium 163
cholesterol, and stroke 183
chorea 136–9
  Huntington's disease 137–8
  paroxysmal 138
chorea-acanthocytosis 138
chronic pain 43–55
  anticonvulsants, antiarrythmics, and local
    anaesthetics 45–6
  central pain 49–50
  destructive neurosurgery 48
  diabetic neuropathy 52–3
  drugs acting on NMDA receptors 46
  management of 44
  muscle relaxants 46
  neuroleptics 45
  physiology of 43
  primary analgesics 44–5
  reflex sympathetic dystrophy 53–4
  spinal cord stimulation 48–9
  trigeminal neuralgia 51–2
  see also pain

cingulate gyrus seizures 66
claudication, neurogenic 203
clinical
  guidelines 417–19, 421
  research *see* research
  scientists 386
clobazam, for epilepsy 81
clonazepam, for epilepsy 81
clonic seizures 67
clonidine, headache 102
cochlear implants 35–6
cognitive rehabilitation 316–17
  attention 317
  memory 317
  neglect and perceptual problems 317
  problem solving and executive functions
    317
colour vision, abnormal 3
commissioners, activities of 402–13
  contracting 402
  finance 410
  health care needs assessment 403
  health service agreements 408–12
  purchasing 402
  quality specification 409
  service and financial framework 407–8
  services to be provided 408
  volume of work 408
  see also health care needs assessment
commissioning 399–415
  and accessing aids 314
  commissioning strategy 407
  and the NHS 399–415
  issues in neurology 413–14
  overview of 401
  see also health care needs assessment
communication
  of doctor 441–50
  and outreach service 452
communication aids 313–14
  commissioning and accessing aids 314
  direct select aids 313
  encoding aids 314
  scanning aids 313
computed tomography scan *see* CT scan
confusion, and palliative care 375
constipation, and palliative care 375
consultants 430–2
consultation 441–50
  diagnosis, impact of 443–7
  drug regime 444–5
  healing approach 441–2, 448
contracting, and the NHS 395–7
contractures 319–20
conversion disorder 298–30, 305
  management of 300
  recognition of 299
Co-ordinated Care Working Party 459
copolymer 1, multiple sclerosis 118
copper concentration, Wilson's disease
    131–2
cortical blindness 18
corticosteroids, multiple sclerosis 115
cost–benefit concept, for elderly 264
Creutzfelt–Jakob disease 140
cricopharyngeal myotomy 341
crisis intervention 453

CT scan
  for epilepsy 72
  stroke 184
Cu/Zn superoxide dismutase gene 256
cuirasse 339
cyanide, toxic optic neuropathy 7–8
cyclophosphamide, multiple sclerosis 116
cyclosporin A, multiple sclerosis 116
cytogenetics laboratory 248

dantrolene
  multiple sclerosis 120
  muscle spasticity 351
DDAVP 358
death
  anxiety and depression 375
  bereavement 380
  confusion 375
  constipation 375
  decisions in treatment 377–8
  disability, fear of 376
  dysphagia 374
  dyspnoea 374
  emotional concerns 375–6
  family concerns 377–8
  incontinence 374–5
  interdisciplinary team care 378
  mental deterioration, fear of 376
  muscle spasm 374
  pain 374
  palliative care 378–9
  patient concerns 373–7
  pressure sores 375
  seizures 374
  spiritual concerns 376–7
decubitus ulcers 320–1
deep vein thrombosis 188
delirium
  alleviating symptoms 163–4
  causes of 164
  comparison with schizophrenia and disso-
    ciative disorders 163
  management of 161–4
  recognizing 161–2
dementia 164–70, 271–2
  behaviour disorders 168–9
  classification 165
  and driving 369–70
  drug treatment 168
  emotional problems 168
  features of 166–7
  intracranial lesions 166
  management 167
  normal pressure hydrocephalus 166
  prevention of cerebrovascular illness 169
  pseudodementia 166
  reality orientation 169
  reminiscence therapy 169
  senile dementia 170
  validation therapy 169–70
demyelinating optic neuritis, steroid treat-
    ment of 4
dental pain 96–7
dentato-rubro-pallido-luysian atrophy 137,
    138, 140
depression 303, 317
  palliative care 375

descending supraspinal influences
muscle spasticity 347–8
detrusor hypokinesia 357
detrusor instability 357
diabetes, symptomatic dystonia 134
diabetes mellitus, and stroke 183
diabetic amyotrophy 209–10
diabetic neuropathy 52–3
diagnosis, impact of 443–7, 452
see also healing approach, outreach service
diazepam, for epilepsy 81, 82
diet
ethnic 286
multiple sclerosis 119
Parkinson's disease 155–6
direct select aids 313
disability, fear of 376
Disabled Living Foundation 459
disc herniation
cervical 211
lumbar 211–12
thoracic 211
disinhibition 317
dissection, of carotid and vertebral arteries
189
dissociative disorders, comparison with
delirium 163
dizziness 21–9
DNA, genetic sequencing 251–2
doctor–patient consultation 441–50
dopamine
agonists 149
see also levodopa
dorsolateral frontal seizures 66
driving 367–70
cerebrovascular disease 369
dementia 369–70
epilepsy 72–3, 368–9
giddiness 369
migraine 369
multiple sclerosis 120, 369
Parkinson's disease 370
physical disabilities 370
sleepiness, excessive 369
visual disturbance 2–3, 370
drug-induced dysfunction, sexual dysfunction in 364
drug treatment 444–5
bladder disorders 358
delirium 164
dementia 168
epilepsy 77–82
Huntington's disease 137–8
meningitis 237
motor neurone disease 175
muscle spasticity 350–2
pain 374
and respiration 337
teratogenicity of 78
toxicity of 78
see also pharmaceutical industry
Duchenne muscular dystrophy, hereditability
of 251, 253–4
dysarthria 313
dysphagia
airway protection 315
assessment 314

causes of 328–9, 331–6, 342
clinical assessment of 331–6
deglutition 328–9
enteral nutrition 314–15
intubation 340–1
management of 336–41
neural control 329
and nutrition 314–15
palliative care 374
sialorrhoea 315
and stroke 188
surgery 341
symptomatic 340
dyspnoea, palliative care 374
dystonia
acute 135–6
cervical 136
idiopathic torsion 132–3
laryngeal 136
oromandibular 136
symptomatic 133–5

echocardiography, for stroke 184
education
of patients 454
and self-help groups 457–60
EEG, value of in epilepsy 71
elderly 259–74
abuse of 170–1
acute care 263
ageing process 261–2
cerebrovascular disease 270–1
changing demography 259–60
co-ordination 262
cost–benefit concept 264
dementia and cognitive impairment
271–2
diagnosis 262–3
disease prevalence 260–1
epilepsy 269–70
falls 265–6
incontinence 273
investigation 263
longer-term care 264
motor neurone disease 268–9
motor power 262
orthostatic hypotension 266
Parkinson's disease 267
peripheral neuropathy 272–3
reflexes and primitive signs 262
rehabilitation 263–4
sensory examination 261–2
terminal care 264–5
test assessments 262
EMLA, for chronic pain 46
emotional concerns, and palliative care
375–6
emotional lability 317
encephalitis 240–3
AIDS 241–2
clinical features 240–1
herpes simplex encephalitis 241
malaria 242–3
management 241
rabies 241
viral 292
encoding aids 314

enteral nutrition 314–15
ependymomas 221–3
epilepsia partialis continua 66
epilepsy
absence seizure 67
accidental injury 74
carbamazepine 80
care in 76
classification of 60–1
clobazam 81
clonazepam 81
clonic seizures 67
confusion with pseudoseizures 63–4
confusion with syncope 62–3
diagnosis 60–4, 72
diazepam 81, 82
and driving 72–3, 368–9
drug therapy 77–82
drugs, toxicity of 78
eclampsia 83
EEG, value of 71
in the elderly 269–70
epidemiology 60
epilepsia partialis continua 66
and ethnic groups 293
ethosuximide 81
febrile seizures 69
focal seizures 59
frontal lobe seizures 65–6
gabapentin 81
generalized seizures 59
genetic epilepsies 70
implications of to patient 72, 75
labour and post-partum period 74
lamotrigine 81
Landau–Kleffner syndrome 69
Lennox–Gastaut syndrome 68
monitoring therapy 79
mortality in 74
myoclonic seizure 67, 140
with myoclonic-astatic seizures 69
neonatal seizures 67–8
occipital lobe seizure 66
oxcarbazepine 81
parietal lobe seizure 66
partial seizures 64–6
phenobarbitone 81, 82
phenytoin 81, 82
post-traumatic seizures 70–1
pregnancy 73–4
prognosis 76–7
psychiatric disorders 75
as a psychosomatic disorder 308–10
pyridoxine seizures 70
Rasmussen's syndrome 69–70
reflex epilepsies 69
seizures in adolescence 68
seizures in infancy and childhood 68, 69
sodium valproate 78, 81
status epilepticus 82–3
and stroke 188
surgical treatment of 83–5
temporal lobe seizures 64–5
tiagabine 81
tonic seizure 67
topiramate 81
vagal stimulation 85

epilepsy *(cont.)*
    vigabatrin 81–2
    withdrawing therapy 80
    zonisamide 82
ergotamine 149
    headaches 100–1
essential tremor 128, 129
ethnic groups, particular neurological prob-
        lems of 281–96
    African trypanosomiasis 292
    alcoholism 291
    attitudes to acute conditions 284–5
    bacterial and parasitic myositis 292
    Bell's palsy 295
    brain tumour 294
    in Britain 281–2
    cerebrovascular disease 291
    clinic or surgery visits 285
    complaints/litigation 286
    concept of disease 284
    diets of 286
    epilepsy 293
    hospital visiting 286
    Huntington's chorea 295
    Japanese encephalitis 290
    kuru 290
    language 283–4
    lepromatous neuropathy 293
    Marchiafava–Bignami disease 291
    mental handicap 294
    migraine 294
    multiple sclerosis 290
    neurofibromatosis 294–5
    neurological sarcoidosis 292–3
    oculopharyngeal muscular dystrophy 291
    pernicious anaemia 290
    politics 286
    practical considerations 295
    religious belief about disease 286–9
    response to chronic disorders 285
    terminology 282–3
    tropical myeloneuropathy 291–2
    tuberculous meningitis 292
    viral encephalitis 292
ethosuximide, for epilepsy 81
European Parkinson's Disease Association
        461
expiration 325–6
extradural abscess 244–5
extratemporal surgery, for epilepsy 84

facial pain 96–7
facioscapulohumeral muscular dystrophy,
        hereditability of 255
falls 37–40, 265–6
    investigation 38–40
    management 40
    risk factors 38
    see also auditory disorders, vestibular prob-
        lems
familial convulsions, benign 70
family concerns, and palliative care 377–8
fatique syndromes 304
febrile seizures 69
fibromuscular dysphasia 190
flecainide, for chronic pain 46
fluorescent-*in-situ* hybridization 248

follow-up clinic 471–2
fragile-X syndrome 251
frontal lobe epilepsy 65–6

GABA receptor 351
gabapentin, for epilepsy 81
gamma globulin, multiple sclerosis 115
genetic
    counselling 247–57
    epilepsies 70
genetics unit, value of 247–57
    analysis of mutations 249–50
    cytogenetics laboratory 248
    molecular diagnostics laboratory 248
    multifactorial conditions 256
    mutations easy to recognize 250–1
    trinucleotide repeats 251
gerebellar tremor 129–30
Gerstmann–Straussler syndrome 140
giant cell arteritis 14
giddiness, and driving 369
Gilles de la Tourette syndrome 142
glaucoma 17
glioma
    brainstem 221
    low grade, of cerebral hemisphere 216
    malignant, of cerebral hemispheres
        214–16
    optic nerve compression 11
glossopharyngeal breathing 339
gluten-free diet, and multiple sclerosis 119
glycerol rhizotomy, and trigeminal neuralgia
        52
Golgi tendon organs, muscle spasticity 346
growth hormone 219
Guillain–Barré syndrome 105–6, 209, 273

haematomata, spinal 202
haemodynamic amaurosis fugax 181
haemorrhage
    cerebral 179–93
    spinal subarachnoid 202
hallucinations, temporal lobe epilepsy 64–5
halogenated hydroxyquinolones 8
haloperidol 164, 169
    tics 141
Hangman's fracture 198
headache 93–103
    analgesics 101–2
    arteriovenous malformations 95–6
    benign intracranial hypertension 94–5
    blood pressure 97–8
    cluster headache 100–1
    epidemiology 98–9
    facial and dental pain 96–7
    hydrocephalus 94
    mass lesions 93–4
    mechanisms of 99–100
    meningitis 97
    migraine 98–9
    neck pain 96
    neuralgia 97
    prophylactic medication 102
    serotonin 99, 100
    sinusitis 96
    subarachnoid haemorrhage 97
    temporal arteritis 96
healing approach 441–2, 448

health care needs assessment 403–7
    available resources 406
    comparative assessment 404
    corporate assessment 405
    costs 404
    epidemiology 403
    outcome of 405–6
    pitfalls in 405
    priority setting 406–7
    quality of care 404
    see also commissioning
health care resource groups 411
Health Improvement Programme 399
health service agreements 408–13
    activity monitoring 412
    finance 410, 412
    meetings 412
    quality 409, 412
    services to be provided 408
    types of 410–12
    variance in 412–13
    volume of work 408
    waiting times 412
hearing impairment 29–36
    cochlear implants 35–6
    hearing aids 34–5
    investigation 30
    management 30–3
hemianopia 1–2
hemifacial spasm, botulinum toxin 136
hemiplegic gait 353
hemispherectomy, for epilepsy 84
hereditary diseases 247–57
    see also named diseases
hereditary motor and sensory neuropathy *see*
        Charcot–Marie–Tooth disease
herpes
    herpes simplex encephalitis 241
    pain after 50–1
    see also zoster
heterotopic ossification 320
HIV
    encephalitis 241–2
    transverse myelopathy 209
homonymous hemianopia 1
Horner's syndrome 179, 180, 189, 210
hospices 379
house officers 427–8
Huntington's disease 137–8, 308
    drug treatment 137–8
    and ethnic groups 295
    hereditability of 251, 254–5
hydrocephalus 94
    bladder and bowel disorders 356
hyperalgesia 43
hyperbaric oxygen, multiple sclerosis 118
hyperkinesia 127–43
hyperpathia 43
hyperprolactinaemia 219
hypertension and stroke 183, 185
hypochondriasis 302
hypotension, orthostatic 266
hysterical tremor 130

idiopathic intracranial hypertension 16
image-guided surgery, intracranial tumours
        213–14

imipramine 45
immunostimulation, multiple sclerosis
    117
inanition 317
incontinence 273
    palliative care 374–5
infancy
    seizures in 68
    spasms 68
infectious diseases 233–45
    see also named diseases
information, and self-help groups 457–60
infratentorial tumours 220–3
    acoustic neuromas 220
    brainstem gliomas 221
    ependymomas 221–3
inspiration 325–6
interdisciplinary team care, palliative care
    378
interferons, multiple sclerosis 117–18
internal carotid artery syndrome 271
International Classification of Impairments,
    Disabilities and Handicaps 311
intracerebral haemorrhage 190
intracranial hypertension 16
    benign 94–5
intracranial suppuration 243–5
    brain abscess 243–4
    extradural abscess 244–5
    subdural empyema 244
intracranial tumours
    image-guided surgery 213–14
    pre-operative ultrasound 213
    stereotactic craniotomy 213
intrathecal medications, and multiple
    sclerosis 120–1
intubation 340–1
involuntary movements 127–43
    acute dystonia 135–6
    athetosis 139
    ballism 139
    chorea 136–9
    drug-induced parkinsonism 135
    essential tremor 128, 129
    gerebellar tremor 129–30
    hysterical tremor 130
    idiopathic torsion dystonia 132–3
    myoclonus 139–41
    neuropathic tremor 130
    parkinsonian tremor 128–9
    physiological tremor 127
    stereotypies 142
    symptomatic dystonia 133–5
    task-specific tremor 130
    thyrotoxic tremor 128
    tics 141–2
    Wilson's disease tremor 131–2
iron lung 339
ischaemia *see* stroke
isoniazid, multiple sclerosis 121

Janz syndrome 68
Japanese encephalitis, and ethnic groups
    290
Jefferson fracture 198
Jervell and Lange–Neilsen syndrome,
    confused with epilepsy 62

Kennedy's disease 173
kuru, and ethnic groups 290
kyphoscoliosis, and respiration 337

labour, and epilepsy 74
lacunar stroke 180–1
lamotrigine, for epilepsy 81
Landau–Kleffner syndrome 69
laryngeal dystonia 136
lay societies *see* self-help groups
L-dopa *see* levodopa
Leber's hereditary optic neuropathy 4–5
Lennox–Gastaut syndrome 68
lepromatous neuropathy, and ethnic groups
    293
Leriche syndrome 201
levodopa 129, 146, 149, 151–2, 156, 267
    idiopathic torsion dystonia 133
Lhermitte's phenomenon 211
lignocaine, for chronic pain 46
local anaesthetics, for chronic pain 45–6
lorazepam, status epilepticus 82
Lyme disease 209
    meningitis 240
lymphoid irradiation, multiple sclerosis 117

magnesium sulphate, for eclampsia 83
magnetic resonance angiography, and stroke
    186–7
magnetic resonance imaging *see* MRI
malaria, and encephalitis 242–3
malingering and factitious disorders 303
Marchiafava–Bignami disease, and ethnic
    groups 291
mass lesions 93–4
medical education
    clinical students 425–7
    continuing 422
    neurological consultants 430–2
    and the patient 425–32
    pre-clinical students 425
    senior house officers 427–8
    trainee neurologists and specialist
        registrars 429
medical literature 419
medical students 425–7
memory 317
    deficits 166
    loss 272
Ménière's disease 23, 26, 28
meningiomas 217–18
    optic nerve compression 12
meningitis 97, 203–5, 234–40
    brain abscess 243–4
    clinical features 235–6
    communication 238
    drug treatment 237
    encephalitis 240–3
    extradural abscess 244–5
    management 236–7
    spirochaetes 240
    subdural empyema 244
    tuberculosis 238–40
mental deterioration, fear of 376
mental handicap, and ethnic groups 294
mesial temporal sclerosis 65
methylprednisolone, optic neuritis 3

metoclopramide
    acute dystonia 135
    headache 101
mexiletene, for chronic pain 46
middle cerebral syndromes 271
migraine 26–7, 98–9
    and driving 369
    and ethnic groups 294
mitochondrial disease, hereditability of 256
mitoxantrone, multiple sclerosis 116
molecular diagnostics laboratory 248
monosynaptic segmental stretch reflex 346
motor neurone disease 173–7, 268–9
    clinical trails 176
    diagnosis 173–4
    drug treatment 175
    feeding gastrostomy 175–6
    genetic testing and counselling 176
    improved management of 437
    investigations 268–9
    management 174–5, 269
    prognosis 175
    surgery 175
    terminal care 176
Motor Neurone Disease Association 458
motor paralytic bladder 357
MRCP examination 427–8
MRI
    for epilepsy 72, 85
    multiple sclerosis 112
    optic nerve compression 11
multidisciplinary team 433–8
    acceptability to clients 435–6
    activity of 435
    continuity of care 436
    cost 438
    development of professional expertise
        437
    education in self-help 436
    general practitioner 435
    growing demand for 438
    hospital–community divide 433
    improved contacts with voluntary societies
        437
    improved job satisfaction of team 437
    improved management of motor neurone
        disease 437
    improved telling of the diagnosis 436
    improved use of resources 437–8
    involving patient and family 435
    less hierarchy 435
    nursing input 434
    outpatient team 433
    reputation and standards 438
    support and information 436
    plus a therapist and dietitian 434
multiple sclerosis 111–23
    acute exacerbation, treatment of 115–16
    ataxia 121
    azathioprine 116
    baclofen 120
    benzodiazepines 120
    bladder and bowel disorders 356, 363
    copolymer 1 118
    cyclophosphamide 116
    cyclosporin A 116
    dantrolene sodium 120

multiple sclerosis (*cont.*)
  diagnosis 112
  diet 119
  and driving 120, 369
  in the elderly 112
  and ethnic groups 290
  fatigue 121–2
  general symptomatic treatment 119
  geographical factors 111
  gluten-free diet 119
  hyperbaric oxygen 118
  immunostimulation 117
  immunosuppression 116
  interferons 117–18
  intrathecal medications 120–1
  lymphoid irradiation 117
  mitoxantrone 116
  optic neuritis 3–4
  paroxysmal symptoms, inhibition of 119
  physiotherapy 120
  and pregnancy 112
  restoration of conduction 119
  sexual problems in 363
  spasticity 119–20
  support in 113–14
  tizanidine 120
  transfer factor 117
  treatment 114–22
  urinary symptoms 122
  in the young 112
multisensory dizziness syndrome 22
Munchhausen syndrome 305–6
muscle spasm, and palliative care 374
muscle spasticity 345–54
  adult hemiplegic gait 353
  alpha-skeletomotor neurone 346
  assessment of 348–9
  baclofen 351
  benzodiazepines 350
  botulinum toxin 352
  and contractures 319–20
  dantrolene 351
  descending supraspinal influences 347–8
  goal-setting 349
  interventions 349–50
  monosynaptic segmental stretch reflex 346
  nerve blocks 351
  orthotic interventions 353
  physical measures 350
  physiology 346–8
  prevention 350
  spastic diplegic gait 353
  spinal interneurones 347
  surgery 352
myalgic encephalopathy and fatigue syndromes 304
myasthenia gravis 108–9
myeloneuropathy, tropical, and ethnic groups 291–2
myoclonic-astatic seizures, epilepsy with 69
myoclonus 139–41
  epileptic 140
  and extrapyramidal disease 141
  and infections 140
  metabolic 139–40
  non-spinal segmental 141

  physiological 139
  post-hypoxic 140
  seizure 67
  spinal 141
myositis, bacterial and parasitic 292

naratriptan, headache 102
nasogastric tube 341
National Health Service 391–7
  change in medical profession 392
  changes in 391
  and commissioning 399–415
  contracting 395–7
  coping 397
  organizational structure of 400
  the provider 393–5
  the purchaser 392–3
  and research and development 417–19
National Patient Charter Standards 409
neck pain 96
neonatal seizures 67–8
nerve blocks, and muscle spasticity 351
nerve injury, chronic pain 43–55
neuralgia 97
neuralgic amytrophy 210
Neuro-care Team 433–8, 459
neurofibromatosis
  and ethnic groups 294–5
  hereditability of 255
neurogenic claudication 203
neuroleptics
  for chronic pain 45
  risks of 135
Neurological Charities Group 460
neurological sarcoidosis, and ethnic groups 292–3
neurologist
  centre-based 386
  clinical scientists 386
  district general hospital-based 385
  general neurological practice 383–4
  inpatient neurological services 385
  leadership role 388
  outcome measures 387–8
  postgraduate education 386–7
  range of functions 383–5
  regional centres 385–6
  research 387–8
  subspecialty services 385
  undergraduate education 386
neurology
  hypochondriasis 302
  myalgic encephalopathy and fatigue syndromes 304
  pseudoseizures 304–7
  relation with psychology 297–310
  somatization disorder 301–2
  somatoform disorders 298–301
neuromuscular disease 105–9
  Guillain–Barré syndrome 105–6
  hereditary motor and sensory neuropathy 106–7
  myasthenia gravis 108–9
  polymyositis 107–8
neuropathic tremor 130
neuropsychiatry 297–310
  affective disorder 303

  alcohol abuse 304
  anxiety 304
  hypochondriasis 302
  malingering and factitious disorders 303
  myalgic encephalopathy and fatigue syndromes 304
  pseudoseizures 304–7
  psychosomatic disorder 308
  psychotic illness 304
  somatization disorder 301–2
  somatoform disorders 298–301
neuro-rehabilitation 311–21
  assisted ventilation 315–16
  behavioural problems 317–18
  cognitive rehabilitation 316–17
  heterotopic ossification 320
  mechanisms of recovery 311–12
  nutrition and dysphagia 314–15
  persistent vegetative state 316
  physiotherapy 319
  skin care: decubitus ulcers 320–1
  spasticity and contractures 319–20
  speech therapy and communication aids 313–14
  time of recovery 312–13
  urinary continence 318
neurosurgery, for chronic pain 48
NHS *see* National Health Service
NMDA receptors, drugs acting on in chronic pain 46
N-methyl-D-aspartate *see* NMDA
non-arteritic anterior ischaemic optic neuropathy 13–14
non-steroidal anti-inflammatory drugs *see* NSAIDs
NSAIDs 374
  chronic pain 44–5
  headache 101
  post-herpetic neuralgia 50
nutrition
  airway protection 315
  and dysphagia 314–15
  enteral nutrition 314–15
  motor neurone disease 175–6
  nasogastric tube 341
  Parkinson's disease 155–6
  percutaneous endoscopic gastrostomy 315, 341
  sialorrhoea 315
nutritional neuropathy 6–9
nystagmus, vestibular problems 24–5

obsessive-compulsive disorder 142
obstructive sleep apnoea 338
occipital lobe seizure 66
oculopharyngeal muscular dystrophy, and ethnic groups 291
ophthalmologist 1
opioids 374
  for chronic pain 45
  post-herpetic neuralgia 50–1
opsoclonus 141
optic chiasm, disorders of 16–17
optic nerve disorders 3–13
  higher visual disorders 17–20
  Leber's hereditary optic neuropathy 4–5
  optic chiasm, disorders of 16–17

optic nerve compression 11–13
   optic neuritis 3
   papilloedema 15–16
   toxic and nutritional neuropathy 6–9
   traumatic optic neuropathy 9–11
   vascular disorders 13–15
optic neuritis 3
   colour vision 3
   demyelinating optic neuritis, treatment
      of 4
orbitofrontal seizures 66
oromandibular dystonia 136
orthostatic hypotension 266
orthotic interventions 353
otoscopy, vestibular problems 24
outpatient services 463–77
   changes to outpatient session 475
   the clinic session 467–72
   duration of clinics 468–9
   follow-up clinic 471–2
   manpower 472–4
   number of patients per session 469–71
   number of sessions per week 468
   one-stop clinics 476
   proposed changes to the system 474–7
   specialist clinics 468
   specialist nurses 476
   waiting lists 464–7, 475
outreach service 451–5
   carers 453
   communication 452
   crisis intervention 453
   education 454
   help with diagnosis 452
   respite 454
   role of 451–2
oxcarbazepine, for epilepsy 81
oxybutynin 358

papilloedema 15–16
pain
   and palliative care 374
   see also chronic pain
palatal myoclonus 141
papaverine 362
parietal lobe seizure 66
Parkinson's disease 145–57, 267
   antimuscarinic agents and amantadine
      150
   assessment, methods of 147
   bladder and bowels 156
   catechol-*O*-methyl transferase inhibitors
      150
   diagnosis and impact of 146, 441–5
   dopamine agonists 149
   and driving 370
   drug-induced 135
   drug therapy 149, 151–2, 156
   early treatment 150–4
   faecal incontinence 360
   feeding and nutrition 155–6
   goal-setting 147
   independence and lifestyle 152–3
   levodopa 129, 146, 149, 151–2, 156, 267
   mood disturbance 153–4
   multidisciplinary team 434, 436
   palliative care 157

physical impairments and disabilities 145
physiological factors 145–6
posture, mobility, and falling 154–5
preventative measures 152
progression of disease 154, 445–7
respiration 156
selegiline 150
services for 148
sexual function 153
sleep 154
support and management 150, 152
surgical treatment 157
symptomatic dystonia 134
therapy 148
tremor 128–9
urinary and bowel problems 363–4
Parkinson's Disease Society 457–61
Parkinson's plus syndromes 267
paroxysmal chorea 138
patient–doctor relationship 441–50
Patient's Charter 465
penicillamine, Wilson's disease 131–2
penicillin, meningitis 237
perceptual problems 317
percutaneous endoscopic gastrostomy 315,
   341
pergolide 149
peripheral nervous system lesions, bladder
   and bowel disorders 356
peripheral neuropathy 272–3
   bladder, bowel and sexual problems in
      364
pernicious anaemia, and ethnic groups
   290
PET, for epilepsy 85
petit mal seizure 67
pharmaceutical industry, research and
   development 418–19
phenobarbitone, for epilepsy 81, 82
phenothiazine 164
   acute dystonia 135
   Parkinson's disease 135
   symptomatic dystonia 134
   tics 141
phenytoin, epilepsy 80, 81, 82, 270
physiological tremor 127
physiotherapy 319
   multiple sclerosis 120
pituitary tumours 218–20
   prolactinomas 219
pizotifen, headache 102
plasma exchange, multiple sclerosis 115
point mutations 252
polycythemia rubra vera, and chorea 138
polymyositis 107–8
positron emission tomography *see* PET
postgraduate education, and the neurologist
   386–7
post-herpetic neuralgia 50–1
post-hypoxic action myoclonus 140
post-partum, and epilepsy 74
post-traumatic seizures 70–1
post-traumatic stress disorder 305
prednisolone
   multiple sclerosis 115
   optic neuritis 3
pregnancy, and epilepsy 73–4

pressure sores, palliative care 375
primary care group 399
primary motor area seizure 66
problem solving and executive functions
   317
progressive bulbar palsy 268
progressive muscular atrophy 268
propofol, status epilepticus 83
propranolol
   for chronic pain 47
   headache 102
pseudoseizures 304–7
   confusion with epilepsy 63–4
psychiatry
   affective disorder 303
   alcohol abuse 304
   anxiety 304
   epilepsy 75
   hypochondriasis 302
   malingering and factitious disorders 303
   myalgic encephalopathy and fatique
      syndromes 304
   pseudoseizures 304–7
   psychosomatic disorder 308
   psychotic illness 304
   relation with neurology 297–310
   somatization disorder 301–2
   somatoform disorders 298–301
psychosomatic disorder 308
psychotic illness 304
pulmonary embolism 338
pyridoxine seizures 70

rabies 241
Ramsay–Hunt syndrome 140
Rasmussen's syndrome 69–70
reflex epilepsies 69
reflex neuropathic bladder 357
reflex sympathetic dystrophy 53–4
regional centres 419
   and the neurologist 385–6
research
   centrally organized information systems
      421–2
   and changes in practice 417–23
   continuing medical education 422
   medical literature 419
   and the neurologist 387–8
   problem-directed research 419–21
   regional centres 419
   specialist associations 422
   summarizing data and clinical guidelines
      421
   who should do research 421
respiratory disorders 325–42
   breathing aids 338–9
   causes 334–6
   clinical assessment of 329–32
   inspiration and expiration 325–6
   management of 336–41
   neural control 326
   respiratory failure 326–7
   respiratory muscle strength 328
   sleep 327–8
respite 454
retina, vascular disorders of 14
Rett syndrome 142

Rickettsia, meningitis 240
Romano–Ward syndrome, confused with
     epilepsy 62
Romford Neuro-care Team 433–8, 459

sarcoidosis 6
scanning aids 313
schizophrenia 317
     comparison with delirium 163
seborrhoeic dermatitis 321
Segawa disease 133
seizures, palliative care 374
selegiline 150
self-help groups 457–62
     empowerment of the individual 461
     fundraising 461
     medical research 460
     welfare, information and education
          457–60
     working with government and other
          voluntary organizations 460–1
sensory paralytic bladder 357
serotonin, and headaches 99, 100
service and financial framework 407–8
sexual dysfunction 360–2
     drug-induced dysfunction 364
     intracorporal injection 362
     management of impaired erection 362
     multiple sclerosis 363
     orgasm 362
     penile erection 361–2
     peripheral neuropathy 364
     spinal cord injury 363
shingles 210
sialorrhoea 315
sildenafil 362
single photon emission computerized
     tomography *see* SPECT
sinus, optic nerve compression 12
sinusitis 96
skin care 320
sleep 327–8
     excessive, and driving 369
sleeping sickness, and ethnic groups 292
smoking
     and stroke 183
     toxic optic neuropathy 7–8
sodium valproate
     for chronic pain 46
     for epilepsy 78, 81
somatization disorder 301–2
somatoform disorders 298–301
spastic diplegic gait 353
spasticity *see* muscle spasticity
specialist
     associations 422
     clinics 452–3, 468
     nurses 476
SPECT, for epilepsy 85
speech therapy 313–14
sphincter-detruser dyssynergia 357
spinal arteriovenous malformations 202–3
spinal cord diseases and injury 197–212
     acute transverse myelopathy 206–9
     arachnoiditis 205
     bladder and bowel disorders 356
     Brown–Sequard syndrome 200

cervical spondylosis 211
diabetic amytrophy 209–10
disc herniations 211
external trauma 198–9
Guillain–Barre syndrome 209
haematomata 202
haemorrhage 202
high cervical compression 197–8
high cervical lesions 197
Lhermitte's phenomenon 211
meningitis 203–5
myoclonus 141
neuralgic amytrophy 210
neurogenic claudication 203
sexual problems in 363
shingles 210
spinal arteriovenous malformations
     202–3
spinal cord laceration 199
spinal epidural abscesses 205–6
subarachnoid haemorrhage 202
subdural haematomata 202
syringomyelia 199–200
thoracic outlet syndromes 210
torticollis 211
traumatic lesions within 199
tumours *see* spinal tumours
vascular anatomy 200
vascular disorders 200–2
whiplash injury 206
spinal cord stimulation, for chronic pain
     48–9
spinal epidural 202
spinal interneurones, muscle spasticity 347
spinal tumours 206
     spinal astrocytomas 223–4
     spinal ependymomas 224–5
spinothalamic tract 44
spiritual concerns, and palliative care 376–7
spirochaetes, meningitis 240
spondylosis 96
status epilepticus 82–3
     diazepam 82
     lorazepam 82
     phenobarbitone 82
     phenytoin 82
     propofol 83
     thiopentone 83
stereotactic craniotomy 213
steroid treatment
     chronic pain 47
     giant cell arteritis 14
     multiple sclerosis 115
     myasthenia gravis 108–9
     optic neuritis 3, 6
     polymyositis 108
     temporal arteritis 96
Strachan's syndrome 8
stroke 179–93, 200
     accuracy of diagnosis 182–3
     acute stroke/rehabilitation 185
     age 183
     border zone infarcts 181
     cardiac disease 183
     care of 191–3
     carotid 179
     cerebral haemorrhage 190

cholesterol 183
diabetes mellitus 183
dysphagia 188
emotional aspects 188
epilepsy 188
fibromuscular dysphasia 190
hypertension 183
intracerebral haemorrhage 190
investigations 183–8
lacunar 180–1
pain after 49
smoking 183
subarachnoid haemorrhage 190–1
subclavian steal syndrome 181
surgical treatment 186–7
thalamic pain 188
timing and pathogenesis 181–2
transient ischaemic attack 179–93
vascular risk factors 185
vertebrobasilar 180
in young people 188–91
subarachnoid haemorrhage 97, 190–1
subclavian steal syndrome 181
subdural empyema 244
subpial transections, for epilepsy 84
sulpiride, Huntington's disease 137
sumatriptan, headaches 100, 101–2, 103
supplementary motor area seizure 66
suprasellar tumour, treatment of 17
supratentorial tumours 214–20
     cerebral metastases 217
     gliomas 214–16
     meningiomas 217–18
     pituitary tumours 218–20
surgery
     callosotomy 84
     destructive neurosurgery for chronic pain
          48
     dysphagia 351
     for epilepsy 83–4
     motor neurone disease 175
     muscle spasticity 352
     neurosurgery for chronic pain 48
     tumours, and image-guided surgery
          213–14
     see also type of
swallowing *see* dysphagia
sympathetic blocks
     for chronic pain 47
     reflex sympathetic dystrophy 54
syncope, confused with epilepsy 62–3
syphilis, meningitis 240
syphilitic labyrinthitis 27
syringomyelia 199–200
systemic lupus erythematosus, and chorea
     138

tachypnoea 330
tardive myoclonus 135
technical development, and changes in
     practice 417–23
     medical literature 419
     problem-directed research 419–21
     regional centres 419
temporal arteritis 96
temporal lobe epilepsy 64–5
     surgery for 83–4

terminal care for elderly 264–5
tetrabenazine, Huntington's disease 137
tetrahydroaminoacridine, dementia 168
thalamic pain, and stroke 188
thiopentone, status epilepticus 83
thoracic outlet syndromes 210
thyrotoxic tremor 128
thyrotoxicosis, chorea 138
tiagabine, for epilepsy 81
ticlopidine 186
tics 141–2
tinnitus 21, 36–7
    investigation 37
    management 37
    pathophysiology 36–7
    see also falls
tizanidine, multiple sclerosis 120
tocainide, for chronic pain 46
tonic seizure 67
topiramate, for epilepsy 81
torticollis 211
toxic neuropathy 6–9
tracheostomy 316
transcultural aspects of neurology 281–6
transcutaneous electrical nerve stimulation,
        for chronic pain 47–8
transfer factor, and multiple sclerosis 117
transient ischaemic attack
    care of 191
    and stroke 179–93
    see also stroke
traumatic optic neuropathy 9–11
tremor 127–32
    essential 128, 129
    gerebellar 129–30
    hysterical 130
    multiple sclerosis 121
    neuropathic 130
    parkinsonian 128–9
    physiological 127
    task-specific 130
    thyrotoxic 128
    Wilson's disease 131–2

tricyclic antidepressants, headache 102
trigeminal neuralgia 51–2
trypanosomiasis, and ethnic groups 292
tuberculosis meningitis 238–40
    and ethnic groups 292
tumour
    acoustic neuromas 220
    of the brain, and ethnic groups 294
    brainstem gliomas 221
    cerebral metastases 217
    controversies in management of 213–25
    ependymomas 221–3
    gliomas 214–16
    image-guided surgery 213–14
    intracranial, surgical techniques
        213–14
    mass lesions 94
    meningiomas 217–18
    myasthenia gravis 108–9
    optic nerve compression 11–13
    pituitary tumours 218–20
    pre-operative ultrasound 213
    spinal 206
    spinal astrocytomas 223–4
    spinal ependymomas 224–5
    stereotactic craniotomy 213
    suprasellar 17
Tunnicliffe jacket 339

ultrasound, intracranial tumours 213
undergraduate education, and the neuro-
        logist 386
uninhibited neuropathic bladder 357, 358
upper motor neurone syndrome 345
urinary continence 318

vagal stimulation, for epilepsy 85
varicella virus, shingles 210
vegetative state 316
vertebrobasilar syndromes 180, 271
vertigo 23, 27
vestibular problems 21–9
    clinical assessment 22–5

drug therapy 28
    management 25–7
    pathophysiology 21–2
    physical exercise regimes 27–8
    psychological support 28
    surgical treatment 29
    see also falls
vigabatrin, for epilepsy 81–2
viral encephalomeningitis 204
vision, loss because of neurological disease
        1–20
    and driving 2–3, 370
    optic nerve disorders 3–13
    see also optic
vitamin B deficiency, toxic optic neuropathy
        6–7
vitamin K, pregnancy and epilepsy 74
von Hippel–Lindau disease, hereditability of
        253

waiting lists 464–7, 475
    allocating appointments 466
    extra clinics 467
    private practice 471
    structure of 465
warfarin, stroke 186
weight gain, and respiration 337
welfare, and self-help groups 457–60
Wernicke's encephalopathy 163
West syndrome 68
whiplash injury 206
Wilson's disease tremor 131–2
Winged Fellowship Trust 458

yohimbine 362

zinc, Wilson's disease 132
zolmitriptan, headache 102
zonisamide, for epilepsy 82
zoster virus
    and shingles 210
    spinal 208
    see also herpes